Basic Skills in

INTERPRETING LABORATORY DATA

Third Edition

Mary Lee, Pharm.D., BCPS, FCCP
Dean and Professor of Pharmacy Practice
Midwestern University
Chicago College of Pharmacy
Downers Grove, Illinois

American Society of Health–System Pharmacists®
Bethesda, Maryland

Any correspondence regarding this publication should be sent to the publisher, American Society of Health-System Pharmacists®, 7272 Wisconsin Avenue, Bethesda, MD 20814, attn: Special Publishing. Produced in conjunction with the ASHP Publications Production Center.

The information presented herein reflects the opinions of the contributors and reviewers. It should not be interpreted as an official policy of ASHP or as an endorsement of any product.

Drug information and its applications are constantly evolving because of ongoing research and clinical experience and are often subject to professional judgment and interpretation by the practitioner and to the uniqueness of a clinical situation. The editor, authors, and ASHP have made every effort to ensure the accuracy and completeness of the information presented in this book. However, the reader is advised that the publisher, authors, contributors, editors, and reviewers cannot be responsible for the continued currency or accuracy of the information, for any errors or omissions, and/or for any consequences arising from the use of the information in the clinical setting.

Acquisition Editor: Cynthia Reilly
Editorial Project Manager: Dana A. Battaglia
Project Editor: Kristin C. Eckles
Cover and page design: David A. Wade

ASHP is the 30,000-member national professional association representing pharmacists who practice in hospitals and health systems. ASHP members practice across the continuum of care, including acute care, long-term care, home care, and ambulatory care. ASHP believes the mission of pharmacists is to help people make the best use of medicines. For more information about ASHP or ASHP products, call ASHP Customer Service at 301-657-4383 or browse our web site at www.ashp.org.

ISBN: 1-58528-059-3

CONTENTS

DEDICATION

This book is dedicated to my parents who gave me the gift of a college education
and to Scott Traub, who had the vision to create this text
and the fortitude to edit the first two editions.
I would also like to acknowledge all of the contributing authors
and reviewers, all of whom are exemplary teachers
committed to the education of health professional students.

INTRODUCTION

This book familiarizes pharmacists and allied health care providers with the fundamentals of interpreting clinical laboratory test results. Most of the tests discussed are performed in the clinical laboratory and involve biochemistry. Pulmonary function tests, some cardiac tests (e.g., electrocardiogram), and selected radiologic tests are exceptions. They are included because of their importance in diagnosis and in the selection and monitoring of drug therapy. The scope of this book is limited to tests that are routinely available at most laboratories and hospitals. With few exceptions, investigational or research assays are not included.

This book is geared primarily to the entry to midcareer, general practitioner who has had only limited experience working with laboratory test results, but who wants to develop skills in this area. A glossary of *contextual* definitions is included (Appendix C) to help readers who do not have an extensive medical vocabulary. The pharmacy or allied health student also may find this book useful as a primary text in a clinical laboratory data course or as a reference for a therapeutics or diagnostics course.

Chapters and discussions are organized primarily by disease or organ system; however, some sections use a "test" perspective (e.g., Chapters 14, 16, and 17). Consequently, some tests are described in more than one chapter. To minimize redundancy, each chapter covers only pertinent aspects of such tests but interchapter referrals are given. In addition, comprehensive indexing allows the reader to locate various clinical applications and interpretations of these tests easily.

Readers must have a basic knowledge of anatomy and physiology, at least as they relate to the mechanisms behind the changes in test results. Therefore, chapters on tests related to specific organ systems or diseases (Chapters 8–19) are prefaced with pertinent anatomy and physiology.

As its title implies, this book emphasizes the *interpretation* of laboratory test results as opposed to the (1) chemical or procedural aspects of assays or (2) decisions regarding appropriate test selection. All chapters begin with learning objectives. Chapters 1 and 2 cover fundamental definitions, concepts, and technologies relating to laboratory testing and should facilitate comprehension of subsequent chapters. Chapters 4–6 deal with drugs and are written from a test viewpoint. Chapters 7–19 cover common laboratory tests to assess functional status of and gain information on various organ systems.

All material from the first edition has been updated and expanded. Unlike the first edition, *all* chapters (except Chapters 2 and 4) include case studies and real-life practical examples of interpreting test results. Although his book is not a "therapeutics" text, the authors have been encouraged to use drug therapy-related examples to reinforce important points or concepts concerning interpretation of a laboratory test. This emphasis is based on the assumption that many readers already have a sound knowledge base in the drug area and will be able to integrate the new knowledge more easily in this context.

New to this edition are QuickView charts for pertinent tests. These charts provide a "snapshot" of important clinical information, including reference ranges for adults and pediatrics, "critical" values, major tissue or organ locations of natural substances and whether the substances have inherent physiological activity, major causes and mechanisms of "true" abnormal (high, positive, or low) results, time course (after insult) of positive or high tests (i.e., time to onset, peak, and normalization of result), signs and symptoms associated with high (or positive) and low values, diseases and drugs monitored with the test, and significant in vitro drug interferences.

The index entries now include codes for readers to quickly identify whether the information is part of a table (t), figure (f), minicase (mc), or glossary (g).

Mary Lee, Pharm.D., BCPS, FCCP, *Editor*

PREFACE

As with the two previous editions, this third edition of *Basic Skills in Interpreting Laboratory Data* provides information about common laboratory tests used to screen or diagnose diseases, monitor the effectiveness and safety of treatment, or assess disease severity. Each laboratory test is described in terms of its uses, how the lab test relates to the pathophysiology of the disease, how to interpret the lab test results, and causes for abnormal lab test results. This information will be useful for pharmacists caring for patients and for students who are learning how to use laboratory tests to assess a patient's response to drug treatment. The authors have focused on making this information clear, relevant, convenient, and practical. It is for this reason that only the most commonly used laboratory tests are included. In addition, minicases and extended cases are presented to illustrate how a particular laboratory test is used in the management of patients. Additionally, quickview tables are expeditious short cuts to finding information about the meaning of an abnormal lab test result.

The third edition has some useful new chapters on tumor markers and tests used in pediatric patients. In addition, some chapters have been extensively rewritten and updated to include some of the newest laboratory tests (e.g., chapters on infectious diseases and therapeutic drug monitoring). The extended patient cases are excellent practice problems for pharmacy students. Keys are provided so that students can double check their thought process.

On behalf of the contributing authors and reviewers, we hope that this text becomes a valuable resource in your library.

Mary Lee, Pharm.D., BCPS, FCCP, *Editor*
2004

CONTRIBUTORS

Jill S. Burkiewicz, Pharm.D., BCPS
Assistant Professor, Department of
 Pharmacy Practice
Chicago College of Pharmacy
Midwestern University
Downers Grove, Illinois

Lingtak-Neander Chan, Pharm.D.,
 BCNSP
Clinical Assistant Professor
Departments of Pharmacy Practice
 and Medicine
Colleges of Pharmacy and Medicine
University of Illinois at Chicago
Chicago, Illinois

Peter A. Chyka, Pharm.D., DABAT,
 FAACT
Professor, Department of Pharmacy
University of Tennessee,
 Health Science Center
Memphis, Tennessee

Thomas J. Comstock, Pharm.D.
Associate Professor of Pharmacy
School of Pharmacy
Medical College of Virginia
Virginia Commonwealth University
Richmond, Virginia

Wafa Y. Dahdal, Pharm.D., BCPS
Associate Professor, Pharmacy Practice
Chicago College of Pharmacy
Midwestern University
Downers Grove, Illinois

Sharon M. Erdman, Pharm.D.
Assistant Director
Anti-Infective Scientific Liaisons
Clinical Communications
Ortho-McNeil Pharmaceutical, Inc.
Raritan, New Jersey

Joshua D. Farkas, M.S.
Joan and Sanford Weill Medical College
Cornell University
New York, New York

Paul Farkas, M.D.
Chief of Gastroenterology
Mercy Hospital
Assistant Clinical Professor
Tufts University Medical School
Springfield, Massachusetts

Rebecca S. Finley, Pharm.D., M.S.
Professor and Chair
Department of Pharmacy Practice and
 Pharmacy Administration
Philadelphia College of Pharmacy
University of the Sciences in Philadelphia
Philadelphia, Pennsylvania

James. B. Groce III, Pharm.D., CACP
Associate Professor of Pharmacy
Campbell University School of Pharmacy
Buies Creek, North Carolina
Clinical Assistant Professor of Medicine
UNC School of Medicine
Chapel Hill, North Carolina
Clinical Pharmacy Specialist-
 Anticoagulation
Department of Pharmacy
The Moses H. Cone Memorial Hospital
Greensboro, North Carolina

Thomas G. Hall, Pharm.D.
Director, Department of Pharmacy
Pharmacy Department
Missouri Baptist Medical Center
Saint Louis, Missouri
Associate Professor, Pharmacy Practice
Saint Louis College of Pharmacy
Saint Louis, Missouri

Paul R. Hutson, Pharm.D.
Associate Professor, Pharmacy Practice
University of Wisconsin School of
 Pharmacy
Madison, Wisconsin

Douglas K. Hyde, M.D.
Western Massachusetts Gastrointestinal
 Associates
Springfield, Massachusetts
Clinical Instructor
Tufts University School of Medicine
Boston, Massachusetts

Donna M. Kraus, Pharm.D.
Associate Professor of Pharmacy Practice
Departments of Pharmacy Practice
  and Pediatrics
Colleges of Pharmacy and Medicine
University of Illinois at Chicago
Chicago, Illinois

Alan Lau, Pharm.D.
Professor, Pharmacy Practice
College of Pharmacy
University of Illinois at Chicago
Chicago, Illinois

Mary Lee, Pharm.D., BCPS, FCCP
Dean and Professor of Pharmacy Practice
Chicago College of Pharmacy
Midwestern University
Downers Grove, Illinois

Julie B. Leumas, BS, MT(ASCP)SH
Product Manager for Oncology Products
TriPath Oncology
Durham, North Carolina

Janis J. MacKichan, Pharm.D.
Professor and Chair, Department of
  Pharmacy Practice
Chicago College of Pharmacy
Midwestern University
Downers Grove, Illinois

Steven J. Melnick, Ph.D., M.D.
Chief, Department of Clinical Pathology
  and Clinical Laboratories
Miami Children's Hospital
Miami, Florida

Gary Milavetz, Pharm.D., FCCP
Associate Professor of Pharmacy
Division of Clinical and Administrative
  Pharmacy
College of Pharmacy
The University of Iowa
Iowa City, Iowa

Keith A. Rodvold, Pharm.D., FCCP, BCPS
Professor of Pharmacy Practice
Associate Professor of Medicine
  in Pharmacy
Colleges of Pharmacy and Medicine
University of Illinois at Chicago
Chicago, Illinois

Terry L. Schwinghammer, Pharm.D.,
  FASHP, FCCP, BCPS
Professor of Pharmaceutical Sciences
University of Pittsburgh School of
  Pharmacy
Ambulatory Care Pharmacist
University of Pittsburgh Medical Center
Pittsburgh, Pennsylvania

Mary E. Teresi, Pharm.D.
Director, Pediatric Allergy/Pulmonary
  Clinical Trials
Coordinator, CFF-TDN, Iowa City Center
Department of Pediatrics
University of Iowa
Iowa City, Iowa

Karen J. Tietze, Pharm.D.
Professor of Clinical Pharmacy
Philadelphia College of Pharmacy
University of the Sciences in Philadelphia
Philadelphia, Pennsylvania

Eva M. Vivian, Pharm.D., BCPS, CDE,
  BC-ADM
Associate Professor of Pharmacy Practice
College of Pharmacy
Western University of Health Sciences
Pomona, California

Kandace V. Whitley, Pharm.D.
Primary Care Specialty Resident
Kaiser Permanente Colorado Region
Denver, Colorado

REVIEWERS

Ann Amerson, Pharm.D.

J. Edward Bell, Pharm.D.

Eric Boyce, Pharm.D.

Bradley C. Cannon, Pharm.D.

Swati (Rina) Desai, Pharm.D.

Art Jacknowitz, Pharm.D.

Timothy Todd, Pharm.D.

William Spruill, Pharm.D.

Amy W. Valley, Pharm.D.

Kimberly Zientara, Pharm.D.

Chapter 1

DEFINITIONS AND CONCEPTS

Karen J. Tietze

Laboratory testing is used to detect disease, guide treatment, monitor response to treatment, and monitor disease progression. However, it is an imperfect science. Laboratory testing may fail to identify abnormalities that are present (false negatives) or identify abnormalities that are not present (false positives). This chapter defines terms used to describe and differentiate laboratory tests and describes factors that must be considered when assessing and applying laboratory test results.

OBJECTIVES

After completing this chapter, the reader should be able to

1. Distinguish between invasive and noninvasive laboratory tests.
2. Distinguish between quantitative, qualitative, and semiqualitative laboratory tests.
3. Differentiate between sensitivity and specificity and calculate and assess these parameters.
4. Differentiate between accuracy and precision.
5. Define reference range and identify factors that affect a reference range.
6. Identify potential sources of laboratory errors and state the impact of these errors in the interpretation of laboratory tests.
7. Compare and contrast the advantages and disadvantages of the Système Internationale.
8. Discuss the pros and cons of point-of-care and at-home laboratory testing.
9. Identify patient-specific factors that must be considered when assessing laboratory data.
10. Describe a rational approach to interpreting laboratory results.

DEFINITIONS

Many terms are used to describe and differentiate laboratory test characteristics and results. The clinician should recognize and understand these terms before assessing and applying test results to individual patients.

Invasive vs. Noninvasive Tests

A noninvasive test is a procedure that examines fluids or other substances (e.g., urine and exhaled air) obtained without using a needle, tube, device, or scope to penetrate the skin or enter the body. An invasive test is a procedure that examines fluids or tissues (e.g., venous blood and skin biopsy) obtained by using a needle, tube, device, or scope to penetrate the skin or enter the body. Invasive tests pose some risk to the patient (e.g., pain and bruising associated with venipuncture) and are less convenient than noninvasive tests.

Specimen

A specimen is a sample (e.g., whole blood, venous blood, arterial blood, urine, stool, sputum, sweat, gastric secretions, exhaled air, gastric secretions, cerebrospinal fluid, or tissues) that is used for laboratory analysis. Plasma is the watery acellular portion of blood. Serum is

---

This chapter is based, in part, on the second edition chapter titled "Definitions and Concepts," which was written by Scott L. Traub.

the liquid that remains after the fibrin clot is removed from plasma. While some laboratory tests are performed only on plasma (e.g., renin activity and adrenocorticotropic hormone concentration) or serum (e.g., serum electrophoresis and acetaminophen concentration), other laboratory tests can be performed on either plasma or serum (e.g., aldosterone, potassium, and sodium concentrations).

Analyte

The analyte is the substance measured by the assay. Some substances, such as phenytoin and calcium, are bound extensively to proteins such as albumin. Although the unbound fraction elicits the physiological or pharmacological effect (bound substances are inactive), most routine assays measure the *total* substance (bound plus unbound). The free fraction may be assayable, but the assays are not routine. Therefore, the reference range for total and free substance may be quite different. For example, the reference range is 10–20 µg/mL for total phenytoin, 1–2 µg/mL for free phenytoin, 8.2–10.2 mg/dL for total serum calcium, and 4.60–5.08 mg/dL for free (also called ionized) calcium.

Some analytes exist in several forms and each has a different reference range. These forms are referred to as fractions, subtypes, subforms, isoenzymes, or isoforms. Results for the total and each form are reported. For example, bilirubin circulates in conjugated and unconjugated subforms. Direct bilirubin refers to the sum of the conjugated plus the delta forms; indirect bilirubin refers to the unconjugated form. Lactate dehydrogenase (LDH) is separated electrophoretically into five different isoenzymes: LDH_1, LDH_2, LDH_3, LDH_4, and LDH_5. Creatine kinase (CK) exists in three isoforms: CK1, CK2, and CK3.

Quantitative Tests

A quantitative test is a test whose results are reported as an exact numeric measurement (usually a specific mass per unit measurement) and assessed in context of a reference range of values. For example, serum potassium is reported in milliequivalents per liter, creatinine clearance is reported in milliliters per minute, and lactate dehydrogenase is reported in units per liter.

Qualitative Tests

A qualitative test is a test whose results are reported as either positive or negative without further characterization of the degree of positivity or negativity. Exact quantities may be measured in the lab but are still reported qualitatively using predetermined ranges. For example, a serum or urine pregnancy test is reported as either positive or negative; a bacterial wound culture is reported as either positive for one or more specific microorganisms or reported as no growth; a urine toxicology drug screen is reported as either positive or negative for specific drugs; and an acid-fast stain for *Mycobacterium* is reported as either positive or negative.

Semiquantitative Tests

A semiquantitative test is a test whose results are reported as either negative or with varying degrees of positivity but without exact quantification. For example, urine glucose and urine ketones are reported as negative or 1+, 2+, 3+; the higher numbers represent a greater amount of the measured substance in the urine but not a specific concentration.

Sensitivity

The sensitivity of a test refers to the ability of the test to identify positive results in patients who actually have the disease (true positive rate).[1,2] Sensitivity assesses the proportion of true positives disclosed by the test (Table 1-1). A test is completely sensitive (100% sensitivity) if it is positive in every patient who actually has the disease; the higher the sensitivity, the lower the chance of a false-negative result, and the lower the sensitivity, the higher the chance of a false-negative result. However, a highly sensitive test is not necessarily a highly specific test (see below).

Highly sensitive tests are preferred when the consequences of not identifying the disease are serious; less sensitive tests may be acceptable if the consequence of a false-negative is not high or if low sensitivity tests are combined with other tests. For example, inherited phenylalanine hydroxylase deficiency (phenylketonuria or PKU) results in increased phenylalanine concentrations. High phenylalanine concentrations damage the central nervous system and are associated with mental retardation. Mental retardation is preventable if PKU

TABLE 1-1	SCREENING TEST RESULT	DISEASED	NOT DISEASED	TOTAL
	Positive	TP	FP	TP + FP
	Negative	FN	TN	FN + TN
	Total	TP + FN	FP + TN	TP + FP + FN + TN

Sensitivity = [TP ÷ (TP + FN)] x 100%.
Specificity = [TN ÷ (FP + TN)] x 100%.
TP = diseased persons detected by test (true positives).
FP = nondiseased persons positive to test (false positives).
FN = diseased persons not detected by test (false negatives).
TN = nondiseased persons negative to test (true negatives).

Table 1-1. Calculation of Sensitivity and Specificity

is diagnosed and dietary interventions initiated before 30 days of age. The phenylalanine blood screening test, used to screen newborns for PKU, is a highly sensitive test with only a 0.3% chance of missing a positive case when infants are screened between 48–72 hr following birth.[3] In contrast, the prostate-specific antigen (PSA) test, a test commonly used to screen men for prostate cancer, is not a very sensitive test when used alone. During the Physicians' Health Study, PSA sensitivity for the entire 10-year follow-up period was only 46% for total prostatic cancer cases.[4] Thus, PSA cannot be relied upon as the sole prostatic cancer screening method.

Sensitivity also refers to the range over which a quantitative assay can accurately measure the substance being measured. In this context, a sensitive test is one that can measure low levels of the substance; an insensitive test cannot measure low levels of the substance accurately. For example, a digoxin assay with low sensitivity might measure digoxin concentrations as low as 0.7 ng/mL. Concentrations below 0.7 ng/mL would not be measurable and would be reported as "less than 0.7 ng/mL" whether the digoxin concentration was 0.69 ng/mL or 0.1 ng/mL. An insensitive digoxin assay would not differentiate between medication nonadherence (a serum concentration of 0 ng/mL) and low concentrations associated with inadequate dosage regimens.

Specificity

Specificity refers to the percent of negative results in people without the disease (true negative rate).[1,2] Specificity assesses the proportion of true negatives disclosed by the test (Table 1-1); the lower the specificity, the higher the chance of a false-positive result. A test with a specificity of 95% for the disease in question indicates that the disease will not be detected in 5% of people with the disease. Tests with high specificity are best for confirming a diagnosis because the tests are rarely positive in the absence of the disease. Several newborn screening tests (e.g., phenylketonuria, galactosemia, biotinidase deficiency, congenital hypothyroidism, and congenital adrenal hyperplasia) have specificity levels above 99%.[5] In contrast, the PSA test is an example of a test with low specificity. The prostate-specific antigen is specific for the prostate but not specific for prostatic carcinoma. Urethral instrumentation, prostatitis, urinary retention, prostatic needle biopsy, and digital rectal exam elevate the PSA. The erythrocyte sedimentation rate (ESR) is another nonspecific test; infection, inflammation, and plasma cell dyscrasias increase the ESR.

Specificity as applied to quantitative laboratory tests refers to the degree of cross-reactivity of the analyte with other substances in the sample. For example, vitamin C cross-reacts with glucose in some urine tests (e.g., Clinitest®), falsely elevating the urine glucose test result. Quinine may cross-react with or be measured as quinidine is some assays, falsely elevating the reported quinidine concentration.

TABLE 1-2

SENSITIVITY AND SPECIFICITY (%)	PREVALENCE (%)	PREDICTIVE VALUE OF POSITIVE TEST (%)
95	0.1	1.9
	1	16.1
	2	27.9
	5	50
	50	95
99	0.1	9
	1	50
	2	66.9
	5	83.9
	50	99

Predictive value of positive test = [TP ÷ (TP + FP)] x 100%.
Predictive value of negative test = [TN ÷ (TN + FN)] x 100%.
Disease prevalence = (TP + FN) ÷ number of patients tested.
TP = diseased persons detected by test (true positives).
FP = nondiseased persons positive to test (false positives).
FN = diseased persons not detected by test (false negatives).
TN = nondiseased persons negative to test (true negatives).

Table 1-2. Relationship of Sensitivity, Specificity, Disease Prevalence, and Predictive Value of Positive Test

Predictive Value

The predictive value, derived from a test's sensitivity, specificity, and prevalence (incidence) of the disease in the population being tested, is used to assess a test's reliability (Table 1-2). As applied to a positive test result, the predictive value indicates the percent of positives that are true positives. For a test with equal sensitivity and specificity, the predictive value of a positive result increases as the incidence of the disease in the population increases. For example, the glucose tolerance test has a higher predictive value for diabetes in women who are pregnant than in the general population. A borderline abnormal serum creatinine concentration has a higher predictive value for kidney disease in patients in a nephrology unit than in patients in a general medical unit. The lower the prevalence of disease in the population tested, the greater the chance that a positive test result is in error. The predictive value may also be applied to negative results. As applied to a negative test result, the predictive value indicates the percent of negatives that are true negatives (refer to Minicase 1).

Accuracy and Precision

Accuracy and precision are important laboratory quality control measures. Laboratories are expected to test analytes with accuracy and precision and to document the quality control procedures. Accuracy of a quantitative assay is usually measured in terms of an analytical performance, which includes accuracy and precision (see below). Accuracy is defined as the extent to which the mean measurement is close to the true value. A sample spiked with a known quantity of an analyte is measured repeatedly; the mean measurement is calculated. A highly accurate assay means that the repeated analyses produce a mean value that is the same as or very close to the known spiked quantity. Accuracy of a qualitative assay is calculated as the sum of the true positives (TP) and true negatives (TN) divided by the number of sample tested (accuracy = [(TP + TN) ÷ number of samples tested] × 100%). Precision refers to assay reproducibility (i.e., the agreement of results when the specimen is assayed many times). An assay with high precision means that the results are likely to be correct.

Reference Range

The reference range is a statistically-derived numerical range obtained by testing a sample of the individuals assumed to be healthy. The upper and lower limits of the range are not absolute (i.e., normal vs. abnormal), but rather points beyond which the probability of therapeutic significance begins to increase. The term *reference range* is preferred over the term *normal range*.[6] The reference population is assumed to have a Gaussian distribution with 68% of the values within one standard deviation (SD) above and below the mean, 95% within ±2 SD, and 99.7% within ±3 SD (Figure 1-1).

MINICASE 1

IN 2000 PATIENTS WITH CHEST PAIN severe and persistent enough to bring them into the emergency room, a derivative test was conducted for the early diagnosis of acute myocardial infarction (AMI), the $LDH_1:LDH_{total}$ ratio. Investigators stated that an $LDH_1:LDH_{total}$ ratio of at least 0.4 (≥40%) was "diagnostic" of an AMI in this setting. A typical reference range for LDH_{total} is 100–250 IU/L; for LDH_1 it is 25–85 IU/L. Therefore, an LDH_{total} of 200 IU with an LDH_1 of 80 IU (ratio = 0.4) would be consistent with an AMI even though neither test alone is outside the reference range. An LDH_{total} of 350 IU with an LDH_1 of 160 IU (ratio = 0.46), along with chest pain, would be diagnostic of an AMI. An $LDH_1:LDH_{total}$ ratio of at least 0.4 was considered a positive ratio.

Question: After reviewing the following results, what conclusions can be made about the clinical performance of this test?

	12–24 hr after onset of chest pain (# patients)	24 hr–5 days after onset of chest pain (# patients)
True Positives	1200	1350
False Positives	75	35
True Negatives	600	550
False Negatives	125	65

Discussion: Calculate sensitivity, specificity, predictive value of a positive test, and the predictive value of a positive and negative test for each time period.

- 12–24 hr:

  Sensitivity = (TP ÷ [TP + FN]) x 100% = (1200 ÷ [1200 + 125]) x 100% = 90.6%.

  Specificity = (TN ÷ [FP + TN]) x 100% = (600 ÷ [75 + 600]) x 100% = 88.9%.

  Predictive value of positive test = (TP ÷ [TP + FP]) x 100% = (1200 ÷ [1200 + 75]) x
     100% = 94%.

  Predictive value of negative test = (TN ÷ [TN + FN]) x 100% = (600 ÷ [600 + 125]) x
     100% = 82.8%.

- 24 hr–5 days:

  Specificity = (TN ÷ [FP + TN]) x 100% = (550 ÷ [35 + 550]) x 100% = 94%.

  Sensitivity = (TP ÷ [TP + FN]) x 100% = (1350 ÷ [1350 + 65]) x 100% = 95.4%.

  Predictive value of positive test = (TP ÷ [TP + FP]) x 100% = (1350 ÷ [1350 + 35]) x
     100% = 97.5%.

  Predictive value of negative test = (TN ÷ [TN + FN]) x 100% = (550 ÷ [550 + 65]) x
     100% = 89.4%.

The $LDH_1:LDH_{total}$ appears to have excellent clinical performance in diagnosing an AMI 12–24 hr after the onset of chest pain. The clinical performance is even better in patients tested 24 hr–5 days after the onset of chest pain, since the numbers of false positives and false negatives decline.

The reference range, usually established as the mean or average value plus or minus two standard deviations, represents the range of values where 95% of individuals within the reference population fall. Acceptance of the mean ±2 SD means that one in 20 normal individuals will have test results outside the reference range (2.5% have values below the lower limit of the reference range, and 2.5% have values above the lower limit of the reference range). Accepting a wider range (e.g., ±3 SD) includes a larger percentage (97.5%) of normal individuals but increases the chance of including individuals with values only slighter outside of a more narrow range, thus decreasing the sensitivity of the test.

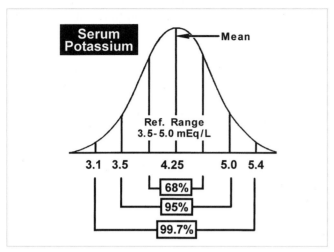

Figure 1-1. Gaussian (random) value distribution with a visual display of the area included within increments of standard deviation (SD) above and below the mean: ±1 SD = 68% of total values; ±2 SD = 95% of total values; and ±3 SD = 99.7% of total values.

Some laboratory tests are either negative or positive and without a reference range. In other words, any positivity is considered abnormal. For example, any amount of serum acetone, porphobilinogen, or alcohol is considered abnormal. The presence of glucose, ketones, blood, bile, or nitrate in urine is abnormal. The results of the Venereal Disease Research Laboratory (VDRL) test, the Lupus Erythematosus (LE) prep test, tests for red blood cell sickling and the malaria smear are either positive or negative.

Factors That Influence the Reference Range

Many factors influence the reference range. Reference ranges may differ between labs depending on analytical technique, reagent, and equipment. The initial assumption that the sample population is normal may be false. For example, the reference range is inaccurate if too many individuals with covert disease (i.e., no signs or symptoms of disease) are included in the sample population. Failure to control for physiologic variables (e.g., age, gender, ethnicity, body mass, diet, posture, and time of day) introduces many unrelated factors and may result in an inaccurate reference range. Reference ranges calculated from nonrandomly distributed (non-Gaussian) test results or from a small number of samples may not be accurate.

Reference ranges may change as new data regarding disease and treatment data are published. For example, the National Cholesterol Education Program's (NCEP) Third Report of the Expert Panel on Detection, Evaluation, and Treatment of High Blood Cholesterol in Adults (Adult Treatment Panel III or ATP III), released in 2001, includes recommendations to lower and more closely space reference range cut-off points for low density lipoprotein C (LDL-C), high density lipoprotein C (HDL-C), and triglycerides (TG).[7]

Critical Value

The term *critical value* refers to a result that is far enough outside the reference range that it indicates impending morbidity (e.g., potassium <2.5 mEq/L). Because laboratory personnel are not in a position to consider mitigating circumstances, a responsible member of the health care team is notified immediately upon discovery of a critical value test result. Critical values may not always be so critical, however, because the reference range varies for the reasons discussed above.

LABORATORY TEST RESULTS

Units Used in Reporting Laboratory Results

Laboratory test results are reported with a variety of units. For example, four different units are used to report serum magnesium concentration (1.0 mEq/L = 1.22 mg/dL = 0.5 mmol/L = 12.2 mg/L). Additionally, the same units may be reported in different ways. For example, mg/dL, mg/100 mL, and mg% are equivalent units. Enzyme activity is usually reported in terms of units, but the magnitude varies widely and depends on the methodology. Rates are usually reported in volume per unit of time (e.g., creatinine clearance is measured in mL/min or L/hr), but erythrocyte sedimentation rate is reported in mm/hr and coagulation test results are reported in seconds or minutes. This lack of standardization is confusing and may lead to misinterpretation of the test results.

The International System of Units (Système Internationale d'Unités, or SI) was created about 40 years ago in an attempt to standardize quantitative units worldwide.[8] The SI system specifies units, abbreviations, superscripts, subscripts, punctuation, and use of decimal points. Seven basic independent units and abbreviations were designated: length (meter, m), mass (kilogram, kg), time (seconds, s), electric current (ampere, A), temperature (kelvin, K), luminous intensity (candela, cd), and concentration of a substance in a body fluid (mol L^{-1}). Some derived units were also designated (volt, V, A^{-1} m^2 kg s^{-3}). In the late 1980s, several major medical journals announced that units should be expressed in SI units.[9,10] But the change was not accepted. Clinicians and the general population continue to think about drug dosages and concentrations in terms of conventional units (milligrams) rather than molar units.[11] It would take a major societal shift for everyone to relate to serum cholesterol as mmol per liter rather than mg per deciliter (e.g., 4.14 mmol L^{-1} vs. 160 mg per deciliter).

Rationale for Ordering Laboratory Tests

Laboratory tests are performed with the expectation that the results will

1. Discover occult disease.
2. Confirm a suspected diagnosis.
3. Differentiate among possible diagnoses.
4. Determine the stage or activity of a disease.
5. Detect disease recurrence.
6. Assess the effectiveness of therapy.
7. Guide the course of therapy.

Laboratory tests are categorized as *screening* or *diagnostic* tests. Screening tests, performed in individuals without signs or symptoms of disease, detect disease early when interventions (e.g., lifestyle modifications, drug therapy, and surgery) are likely to be effective. Features of screening tests are listed in Table 1-3. Examples of screening tests include the Papanicolaou smear, lipid profile, prostate-specific antigen, fecal occult blood, tuberculin skin test, sickle cell tests, blood coagulation tests, and serum chemistries. Screening tests may be performed on healthy outpatients (e.g., ordered by the patient's primary care provider or performed during public health fairs) or on admission to an acute care facility (e.g., prior to scheduled surgery). Screening laboratory tests offered at health fairs often include blood chemistry, serum cholesterol, hematocrit, fecal occult blood, and sickle cell tests.[13] Preoperative laboratory tests often include platelets, clotting time assessment, hemoglobin, white blood cell count, electrolytes, and glucose.[14] Abnormal screening tests are followed by more specific tests to confirm the abnormality.

TABLE 1-3

FEATURE	SCREENING TEST	DIAGNOSTIC TEST
Simplicity of test	Fairly simple	More complex
Target population	Individuals without signs or symptoms of the disease	Individuals with signs or symptoms of the disease
Ordered by	Nonphysician providers and physicians	Physicians
Characteristic	High sensitivity	High specificity
Disease characteristics	Relatively common	Common or rare
Test characteristics	Acceptable to population	Acceptable to individual

Compiled from Reference 12.

Table 1-3. Comparative Features of Screening and Diagnostic Laboratory Tests

Screening tests need to be cost-effective and population-appropriate. A new statistical term, the number needed to screen, has been proposed to assess screening cost-effectiveness. The number needed to screen is defined as "the number of people that need to be screened for a given duration to prevent one death or one adverse event."[15] For example, screening for dyslipidemias produces a large clinical benefit (i.e., one death in 5 years can be prevented by screening 418 people)[15] whereas screening for anemia has little clinical benefit.[13]

Diagnostic tests are performed in individuals with signs or symptoms of disease, a history suggestive of a specific disease or disorder, or an abnormal screening test. Diagnostic tests are used to confirm a suspected diagnosis, differentiate among possible diagnoses, determine the stage of activity of disease, detect disease recurrence, and assess and guide the therapeutic course. Diagnostic test features are listed in Table 1-3. Examples of diagnostic tests include blood cultures, serum troponin, kidney biopsy, and the cosyntropin test.

Many laboratories group a series of related tests (screening and/or diagnostic) into a set called a *profile*. For example, the panel-7 (Chem-7, SMA-7) profile includes common serum electrolytes (sodium, potassium, chloride, and carbon dioxide content), blood urea nitrogen, serum creatinine, and glucose. A 12-test profile (panel-12, Chem-12, and SMA-12) includes 12 of the following tests: electrolytes, creatinine, calcium, phosphorous, glucose, blood urea nitrogen, uric acid, total protein, albumin, cholesterol, total bilirubin, aspartate aminotransferase, lactate dehydrogenase, and alkaline phosphatase. Grouped together for convenience, some profiles may be less costly to perform than the sum of the cost of each individual test. However, profiles may generate unnecessary patient data. Attention to cost is especially important in the current cost-conscious era. A test should not be done if it is unnecessary, redundant, or provides suboptimal clinical data (e.g., non-steady-state serum drug concentrations). Before ordering a test, the clinician should consider the following questions:

1. Was the test recently performed so that the result has not significantly changed?
2. Were other tests performed that provide the same information?
3. Can the needed information be estimated with adequate reliability from existing data?

For example, creatinine clearance can be estimated using age, height, weight, and serum creatinine rather than measured from a 24-hr urine collection. Serum osmolality can be calculated from electrolytes and glucose rather than measured directly. Additionally, a clinician should ask, "What will I do if results are positive or negative (or absent or normal)?" If the test result will not aid in clinical decisions or change the diagnosis, prognosis or treatment course, the benefits from the test are not worth the cost of the test.

Factors That Influence Laboratory Test Results

Laboratory results may be inconsistent with patient signs, symptoms, or clinical status. Before accepting laboratory test results at face value, clinicians must consider the numerous laboratory- and patient-specific factors that influence the laboratory test results (Table 1-4). For most of the major tests discussed in this book, a QuickView chart summarizes information helpful in interpreting results. Figure 1-2 depicts the format and content of a typical QuickView chart.

Laboratory-Specific Factors

Laboratory errors are uncommon but may occur. Defined as a test result that is not the true result, *laboratory error* most appropriately refers to inaccurate results that occur because of an error made by laboratory personnel or equipment. However, laboratory error is sometimes used to refer to accurate results rendered inaccurate by specimen-related issues. Laboratory errors should be suspected if one or more of the following situations occurs:

1. An unusual intrapatient trend develops.
2. The magnitude of error is great.
3. The result is not in agreement with a confirmatory test result.
4. The result is inconsistent with clinical signs or symptoms or other patient-specific information.

True laboratory errors (inaccurate results) are caused by one or more laboratory processing or equipment errors, such as deteriorated reagents, calibration errors, calculation errors, misreading the results, computer entry or other documentation errors, or improper sample preparation. For example, incorrect entry of thromboplastin activity (International Sensitivity Index, ISI) when calculating the International Normalized Ratio (INR) results in accurately assayed but incorrectly reported INR results.

Accurate results may be rendered inaccurate by one or more specimen-related problems. Improper specimen handling prior to or during transport to the laboratory may alter analyte concentrations between the time the sample was obtained from the patient and the time the sample was analyzed in the laboratory.[16] For example, arterial blood withdrawn for blood gas analysis must be transported on ice to prevent continued in vitro changes in pH, $PaCO_2$, and PaO_2. Failure to remove the plasma or serum from the clot within 4 hr of obtaining blood for serum potassium analysis may elevate the reported serum potassium concentration. Red blood cell hemolysis elevates the serum potassium and phosphate concentrations. Failure to refrigerate samples may cause falsely low concentrations of serum enzymes (e.g., creatine kinase). Prolonged tourniquet time may hemoconcentrate analytes, especially highly protein bound analyte (e.g., calcium).

Patient-Specific Factors

Laboratory test values cannot be interpreted in isolation of the patient. Numerous age-related (e.g., age and renal function) and other patient-specific factors (e.g., time of day, posture) as well as disease-specific factors (e.g., time course) affect lab results. The astute clinician places the lab value in context of all that is known about the patient when interpreting individual lab values.

Time course. Incorrectly timed laboratory tests produce misleading lab results. Disease states, normal physiologic patterns, pharmacodynamics, and pharmacokinetics time courses must be considered when interpreting lab values. For example, digoxin has a prolonged distribution phase. Digoxin serum concentrations obtained before tissue distribution is complete do not accurately reflect true tissue drug concentrations. Post-myocardial infarction enzyme patterns are an example of a more complex and prolonged post-event time course. Creatinine kinase elevates about 6 hr following myocardial infarction (MI) and returns to baseline about 48–72 hr after the MI. Lactate dehydrogenase elevates about 12–24 hr following MI and returns to baseline about 10 days after the MI. Troponin elevates a few hours following MI and returns to baseline in about 5–7 days. Serial samples are used to assess myocardial damage.

Lab samples obtained too early or too late may miss critical changes and lead to incorrect assessments. For example, cosyntropin (synthetic ACTH) tests adrenal gland responsiveness. The baseline 8 a.m. plasma cortisol is compared to the stimulated plamsa cortisol obtained 30 and 60 min following injection of the drug. Incorrect timing leads to incorrect results. The sputum acid-fast bacillus (AFB) smear may become AFB-negative with just a few doses of antituberculous drugs, but the sputum culture may remain positive for several weeks. Expectations of a negative sputum culture too early in the time course may lead to the inappropriate addition of unnecessary antituberculous drugs.

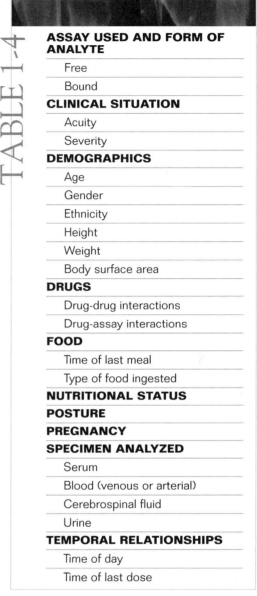

TABLE 1-4

ASSAY USED AND FORM OF ANALYTE
Free
Bound
CLINICAL SITUATION
Acuity
Severity
DEMOGRAPHICS
Age
Gender
Ethnicity
Height
Weight
Body surface area
DRUGS
Drug-drug interactions
Drug-assay interactions
FOOD
Time of last meal
Type of food ingested
NUTRITIONAL STATUS
POSTURE
PREGNANCY
SPECIMEN ANALYZED
Serum
Blood (venous or arterial)
Cerebrospinal fluid
Urine
TEMPORAL RELATIONSHIPS
Time of day
Time of last dose

Table 1-4. Factors That Influence Assessment of Laboratory Results

PARAMETER	DESCRIPTION	COMMENTS
Common reference ranges		
Adults	Reference range in adults	Variability and factors affecting range
Pediatrics	Reference range in children	Variability, factors affecting range, age grouping
Critical value	Value beyond which immediate action usually needs to be taken	Disease-dependent factors; relative to reference range; value is a number or multiple of upper normal limit
Natural substance?	Does substance exist naturally in the body?	Is it formed only under abnormal circumstances?
Inherent activity?	Does substance have any physiological activity?	Description of activity and factors affecting activity
Location		
Production	Is substance produced? If so, where?	Factors affecting production
Storage	Is substance stored? If so, where?	Factors affecting storage
Secretion/excretion	Is substance secreted or excreted? If so, where/how?	Factors affecting secretion or excretion
Major causes of...		
High-positive results	Major causes	Modification of circumstances/other related causes
Associated signs and symptoms	Major signs and symptoms with high or positive result	Modification of circumstances/other related signs and symptoms
Low-positive results	Major causes	Modification of circumstances/other related causes
Associated signs and symptoms	Signs and symptoms associated with low result	Modification of circumstances/other related signs and symptoms
After insult, time to...		
Initial elevation or positive result	Minutes, hours, days, weeks	Assumes acute insult/modification of circumstances
Peak values	Minutes, hours, days, weeks	Assumes insult not removed/modification of circumstances
Normalization	Minutes, hours, days, weeks	Assumes insult removed and nonpermanent damage/modification of circumstances
Drugs often monitored with test	List of typical drugs	Suggested monitoring frequency/other (less typical) drugs
Causes of spurious results	List of common causes	Modification of circumstances/assay specific?

Figure 1-2. Contents of a typical QuickView chart.

Non-steady-state drug concentrations are difficult to interpret; inappropriate dosage adjustments (usually inappropriate dosage increases) may occur if the clinician fails to recognize that a drug has not reached steady-state concentrations. Although non-steady-state drug concentrations may be useful when assessing possible drug toxicity (e.g., overdose situations and new onset adverse drug events), all results need to be interpreted in context of the drug's pharmacokinetics. Absorption, distribution, and elimination may change with changing physiology. For example, increased/decreased hepatic or renal perfusion may affect the clearance of a drug. Some drugs (e.g., phenytoin) have very long half-lives; constantly changing hemodynamics during the hospital course prevents the drug from reaching steady-state.

Age. Age influences many physiologic systems. Age-related changes are well-described for neonates and young children, but less data are available for the elderly and the very elderly (usually described as ≥75 years of age). Age influences some but not all lab values; not all changes are clinically significant.

Pediatric reference ranges often reflect physiologic immaturity, with lab values approaching those of healthy adults with increasing age. For example, the complete blood count (CBC) (hemoglobin, hematocrit, red blood cell count, and red cell indices) ranges are greatly dependent on age with different values reported for premature neonates, term neonates, and young children. The fasting blood glucose reference range in premature neonates is approximately 40–65 mg/dL compared to 60–115 mg/dL for children 2 years of age and older and 115–140 mg/dL for adults. The serum creatinine reference range for children 1–5 years of age differs from the reference range for children 5–10 years of age (0.3–0.5 mg/dL vs. 0.5–0.8 mg/dL). Reference ranges for children are well-described because it is relatively easy to identify age-differentiated populations of healthy children. Most laboratory reference texts provide age-specific reference values.

Geriatric reference ranges are more difficult to establish because of physiologic variability with increasing age and the presence of symptomatic and asymptomatic disease states that influence reference values. Diet (e.g., malnutrition) also influences some lab results. Some physiologic functions (e.g., cardiac, pulmonary, and renal and metabolic functions) progressively decline with age, but each organ declines at a different rate.[17] Other physiologic changes associated with aging include decreased body weight, decreased height, decreased total body water, increased extracellular water, increased fat percentage, and decreased lean tissue percentage; cell membranes may leak.[17] Published studies sometimes lead to contradictory conclusions due to differences in study methodology (e.g., single point vs. longitudinal evaluations) and populations assessed (e.g., nursing home residents vs. general population). Little data are available for very elderly (≥75 years of age). Most laboratory reference texts provide age-specific reference values.

TABLE 1-5.

NO CHANGE
Amylase
Lipase
Hemoglobin
Hematocrit
Red blood cell count
Red blood cell indices
Platelet count
White blood cell count and differential
Serum electrolytes (sodium, potassium, chloride, bicarbonate, magnesium)
Coagulation
Total iron binding capacity
Thyroid function tests (thyroxine, T_3 resin uptake)
Liver function tests (AST, ALT, LDH)
SOME CHANGE (UNCLEAR CLINICAL SIGNIFICANCE)
Alkaline phosphatase
Erythrocyte sedimentation rate
Serum albumin
Serum calcium
Serum uric acid
Thyroid function tests (thyroid stimulating hormone, triiodothyronine)
CLINICALLY SIGNIFICANT CHANGE
Arterial oxygen pressure
2-hr postprandial glucose
Serum lipids (total cholesterol, low-density lipoprotein, triglycerides)
NO CHANGE BUT CLINICALLY SIGNIFICANT
Serum creatinine

Table 1-5. Laboratory Testing: Tests Affected by Old Age[17-21]

Despite the paucity of data and difficulties imposed by different study designs and study populations, there is general consensus that some laboratory reference ranges are unchanged in the elderly, some laboratory reference ranges are different in the elderly (but the clinical significance of the differences are uncertain), and some laboratory references ranges are significantly different in the elderly (Table 1-5). For example, decreased lean muscle mass with increased age results in decreased creatinine production. Decreased renal function is associated with decreased creatinine elimination. Taken together, the serum creatinine reference range in the elderly is not different from younger populations though creatinine clearance clearly declines with age.

Significant age-related changes are reported for the 2-hr postprandial glucose test, serum lipids, and arterial oxygen pressure (Table 1-5). The 2-hr postprandial glucose increases by about 5–10 mg/dL per decade. Progressive ventilation-perfusion mismatching from loss of elastic recoil with increasing age causes progressively decreased arterial oxygen pressure with

MINICASE 2

NORMA S., A 78-YEAR-OLD FEMALE nursing home resident, suffered a minor stroke about 5 weeks ago. Her neurological deficits improved to only residual weakness on her left side. She returned from an acute care hospital 12 days ago. Since that time, Norma S. has not been eating much and has been drinking even less. She has a history of chronic iron and folate deficiency anemia with her usual Hgbs around 10 g/dL (reference range: 12–16 g/dL), Hcts around 30% (reference range: 37–47%), iron concentrations around 35 µg/dL (reference range: 40–160 µg/dL), and folates less than 1–3 ng/mL (reference range 4–15 ng/mL).

Norma S. takes daily iron and folate supplements as well as many other drugs. Her blood pressure has remained stable, but her heart rate has increased from 70s to 90s over the past 5–7 days. Her mucous membranes became dry, her skin turgor diminished, and her urine output decreased over that same time period. A complete blood count is ordered. Tests results indicate a Hgb of 13 and a Hct of 40. Her BUN is 40 mg/dL (reference range: 8–20 mg/dL), and sodium is 145 mEq/L (reference range: 136–145 mEq/L).

Question: Has the patient's anemia resolved? What is happening here?

Discussion: An astute clinician should realize that the Hgb, Hct, BUN, and possibly sodium concentrations have become temporarily hemoconcentrated because the patient is dehydrated. Thirst mechanisms sometimes are disrupted after a stroke. Her dry mucous membranes, decreased skin turgor and urine output, and increased heart rate are all consistent with dehydration. As the patient is rehydrated, the Hgb and Hct values should fall below the reference range to her usual baseline.

If the patient is overhydrated, the opposite scenario can occur. Of course, assay interference by drugs, metabolites, and other foreign substances (as well as laboratory error) should always be kept in mind. If hemoconcentration had not been so apparent, laboratory error and interferences might be considered. In that case the test should be repeated.

---

increasing age. Cholesterol progressively increases from age 20 years reaching a plateau in the 5th to 6th decade in men and in the 6th to 7th decade in women followed by progressive decline. LDL and TG follow a similar pattern, though TG appears to progressively increase in women.

Genetics, ethnicity, and gender. Inherited ethnic and/or gender differences are identified for some laboratory tests. For example, the hereditary anemias (e.g., thalassemias and sickling disorders such as sickle cell anemia) are more common in individuals with African, Mediterranean, Middle Eastern, India, and southeast Asia ancestry.[22] Glucose-6-phosphate dehydrogenase (G6PD) deficiency is an example of an inherited sex-linked (X-chromosome) enzyme deficiency found primarily in men of African and Mediterranean ancestry.[23] The A-G6PD variant occurs mostly in Africans and affects about 13% of African American males and 3% of African American females in the United States. The Mediterranean G6PD variant, associated with a less common but more severe enzyme deficiency state, occurs mostly in individuals of Greek, Sardinian, Kurdish, Asian and Sephardic Jewish ancestry.

Other enzyme polymorphisms influence drug metabolism.[24,25] The cytochrome P450 (CYP450) superfamily consists of >100 isoenzymes with selective but overlapping substrate specificity. The genetically-linked absence of an enzyme may lead to drug toxicity secondary to drug accumulation or lack of drug effect if the parent compound is an inactive prodrug (e.g., codeine). Some individuals are poor metabolizers while some are hyperextensive metabolizers. At least 16 CYP2D6 variants have been identified with definite ethnic differences. CYP3A4, the most abundant CYP450 hepatic enzyme, mediates about half of all drug oxidative reactions and is also present in the gut epithelium. There is approximately a 10-fold difference in individual CYP3A4 metabolic activity, accounting for wide differences in the metabolism of drugs such as cyclosporine and theophylline.

Additional enzyme polymorphisms include pseudocholinesterase deficiency, phenytoin hydroxylation deficiency, inefficient N-acetyltransferase activity, inefficient or rapid debrisoquine hydroxylase activity, and diminished thiopurine methyltransferase activity. Approximately 50% of Caucasians and Africans are slow acetylators. Other examples of genetic polymorphisms include variations in the ß$_2$-adrenoceptor gene that appear to influence response to sympathomimetic amines[26] and P-glycoprotein (P-gp), a drug transport pump.

Biologic rhythms. A circadian rhythm is a 24-hr endogenously generated cycle.[27] Hypothalamic suprachiasmatic nuclei, modified by direct retinal input, function as the biologic clock.[27] Well-described human circadian rhythms include body temperature, cortisol production, melatonin production, and hormonal production (gonadotropin, testosterone, growth hormone, and thyrotropin). Platelet function, cardiac function, and cognition also follow a circadian rhythm.[27]

Other laboratory parameters follow circadian patterns. For example, statistically significant circadian rhythms have been reported for creatine kinase, alanine aminotransferase, gamma glutamyl transferase, lactate dehydrogenase, and some serum lipids.[28,29] Glomerular filtration has a circadian rhythm.[30] Amikacin, almost completely excreted via glomerular filtration, has been reported to have a diurnal variation.[31] Though the clinical significance of diurnally variable laboratory results is not well understood, diurnal variability should be considered when assessing laboratory values. Obtaining laboratory results at the same time of day (e.g., routine 7 a.m. blood draws) minimizes variability due to circadian rhythms. Different results obtained at different times of the day may be due to circadian variability rather than acute physiologic changes.

Other well-described biologic rhythms include the monthly rhythms of follicle stimulating hormone, luteinizing hormone, and progesterone production. Seasonal rhythms have been described for cholesterol and 25-hydroxycholecalciferol.[21]

Drugs. The four generally accepted categories of drug-laboratory interactions include methodological interference, drug-induced end-organ damage, direct pharmacologic effect, and a miscellaneous category.

Many drugs interfere with analytical methodology. Drugs that discolor the urine interfere with fluorometric, colorimetric, and photometric tests and mask abnormal urine colors. For example, amitriptyline turns the urine a blue-green color and phenazopyridine and rifampin turn the urine an orange-red color. Other drugs directly interfere with the laboratory assay. For example, high doses of ascorbic acid (greater than 500 mg/day) cause false-negative stool occult blood tests as well as false-negative urine glucose oxidative glucose tests. Some drugs interfere with urinary fluorescence tests for urine catecholamines by producing urinary fluorescence themselves (e.g., ampicillin, chloral hydrate, and erythromycin).

Direct drug-induced end-organ damage (e.g., kidney, liver, and bone marrow) change the expected lab results. For example, amphotericin B causes renal damage evidenced by increased serum creatinine and bone marrow suppressants such as doxorubicin and bleomycin cause thrombocytopenia. Some drugs alter laboratory results as a consequence of a direct pharmacologic effect. For example, thiazide and loop diuretics increase serum uric acid by decreasing uric acid renal clearance or tubular secretion. Narcotics, such as codeine and morphine sulfate, increase serum lipase by inducing spasms of the sphincter of Oddi. Urinary specific gravity is increased in the presence of dextran. Other examples of drug-lab interactions include drugs that cause a positive direct Coombs' test (e.g., isoniazid, sulfonamides, and quinidine), drugs that cause a positive antinuclear antibody test (e.g., penicillins, sulfonamides, and tetracyclines), and drugs that inhibit bacterial growth in blood or urine cultures (e.g., antibiotics).

Thyroid function tests are a good example of the complexity of potential drug-induced laboratory test changes.[32] Thyroxine (T_4) and triiodothyronine (T_3) are displaced from binding proteins by salicylates, heparin and high-doses of furosemide. Free T_4 initially increases, but chronic drug administration results in decreased T_4 with a normal thyroid stimulating hormone. Phenytoin, phenobarbital, rifampin, and carbamazepine stimulate thyroid hormone hepatic metabolism, resulting in decreased serum hormone concentration. Amiodarone, high-dose beta-adrenergic blocking drugs, glucocorticosteroids, and some iodine contrast dyes interfere with the conversion of T_4 to T_3. Ferrous sulfate, aluminum hydroxide, sucralfate, colestipol, and cholestyramine decrease thyroxine absorption. Somatostatin, octreotide, and glucocorticosteroids suppress thyroid stimulating hormone production.

Pregnancy. Pregnancy is a normal physiologic condition that alters the reference range for many laboratory tests.[33–36] Normal pregnancy increases serum hormone concentrations (e.g., estrogen, testosterone, progesterone, human chorionic gonadotropin, prolactin, corticotropin releasing hormone, adrenocorticotropic hormone, cortisol, and atrial natriuretic hormone). The plasma volume increases by about 45%, resulting in a relative hyponatremia (e.g., serum sodium decreased by about 5mEq/L) and modest decreases in hematocrit. The metabolic adaptations to pregnancy include increased red blood cell mass and altered carbohydrate (e.g., 10–20% decrease in fasting blood glucose) and lipid (e.g., 300% increase in triglycerides and a 50% increase in total cholesterol) metabolism. Pregnancy changes the production and elimination of thyroid hormones, resulting in different values at different times over the course of pregnancy.[32] For example, thyroxine binding globulin increases during the first trimester but pregnancy-associated accelerated thyroid hormone metabolism occurs later in the pregnancy. Other physiologic changes during pregnancy include an increased cardiac output (increases by 30–50%), decreased systemic vascular resistance, increased glomerular filtration rate (increases by 40–50%), and hyperventilation resulting in compensated respiratory alkalosis and increased arterial oxygenation.

Other Factors

Organ function, diet, fluid status, patient posture, and altitude affect some laboratory tests.

Organ function. Renal dysfunction may lead to hyperkalemia, decreased creatinine clearance, and hyperphosphatemia. Hepatic dysfunction may lead to reduced clotting factor production with prolonged partial thromboplastin times. Bone marrow dysfunction may lead to pancytopenia.

Diet. Serum glucose and lipid profiles are best assessed in the fasting state. Unprocessed grapefruit juice down-regulates intestinal CYP3A4 and increases the bioavailability of some orally administered drugs.

Fluid status. Dehydration is associated with a decreased amount of fluid in the bloodstream; all blood constituents (e.g., sodium, potassium, creatinine, glucose, and blood urea nitrogen) become more concentrated. This effect is called *hemoconcentration*. Although the absolute amount of the substance in the body has not changed, the loss of fluid results in an abnormally high concentration. The converse is true with hemodilution. Relativity must be applied or false impressions may arise (refer to Minicase 2).

Posture. Plasma renin release is stimulated by upright posture, diuretics, and low-sodium diets; plasma renin testing usually occurs after 2–4 weeks of normal sodium diets under fasting supine conditions.

Altitude. At high altitude, hemoglobin initially increases secondary to dehydration. However, hypoxia stimulates erythropoietin production, which in turn stimulates hemoglobin production resulting in increased hemoglobin concentration and increased blood viscosity.[37]

Noncentralized Laboratory Tests

Point-of-Care Testing

Point-of-care testing (POC or POCT), also known as near patient testing, bedside testing, or extra-laboratory testing, is clinician-directed diagnostic testing performed at or near the site of patient care rather than in a centralized laboratory.[38] POC test equipment ranges from small hand-held devices to table-top analyzers. In vitro, in vivo and ex vivo POC testing refer to tests performed near the patient (e.g., fingerstick blood glucose), in the patient (e.g., specialized intra-arterial catheter that measures lactate), and just outside the patient (e.g., intra-arterial catheter attached to an external analyzer), respectively. Although POC testing is not a new concept, recent technological advances (e.g., microcomputerization, miniaturization, biosensor development, and electrochemical advances) have rapidly expanded the variety of available POC tests beyond the traditional urinalysis dipsticks or fingerstick blood glucose monitors. (Table 1-6).

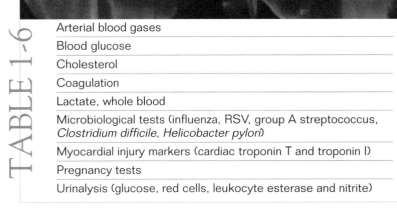

TABLE 1-6	
Arterial blood gases	
Blood glucose	
Cholesterol	
Coagulation	
Lactate, whole blood	
Microbiological tests (influenza, RSV, group A streptococcus, *Clostridium difficile*, *Helicobacter pylori*)	
Myocardial injury markers (cardiac troponin T and troponin I)	
Pregnancy tests	
Urinalysis (glucose, red cells, leukocyte esterase and nitrite)	

Table 1-6. Point-of-Care Tests

The major advantages of POC testing include reduced turn-around time (TAT) and test portability.[38–40] Reduced TAT is especially advantageous in settings where rapidly available laboratory test results may improve patient care (e.g., emergency departments, operating rooms, critical care units, accident scenes, and patient transport). Reduced TAT also enhances patient care in more traditional ambulatory settings by reducing patient and provider time and minimizing delays in initiating therapeutic interventions. Patient care sites without local access to centralized laboratories (e.g., nursing homes, rural physician practices, and military field operations) also benefit from POC testing. Other POC advantages include blood conservation (POC tests usually require drops of blood as opposed to the several milliliters required for traditional testing), less chance of preanalytical error from inappropriate transport, storage or labeling of samples, and overall cost savings. Although the per test cost is usually higher with POC testing, cost analyses must consider the per unit cost of the test as well as other costs such as personnel time, length of stay, and quality of life.

The major disadvantages of POC testing include misuse or misinterpretation of results, loss of centrally-generated epidemiological data, documentation errors, inappropriate test material disposal, and quality assurance issues.[38–40] All laboratory testing must meet the minimum standards established by the Clinical Laboratory Improvement Amendments of 1988 (CLIA-88).[41] Under CLIA-88, tests are categorized based on potential public health risk into one of three groups: waived tests, tests of moderate complexity, and tests of high complexity. The Food and Drug Administration (FDA) categorizes tests and the Health Care Financing Administration (HCFA) manages the financial aspects of the program. Waived tests pose no risk of harm to the patient if used incorrectly or use such simple and accurate methodologies that inaccurate results are unlikely. Many POC tests meet the criteria for waived status but increasingly sophisticated POC tests may be subject to more stringent control. State-specific regulations may be more stringent than federal regulations.

Home-Testing

Home-testing refers to patient-directed diagnostic and monitoring testing usually performed by the patient or family member at home. Many types of nonprescription in vitro diagnostic devices are marketed (Table 1-7). Home glucose monitoring and pregnancy testing are among the most popular home-testing kits. Advantages of home-testing include convenience, cost-

TABLE 1-7

TEST	BODY FLUID TESTED
Bilirubin	Urine
Catalase	Urine
Chloride	Urine
Cholesterol	Whole blood
Drugs of abuse	Urine
Fructosamine	Whole blood
Glucose	Whole blood, urine
Glycosylated hemoglobin	Whole blood
High density lipoprotein	Whole blood
Human immunodeficiency virus	Whole blood
Ketones	Whole blood, urine
Lactate	Whole blood
Menopause	Urine
Nitrates	Urine
Occult blood	Stool, urine
Ovulation prediction	Urine
pH	Urine, vaginal fluid
Pregnancy	Urine
Protein	Urine
Semen analysis	Semen
Triglycerides	Whole blood
Urobilinogen	Urine

Table 1-7. Types of Nonprescription In Vitro Diagnostic Tests

savings (as compared to physician office visit), quickly available results, and privacy. Home monitoring of chronic drug therapy, such as insulin and Coumadin, may give the patient a better sense of control over the disease. Disadvantages include misinterpretation of test results, delays in seeking medical advice, and lack of pre- and post-test counseling and psychological support. In addition, home test kits typically do not provide the consumer with information regarding sensitivity, specificity, precision, or accuracy. Consumers should read and follow the test instructions to minimize testing error.

Guidelines for Interpreting Laboratory Results

Laboratory results must be interpreted in context of the patient and the limitations of the laboratory test. However, a laboratory result is only one piece of information; diagnostic and therapeutic decisions cannot be made on the basis of one piece of information. Clinicians typically give more weight to the presence or absence of signs and symptoms associated with the medical problem rather than to an isolated laboratory report. For example, an asymptomatic patient with a serum potassium concentration of 3 mEq/L (reference range: 3.5–5.0 mEq/L) should not cause as much concern as a patient who has a concentration of 3.3 mEq/L but is symptomatic. Tests for occult disease, such as colon cancer, cervical cancer, and hyperlipidemia, are exceptions to this logic because, by definition, the patients being tested are asymptomatic. Baseline results, rate of change, and patterns should be considered when interpreting laboratory results.

Baseline Results

Baseline studies establish relativity and are especially useful when reference ranges are wide or when reference values vary significantly among patients. For example, lovastatin and other HMG-CoA reductase inhibitors cause myopathy and liver dysfunction in a small percentage of patients. The myopathy is symptomatic (muscle pain or weakness) and elevates CK concentrations. The drug-induced liver dysfunction is asymptomatic and causes elevated AST and ALT. Most clinicians establish a pretreatment baseline profile including CK, AST, and ALT before periodically monitoring to identify potential drug-induced toxicity. CK has a wide reference range (50–200 U/L); establishment of a baseline allows the clinician to identify early changes, even within the reference range. The baseline value is also used to establish relative therapeutic goals. For example, the activated partial thromboplastin time (aPTT) is used to assess patient response to heparin anticoagulation. Therapeutic targets are expressed in terms of how much higher the patient's aPTT is compared to the baseline control (e.g., 2 times control).

Lab Value Compared to Reference Range

Not all lab values above the upper limit of normal (ULN) require intervention. Risk-to-benefit considerations may require that some evidence of drug-induced organ damage is acceptable given the ultimate benefit of the drug. For example, a 6-month course of combination drug therapy including isoniazid, a known hepatotoxin, is recommended for treatment of latent tuberculosis.[42] The potential benefit of at least 6 months of therapy (i.e., lifetime protection from tuberculosis in the absence of reinfection) means that clinicians are willing to accept some evidence of liver toxicity with continued drug therapy (e.g., isoniazid is continued until AST is greater than 5 times the ULN in asymptomatic individuals).

Rate of Change

The rate of change of a laboratory value provides the clinician with a sense of risks associated with the particular signs and symptoms. For example, a patient whose red blood cell (RBC) count falls from 5 to 3.5 million/mm³ over several hours is more likely to be symptomatic and need immediate therapeutic intervention than if the decline took place over several months.

Isolated Results vs. Trends

An isolated abnormal test result is difficult to interpret. However, one of several values in a series of results or similar results from the same test performed at two different times suggests a pattern or trend. For example, a random serum glucose concentration of 300 mg/dL (reference range ≤200 mg/dL in adults) might cause concern unless it was known that the patient was admitted to the hospital last night for treatment of diabetic ketoacidosis with random serum glucose of 960 mg/dL. A series of lab values adds perspective to an interpretation but may increase overall costs.

Spurious Results

A spurious lab value is a false lab value. The only way to differentiate between an actual and a spurious lab value is to interpret the value in context of what else is known about the patient. For example, a serum potassium concentration of 5.5 mEq/L (reference range: 3.5–5.0 mEq/L) in the absence of significant electrocardiographic changes (i.e., wide, flat p waves, wide QRS complexes, and peaked T waves) and risk factors for hyperkalemia (i.e., renal insufficiency) is most likely a spurious value. Possible causes of falsely elevated potassium, such as hemolysis, acidosis, and lab error, have to be ruled out before accepting that the elevated potassium accurately reflects the patient's actual serum potassium. Repeat testing of suspected spurious lab values increases the cost of patient care but may be necessary to rule out an actual abnormality.

Future Trends

Point-of-care testing will progress and become more widely available as advances in miniaturization produce smaller and more portable analytical devices. Real-time, in vivo POC testing may become standard in many patient care areas. Laboratory test specificity and sensitivity will improve with more sophisticated testing. Genetic testing (laboratory analysis of human DNA, RNA, chromosomes, and proteins) will undergo rapid growth and development in the next few decades; genetic testing will be able to predict an individual's risk for disease, identify carriers of disease, establish diagnoses, and provide prognostic data. Genetic links for a diverse group of diseases including cystic fibrosis, Down syndrome, Huntington's disease, breast cancer, Alzheimer's disease, schizophrenia, phenylketonuria, and familial hypercholesterolemia are established. Screening may be antenatal (e.g., Down syndrome), neonatal (e.g., phenylketonuria and cystic fibrosis), and in adults when familial risk factors become known (e.g., Huntington's disease, colon caner, and breast cancer).[43] Some preliminary studies suggest that in the not so distant future genetic testing may even enable genetically-based targeted drug therapy.[44] The clinical validity (sensitivity, predictive value) of each test will need to be proven and systems established to provide adequate pre- and post-test counseling and protect patient confidentiality.[45]

SUMMARY

Clinical laboratory tests are convenient methods to investigate disease- and drug-related patient issues, especially since knowledge of pathophysiology and therapeutics alone is insufficient to provide high-quality clinical considerations. This chapter should help clinicians appreciate general causes and mechanisms of abnormal test results. However, results within the reference range are not always associated with lack of signs and symptoms. Many factors influence the reference range. Knowing the sensitivity, specificity, and predictive value is important in selecting an assay and interpreting its results. Additionally, an understanding of the definitions, concepts, and strategies discussed should also facilitate mastering information in the following chapters.

REFERENCES

1. Krieg AF, Gambino R, Galen RS. Why are clinical laboratory tests performed? When are they valid? JAMA. 1975; 233:76–8.
2. Altman DG, Bland JM. Statistics notes. Diagnostic tests I: sensitivity and specificity. Br Med J. 1994; 308:1552.
3. Committee on Genetics. Newborn screening fact sheets. Pediatrics. 1996; 98:473–501.
4. Gann PH, Hennekens CH, Stampfer MJ. A prospective evaluation of plasma prostate-specific antigen for detection of prostatic cancer. JAMA. 1995; 273:289–94.
5. Kwon C, Farrell PM. The magnitude and challenge of false-positive newborn screening test results. Arch Pediatr Adolesc Med. 2000; 154:714–8.
6. Solberg HE. Approved recommendation (1986) on the theory of reference values. Part 1. The concept of reference values. J Clin Chem Clin Biochem. 1987; 25:337–42.
7. Expert panel on Detection, Evaluation, and Treatment of High Blood Cholesterol in Adults. Executive summary of the third report of the National Cholesterol Education Program (NCEP) Expert Panel on detection, evaluation, and treatment of high blood cholesterol in adults (Adult Treatment Panel III). JAMA. 2001; 285:2486–97.
8. Council on Scientific Affairs. SI units for clinical laboratory data. JAMA. 1985; 253:2553–4.
9. Lundberg GD, Iverson C, Radulescu G. Now read this: the SI units are here. JAMA. 1986; 255:2329–30.
10. Huth EJ. The American shift to medical SI units. Ann Intern Med. 1987; 106;149–50.
11. Campion EW. A retreat from SI units. N Engl J Med. 1992; 327:49.
12. Boardman LA, Peipert JF. Screening and diagnostic testing. Clin Obstet Gynecol. 1998; 41:267–74.
13. Berwick DM. Screening in health fairs. JAMA. 1985; 254:1492–8.
14. Kaplan EB, Sheiner LB, Boeckmann AJ, et al. The usefulness of preoperative laboratory screening. JAMA. 1985; 253:3576–81
15. Rembold CM. Number needed to screen: development of a statistic for disease screening. Br Med J. 1998; 317:307–12.
16. Narayanan S. The preanalytic phase. An important component of laboratory medicine. Am J Clin Pathol. 2000; 113:429–52.
17. Coodley EL, Coodley GO. Laboratory changes associated with aging. Hospital Physician. 1993; Jan:12–18, 25–31.
18. Tietz NW, Wekstein DR, Shuey DF, et al. A two-year longitudinal reference range study for selected serum enzymes in a population more than 60 years of age. J Am Geriatr Soc. 1984; 32:563–70.
19. Kelso T. Laboratory values in the elderly. Are they different? Emerg Med Clinics North America. 1990; 8:241–54.
20. Duthie EH, Abbasi AA. Laboratory testing: current recommendations for older adults. Geriatrics. 1991; 46:41–50.
21. Fraser CG. Age-related changes in laboratory test results. Clin Pharmacol. 1993; 3:246–57.
22. Weatherall DJ. ABC of clinical haematology. The hereditary anaemias. Br Med J. 1997; 314:492–6.
23. Beutler E. G6PD deficiency. Blood. 1994; 84:3613–36.
24. Caraco Y. Genetic determinants of drug responsiveness and drug interactions. Ther Drug Monit. 1998; 20:517–24.
25. Roden D. Genetic determinants of drug metabolism. In: UpToDate Clinical Reference Library. Wellesley, MA: UpToDate Release 10.1; 2002.
26. Martinez FD, Graves PE, Baldini MJ, et al. Association between genetic polymorphisms of the β2-adrenoceptor and response to albuterol in children with and without a history of wheezing. J Clin Invest. 1997; 100:3184–8.
27. Rivkees SA. Mechanisms and clinical significance of circadian rhythms in children. Curr Opinion Pediatr. 2001; 13:352–7.
28. Rivera-Coll A, Fuentes-Arderiu X, Diez-Noguera A. Circadian rhythms of serum concentrations of 12 enzymes of clinical interest. Chronobiology International. 1993; 10:190–200.
29. Rivera-Coll A, Fuentes-Arderiu X, Diez-Noguera A. Circadian rhythmic variations in serum concentrations of clinically important lipids. Clin Chemistry. 1994; 40:1549–53.
30. Koopman MG, Koonen GCM, Krediet RT, et al. Circadian rhythm of glomerular filtration rate in normal individuals. Clin Sci. 1989; 77:105–11.

31. Bleyzac N, Allard-Latour B, Laffont A, et al. Diurnal changes in the pharmacokinetic behavior of amikacin. *Ther Drug Monit.* 2000; 22:307–12.

32. Brent GA. Maternal thyroid function: interpretation of thyroid function tests in pregnancy. *Clin Obstet Gynecol.* 1997; 40:3–15.

33. McClamrock HD. Androgen production and metabolism in normal pregnancy. In: *UpToDate Clinical Reference Library.* Wellesley, MA: UpToDate Release 10.1; 2002.

34. Lampert MB, Lang RM, Rose BD. Renal function in pregnancy. In: *UpToDate Clinical Reference Library.* Wellesley, MA: UpToDate Release 10.1; 2002.

35. Petraglia F, D'Antonio D. Maternal endocrine and metabolic adaptation to pregnancy. In: *UpToDate Clinical Reference Library.* Wellesley, MA: UpToDate Release 10.1; 2002.

36. Foley MR. Maternal cardiovascular adaptation to pregnancy. In: *UpToDate Clinical Reference Library.* Wellesley, MA: UpToDate Release 10.1; 2002.

37. Peacock AJ. ABC of oxygen: oxygen at high altitude. *Br Med J.* 1998; 317:1063–6.

38. Kost GJ, Ehrmeyer SS, Chernow B, et al. The laboratory-clinical interface: point-of-care testing. *Chest.* 1999; 115:1140–54.

39. Mor M, Waisman Y. Point-of-care testing: a critical review. *Ped Emerg Care.* 2000; 16:45–8.

40. Price CP. Point of care testing. *Br Med J.* 2001; 322:1285–8.

41. Medicare, Medicaid, and CLIA Programs. Extension of Certain Effective Dates for Clinical Laboratory Requirements Under CLIA: final rule. *Federal Register.* 1998; 63:55031–4.

42. Small PM, Fujuwara I. Medical progress: management of tuberculosis in the United States. *N Engl J Med.* 2001; 345:189–200.

43. Emery J, Hayflick S. The challenge of integrating genetic medicine into primary care. *Br Med J.* 2001; 322:1027–30.

44. Aithal GP, Day CP, Kesteven PJ, et al. Association of polymorphisms in the cytochrome P450 CYP2C9 with warfarin dose requirement and risk of bleeding complications. *Lancet.* 1999; 353:717–9.

45. Holtzman NA, Shapiro D. The new genetics: genetic testing and public policy. *Br Med J.* 1998; 316:852–6.

BIBLIOGRAPHY

Bakerman S, Bakerman P, Strausbauch P. *ABC's of Interpretive Laboratory Data.* 4th ed. Myrtle Beach, SC: Interpretive Laboratory Data; 2002.

Fischbach F. *A Manual of Laboratory & Diagnostic Tests.* 6th ed. Philadelphia, PA: J. B. Lippincott; 1996.

Jacobs DS. *Laboratory Test Handbook.* 4th ed. AACC Press; 1996.

Jacobs DS, DeMott WR, Grady HJ, et al. *Laboratory Test Handbook: Concise with Disease Index.* Hudson, OH: Lexi-Comp, Inc.; 1996.

Kraemer HC. *Evaluating Medical Tests.* Newbury Park, CA: Sage Publications; 1992.

Ravel R. *Clinical Laboratory Medicine: Clinical Application of Laboratory Data.* 6th ed. Chicago, IL: YearBook Medical Publisher, Inc.; 1999.

Sacher RA, McPherson RA. *Widman's Clinical Interpretation of Laboratory Tests.* 10th ed. Philadelphia, PA: F. A. Davis; 1991.

Speicher CE. *The Right Test: A Physician's Guide to Laboratory Medicine.* Philadelphia, PA: W. B. Saunders; 1998.

Wallach J. *Interpretation of Diagnostic Tests.* 7th ed. Boston, MA: Little, Brown; 2000.

Chapter **2**

INTRODUCTION TO COMMON LABORATORY ASSAYS AND TECHNOLOGY

Steven J. Melnick

Clinical laboratory data are used in the diagnosis and treatment of disease. The performance of laboratory tests involves clinical chemistry methodologies to identify and/or quantify clinically important endogenous or exogenous substances. Other laboratory methods—in the areas of hematology, microbiology, and molecular pathology—are used to evaluate a wide range of biological parameters. Although clinicians do not usually perform laboratory tests, they still need an introduction to and a basic understanding of the common methods and techniques. This chapter provides an introduction to these techniques.

Early methods for identification and separation of analytes included flame photometry and paper chromatography. Although recent technological advances have increased the sophistication and complexity of laboratory methodologies, many procedures still rely on the basic principles of those two tests: (1) changes in color or light absorbance and (2) various solubility and polarity characteristics. Even new developments in molecular biology and immunobiology utilize these principles in some test steps.

This chapter reviews the principles and applications of some common laboratory tests as well as their advantages and disadvantages.

OBJECTIVES

After completing this chapter, the reader should be able to

1. List the primary analytes of ion-selective electrodes (ISE).
2. Explain the principles behind turbidimetry and nephelometry.
3. List the basic components of a spectrophotometer and describe the purpose of each.
4. Describe the major electrophoresis techniques and their applications.
5. Compare gas and high-performance (or pressure) liquid chromatography (HPLC) with respect to equipment and methodology.
6. Explain the methodological basis of immunoassays.
7. List common tests using agglutination.
8. Compare and contrast radioimmunoassay (RIA), enzyme-linked immunosorbent assay (ELISA), enzyme-multiplied immunoassay technique (EMIT), and fluorescent polarization immunoassay (FPIA) with respect to methods and tests performed.
9. Describe the basic components of a mass spectrometry system.
10. Compare the commonly used cytometry systems.
11. Describe the purpose of the polymerase chain reaction (PCR).
12. Describe the role and fundamental elements of laboratory automation.

PHOTOMETRY

Photometry is used to identify and/or quantify a given substance by measuring the light absorbed or emitted at a characteristic spectral region upon excitation by a specific narrow wavelength of light. In clinical laboratory instruments, the range of wavelengths measured is between 150 and 2500 nm, corresponding to the low ultraviolet (UV) to the near infrared (IR) region.[1] Photometric devices are classified by the source of light that is measured (i.e., whether the light is absorbed or emitted by either molecules or atoms). The four types of instruments are molecular absorption, atomic emission (flame photometers), atomic absorption, and molecular emission spectrophotometers (fluorometers).

Molecular Absorption Spectrophotometry

Molecular absorption spectrophotometers, usually referred to as spectrophotometers, are commonly employed in conjunction with other methodologies, such as nephelometry and enzyme immunoassay (EIA) (e.g., to quantify the reaction produced by an immunoassay), because of their rapidity, ease of use, and relatively high specificity. The high specificity achieved with spectrophotometry is obtained by an analyte reacting with various substances that produce colorimetric reactions. The specificity can be further enhanced by first isolating the analyte.

The basic components of the two types of spectrophotometers (single and double beam) are depicted in Figure 2-1. Light from a source (I) (e.g., a tungsten bulb or laser) passes through an entrance slit that minimizes stray light. Specific wavelengths of light are isolated by a monochromator (II). The selected wavelength then passes through the exit slit and illuminates the analytical cell (cuvette) containing the test solution (III).

After passing through the test solution the light strikes a detector, usually a photomultiplier tube (IV).[1] This tube amplifies the electronic signal, which is then sent to a recording device (V). The result is compared with a standard curve to yield a specific concentration of analyte.

The double-beam instrument is designed to compensate for changes in absorbance of the reagent blank and light source intensity. It utilizes a mirror (VI) to split the light from a single source into two beams, one passing through the test solution and one through the reagent blank. By doing so, it automatically corrects optical errors as the wavelength changes.

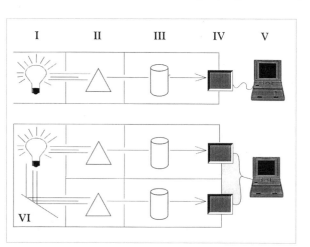

Figure 2-1. Schematic of single-beam (upper portion) and double-beam (lower portion) spectrophotometers. I = radiant light source; II = monochromator; III = analytical cuvette; IV = photomultiplier; V = recording device; VI = mirror.

Most measurements are made in the visible range of the spectrum, with some in the ultraviolet and infrared ranges. The greatest sensitivity is achieved by selecting the wavelength of light in the range of maximum absorption. If substances are known to interfere at this wavelength, measurements may be made at a different one in the absorption spectrum. This procedure allows detection of the analyte of interest with minimal interference from other endogenous or exogenous substances.

Atomic Emission and Atomic Absorption Spectrophotometry

Atomic emission (flame photometry) and atomic absorption spectrophotometry are rarely used in modern clinical laboratories. Concentrations of elements such as sodium, potassium, and lithium were classically determined by flame photometry. This technique is based on the elementary quantum principle that electrons in an atom are excited to a higher energy level by heat. The electrons, being unstable in this state, return to a lower energy state. In doing so, the excess energy is liberated as photons in the visible light range.

Usually, multiple energy levels are involved and the resulting spectral patterns are characteristic of each element. When conditions are held constant, the concentration of each ion is proportional to the light intensity at its characteristic wavelength.

Atomic absorption spectrophotometry is confined mainly to specialized toxicology laboratories. Unlike flame photometry, the element that is analyzed by this technique is not appreciably excited. Rather, the element is dissociated from its chemical bonds. In this state, the element is in its lowest energy state and capable of absorbing energy in a narrow range that corresponds to its line spectrum.[2] Atomic absorption spectrophotometers are much more sensitive than flame photometers and more specific since the light sources used (hollow cathode lamps) emit at wavelengths that are specific for the element being measured.[2]

Molecular Emission Spectrophotometry

Molecular emission spectrophotometry is usually referred to as molecular luminescence spectroscopy or fluorometry. This technology is based upon the principles of luminescence, which is an energy exchange process that occurs when electrons absorb electromagnetic radiation and then return from this excited energy level to a lower level. Three types of fluorescence phenomena—fluorescence, phosphorescence, and chemiluminescence—form the basis of this very sensitive clinical laboratory instrumentation.

Fluorescence results from a three-stage process that occurs in certain molecules known as fluorophores. The first stage involves the absorption of radiant energy by an electron in the ground state creating an excited singlet state. During the very short lifetime of this state (order of nanoseconds), energy from the electronic-vibrational excited state is partially dissipated through a radiationless transfer of energy that results from interactions with the molecular environment and leads to the formation of an relaxed excited singlet state. This is followed by relaxation to the electronic ground state by the emission of radiation (fluorescence). Because energy is dissipated, the energy of the emitted photon is lower and the wavelength is longer than the absorption photon. The difference between these two energies is known as Stokes shift. This principle is the basis for the sensitivity of the different fluorescence techniques since the emission photons can be detected at a different wavelength band than the excitation photons. Consequently, the background is lower than with absorption spectrophotometry where the transmitted light is detected against a background of incident light at the same wavelength.[3]

The phenomenon of *phosphorescence* is similar to fluorescence since it also results from the absorption of radiant energy by a molecule. However, it is also a competitive process. Unlike fluorescence, which results from a singlet-singlet transition, phosphorescence results from a triplet-singlet transition. When a pair of electrons occupies a molecular orbital in the ground or excited state, a singlet state is created. In a singlet state, the electrons must have opposite spins because of the Pauli exclusion principle, and only one magnetic moment is derived from this state. When the electrons are no longer paired, three different arrangements are possible, each with a different magnetic moment. This is referred to as a *triplet state*. The electronic energy of a triplet state is lower than a singlet state. Therefore, when the relaxed excited singlet state overlaps with a higher triplet state, energy may be transferred through a process called *intersystem crossing*. As in the case of an excited singlet state, energy may be dissipated through several radiationless mechanisms to the electronic ground state. However, when a triplet-singlet transition occurs, the result is phosphorescence. The probability of this type of transition is much lower than a singlet-singlet transition (fluorescence), and the emission wavelength and decay times are also longer than for fluorescence emission. Because the various forms of radiationless energy transfer compete so effectively, phosphorescence is generally limited to molecules (e.g., many aromatic and organometallic compounds) at very low temperatures or in highly viscous solutions.[3,4]

The phenomenon of *chemiluminescence* is also similar to that of fluorescence in that it results from light emitted from an excited singlet state. However, unlike both fluorescence and phosphorescence, the excitation energy is caused by a chemical or electrochemical reaction. The energy is typically derived from the oxidation of an organic compound (e.g., luminol, luciferin, and acridinium ester). The light is derived from the excited products that are formed in the reaction.

Different instruments have been developed that use these basic principles of luminescence. These devices use similar basic components along the following pathway: a light source (laser or mercury arc lamp), an excitation monochromator, a sample cuvette, an emission monochromator, and a photodetector.[1] While the principles of these instruments are relatively straightforward, various modifications have been developed for specific applications.

An important example is fluorescent polarization in fluorometers. Fluorescent molecules (fluorophores) become excited by polarized light when the plane of polarization is parallel to their absorption transition vector, provided the molecule remains relatively stationary throughout the excited state. If the molecules rotate rapidly, light will be emitted in a different plane than the excitation plane. The intensity of light emitted by the molecules in the excitation polarization plane and at 90° permits the fluorescence polarization to be measured (fluorometry). The degree to which the emission intensity varies between the two planes of polarization is a function of the mobility of the fluorophore. Large molecules move slowly during the excited state and will remain highly polarized. Small molecules that rotate faster will emit light that is depolarized relative to the excitation plane.[4]

One of the most common applications of fluorescence polarization is competitive immunoassays, used to measure a wide range of analytes including therapeutic and illicit drugs, hormones, enzymes, and other commonly measured analytes in the clinical laboratory. This important methodology involves the addition of a known quantity of fluorescent-labeled analyte molecules to a serum-antibody (specific to the analyte) mixture. The labeled analyte will emit depolarized light because its motion is not constrained. However, when it binds to an antibody, its motion will decrease and the emitted light will be more polarized. When an unknown quantity of an unlabeled analyte is added to the mixture, competitive binding for the antibody will occur and reduce the polarization of the labeled analyte. By using standard curves of known drug concentrations vs. polarization, the concentration of the unlabeled analyte can be determined.[4]

Another important application of fluorometry is flow cytometry. This technology is discussed in the cytometry section. Like many modern laboratory instruments, flow cytometry involved the application of multiple physical, chemical, and biological principles and is, therefore, best addressed in a separate category.

TURBIDIMETRY AND NEPHELOMETRY

When light passes through a solution in a cuvette, it can be either absorbed or scattered. Turbidimetry is a simple technique for measuring the percent transmittance of light due to particles such as immune complexes. Nephelometry is also commonly used in immunoglobulin assays.

The major advantage of turbidimetry is that measurements can be made with common laboratory instruments such as a spectrophotometer. Errors associated with this method center around sample and reagent preparation. Since the amount of light blocked depends on both the concentration and size of each particle, differences in particle size between the sample and the standard result in error. The length of time between sample preparation and measurement should be consistent since particles settle to varying degrees, allowing more or less light to pass. Large concentrations are necessary because this test measures small differences in large numbers.

Nephelometry is similar to turbidimetry. The main differences are that (1) the light source is usually a laser and (2) the detector to measure scattered light is at a right angle to the incident light. The scattered light is a function of the size and number of particles in the beam. Nephelometric measurements are more precise than turbidimetric ones since the smaller signal generated for low analyte concentrations is more easily detected against a very low background.[5] Because antigen-antibody complexes are easily detected by this method, it is commonly employed in combination with EIA (discussed later).

REFRACTOMETRY

The principle whereby light bends as it passes through different media is the basis of refractometry. Refractivity, the ability of a liquid to bend light, depends upon several factors: the wavelength of the incident light, the temperature, the physical characteristics of the medium, and the solute concentration in the medium. Refractometers, by keeping constant the first three parameters, permit the measurement of the total solute concentration of a liquid. These instruments are particularly useful, especially as a rapid screening test because no chemical reactions are required.[1]

Refractometers are frequently used to measure the total dissolved plasma solids (most of which is protein) and the urine specific gravity. The basic design of refractometers is relatively unchanged since development over 100 years ago. The main advancement has been to incorporate an electric heater to maintain a constant temperature. In a refractometer, light is passed through the sample and then a series of prisms. The refracted light is projected on a reticle or scale against the eyepiece. The scale is calibrated for grams per deciliter of serum protein or for the specific gravity of urine. In the eyepiece, a sharp line of demarcation is apparent and represents the boundary between the sample and distilled water. In the case of serum or plasma samples, the refraction angle is produced by the total dissolved solids. Although proteins are the predominant solute, other substances such as electrolytes, glucose, lipids, and urea contribute to the refraction angle. Therefore, the measurement made on serum or plasma is not identical to the true protein concentration. The various instruments in use rely on the assumption that the nonprotein solutes contribute to the total solutes in a predictable manner.[6]

OSMOMETRY

In a strict sense, osmometry is the measurement of osmotic pressure. However, in the clinical laboratory the osmometer reading is interpreted as a measure of total concentration of solute particles. Clinically, osmometers are used to measure the osmolality of biological fluids such as serum, plasma, and urine. As osmotically active particles are dissolved in a solvent (water, in the case of these biological fluids), four physical properties of the pure solvent (water) are affected: the osmotic pressure is increased, the vapor pressure is decreased, the boiling point is increased, and the freezing point is decreased. Since each property is related, they can be expressed mathematically in terms of the others (colligative properties) and to osmolality. Consequently, several methods can be used to measure osmolality including freezing-point depression, colloid osmotic pressure, and vapor pressure osmometry.[7]

The most commonly used devices to measure osmolality or other colligative properties of a solution are *freezing-point depression* osmometers. These simple devices consist of a sample chamber with a stirrer and a thermistor, a cooling chamber containing antifreeze, and a potentiometer with a direct readout. The sample is rapidly cooled several degrees below its freezing point in the cooling chamber. The sample is stirred to initiate freezing of the supercooled solution. When the freezing point of the solution is reached (the point where the rate of the heat of fusion released by ice formation comes into equilibrium with the rate of heat removal by the cooling chamber), the osmolality can be calculated.[1]

It is often important to measure the *colloid osmotic pressure* (COP), a direct measure of the contribution of plasma proteins to the osmolality. Because of the large molecular weight of plasma proteins, their contribution to the total osmolality is very small as measured by freezing-point depression and vapor pressure osmometers. Since a low colloid osmotic pressure favors a shift of fluid from the intravascular compartment to the interstitial compartment, measurement of the COP is particularly important in monitoring the intravascular volume. This helps to guide fluid therapy in different circumstances to prevent peripheral and pulmonary edema.

The COP osmometer, also known as a membrane osmometer, consists of two fluid-filled chambers separated by a semipermeable membrane. One chamber is filled with a colloid-free physiologic saline solution that is in contact with a pressure transducer. When the plasma or serum is placed in the sample chamber, fluid moves by osmosis from the saline chamber to the sample chamber, thus causing a negative pressure to develop in the saline chamber. This pressure is the COP.[7]

The *vapor pressure* osmometer is not commonly used in the clinical laboratories because it is less precise that the freezing-point depression osmometer.[8] The reasons include the poorer coefficient of variation in interlaboratory comparisons, nonlinear responses in certain ranges, and the inability to include the measurement of osmolality to the contributions of volatile solutes.

ELECTROCHEMISTRY

In the broadest context, electrochemistry involves the study of charge-transfer phenomena. However, the analytic electrochemical techniques used in the clinical laboratory involve the measurement of the current or voltage produced by the activity of different ion species. These analytic techniques are based on the fundamental electrochemical phenomenon of potentiometry, coulometry, voltammetry, and conductometry.

Potentiometry

Potentiometry involves the measurement of electrical potential differences between two electrodes in an electrochemical cell at zero current flow. This electrochemical method uses the Nernst equation, which relates the potential to the concentration of an ion in solution, to measure analyte concentrations.[9] Each electrode or half-cell in an electrochemical cell consists of a metal conductor that is in contact with an electrolyte solution. One of the electrodes is a reference electrode with a constant electric potential, the other is the measuring or indicator electrode. The boundaries between the ion conductive phases in the cell determine the type of potential gradients that exist between the electrodes and are defined as redox (oxidation reduction), membrane, and diffusion potentials.

The redox potential occurs when the two electrolyte solutions in the electrochemical cell are brought into contact with each other by a salt bridge so that the two solutions can be brought into equilibrium. A potentiometer may be used to measure the potential difference between the two electrodes. This is known as the *redox potential difference* because the reaction involves the transfer of electrons between substances that accept electrons (oxidant) and substances that donate electrons (reductant). Junctional potentials rather than redox potentials occur when either a solid-state or liquid interface exists between the ion conductive phases. These produce membrane or diffusion potentials respectively. In each case the concentration of an ion in solution can be measured using the Nernst equation, which relates the electrode potential to the activity of the measured ions in the test solution[1]:

$$E = E^0 - (0.059/z)\log (C_{red}/C_{ox})$$

where E = the total potential (in mV), E^0 = is the standard reduction potential, z = the number of electrons involved in the reduction reaction, C_{red} = the molar concentration of the ion in the oxidized form, and C_{ox} = the molar concentration of the ion in the reduced form.

Ion-selective electrodes (ISE) consisting of a membrane that separates the reference and test electrolyte solutions are very selective and sensitive for the ions that they measure. For this reason further discussion on potentiometry will focus on these types of electrodes.

The ISE method, having comparable or better sensitivity than flame photometry, has become the principal test for determining urine and serum electrolytes in the clinical labo-

TABLE 2-1

ASSAY	ANALYSIS TIME (MIN)	COMMON TESTS	USE
ISE	6–18	Electrolytes, (sodium potassium, chloride, calcium, lithium, total carbon dioxide)	Primary testing method
GC	30	Toxicologic screens, organic acids, drugs (e.g., benzodiazepines and tricyclic antidepressants [TCAs])	Primary testing method
HPLC	30	Toxicologic screens, vanilmandelic acid, hydroxyvanilmandelic acid, amino acids, drugs (e.g., indometh-acin, steroids, cyclosporin)	Primary and secondary or confirmatory testing methods
RIA	15	Endocrinology (e.g., thyroid) and drugs (e.g., digoxin)	Secondary or confirmatory testing method
ELISA	0.1–0.3	Serologic tests (e.g., antinuclear antibody, rheumatoid factor, hepatitis B, cytomegalovirus, and human immunodeficiency virus antigens)	Primary testing method
EMIT	0.1–0.3	General chemistries (e.g., albumin, blood urea nitrogen [BUN], creatine, glucose, cholesterol, bilirubin, total protein) and enzymes (e.g., acid and alkaline phosphatase, amylase, creative kinase)	Primary testing method
		Coagulation (e.g., antithrombin III, fibrinogen, degradation products, heparin, plasminogen)	
		Therapeutic drug monitoring (e.g., aminoglycosides, vancomycin, digoxin, antiepileptics, antiarrhythmics, theophylline)	
		Toxicology (acetaminophen, salicylate, barbiturates, TCAs, amphetamines, cocaine, opiates)	
FPIA	0.1–0.2	Therapeutic drug monitoring (e.g., aminoglycosides, vancomycin, antiepileptics, antiarrhythmics, theophylline, methotrexate, digoxin, cyclosporine)	Primary testing method
		General chemistries (e.g., thyroxine, triiodothyronine, cortisol, amylase, BUN, lactate dehydrogenase, creatinine, glucose, cholesterol, iron)	
PCR	0.1–0.2	Microbiologic and virologic markers of organisims and genetic markers	Primary testing method

Table 2-1 Routine Tests Performed by Common Laboratory Assays

ratory. Typically, ion concentrations such as sodium and potassium are measured using this method (Table 2-1).

The principle of ISE involves the generation of a small electrical current when a particular ion comes in contact with an electrode. The electrode selectively binds the ion to be measured. To measure the concentration, the circuit must be completed with a reference electrode. The three types of electrodes are

1. Ion-selective glass membranes.
2. Solid-state electrodes.
3. Liquid ion-exchange membranes.

As shown in Figure 2-2, ion-selective glass membranes preferentially allow hydrogen (H^+), sodium (Na^+), and ammonium (NH_4^+) ions to cross a hydrated outer layer of glass. The H^+ glass electrode or pH electrode is the most common electrode for measuring H^+. However, electrodes for Na^+, K^+, Li^+, and NH_4^+ are available. An electrical potential is created when these ions diffuse across the membrane.

Solid-state electrodes consist of halide-containing crystals for measuring specific ions. An example is the silver–silver chloride electrode for measuring chloride.[1] Liquid ion-exchange membranes contain a water-insoluble, inert solvent that can dissolve an ion-selective carrier. Ions outside the membrane produce a concentration-related potential with the ions bound to the carrier inside the membrane.[1]

The electrodes are separated from the sample by a liquid junction or salt bridge. Since the liquid junction generates its own voltage at the sample interface, it is a source of error. This error is overcome by adjusting the composition of the liquid junction.[10] Another source of error is the selectivity of the electrode. Therefore, careful electrode selection is important. Overall, this method is simple to use and more accurate than flame photometry for samples having low plasma water due to conditions such as hyperlipoproteinemia.[11] Furthermore, ion-selective electrodes are relatively inexpensive and simple to use compared to other techniques and have an extremely wide range of applications and wide concentration range. They are also very useful in biomedical applications because they can measure the activity of the ion directly in addition to the concentration.

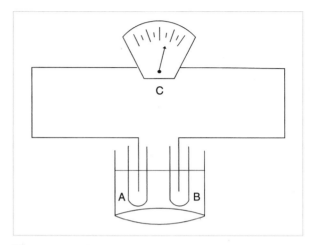

Figure 2-2. The pH meter is an example of a test that uses ISE to measure the concentration of hydrogen ions. An electric current is generated when hydrogen ions come in contact with the ISE (A). The circuit is completed through the use of a reference electrode (B) submerged in the same liquid as the ISE (also known as the liquid junction). The concentration can then be read on a potentiometer (C).

Coulometry

Coulometry is an analytical method for measuring an unknown concentration of an analyte in solution by completely converting the analyte from one oxidation state to another. This is accomplished through a form of titration where a standardized concentration of the titrant is reacted with the unknown analyte and, thus, requires no chemical standards or calibration. The point at which all of the analyte has been converted to the new oxidation state is called the *endpoint* and is determined by some type of indicator that is also present in the solution.

The basis of this technique is Faraday's law, which relates the quantity of electric charge generated by an amount of substance produced or consumed in the redox process and is expressed as

$$znF = It = Q$$

where z is the number of electrons involved in the reaction, n is the quantity of the analyte, F is Faraday's constant (96,487 C/mol), Q is the amount of charge that passes through the cell, I is the current, and t is time. The chloridometer is a common instrument that employs this method.[1] These instruments may be used to measure the chloride ion concentration in sweat, urine, and CSF samples. The device uses a constant current across two silver electrodes. The Ag^+ ions that are generated at a constant rate react with the Cl^- ions in the sample. The reaction that produces insoluble AgCl ceases once excess Ag^+ ions are detected by an indicator and reference electrodes. Since the quantity of Ag^+ ions generated is known, the quantity of Cl^- ions may be calculated using Faraday's law.

Voltammetry

Voltammetry encompasses a group of electrochemical techniques in which a potential is applied to an electrochemical cell with the simultaneous measurement of the resulting current. By varying the potential of an electrode, it is possible to oxidize and reduce analytes in solution. At more positive potentials, the electrons within the electrode become lower in energy and the oxidation of species in solution becomes more likely. At lower potentials, the opposite occurs. By monitoring the current of an electrochemical cell at varying electrode potentials, it is possible to determine several characteristics of the solution species such as concentration, reaction kinetics, and thermodynamic parameters.[7]

This technique differs from potentiometry in a number of important ways. Voltammetric techniques use an externally applied force (potential) to generate a signal (current) in a way that would not normally occur, whereas in potentiometric techniques the analytical signal is produced internally through a redox reaction. The electrode arrangement is also quite different between the two techniques. In order to analyze both the potential and the resulting current, three electrodes are employed in voltammetric devices. The three electrodes include the working, auxiliary, and reference electrodes, which (when connected through a voltmeter) permit the application of specific potential functions. The measurement of the resulting current can yield results about ionic concentrations, conductivity, and diffusion. The ability to apply different types of potential functions or waveforms has lead to the development of different voltammetric techniques: linear potential sweep polarography, pulse polarography, cyclic voltammetry, and anode stripping voltammetry.[1] These analytical methods, though not commonly used in clinical laboratories, are very sensitive (detection limits as low as the parts per billion range) and are capable of multielement studies.

Conductometry

Conductometry is the measurement of current flow (proportional to conductivity) between two nonpolarized electrodes of which a known potential is established. Because the conductivity in aqueous solutions is a function of the electrolyte concentration, conductance techniques are often used to assess water purity. Clinical applications include urea estimation through the measurement of the rate-of-change of conductance that occurs with the urease-catalyzed formation of NH_4^+ and HCO_3^-. The technique is limited at low concentrations because of the high conductance of biological fluids. Perhaps the most important application of impedance (inversely proportional to conductance) measurements in the clinical laboratory involves the Coulter principle for the electronic counting of blood cells. This method is discussed in detail in the cytometry section.

ELECTROPHORESIS

Electrophoresis is the process of moving charged molecules in solution or a support medium under the influence of an electrical field. The movement of molecules in an electrical field is dependent on their charge, shape, and size, making electrophoresis an important methodology for molecular separations.[12] Because biomolecules are often water-soluble and charged, this relatively simple analytical tool has become one of the most important techniques for molecular separation in the clinical laboratory. The primary application of electrophoresis is the analysis and purification of very large molecules such as proteins and nucleic acids. However, it can also be applied to smaller molecules, including charged sugars, amino acids, peptides, nucleotides, and simple ions. Through the proper selection of the medium for electrophoretic separations, extremely high resolution and sensitivity of separation can be achieved. Electrophoretic systems are usually combined with highly sensitive detection methods to monitor and analyze the separations that suit the specific application.[13]

The basic electrophoresis apparatus consists of a high voltage supply, electrodes, a buffer, and a support for the buffer or a capillary tube. Supports for the buffer include filter paper, cellulose acetate membranes, agarose, and polyacrylamide gels. When an electrostatic force is applied across the electrophoresis apparatus, the charged molecules will migrate to the anode or the cathode of the system depending on their charge. The force that acts on these molecules is proportional to the net charge on the molecular species and the applied voltage (electromotive force). This relationship is expressed as

$$F = qE/d$$

where F is the force exerted on the charged molecule, q is its net charge, E is the electromotive force, and d is the distance across the electrophoretic medium.[14]

While this relationship is very simple, the phenomenon of electrophoresis is considerably more complex. The molecules are dissolved in a buffer that contains electrolytes in order to carry the applied current and fix the pH. The mobility of the molecules will be affected locally by the charge of the electrolytes, the viscosity of the medium, and their size and degree of asymmetry. These factors have been shown to be related by the following equation:

$$\mu = q/6\pi\eta r$$

where μ is the electrophoretic mobility of the charged molecule, η is the viscosity of the medium, and r is the ionic radius.[14]

The conditions in which this process occurs are further complicated by the use of a support medium, which is necessary to minimize diffusion and convective mixing of the bands (caused by the heated current flowing through the buffer). The media used include polysaccharides (cellulose and agarose) and synthetic media such as polyacrylamide. The porosity of these media will, to a large extent, determine the resistance to movement for different ionic species. Therefore, the type of support medium used depends on the application.

The many factors that affect the process of electrophoresis are controllable to provide the optimal resolution for the specific application. The main types of electrophoresis techniques used in both clinical and research laboratories include cellulose acetate, agarose gel, polyacrylamide gel, isoelectric focusing, two-dimensional (2D), and capillary electrophoresis.

Gel Electrophoresis

Cellulose Acetate and Agarose Gel Electrophoresis

Cellulose acetate and agarose gel electrophoresis are commonly used for both serum protein and hemoglobin separation. Serum protein electrophoresis is often used as a screening procedure for the detection of various pathologic states, such as inflammation, protein loss, monoclonal gammopathies, and other dysproteinemias. In practice, the electrophoresis apparatus, cellulose acetate and agarose gels, and reagents are obtained from commercial suppliers for this specific application. Once the bands are separated, specific stains are used to visualize them. Densitometry is typically used to quantify each band. When a monoclonal immunoglobulin pattern is identified, another technique, immunofixation electrophoresis, is used to quantify the immunoglobulins IgG, IgA, IgM, κ, and λ. Once these proteins are separated on an agarose gel, specific antibodies directed at the immunoglobulins are added. The sample is then fixed and stained to visualize and quantify the bands.[15] Separation of proteins may also be accomplished with isoelectric focusing where the proteins migrate through a stable pH gradient with the pH varying in the direction of migration. Each protein moves to its isoelectric point (i.e., the point where the protein's charge becomes zero and migration ceases). This technique is often used for separation of isoenzymes and hemoglobin variants.

Hemoglobin electrophoresis remains a cost effective method for the screening of hemoglobin variants. The hemoglobins are separated on a cellulose acetate membrane at an alkaline pH (8.6) and on an agarose gel at an acid pH (6.2). Electrophoresis at both pH conditions is performed for optimal resolution of comigrating hemoglobin bands that occur at either of the pH conditions. For example, hemoglobin S, which comigrates with hemoglobins D and G at pH 8.6, can be separated at pH 6.2. The choice of support media is determined by the resolution of the hemoglobin bands that are achieved. Following electrophoresis, the bands are stained for visualization and the relative proportions of the hemoglobins are obtained by densitometry.[16]

Electrophoresis is an important technique that is used in the molecular pathology laboratory. It is a powerful yet reasonably inexpensive method to separate DNA, RNA, and protein fragments. Three common techniques used are Southern, Northern, and Western blots. These techniques differ in the target molecules that are separated. Southern blots separate DNA that is cut with restriction endonucleases and then identified with a labeled (usually radioactive) DNA probe; Northern blots separate fragments of RNA that are probed with labeled DNA or RNA; and Western blots separate proteins that are probed with radioactive or enzymatically-tagged antibodies.

Each method involves a series of steps that lead to the detection of the various targets. Following electrophoresis, typically performed with an agarose or polyacrylamide gel, the molecules are transferred to a solid support where they will remain during the probe hybridization, washing, and detection stages of the assay. The DNA, RNA, or protein in the gel may be transferred onto nitrocellulose paper through electrophoresis or capillary blotting. In the former method the molecules, by virtue of their negative charge, are transferred by electrophoresis. The latter method involves layering the gel on wet filter paper with the nitrocellulose paper on top. Dry filter paper is placed on the nitrocellulose paper and the molecules are transferred with the flow of buffer from the wet to dry filter paper via capillary action. Following the transfer, the nitrocellulose paper is soaked in a blocking solution containing high concentrations of DNA, RNA, or protein. This prevents the probe from randomly sticking to the paper during hybridization. During the hybridization stage, the labeled DNA, RNA, or antibody is incubated with the blot where binding with the molecular target occurs. The probe-target hybrids are detected following a wash step to remove any unbound probe.

Two-Dimensional Electrophoresis

Two-dimensional electrophoresis (2-D electrophoresis) is a powerful and widely used method for the analysis of complex protein mixtures extracted from cells, tissues, or other biological samples. Proteins are sorted according to two independent properties: isoelectric focusing, which separates proteins according to their isoelectric points, and SDS-polyacrylamide gel electrophoresis, which separates proteins according to their molecular weights. Each spot on the resulting two-dimensional array corresponds to a single protein species in the sample.[18] Using this technique, thousands of different proteins can be separated, quantified, and characterized. This technology has many research applications especially in the field of proteomics, which includes the large scale screening and cataloging of proteins in biological systems.

These relatively simple techniques have led to many important diagnostic tests in all fields of medicine. Routine diagnostic applications for this technology exist for infectious diseases, malignancies, genetic diseases, paternity testing, forensic analysis, and tissue typing for transplantation.

Capillary Electrophoresis

Capillary electrophoresis (CE) is a relatively new and diversified analytical technique that includes such methods as capillary zone electrophoresis, capillary gel electrophoresis, capillary chromatography, capillary isoelectric focusing, micelle electrokinetic capillary chromatography, and capillary isotachophoresis. While primarily a research tool, this technique is entering the clinical laboratory because of its rapid and high-efficiency separation power, diverse applications, and potential for automation. The possibility of this becoming an important technology in the clinical laboratory is illustrated by its use in the separation and quantification of a wide spectrum of biological components ranging from macromolecules (proteins, lipoproteins, and nucleic acids) to small analytes (amino acids, organic acids, or drugs).

Capillary electrophoresis apparatus consists of a small-bore, silica-fused capillary (25–75 µm), approximately 50–100 cm in length, connected to a detector at one end and via buffer reservoirs to a high-voltage power supply (25–35kV).[17] Because the small capillaries efficiently dissipate the heat, high voltages can be used to generate intense electric fields across the capillary to produce highly efficient separations with short separation times. In a CE separation, a very small amount of sample (0.1 to 10 nL) is required. When the sample solution is injected into the apparatus, the molecules in the solution migrate through the capillary due to its charge in an electric field (electrophoretic mobility) or due to a phenomenon known as the *electroosmotic force* (EOF). The negatively charged surface of the silica capillary attracts positively-charged ions in the buffer solution, which in turn migrate toward the cathode and carry solvent molecules in the same direction. The overall movement of the solvent is called *electroosmotic flow*. The separated proteins are eluted from the cathode end of the capillary. Quantitative detectors such as fluorescence, absorbance, electrochemical detectors, and mass spectrometry can be used to identify and quantify the proteins in the solution in amounts as little as 10^{-20} mol of substance in the injected volume.[17]

Capillary Zone Electrophoresis

Capillary zone electrophoresis (CZE) is the most widely-used mode of CE and is used for the separation of both anionic and cationic solutes in a single analysis. In CZE the anions and cations migrate in different directions, but they both rapidly move toward the cathode due to EOF, which is usually significantly higher than the solute velocity. Therefore, all molecules, regardless of their charge, will migrate to the cathode. In this way the negative, neutral, and positive species can be detected and separated. Common clinical applications include high throughput separation of serum and urine protein and hemoglobin variants. No doubt other applications will become more commonplace. However, these systems are expensive, and conventional methods can suffice.

Capillary Gel Electrophoresis

Capillary gel electrophoresis (CGE) is the CE-analog of traditional gel electrophoresis and is used for the size-based separation of biological macromolecules such as oligonucleotides, DNA restriction fragments, and proteins. The separation is performed by filling the capillary with a sieve-like matrix such as polyacrylamide or agarose to reduce the EOF. Therefore, larger molecules such as DNA will move more slowly resulting in better separation. This and the other methods of CE are primarily used in research.

DENSITOMETRY

Densitometry is essentially a specialized form of spectrophotometry used to evaluate electrophoretic patterns. Densitometers can perform measurements in an absorbance optical mode and a fluorescence mode, depending on the type of staining of the electrophoretic pattern. An absorbance optical system consists of a light source, filter system, a movable carriage to scan the electrophoretic medium, an optical system, and a photodetector (silicon photocell) to detect light in the absorbance mode. When a densitometer is operated in the absorbance mode, an electrophoretic pattern located on the carriage system is moved across a focused beam of incident light. After the light passes through the pattern, it is converted to an electronic signal by the photocell to indicate the amount of light absorbed by the pattern. The absorbance is proportional to the sample concentration. The filter system provides a narrow band of visible light to provide better sensitivity and resolution of the different densities. This mode of operation is commonly used to evaluate hemoglobin and protein electrophoresis patterns and molecular diagnostics applications including 1D, 2D, DNA, RNA, and PCR gel electrophoresis bands, dot blots, slot blots, image analysis, and chromosome analysis.

The fluorescence mode is used in the case of electrophoretic patterns that fluoresce when radiated by UV light (340 nm). Densitometers used in this mode include a UV light source and a photomultiplier tube instead of the silicon photocell. When the pattern located on the carriage moves across a focused beam of UV light, the pattern absorbs the light and emits visible light. The light is focused by a collection of lenses onto a UV blocking filter and then to a photomultiplier tube where the visible light is converted into an electronic signal that is proportional to the intensity of the light.

In each case the electrophoretic patterns are evaluated by comparison of peak heights or peak areas of the sample and the standards. Current densitometry systems employ sophisticated software to provide analysis of the signal intensities with high resolution and sensitivity.[1]

CHROMATOGRAPHY

Chromatography is used primarily for separation and identification of various compounds. Three types of chromatography are routinely used in the clinical laboratory: thin layer chromatography, gas chromatography (GC), and high-performance (or pressure) liquid chromatography (HPLC). Although paper chromatography was used at one time, it is seldom employed today.

Because chromatographic assays require more time for specimen preparation and performance, they are usually performed only when another assay type is not available or when interferences are suspected with an immunoassay. Chromatographic assays do not require premanufactured antibodies and, therefore, afford better flexibility than an immunoassay.

Paper Chromatography

The principle behind paper chromatography is simple and applies in all forms of chromatography. However, quantification of a substance is not possible with this method.

A drop of the sample is placed at the bottom of a piece of chromatography paper and allowed to dry. The paper is then hung in a chromatography jar so that the bottom edge contacts a solvent. Each component, having a different solubility and polarity, migrates toward the top of the paper as the solvent moves by capillary action. After separation is complete (12–24 hr), the paper is sprayed with a developing solution. Various fractions can be identified by how far they migrated on the paper.

Thin Layer Chromatography

Thin layer chromatography is used for drug screening and analysis of clinically important substances such as oligosaccharides and glycosaminoglycans (e.g., dermatan sulfate, heparan sulfate, and chondroitin sulfate). The principles of thin layer chromatography are identical to those of paper chromatography, except that a thin layer of gel (sorbent) applied to glass or plastic, forming the stationary phase, is used in place of paper. The sorbent may be composed of silica, alumina, polyacrylamide, or starch. The choice of sorbent depends upon the specific application since compounds have different relative affinities for the solvent (mobile phase) and the stationary phase. These factors affect the separation of a mixture into the different components. Silica gel is the most commonly used sorbent because it may be used to separate a broad range of compounds. These include amino acids, alkaloids, sugars, fatty acids, lipids, and steroids. Thin layer chromatography is used for

- Identification and separation of multiple components of a sample in a single step.
- Initial component separation prior to analysis by another technique.

Unlike paper chromatography, quantification of various substances is possible because each spot can be scraped off and analyzed individually.[1] While thin layer chromatography is a useful screening technique, it has lower sensitivity and resolution than either gas or high-performance chromatography. Another disadvantage, as with gas and high-performance chromatography, is that someone with skill and expertise must interpret the results.

Gas Chromatography

Gas chromatography (GC) is used to identify and quantify volatile substances such as alcohols, steroids, and drugs in the picogram range (Table 2-1). This technique is based on the principles of paper and thin layer chromatography but has better sensitivity. Instead of a solvent, GC uses an inert gas (e.g., nitrogen or helium) as a carrier for the volatile substance. A column packed with inert material, coated with a thin layer of a liquid phase, is substituted for paper or gel.

The sample is injected into the column (contained in a heated compartment) where it is immediately volatilized and picked up by the carrier gas. Heating at precise temperature gradients is essential for good separation of the analytes. The gas carries the sample through the column where it contacts the liquid phase, which has a high boiling point. Analytes with lower boiling points migrate faster than those with higher boiling points, thus fractionating the sample components.

When the sample leaves the column, it is exposed to a detector. The most common detector consists of a hydrogen flame with a platinum loop mounted above it. When the sample is exposed to the flame, ions collect on the platinum loop and generate a small current. This current is amplified by an electrometer, and the signal is sent on to an integrator or recorder.

The recorder produces a chromatogram with various peaks being recorded at different times. Because each sample component is retained for a different length of time, the peak produced at a particular retention time is characteristic for a specific component (Figure 2-3). The amount of each component present is determined by the area of the characteristic peak or by the ratio of the peak heights calibrated against a standard curve.

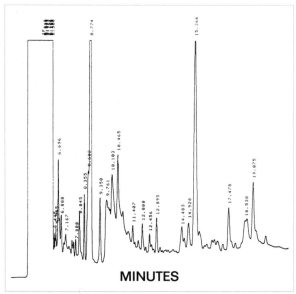

MINUTES

Figure 2-3. Gas chromatogram. Area under the curve or peak height of an analyte (e.g., drug or toxin) is compared to the area under the curve or peak height of an internal standard, and then the ratio is calculated. This ratio is compared to a standard curve of peak area ratios to give the concentration of the analyte.

This technique has many advantages, including high sensitivity and specificity. However, it requires sophisticated and expensive equipment. In addition, one or more compounds may produce peaks with the same retention time as the analyte of interest. If such interference is suspected, the temperature and/or composition of the liquid phase can be adjusted for better peak resolution.

High-Performance Liquid Chromatography

High-performance liquid chromatography (HPLC) has been used for toxicologic screening and to measure various drugs (Table 2-1). Its basic principles are similar to those of GC, but it is useful for nonvolatile or heat-sensitive substances. Instead of gas, HPLC utilizes a liquid solvent (mobile phase) and a column packed with a stationary phase, usually with a porous silica base. The mobile phase is pumped through the column under high pressure to decrease the assay time.

The sample is injected onto the column at one end and migrates to the other end in the mobile phase. Various components move at different rates, depending on their solubility characteristics and the amount of time spent in the solid vs. liquid phases. As the mobile phase leaves the column, it passes through a detector that produces a peak proportional to the concentration of each sample component. The detector is usually a spectrophotometer with variable wavelength capability in the ultraviolet and visible ranges.

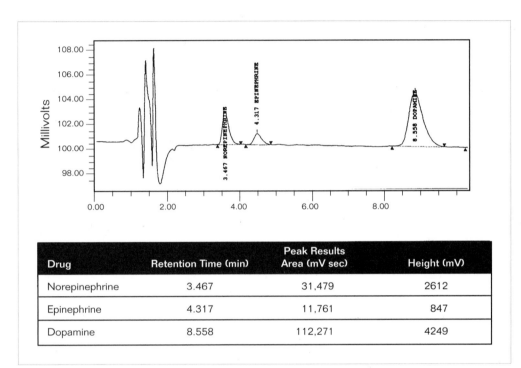

Drug	Retention Time (min)	Peak Results Area (mV sec)	Height (mV)
Norepinephrine	3.467	31,479	2612
Epinephrine	4.317	11,761	847
Dopamine	8.558	112,271	4249

Figure 2-4. HPLC chromatogram. Appearance of this chromatogram is similar to the gas chromatogram, and area or peak height ratio is used to quantify the analyte in a sample.

A signal from the detector is sent to a recorder or integrator, which plots peaks for each component as it elutes from the column (Figure 2-4). Once again, each component has its own characteristic retention time so each peak represents a specific component. As with GC, interferences may occur with compounds of similar structure or solubility characteristics; the peaks may fall on top of each other. Better resolution can be obtained by using a column packing with different characteristics or by changing the composition and/or pH of the mobile phase.

Compounds are identified by their retention times and quantified either by computing the area of the peak or by comparing the peak height or area to an internal standard to obtain a peak height or peak area ratio. This ratio is then used to calculate a concentration by comparison to a predetermined standard curve.

Although HPLC offers both high sensitivity and specificity, it requires specialized equipment and personnel. Furthermore, since the substance being determined is usually in a body fluid (e.g., urine or serum), one or more extraction steps are needed to isolate it. Another concern is that since many assays require a mobile phase composed of volatile and possibly toxic solvents, federal guidelines (Occupational Safety and Health Administration) must be followed. In addition, assays developed for commercial use may be costly since modifications to published methods are almost always required.

IMMUNOASSAYS

Immunoassays are all based on the reaction between an antigenic determinant or hapten (e.g., drug) and a labeled antibody. The label may consist of a radioisotope, an enzyme or enzyme substrate, a fluorophore, or a chromophore. The reaction may be measured by several detection methods including liquid scintillation, ultraviolet absorbance, fluorescence, fluorescent polarization, and turbidimetry or nephelometry. Serum drug concentrations are usually measured using immunoassays.

Immunoassays can be divided into two general categories: heterogeneous and homogeneous. In heterogeneous assays, the free and bound portions of the determinant must be separated before either or both portions can be assayed. This separation can be accomplished by various methods including protein precipitation, double antibody technique, adsorption of free drug, and removal by immobilized antibody on a solid phase.

Homogeneous assays do not require a separation step and, therefore, can be easily automated. The binding of the labeled hapten to the antibody alters its signal in a way (color change or reduction in enzyme activity) that can then be used to measure the analyte concentration. Homogeneous assays are also suited to stat tests due to their rapid turnaround time.

Early immunoassays used polyclonal antibodies, generated as a result of an animal's natural immune response. Typically, an antigen is injected into an animal. The animal's immune system then recognizes the material as foreign and produces antibodies against it. These antibodies are then isolated from the blood.

Many different antibodies may be generated in response to a single antigen. The numbers as well as the specificities of the antibodies depend on the size and number of antigenic sites on the antigen. In general, the larger and more complex the antigen (e.g., cell or protein), the more antigenic sites it has and the greater the variety of antibodies formed.

Although polyclonal antibodies have been used successfully, both specificity and response may vary greatly because of their heterogeneous nature. The result is a high degree of cross-reactivity with similar substances. To address this problem, monoclonal antibodies have been developed.

Prior to 1975, the only monoclonal antibodies available were from patients with malignant plasma cells. However, in 1975 a technique was developed to make monoclonal antibodies in the laboratory.[19] The technique is based on the fusion of

- Genetic material from plasma cells that produce antibody but cannot reproduce.
- Myeloma cells that do not produce antibody but can reproduce.

The plasma cells and myeloma cells are cultured together, resulting in a mixture of both parent cells and a hybrid cell. This hybrid cell produces the specific antibody and reproduces.

The mixture is incubated in a special medium, which kills the parent cells and leaves only the hybrid antibody-producing cells alive. The hybrid cells can then be grown using conventional cell culture techniques, resulting in large amounts of the monoclonal antibody. The development of monoclonal antibodies has allowed for high sensitivity and specificity in immunoassay technology.

Radioimmunoassay

As with flame photometry, radioimmunoassay (RIA) is rarely used in the modern clinical laboratory and is largely discussed from a historical perspective. RIA, a heterogeneous immunoassay, was developed in the late 1950s[20] and has been primarily used in endocrinology (Table 2-1). This technique takes advantage of the fact that certain atoms can be either incorporated directly into the analyte's structure or attached to antibodies. The primary atoms used in the clinical laboratory fall into two classes: gamma emitters and beta emitters.

Gamma emitters (^{125}I and ^{57}Co) are generally incorporated into compounds such as thyroid hormone and cyanocobalamin (vitamin B_{12}).[5] These isotopes can be counted directly with standard gamma counters that utilize a sodium iodide–thallium crystal. When the gamma ray hits the crystal, it gives off a flash of light. This light, in turn, stimulates a photomultiplier tube to amplify the signal.

Beta emitters (^{14}C and ^{3}H) are primarily used to measure steroid concentrations.[5] Beta rays cannot be counted directly since endogenous substances tend to absorb the radiation. Therefore, this technique requires a scintillation cocktail with an organic compound capable of absorbing the beta radiation and reemitting it as a flash of light. This light is then amplified by a photomultiplier tube and counted.

RIA is extremely sensitive and has been made more specific with the introduction of monoclonal antibodies. Unfortunately, this technique also has several significant disadvantages[5]:

- A short shelf-life for labeled reagents is a source of increased cost.
- Lead shielding is required, making the instrument heavy and bulky.
- Strict recordkeeping is required, resulting in a higher workload.
- Monitoring of personnel for radiation exposure.
- Special licensing is required.
- Waste disposal requires additional costs to comply with government regulations.

Since EIAs have none of these problems, the clinical use of RIA has decreased in recent years.

Agglutination

The simplest immunoassay is agglutination. Typical tests that can be performed using this assay include human chorionic gonadotropin, rheumatoid factor, antigens from infectious agents such as bacteria and fungi, and antinuclear antibodies (ANA). The agglutination reaction, used to detect either antigens or antibodies, results when multivalent antibodies bind to antigens with more than one binding site.

The reaction occurs through the formation of cross-linkages between antigen and antibody particles. When enough complexes form, clumping results and a visible mass is formed (Figure 2-5). Since the reaction depends on the number of binding sites on the antibody, the greater the number, the better the reaction. For example, immunoglobulin M produces better agglutination than immunoglobulin G because it has more binding sites.

The agglutination reaction is also affected by other factors[20]:

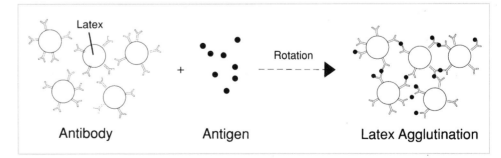

Figure 2-5. Schematic of latex agglutination immunoassay. The specimen (cerebrospinal fluid, serum, etc.) contains the analyte (in this case, antigens to bacteria) that causes an easily readable reaction (adapted, with permission, from Power DA, McCuen PJ, eds. *Manual of BBI Products and Laboratory Procedures*. Cockeysville, MD: Becton Dickinson Microbiology Systems; 1998:77).

- Avidity and affinity of antibody.
- Number of binding sites on antigen as well as antibody.
- Relative concentrations of antigen and antibody.
- z-Potential (electrostatic interaction that causes particles in solution to repel each other).
- Viscosity of medium.

The two types of agglutination reactions are (1) direct and (2) indirect. Direct agglutination occurs when the antigen and antibody are mixed together, resulting in visible clumping. An example of this reaction is the test for *Salmonella typhi* antibody.

Indirect agglutination (also known as passive or particle agglutination) uses a carrier for either the antibody or antigen. Originally, erythrocytes were selected as the carrier (as described for hemolytic anemia tests). However, latex-coated particles are now commonly used, and the latex agglutination method is simpler and less expensive than the erythrocyte immunoassay. In addition, latex particles allow titration of the amount of antibody bound to the latex particle, thus reducing variability. Other advantages include a rapid performance time with no separation step, allowing full automation. Disadvantages include expensive equipment and lower sensitivity than either RIA or EIA. The use of an automated particle counter increases the sensitivity of the test 10–1000 times.[21]

Enzyme Immunoassays

Enzyme immunoassays (EIA) employ enzymes as labels for specific analytes. When antibodies bind to the antigen-enzyme complex, a defined reaction occurs (e.g., color change, fluorescence, radioactivity, or altered activity). This altered enzyme activity is used to quantitate the analyte.

The advantages of EIA include commercial availability at a relatively low cost, long shelf life, good sensitivity, automation, and none of the specific requirements mentioned for RIA.

Enzyme-Linked Immunosorbent Assay

Enzyme-linked immunosorbent assay (ELISA) is a heterogeneous EIA. This assay employs the same basic principles as RIA, except that enzyme activity rather than radioactivity is measured. This assay is commonly used to determine antibodies directed against a wide range of antigens such as rheumatoid factor, hepatitis B antigen, and bacterial and viral antigens in the serum (Table 2-1).

In a competitive ELISA assay, the specific antibody is adsorbed to a solid phase. Enzyme-labeled antigen is incubated together with the sample and the antibodies attached to the solid phase. After a specified time, an equilibrium is reached and the solid phase is washed with buffer. Then the reaction is stopped, and the reaction product is measured with a spectrophotometer or fluorometer.

Enzyme-Multiplied Immunoassay

Enzyme-multiplied immunoassay (EMIT) is a homogeneous EIA; enzyme is used as a label for a specific analyte (e.g., a drug). Many drugs commonly assayed using EMIT are also measured by fluorescence polarization immunoassay (FPIA) (e.g., digoxin, quinidine, procainamide, N-acetylprocainamide, and aminoglycoside antibiotics) as are substances like blood urea nitrogen (BUN) and creatinine (Table 2-1).

With the EMIT assay, the enzyme retains its activity after attaching to the analyte. For example, to determine a drug concentration, an enzyme is conjugated to the drug and incubated with antidrug antibody. As shown in Figure 2-6, the test drug (D) is covalently bound to an enzyme that retains its activity and acts as a label. When this complex is combined with antidrug antibody, the en-

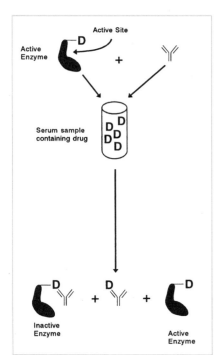

Figure 2-6. EMIT. This assay is used in quantifying the drug concentration in a serum sample, as described in the text.

zyme is inactivated. If the antibody and enzyme-bound drug are combined with serum that contains unbound drug, competition occurs. Since the amount of antidrug antibody is limited, the free drug in the sample and the enzyme-linked drug compete for binding to the antibody. When the antibody binds to the enzyme-linked drug, enzyme activity is inhibited. The result is that the serum drug concentration is proportional to the amount of active enzyme remaining. Since no separation step is required, this assay can be automated.

Fluorescent Polarization Immunoassay

Fluorescent polarization immunoassay (FIPA), the most common form of immunoassay, is used to measure concentrations of many clinical chemistries such as BUN and creatinine. It is also commonly employed for determining serum drug concentrations of aminoglycoside antibiotics, vancomycin, and theophylline (Table 2-1).

Molecules having a ring structure and a large number of double bonds, such as some aromatic compounds, can fluoresce when excited by a specific wavelength of light. These molecules must have a particular orientation with respect to the light source for electrons to be raised to an excited state. When the electrons return to their original lower energy state, some light is reemitted as a flash with a longer wavelength than the exciting light. Fluorescent immunoassays take advantage of this property by conjugating an antibody or analyte to a fluorescent molecule. The concentration can be determined by measuring either the degree of fluorescence or, more commonly, the decrease in the amount of fluorescence present.[5,21]

In FPIA, a polarizing filter is placed between the light source and the sample and between the sample and the detector. The first filter assures that the light exciting the molecules is in a particular orientation; the second filter assures that only fluorescent light of the appropriate orientation reaches the detector.

The fluorescent polarization of a small molecule is low because it rotates rapidly and is not in the proper orientation long enough to give off an easily detected signal. To decrease this molecular motion, the molecule is complexed with an antibody. Since this larger complex rotates at a slower rate, it stays in the proper orientation to be excited by the incident light.

When unlabeled analyte is mixed with a fixed amount of antibody and fluorescent-labeled analyte, a competitive binding reaction occurs between the labeled and unlabeled analytes. The result is a decrease in fluorescence. Thus, the concentration of unlabeled analyte is inversely proportional to the amount of fluorescence.[21]

Because of their simplicity, automation, and low cost, assays have been developed with relatively high sensitivity for many drugs (e.g., antiepileptics, antiarrhythmics, and antibiotics). The primary difficulty is interference from endogenous substances (lipids and bilirubin) or metabolites of the drugs.

MASS SPECTROMETRY

Mass spectrometry involves the fragmentation and ionization of molecules in the gas phase according to their mass to charge ratio (m/z). The resulting mass fragments are displayed on a mass spectrum, or a bar graph, that plots the relative abundance of an ion vs. its m/z ratio. Since the mass spectrum is characteristic of the parent molecule, an unknown molecule can be identified by comparing its mass spectrum with a library of known spectra to identify the compound.

A wide array of mass spectrometry systems has been developed to meet the increasing demands of the biomedical field. However, the basic principles and components of mass spectrometers are essentially the same. These include an inlet unit, an ion source, a mass analyzer, an ion detector, and a data/recording system. Compounds introduced into a mass spectrometer (MS) must first be isolated. This is accomplished with separation techniques such as gas chromatography (GC), liquid chromatography (LC), and capillary electrophoresis, which are used in tandem with mass spectrometers. In a GC/MS system an interface between the GC and MS components, which restricts the gas flow from the GC column into the mass spectrometer, is required to prevent a mismatch in the operating pressures between the two instruments. The unit must also be heated to maintain the volatile compounds in the vapor state and remove most of the carrier gas from the GC effluent entering the ion source unit.[22]

Ionization Methods

The ionization of the molecules introduced into a MS is accomplished by several methods. In each case, the ion sources are maintained at high temperatures and high vacuum conditions necessary for ionizing vaporized molecules. The *electron ionization* (EI) method, a form of gas-phase ionization, consists of a beam of high energy electrons that bombard the incoming gas molecules. The energy used is sufficiently high to not only ionize the gas molecules but also cause them to fragment through the breaking of their chemical bonds. This process yields ion fragments in addition to intact molecular ions that appear in the mass spectra. The EI method is most useful for low molecular weight compounds (<400 daltons) because of problems with excessive fragmentation and thermal decomposition of large molecules during vaporization.[23,24] Therefore, EI is typically used in GC/MS systems that are suitable for applications including the analysis of synthetic organic chemicals, hydrocarbons, pharmaceutical compounds, organic acids, and drugs of abuse.

Chemical ionization (CI) is another form of gas-phase ionization. This technique is a less energetic technique than EI because the sample molecule is ionized by a reagent such as methane or ammonia that is first ionized by an electron beam. Less fragmentation is produced by this method making it useful for determining the molecular weights of compounds and for enhancing the abundance of intact molecular ions.

Electrospray ionization (ESI), a form of atmospheric pressure ionization, generates ions directly from solution permitting it to be used in combination with high-performance liquid chromatography and capillary electrophoresis systems. This method involves the creation of a fine spray in the presence of a strong electric field. As the droplets become declustered, the force of the surface tension of the droplet is overcome by the mutual repulsion of like charges, allowing the ions to leave the droplet and enter the mass analyzer. This technique will yield multiple ionic species especially for high molecular weight ions that have a large distribution of charge states, thus making this a very sensitive technique for small, large, and labile molecules.[25] This ionization method is well-suited for the analysis of peptides, proteins, carbohydrates, DNA fragments, and lipids.

Other common ionization techniques include fast atom bombardment (FAB), which uses high velocity atoms such as argon to ionize molecules in a liquid or solid, and matrix assisted laser desorption/ionization (MALDI), which uses high energy photons to ionize molecules embedded on a solid organic matrix.[25]

Mass Analyzers

Following ionization, the gas phase ions enter the mass analyzer. This component of the mass spectrometer separates the ions by their m/z ratios. Commonly used mass analyzers include the double-focusing magnetic sector analyzer, quadrupole, quadrupole ion trap mass spectrometers, and tandem mass spectrometers. The magnetic sector mass spectrometer uses a magnetic field perpendicular to the direction of the ion motion to deflect the ions into a circular path with a radius dependent upon the m/z ratio and the velocity of the ion. The detector will then separate the ions by their m/z ratios. However, since the kinetic energy (or velocity) of the molecules leaving the ion source is not necessarily constant, the path radii will become dependent on the velocity and the m/z ratio. To enhance the resolution, an electrostatic analyzer or electric sector is used to allow molecules with only a specific kinetic energy to pass through its field. That is, for a particular kinetic energy, the radius of curvature is directly related to the m/z ratio. This type of analyzer is commonly used in combination with EI and FAB ionization systems.

Quadrupole mass spectrometers act as a filter for molecules or fragments with a specific m/z ratio. This is accomplished by using four equally spaced parallel rods with direct current (DC) and radio-frequency (RF) potentials on opposing rods of the quadrupole. The field produced is along the x- and y- axis. The radio frequency oscillation causes the ions to be attracted or repelled by the rods. Only ions with a specific m/z ratio will have a trajectory along the z-axis, allowing them to pass to the detector while others will be trapped by the rods of the quadrupole. By varying the RF field, other m/z ranges are selected, thus resulting in the mass spectrum.[24] The quadrupole mass spectrometer, commonly combined with the EI ionization system, is perhaps the most commonly used type of mass spectrometer because of its relatively low cost, ability to analyze up to high m/z ratios (up to 3000), and its compatibility with ESI ionization systems.

The *ion trap analyzer* is another form of a quadrupole mass spectrometer, consisting of a ring electrode to which an RF voltage is applied to two end caps at ground potential. This arrangement generates a quadrupole field trapping ions that are injected into the chamber or are generated within it. As the RF field is scanned, ions with specific and successive m/z ratio are ejected from the trap to the ion detector through holes in the caps.[24] The quadrupole ion trap mass spectrometer is regarded for its high sensitivity and compact size.

Tandem mass spectrometry is a technique that uses multiple stages of mass analysis on subsequent generations of ion fragments. This is accomplished by preselecting an ion from the first analysis and colliding it with an inert gas such as argon or helium to induce further fragmentation of the ion. The next stage involves analysis of the fragments generated by an earlier stage. The abbreviation MS^n is applied to the stages, which analyze fragments beyond the initial ions (MS) to the first generation of ion fragments (MS^2) and subsequent generations (MS^3, MS^4, and ...). These techniques can be tandem in space (two or more instruments) or tandem in time. In the former case, many combinations have been used for this type of analysis. In the later cases, quadrupole ion trap devices are often used and can achieve multiple MS^n measurements.[26] Tandem mass analysis is primarily used to obtain structural information such as peptides sequences, small DNA/RNA oligomers, fatty acids, and oligosaccharides. Other mass analyzers such as time-of-flight and Fourier transform mass spectrometers are not commonly used for clinical applications.

Ion Detector

The ion detector is the final element of the mass spectrometer. Once an ion passes through the mass analyzer, a signal is produced in the detector. The detector consists of an electron multiplier that converts the energy of the ion into a cascade of secondary electrons (similar to a photomultiplier tube), resulting in about a million-fold amplification of the signal. Due to the rapid rate at which data is generated, computerized data systems are indispensable components of all modern mass spectrometers. The introduction of rapid processors, large storage capacities, and spectra databases has lead to automated high throughput. Miniaturization of components has also led to the development of bench-top systems practical for routine clinical laboratory analysis. Clinical applications include newborn screening for metabolic disorders, hemoglobin analysis, and drug testing. Pharmaceutical applications include drug discovery, pharmacokinetics, and drug metabolism.

CYTOMETRY

Cytometry may be defined as a process of measuring physical, chemical, or other characteristics of cells or other biological particles. While this definition usually encompasses the fields of flow cytometry and cellular image analysis, many additional methods are now used to study the vast spectrum of cellular properties. Consequently, the term *cytomics* has been introduced. This term may be defined as the science of cell-based analysis that integrates genomics and proteomics with dynamic functions of cells and tissues. The technology used includes techniques discussed in this chapter, such as flow cytometry and mass spectrometry, and others that are beyond the scope of this chapter.

Flow Cytometry

Flow cytometry is the technology used to measure properties of cells as they move or flow in liquid suspension.[27] The hematology analyzer, a common form of flow cytometry system, also incorporates the principles of impedance, absorbance, and laser light scatter to measure cell properties. Instruments generally referred to as *flow cytometers* are based on the principles of laser-induced fluorometry and light scatter. The terminology can become confusing since various conventions have taken root over the years. However, regardless of the principles of detection or measurement, the term flow cytometry may in general be applied to technologies that rely on cells moving in a fluid steam for analysis.

The basis of cell counting and sizing in hematology analyzers is the Coulter principle. This technique, first developed by Wallace H. Coulter in 1947 and patented in 1953, relates counting and sizing of particles to changes in electrical impedance across an aperture in a conductive medium, which is created when a particle moves through it. The basic system consists of a smaller chamber within a larger chamber, both filled with a conductive medium and each with one electrode across in which a constant DC current is applied. The fluids within each chamber communicate through a small aperture (≤ 100 μm) or sensing zone. When a nonconductive particle or cell passes through the aperture, it displaces an equivalent volume of conductive fluid. This increases the conductance and creates a voltage pulse for each cell counted, the intensity of which is proportional to the cell volume.[9]

In hematology analyzers, blood is separated into two volumes for measurement. One volume is mixed with a diluent and delivered to a chamber where platelet and erythrocyte counts are performed. Particles with volumes between 2 and 20 fL are counted as platelets, and particles with volumes >36 fL are counted as erythrocytes. The other volume is mixed with a diluent, and an erythrocyte lysing reagent is used to permit leukocyte (>36 fL) counts to be performed. The number of cells in this size range may be subtracted from the erythrocyte count performed in the other chamber.

Modern hematology analyzers employ additional technologies to enhance the resolution of blood cell analysis. Radiofrequency energy is used to assess important information about the internal structure of cells such as nuclear volume. Laser light scatter is used to obtain information about cell shape and granularity. The combination of these and other technologies such as light absorbance (for hemoglobin measurements) provide accurate blood cell differentials, counts, and other important blood cell indices. These basic principles are common to many of hematology analyzers used in clinical laboratories. However, each uses different proprietary detection, measurement, and software systems and ways of displaying this data.[1]

Flow cytometers incorporate the principles of fluorometry and light scatter to the analysis of particles or cells that pass within a fluid stream. This technology provides multiparametric measurements of intrinsic and extrinsic properties of cells. Intrinsic properties, including cell size and cytoplasmic complexity, are properties that can be assessed directly by light scatter and does not require the use of any type of probe. Extrinsic cellular properties, such as cell surface or cytoplasmic antigens, enzymes or other proteins, and DNA/RNA, require the use of a fluorescent dye or probe to label the components of interest and a laser to induce the fluorescence (older systems used mercury arc lamps as a light source) to be detected.

The basic flow cytometer consists of four types of components: fluidics, optics, electronics, and data analysis. *Fluidics* refers to the apparatus that directs the cells in suspension to the flow cell where they will be interrogated by the laser light. Fluidics systems use a combination of air pressure and vacuum to create the conditions that allow the cells to pass the flow chamber in single file. The optical components include the laser (or other light source), flow chamber, monochromatic filters, dichroic mirrors, and lenses. These are used to direct the scattered or fluorescent light to detectors, which measure the signals that are subsequently analyzed.[27]

The light scattered by the cell when it reaches the flow chamber is used to measure its intrinsic properties. The forward angle light scatter (FALS) is detected by a diode and reflects the size of the passing cell. The right-angle light scatter (RALS) is detected by a photomultiplier tube and is a function of the cytoplasmic complexity of the cell. The analysis of extrinsic properties is more complicated. The measurement of DNA or RNA, for example, requires the use of intercalating nucleic acid dyes such as propridium iodide. The detection of antigenic determinants on cells can be performed with fluorescent-labeled monoclonal antibodies (MAB) directed at these antigens. In each case the principle of detection involves the use of laser light to excite the fluorescent dye and detect its emitted signal. Fluorescent dyes are characterized by their excitation (absorption) and emission wavelength spectra and by the difference between the maxima of these spectra or Stokes shift (discussed in the spectrophotometry section). These properties permit the use of multiple fluorescent probes on a single cell.

To illustrate the operation of a flow cytometer, consider a four-color, six-parameter (FALS and RALS) configuration (Figure 2-7).[28] An argon gas laser with a wavelength of 488 nm is commonly used because it simultaneously excites several different dyes that possess different emission wavelengths. Fluorochromes conjugated with monoclonal antibodies (MoAb) that may be used include fluorescein isothyocyanate (FITC), phycoerythrin (PE), energy coupled dye (ECD), and Cy5PE (tandem dye composed of the carbocyanine derivative Cy5 and PE) with

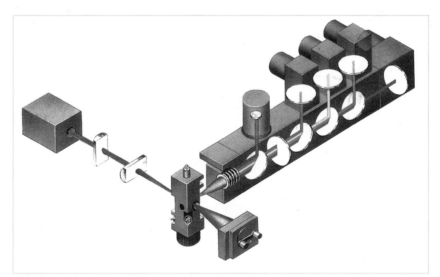

Figure 2-7. Schematic of a four-color flow cytometry system. The laser beam is focused onto the flow cell through which the cell suspension is directed. Scattered light is detected by the forward and side scatter detectors. Emitted light from specific monoclonal antibodies labeled with fluorochromes; FITC, PE, ECD, and CY5PE are detected at PMT's FL1–FL4 respectively. Appropriate dichroic long pass filters direct the specific wavelength of light through a narrow band pass filter and then to the appropriate PMT (provided courtesy of Beckman Coulter, Inc.).

peak emission wavelengths of approximately 520, 578, 613, and 670 nm, respectively. The emitted light at each of these wavelengths is detected at an angle of 90°. The array of optical filters selects light in each wavelength region and directs it to a different photomultiplier tube where it is detected, amplified, and converted into an electronic signal. This measurement can be made on thousands of cells in a matter of seconds. The result is a histogram that identifies distinct cell populations based on light scatter and extrinsic properties. In the case of blood, a histogram will distinguish lymphocytes, monocytes, and granulocytes by light scatter. The B cell, T cell, T cell subsets, and natural killer cell populations can all be distinguished.

This important method of cell analysis has found many applications in medicine making it a relatively common clinical laboratory instrument. Flow cytometry is routinely used to assist in the diagnosis of leukemia and lymphoma, derive prognostic information in these and other malignancies, monitor immunodeficiency disease states such as HIV/AIDS, enumerate stem cells (CD34) and reticulocytes, and assess various functional properties of cells.

Image Cytometry

Image cytometry is a form of cytometry that encompasses a class of instruments and techniques used to analyze tissue specimens or individual cells. The basic components of an image cytometry system are a microscope, camera, computer, and monitor. This basic description does not capture the variations and complexity of these systems, which are beyond the scope of this chapter. However, the essence of these instruments is the ability to acquire images in two or three (confocal microscopy) dimensions to study the distribution of various components within cells or tissues. The high optical resolution of these systems is an important determinant in obtaining morphometric information and precise data about cell and tissue constituents through the use of fluorescence/absorbance-based probes, as in flow cytometry.[29] Specific applications of image cytometry generally involve unique methods of cell or tissue preparation and other modifications. This lends to the versatility of this technology, which yields such applications as the measurement of DNA content in nuclei to assess prognosis in cancer and the detection of specific nucleic acid sequences to diagnose genetic disorders.

In Situ Hybridization

Among the methods of image cytometry, in situ hybridization is perhaps the most commonly used in the clinical laboratory, particularly in molecular cytogenetics laboratories. In situ hybridization is used to localize nucleic acid sequences (entire chromosomes or parts, including genes) in cells or tissues through the use of probes, which consist of a nucleic acid sequence that is complementary to the target sequence and labeled in some way that makes the hybridized sequence detectable. These principles are common to all methods of in situ hybridization, but they differ in the type of probe that is used. Radioactive probes may be used for this application. However, because their spatial resolution is limited, detection and artifacts are often produced. Fluorescent probes, which provide excellent spatial resolution, have become a preferred method of in situ hybridization for many applications.

Fluorescent in situ hybridization (FISH) is a powerful technique for detecting genes and genetic anomalies and monitoring different diseases at the genetic level. This technique involves the use of a system of coupled antibodies and fluorochromes similar to those used with flow cytometry. The probe, which is the complementary nucleic acid sequence, is incorporated with a fluorescent molecule or antigenic site to which fluorescently labeled antibodies may be directed (biotin-avidin system). When the two strands of DNA are separated through heating (denaturation), the labeled probe can hybridize the target sequence. Fluorescent microscopes are used to visualize the hybridized sequences. An appropriate arrangement of filters is used to direct the relevant wavelength of light from the light source to excite the fluorescent molecule on the probe. All but the emission wavelength of light is blocked with a special filter permitting the signal from the probe to be visualized.[30]

NUCLEIC ACID AMPLIFICATION

Nucleic acid amplification technologies have revolutionized molecular diagnostic testing. Polymerase chain reaction (PCR) is the most frequently used of these technologies. However, several other techniques are beginning to emerge in the clinical laboratory and are worthy of note. These include ligase chain reaction (LCR), transcription mediated amplification (TMA), branched DNA amplification, and nucleic acid sequence-based amplification (NASBA).

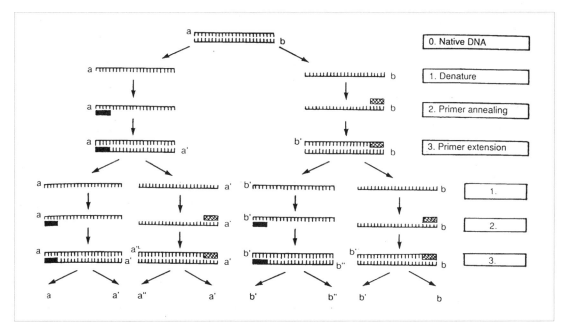

Figure 2-8. Schematic of the three steps in the PCR amplification of a specific DNA sequence, as described in the text (adapted from Reference 32).

PCR is used principally for detecting microbiologic organisms and genetic diseases (Table 2-1). Microorganisms identified by this process include chlamydia, cytomegalovirus (CMV), Epstein-Barr virus, human immunodeficiency virus (HIV), mycobacteria, and herpes simplex virus. Although the number of organisms that can be identified is limited at present, this list is growing. Furthermore, PCR can often identify organisms with greater rapidity and sensitivity than conventional methods.

Genetic diseases diagnosed using PCR include a-1-antitrypsin deficiency, cystic fibrosis, sickle cell anemia, fragile X syndrome, Tay-Sachs disease, drug-induced hemolytic anemia, and von Willebrand's disease. In addition, cancer research has benefited from PCR through the diagnosis of various cancers (e.g., chronic myeloid leukemia and pancreatic and colon cancers) as well as through the detection of residual disease after treatment.[31] This technique is used to amplify specific DNA and RNA sequences enzymatically.

PCR takes advantage of the normal DNA replication process. In vivo, DNA replicates when the double helix unwinds and the two strands separate. A new strand forms on each separate strand through the coupling of specific base pairs (e.g., adenosine with thymidine and cytosine with guanosine). The PCR cycle is similar and consists of three separate steps (Figure 2-8) [21]:

1. Denaturation—the two strands of DNA are thermally separated.
2. Primer annealing—sequence-specific primers are allowed to hybridize to opposite strands flanking the region of interest by decreasing the temperature.
3. Primer extension—DNA polymerase then extends the hybridized primers, generating a copy of the original DNA template.

The efficiency of the extension step can be increased by raising the temperature. Typical temperatures for the three steps are 201.2 °F (94 °C) for denaturation, 122–149 °F (50–65 °C) for annealing, and 161.6 °F (72 °C) for extension. Since the entire cycle is completed in only about 3 min,[32] many cycles can occur within a short time, resulting in the exponential production of millions of copies of the target sequence.

The genetic material is then identified by agarose gel electrophoresis. While not truly a chromatographic technique, gel electrophoresis utilizes principles similar to thin layer chromatography in that the migration of bands is similar to the migration of spots. An electric current is applied to facilitate DNA migration, and the gene is identified by the distance it migrates through the gel.

One potential disadvantage of this method is contamination of the amplification reaction with products of a previous PCR (carryover), exogenous DNA, or other cellular material. Contamination can be reduced by prealiquoting reagents, using dedicated positive-displacement pipettes, and physically separating the reaction preparation from the area where the product is analyzed. In addition, multiple negative controls are necessary to monitor for contamination.

LABORATORY AUTOMATION

Laboratory automation can be defined as a mechanized analytical process, including any device, software, or system configuration that improves the efficiency of the laboratory.[33] This concept commonly applies to mechanization of basic manual laboratory techniques or procedures such as those addressed throughout this chapter.

Many different automated systems are used on clinical laboratory testing to analyze patient specimens. However, they generally involve the same basic steps that are usually performed sequentially:

1. Identification.
2. Preparation.
3. Handling, transport, and delivery.
4. Processing.
5. Reagent handling and storage.
6. Reagent delivery.
7. Chemical reaction phase.
8. Measurement.
9. Signal processing and data handling.
10. Information transfer.

The specimen identification and preparation steps of this process are usually manual. However, this is beginning to change as advances in bar coding and robotic technologies begin to emerge. Using the example of a chemistry analyzer, the next stage in the process involves the presentation of the specimen (usually serum) to the analyzer. Some analyzers can sample the serum directly from the collection tubes, while others require the use of specially designed cups or tubes.

Introduction of the specimen occurs through aspiration in continuous-flow systems or by pipetting in discrete processing systems. In continuous flow systems, each specimen passes through the same continuous stream and is subjected to the same analytical reactions. Specimens analyzed in discrete systems have their own physical and chemical space. During the delivery of the specimen to the reaction chamber, carryover between specimens may occur and lead to contamination. This problem has been minimized through the proper selection of probe materials, surface conditions, and the use of flushing systems.

While the sample is being processed, the reagents used in the chemical reactions are stored as required and identified by bar code labels. Reagents are used to cause a chemical reaction that results in the indirect detection of an analyte or to separate the analyte contained in the sample. Reagents may be liquid or dry and may require mixing when multiple reagents are combined. This process, depending upon the compound being measured, is managed by the reagent delivery system. Automated chemistry analyzers rely on principles of the photometry that have been addressed in earlier sections of this chapter. They include absorbance/transmittance photometry, fluorometry, and chemiluminescence. Many enzymes, therapeutic drugs, hormones, and other analytes are measured in with these principles. Electrochemical methods such as ISE are also employed for the measurement of electrolytes.[33]

All modern automated analyzers rely upon computers and sophisticated software to perform signal and data processing functions. The analogue signals from the detectors are converted into digital form for processing. Different data acquisition, calculation (statistics on patient or control values and subtraction of blank response), monitoring (linearity and quality control), and display (acquisition and collation of patient results and warning messages) functions are routinely performed by these instruments. The automated transfer of information does not end at this stage. While printed reports are almost always produced, these instruments are more commonly interfaced (uni- and bidirectional) with a laboratory information system (LIS) that is part of a comprehensive information system within and often beyond the walls of a hospital or commercial laboratory. Advanced LIS functionalities include the monitoring and control of many laboratory processes such as mapping orders to processing and work areas, repeat and reflex testing, tracking samples and results through the system, and storage and retrieval of specimens.

The trend toward automation in the clinical laboratory is, in part, motivated by the drive toward higher productivity and cost efficiency.[34] In its broadest sense, laboratory automation encompasses all processes in the lab from receipt of the specimen to the reporting of results. A total laboratory automation (TLA) system consists of several instruments, consolidated analyzers, and individual or integrated workcells (automated devices that address a specific task) that are coupled to a specimen management and transportation system (track or conveyer system) as well as to a process control software that automates each stage of the system.[35] While TLA is well-suited for high volume laboratories, it is unaffordable for most small or mid-sized hospital or reference laboratories. Modular automation represents an accessible form of automation for most laboratories. This involves consolidating and integrating analyzers, independent work cells, and both preanalytic and postanalytic systems in a manner that allows for independent operation or integration with other components. Modular devices include specimen loaders and unloaders, decappers, centrifuges, and aliquoters.[34]

The emerging discipline of informatics is also a fundamental component of laboratory automation. As purveyors of information, clinical laboratories provide relevant clinical information (not just data) to physicians and other healthcare professionals in an efficient manner. Informatics in the laboratory involves the manipulation of collected data for the purposes of problem solving and decision making in healthcare. Modern laboratory information systems (LIS) and other tools have the capability of trending and analyzing data in a variety of ways that enhance patient care. The ability to convey such information expeditiously through an intranet or the internet is becoming as indispensable a function of the laboratory as performing the tests themselves.

The centralized core laboratory in the future will represent the center of information management for hospital-based medicine and the community and will house automated laboratory systems capable of controlling process flow and performing high volume and esoteric testing.[36] In parallel with the development of the highly automated core laboratory, technological advances in miniaturization of analyzers will make point-of-care testing an essential and complementary tool for the diagnosis and treatment of disease.

POINT-OF-CARE TESTING

Point-of-care testing may be considered any laboratory testing that exists outside the walls of the central laboratory. These sites include the clinics, a rapid-response setting (community, physician's office, emergency room, or hospital ward), a patient's bedside, or a patient's home. Currently, hand-held analyzers are capable of measuring many common analytes (electrolytes, blood gases, pH, BUN, creatinine, lactate, glucose, lipids, coagulation factors, hemoglobin, and hematocrit).[37]

The principle technology that underlies these analytical devices is biosensor systems. Biosensors are electronic devices that consist of two components: a bioreceptor and a transducer. The bioreceptor is a molecule such as an antibody, enzyme, receptor protein, or nucleic acid that recognizes the target analyte. The interaction between the bioreceptor and the target analyte generates a chemical species or other physiochemical change measurable by electrochemical methods. The transducer detects this change and converts it into a measurable signal proportional to the concentration of the analyte. Common transducers used in these systems are based upon amperometry (measurement of H_2O_2 and O_2), potentiometry (measurement of pH and ions), and photometry using optical fibers (measure changes in refractive index).[9] The bioreceptors used are generally antibody-based or enzyme. Because both components are integrated into one sensor, reagents are not required in contrast to conventional assays where multiple steps and reagents are used.

This rapidly evolving technology continues to yield new applications that include DNA microchips. This technology represents the integration of multiple biosensors with DNA microarrays, providing rapid analysis for genetic diseases, measurements of gene expression, detection of infectious agents, and drug screening. With further advances in microfabrication technology, the role of point-of-care testing will continue to expand as will the amount of information. The role of a centralized clinical laboratory of the future will likely diminish to a point where only esoteric testing is performed.[38,39] The primary function of the laboratory will be focused on informatics.

SUMMARY

This chapter presents a brief overview of the more common and emerging laboratory assay methodologies, including their potential advantages and problems. A number of these methodologies—flame photometry, paper chromatography, and RIA—are discussed primarily to provide a historical basis and description of the simple principles on which the more complex methods are based.

Due to its simplicity and improved sensitivity, ISE has replaced flame photometry as the principal method for measuring serum and urine electrolytes. Some methods, including turbidimetry, nephelometry, and spectrophotometry, are used in conjunction with other tests such as the immunoassay. With these methods, concentrations of substances such as immune complexes can be determined.

Chromatography is one of the mainstays of the laboratory for drug detection. The two principal forms of chromatography are liquid and gas. Both types are similar in that they depend on differences in either solubilities or boiling points, respectively, to separate different analytes in a sample. Another group of important tests is the immunoassays: EIA, EMIT, ELISA, and FPIA. All of these methods depend on an immunologically mediated reaction that increases sensitivity and specificity. These assays are commonly used to determine routine clinical chemistries and drug concentrations. Finally, PCR—a relatively new technology—is used to amplify specific DNA and RNA sequences, primarily in the areas of microbiology and detection of genetic diseases.

The rapid technological advancement of laboratory instrumentation has led to the implementation of new and enhanced clinical laboratory methodologies, including mass spectrometry, cytometry, laboratory automation, and point-of-care testing. While laboratory medicine endeavors to keep pace with the burgeoning developments in biomedical sciences, especially with an increase in the sophistication of the tests, it is essential that today's clinicians have a basic understanding of the more common and esoteric tests in order to select the most appropriate one in each case. All of these developments will translate directly into improved patient care.

REFERENCES

1. Nguyen AN, Sunheimer RL, Henry JB. Principles of instrumentation. In: Henry JB, ed. *Clinical Diagnosis and Management.* 20th ed. Philadelphia, PA: W. B. Saunders; 2001: 60–78.

2. Evenson MA. Photometry. In: Burtis CA, Ashwood ER, eds. *Clinical Chemistry.* 2nd ed. Philadelphia, PA: W. B. Saunders; 1994: 104–58.

3. Wehry EA. Molecular fluorescence and phosphorescence spectrometry. In: Settle FA, ed. *Handbook of Instrumental Techniques for Analytical Chemistry.* Upper Saddle River, NJ: Prentice-Hall; 1997: 507–39.

4. Tiffany TO. Fluorometry, nephelometry, and turbidimetry. In: Burtis CA, Ashwood ER, eds. *Clinical Chemistry.* 2nd ed. Philadelphia, PA: W. B. Saunders; 1994: 132–58.

5. Moore RE. Immunochemical methods. In: McClatchey KD, ed. *Clinical Laboratory Medicine.* 1st ed. Baltimore, MD: Williams & Wilkins; 1994: 213–38.

6. George JW, O'Neill SL. Comparison of refractometer and biuret methods for total protein measurement in body cavity fluids. *Vet Clin Pathol.* 2001; 30:16–8.

7. Freier ES. Osmometry. In: Burtis CA, Ashwood ER, eds. *Clinical Chemistry.* 2nd ed. Philadelphia, PA: W. B. Saunders; 1994: 184–90.

8. Juel R. Serum osmolality, a CAP survey analysis. *Am J Clin Pathol.* 1977; 68(suppl):165–69.

9. Durst RA, Siggaard-Andersen. Electrochemistry. In: Burtis CA, Ashwood ER, eds. *Clinical Chemistry.* 2nd ed. Philadelphia, PA: W. B. Saunders; 1994: 159–83.

10. Burnett W, Lee-Lewandrowski E, Lewandrowski K. Electrolytes and acid base balance. In: McClatchey KD, ed. *Clinical Laboratory Medicine.* 1st ed. Baltimore, MD: Williams & Wilkins; 1994: 331–54.

11. Ladenson JH, Apple FS, Koch DD. Misleading hypo-natremia due to hyperlipemia: a method-dependent error. *Ann Intern Med.* 1981; 95:707.

12. Southern EM. Detection of specific sequences among DNA fragments separated by gel electrophoresis. *J Mol Biol.* 1975; 98:503–17.

13. Hoefer Scientific Instruments. *Protein Electrophoresis Applications Guide* (1994). http://www.seas.upenn.edu /belab/ ReferenceFiles/hofferelectrobook.pdf.

14. Chang R. *Physical Chemistry with Applications to Biological Systems.* New York, NY: MacMillan; 1977.

15. Silverman LM, Christenson RH. Amino acids and proteins. In: Burtis CA, Ashwood ER, eds. *Clinical Chemistry.* 2nd ed. Philadelphia, PA: W. B. Saunders; 1994: 625–734.

16. Fairbanks VF, Klee GG. Biochemical aspects of hematology. In: Burtis CA, Ashwood ER, eds. *Clinical Chemistry.* 2nd ed. Philadelphia, PA: W. B. Saunders; 1994: 1974–2072.

17. Epstein E, Karcher RE. Electrophoresis. In: Burtis CA, Ashwood ER, eds. *Clinical Chemistry.* 2nd ed. Philadelphia, PA: W. B. Saunders; 1994: 191–205.

18. Görg A., Postel W., Günther S. The current state of two-dimensional electrophoresis withimmobilized pH gradients. *Electrophoresis.* 1988; 9:531–46.

19. Kohler G, Milstein C. Continuous cultures of fused cells secreting antibody of predefined specificity. *Nature.* 1975; 256:445–97.

20. Berson SA, Yalow RS, Bauman A, et al. Insulin I131 metabolism in human subjects: demonstration of insulin binding globulin in the circulation of insulin treated subjects. *J Clin Invest.* 1956; 35:170.

21. Nakamura RM, Tucker ES, Carlson IH. Immunoassays in the clinical laboratory. In: Henry JB, ed. *Clinical Diagnosis and Management,* 18th ed. Philadelphia, PA: W. B. Saunders; 1991: 848–84.

22. Kitson FG, Larsen BS, McEwen CN. *Gas Chromatography and Mass Spectrometry: a Practical Guide.* San Diego, CA: Academic Press; 1996.

23. Siuzdak G. *Mass Spectrometry for Biotechnology.* San Diego, CA: Academic Press; 1996.

24. Bowers LD, Ullman MD, Burtis CA. Chromatography. In: Burtis CA, Ashwood ER, eds. *Clinical Chemistry,* 2nd ed. Philadelphia, PA: W. B. Saunders; 1994: 206–55.

25. Van Bramer SE. An introduction to mass spectrometry (1997). Available at: http://science.widener.edu/svb/ massspec/massspec.pdf.

26. Busch KL, Glish GL, McLuckey SA. *Mass Spectrometry/Mass Spectrometry: Techniques and Applications of Tandem Mass Spectrometry.* New York, NY: VCH Publishers, Inc.; 1988.

27. Melnick SJ. Acute lymphoblastic leukemia. *Clin Lab Med.* 1999; 19:169–86.

28. Alamo AL, Melnick SJ. Clinical applications of four and five-color flow cytometry lymphocyte subset immunophenotyping. *Comm Clin Cytometry.* 2000; 42:363–70.

29. Raap AK. Overview of fluorescent in situ hybridization techniques for molecular cytogenetics. *Current Protocols in Cytometry.* 1997; 8.1.1–8.1.6.

30. Wilkinson DG. Chapter 1: The theory and practice of in situ hybridization. In: Wilkinson DG, ed. *In Situ Hybridization—A Practical Approach.* Oxford: Oxford University Press; 1992: 1–13.

31. Erlich HA, Gelfand D, Sninsky JJ. Recent advances in the polymerase chain reaction. *Science.* 1991; 252:1643–51.

32. Remick DG. Clinical applications of molecular biology. In: McClatchey KD, ed. *Clinical Laboratory Medicine.* 1st ed. Baltimore, MD: Williams & Wilkins; 1994: 165–74.

33. Maclin E, Young DS. Automation in the clinical laboratory. In: Burtis CA, Ashwood ER, eds. *Clinical Chemistry.* 2nd ed. Philadelphia, PA: W. B. Saunders; 1994: 313–82.

34. Zakowski J, Powell D. The future of automation in clinical laboratories. *In Vitro Diagnostics Technology.* 1999; July:48.

35. Felder RA. Automation: survival tools for the hospital laboratory. Paper presented at: The Second International Bayer Diagnostics Laboratory Testing Symposium; July 17, 1998; New York, NY. Available at: http://marc.med.virginia.edu/pdfs/lib_automation.html.

36. Felder RA, Graves S, Mifflin T. Increasing the relevance of laboratory medicine in the next century. *Medical Laboratory Observer*. 1999; July:20.

37. Imants RL. Microfabricated biosensors and microanalytical systems for blood analysis. *Acc Chem Res*. 1998; 31:317–24.

38. Ouellette J. Biosensors: microelectronics marries biology. *The Industrial Physicist*. 1998; September:11.

39. Wang J. Survey and summary from DNA biosensors to gene chips. *Nucleic Acids Research*. 2000; 28:3011–6.

Chapter **3**

INTERPRETING PEDIATRIC LABORATORY DATA

Donna M. Kraus

The interpretation of laboratory data in the pediatric patient population can be complex. Compared to adults, the pediatric population is much more dynamic. Alterations in body composition, organ function, and physiologic activity accompany the normal processes of maturation and growth that occur from birth through adolescence. These alterations can result in different normal reference ranges in pediatric patients for various laboratory tests. Pediatric patients not only have different normal laboratory values compared to adults, but normal laboratory values may differ in various pediatric age groups. It is important for the clinician to understand the reasons for these different, commonly accepted reference ranges and to use age-appropriate reference ranges when providing pharmaceutical care to pediatric patients.

The measurement of substances in neonates, infants, and young children is further complicated by the patient's smaller physical size and difficulty in obtaining blood and urine samples. The smaller blood volume in these patients requires blood samples to be smaller and, thus, special microanalytical techniques must be used. Additionally, in the neonate, substances that normally occur in higher amounts in the blood—such as bilirubin, lipids, and hemoglobin—may interfere with certain assays. This chapter will briefly review pertinent general pediatric principles and focus on the different age-related factors that must be considered when interpreting commonly used laboratory data in pediatric patients.

OBJECTIVES

After completing this chapter, the reader should be able to

1. Define the various pediatric age group terminology.
2. Discuss general pediatric considerations as they relate to blood sampling.
3. Describe how pediatric reference ranges are determined.
4. Discuss the age-related physiologic differences that account for the variations by age in the normal reference ranges for serum sodium, potassium, bicarbonate, calcium, phosphorus, and magnesium.
5. List common pediatric causes of abnormalities in the electrolytes and minerals listed above.
6. Explain why age-related differences in serum creatinine and kidney function tests occur.
7. Discuss the age-related differences that occur in serum albumin, liver enzyme tests, and bilirubin.
8. Describe what is meant by the physiologic anemia of infancy and explain how it occurs.

GENERAL PEDIATRIC CONSIDERATIONS

Knowledge of pediatric age group terminology is important to better understand age-related physiological differences and other factors that may influence the interpretation of pediatric laboratory data. These terms are defined in Table 3-1 and will be used throughout this chapter.

TABLE 3-1

Gestational age (GA)	The time from conception until birth. More specifically, gestational age is defined as the number of weeks from the first day of the mother's last menstrual period (LMP) until the birth of the baby. Gestational age at birth is assessed by the date of the LMP and by physical exam (Dubowitz score).
Postnatal age (PNA)	Chronological age since birth
Postconceptional age (PCA)	Age since conception. Postconceptional age is calculated as gestational age plus postnatal age (PCA = GA + PNA).
Neonate	A full-term newborn 0–4 weeks postnatal age. This term may also be applied to a premature neonate whose postconceptional age (PCA) is 42–46 weeks.
Premature neonate	Neonate born at <38 weeks gestational age
Full-term neonate	Neonate born at 38–42 weeks (average ~40 weeks) gestational age
Infant	1 month to 1 year of age
Child/Children	1–12 years of age
Adolescent	13–18 years of age
Adult	>18 years of age

^a*Reproduced, with permission, from Reference 1.*

Table 3-1. Definition of Age Group Terminology[a]

The interpretation of any patient's laboratory data must be viewed in light of the patient's clinical status. This includes the patient's symptoms, physical signs of disease, and physiologic parameters, such as respiratory rate, heart rate, and blood pressure. For example, an elevated $PaCO_2$ from an arterial blood gas may be clinically more significant in a patient who is extremely tachypneic (perhaps indicating impending respiratory failure) compared to a patient whose respiratory rate is mildly elevated. Thus, it is important to know the relative differences in physiologic norms that occur in the various pediatric age groups.

Normal respiratory rates are higher in neonates and young infants compared to children, adolescents, and adults. The average respiratory rate of a newborn is 60 breaths/min at 1 hr after birth, but 30–40 breaths/min at greater than 6 hr after birth. Mean respiratory rates of infants and young children <2 years of age (25–30 breaths/min) continue to be higher than in children 3–9 years of age (20–25 breaths/min) and adolescents (16–20 breaths/min).[1]

Normal heart rates follow a similar pattern with higher heart rates in neonates and young infants, which then slowly decrease with increasing age through adolescence. For example, the mean heart rate of a newborn on the first day of life is 123 beats/min and that of a 1-month-old infant is 149 beats/min, while the mean heart rate for a 1 year old is 119 beats/min and that of a 12 year old is 85 beats/min.[2]

In pediatric patients, normal blood pressure values vary according to age, gender, and percentile height of the patient.[3,4] Blood pressures are lower in neonates and increase throughout infancy and childhood. For example, typical blood pressures for a full-term newborn would be in the range of 65–95 systolic and 30–60 diastolic. The normal blood pressure (blood pressure <90th percentile) for a 1-year-old girl of average height would be less than 100/54, while that of a 15-year-old girl of average height would be less than 124/79. Blood pressures are slightly different for girls compared to boys and are higher in taller children. Appropriate references should be consulted to obtain normal blood pressure values when providing clinical care to pediatric patients.[1,3,4]

In addition to age-related physiologic differences in respiratory rates, heart rates, and blood pressures, age-related changes in body composition (e.g., fluid compartments), cardiac output, organ perfusion, and organ function also exist. These age-related changes may result in different normal laboratory values for pediatric patients compared to adults. Being aware of the normal laboratory values for age is important for proper monitoring of efficacy and toxicity of pediatric drug therapy.

Pediatric Blood Sampling

The smaller physical size of pediatric patients makes the obtainment of blood samples more difficult. In general, venipuncture techniques used in adults can be utilized in older children and adolescents. However, vacuum containers used for blood sampling may collapse the small veins of younger children and are not recommended in these patients.[5] Capillary puncture (also called microcapillary puncture or skin puncture) is used in patients with small or inaccessible veins. Thus, it is the blood sampling method of choice for premature neonates, neonates, and young infants. Since this method also helps preserve total blood volume, it may also be beneficial to use in infants and small children who require multiple blood tests.[6]

The physical sites that are used for capillary puncture include the heel, finger, great toe, and ear lobe.[5,6] The preferred site in neonates is the medial or lateral portion of the plantar surface of the heel. The medial surface of the great toe may also be used. The central area of the foot is avoided because of the risk of damage to the calcaneus bone, tendons, nerves, and cartilage. Heelsticks are often used in neonates and younger infants, while fingersticks may be used in children and adults. The earlobe is never used for capillary puncture for neonates and infants but may be used as a "site of last resort" in older children and adults.[6]

Since capillary and venous blood are similar in composition, the capillary puncture method may be used to obtain samples for most chemistry and hematology tests.[6] However, differences may occur between venous and capillary blood for certain substances such as glucose, calcium, potassium, and total protein. For example, glucose concentrations may be 10% higher when the sample is collected by capillary puncture compared to venipuncture.[5] In addition, improper capillary puncture sample collection may result in hemolysis or introduction of interstitial fluid into the specimen. This may result in higher concentrations for potassium, magnesium, lactate dehydrogenase, and other substances. Therefore, using the proper procedure to collect blood by the capillary puncture method is essential. It is also important that the site of capillary puncture be warmed prior to sample collection, especially for blood gas determinations.[5] Complications of capillary puncture include infection, hematoma, and bruising.

The size of the blood sample is an important issue to the pediatric clinician. Compared to adults, pediatric patients have a much smaller total blood volume (Table 3-2). For example, a full-term newborn of average weight (3.4 kg) has an approximate total blood volume of 78–86 mL/kg, or about 265–292 mL total.[1,7] However, a 70 kg adult has as estimated total blood volume of 68–88 mL/kg or 4760–6160 mL total. If a standard 10 mL blood sample were to be drawn from a pediatric patient, it would represent a much higher percent of total blood volume compared to an adult. Therefore, the smaller total blood volume in pediatric patients requires blood sample sizes to be smaller. This issue is further complicated in newborns because their relatively high hematocrit (approximately 60% or higher) decreases the yield of serum or plasma from the amount of blood collected. Microanalytical techniques have reduced the required size of blood samples. However, critically ill, pediatric patients

TABLE 3-2

AGE	EXAMPLE WEIGHT (kg) [AGE]	APPROXIMATE TOTAL BLOOD VOLUME (mL/kg)[b]	ESTIMATED TOTAL BLOOD VOLUME (mL)
Premature infant	1.5	89–105	134–158
Term newborn	3.4	78–86	265–292
1–12 months	7.6 [6 months]	73–78	555–593
1–3 years	12.4 [2 years]	74–82	918–1017
4–6 years	18.2 [5 years]	80–86	1456–1565
7–18 years	45.5 [13 years]	83–90	3777–4095
Adults	70.0	68–88	4760–6160

[a] Reproduced, with permission, from Reference 1.
[b] Approximate total blood volume information compiled from Reference 7.

Table 3-2. Total Blood Volume[a]

may require multiple or frequent blood sample determinations. Thus, it is essential to plan pediatric laboratory tests, especially in the neonate and premature neonate, to avoid excessive blood drawing.

Substances that normally occur in higher amounts in the blood of neonates, such as bilirubin, lipids, and hemoglobin, may interfere with certain assays. Hyperbilirubinemia may occur in premature and term neonates. High bilirubin concentrations may produce falsely low creatinine or cholesterol values when measured by certain analytical instruments.[5] Neonates, especially those that are born prematurely, may have lipemia when receiving intravenous fat emulsions. Lipemia may interfere with spectrophotometric determinations of any substance or with flame photometer determinations of potassium and sodium. Newborns have higher hemoglobin values and hemoglobin may interfere with certain assays. For example, hemolysis and the presence of hemoglobin may interfere with bilirubin measurements. Therefore, it is important to ensure that the assay methodology selected for measurement of substances in neonatal serum or plasma is not subject to interference from bilirubin, lipids, or hemoglobin.

Pediatric Reference Ranges

Various methods can be used to determine reference ranges, and each method has its own advantages and disadvantages. In adults, reference ranges are usually determined by obtaining samples from known healthy individuals. The frequency distribution of the obtained values are assessed and the extreme outliers (e.g., 0–2.5th percentile and 97.5–100th percentile) are excluded. This leaves the values of the 2.5–97.5th percentiles to define the reference range.[8] However, it also labels the 0–2.5th percentile and 97.5–100th percentile values from the healthy individuals as being outside of the reference range. If the frequency distribution of the obtained values fall in a bell-shaped or Gaussian distribution, then the mean (or average) value plus or minus two standard deviations (SD) can then be used to define the reference range. The mean value plus or minus 2 SD includes 95% of the sample. This method labels 5% of the healthy individuals as having values that fall outside of the reference range.

In the pediatric population, however, one cannot easily obtain blood samples from known healthy individuals. Large sample sizes of healthy pediatric individuals that include an appropriate age distribution from birth to 18 years of age would be required. Furthermore, it may be considered unethical to obtain blood samples from healthy pediatric patients when these individuals cannot legally give informed consent and there is no direct benefit to these individuals of obtaining the blood sample. Therefore, many pediatric reference ranges are determined by using results of tests from hospitalized sick pediatric patients and applying special statistical methods.[8] The statistical methods are designed to remove outliers and to distinguish the normal values from the values found in the sick patients. Obviously, problems in determining the true reference range may arise, especially when overlap between values from the diseased and nondiseased population occurs.

As in adults, many factors can influence the pediatric reference range including the specific assay methodology used, type of specimen analyzed, specific population studied, nutritional status of the individual, time of day the sample is obtained, timing of meals, medications taken, and specific patient demographics (age, sex, height, weight, and body surface area). These factors, if not properly identified, may also influence the determination of reference ranges. In addition, since pediatric reference ranges are typically established in hospitalized patients, concomitant diseases may also influence the determination of the specific reference range being studied. All of these factors, plus the greater heterogeneity (variance) observed in the pediatric population makes the determination of pediatric reference ranges more complex.

Pediatric studies that define reference ranges may not always give detailed information about factors that may have influenced the determination of the specific pediatric reference range. Furthermore, due to the variation in influencing factors, most published pediatric reference ranges are not in exact agreement with each other.[1,2,8–16] Some studies report reference ranges by age for each year, others by various age groups, and others only by graphic display. Thus, it makes it very difficult to ascertain standard values for pediatric reference ranges and to apply published pediatric reference ranges to one's own patient population.

The reference ranges listed in this chapter reflect a compilation from various sources and are meant to be general guidelines. Clinicians should consult with their institution's laboratory to determine the specific age-appropriate pediatric reference ranges to be used in their patient population.

Pediatric Clinical Presentation

In general, the clinical symptoms of laboratory abnormalities in pediatric patients are similar to those symptoms observed in adults. However, certain manifestations of symptoms may be different in pediatric patients. For example, central nervous system irritability due to electrolyte imbalances (such as hypernatremia) may manifest as a high-pitched cry in infants. Hypocalcemia, which may also cause seizure activity in adults, is more likely to manifest as seizures in neonates and young infants due to the immaturity of the central nervous system. Neonates may also have nonspecific or vague symptoms for many disorders. For example, neonates with sepsis, or with hypocalcemia, may have poor feedings, lethargy, and vomiting. In addition, young pediatric patients are unable to communicate symptoms they may be experiencing. Thus, although symptoms of laboratory abnormalities in pediatric patients are important, oftentimes the correct diagnosis relies on the physical exam and appropriate laboratory tests.

SERUM ELECTROLYTES AND MINERALS

The homeostatic mechanisms that regulate fluid, electrolyte, and mineral balance in adults also apply to the pediatric patient. However, several important age-related differences exist. Compared to adults, neonates and young infants have alterations in body composition and fluid compartments; increased insensible water loss; immature (decreased) renal function; and variations in the neuroendocrine control of fluid, electrolyte, and mineral balance.[17] In addition, fluid, electrolyte, and mineral intake are not controlled by the individual (i.e., the neonate or young infant) but are controlled by the individual's caregiver. These age-related physiologic differences can result in alterations in the pediatric reference range for several electrolytes and minerals and can influence the interpretation of pediatric laboratory data.

A large percent of the human body is comprised of water. Total body water (TBW) can be divided into two major compartments, intracellular water (ICW) and extracellular water (ECW).

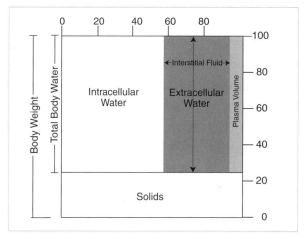

Figure 3-1. Distribution of body water in a term newborn infant. (Reproduced, with permission, from Reference 17, page 346.)

The ECW consists of the interstitial water and the intravascular water (or plasma volume) (see Figure 3-1). Both TBW and ECW, when expressed as a percentage of body weight, are increased in the fetus and the newborn (especially the premature neonate) and decrease during childhood with increasing age (Figure 3-2).[18,19] The TBW of a fetus is 94% during the first month of gestation and decreases to 75% in a full-term newborn. The TBW of a preterm newborn may be 80%. The TBW decreases to approximately 60% by 6–12 months of age and to 55% in an adult. ECW is about 44% in a full-term newborn, 30% in a 3–6-month-old

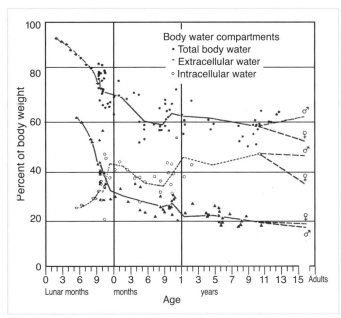

Figure 3-2. Changes in body water from early fetal life to adult life. (Reproduced, with permission, from Reference 18, page 8.)

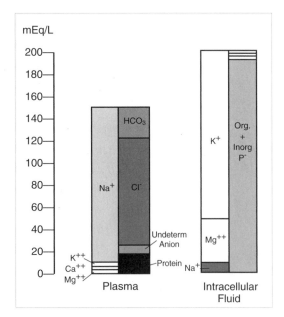

Figure 3-3. Ion distribution in the blood plasma, which represents extracellular fluid, and in the intracellular fluid compartment. (Reproduced, with permission, from Reference 17, page 346.)

infant, 25% in a 1 year old, and 19% in an adult.[18,19] The decrease in TBW that is seen after birth is largely due to a contraction (or mobilization) of the ECW compartment. This mobilization is, most likely, the result of an increase in renal function that is seen after birth. ICW is lower at birth, increases slowly after birth, and is greater than ECW by about 3 months of age. It is important to note that the intake of water and electrolytes can influence these post-natal changes in TBW and the distribution between ECW and ICW.[17]

The electrolyte composition of ECW vs. ICW is very different (Figure 3-3). Sodium is the major cation found in the intravascular (plasma volume) of the ECW. Potassium, calcium, and magnesium make up a much smaller amount of the intravascular cations. Chloride is the primary intravascular anion and bicarbonate, protein, and other anions comprise the balance. The electrolyte composition of the interstitial component of ECW is similar to the intravascular composition but protein content is lower. Potassium and magnesium are the major cations found in ICW. Phosphate (organic and inorganic) is the primary intracellular anion, and bicarbonate makes up a smaller amount.[17]

These compositional differences in ECW and ICW, along with the age-related differences in the amounts of these water compartments, can result in maturational differences in the amount of electrolytes per kg of body weight. For example, since premature neonates have a larger ECW compartment and ECW contains a higher amount of sodium and chloride, premature neonates contain a higher amount of sodium and chloride per kilogram of body weight compared to term neonates.[17] These principles are important to keep in mind when managing neonatal fluid and electrolyte therapy. One must also remember that the management of fluid and electrolyte therapy in the mother during labor can result in alterations in the newborn's fluid and electrolyte status. For example, if the mother is given too much fluid (i.e., too much free water) during labor, the newborn may be born with hyponatremia.[20]

Insensible water loss is the water that is lost via evaporation from the skin and through the respiratory tract.[17] Knowledge of the factors that influence insensible water loss in pediatric patients is important to estimate appropriate water intake and to assess electrolyte imbalances that may occur. Compared to adults, neonates and young infants have an increase in the amount of insensible water loss. This is primarily due to their increased surface area to body weight ratio and higher respiratory rate. Smaller newborns and those born at a younger gestational age have an even higher insensible water loss. This is related to their immature (thinner) skin, greater skin blood flow, and larger TBW. Many other factors increase insensible water loss, such as the environmental and body temperature, radiant warmers, phototherapy, motor activity, crying, and skin breakdown or injury. Congenital skin defects, such as gastroschisis, omphalocele, or neural tube defects will also increase insensible water loss. The use of high inspired or ambient humidity, plastic heat shields or blankets, occlusive dressings, and topical waterproof agents will decrease insensible water loss.

The primary functions of the kidney (glomerular filtration, tubular secretion, and tubular reabsorption) are all decreased in the newborn, especially in the premature newborn, compared to adults. These functions increase with gestational age at birth and with postnatal age. The decreased glomerular and tubular functions in the neonatal kidney result in differences in how the neonate handles various electrolyte loads and differences in the normal reference ranges for several electrolytes, as described below.

Sodium

Normal range,[21] premature neonates (at 48 hr of life):
128–148 mEq/L or 128–148 mmol/L;
newborns: 133–146 mEq/L or 133–146 mmol/L;
infants: 139–146 mEq/L or 139–146 mmol/L;
children: 138–145 mEq/L or 138–145 mmol/L;
adults: 136–145 mEq/L or 136–145 mmol/L

Sodium is primarily excreted via the kidneys, but it is also excreted via stool and sweat.[22] Usually, unless diarrhea occurs, sodium loss in the stool is minimal. In children with cystic fibrosis, aldosterone deficiency, or pseudohypoaldosteronism, the sodium concentration in sweat is increased and higher sweat losses may contribute to or cause sodium depletion.

In neonates and young infants, the renal handling of sodium is altered compared to adults.[23,24] Differences in tubular reabsorption, aldosterone concentrations, and patterns of renal blood flow help to maintain a positive sodium balance, which is required for growth. In the neonate, sodium reabsorption is decreased in the proximal tubule but increased in the distal tubule. Aldosterone increases sodium reabsorption in the distal tubules, and plasma concentrations of renin, angiotensin II, and aldosterone are all increased in neonates. This increase in aldosterone may be a compensatory mechanism to help increase sodium reabsorption in the distal tubule. The pattern of renal blood flow is also different in the neonate. In adults, a larger amount of renal blood flow goes to the cortical area of the kidneys. However, in the neonate, the majority of renal blood flow goes to the medullary area, which is more involved with sodium conservation than excretion. These factors help the neonatal kidney to retain sodium but also result in the neonate having a decreased ability to excrete a sodium load. Therefore, if an excessive amount of sodium is administered to a neonate, it will result in sodium retention with subsequent water retention and edema.

Although most infants are in a positive sodium balance, very low birth weight infants (birth weight <1.5 kg) are usually in a negative sodium balance.[23] This is due to their very immature kidneys and the larger amounts of sodium that are lost in the urine. These infants are at a higher risk of sodium imbalance and may require higher amounts of sodium, especially during the first weeks of life.

Compared to adults, pediatric patients may be more susceptible to imbalances of sodium and water. This may be due to their higher amount of TBW and the common pediatric occurrence of causative factors such as diarrhea and dehydration.

Hyponatremia

In infants and children, hyponatremia is defined as a serum sodium less than 135 mEq/L,[22] although slightly lower values would be considered acceptable for premature neonates and newborns. As in adults, hyponatremia occurs in pediatric patients when the ratio of water to sodium is increased. This may occur with low, normal, or high amounts of sodium in the body; likewise, the amount of water in the body may be low (hypovolemic), normal (euvolemic), or high (hypervolemic). The causes of hyponatremia in pediatric patients are the same as in adults (see Chapter 7). However, certain causes may be more commonly seen in children.

In hypovolemic hyponatremia, both sodium and water have been lost from the body, but a higher proportion of sodium has been lost. The most common cause of hypovolemic hyponatremia in children is diarrhea due to gastroenteritis.[22] Emesis can also cause hyponatremia if hypotonic fluids are administered, but most children with emesis have either a normal serum sodium or hypernatremia. In addition to gastrointestinal losses, hypovolemic hyponatremia may also occur from losses of sodium through the skin (e.g., excessive sweating or burns), third space losses, and renal losses.

Renal sodium loss can occur in the pediatric population from a number of causes including thiazide or loop diuretics, osmotic diuresis, cerebral salt wasting, and hereditary or acquired kidney diseases. Cerebral salt wasting is thought to be due to hypersecretion of atrial natriuretic peptide, which causes renal salt wasting. This condition is usually seen in patients with central nervous system disorders such as head trauma, brain tumors, hydrocephalus, and neurosurgery.[25] Hereditary kidney diseases that can cause hypovolemic hyponatremia include juvenile nephronophthisis, autosomal recessive polycystic kidney disease, proximal (type II) renal tubular acidosis, 21-hydroxylase deficiency, and pseudohypoaldosteronism type I. Patients with congenital adrenal hyperplasia due to 21-hydroxylase deficiency have an absence of aldosterone. Aldosterone is needed for sodium retention and potassium and acid excretion in the kidneys. The lack of aldosterone in these patients produces hyponatremia, hyperkalemia, and metabolic acidosis. Patients with pseudohypoaldosteronism have elevated aldosterone serum concentrations, but the kidneys do not respond properly to aldosterone. A lack of response to aldosterone by the renal tubules may also occur in children with a urinary tract obstruction and/or acute urinary tract infection and result in hyponatremia.[22]

In euvolemic hyponatremia, patients have no real evidence of volume depletion or volume overload.[22] Usually, these patients have a slight decrease in total body sodium with an excess of TBW. Although some patients may have an increase in body weight (indicating volume overload), patients often appear clinically normal or have subtle signs of fluid overload. Causes of euvolemic hyponatremia include syndrome of inappropriate antidiuretic hormone (SIADH), glucocorticoid deficiency, hypothyroidism, and water intoxication. SIADH is not common in children but may occur in patients with central nervous system disorders or lung disease and tumors. Certain medications can cause an increase in ADH secretion or effect and are reviewed in Chapter 7.

Dilutional hyponatremia may commonly occur in hospitalized children who receive relatively large amounts of free water (e.g., hypotonic intravenous solutions). This may even occur when medications are diluted in 5% dextrose in water, for example, and administered as 50 or 100 mL intravenous rider bags or piggyback riders. Neonates and young infants are more prone to this water overload (due to their lower GFR and limited ability to excrete water), and, thus, should receive medications diluted in smaller volumes of IV fluid. Other causes of hyponatremia due to water intoxication in pediatric patients include administration of diluted infant formula, tap water enemas, infant swimming lessons, forced water intake (child abuse), and psychogenic polydipsia.[22]

In hypervolemic hyponatremia, both sodium and water are increased in the body, but there is a greater increase in water than sodium. Hypervolemic hyponatremia is typically observed in patients with CHF, cirrhosis, nephrotic syndrome, and chronic renal failure. It may also occur in patients with hypoalbuminemia or in patients with capillary leak syndrome due to sepsis.[22] These conditions decrease the patient's effective blood volume, either due to poor cardiac function or third spacing of fluid. The compensatory mechanisms in the body sense this decrease in blood volume; ADH and aldosterone are secreted and cause retention of water and sodium in the kidneys. A decrease in serum sodium occurs because the intake of water in these patients is greater than their sodium intake and ADH decreases water excretion.

Hypernatremia

In general for pediatric patients, hypernatremia is defined as a serum sodium concentration greater than 145 mEq/L. As in adults, hypernatremia occurs in pediatric patients when the ratio of sodium to water is increased. This may occur with low, normal, or high amounts of sodium in the body. Hypernatremia may occur with excessive sodium intake, excess water loss, or a combination of water and sodium loss when the water loss exceeds the sodium loss.[22]

Excessive sodium intake or sodium intoxication may occur due to improperly mixed infant formulas, excess sodium bicarbonate administration, intravenous hypertonic saline solutions, intentional salt poisoning (e.g., child abuse), and ingestion of sodium chloride or seawater.[22]

Neonates, especially premature newborns, and young infants can develop hypernatremia from excessive sodium due to the decreased ability of immature kidneys to excrete a sodium load. This becomes a problem especially in the premature neonate when intravenous sodium bicarbonate is used to correct a metabolic acidosis.

Excess water loss resulting in hypernatremia may occur in pediatric patients due to diabetes insipidus, increased insensible water losses, or inadequate intake. Diabetes insipidus can be of central or nephrogenic origin and either type can be acquired or congenital. Certain drugs may cause diabetes insipidus (see Chapter 7).

Neonates may be predisposed to hypernatremia from increased insensible water losses, especially during the first few days of life. A normal physiologic contraction of the ECW occurs after birth, resulting in a net loss of water and sodium. In term infants, this may result in a weight loss of 5–10% during the first week of life. In premature newborns, the weight loss may be 10–20%. This water loss, plus the relatively large and variable insensible water loss in neonates, can complicate the assessment of fluid and sodium balance. More premature newborns may be at higher risk for hypernatremia, as they have a more pronounced contraction of ECW and higher insensible water loss.[26] The use of radiant warmers and phototherapy (used to treat hyperbilirubinemia) will further increase insensible water loss.

Inadequate water intake can also cause hypernatremia in pediatric patients. This may be due to the caregiver not administering enough fluids (e.g., child neglect or abuse, or ineffective breast-feeding). Ineffective breast-feeding may result in severe hypernatremic dehydration. Rarely, inadequate intake may be due to adipsia (absence of thirst).[22]

Hypernatremia, due to water losses greater than sodium losses, occurs in patients with water and sodium losses through the gastrointestinal tract (e.g., diarrhea, emesis, nasogastric suctioning, and osmotic cathartics), skin (e.g., burns and excessive sweating), and kidneys (e.g., diabetes mellitus, chronic kidney disease, osmotic diuretics, and acute tubular necrosis [polyuric phase]). Hypernatremia is most likely to occur in infants or children with diarrhea who also have inadequate fluid intake due to anorexia, emesis, or lack of access to water.

It should be noted that due to the immaturity of the blood vessels in their central nervous system, premature neonates are especially vulnerable to the adverse effects of hypernatremia (e.g., intracranial hemorrhage). These patients are also at greater risk of adverse central nervous system effects if an elevated serum sodium is corrected too rapidly. Thus, maintaining a proper sodium balance in these patients is extremely important.

Potassium

Normal range,[10,21] for premature neonates (at 48 hr of life):
3.0–6.0 mEq/L or 3.0–6.0 mmol/L;
newborns: 3.7–5.9 mEq/L or 3.7–5.9 mmol/L;
infants: 4.1–5.3 mEq/L or 4.1–5.3 mmol/L;
children: 3.4–4.7 mEq/L or 3.4–4.7 mmol/L;
adults: 3.5–5.0 mEq/L or 3.5–5.0 mmol/L

Potassium is the major intracellular cation, and less then 1% of total body potassium is found in the plasma.[22] However, small changes in serum potassium can have large effects on cardiac, neuromuscular, and neural function. Thus, appropriate homeostasis of extracellular potassium is extremely important. Insulin, aldosterone, acid-base balance, and renal function all play important roles in the regulation of serum potassium. Serum potassium can be lowered quickly when potassium shifts intracellularly or more slowly via elimination by the kidneys.

The kidney is the primary organ that regulates potassium balance and elimination. Potassium undergoes glomerular filtration and almost all filtered potassium is then reabsorbed in the proximal tubule. Urinary excretion of potassium, therefore, is dependent on distal potassium secretion by the collecting tubules. Neonates and young infants, however, have a decreased ability to secrete potassium via the collecting tubules. Thus, the immature kidneys tend to retain potassium. This results in a positive potassium balance, which is required for growth (potassium is incorporated intracellularly into new tissues).[23,24] Potassium retention by the immature kidneys also results in higher serum potassium concentrations compared to the adult.[24]

Hypokalemia

Hypokalemia is defined as a serum potassium concentration <3.5 mEq/mL. As in adults, a low serum potassium may occur in pediatric patients due to an intracellular shift of potassium, decreased intake, or increased output (from renal or extrarenal losses). An intracellular shift of potassium may be seen with alkalosis, beta-adrenergic stimulation, or insulin treatment. Endogenous beta-adrenergic agonists (such as epinephrine released during stress) and exogenously administered beta-agonists (such as albuterol) stimulate the cellular uptake of potassium. Other causes of an intracellular shift of potassium seen in pediatric patients include overdoses of theophylline, barium intoxication, and glue sniffing (toluene intoxication).

Most cases of hypokalemia in children are related to extrarenal loses of potassium due to gastroenteritis and diarrhea.[22] Hypokalemia due to diarrhea is usually associated with a metabolic acidosis, since bicarbonate is also lost in the stool. Adolescent patients with eating disorders may be hypokalemic due to inadequate intake of potassium, for example, in patients with anorexia nervosa. Adolescents with bulimia or laxative abuse may also have significant extrarenal loses of potassium.

Many causes of hypokalemia due to renal potassium loss exist. Medications commonly used in the pediatric population that are associated with hypokalemia due to renal potassium loss include loop and thiazide diuretics, corticosteroids, amphotericin B, and cisplatin (see Chapter 7). Cushing's syndrome, hyperaldosteronism, and licorice ingestion may also cause hypokalemia via this mechanism.

In the pediatric population, other causes of increased renal potassium loss, such as hereditary diseases, must be considered. Remember that many hereditary diseases are first diagnosed during infancy and childhood. Renal tubular acidosis (both distal and proximal types) may present with hypokalemia and metabolic acidosis. Patients with cystic fibrosis have greater losses of chloride in sweat. This may lead to metabolic alkalosis, low urine chloride, and hypokalemia. Certain forms of congenital adrenal hyperplasia may also lead to increased renal potassium excretion and hypokalemia. Other inherited renal diseases that are due to defects in renal tubular transporters, such as Bartter's syndrome, may result in metabolic alkalosis, hypokalemia, and high urine chloride. Thus, unlike the adult population, hereditary diseases need to be considered when certain electrolyte abnormalities are not explained by common causes.

Hyperkalemia

In infants, children, and adults, hyperkalemia is defined as a serum potassium greater than 5.0 mEq/L. Since a normal serum potassium is slightly higher in neonates and preterm infants, hyperkalemia is defined as a serum potassium greater than 6.0 mEq/L in these patients. Hyperkalemia is one of the most alarming electrolyte imbalances because it has the potential to cause lethal cardiac arrhythmias.

As in adults, hyperkalemia in pediatric patients may be due to increased intake, an extracellular shift of potassium, or decreased renal excretion (see Chapter 7). Factitious hyperkalemia is very common in pediatric patients, due to the difficulty in obtaining blood samples. Hemolysis often occurs during blood sampling and potassium is released from red blood cells in sufficient amounts to cause falsely elevated test results.

Hyperkalemia may occur due to extracellular shifts of potassium. During a metabolic acidosis, hydrogen ions move into the cells (down a concentration gradient), and in exchange, potassium ions move out of the cells into the extracellular (intravascular) space. This shift leads to a significant increase in serum potassium.

In older patients with fully developed (normal) renal function, hyperkalemia rarely results from increased intake alone. However, this may occur in patients receiving large amounts of oral or intravenous potassium or in patients receiving rapid or frequent blood transfusions (due to the potassium content of blood).[22] In patients with immature renal function or in those with renal failure, increased intake of potassium can also lead to hyperkalemia due to decreased potassium excretion.

Decreased renal excretion of potassium is the most common cause of hyperkalemia. Decreased potassium excretion occurs in patients with immature renal function, renal failure, primary adrenal disease, hyporeninemic hypoaldosteronism, renal tubular disease, and with certain medications.[22] Hyperkalemia is the most common life-threatening electrolyte imbalance seen in neonates. Due to the decreased ability of immature kidneys to excrete potassium, neonates, particularly premature neonates, may be predisposed to hyperkalemia. These patients also cannot tolerate receiving extra potassium. Hyperkalemia can be seen in premature infants, during the first 3 days of life, even when exogenous potassium is not given and when renal dysfunction is absent.[26] A rapid elevation in serum potassium is seen within the first day of life in the more immature newborns. This hyperkalemia, which can be life-threatening, may be due to a shift of potassium from the intracellular space to the extracellular (intravascular) space, immaturity of the distal renal tubules, and a relative hypoaldosteronism.[27]

Acute or chronic renal failure in pediatric patients will decrease potassium excretion and may result in hyperkalemia. Several inherited disorders may also cause decreased potassium excretion and hyperkalemia in pediatric patients including certain types of congenital adrenal hyperplasia (e.g., 21-hydroxylase deficiency), aldosterone synthase deficiency, sickle cell disease, and pseudohypoaldosteronism (types I and II).[22] Medications used in pediatric patients that may also cause hyperkalemia include angiotensin-converting enzyme inhibitors, potassium-sparing diuretics, nonsteroidal anti-inflammatory agents, trimethoprim, and cyclosporine.

Serum Bicarbonate (Total Carbon Dioxide)

Normal range,[21,24] for preterm infants: 16–20 mEq/L or 16–20 mmol/L;
full-term infants: 19–21 mEq/L or 19–21 mmol/L;
infants–children 2 years of age: 18–28 mEq/L or 18–28 mmol/L;
children >2 years and adults: 24–30 mEq/L or 24–30 mmol/L

The total carbon dioxide concentration actually represents serum bicarbonate, the basic form of the carbonic acid-bicarbonate buffer system (i.e., a low serum bicarbonate may indicate an acidosis; see Chapter 7). In addition to the buffer systems, the kidneys also play an important role in acid-base balance. The proximal tubule reabsorbs 85–90% of filtered bicarbonate. The distal tubule is responsible for the net secretion of hydrogen ions and urinary acidification.[28] Compared to adults, neonates have a decreased capacity to reabsorb bicarbonate in the proximal tubule, and, therefore, a decreased renal threshold for bicarbonate (the renal threshold is the serum concentration at which bicarbonate appears in the urine). The mean renal threshold for bicarbonate in adults is 24–26 mEq/L but only 18 mEq/L in the premature infant and 21 mEq/L in the term neonate. The renal threshold for bicarbonate increases during the first year of life and reaches adult values by about 1 year of age. Neonates also have a decreased function of the distal tubules to secrete hydrogen ions and to acidify urine. The ability to acidify urine increases to adult values by about 1–2 months of age.[24,28] The neonate's decreased renal capacity to reabsorb bicarbonate and excrete hydrogen ions results in lower normal values for serum bicarbonate and blood pH. In addition, the neonate is less able to handle an acid load or to compensate for acid-base abnormalities.

It should be noted that for multiple reasons, the full-term newborn is in a state of metabolic acidosis immediately after birth (arterial pH 7.11–7.36).[11] The blood pH increases to more normal values within 24 hr, mostly due to increased excretion of carbon dioxide via the lungs.[24]

Calcium

Total serum calcium—normal range[11] for newborns: 3–24 hr old:
9.0–10.6 mg/dL or 2.3–2.65 mmol/L; 24–48 hr old: 7.0–12.0 mg/dL or 1.75–3.0 mmol/L;
4–7 days old: 9.0–10.9 mg/dL or 2.25–2.73 mmol/L;
children: 8.8–10.8 mg/dL or 2.2–2.7 mmol/L;
adolescents and adults: 8.4–10.2 mg/dL or 2.1–2.55 mmol/L

Ionized calcium—normal range for newborns: 3–24 hr old: 4.3–5.1 mg/dL or 1.07–1.27 mmol/L;
24–48 hr old: 4.0–4.7 mg/dL or 1.00–1.17 mmol/L;
infants, children, adolescents, and adults: 4.8–4.92 mg/dL or 1.12– 1.23 mmol/L

Calcium plays an integral role in many physiologic functions including muscle contraction, neuromuscular transmission, blood coagulation, bone metabolism, and regulation of endocrine functions (see Chapter 13). The great majority of calcium in the body (99%) is found in the bone, primarily as hydroxyapatite. Due to the growth that occurs during infancy and childhood, bone mass increases faster than body weight.[22] This increase in bone mass requires a significant increase in total body calcium. The increased calcium requirement is reflected in the higher recommended daily allowances (per kg body weight) in pediatric patients compared to adults.

Calcium regulation in the body has two main goals.[22] First, serum calcium must be tightly regulated to permit the normal physiologic functions in which calcium plays a role. Second, calcium intake must be adequate to permit appropriate bone mineralization and skeletal growth. It is important to remember that bone mineralization may be sacrificed (i.e., calcium may be released from the bone) in order to allow maintenance of a normal serum calcium concentration.

As in adults, serum calcium in pediatric patients is regulated by a complex hormonal system that involves vitamin D, serum phosphate, parathyroid hormone (PTH), and calcitonin. Briefly, calcium is absorbed in the gastrointestinal tract, primarily via the duodenum and jejunum.[22] Although some passive calcium absorption occurs when dietary intake is high, most gastrointestinal absorption of calcium occurs via active transport that is stimulated by 1,25-dihydroxyvitamin D. This occurs especially when dietary intake is low. Calcium excretion is controlled by the kidneys and influenced by multiple hormonal mediators (e.g., PTH, 1,25-dihydroxyvitamin D, and calcitonin). In the mature kidneys, approximately 99% of filtered calcium is reabsorbed by the tubules with the majority (>50%) absorbed by the proximal tubules. Calcium is also absorbed in the loop of Henle, distal tubule, and collecting ducts.

During the first week of life, urinary calcium excretion is inversely related to gestational age (i.e., more premature infants will have a greater urinary calcium excretion).[24] Compared to adults, urinary calcium excretion is higher in neonates and preterm infants. The urinary calcium-to-creatinine ratio is 0.11 in adults but may be greater than 2 in premature neonates and ranges from 0.05–1.2 in full-term neonates during the first week of life. This high rate of calcium excretion may be related to the immaturity of the renal tubules and may contribute (along with other factors) to neonatal hypocalcemia (see below). In addition, certain medications that are commonly administered to neonates and premature infants, such as furosemide, dexamethasone, and methylxanthines, further increase urinary calcium excretion. These medications may also increase the risk for hypocalcemia as well as nephrocalcinosis and nephrolithiasis.[24]

Measurement of Calcium

Total serum calcium measures all three forms of extracellular calcium: complex bound, protein bound, and ionized. However, ionized calcium is the physiologically active form. Usually a parallel relationship exists between the ionized and total serum calcium concentrations. However, in patients with alterations in acid-base balance or serum proteins, the ionized serum calcium is affected and measurements of total serum calcium no longer reflect the ionized serum concentration. Neonates have lower serum concentrations of protein (including albumin) and may be acidotic. This results in a lower total serum calcium concentration for a given ionized plasma concentration.[26] Although equations exist to adjust total serum calcium measurements for low concentrations of serum albumin, these equations have limitations and may not be precise. Therefore, ionized calcium should be measured in neonates (if micro-techniques are available) and other pediatric patients with hypoalbuminemia or acid-base disorders.

Hypocalcemia

As in adults, hypocalcemia may occur in pediatric patients due to a variety of causes including inadequate calcium intake, hypoparathyroidism, vitamin D deficiency, renal failure, redistribution of plasma calcium (e.g., hyperphosphatemia and citrated blood transfusions), and hypomagnesemia. Hypocalcemia may also occur due to lack of organ response to PTH (e.g., pseudohypoparathyroidism) and in the neonate due to other specific causes.

In the pediatric population, hypocalcemia most commonly occurs in neonates. "Early neonatal hypocalcemia" occurs during the first 72 hr of life and may be due to several factors. During fetal development, a transplacental active transport process maintains a higher calcium concentration in the fetus compared to the mother. After birth, this transplacental process suddenly stops. Serum calcium concentrations then decrease, even in healthy full-term newborns, reaching a nadir at 24 hr.[22] The high serum calcium concentrations in utero may also suppress the fetus' parathyroid gland. Thus, early neonatal hypocalcemia may also be due to a relative hypoparathyroidism in the newborn. In addition, newborns may have a decreased response to PTH.

Early neonatal hypocalcemia is more likely to occur in premature and low birth weight newborns. It also occurs more commonly in infants of diabetic mothers, infants with intrauterine growth retardation, and in newborns who have undergone prolonged difficult deliveries. Inadequate calcium intake in critically ill newborns also contributes to hypocalcemia.

"Late neonatal hypocalcemia," which usually presents during the first 5–10 days of life, is caused by a high phosphate intake. It is much less common than early neonatal hypocalcemia, especially since the phosphorus content of infant formulas was decreased. It may however, still occur if neonates are inappropriately given whole cow's milk. Cow's milk has a high phosphate load, which can cause hyperphosphatemia and secondary hypocalcemia in the neonate.

Hypocalcemia may also occur in neonates born to mothers with hypercalcemia. The maternal hypercalcemia is usually due to hyperparathyroidism. In utero suppression of the fetal parathyroid gland can lead to hypoparathyroidism and hypocalcemia in the neonate.

Hypocalcemia due to inadequate dietary calcium intake rarely occurs in the United States but can occur if infant formula or breast milk is replaced with liquids that contain lower amounts of calcium. Hypocalcemia may be iatrogenically induced if inadequate amounts of calcium are administered in hyperalimentation solutions. Adequate amounts of calcium and phosphorus may be difficult to deliver to preterm neonates due to their high daily requirements and limitations of calcium and phosphorus solubility in hyperalimentation solutions. Certain pediatric malabsorption disorders, such as celiac disease, may also cause inadequate absorption of calcium and vitamin D.

Hypoparathyroidism can be caused by many genetically inherited disorders, such as the DiGeorge syndrome, X-linked hypoparathyroidism, or PTH gene mutations.[22] These and other syndromes must be considered when pediatric patients present with hypoparathyroidism.

In pediatric patients with vitamin D deficiency, hypocalcemia occurs primarily due to decreased intestinal absorption of calcium. The lower amounts of calcium in the blood stimulate the release of PTH from the parathyroid gland. PTH then prevents significant hypocalcemia via several different mechanisms. It causes bone to release calcium, increases urinary calcium reabsorption, and increases the activity of 1-alpha-hydroxylase in the kidneys (the enzyme that converts 25-hydroxyvitamin D into 1, 25-dihydroxyvitamin D, the active form of vitamin D). Hypocalcemia only develops after these compensatory mechanisms fail. In fact, most children with vitamin D deficiency present with rickets before they develop hypocalcemia.[22] In addition to elevated PTH concentrations, children with vitamin D deficiency will have an elevated serum alkaline phosphatase concentration (due to increased osteoclast activity) and a low serum phosphorus (secondary to decreased intestinal absorption and decreased reabsorption in the kidneys), all due to the effects of PTH.

Vitamin D deficiency may be due to several factors including inadequate intake, lack of exposure to sunlight, malabsorption, or increased metabolism of vitamin D (e.g., from medications such as phenobarbital and phenytoin). Generally, patients may have more than one of these factors. For example, institutionalized children (who are not exposed to sunlight) receiving chronic anticonvulsant therapy may be at a greater risk for developing vitamin D deficiency and rickets. Vitamin D deficiency may also occur with liver disease (failure to form 25-hydroxyvitamin D in the liver) and with renal failure (failure to form the active moiety, 1,25-dihydroxyvitamin D, due to a loss of activity of 1-alpha-hydroxylase in the kidneys).

Genetic disorders, such as vitamin D-dependent rickets, may also cause hypocalcemia. The absence of the enzyme, 1-alpha-hydroxylase, in the kidneys occurs in children with vitamin D-dependent rickets type 1. Therefore, these children cannot convert 25-hydroxyvitamin D to its active form. Children with vitamin D-dependent rickets type 2 have a defective vitamin D receptor, which prevents the normal response to 1,25-dihydroxyvitamin D.[22]

Hypocalcemia also occurs when patients receive citrated blood transfusions or exchange transfusions (citrate is used to anticoagulate blood). Citrate forms a complex with calcium and decreases the ionized calcium concentration. This may result in symptoms of hypocalcemia. Pediatric patients at highest risk include those receiving multiple blood transfusions or exchange transfusions, such as neonates treated for hyperbilirubinemia and older children treated for sickle cell crisis. It should be noted that the total serum calcium concentration in these patients can be normal or even elevated, because the calcium-citrate complex is included in the measurement.[22]

Hypercalcemia

Hypercalcemia is an uncommon pediatric electrolyte disorder. As in adults, it may be caused by excess PTH, excess vitamin D, excess calcium intake, excess renal reabsorption of calcium, increased calcium released from the bone, and miscellaneous factors, such as hypophosphatemia or adrenal insufficiency.[22] Causes of hypercalcemia that are of particular interest in pediatric patients include neonatal hyperparathyroidism, hypervitaminosis D, excessive calcium intake, malignancy associated hypercalcemia, and immobilization. Also, several genetic syndromes and disorders may cause hypercalcemia.

Neonatal hyperparathyroidism, an autosomal recessive disorder, can be severe and life-threatening.[22] Typically, these patients have defective calcium sensing receptors in the parathyroid gland. Normally, high serum calcium concentrations would be sensed by the parathyroid gland, and PTH levels would then decrease. In these patients, however, the parathyroid gland cannot sense the high serum calcium concentrations, and PTH continues to be released. This further increases serum calcium concentrations. Transient secondary neonatal hyperparathyroidism occurs in neonates born to mothers with hypocalcemia. Maternal hypocalcemia leads to hypocalcemia in the fetus with secondary hyperparathyroidism. These neonates may be born with skeletal demineralization and bone fractures. Hypercalcemia in these patients usually takes days to weeks to resolve.

Excessive intake of vitamin D or calcium may also cause hypercalcemia. Typically, this may occur in children who are being treated with vitamin D and calcium with excessive doses. Excess calcium in hyperalimentation solutions commonly results in hypercalcemia.

Compared to adults, hypercalcemia from immobilization occurs more frequently in children, especially adolescents.[22] This is due to a higher rate of bone remodeling in these patients. Immobilization of children and adolescents may be required due to specific injuries such as leg fractures, spinal cord paralysis, burns, or other severe medical conditions. In children with leg fractures requiring traction, hypercalcemia usually occurs within 1–3 weeks. Immobilization may also result in isolated hypercalciuria, which may result in nephrocalcinosis, kidney stones, or renal insufficiency.

Phosphorus

Normal range[22] for newborns: 0–5 days old: 4.8–8.2 mg/dL or 1.55–2.65 mmol/L;
1–3 years: 3.8–6.5 mg/dL or 1.25–2.10 mmol/L;
4–11 years: 3.7–5.6 mg/dL or 1.20–1.80 mmol/L;
12–15 years: 2.9–5.4 mg/dL or 0.95–1.75 mmol/L;
16–19 years: 2.7–4.7 mg/dL or 0.90–1.50 mmol/L;
adults: 2.6–4.5 mg/dL or 0.84–1.45 mmol/L

Phosphorus is the primary intracellular anion and plays an integral role in cellular energy and intracellular metabolism. It is also a component of phospholipid membranes and other cell structures. The great majority of phosphorus in the body (85%) is found in the bone, while <1% of phosphorus is found in the plasma. Like calcium, phosphorus is essential for bone mineralization and skeletal growth. During infancy and childhood, a positive phosphorus balance is required for proper growth to allow adequate amounts of phosphorus to be incorporated into bone and new cells. The higher phosphorus requirement that is needed to facilitate growth may help explain the higher serum concentrations seen in the pediatric population compared to adults.

The kidney is the primary organ that regulates phosphorus balance. Approximately 90% of plasma phosphate is filtered by the glomerulus with the majority being actively reabsorbed at the proximal tubule. Some reabsorption also occurs more distally, but phosphate is not significantly secreted along the nephron.[22] Unlike other active transport systems, phosphate reabsorption, both proximal and distal, is greater in the neonatal kidney compared to adults.[24,28] Thus, the neonatal kidney tends to retain phosphate, perhaps as a physiologic adaptation to the high demands for phosphate that are required for growth. Neonatal renal phosphate reabsorption may be regulated by growth hormone.[28]

Hypophosphatemia

As in adults, hypophosphatemia may occur in pediatric patients due to several causes including increased renal excretion, decreased phosphate or vitamin D intake, or intracellular shifting. Causes of excessive renal phosphorus excretion in pediatric patients include hyperparathyroidism, metabolic acidosis, diuretics, glucocorticoids, and inherited disorders such as hypophosphatemic rickets.

Inadequate dietary phosphate intake is an unusual cause of hypophosphatemia in adults. However, infants are more predisposed to nutritional hypophosphatemia due to their higher phosphorus requirements.[22] The phosphorus requirements of premature infants are even higher due to their rapid skeletal growth. If premature infants are fed regular infant formula (instead of premature infant formula that contains additional calcium and phosphorus) phosphorus deficiency and rickets may occur. Inadequate vitamin D intake and genetic causes of vitamin D deficiency (e.g., vitamin D-dependent rickets type 1) can also result in hypophosphatemia in pediatric patients.

Hypophosphatemia due to intracellular shifting of phosphorus occurs with processes that stimulate intracellular phosphorus utilization. For example, high serum levels of glucose will stimulate insulin. Insulin then enables glucose and phosphorus to move into the cell, where phosphorus is used during glycolysis. Intracellular shifting of phosphorus also occurs during anabolism, for example, in patients receiving hyperalimentation and during refeeding in those with protein-calorie malnutrition (e.g., severe anorexia nervosa). The high anabolic (growth) rate in infants (especially premature infants) and children make them more susceptible to hypophosphatemia when adequate amounts of phosphate are not supplied in the hyperalimentation solution. Hypophosphatemia, due to refeeding malnourished children, usually occurs within 5 days of refeeding. It may be prevented by a more gradual increase in nutrition and with phosphate supplementation.[22]

Hyperphosphatemia

Hyperphosphatemia in pediatric patients may be caused by decreased excretion of phosphorus, increased intake of phosphate or vitamin D, or a shift of intracellular phosphate to extracellular fluid. The most common cause of hyperphosphatemia in the pediatric population is decreased excretion of phosphorus due to renal failure. Excessive phosphorus intake in pediatric patients (especially in those with renal dysfunction or in neonates whose renal function is normally decreased due to immaturity) is a common cause of hyperphosphatemia.[22] Hyperphosphatemia may also occur if neonates are inappropriately given whole cow's milk. As previously mentioned, cow's milk contains a high phosphate load, which can cause hyperphosphatemia and secondary hypocalcemia in the neonate. Administration of sodium phosphorus laxatives or enemas to infants and children may also result in excessive phosphate intake. In addition, the pediatric dosing of phosphate supplements may be confusing to some due to the multiple salts available and multiple units of measure. This may result in unintentional overdoses with resultant hyperphosphatemia.

Magnesium

Normal range[22] for newborns: 0–6 days old: 1.2–2.6 mg/dL or 0.48–1.05 mmol/L;
7 days–2 years: 1.6–2.6 mg/dL or 0.65–1.05 mmol/L;
2–14 years: 1.5–2.3 mg/dL or 0.60–0.95 mmol/L

Magnesium plays an important role in neuromuscular function and is a required cofactor for many enzymatic systems in the body. Approximately 50% of magnesium is located in bone with one-third being slowly exchangeable with extracellular fluid. About 45% of magnesium is found in the intracellular fluid with only 5% in extracellular fluid. The kidney is the primary organ responsible for magnesium excretion. Approximately 95–97% of filtered magnesium is reabsorbed; 15% in the proximal tubule, 70% in the thick ascending limb of Henle, and 5–10% in the distal tubule.[22] In the neonate, reabsorption of magnesium may be increased in the proximal tubule. Thus, the immature neonatal kidney tends to retain magnesium compared to adults.[24] This results in slightly higher normal values for serum magnesium in neonates and infants compared to older children and adults. In fact, serum magnesium concentrations in the newborn have been shown to be inversely related to gestational age at birth and postconceptional age. In other words, more immature neonates will have slightly higher serum magnesium concentrations.[29,30]

Hypomagnesemia

Hypomagnesemia occurs in pediatric patients due to excessive renal or gastrointestinal losses, decreased gastrointestinal absorption, decreased intake, and specific neonatal causes.[22] Hypomagnesemia may occur in neonates due to several maternal causes. Maternal diuretic use, laxative overuse or abuse, diabetes, or decreased intake due to vomiting during pregnancy may cause maternal hypomagnesemia and lead to hypomagnesemia in the newborn.[31] Hypomagnesemia also commonly occurs in neonates with intrauterine growth retardation (due to deficient placental transfer of magnesium) and in neonates who receive exchange transfusions with citrated blood.

Excessive renal losses of magnesium may be due to a variety of reasons. Of particular pediatric concern is the use of medications (e.g., diuretics, amphotericin, and cisplatin) that may cause magnesium wasting. Hypomagnesemia may also occur due to rare hereditary renal magnesium-losing syndromes, such as Bartter's syndrome and autosomal recessive renal magnesium wasting syndrome.

Excessive gastrointestinal losses of magnesium may occur in pediatric patients with diarrhea or large losses of gastric contents (e.g., emesis or nasogastric suction). Decreased gastrointestinal absorption of magnesium may occur in patients with short gut syndrome. These patients have had a portion of their small bowel removed, which results in poor intestinal absorption. Other important pediatric gastrointestinal diseases that may result in hypomagnesemia include cystic fibrosis, inflammatory bowel disease, and celiac disease.[22]

Poor magnesium intake may also result in hypomagnesemia. Although this rarely occurs in children fed orally, it may occur in hospitalized children receiving inadequate amounts of magnesium in intravenous fluids or hyperalimentation. Hypomagnesemia can also occur during the refeeding of children with protein-calorie malnutrition (e.g., severe anorexia nervosa). These patients have low magnesium reserves but a high requirement of magnesium during cellular growth during refeeding.[22]

Hypermagnesemia

As in adults, the most common cause of hypermagnesemia in pediatric patients is renal dysfunction. However, in neonates, the most common cause is the intravenous infusion of magnesium sulfate in the mother for the treatment of preeclampsia or eclampsia.[22,31] The high levels of magnesium in the mother are delivered transplacentally to the fetus. Neonates and young infants are also more prone to hypermagnesemia, due to their immature renal function. Thus, these patients cannot easily tolerate a magnesium load. Other common pediatric causes of hypermagnesemia include excessive intake due to magnesium containing antacids, laxatives, or enemas.

AGE-RELATED DIFFERENCES IN KIDNEY FUNCTION TESTS

Serum Creatinine

Normal range[11] for newborns: 0.3–1.0 mg/dL or 27–88 μmol/L; infants: 0.2–0.4 mg/dL or 18–35 μmol/L; children: 0.3–0.7 mg/dL or 27–62 μmol/L; adolescents: 0.5–1.0 mg/dL or 44–88 μmol/L; adult males: 0.6–1.2 mg/dL or 53–106 μmol/L; adult females: 0.5–1.1 mg/dL or 44–97 μmol/L

Serum creatinine is a useful indicator of renal function and can be used to estimate glomerular filtration rate (GFR). Creatinine is generated from the metabolism of creatine and creatine phosphate, a high-energy biochemical important in muscle activity. Creatinine is produced in muscles, released into the extracellular fluid, and excreted by the kidneys. Excretion of creatinine is primarily via glomerular filtration, but a smaller amount undergoes tubular secretion. The amount of creatinine that is secreted by the tubules increases in patients as GFR decreases. Thus, creatinine clearance will overestimate the actual GFR in patients with renal insufficiency.[32]

In pediatric patients, three major factors influence the serum creatinine concentration: the patient's muscle mass per unit of body size, their GFR, and (in newborns) the exogenous (maternal) creatinine load.[33] At birth, the newborn's serum creatinine reflects the maternal serum creatinine. Since serum creatinine crosses the placenta, if a pregnant woman has an elevated serum creatinine, then the concentration of creatinine in the fetus will also be elevated. In fact, the plasma creatinine concentration of umbilical cord blood is almost equal to the creatinine concentration in the mother.[26] In full-term newborns, serum creatinine may increase slightly, shortly after birth, due to the contraction of the ECW compartment.[33] Serum creatinine then decreases over the first few days of life and usually reaches 0.4 mg/dL by about 10 days of age.[24,33] The apparent half-life of this postnatal decrease in serum creatinine is about 2.1 days in normal full-term infants and is due to the ongoing maturation of the kidneys and progressive increase in GFR. Serum creatinine is higher at birth in premature newborns compared to full-term newborns, and the postnatal decrease in serum creatinine may occur more slowly. This is due to the preterm newborn's more immature kidneys and lower GFR.[26]

Compared to adults, pediatric patients have a lower muscle mass per unit of body size. Since the production of creatinine is dependent on muscle mass, this results in significantly lower normal values for serum creatinine for neonates, infants, and children. The percentage of muscle mass differs with various pediatric age groups and increases with age from birth through young adulthood.[33] This increase in muscle mass accounts for the increase in the normal values for serum creatinine with increasing age (see normal values for serum creatinine above).

Creatinine excretion is dependent on GFR and, as in adults, serum creatinine will become elevated in pediatric patients with renal dysfunction. For example, an infant with a serum creatinine of 0.8 mg/dL (twice the normal value for age) will have approximately a 50% decrease in GFR. Using the age-appropriate normal values to interpret serum creatinine is essential. In the above example, a serum creatinine of 0.8 mg/dL (which would be considered normal in an adult) denotes significant renal dysfunction in younger patients. Correct interpretation of serum creatinine values is extremely important because the doses of fluids, many electrolytes, and medications that are renally eliminated will need to be adjusted. Misinterpretation of serum creatinine (e.g., not recognizing renal dysfunction) can result in serious and potentially fatal fluid and electrolyte imbalances and overdosing of medications.

It is also important to note that certain medications and endogenous substances (e.g., bilirubin, lipemia, and hemolysis) may interfere with the determination of serum creatinine.[5,10] This interference may especially be a problem in the neonatal population, since neonates often have hyperbilirubinemia or lipemia, and blood sampling in neonates often results in hemolysis.

Age-Related Physiologic Development of Renal Function

Compared to adults, a newborn's kidneys are anatomically and functionally immature. The primary functions of the kidney (glomerular filtration, tubular secretion, and tubular reabsorption) are all decreased in the full-term newborn. These renal functions are even further decreased in the premature infant. After birth, glomerular and tubular renal function increase (i.e., mature) with postnatal age. During the first 2 years of life, kidney function matures to adult levels and in the following order: (1) glomerular filtration, (2) tubular secretion, and (3) tubular reabsorption. The interpretation of pediatric kidney functions tests can be better understood if one knows how each kidney function matures during the first 2 years.

Glomerular filtration. In the fetus, nephrogenesis (i.e., the formation of new nephrons) begins at 8 weeks gestation and continues until about 36 weeks of gestation.[35] Although the number of adult nephrons (~1 million) is reached at this time, the nephrons are smaller and not as functionally mature as the nephrons found in an adult kidney.[23] After 36 weeks of gestation, no new nephrons are formed. However, renal mass continues to increase due to the increase in renal tubular growth. GFR is very low in the young fetus but gradually increases during gestation (Figure 3-4). Before 36 weeks of gestation, the increase in GFR is primarily due to nephrogenesis and the increase in the number of new glomeruli. From 36 weeks of gestation until birth, a much smaller increase in GFR occurs as renal mass and kidney function increase.[36]

At birth, GFR increases dramatically compared to what it was in utero (Figure 3-4). This dramatic increase in GFR, which occurs at birth and continues during the early postnatal period, is due to several important hemodynamic and physiologic changes. Cardiac output and systemic blood pressure increase at birth and a significant decrease in renal vascular resistance occurs. These changes result in an increase in renal blood flow

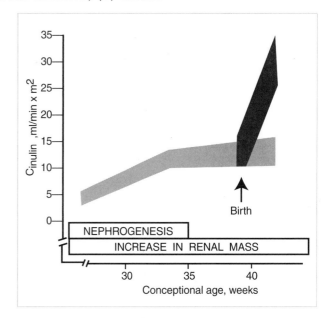

Figure 3-4. Maturation of GFR in relation to conceptional age. (Reproduced, with permission, from Guignard JP. The neonatal stressed kidney. In: Gruskin AB, Norman ME, eds. *Pediatric Nephrology: Proceedings of the Fifth International Pediatric Nephrology Symposium*. Presented at: The Fifth International Pediatric Nephrology Symposium; October 6–10, 1980; Philadelphia, PA; The Hague: Martinus Nijhoff Publishers;1981: 507.)

and effective glomerular filtration pressure. In addition, alterations in the pattern of renal blood flow distribution occur and the permeability of the glomerular membrane and surface area available for filtration increase.[23,35,36] All of these changes help to increase GFR.

Despite the increase in GFR that occurs during this time, GFR is still very much decreased in comparison to adults. As determined by creatinine or inulin clearance, the GFR in a full-term newborn is only 10–15 mL/min/m² (2–4 mL/min). GFR then doubles by 1–2 weeks of age to 20–30 mL/min/m² (8–20 mL/min).[35] Adult values of GFR are approached by about 6–12 months of age (70–90 mL/min/m²).[32,35] Compared to full-term newborns, the GFR in premature newborns is much lower at birth (5–10 mL/min/m² or 0.7–2 mL/min) and increases at a less dramatic rate during the first 1–2 weeks after birth (10–12 mL/min/m² or 2–4 mL/min).[35] After the first postnatal week, the rate of increase in GFR is comparable in preterm and full-term infants, but the actual GFR value is still lower in preterm infants.

Renal tubular function. Tubular secretion and reabsorption are both decreased in the full-term newborn. This is due to the small size and mass of the renal tubules, decreased peritubular blood flow, and immature biochemical processes that supply energy for active transport. In addition, full-term newborns have a limited ability to concentrate urine and have lower urinary pH values.[35] In the preterm newborn, renal tubular functions are further decreased. Limitations of the newborn's tubular function with respect to the renal handling of serum electrolytes are listed above within the discussion section of each serum electrolyte.

Tubular secretion transports certain electrolytes and medications from the peritubular capillaries into the lumen of the renal tubule. At birth, tubular secretion is only 20–30% of adult values and slowly matures by about 8 months of age. Tubular reabsorption, which is also decreased at birth, may not fully mature until 1–2 years of age. Thus, during infancy, a glomerulotubular imbalance occurs, with GFR maturing at a faster rate than renal tubular function.

The decreased renal function in newborns and the maturational changes in GFR and tubular function that occur throughout early infancy have important implications for the interpretation of laboratory data. For example, one must remember that even with a normal serum creatinine for age, neonates and infants still have decreased renal function compared to adults. This decreased renal function must be taken into account, especially in the very young, when dosing electrolytes or medications that are eliminated by the kidneys. In addition, as in adults, certain medications, diseases, and medical conditions (such as hypoxic events that may occur in newborns) may cause further decreases in renal function.

Standardization of Creatinine Clearance (CrCl)

Creatinine clearance can be expressed using several different units of measure, including mL/min, mL/min/m², or mL/min/1.73 m². To better compare the creatinine clearance of patients of different body sizes, creatinine clearance is most commonly standardized to the body surface area of an average sized adult (1.73 m²). Thus, creatinine clearance is most commonly measured as mL/min/1.73 m². Using these units is especially helpful in pediatric patients where a large range of body sizes occur. For example, the average body surface area ranges from 0.25 m² in a full-term newborn to 1.34 m² in a 12 year old.[1] Expressing creatinine clearance in mL/min or even mL/min/m² over this wide of a range of body surface areas would give an extremely wide range of values.

Estimating Body Surface Area in Pediatric Patients

Body surface area can be estimated using several different methods. In pediatrics, body surface area is most commonly estimated using standard nomograms or equations and the patient's measured height and weight.[1] Two equations are commonly used in pediatrics, an older equation (the DuBois formula)[37]

$$BSA \ (m^2) = Wt \ (kg)^{0.425} \times Ht \ (cm)^{0.725} \times 0.007184 \tag{1}$$

and a more simplified equation.[38]

$$BSA \ (m^2) = \text{the square root of } ([\ Ht \ (cm) \times Wt \ (kg)]/3600) \tag{2}$$

Estimation of the patient's body surface area is required in order to calculate creatinine clearance from a urinary collection.

Determination of CrCl from a Urinary Creatinine Collection

The same equation that is used in adults can be used in pediatric patients to calculate creatinine clearance from a timed urine collection. The following equation is used:

$$CrCl = UV/P \times 1.73/BSA \tag{3}$$

where CrCl is in units of mL/min/1.73m²; U is the urinary creatinine concentration in mg/dL; V (mL/min) is the total urine volume collected in milliliters divided by the duration of the collection in minutes; P is the serum creatinine concentration in mg/dL; and BSA is the patient's body surface area in m².

Ideally, urine should be collected over a 24-hr period. However, a full 24-hr collection period is very difficult in pediatric patients, especially in those who do not have full control over their bladder and do not have a urinary catheter in place. Thus, shorter collection periods (e.g., 8 or 12 hr) are sometimes used. Urinary specimen bags can be placed to collect urine in neonates and infants, but incomplete collection due to leakage of urine often occurs. The incomplete collection of urine will result in an inaccurate calculation of creatinine clearance.

With any urine collection for creatinine determination, it is important to have the patient empty their bladder and discard this specimen before beginning the urine collection. All urine during the time period should be collected, including the urine that would be voided at the end of the collection period. A serum creatinine is usually obtained once during the urinary collection period (ideally at the midpoint) if the patient has stable renal function. If the patient's renal function is changing, then two serum creatinine samples (one at the beginning of the urine collection and one at the end of the urine collection) may be obtained. The average serum creatinine can then be used in the above equation.[2]

Due to the inherent problems of collecting a 24-hr urine sample from pediatric patients and receiving inaccurate calculations, creatinine clearance (or GFR) is often estimated using prediction equations that consider the patient's age, height, gender, and serum creatinine (see below). In fact, using a 24-hr timed urine specimen to calculate creatinine clearance has been shown to be no more reliable (and often less reliable) than using equations based on serum creatinine.[39] Therefore, the National Kidney Foundation recommends that GFR should be estimated in children and adolescents using prediction equations, such as the one by Schwartz.[33] A timed urine collection (e.g., 24-hr sample) may be useful for (1) estimations of GFR in patients with decreased muscle mass (e.g., muscle wasting, malnutrition, or amputation) or in those receiving special diets (e.g., vegetarian diets or creatine supplements), (2) assessments of nutritional status or diets, and (3) evaluations for the need to start dialysis.[39]

Estimating CrCl from Serum Creatinine

Several methods are used in adults to estimate creatinine clearance from a serum creatinine. These equations cannot be used in pediatrics because pediatric patients have a different ratio of muscle mass to serum creatinine. In addition, the amount of pediatric muscle mass per body weight changes over time. Adult equations are based on adult muscle mass and adult urinary creatinine excretion rates. Thus, the use of adult equations in pediatric patients will result in erroneous calculations.

Several predictive equations have been developed to estimate creatinine clearance in pediatric patients. One simple equation was developed for use in children 1–18 years of age with stable serum creatinine[40]:

$$CrCl \ (mL/min/1.73 \ m^2) = 0.48 \times Height \ (cm)/Scr \ (mg/dL) \tag{4}$$

This equation was found to be clinically useful in predicting CrCl in children. However, it may be less accurate in children with a height <107 cm.[41]

Another equation, developed by Schwartz, is more commonly used to estimate GFR in pediatric patients,[33]

$$GFR \ (mL/min/1.73 \ m^2) = k \times Length(cm)/Scr \ (mg/dL) \tag{5}$$

where k is a constant of proportionality. In patients with stable renal function, k is directly related to the muscle component of body weight, which correlates well with the daily rates of urinary creatinine excretion. Since the percentage of muscle mass per body weight varies for different age groups, a different value for k must be used for different age groups. In addition to age, the value of k will be affected by body composition, thus, the values for k listed in Table 3-3 should be used in pediatric patients with average build.

The above equations may not be accurate in certain pediatric populations, including those patients with unstable renal function, abnormal body habitus (e.g., obesity or malnutrition), decreased muscle mass (e.g., cardiac patients), severe chronic renal failure, or insulin dependent diabetes.[33,42] If clinically indicated, creatinine clearance should be determined by a timed urine collection in these patients.

TABLE 3-3

AGE GROUP	MEAN k VALUE
Low birth weight infants ≤1 year	0.33
Full-term infants ≤1 year	0.45
Children 2–12 years	0.55
Females 13–21 years	0.55
Males 13–21 years	0.70

[a]Modified from Reference 33.

Table 3-3. Mean Values of k by Age Group[a]

AGE-RELATED DIFFERENCES IN LIVER FUNCTION TESTS

Serum Albumin

Normal range[8] for newborns: 0–5 days old, body weight <2.5 kg: 2.0–3.6 g/dL or 20–36 g/L;
0–5 days old, body weight >2.5 kg: 2.6–3.6 g/dL or 26–36 g/L;
1–3 years: 3.4–4.2 g/dL or 34–42 g/L;
4–6 years: 3.5–5.2 g/dL or 35–52 g/L;
7–19 years: 3.7–5.6 g/dL or 37–56 g/L

Serum proteins, including albumin, are synthesized by the liver. Thus, measurements of serum total protein, albumin, and other specific proteins are primarily a test of the liver's synthetic capability. Maturational differences in the liver's ability to synthesize protein help determine the normal range for serum albumin concentrations. The liver of the fetus is able to synthesize albumin beginning at approximately 7–8 weeks gestation. However, the predominant serum protein in early fetal life is alpha-fetoprotein. As gestation continues, the concentration of albumin increases, while alpha-fetoprotein decreases. At approximately 3–4 months of gestation, the fetal liver is able to produce each of the major serum protein classes. However, serum concentrations are much lower than those found at maturity.[43]

At birth, the newborn liver is anatomically and functionally immature. Due to immature liver function and a decreased ability to synthesize protein, full-term neonates have decreased concentrations of total plasma proteins, including albumin, gamma globulin, and lipoproteins. Concentrations in premature newborns are even lower, with serum albumin levels as low as 1.8 g/dL.[11] Adult serum concentrations of serum albumin (~3.5 g/dL) are reached only after several months of age. Conditions that cause abnormalities in serum albumin in pediatric patients are the same as in adults and can be reviewed in Chapter 12.

Liver Enzymes

Alanine aminotransferase (ALT, also called SGPT)—normal range[2] for infants: <54 U/L; children and adults: 1–30 U/L

Aspartate aminotransferase (AST, also called SGOT)—normal range for newborns and infants: 20–65 U/L; children and adults: 0–35 U/L

Alkaline phosphatase—normal range for infants: 150–420 U/L; children 2–10 years: 100–320 U/L; males 11–18 years: 100–390 U/L; females 11–18 years: 100–320 U/L; adults: 30–120 U/L

Lactate dehydrogenase—normal range for neonates: 160–1500 U/L; infants: 150–360 U/L; children: 150–300 U/L; adults: 0–220 U/L

The normal reference ranges for liver enzymes are higher in pediatric patients compared to adults. This may be due to the fact that the liver makes up a larger percentage of total body weight in infants and children compared to adults. For certain enzymes, such as alkaline phosphatase, the higher normal concentrations in childhood represent higher serum concentrations of an isoenzyme from another source (i.e., other than liver). Approximately 80% of alkaline phosphatase originates from liver and bone. Smaller amounts come from the intestines, kidneys, and placenta. Normally, growing children have a higher osteoblastic activity during bone growth and an influx into serum of the alkaline phosphatase isoenzyme from bone.[10] Thus, the higher normal concentrations of alkaline phosphatase in childhood primarily represent a higher rate of bone growth. After puberty, the liver is the primary source of serum alkaline phosphatase.

One must keep these age-related differences in mind when interpreting liver enzyme test results. For example, an isolated increase in alkaline phosphatase in a rapidly growing adolescent—whose other liver function tests are normal—would not indicate hepatic or biliary disease but merely a rapid increase in bone growth.

As in adults, increases in AST and ALT in pediatric patients are associated with hepato-cellular injury, while elevations of alkaline phosphatase are associated with cholestatic disease (see Chapter 12). Cholestasis and bone disorders (such as osteomalacia and rickets) are common causes of elevated serum alkaline phosphatase concentrations in pediatric patients.

Bilirubin

Total bilirubin, premature neonates—normal range[2] for 0–1 day old: <8 mg/dL or <137 μmol/L; 1–2 days old: <12 mg/dL or <205 μmol/L; 3–5 days old: <16 mg/dL or <274 μmol/L; >5 days old: <2 mg/dL or <34 μmol/L

Total bilirubin, full-term neonates—normal range for 0–1 day old: <6 mg/dL or <103 μmol/L; 1–2 days old: <8 mg/dL or <137 μmol/L; 3–5 days old: <12 mg/dL or <205 μmol/L; >5 days old: <1 mg/dL or <17 μmol/L; adults: 0.1–1.2 mg/dL or 1.7–20.5 μmol/L

Conjugated bilirubin—normal range: 0–0.4 mg/dL or 0–8 μmol/L

To better understand the age-related differences in serum bilirubin concentrations, a brief review of bilirubin metabolism is needed. Bilirubin is a breakdown product of hemoglobin. Hemoglobin, which is released from senescent or hemolyzed red blood cells, is degraded by heme oxygenase into iron, carbon monoxide, and biliverdin. Biliverdin undergoes reduction by biliverdin reductase to bilirubin. Unconjugated bilirubin then enters the liver and is conjugated with glucuronic acid to form conjugated bilirubin, which is water soluble. Conjugated bilirubin is excreted in the bile and enters the intestines, where is it broken down by bacterial flora to urobilinogen. However, conjugated bilirubin can also be deconjugated by bacteria in the intestines and reabsorbed back into the circulation.[44]

Compared to adults, newborns have higher concentrations of bilirubin. This results from a higher production of bilirubin in the neonate and a decreased ability to excrete it. A higher rate of production of bilirubin occurs in newborns due to the shorter life span of neonatal red blood cells and the higher initial neonatal hematocrit. The average RBC life span is only 65 days in very premature neonates and 90 days in full-term neonates, compared to 120 days in adults.[45] In addition, full-term neonates have a mean hematocrit of about 50%, compared to adult values of approximately 33%. The shorter RBC life span plus the higher hematocrit both increase the load of unconjugated bilirubin to the liver. Newborn infants, however, have a decreased ability to eliminate bilirubin. The activity of neonatal uridine diphosphate glucuronosyltransferase, the enzyme responsible for conjugating bilirubin the in liver, is decreased. In addition, newborns lack the intestinal bacteria needed to breakdown conjugated bilirubin into urobilinogen. However, the newborn's intestine does contain glucuronidase, which can deconjugate bilirubin and allow unconjugated bilirubin to be reabsorbed back into the circulation (enterohepatic circulation). This enterohepatically reabsorbed bilirubin further increases the unconjugated bilirubin load to the liver.

Due to these limitations in bilirubin metabolism, a "physiologic jaundice" commonly occurs in newborns. Typically in full-term neonates, high serum bilirubin concentrations occur in the first few days of life, with a decrease over the next several weeks to values seen in adults. High bilirubin concentrations may occur later in premature newborns, up to the first week of life, and are usually higher and persist longer than in full-term newborns.

Pathologic jaundice may occur in newborns due to many reasons, including increased production of bilirubin, decreased uptake of unconjugated bilirubin into the liver, decreased conjugation of bilirubin in the liver, and increased enterohepatic circulation of bilirubin.[44] Increased production of bilirubin may occur with RBC hemolysis due to blood group incompatibilities, enzyme deficiencies of the erythrocytes, erythrocyte structural defects (e.g., spherocytosis), or in infants of certain racial or ethnic groups (e.g., Asian, Native American, and Greek islander). Certain genetic disorders may cause neonatal hyperbilirubinemia. For example, patients with Gilbert's syndrome have decreased hepatic uptake of bilirubin and infants with Crigler-Najjar syndrome have a deficiency of uridine diphosphate glucuronosyltransferase, the enzyme that is responsible for conjugation of bilirubin in the liver. Breast-feeding is also associated with neonatal hyperbilirubinemia and jaundice. Newborns who are exclusively breast-fed, not feeding well, or not being enterally fed (i.e., newborns who are not taking anything by mouth) may have increased intestinal reabsorption of bilirubin that can cause or worsen hyperbilirubinemia. Breast-feeding may also increase bilirubin concentrations by other mechanisms. Breast milk may contain substances that decrease the conjugation of bilirubin by inhibiting the enzyme, uridine diphosphate glucuronosyltransferase.

Appropriate monitoring of serum bilirubin is very important in neonates, as high concentrations of unconjugated bilirubin can cause bilirubin encephalopathy or kernicterus (i.e., deposits of bilirubin in the brain). The neurotoxic effects of bilirubin are serious and potentially lethal. Clinical features of acute kernicterus include poor sucking, stupor, seizures, fever, hypotonia, hypertonia, opisthotonus, and retrocollis. Neonates who survive may develop mental retardation, delayed motor skills, movement disorders, and sensorineural hearing loss. Phototherapy and exchange transfusion are common treatments for neonatal hyperbilirubinemia.[44]

AGE-RELATED DIFFERENCES IN HEMATOLOGIC TESTS

Erythrocytes

Mean values and lower limit of normal (minus 2 standard deviations)[12]:

Red Blood Cell Count

Birth (cord blood): 4.7 (3.9) x 10^{12} cells/L; newborns 1–3 days old: 5.3 (4.0) x 10^{12} cells/L;
1 week: 5.1 (3.9) x 10^{12} cells/L; 2 weeks: 4.9 (3.6) x 10^{12} cells/L;
1 month: 4.2 (3.0) x 10^{12} cells/L; 2 months: 3.8 (2.7) x 10^{12} cells/L;
3–6 months: 3.8 (3.1) x 10^{12} cells/L; 0.5–2 years: 4.5 (3.7) x 10^{12} cells/L;
2–6 years: 4.6 (3.9) x 10^{12} cells/L; 6–12 years: 4.6 (4.0) x 10^{12} cells/L;
12–18 years, female: 4.6 (4.1) x 10^{12} cells/L; 12–18 years, male: 4.9 (4.5) x 10^{12} cells/L;
18–49 years, female: 4.6 (4.0) x 10^{12} cells/L; 18–49 years, male: 5.2 (4.5) x 10^{12} cells/L

Hemoglobin

Birth (cord blood): 16.5 (13.5) g/dL; newborns 1–3 days old: 18.5 (14.5) g/dL;
1 week: 17.5 (13.5) g/dL; 2 weeks: 16.5 (12.5) g/dL;
1 month: 14.0 (10.0) g/dL; 2 months: 11.5 (9.0) g/dL;
3–6 months: 11.5 (9.5) g/dL; 0.5–2 years: 12.0 (10.5) g/dL; 2–6 years: 12.5 (11.5) g/dL;
6–12 years: 13.5 (11.5) g/dL; 12–18 years, female: 14.0 (12.0) g/dL;
12–18 years, male: 14.5 (13.0) g/dL; 18–49 years, female: 14.0 (12.0) g/dL;
18–49 years, male: 15.5 (13.5) g/dL

Hematocrit

Birth (cord blood): 51 (42)%; 1–3 days old: 56 (45)%;
1 week: 54 (42)%; 2 weeks: 51 (39)%; 1 month: 43 (31)%; 2 months: 35 (28)%;
3–6 months: 35 (29)%; 0.5–2 years: 36 (33)%; 2–6 years: 37 (34)%;
6–12 years: 40 (35)%; 12–18 years, female: 41 (36)%; 12–18 years, male: 43 (37)%;
18–49 years, female: 41 (36)%; 18–49 years, male: 47 (41)%

Compared to adults, normal newborn infants have higher hemoglobin and hematocrit values. For example, the mean hemoglobin value in a full-term newborn on the first day of life is 18.5 g/dL, compared to 15.5 g/dL in adult males. Hemoglobin and hematocrit start to decrease within the first week of life and reach a minimum level at 8–12 weeks in term infants and by 6 weeks of age in premature infants.[46] This normal decrease in hemoglobin and hematocrit is called the *physiologic anemia of infancy*. This physiologic anemia is normochromic and microcytic and is accompanied by a low reticulocyte count. Physiologic anemia of infancy does not require medical treatment.

The age-related changes in hemoglobin that occur during the first few months of life are due to several reasons. In utero, a low arterial pO_2 exists, which stimulates the production of erythropoietin in the fetus. This results in a high rate of erythropoiesis and accounts for high levels of hemoglobin and hematocrit that exists at birth. At birth, pO_2 and oxygen content of blood significantly increase with the newborn's first breaths. The higher amount of oxygen that is available to the tissues will down-regulate erythropoietin production and decrease the rate of erythropoiesis.[47] Without the stimulation of erythropoietin to produce new red blood cells, hemoglobin concentrations decrease as aged red blood cells are removed from the circulation. The shorter life span of neonatal red blood cells (90 days vs. 120 days in adults) also contributes to the decline in hemoglobin.

Hemoglobin continues to decline in full-term infants until 8–12 weeks of age when values reach 9–11 g/dL. These levels of hemoglobin result in lower amounts of oxygen deliv-

TABLE 3-4

	MCV f/L	MCH pg/cell	MCHC g/dL
Birth (cord blood):	108 (98)	34 (31)	33 (30)
1–3 days old:	108 (95)	34 (31)	33 (29)
1 week old:	107 (88)	34 (28)	33 (28)
2 week old:	105 (86)	34 (28)	33 (28)
1 month old:	104 (85)	34 (28)	33 (29)
2 month old:	96 (77)	30 (26)	33 (29)
3–6 months:	91 (74)	30 (25)	33 (30)
0.5–2 years:	78 (70)	27 (23)	33 (30)
2–6 years:	81 (75)	27 (24)	34 (31)
6–12 years:	86 (77)	29 (25)	34 (31)
12–18 years: Female:	90 (78)	30 (25)	34 (31)
Male:	88 (78)	30 (25)	34 (31)
18–49 years:	90 (80)	30 (26)	34 (31)

ª Adapted from Reference 12.

Table 3-4. Red Blood Cell Indices by Age: Mean values and lower limits of normal (minus 2 standard deviations)ª

ery to the tissues. Usually at this point, oxygen requirements exceed oxygen delivery and the relative hypoxia stimulates the production of erythropoietin. Erythropoiesis then increases and the reticulocyte count and hemoglobin concentrations begin to rise.

It is important to remember that the iron from the aged red blood cells that were previously removed from the circulation has been stored. The amount of this stored iron is usually adequate to meet the requirements of hemoglobin synthesis.

In premature infants, the physiologic anemia occurs sooner than in full-term infants and the nadir of the hemoglobin concentrations is lower (e.g., 7–9 g/dL).[47] This can be explained by the even shorter life span of the premature infant's red blood cells (65 days vs. 90 days in full-term newborns) and by the inadequate synthesis of erythropoietin in response to anemia. Thus, anemia of prematurity may require treatment with recombinant human erythropoietin and iron.

Differences in red blood cell indices also exist for different pediatric ages. For example, compared to adults, newborns have larger erythrocytes (mean MCV of 108 fL, compared to an adult value of 90 fL). Mean values and the lower limits of normal for red blood cell indices according to different ages are listed in Table 3-4.

Causes of the various types of anemias in pediatric patients are similar to the causes in adults. Of particular pediatric note is the iron deficiency anemia that occurs in infants who are fed whole cow's milk. The iron in whole cow's milk is less bioavailable and may cause inadequate iron intake. However, some infants receiving whole cow's milk develop severe iron deficiency due to chronic intestinal blood loss. The blood loss is thought to be due to intestinal exposure to a specific heat-labile protein. Decreasing the amount of whole cow's milk to ≤1 pint per day, heating the milk, or feeding evaporated milk or a milk substitute will decrease the loss of blood.[47]

In pediatric patients with anemia, genetic disorders that produce inadequate RBC production (e.g., Diamond-Blackfan anemia), hemolytic anemias (e.g., hereditary spherocytosis), or hemoglobin disorders (e.g., sickle cell disease) must also be considered.

Leukocytes

White Blood Cell Count

Normal range[48] for newborns at birth: 9.0–30.0 x 10³ cells/mm³;
2 weeks: 5.0–21.0 x 10³ cells/mm³;
3 months: 6.0–18.0 x 10³ cells/mm³; 0.5–6 years: 6.0–15.0 x 10³ cells/mm³; 7–12 years:
4.5–13.5 x 10³ cells/mm³; adults: 5.0–10.0 x 10³ cells/mm³

Normal white blood cell counts are higher in neonates and infants compared to adults. Typically in adults, an elevated WBC may indicate infection. However, in neonates and infants with a systemic bacterial infection, the WBC count may be increased, decreased, or

TABLE 3-5

| | MEAN VALUES | | | |
	NEUTROPHILS	LYMPHOCYTES	EOSINOPHILS	MONOCYTES
Birth:	61%	31%	2%	6%
2 weeks:	40%	63%	3%	9%
3 months:	30%	48%	2%	5%
0.5–6 years:	45%	48%	2%	5%
7–12 years:	55%	38%	2%	5%
Adult:	55%	35%	3%	7%
[a] Adapted from Reference 48.				

Table 3-5. White Blood Cell Differential by Age[a]

within the normal range. Neonates have a lower storage pool of neutrophils and an overwhelming infection may deplete this pool and cause neutropenia.[46] Therefore, while an increase in WBCs is a nonspecific finding in neonates (i.e., it may occur in many conditions other than sepsis), neutropenia is a highly significant finding and may be the first abnormal laboratory result that indicates neonatal bacterial infection.

In addition to the age-related differences in total WBC count, the age-related differences in WBC differential also need to be taken into consideration when interpreting laboratory results (Table 3-5).

Platelet Count
Normal range[11] for newborns: 84,000–478,000/mm³; adults: 150,000–400,000/mm³

Compared to adults, the normal platelet count in the newborn may be lower. Adult values are reached after 1 week of age. Platelet counts are discussed in detail in Chapter 15.

SUMMARY

Interpreting pediatric laboratory data can be complex. Age-related differences in normal reference ranges occur for many common laboratory tests. These differences may be due to changes in body composition and the normal anatomic and physiologic maturation that occurs throughout childhood. Changes in various body compartments, the immature function of the neonatal kidney, and the increased electrolyte and mineral requirements necessary for proper growth, help to explain many age-related differences in serum electrolytes and minerals. Alterations in skeletal muscle mass and the pattern of kidney function maturation account for the various age-related differences in serum creatinine and kidney function tests. Neonatal hepatic immaturity and subsequent maturation help to explain the age-related differences in serum albumin, liver enzymes, and bilirubin. Likewise, the immature hematopoietic system of the newborn and its maturation account for the age-related differences in various hematologic tests.

This chapter also reviews several general pediatric considerations including differences in physiologic parameters, pediatric blood sampling considerations, and the determination of pediatric reference ranges. Interpretation of pediatric laboratory data must take into account the various age-related differences in normal values. If these differences are not taken into consideration, inappropriate diagnoses and treatment may result.

REFERENCES

1. Taketomo CK, Hodding JH, Kraus DM. *Pediatric Dosage Handbook*. 10th ed. Hudson, OH: Lexi-Comp, Inc.; 2003.
2. Siberry GK, Iannone R, eds. *The Harriet Lane Handbook*. 15th ed. St. Louis, MO: Mosby; 2000.
3. Task force on blood pressure control in children. Report of the second task force on blood pressure control in children – 1987. *Pediatrics*. 1987; 79:1–25.
4. Update on the 1987 Task Force Report on High Blood Pressure in Children and Adolescents: a working group report from the National High Blood Pressure Education Program. National High Blood Pressure Education Program Working Group on Hypertension Control in Children and Adolescents. *Pediatrics*. 1996; 98:649–58.
5. Hicks JM. Pediatric clinical biochemistry: why is it different? In: Soldin SJ, Rifai N, Hicks JM, eds. *Biochemical Basis of Pediatric Disease*. 2nd ed. Washington DC: AACC Press; 1995: 1–17.
6. Malarkey LM, McMorrow ME. Specimen collection procedures. In: *Nurses Manual of Laboratory Tests and Diagnostic Procedures*. 2nd ed. Philadelphia, PA: W. B. Saunders; 2000: 16–36.
7. Nathan DG, Orkin SH, eds. *Nathan and Oski's Hematology of Infancy and Childhood*. 5th ed. Philadelphia, PA: W. B. Saunders; 1998.
8. Soldin SJ, Brugnara C, Hicks JM, eds. *Pediatric Reference Ranges*. 3rd ed. Washington DC: AACC Press; 1999.
9. Malarkey LM, McMorrow ME. *Nurses Manual of Laboratory Tests and Diagnostic Procedures*. 2nd ed. Philadelphia, PA: W. B. Saunders; 2000.
10. Jacobs DS, DeMott WR, Oxley DK. *Laboratory Test Handbook*. 5th ed. Hudson, OH: Lexi-Comp, Inc.; 2001.
11. Nicholson JF, Pesce MA. Reference ranges for laboratory tests and procedures. In: Behrman RE, Kliegman RM, Jenson HB, eds. *Nelson Textbook of Pediatrics*. 17th ed. Philadelphia, PA: W. B. Saunders; 2004.
12. Osberg IM. Chemistry and hematology reference (normal) ranges. In: *Current Pediatric Diagnosis and Treatment*. 16th ed. New York, NY: Lange Medical Books/McGraw-Hill; 2003.
13. Gomez P, Coca C, Vargas C, et al. Normal reference-intervals for 20 biochemical variables in healthy infants, children, and adolescents. *Clin Chem*. 1984; 30:407–12.
14. Burritt MF, Slockbower JM, Forsman RW, et al. Pediatric reference intervals for 19 biological variables in healthy children. *Mayo Clin Proc*. 1990; 65:329–36.
15. Jagarinec N, Flegar-Mestric Z, Surina B, et al. *Clin Chem Lab Med*. 1998; 36:327–37.
16. Cherian AG, Hill JG. Percentile estimates of reference values for fourteen chemical constituents in sera of children and adolescents. *AJCP*. 1978; 69:24–31.
17. Bell EF, Oh W. Fluid and electrolyte management. In: Avery GB, Fletcher MA, MacDonald MG, eds. *Neonatology: Pathophysiology and Management of the Newborn*. 5th ed. Philadelphia, PA: Lippincott Williams & Wilkins; 1999.
18. Friis-Hansen B. Water distribution in the foetus and newborn infant. *Acta Paediatr Scand*. 1983; 305:7–11.
19. Friis-Hansen B. Changes in body water compartments during growth. *Acta Paediatr*. 1957; 110 (suppl):1–68.
20. Tarnow-Mordi WO, Shaw JC, Liu D, et al. Iatrogenic hyponatremia of the newborn due to maternal fluid overload: a prospective study. *Br Med J*. 1981; 283:639–42.
21. Malarkey LM, McMorrow ME. Serum electrolytes. In: *Nurses Manual of Laboratory Tests and Diagnostic Procedures*. 2nd ed. Philadelphia, PA: W. B. Saunders; 2000: 82–103.
22. Greenbaum LA. Electrolytes and acid-base disorders. In: Behrman RE, Kliegman RM, Jenson HB, eds. *Nelson Textbook of Pediatrics*. 17th ed. Philadelphia, PA: W. B. Saunders; 2004.
23. Blackburn ST. Renal function in the neonate. *J Perinat Neonatal Nurs*. 1994; 8:37–47.
24. Brion LP, Satlin LM, Edelmann CM. Renal disease. In: Avery GB, Fletcher MA, MacDonald MG, eds. *Neonatology: Pathophysiology and Management of the Newborn*. 5th ed. Philadelphia, PA: Lippincott Williams & Wilkins; 1999.
25. Breault DT, Majzoub JA. Other abnormalities of arginine vasopressin metabolism and action. In: Behrman RE, Kliegman RM, Jenson HB, eds. *Nelson Textbook of Pediatrics*. 17th ed. Philadelphia, PA: W. B. Saunders; 2004.
26. Lorenz JM. Assessing fluid and electrolyte status in the newborn. *Clinical Chemistry*. 1997; 43:205–10.
27. Papageorgiou A, Bardin CL. The extremely low birth weight infant. In: Avery GB, Fletcher MA, MacDonald MG, eds. *Neonatology: Pathophysiology and Management of the Newborn*. 5th ed. Philadelphia, PA: Lippincott Williams & Wilkins; 1999.
28. Jones DP, Chesney RW. Development of tubular function. *Clinics in Perinatology*. 1992; 19:33–57.
29. Stigson L, Kjellmer I. Serum levels of magnesium at birth related to complications of immaturity. *Acta Paediatr*. 1997; 86: 991–4.
30. Ariceta G, Rodriguez-Soriano J, Vallo A. Magnesium homeostasis in premature and full-term neonates. *Pediatr Nephrol*. 1995; 9:423–7.
31. Geven WB, Monnens LA, Willems JL. Magnesium metabolism in childhood. *Mimer Electrolyte Metab*. 1993; 19:308–13.
32. Davis ID, Avner ED. Introduction to glomerular diseases. In: Behrman RE, Kliegman RM, Jenson HB, eds. *Nelson Textbook of Pediatrics*. 17th ed. Philadelphia, PA: W. B. Saunders; 2004.
33. Schwartz GJ, Brion LP, Spitzer A. The use of plasma creatinine concentration for estimating glomerular filtration rate in infants, children, and adolescents. *Pediatric Clinics of North America*. 1997; 34:571–90.
34. Bueva A, Guignard JP. Renal function in preterm neonates. *Pediatric Research*. 1994; 36:572–7.
35. Alcorn J, McNamara PJ. Ontogeny of hepatic and renal systemic clearance pathways in infants: part 1. *Clin Pharmacokinet*. 2002; 41:959–98.
36. Guignard JP. Renal function in the newborn infant. *Pediatr Clin North Am*. 1982; 29:777–90.

37. DuBois D, Dubois EF. A formula to estimate the approximate surface area if height and weight be known. *Arch Intern Med*. 1916; 17:863–71.

38. Mosteller RD. Simplified calculation of body-surface area. *New Engl J Med*. 1987; 317:1098.

39. Hogg RJ, Furth S, Lemley KV, et al. National Kidney Foundation's kidney disease outcomes quality initiative clinical practice guidelines for chronic kidney disease in children and adolescents: evaluation, classification, and stratification. *Pediatrics*. 2003; 111:1416–21.

40. Traub SL, Johnson CE. Comparison of methods of estimating creatinine clearance in children. *Am J Hosp Pharm*. 1980; 37:195–201.

41. DeAcevedo LH, Johnson CE. Estimation of creatinine clearance in children: comparison of six methods. *Clin Pharm*. 1982; 1:158–61.

42. Waz WR, Feld LG, Quattrin T. Serum creatinine, height, and weight do not predict glomerular filtration rate in children with IDDM. *Diabetes Care*. 1993; 16:1067–70.

43. Bates MD, Balistreri WF. Development and function of the liver and biliary system. In: Behrman RE, Kliegman RM, Jenson HB, eds. *Nelson Textbook of Pediatrics*. 17th ed. Philadelphia, PA: W. B. Saunders; 2004.

44. Dennery PA, Seidman DS, Stevenson DK. Neonatal hyperbilirubinemia. *N Engl J Med*. 2001; 344:581–90.

45. Lockitch G. Beyond the umbilical cord: interpreting laboratory tests in the neonate (review). *Clin Biochem*. 1994; 27:1–6.

46. Doyle JJ, Schmidt B, Blanchette V, et al. In: Avery GB, Fletcher MA, MacDonald MG, eds. *Neonatology: Pathophysiology and Management of the Newborn*. 5th ed. Philadelphia, PA: Lippincott Williams & Wilkins; 1999.

47. Glader B. Physiologic anemia of infancy. In: Behrman RE, Kliegman RM, Jenson HB, eds. *Nelson Textbook of Pediatrics*. 17th ed. Philadelphia, PA: W. B. Saunders; 2004.

48. Glader B. The anemias. In: Behrman RE, Kliegman RM, Jenson HB, eds. *Nelson Textbook of Pediatrics*. 17th ed. Philadelphia, PA: W. B. Saunders; 2004

Chapter **4**

DRUG INTERFERENCE WITH TEST RESULTS

Mary Lee

Through a variety of mechanisms, drugs can interfere with laboratory test results. If the clinician who has ordered the laboratory test is not aware that the drug has altered the results of the test, inappropriate management of the patient may follow including unnecessary hospitalization, extra office visits, or additional laboratory tests—all of which may increase the cost of health care. This chapter addresses this situation and provides resources that can be used by the pharmacist to provide information for better interpretation of laboratory tests when a drug is suspected to cause an interference with test results.

OBJECTIVES

After completing this chapter, the reader should be able to

1. Compare and contrast in vivo and in vitro drug interferences with laboratory tests.
2. Identify a suspected drug-laboratory test interference in a logical, systematic manner given a drug and a laboratory test.
3. Describe options for managing situations of clinically significant drug-laboratory test interferences.
4. List key literature resources about drug-laboratory test interferences.
5. Describe a systematic method to search and identify medical literature relevant to a particular clinical situation.

IN VIVO AND IN VITRO DRUG INTERFERENCES[1]

When a drug interferes with a laboratory test result, it alters the lab value. Mechanisms for drug interference of clinical laboratory tests can be classified as either in vivo or in vitro. *In vivo* drug effects can also be called biological and can be subclassified as pharmacological or toxicological. In contrast, the term *in vitro* is used synonymously with *analytical* or *methodical*.

In vivo interferences account for most effects of drugs on laboratory tests.[2]

In Vivo Interference

An in vivo interference is an actual change in the analyte concentration or activity prior to collection and analysis. The assay measurement is true and accurate and reflects a change in the measured substance that has occurred in the patient. Therefore, an in vivo interference will always change a laboratory test result, independent of the assay methodology. A drug can produce an in vivo interference in several ways. By a direct extension of its pharmacological effects, a drug can produce changes in some lab test results. For example, thiazide and loop diuretics will commonly cause increased renal elimination of potassium. Therefore, decreased serum potassium levels can occur in treated patients. In these patients, hypokalemia is true and accurate. Similarly, increased blood glucose levels can occur after treatment with thiazide and loop diuretics, diazoxide, corticosteroids, and oral contraceptives

Other drugs produce changes in lab test results by producing in vivo toxicological effects. As the drug damages a particular organ system, abnormal laboratory tests may be one of the first signs of the problem. For example, as isoniazid and rifampin produce hepatotoxicity, elevated hepatic transaminases will herald the onset of liver inflammation. Similarly, as a prolonged course of high-dose aminoglycoside antibiotic causes acute renal failure, serum creatinine and serum aminoglycoside levels will increase steadily. In the face of quinidine-induced hemolytic anemia, intracellular red blood cell contents will spill out into plasma, thereby increasing serum potassium, magnesium, and creatine kinase levels.

In Vitro Interference

Drugs in a subject's body fluid or tissue can directly interfere with a clinical laboratory test during the in vitro analytical process. This type of drug-laboratory test interaction is highly dependent on the laboratory test methodology, as the reaction may occur with one specific assay method but not another. For example, some beta-lactam antibiotics in adequate concentrations will deactivate aminoglycosides if allowed adequate contact time in the same test tube and, as a result, will lower measured aminoglycoside levels. In addition, substances that are prepackaged in or added to the in vitro system before or after sample collection can cause laboratory test interference in vitro. As an example, test tubes sometimes contain heparin or fluoride. Heparin can interfere with aminoglycoside assays, and fluoride can cause false increases in BUN when measured by the Ekatchem assay.

In addition, some drugs can indirectly interfere with a clinical laboratory test during the in vitro analytical process. In this case, the drug can produce changes in endogenous biochemicals (e.g., lipids or bilirubin). The concentration of endogenous substances usually must be well above normal levels before it significantly influences an assay. A common example is a patient with drug-induced hepatotoxicity who is jaundiced and has a bilirubin of 10 mg/dL. Icteric blood samples cause many immunologically-based drug concentration assays to generate spurious results or interfere with peroxidase-catalyzed assays used for measuring glucose or cholesterol.[3] Alternatively, the drug may cause discoloration of the body fluid specimen, which may interfere with colorimetric, photometric, or fluorometric laboratory-based assay methods. For example, phenazopyridine causes an orange-red discoloration of urine that interferes with selected tests in a urinalysis. Amitriptyline and methylene blue can produce a blue-green or blue, respectively, discoloration of urine. These can be detected visually and appropriate attribution of the abnormality should be made by knowledgeable clinicians.

Common mechanisms by which drugs cause in vitro interferences with laboratory tests include

1. Drug reacts with reagent to form a chromophore (e.g., cefoxitin or cephalothin) with Jaffe-based creatinine assay.
2. Drug reacts with immunoassay's antibody that is intended to be specific for the analyte. For example, caffeine cross-reacts in the theophylline assay; digitoxin, digoxin metabolites, and antigen-binding fragments derived from anti-digoxin antibodies (used for treating digoxin intoxication) cross-react with the digoxin assay.
3. Drug alters the specimen pH (usually urine) so that reagent reactions are inhibited or enhanced. For example, acetazolamide produces an alkaline urinary pH that causes a false-positive proteinuria with reagent dip strips.
4. Drug has chemical properties similar to the analyte. For example, patients who receive radiographic contrast media, which contain iodine, may exhibit altered laboratory values for protein-bound iodine.
5. Drug chelates with an enzyme activator or reagent used in the in vitro laboratory analysis.
6. Drug absorbs at the same wavelength as the analyte. For example, methotrexate interferes with analytic methods using an absorbance range of 340–410 nm.

MINICASE 1

A 60-YEAR-OLD FEMALE PATIENT has congestive heart failure, which is treated with digoxin. She has also suffered from asthma for many years and is admitted for an exacerbation of this condition. At the time of admission, her serum potassium and digoxin levels are 4.2 mEq/L and 1.0 ng/mL, respectively. After admission, her asthma is treated with subcutaneous albuterol, and she responds well to the treatment. A repeat serum potassium level is 2.6 mEq/L.

Question: What is the cause of hypokalemia in this patient? Should hypokalemia be treated? Should this patient receive potassium supplementation chronically?[2]

Discussion: The likelihood of digoxin cardiac toxicity is increased in patients with hypokalemia. Therefore, hypokalemia should be treated. The most likely cause of hypokalemia is albuterol. When administered systemically, albuterol causes potassium to shift from the plasma compartment to the intracellular compartment. As a result, the plasma potassium level decreases. When albuterol's effects dissipate, the plasma potassium level should normalize. Therefore, in the absence of any other disorders or drugs, which could cause hypokalemia, this patient will not require any chronic potassium supplementation.[22,23]

In addition to the parent drug, other drug-related components may cause significant interferences with laboratory tests. Metabolites of drugs or inactive ingredients of some drug products may influence assay results. Inactive ingredients include excipients such as lactose or starch, preservatives, colorants, or flavoring agents. Although most manufacturers do report the inactive ingredients in their products, little systematic research has been performed to assess the impact of these substances on laboratory tests. Compounding these factors, many laboratory test interferences are concentration-related and many drug metabolites and their usual plasma concentrations have yet to be identified. Therefore, systematic study of all of these potential causes of interactions is difficult to conduct and not available in most cases.[3]

Simultaneous In Vitro and In Vivo Effects

Some drugs can affect an analyte both in vivo and in vitro. In these rare situations, interpretation is extremely difficult because the degree of impact in each environment cannot be easily determined. The prototypic example involves reaction of aminoglycosides with penicillins, which leads to a loss of antibacterial activity in vivo and can decrease measured aminoglycoside concentrations and antibacterial activity in vitro. Although this inactivation mechanism is unclear, it seems to involve the formation of an adduct between the aminoglycoside and beta-lactam ring of the penicillins. Although only this interaction is discussed here, the concepts can be extrapolated to other drugs.

In vitro, carbenicillin is the most potent inactivator of aminoglycosides when compared to the other penicillins; tobramycin is the most susceptible when compared to the other aminoglycosides; and amikacin and netilmicin are degraded the least. Refrigeration does not significantly slow the reaction, but centrifugation with freezing does. Unreasonably low aminogycoside concentrations in patients receiving concomitant high-dose penicillins should alert the practitioner to this in vitro interaction.[4–6]

In vivo, inactivation of aminoglycosides by penicillins is a problem primarily in patients with renal failure. With normal renal function, these antibiotics are excreted at a rate faster than their interaction rate. In one study, the in vivo inactivation rate constant of gentamicin in patients with renal failure receiving carbenicillin was 0.025 hr^{-1}. The inactivation rate constant was defined as the difference between the elimination rate constant for gentamicin alone and that for its combination with carbenicillin. Thus, in renal failure patients, carbenicillin apparently eliminates gentamicin at the same rate as do the kidneys. The change corresponded to a shortening of the gentamicin half-life from 61.6 to 19.6 hr after carbenicillin was added. Fortunately, carbenicillin is rarely used today.

The effect of penicillins on aminoglycosides can be minimized several ways[6]:

1. To eliminate in vitro problems, the sample can be centrifuged and frozen soon after it is drawn.
2. Antibiotics with a lesser interaction (amikacin and piperacillin or a cephalosporin) can be used.
3. Administration times can be separated or blood can be drawn just before the next scheduled penicillin dose to decrease the penicillin concentration in the specimen tube, the concentration-exposure time (in vivo), and, thus, the degradation time.

This last maneuver would be less applicable in patients with renal failure, particularly if the pencillin dose were not adjusted. However, decreasing the daily penicillin dose according to renal function and required serum concentration would make testing more accurate even for these patients.

IDENTIFYING DRUG INTERFERENCES

Incidence of Drug Interferences

The true incidence of drug interferences with laboratory tests is unknown. This is because many situations probably go undetected. However, as the number of laboratory tests and drugs on the US commercial market increase, it is likely that the number of cases of in vivo interferences will also increase.[3,7]

As a reflection of this, consider the number of drug-laboratory test interferences reported by D. S. Young, author of one of the classic literature references on this topic. In the first edition of Effects of Drugs on Clinical Laboratory Tests, published in the journal *Clinical Chemistry* in 1972, 9000 such interactions were included. In the second edition of the same publication, which was published in 1975, 16,000 such interactions were reported.[8,9]

As for in vitro interferences, the number of drug-laboratory test interferences may be moderated over time because of newer, more specific laboratory test methodologies that minimize cross-reactions with drug metabolites or drug effects on reagents or laboratory reactions.[10,11] In addition, manufacturers of commonly used laboratory equipment systematically study the effects of drugs on assay methods.[12] Therefore, this information is often available to clinicians who confront problematic laboratory test results in patients. This increased awareness reduces the number of patients who are believed to have experienced newly reported drug-laboratory test interferences.

Suspecting a Drug Interference

A clinician should suspect a drug-laboratory test interference when an inconsistency appears among related test results or between test results and the clinical picture. Specifically, clinicians should become suspicious whenever

1. Test results do not correlate with the patient's signs, symptoms, or medical history.
2. Results of different tests—assessing the same organ anatomy or organ function or the drug's pharmacology—conflict with each other.
3. Results from a series of the same test vary greatly over a short period of time.
4. Results from a series of the same test change in the wrong direction.

No Correlation with Patient's Signs, Symptoms, or Medical History

As emphasized elsewhere in this book, when test results do not correlate with signs, symptoms, or medical history of the patient, the signs and symptoms should be considered more strongly than the test results. This rule is particularly true when test results are being used to confirm suspicions raised by the signs and symptoms in the first place or when the test results are being used as surrogate markers or indirect indicators of underlying pathology.

For example, serum creatinine is used in various formulae to approximate the glomerular filtration rate, which is used to assess the kidney's ability to make urine. However, actual urine output and measurement of urinary creatinine excretion is a more accurate method of assessing overall renal function. If a patient's serum creatinine has increased from a baseline of 1 mg/dL to 5 mg/dL over a 3-day period but the patient has had no change in urine output, urinary creatinine excretion, or serum electrolyte levels, then the serum creatinine level may be elevated because of a drug interference with the laboratory test.

Similarly, if a patient has a total serum bilirubin of 6 mg/dL but the patient is not jaundiced or does not have scleral icterus, then a drug interference with the laboratory test should be considered.

Conflicting Test Results

Occasionally, pharmacological effects of a drug or results of two tests that assess the same organ anatomy or function conflict with each other. For example, a presurgical test screen shows a serum creatinine of 4.2 mg/dL in an otherwise healthy 20-year old patient with a BUN of 8 mg/dL. Usually, if a patient had true renal impairment, BUN and serum creatinine would likely be elevated in tandem. Thus, in this patient, a drug interference with the laboratory test was suspected. Further investigation revealed that the patient received cefoxitin shortly before blood was drawn for the lab test. Cefoxitin can falsely elevate serum creatinine concentrations. Thus, the elevated serum creatinine is likely due to drug interference not to renal failure. To confirm that this is the case, cefoxitin should be discontinued and the serum creatinine repeated after that. If due to the drug, the elevated serum creatinine should return to the normal range.[13]

Varying Serial Test Results

Prostate specific antigen (PSA) is a tumor marker for prostate cancer. It is produced by glandular cells of the prostate. Whereas the normal serum level is ≤4 ng/mL in a patient without prostate cancer, the level is typically elevated in patients with prostate cancer. However, it is not specific for prostate cancer. Elevated PSA serum levels are also observed in patients with benign prostatic hyperplasia, prostatitis, or following instrumentation of the prostate. A 70-year-old male patient with stage C (locally invasive) prostate cancer has a PSA of 20 ng/mL and has decided to undergo no treatment. Four serial PSA tests over the course of 1 year and done at 3-month intervals show no change. Despite the absence of any changes on pelvic computerized axial tomography, bone scan, or chest x-ray, his PSA is 10 ng/mL at his most recent office visit. After a careful interview of the patient, it is apparent that he has been using an over-the-counter herbal product, PC-SPES®, which is known to reduce prostate size. It is likely that this drug product caused the change in PSA.[14–16]

Changing Serial Test Results

Leuprolide, a luteinizing hormone-releasing hormone analog, is useful in the management of prostate cancer, which is an androgen dependent tumor. Persistent use of leuprolide causes down-regulation of pituitary luteinizing hormone-releasing hormone (LHRH) receptors, decreased secretion of luteinizing hormone, and decreased production of testicular androgens. A patient with prostate cancer, treated with leuprolide, should experience a sustained reduction in serum testosterone levels from normal (400–1200 ng/dL) to castration levels (less than 50 ng/dL) after 2–3 weeks. However, one of the adverse effects of leuprolide is decreased libido and erectile dysfunction, which is a direct extension of the drug's testosterone-lowering effect. Such a patient may seek medical treatment of sexual dysfunction, and he may be inappropriately prescribed depot testosterone injections. Thus, in this case, depot testosterone injections caused a change in serum testosterone levels in the wrong direction. If serum testosterone levels increase, this should signal a problem with this patient's response to leuprolide.[17]

MANAGING DRUG INTERFERENCES

When a drug is suspected to interfere with a laboratory test, the clinician should collect appropriate evidence to confirm the interaction. Important information includes

1. Establishing a temporal relationship between the change in the laboratory test and drug use. Ensure that the change in the laboratory test occurred after the drug was started or after the drug dose was changed.
2. Ruling out other drugs as causes of the laboratory test change.
3. Ruling out other diseases as causes of the laboratory test change.
4. If possible, discontinuing the causative agent and repeating the test to see if dechallenge results in correction of the abnormal laboratory test.
5. Alternatively, choosing another laboratory test that will provide assessment of the same organ's function but is unlikely to be affected by the drug. Conduct the lab test and compare the results against the original lab test result. Check for dissimilarity or similarity of results.[3]
6. Identifying medical literature that documents the suspected drug-laboratory test interference.
7. Contacting the head of diagnostic labs. They oftentimes maintain or have access to computerized lists of drugs that interfere with laboratory tests.[18,19]

For any particular patient case, it is often not possible to obtain information on all seven of the above items. However, the first four items are key in any suspected drug-laboratory test interference.

LITERATURE RESOURCES

A systematic search of the medical literature is essential for providing the appropriate background information to address steps 2–6. This search will ensure that a complete and comprehensive review—necessary in making an accurate diagnosis—has been done. When searching the literature, it is recommended to use the method originally described by Watanabe et al.[20] and, subsequently, modified by C. F. Kirkwood.[21] Using this technique, the clinician would search tertiary, secondary, and then primary literature.

Tertiary literature includes reference texts and monograph databases (e.g., DRUGDEX), which provide appropriate foundational content and background material essential for understanding basic concepts and historical data relevant to the topic. *Secondary literature*, functioning as a gateway to primary literature, includes indexing and abstracting services (i.e., PubMed and *International Pharmaceutical Abstracts*). *Primary literature* includes case reports, experimental studies, and other non-review types of articles in journals about the topic. These represent the most current literature on the topic. By systematically scanning the literature in this order, the clinician can be sure to have identified and analyzed all relevant literature, which is crucial in developing appropriate conclusions for these types of situations.

Tertiary Literature

Tertiary literature, which contains useful information about drug-lab test interferences, includes the *Physicians' Desk Reference*. Each complete package insert included in this book contains a precautions section that contains information on drug-lab test interferences. However, it is important to note that the *Physicians' Desk Reference* does not include package inserts on all commercially available drugs, nor does it include complete package inserts for all of the products included in the text. Thus, additional resources will need to be checked. The drug monographs in the *AHFS Drug Information*, published by the American Society of Health-System Pharmacists, also contain a section on lab test interferences. Although the information provided is brief, it can be used as an initial screen. *Meyler's Side Effects of Drugs*, although well-referenced, gives limited background information on each drug-laboratory test interference. A new edition is published every 4 years, but it is updated annually in a series of companion books. Thus, to do a complete search through *Meyer's Side Effects of Drugs*, the clinician must go through several volumes. Also, unlike the other two texts, *Meyler's Side Effects of Drugs* is usually only available in drug information centers or medical libraries because of its expense.

One of the most comprehensive compilations of drug-laboratory test interactions is *Effects of Drugs on Clinical Laboratory Tests* by D. S. Young. Although originally published for many years as a special issue of the journal, *Clinical Chemistry,* the book has subsequently been published as a separate text. The book is divided into two sections: a database sorted by laboratory test and a database sorted by drug. This compilation includes pharmacological and analytical effects of drugs on laboratory tests. All entries are referenced, and no attempt is made to analyze the validity of various reports. Thus, a single drug may be reported to cause an increase, decrease, or no change in a laboratory test. No detail is provided on the dosage of drug that produced the interference. Hence, a clinician will need to obtain the original references and evaluate the data independently.

A variety of other books about clinical laboratory tests are listed below. Some are comprehensive references while others are handbooks. All of them provide information about drug-laboratory test interferences. However, the references are more complete than the handbooks. In addition, several comprehensive review articles include more current information about drug-laboratory test interferences.

DRUGDEX, prepared by MICROMEDEX, is available on CD-ROM. For every drug included in the system, information is available in a drug monograph format, and any information about drug-lab test interferences are included in a unique section of the monograph. In addition, for some drugs, drug information questions and answers are included. To access relevant information, the clinician can retrieve information using the name of the drug or the laboratory test.

Books and Handbooks

- Anon. *Physician's Desk Reference 2001*. Montvale, NJ: Medical Economics; 2001.
- Chernecky CC, Berger BJ. *Laboratory Tests and Diagnostic Procedures*. 3rd ed. Philadelphia, PA: W. B. Saunders; 2001.
- Dukes MNG, ed. *Meyler's Side Effects of Drug: An Encyclopedia of Adverse Reactions and Interactions*. 14th ed. Amsterdam: Elsevier; 2000.
- Friedman RB, Young DS. *Effects of Disease on Clinical Laboratory Tests*. 3rd ed. Washington, DC: American Association for Clinical Chemistry; 1997.
- Henry JB. *Clinical Diagnosis and Management by Laboratory Methods*. 20th ed. Philadelphia, PA: W. B. Saunders; 2001.
- Jacobs DS, Demott WR, Oxley DK. *Laboratory Test Handbook: Concise with Disease Index*. 2nd ed. Hudson, OH: Lexi-Comp, Inc.; 2002.
- McEvoy GK. *AHFS Drug Information 2002*. Bethesda, MD: American Society of Health-System Pharmacists; 2002.
- Ravell R. *Clinical Laboratory Medicine*. 6th ed. St. Louis, MO: Mosby; 1995.
- Sacher RA, McPherson RA, Campos JM. *Widmann's Clinical Interpretation of Laboratory Tests*. 11th ed. Philadelphia, PA: F. A. Davis Company; 2000.
- Tietze N. *Clinical Guide to Laboratory Tests*. 3rd ed. Philadelphia, PA: W. B. Saunders; 1995.
- Wallach JB. *Interpretation of Diagnostic Tests: A Synopsis of Laboratory Tests*. Philadelphia, PA: Lippincott Williams & Wilkins; 2000.
- Young DS. *Effects of Drugs on Clinical Laboratory Tests*. 2nd ed. Washington, DC: American Association for Clinical Chemistry; 1997.

Review Articles

- Young DS, Pestancer LC, Gibberman V. Effects of drugs on clinical laboratory tests. *Clin Chem*. 1975; 21:10–432.

This master work is considered the first comprehensive database about drug effects on laboratory tests. Information on 16,000 drug-laboratory test interferences is included. Information can be retrieved using drug name or name of the laboratory test. This superceded the author's 1972 publication on the same topic, and it includes several improvements over the previous manuscript including updated references, some entries include information on the drug dosing regimen used, and a rating of the likelihood of the laboratory test interference occurring after drug use.

- Sher PP. Drug interferences with clinical laboratory tests. *Drugs*. 1982; 24:24–63.

This useful reference provides many tables of drugs known to interfere with various laboratory tests. The data is arranged by laboratory test. So, for many common laboratory tests, summary tables of drugs known to interfere with the particular lab tests are provided. Also, mechanisms for the in vivo and in vitro interactions are described. This reference is dated, so it is useful for older drugs but not for newer agents.

- Sonntag O, Scholer A. Drug interference in clinical chemistry: recommendation of drugs and their concentrations to be used in drug interference studies. *Ann Clin Biochem*. 2001; 38:376–85.

In 1995, 18 clinical laboratory test experts identified 24 commonly used drugs known to interfere with laboratory tests. Usual therapeutic and toxic drug concentrations were identified. Both concentrations of each drug were added in vitro to blood and urine specimens and then various laboratory tests were run on the specimens. Laboratory testing was duplicated in three different laboratories. This review article summarizes drug-laboratory test interactions for over 70 different laboratory tests.

- Kroll MH, Elin RJ. Interference with clinical laboratory analyses. *Clin Chem*.1994; 40(11 Part 1):1996–2005.

An excellent overview of drug-laboratory test interactions, this article discusses how drugs can produce significant interactions and discrepancies caused by in vitro experimental designs (which do not reflect the effect of drug metabolites and their concentrations on outcome). It also provides a summary of useful references (although outdated) on the topic. In addition, a suggested approach to drug-laboratory test interactions is described.

Secondary and Primary Literature

For secondary literature, the main indexing or abstracting service that should be used is PubMed. This allows the clinician to check the literature from thousands of biomedical journals from 1966 to the present. Due to improvements in search capabilities, clinicians can search using text words or words as they might appear in the title or abstract of a journal article. The database will automatically convert that text word to official medical subject headings or accepted indexing terms. As a result, search output is optimized despite the lack of proficiency or experience of the searcher. If the searches represent a combination of concepts, the concepts can be appropriately linked using Boolean logical operators, *or* or *and*. In addition, the database provides links enabling clinicians to locate related articles or order articles online, which enhances search capabilities and convenience in obtaining primary literature articles.

This chapter does not allow a complete tutorial on search strategy development and conducting PubMed searches. However, the reader is encouraged to develop expertise in this area so that he or she can identify current, relevant literature efficiently.

MINICASE 2

A 35-YEAR-OLD FEMALE PATIENT receives ticarcillin 3 g intravenously every 4 hr and gentamicin 100 mg intravenously every 8 hr for urosepsis. Her lean body weight is 70 kg. Prior to the start of the antibiotics, the patient's clinical chemistry tests were normal. Serum sodium was 137 mEq/L, potassium 4.0 mEq/L, BUN 10 mg/dL, and creatinine 1 mg/dL. She is taking no other medications and has no other medical illnesses. After 3 days of antibiotics, routine clinical chemistry tests reveal a serum sodium level of 147 mEq/L, potassium 2.8 mEq/L, and BUN and creatinine are unchanged.

Question: What do you think is causing the laboratory abnormalities? Are hypernatremia and hypokalemia signs of drug-induced nephrotoxicity?

Discussion: This patient's past medical history is consistent with that of a healthy young female with no renal impairment. Since hypernatremia and hypokalemia occurred 3 days after the start of antibiotics, these drugs should be evaluated as possible causes for the lab abnormalities.

Gentamicin nephrotoxicity occurs more often in patients with risk factors for the adverse reaction. The patient does not have risk factors for gentamicin toxicity. Her course of aminoglycoside has been short (less than 7 days), her daily dose appears to be average, and she has normal renal function prior to the start of gentamicin (her estimated creatinine clearance is 87 mL/min). She is not using any other nephrotoxins. Following 3 days of aminoglycoside, her serum creatinine is unchanged, and it is improbable that she has gentamicin nephrotoxicity. However, she is taking large daily doses of ticarcillin, which is commercially available as a disodium salt. Each gram delivers 3 mEq of sodium. Therefore, this patient is receiving 36 mEq of sodium per day in addition to her usual dietary intake of sodium. As disodium ticarcillin is filtered through the glomerulus and passes into the renal tubule, sodium disocciates from ticarcillin. Sodium is reabsorbed from the renal tubule whereas ticarcillin is a nonresorbable anion that is excreted as a dipotassium salt. As a result, the patient develops hypernatremia and hypokalemia. Thus, this patient's electrolyte abnormality is due to ticarcillin and not due to aminoglycoside nephrotoxicity.[24]

SUMMARY

Although the number of drug-laboratory test interferences increases as the number of commercially available drugs increases, improved literature resources that compile information on this topic and improved assay methodologies have helped clinicians in dealing with suspected cases of this problem. Most drug-laboratory test interferences are due to in vivo effects of drugs; that is, the drug's pharmacological or toxic effects produce specific alterations in laboratory values. A drug-laboratory test interference should be suspected whenever a laboratory test result does not match the signs and symptoms in a patient, when the results of different tests—assessing the same organ function or drug effect—conflict with each other, or when a series of the same test vary greatly over a short period of time.

To determine if a drug is interfering with a drug-laboratory test, the clinician should, at a minimum, establish a temporal relationship between the change in the laboratory test and drug use; rule out other drugs and diseases as the cause; and discontinue the drug and repeat the lab test to see if dechallenge results in correction of the abnormal laboratory test. The literature should be checked to see if documentation of the drug-laboratory test interference can be found. The literature search should be systematic to ensure complete literature retrieval. Therefore, the clinician should proceed from the tertiary to the secondary and then to the primary literature. Many helpful literature resources provide relevant information on this topic.

REFERENCES

1. Sher PP. Drug interferences with clinical laboratory tests. *Drugs*. 1982; 24:24–63.
2. Salway JG. Drug interference causing misinterpretation of laboratory results. *Ann Clin Biochem*. 1978; 15:44–8.
3. Kroll MH, Elin RJ. Interference with clinical laboratory analyses. *Clin Chem*. 1994; 49:1996–2005.
4. Pickering LK, Rutherford I. Effect of concentration and time upon inactivation of tobramycin, gentamicin, netilmicin, and amikacin by azlocillin, carbenicillin, mecillinam, mezlocillin, and piperacillin. *J Pharmacol Exp Ther*. 1981; 217:345–9.
5. Chow MS, Quintiliani R, Nightingale CH. In vivo inactivation of tobramycin by ticarcillin. *JAMA*. 1982; 247:658–9.
6. Thompson MI, Russo ME, Saxon BJ, et al. Gentamicin inactivation by piperacillin or carbenicillin in patients with end stage renal disease. *Antimicrob Agents Chemother*. 1982; 21:268–73.
7. Munzenberger P, Emmanuel S. The incidence of drug-diagnostic test interferences in outpatient. *Am J Hosp Pharm*. 1971; 28:786–91.
8. Young DS, Thomas DW, Friedman RB, et al. Effects of drugs on clinical laboratory tests. *Clin Chem*. 1972; 18:1041–1303.
9. Young DS, Pestaner LC, Gibberman V. Effects of drugs on clinical laboratory tests. *Clin Chem*. 1975; 21:1D–432D.
10. Hansen JL, Schneiweiss FN. Drug interference with laboratory value interpretation: a review. *Am J Med Technol*. 1981; 47:183–7.
11. Young DS. Effects of drugs on clinical laboratory tests. *Ann Clin Biochem*. 1997; 34:579–81.
12. Powers DM, Boyd JC, Glick MR, et al. *Interference Testing in Clinical Chemistry*. NCCLS Document. 1986; EP7–P:6(13).
13. Letellier G, Desjarlais F. Analytical interference of drugs in clinical chemistry: II—the interference of three cephalosporins with the determination of serum creatinine concentration by the Jaffe reaction. *Clin Biochem*. 1985; 18:352–6.
14. Van Der Cruijsen-Koeter IW, Wildhagen MF, De Koning HJ, et al. The value of current diagnostic tests in prostate cancer screening. *BJU Int*. 2001; 88:458–66.
15. Small EJ, Frohlich MW, Bok R, et al. Prospective trial of the herbal supplement PS-SPES in patients with progressive prostate cancer. *J Clin Oncol*. 2000; 18:3595–603.
16. Trump DL, Waldstreicher JA, Kolvenbag G, et al. Androgen antagonists: potential role in prostate cancer prevention. *Urology*. 2001; 57(4 suppl 1):64S–7S.
17. Plosker GL, Brogden RN. Leuprorelin. A review of its pharmacology and therapeutic use in prostatic cancer, endometriosis and other sex hormone-related disorders. *Drugs*. 1994; 48:930–67.
18. Gronroos P, Irjala K, Heiskanen J, et al. Using computerized individual medication data to detect drug effects on clinical laboratory tests. *Scan J Clin Lab Invest Suppl*. 1995; 222:31–6.
19. Forsstrom JJ, Gronroos P, Irjala K, et al. Linking patient medication data with laboratory information system. *Int J Biomed Comput*. 1996; 42:111–6.
20. Watanabe AS, McCart G, Shimomura S, et al. Systematic approach to drug information requests. *Am J Hosp Pharm*. 1975; 32:1282–5.
21. Kirkwood CF. Modified systematic approach to answering questions. In: Malone PM, Mosdell KW, Kier KL, et al, eds. *Drug Information: A Guide for Pharmacists*. 2nd ed. Stamford, CT: Appleton & Lange; 2000: 19–30.
22. Greenberg A. Hyperkalemia: treatment options. *Semin Nephrol*. 1998; 18:46–57.
23. Borron SW, Bismuth C, Muszynski J. Advances in the management of digoxin toxicity in the older patient. *Drugs Aging*. 1997; 10:18–33.
24. Neu HC. Carbenicillin and ticarcillin. *Med Clin North Am*. 1982; 66:61–77.

Chapter **5**

SUBSTANCE ABUSE AND TOXICOLOGICAL TESTS

Peter A. Chyka

When substance abuse, poisoning, or overdose is suspected, the testing of biological specimens is crucial for characterizing usage or exposure, monitoring therapy or abstinence, or aiding in diagnosis or treatment. According to the 2001 National Household Survey on Drug Abuse, 15.9 million Americans age 12 years and older (7.1% of the population) reported using an illicit drug in the past month and 12.6% reported illicit drug use during the past year (Table 5-1).[1] Each year an estimated 600,000 drug abuse episodes, not including alcohol alone, are treated in emergency departments (ED),[2] and annually 1.4 million people are arrested for driving under the influence in the United States.[3] In 2001, 11.1% of Americans (25.1 million persons) reported driving under the influence of alcohol at least once during the past year.[1]

Poison control centers document approximately 2 million unintentional and intentional poisonings each year with one-half occurring in children under 6 years of age (Table 5-2).[4] Workplace substance abuse has been estimated to involve 6.3 million (7.7%) full-time workers between the ages of 18 and 49 years with an equal number claiming heavy use of alcohol (Table 5-3).[5] In 1997, about 1.6 million full-time workers were both current illicit drug users and heavy alcohol users. For eighth, tenth, and twelfth grade students, the lifetime prevalence of the use of illicit drugs was 24.5%, 44.6% and 53.0%, respectively, during 2002 from a variety of substances (Table 5-4).[6]

Of adult arrestees in 33 US sites, approximately 64% tested positive for at least one of the following drugs: cocaine, opiates, marijuana, methamphetamine, or phencyclidine.[3] Marijuana was most common in male arrestees, whereas cocaine was most common in women. In 2001, 16.6 million Americans (7.3% of the population) admitted to substance dependence or abuse.[1,2] During 2001, 20,230 people died from poisoning or overdose with 69 deaths (0.3%) occurring in children under 5 years of age.[7]

There is no comprehensive tabulation of all incidents of substance abuse or poisoning, and the available databases have strengths and weaknesses.[8,9] Nevertheless, substance abuse

TABLE 5-1

SUBSTANCE	PAST YEAR (%)	PAST MONTH (%)
Any Illicit Drug	12.6	7.1
Marijuana and Hashish	9.3	5.4
Cocaine	1.9	0.7
Crack	0.5	0.2
Heroin	0.2	0.1
Hallucinogens	2.0	0.6
LSD	0.7	0.1
Phencyclidine (PCP)	0.1	0.0
MDMA (Ecstasy)	1.4	0.3
Inhalants	0.9	0.2
Any Illicit Drug Other Than Marijuana	7.0	3.1
Nonmedical Use of Any		
Psychotherapeutic drug	4.9	2.1
Pain Reliever	3.7	1.6
Tranquilizer	1.6	0.6
Stimulant	1.1	0.5
Methamphetamine	0.6	0.3
Sedative	0.4	0.1

Table 5-1. Americans Age 12 Years or Older Reporting Use of Illicit Drugs during 2001 (Percentage of the Total Population)[1]

TABLE 5-2

ALL EXPOSURES	CHILDREN (UNDER 6 YEARS)	ADULTS (OVER 19 YEARS)	FATALITIES
Analgesics	Cosmetics and personal care products	Analgesics	Analgesics
Cleaning substances	Cleaning substances	Sedative drugs	Sedative drugs
Cosmetics and personal care products	Analgesics	Cleaning substances	Antidepressant drugs
Foreign bodies	Foreign bodies	Antidepressant drugs	Stimulant and street drugs
Plants	Topical drugs	Bites and envenomations	Cardiovascular drugs
Sedative drugs	Plants	Alcohols	Alcohols
Cough and cold drugs	Cough and cold drugs	Food products	Chemicals
Topical drugs	Pesticides	Cosmetics and personal care products	Anticonvulsants
Bites and envenomations	Vitamins	Pesticides	Gases and fumes
Antidepressant drugs	Gastrointestinal drugs	Chemicals	Antihistamine drugs
Pesticides	Antimicrobial drugs	Cardiovascular drugs	Muscle relaxant drugs
Food products	Arts, crafts, and office	Gases and fumes supplies	Hormones and antagonists

[a]In decreasing order of frequency and based on 2,267,979 poison exposures.
[b]Reprinted, with permission, from Reference 4.

Table 5-2. Ranking of Twelve Most Frequent Poison Exposure Categories Reported to US Poison Control Centers during 2001[a,b]

and poisoning are common problems facing health care professionals, law enforcement officials, employers, teachers, family members, and individuals throughout society. The detection and management of these incidents often involves laboratory testing and interpretation of the results. This chapter will focus on urine drug testing and serum drug concentration determinations as a means to aid the management of substance abuse and poisoning.

OBJECTIVES

After completing this chapter, the reader should be able to

1. List the testing methods used in substance abuse and toxicological screening and discuss their limitations.
2. Compare the value of preliminary and confirmatory urine drug tests.
3. Discuss the considerations in interpreting a positive and negative drug screen result.
4. Discuss why interfering substances can cause both false-negative and false-positive results of screening tests.
5. Recognize the value of serum drug concentration in the evaluation and treatment of a patient who has a suspected poisoning or overdose.
6. Describe how the pharmacokinetics of a drug on overdose may affect the interpretation of serum concentrations.
7. Discuss how toxicologic analyses may be helpful in medicolegal situations, postmortem applications, and athletic competition.

TABLE 5-3

SUBSTANCE	PERCENT
Heavy alcohol use[a]	7.6
Marijuana	6.0
Psychotherapeutics	1.5
Cocaine	0.8
Hallucinogens	0.8
Inhalants	0.3
Heroin	0.1
Any illicit drug other than marijuana and alcohol	2.9
Any illicit drug other than alcohol	7.7

[a]Five or more drinks per occasion on 5 or more days.

Table 5-3. Full-Time Workers, 18–49 Years of Age, Reporting Current Illicit Drug Use during 1997 (Percentage of Workers)[5]

URINE DRUG SCREENS

Objectives of Analysis

A drug screen is a qualitative test to determine the presence of a specific substance or group of substances. This determination is also called a *toxicology screen* or *tox screen*. Urine is the specimen of choice, and it is widely used for most situations requiring a drug screen. The collection of urine is generally noninvasive and can be collected following urinary catherization in unresponsive patients. Adequate urine samples of 20–100 mL are easily collected. Most drugs and their metabolites are excreted and concentrated in urine. They are also stable in frozen urine allowing long-term storage for batched analyses or reanalysis. Urine is a relatively clean matrix for analysis due to the usual absence of protein and cellular components, thereby eliminating preparatory steps for analysis.[10–15]

TABLE 5-4

SUBSTANCE	PAST YEAR (%)	EVER (%)
Any illicit drug	41.0	53.0
Marijuana and hashish	36.2	47.8
Cocaine	5.0	7.8
Crack	2.3	3.8
Amphetamines	11.1	16.8
Methamphetamine	3.6	6.7
Hallucinogens	6.6	12.0
LSD	3.5	8.4
Phencyclidine (PCP)	1.1	3.1
MDMA (Ecstasy)	7.4	10.5
Inhalants	4.5	11.7
Androgenic anabolic steroids	2.5	4.0
Heroin	1.0	1.7
Alcohol (to a drunken condition)	50.4	61.6

Table 5-4. Categories of Substances Abused as Claimed by High School Seniors during 2002 Survey (Percentage of Survey Respondents)[6]

A urine drug screen result does not provide an exact determination of how much of the substance is present in the urine. However, concentrations of the substance are measured by urine drug screen assays in the process of determining whether the drug is present in a significant amount to render the test as positive. For each substance, the test has performance standards established by the intrinsic specificity and sensitivity of the analytical process that are linked to regulatory or clinical thresholds, commonly called *cutoff values*. These thresholds are a balance of the actual analytical performance, likelihood for interfering substances, and the potential for false positives, which together suggest that the substance is actually present in the urine. Cutoff values may be set by an individual laboratory to meet regulatory or clinical needs or by purchasing immunoassay kits with the desired cutoff values.

Regulatory cutoff values are typically used to monitor people in the workplace or patients undergoing substance abuse therapy. The Substance Abuse and Mental Health Services Administration (SAMHSA) in the Department of Health and Human Services specifies cutoff values and requires that five categories be routinely included in urine screens (Table 5-5).[16] In hospital and forensic settings, cut-off values are sometimes lowered relative to workplace values in order to detect more positive results, which can serve as an aid in

TABLE 5-5

DRUG	INITIAL TEST (ng/mL)	CONFIRMATORY TEST (ng/mL)
Amphetamines	1000	
Amphetamine		500
Methamphetamine		500[b]
Cocaine metabolites	300	150[c]
Marijuana metabolites	50	15[d]
Opiate metabolites	2000	
Morphine		2000
Codeine		2000
6-Acetylmorphine		10[e]
Phencyclidine	25	25

[a]*Standards issued by Substance Abuse Mental Health Services Administration on November 1, 2001 for urine specimens collected by federal agencies and by employers regulated by the Department of Transportation; check website for changes (http://workplace.samhsa.gov).*
[b]*Specimen must also contain amphetamine at a concentration of 200 ng/mL or more.*
[c]*Metabolite as benzoylecgonine.*
[d]*Metabolite as delta-9-tetrahydrocannabinol-9-carboxylic acid.*
[e]*Test specimen for 6-Acetylmorphine (a specific heroin metabolite) when morphine concentration exceeds 2000 ng/mL.*

Table 5-5. Federal Cutoff Concentrations for Urine Drug Tests[16,a]

verifying or detecting an overdose or poisoning.[12–14,17] Reports of urine drug screen results will often list the cutoff value for a substance and whether the substance was detected at the specified value.

General Analytical Techniques

There is no standardized urine drug screen that employs the same panel of tested drugs, analytical techniques, or turnaround times. There is some commonality among laboratories, but tests differ by individual laboratory. Generally, urine drug screens are categorized by level of sensitivity of the analytical technique (preliminary vs. confirmatory) and by the variety of drugs tested (Tier I or focused vs. Tier II or broad).[11,14,17] Preliminary tests, also known as *initial, provisional,* or *stat* urine drug screens, typically employ one of six currently available immunoassays (EMIT, KIMS, CEDIA, RIA, FPIA, or ELISA) (see Chapter 1).

Clinical laboratories often add several spectrophotometric assays to test for substances, such as salicylates and ethanol, to the panel of immunoassays. Immunoassays can readily be performed on autoanalyzers that are available in most hospitals. These assays are available for many substances of abuse, and results can be reported within 1–2 hr.[13,17] Unfortunately, the result of an immunoassay is preliminary due to compromises in specificity that lead to cross-reactivity, particularly with amphetamines and opiates. A preliminary urine drug screen result cannot stand alone for medicolegal purposes and must be confirmed with another type of analysis that is more specific.[10,11,18] For clinical purposes, some laboratories routinely confirm the results of preliminary drug screens, but others do so only on request of the physician. The need for confirming preliminary test results is based on several factors: whether the result would affect the patient's care; whether the patient is expected to be discharged by the time the results are known; and whether the cost justifies the possible outcome.

Confirmatory techniques are more specific than preliminary tests and utilize another analytical technique.[11,14,17] These tests include high-performance liquid chromatography, gas chromatography, or mass spectrometry, depending on the substances being confirmed (see Chapter 1). The "gold standard" of confirmatory tests is the combination of gas chromatography and mass spectrometry, often referred to as *GC mass spec* or *GC-MS*. Compared to preliminary tests, these techniques are more time consuming, more costly, require greater technical expertise, and require greater time for analysis—often several hours to days. Most hospital clinical laboratories do not have the capability to perform confirmatory tests and must send the specimen to a local reference laboratory or a regional laboratory. Transportation of the specimen will add to the delay in obtaining results. Confirmatory tests are routinely performed for workplace settings and forensic and medicolegal purposes, and the delay is often less critical than in clinical settings.[10,18]

KISHA, A 21-YEAR-OLD COLLEGE STUDENT, is brought to the emergency department by her family because of bizarre behavior. She is having visual hallucinations and is paranoid and jittery. She is clinically dehydrated, tachycardic, and delirious. A stat preliminary urine drug screen is positive for amphetamines.

Question: Is this student abusing amphetamine?

Discussion: Amphetamine abuse is possible, but alternative causes should be considered. Her parents report that Kisha has just completed a week of final exams, is taking a full course load, and is working two jobs. She is described as studious and a compulsive achiever. After 18 hr of supportive therapy, rest, and IV fluids, she is lucid and confesses to using large quantities of nonprescription diet pills and energy drinks to stay awake for 5 days. A targeted confirmatory screen for amphetamines was negative for amphetamines and methamphetamine. Urine drug screens by immunoassay for amphetamines are subject to cross-reactivity with several sympathomimetic amine-type drugs (e.g., pseudoephedrine and ephedrine) and dietary supplements marketed for energy and weight loss, which would cause a false positive for amphetamines.

The inclusion of a substance on a drug screen is also subject to individual laboratory discretion. Workplace and substance abuse monitoring programs are required to test for five categories of substances (marijuana metabolites, cocaine metabolites, opiate metabolites, phencyclidine, and amphetamines) as specified by the Substance Abuse and Mental Health Services Administration,[10] sometimes referred to as the *SAMHSA 5*. Most immunoassay manufacturers design the range of assays to meet this need and offer additional categories that a laboratory may choose to include. The high expense of developing an immunoassay is balanced with the promise of economic recovery with widespread utilization. This economic reality precludes the development of a test for emerging substances of abuse, such as ketamine and gamma hydroxybutyrate, and life-threatening—albeit infrequent—overdoses, such as calcium channel antagonists and beta adrenergic blockers.[17] Techniques used for confirmatory tests would be required to detect many of the substances not included in the panel of the preliminary drug screen.

MINICASE 2

FRANK, A 51-YEAR-OLD MALE, is dropped off at an emergency department in the late evening after he became progressively more unresponsive in a hotel room. His acquaintances do not know his medical history, but eventually admit that he had injected some drugs. They promptly leave the area. Frank is unconscious with some response to painful stimuli and exhibits pinpoint pupils and depressed respirations at 12 breaths/min. His other vital signs are satisfactory. Oxygen administration and intravenous fluids are started. A bedside stat glucose determination yields a result of 60 mg/dL. A 50-mL intravenous bolus of dextrose 50% is administered with no change in his level of consciousness. Naloxone 2 mg is given IV push, and within minutes Frank awakens, begins talking, and exhibits an improved respiratory rate. He admits to injecting several crushed oxycodone tablets that he had dissolved in tap water shortly before he was dropped off at the ED. In addition to routine laboratory assessment, a serum acetaminophen concentration is determined. During the next 24 hr, he receives supportive care in the critical care unit and requires two additional doses of naloxone. He is scheduled for a psychiatric evaluation to assess treatment options for his substance abuse, but he walks out of the hospital against medical advice on the second day. A urine drug screen by immunoassay that was obtained in the ED is reported as positive for opiates, marijuana, and amphetamines on the morning of his second day of hospitalization.

Question: Was a urine drug screen necessary for the immediate care of this patient? How is a urine drug screen helpful in this type of situation?

Discussion: In emergent situations like this one that involve an apparent acute opiate overdose, the results of a urine drug screen are not necessary for immediate evaluation and effective treatment. The symptoms and history clearly indicate that an opiate overdose is very likely. The response to naloxone confirms that an opiate is responsible for the CNS depressant effects. Since immediate treatment was necessary, waiting for the results of the preliminary drug screen, even if it was reported within hours, would not change the use of supportive care, glucose, and naloxone. The urine drug screen may be helpful to confirm the diagnosis for the record and to assist in guiding substance abuse treatment. Several additional issues to be considered in Frank's overall health care include the risk of local or systemic infections from intravenous drug abuse, emboli from undissolved tablet particles, and health effects from abusing multiple drugs. The serum acetaminophen concentration is important in determining cases of intentional drug use (suicide attempt and substance abuse). This practice is particularly important in situations of a multiple drug exposure, an unknown drug exposure, or when acetaminophen may be contained in a multiple-ingredient oral drug product (e.g., analgesics, cough and cold medicines, sleep aids, and nonprescription allergy medicines). A serum specimen is needed because acetaminophen is not part of routine urine drug screens, and serum assays on acetaminophen generally have a quick turnaround time so they can be used clinically to assess the potential severity of the exposure.

Common Applications

The purpose of a urine drug screen depends on the circumstances for its use, the condition of the patient, and the setting of the test. In an emergency department where a patient is being evaluated for a poisoning or overdose, the primary purposes are to verify substances claimed to be taken by the patient and to identify other toxins that could be likely causes of the poisoning or symptoms.[12,13] This is particularly important when the patient has altered mental status and cannot give a clear history or is experiencing nondrug causes of coma, such as traumatic head injury or stroke. The value of routinely performing urine drug screens in the ED for patients who overdose has been questioned. The benefits include having objective evidence of the toxin's presence to confirm the exposure; suggesting alternative toxins in the diagnosis; ruling out a toxin as a cause of symptoms of unknown etiology; and providing medicolegal documentation. The disadvantages include being misled by false-positive results; impractical delays in receiving the results that do not influence therapy; and limited practical value because many poisonings can be recognized by a collection of signs and symptoms.[19]

The American College of Emergency Physicians states in a clinical policy on the immediate treatment of poisonings[20] that "qualitative toxicologic screening tests rarely assist the emergency physician in patient management." Urine drug testing can be important with substances exhibiting delayed onset of toxic symptoms, such as sustained release products, when patients ingest multiple agents, or when patients are found with multiple agents at the scene. Some trauma centers routinely perform urine drug screens on newly admitted patients, but the value of this practice has also been questioned.[21] Suicidal and substance-abusing patients are poor or misleading historians, whereby the amounts, number of substances, and routes of exposure can be exaggerated or downplayed. A urine drug screen may assist in identifying potential substances involved in these cases and lead to specific monitoring or treatment.

In the workplace, the purpose of a urine drug screen may include pre-employment tests, monitoring during work, postaccident evaluation, and substance abuse treatment monitoring.[10,18] Employers who conduct pre-employment urine drug tests will generally make hiring contingent on a negative test result. Many positions in the health care industry require pre-employment drug tests, and some employers perform random tests for employees in positions requiring safety or security as a means to deter drug use and abuse that could affect performance. In addition to random tests, some employers test individuals based on a reasonable suspicion of substance abuse such as evidence of use or possession, unusual or erratic behavior, or arrests for drug-related crimes. For employees involved in a serious accident, employers may test for substances when there is suspicion of use—to determine whether substance abuse was a factor—or as a necessity for legal or insurance purposes. Employees who return to work following treatment for substance abuse are often randomly tested as one of their conditions for continued employment or licensure. In the workplace setting, specific procedures must be followed to ensure that the rights of employees and employers are observed.

The Division of Workplace Programs of the Substance Abuse and Mental Health Services Administration specifies guidelines for procedures, due process and the appeals process, and lists certified laboratories.[10] Two critical elements of workplace drug testing include establishing a chain of custody and control for the specimen and involving a medical review officer to interpret positive test results. The chain of custody starts with close observation of urine collection. Patients are required to empty their pockets, and they are placed in a collection room without running water and where blue dye has been added to the toilet water. These measures minimize the risk of adulteration or dilution of the urine sample. After the urine is placed in the container, the temperature is taken, the container is sealed, and the chain-of-custody documentation is completed. After the chain-of-custody form is completed by everyone in possession of the specimen, it reaches the laboratory where the seal is broken and further procedures are observed. Positive specimens are often frozen for 1 year or longer if requested by the client or if the results are contested by a court. Chain-of-custody procedures are time-consuming and are not typically considered in the clinical management of poisonings and overdoses, but they are important to sustain the validity of the sample and its result in a court of law.[10,18]

JUAN, A 35-YEAR-OLD PHARMACIST, applies for a position at a hospital pharmacy. As part of his pre-employment evaluation, he is asked to provide a urine specimen in a specially designed room for drug testing. His urine sample is positive for opiates and marijuana by immunoassay. His case is referred to the hospital's medical review officer for a review of the findings. The physician orders a confirmatory test on the same urine specimen. The human resources department of the hospital learns from his current employer that he is an above average worker with no history of substance abuse. A check with the law enforcement authorities is negative for any criminal record. The MRO contacts Juan and learns that he was taking acetaminophen and codeine prescribed for pain from suturing of a laceration of his hand for 2 days prior to drug testing. He also routinely takes naproxen for arthritis in his knees. He had forgotten to list the recent use of these drugs on his employment application because his injured hand began to ache while writing.

Question: Has this pharmacist used any drugs or substances that should prevent him from being considered for employment?

Discussion: Consideration of several factors is important in interpreting the urine drug screen result in this case. The job applicant has no obvious symptoms of intoxication and has a good employment record. It is likely that the codeine prescribed for pain control produced the positive opiate result. This drug is being used for a legitimate purpose with a valid prescription. The positive for marijuana is likely from the pharmacist's use of naproxen causing a false-positive result. The confirmatory test by GC-MS was negative for marijuana, but it was positive for codeine and morphine. Codeine is metabolized in part to morphine. The MRO reviewing this applicant's case would likely conclude that the test results are not indicative of opioid abuse and the marijuana immunoassay result was a false positive. If there were concerns about his suitability for employment, Juan may be subjected to an unannounced drug test during his probationary employment period. Acetaminophen and naproxen were not reported as a result, because they were not on the routine assay panel.

A medical review officer is typically a physician trained in this specialty who has responsibility to determine whether the result of the drug test is related to substance abuse.[18,22] The job often involves interviewing the donor; reviewing their therapeutic drug regimen; reviewing possible extraneous causes of a positive result, such as a false-positive result from a prescribed medication or substance interfering with the analytical test; rendering an opinion on the validity of the test result; considering a retest of the donor or the same specimen; reporting the result to the employer; and maintaining confidential records. This individualized interpretation is not only critical because people's careers, reputations, livelihood, and legal status can be affected, but also because it is a regulatory requirement.

Drug screening is also used in the criminal justice system for several purposes such as informing judges for bail-setting and sentencing, monitoring whether specified drug abstinence is being observed, and identifying individuals in need of treatment.[23] For example, a positive drug test at the time of arrest may identify substance abusers who need medical treatment prior to incarceration, which may result in a pretrial release condition that incorporates periodic drug testing. If a defendant is being monitored while on parole or work release, a drug screen can verify that he or she is remaining drug-free. Drug tests in prisons can also assist in monitoring substance use in jail.

The impact of a drug screen result can be profound if it affects decisions of medical care, employment, legal importance, and a person's reputation. In addition, several factors can affect the reliability and interpretation of drug screen results. These issues should be considered when evaluating a drug screen and are described in the following section.

TABLE 5-6

- Androgenic anabolic steroids
- Angiotensin converting enzyme inhibitors
- Animal venoms
- Antidysrhythmic drugs
- Anticoagulant drugs and rodenticides
- Beta-adrenergic agonists
- Beta-adrenergic antagonists
- Calcium channel antagonists
- Carbon monoxide
- Chem-bioterrorism agents
- Clonidine
- Colchicine
- Dietary supplements[a]
- Ergot alkaloids
- Hydrocarbon solvents and inhalants
- Ethylene glycol
- Gamma-hydroxybutyrate
- Heavy metals (lead, arsenic, and mercury)[b]
- Iron
- Lithium
- Methemoglobin producing agents
- Methylphenidate
- Pesticides
- Plant toxins
- Selective serotonin reuptake inhibitors

[a]Those without chemically similar drug counterparts are not detected on a drug screen.
[b]Heavy metals will require a special collection container, collection duration, and assay.

Table 5-6. Drugs and Chemicals Often Not Detected by Routine Drug Screens

Unique Considerations

When a urine drug screen is reported as negative, it does not mean that the drug was not present or not taken—it means that it was not detected. The drug in question may not be part of a testing panel of the particular drug screen (Table 5-6). For example, meperidine, propoxyphene, and pentazocine are not detected on current opioid immunoassays.[13,17] Likewise, the urine may be too dilute for detection of the substance. This may be due renal disease, intentional dilution to avoid detection, or administration of large volumes of intravenous fluids as part of a critically ill patient's care. The urine may have been collected before the drug was excreted, but this is unlikely in symptomatic acute overdoses or poisonings. The time that an individual tests positive (i.e., the drug detection time) depends on pharmacologic factors including dose, route of administration, rates of metabolism and elimination, and analytical factors (e.g., sensitivity, specificity, and accuracy). In some cases, the urine sample may have been intentionally adulterated to mask or avoid detection. This is more common in workplace testing than in critical care settings.

Adulteration of a urine sample either intentionally or unintentionally can lead to negative or false-positive results through several means.[10,24] A freshly voided urine sample may be replaced with a drug-free sample when urine collection is not directly observed. The ingestion of large volumes of water with or without a diuretic may dilute or enhance the elimination of a drug, thereby reducing the concentration of the urine below the assay detection limit. Urine specimens for workplace testing will often be immediately tested for temperature and later tested for creatinine content and specific gravity in order to detect water dilution of the sample.

Adding a chemical to a urine sample may invalidate some test results. Adulteration products that are available through the Internet contain chemicals such as soaps, glutaraldehyde, nitrites, other oxidants, and hydrochloric acid. Depending on the assay method and test, these substances may interfere with absorbance rates, produce false-positive or false-negative results, or oxidize metabolites that are measured in the immunoassay. For example, some chromate- and peroxidase-based oxidizers will degrade 9-carboxy-tetrahydrocannabinol, a principal metabolite of tetrahydrocannabinol, and lead to a negative result for marijuana.[18,24] The effects of adulterants vary with the immunoassay technique and the specific test used by the laboratory; they are not reliable ways to mask drug use. Most adulterants do not affect the GC/MS analysis for drugs in urine, but such a confirmatory step would be ordered only if there was a high suspicion of adulteration. A positive immunoassay result is typically used to justify the use of a confirmatory GC/MS analysis.

A positive drug test can show the presence of specific drugs in urine at the detectable level of the test. It does not indicate the dosage, when the drug was administered, how it was administered, or the degree of impairment. Many drugs can be detected in urine for up to 3 days after being taken and some up to 2 weeks or more (Table 5-7).[11–15,18,25] It is possible for a legitimate substance in the urine to interact with the immunoassay and produce a false-positive result.

Exposure to interfering substances can affect the results of an immunoassay urine drug screen (Table 5-7). A positive immunoassay result for opiates may result from the ingestion of pastries containing poppy seeds because they contain codeine and morphine in small, but sufficient, amounts to render the test positive. The result is a true positive, but not a positive indicator of drug abuse. The immunoassay for amphetamines is prone to false-positive re-

TABLE 5-7

DRUG	DETECTION TIME	POTENTIAL FALSE-POSITIVE AGENTS AND COMMENTS
Amphetamines	2–5 days; up to 2 weeks with prolonged or heavy use	Ephedrine, pseudoephedrine, ephedra (ma huang), phenylephrine, desoxyephedrine, selegiline, chlorpromazine, trazodone, bupropion, desipramine, amantadine, ranitidine, phenylpropanolamine, brompheniramine, methylenedioxymethamphetamine, propylhexedrine, isometheptene, labetalol, fenfluramine, phentermine, isoxsuprine
Barbiturates	Short-acting, 1–7 days; intermediate-acting, 1–3 weeks	Phenobarbital may be detected up to 4 weeks
Benzodiazepines	Up to 2 weeks; up to 6 weeks with chronic use of some agents	Benzodiazepines vary in cross-reactivity, persistence, and detectability; flunitrazepam may not be detected
Cocaine metabolite (benzoylecgonine)	12–72 hr; up to 1–3 weeks with prolonged or heavy use	Cross-reactivity with cocaethylene varies with the assay because assay is directed to benzoylecgonine; false positives from -caine anesthetics and other drugs are unlikely
Lysergic acid diethylamide (LSD)	24–48 hr typically; up to 120 hr possible	
Marijuana metabolite (delta 9-tetrahydrocannabinol-9-carboxylic acid)	7–10 days; up to 1–2 months with prolonged or heavy use	Ibuprofen, naproxen, efavirenz, hemp seed, hemp oil
Methadone	3–14 days	Doxylamine
Opioids	2–3 days typically; up to 6 days with sustained-release formulations; up to 1 week with prolonged or heavy use	Rifampin, some fluoroquinolones, poppy seeds, quinine in tonic water; assay directed toward morphine with varying cross-reactivity for codeine, oxycodone, hydrocodone, and other semisynthetic opioids; synthetic opioids, (e.g., fentanyl, meperidine, methadone, pentazocine, propoxyphene, and tramadol), have minimal cross-reactivity and may not be detected
Phencyclidine	2–10 days; 1 month or more with prolonged or heavy use	Ketamine, dextromethorphan, diphenhydramine, sertraline
Propoxyphene	3–6 days	

[a]Time after which a drug screen remains positive after last use.
[b]Since performance characteristics may vary with the type of immunoassay, manufacturer, and lot, consult the laboratory technician and package insert for the particular test.
[c]Adapted, with permission, from References 11–15, 18, 25.

Table 5-7. Detection Times and Inferring Substances for Immunoassay Urine Drug Screens[a,b,c]

sults from drugs with similar structures such as phenylpropanolamine (a decongestant no longer on the US market), ephedrine, psuedoephedrine, and buproprion.[13,18] The immunoassay manufacturer's package insert should be consulted for information on known interfering substances. In workplace settings, the medical review officer is obligated to assess whether a person's legitimate drug therapy could interfere with the result.

MINICASE 4

DANNY, A 23-YEAR-OLD ASSEMBLY LINE WORKER at a computer manufacturing facility, is examined by the company's physician within an hour of being involved in a workplace accident. She observes a laceration on his left arm, pupil size of 1–2 mm, bilateral ptosis, and recent punctate lesions on the left antecubital fossa. The rest of the physical exam is unremarkable. Danny denies eating poppy seeds, taking any medication or dietary supplement, or having a neurological condition. He has no history of substance abuse in his files. The physician suspects heroin use and orders a focused urine drug test for opiates. Several days later, the laboratory report indicates positive results for morphine, codeine, and 6-acetylmorphine.

Question: Has this employee used a drug or substance that would impair his ability to work? What, if any, substance is likely?

Discussion: This employee has likely used heroin several hours before the accident and several symptoms are consistent with opiate intoxication. Heroin may not be present in sufficient amounts to be detected, in part, because it is metabolized to several compounds such as morphine and 6-acetylmorphine, which are often detected in the urine of heroin users. Since 6-acetylmorphine is only found in urine following heroin use, its presence eliminates other opiates as possible causes of Danny's symptoms. The presence of small amounts of codeine in heroin abusers is likely from contamination of the heroin with codeine and not as a metabolic by-product.

The persistence of the substance in the urine is an important factor in the interpretation of the results (see Table 5-7).[22] For lab results reported as negative, it may indicate that the specimen was obtained too early or too late after exposure to a chemical, thereby producing a urine specimen with insufficient concentration of the drug to lead to a positive result. Drugs with short half-lives, such as amphetamine, may not be detectable several hours after use. A common concern for individuals undergoing workplace testing is the length of time after use that the drug will still be detectable. This will vary with the sensitivity of the assay; whether the assay is directed to the parent drug or the metabolite; whether the drug or its metabolites exhibits extensive distribution to tissues that will affect its half-life; the dose of the drug taken; and whether the drug was used chronically or only once. For example, cocaine is rarely detected in a urine specimen because of its rapid metabolism. Immunoassays are directed to cocaine metabolites, such as benzoylecgonine, which are detected for up to 2 to 3 days after use and up to 8 days with heavy use. The major active component of marijuana, delta-9-tetrahydrocannabinol, is converted to several metabolites of which delta-9-tetrahydrocannabinol-9-carboxylic acid is the agent to which many immunoassays direct their antibodies for the assay.[13,14] This metabolite is distributed to tissues and can be detected for days to weeks after use.[13] Chronic or heavy use can lead to detection up to a month after stopping use.

For clinical applications, the time it takes for the test result to be reported to the clinician after specimen collection, also known as *turnaround time*, can affect the utility of the drug screen.[17] Many hospital laboratories can perform preliminary immunoassay urine drug screens using AutoAnalyzer technology, which is used for common clinical tests or using dedicated desktop analyzers. Results from in-hospital laboratories can often be returned within 2 hr of collection. For many urgent situations such as an acute overdose or poisoning, this

MINICASE 5

SHELLY, A 46-YEAR-OLD SUPERVISOR for a large utility company, had recently conducted an inspection at a nuclear power plant. She then left for a 2-week vacation with a friend. After returning to work, she is asked to submit a urine sample for drug testing because the company performs random drug tests for compliance with regulatory, insurance, and contractual requirements. A week later, the results of the immunoassay are reported as positive for the cocaine metabolite, benzoylecognine. A confirmatory test by GC-MS confirms the immunoassay result. Shelly is asked to report to the company's medical office. During the interview with the physician she denies illicit drug use, but states that she had dental work performed immediately before returning to work from her vacation and that she had received procaine hydrochloride (Novocain) for local anesthesia.

Question: What caused the positive test result for cocaine?

Discussion: This case illustrates a common, but false, explanation for a positive urine screen for cocaine. Shelly apparently believed that any substance with a name ending in -caine must share chemical similarity with cocaine and could be a probable cause of a false-positive result. While interference with immunoassays is possible, a false positive for cocaine with local anesthetics is not likely. The positive result was confirmed by a confirmatory test that is not subject to this type of interference. With the exception of coca leaf tea, foods as a source of interference may also be eliminated as a cause of the positive test result. In Shelly's case, use of cocaine is the most likely explanation for the positive result.

delay may not affect immediate therapy of the victim. The results may lead to later consideration of alternative or additional diagnoses. Most clinics, small hospitals, or specimen collection sites do not possess such capability and must rely on making the specimen a *send out* that is performed at a nearby or regional reference laboratory. The turnaround time from a reference laboratory varies with the laboratory and the need for urgency. Most results for clinical applications are reported within 24–48 hr. However, some results may take up to 3–7 days. In some situations, such as pre-employment workplace testing, this delay is acceptable. The turnaround time for confirmatory testing depends on the laboratory, transportation time from the collection site to the laboratory, the tests being performed or requested, and the need for urgency. The delay could be as short as 24 hr or as long as a month or more, particularly for postmortem samples.

SERUM CONCENTRATIONS

Objectives of Analysis

Quantitative assays determine the concentration of a substance in a biological specimen, typically this involves serum. The availability of serum concentrations for toxins is based on considerations of whether the concentration correlates with an effect; the outcome or need for therapy; the existing use of the assay for another application such as therapeutic drug monitoring; and technical ease of performing the assay. Serum is typically not used for drug screening purposes in clinical or workplace settings.

Many poisonings and overdoses can be adequately managed without quantitative analysis.[9,26,27] A history of the exposure, signs and symptoms, and routinely available clinical tests—such as full blood count, electrolytes, glucose, INR, liver function tests, blood urea nitrogen, serum creatinine, anion gap, serum osmolality and osmolal gap, arterial blood gases, and creatinine kinase—can guide patient management decisions.

Serum concentrations of potential toxins can be complementary to clinical tests or become essential in several situations (Table 5-8).[17,28] A serum concentration can confirm the diagnosis of a poisoning when in doubt or when a quantitative assessment in the serum is important to interpret a qualitative urine drug screen. When there is a relationship between serum concentration and toxicity, a serum concentration can assist in patient evaluation or

TABLE 5-8

ASSAY	INDICATION	TIMING AFTER EXPOSURE	REPEAT SAMPLING	INTERPRETATION
Acetaminophen	Suspected acetaminophen overdose; every intentional overdose where acetaminophen poisoning has not been reliably excluded	At least 4 hr after ingestion	Rarely required unless timing of overdose is uncertain or for sustained-release formulations	Refer to nomogram to assess toxicity and need for N-acetylcysteine; toxic concentrations depend on patient's individual risk factors
Carboxyhemoglobin	Suspected carbon monoxide poisoning or smoke inhalation	Immediate	No	Greater than 20% indicates significant exposure, but there is a poor relationship with severity and outcome
Digoxin	Severe digoxin toxicity and prior to use of digoxin antibodies	Immediate	No	Greater than 2.0 ng/L associated with toxicity, but may be lower with patient risk factors
Ethanol	Undiagnosed coma with widened osmolal gap; prior to anesthesia when ethanol abuse is suspected; assessment for hemodialysis with severe intoxication; monitor ethanol therapy when used as an antidote	Immediate	Every 2–4 hr for monitoring when used as an antidote; repeat following hemodialysis used as treatment for methanol or ethylene glycol poisoning	Target of 100–150 mg/dL when used as an antidote for ethylene glycol or methanol poisoning; greater than 180–200 mg/dL associated with systemic ethanol toxicity in the absence of other agents and in patients without tolerance to ethanol
Iron	Ingestion of greater than 20 mg/kg elemental iron and obtained within 6 hr; symptoms suggesting acute iron toxicity at any time after poisoning	At least 4 hr after overdose	No	Greater than 350–500 µg/dL may be associated with systemic toxicity; greater than 500 µg/dL usually treated with deferoxamine
Lithium	Suspected acute or chronic lithium poisoning	Immediate for suspectd chronic or acute-on-chronic poisoning, or for patients with symptoms suggesting lithium intoxication; after 6 hr for asymptomatic acute overdose	Every 6–12 hr in severe poisoning or following use of a sustained-release formulation until concentrations are falling; after hemodialysis that has been used as treatment for lithium toxicity	Usual therapeutic range 0.6–1.2 mEq/L (mmol/L); varies with the laboratory and patient factors; acute ingestions may achieve high concentrations that may not lead to serious toxicity.
Methemoglobin	Exposure to relevant toxins or sources (e.g., well water) that produce methemoglobinemia	Immediate	Worsening symptoms	Values greater than 20% are associated with hypoxic symptoms but there is poor correlation with clinical severity
Salicylate	Salicylate overdose (acute aspirin dose over 150 mg/kg); ingestion of concentrated methyl salicylate; unidentified poisoning with clinical features suggesting salicylate toxicity (e.g., altered mental status with acid-base disorder)	At least 2 hr if symptomatic; at least 4 hr if asymptomatic	Repeat in 2–4 hr in patients with suspected severe toxicity or enteric-coated aspirin; measurements should be repeated until concentrations are falling	Systemic toxicity usually associated with concentrations greater than 30 mg/dL; severe toxicity usually associated with concentrations greater than 90–100 mg/dL
Theophylline	Signs and symptoms suggesting theophylline toxicity (e.g., vomiting, tremor, tachycardia, seizures)	Immediate if clinical evidence of toxicity is present; at least 4 hr after exposure if asymptomatic	Repeat every 2–4 hr in patients with severe poisoning or concentrations greater than 60 mg/L especially if a sustained-release formulation was ingested	Serious toxicity usually associated with concentrations greater than 35–40 for acute exposures in infants and the elderly; greater than 25–30 mg/L for chronic exposures; greater than 100 mg/L for acute exposures in adults

[a]These concentrations are given for general guidance only. Drug/toxin concentrations may not correlate closely with the severity of poisoning in individual patients and values may vary between laboratories.
[b]Reprinted, with permission, from Reference 28 with adaptations from Reference 29.

Table 5-8. Toxicologically Important Serum Concentrations for Selected Agents[28,a,b]

for medicolegal purposes. When sustained release drug formulations have been ingested, serial serum concentrations can indicate when peak serum concentrations have occurred and whether efforts to decontaminate the gastrointestinal tract with activated charcoal or whole bowel irrigation have been achieved. A serum concentration can also be useful in determining when to reinitiate drug therapy after the drug has caused toxicity. For some agents, serum concentrations can guide the decision to use therapies that are often risky, invasive, or expensive such as antidotes (e.g., N-acetylcysteine, digoxin immune antibody, and fomepizole) or treatments (e.g., hemodialysis and hyperbaric oxygen).

General Analytical Techniques

There is no standardized panel of quantitative serum assays for toxicologic use. Tests differ by individual laboratory, but a set of essential tests has been proposed (Table 5-8).[17,28] Generally, serum concentrations utilize existing technologies (e.g., immunoassay, spectrophotometry, gas chromatography, high-performance liquid chromatography, and atomic absorption spectrometry) that are commonly used for therapeutic drug monitoring (see Chapter 1). Assays for carboxyhemoglobin, methemoglobinemia, and serum cholinesterase activity are available in many hospitals.[17] In most toxicological applications, the specimen is usually 5–10 mL of blood in adults (1–5 mL in children depending on the assay) that has been allowed to clot for several minutes. It is then is centrifuged and the clear serum, which is devoid of red blood cells and coagulants, is aspirated and subjected to analysis or frozen for later analysis. The type of test tube, test tube additive, and quantity of blood necessary should be verified with the laboratory prior to blood collection.

Common Applications

Serum concentrations of several drugs and chemicals can be helpful in the assessment of patients who may be poisoned or overdosed and arrive at a hospital for evaluation and treatment. Although general treatment approaches—such as supportive care, resuscitation, symptomatic care, and decontamination—are performed without the need of serum concentrations, the severity of several toxicities are related to serum concentrations (Table 5-8). A more detailed discussion of the toxicity relationships can be found in toxicology references.[9,26,27] The examples of ethanol, salicylates, acetaminophen, and digoxin demonstrate important principles in the application of serum concentrations to toxicity and therapy.

One of the most widely studied and used concentration test result involves blood, serum, or breath ethanol concentrations. Due to the absence of protein binding and small volume of ethanol distribution, the serum concentration generally correlates with many of the acute toxic effects of ethanol as shown in Table 5-9.[29] Regular ethanol use can lead to tolerance, and ethanol concentrations in excess of 4% (400 mg/dL) can easily be tolerated by some patients (e.g, they can make conversation and exhibit stable vital signs).[30,31] Conversely, uninitiated drinkers, such as small children who ingest household products containing ethanol (e.g., cologne and mouthwash) and those who concurrently ingest other CNS depressants, may have an exaggerated effect. Most acute poison-

TABLE 5-9

BLOOD ETHANOL CONCENTRATION	TOXIC EFFECT OR CONSEQUENCE
0.08% (80 mg/dL)	Federal legal definition for driving impairment
0.15% (150 mg/dL)	Euphoria, loss of critical judgment, slurred speech, incoordination, drowsiness
0.2% (200 mg/dL)	Increased incoordination, staggering gait, slurred speech, lethargy, disorientation, visual disturbances (diplopia, reduced acuity and perception)
0.3% (300 mg/dL)	Loss of motor functions, marked decreased response to stimuli, impaired consciousness, marked incoordination and inability to stand or walk, vomiting and incontinence, possible amnesia of the event
0.4% (400 mg/dL) and higher	Comatose, unresponsive to physical stimuli, absent reflexes, unstable vital signs, shallow and decreased respirations, hypotension, hypothermia, potentially lethal

Table 5-9. Relationship of Blood Ethanol Concentration and Toxic Effects[29,32,33]

ings can be managed with supportive and symptomatic care; an unstable patient with exceedingly high ethanol concentrations may be the rare candidate for hemodialysis.[29]

Ethanol concentrations also have medicolegal applications involving driving or work performance and ethanol intake. By 2004, the minimum legal threshold for driving under the influence of ethanol intoxication in the United States will be established at blood ethanol concentrations of 0.08% (equivalent to 0.08 g/dL or 80 mg/dL).[32,33] Some states will use 0.1% up to that time. This value can be determined at the scene or at bedside by a breath alcohol test.[34] The breath alcohol test is based on the assumption that equilibrium exists between ethanol in the blood supply of the lung and the alveolar air at a relatively uniform partition ratio. A number of variables can affect this relationship such as temperature, hematocrit, and sampling technique. The National Highway Traffic and Safety Administration publishes a list of breath alcohol testing devices that conform to their standards (www.nhtsa.gov).

Since ethanol concentrations are reported in several different units for either serum or blood, verification of these issues can be important.[17,35] Further, many hospital-based laboratories perform ethanol determinations on serum and use the units of mg/dL vs. forensic situations that typically use blood and report the value as %, g% or g/dL (all of which are equivalent expressions). Serum concentrations of ethanol are greater than blood concentrations by a median factor of 1.2, which varies with the hematocrit value because of the greater water content of serum compared to whole blood.[13,17] Although legal standards are written in terms of whole blood concentrations, this difference is without clinical significance.

Ethanol is also used as a drug to treat poisonings by methanol (blindness, acidosis, and death) and ethylene glycol (acidosis, renal failure, and death) in order to achieve a consistent concentration near 100 mg/dL.[27] Serial serum ethanol concentrations are obtained to assure that sufficient quantities have been administered to prevent severe toxicities of methanol and ethylene glycol (during therapy, hemodialysis removes ethanol while also removing methanol and ethylene glycol).

An early attempt to correlate serum drug concentrations with acute toxicity over time involved the Done nomogram for salicylate poisoning.[36] Categories of toxicity (mild, moderate, and severe) were demarcated on a semilogrithmic plot of serum salicylate vs. time after ingestion as an aid to interpreting serum concentrations. Given the limited knowledge available at the time, the nomogram was based on several assumptions (zero-order kinetics and back extrapolation of single concentrations to time zero) that were later proven to be false. The nomogram did not guide therapy to any great extent and was not confirmed to be clinically useful in subsequent studies.[37]

Clinical findings such as vital signs, electrolytes, anion gap, and arterial blood gases, which have quick turnaround times in most hospitals, are more direct indicators of salicylate toxicity and are now preferred to the Done nomogram. A patient, with exceedingly high serum salicylate concentrations (in excess of 100 to 120 mg/dL) who is unresponsive to supportive and symptomatic therapy, may benefit from hemodialysis to remove salicylate from the body. Elderly and very young patients with unexplained changes in consciousness, acid-base balance, and respiratory rate who present to an ED could be suffering from unrecognized acute or chronic salicylate poisoning.[38,39] A routine serum salicylate concentration in such patients could determine the contribution of excessive salicylate to their symptoms.

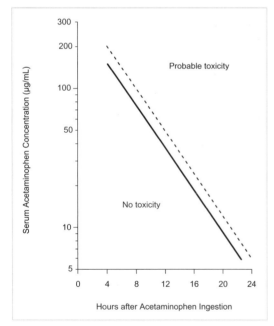

Figure 5-1. Nomogram for prediction of acetaminophen hepatoxicity following acute overdose from nonslow-release oral dosage forms. The lower line (starting at 150 µg/mL at 4 hr) allows a margin for error and should be used as a guide as to whether treatment with N-acetylcysteine is necessary. (Reprinted, with permission, from Reference 40.)

Serum acetaminophen concentrations following acute, large ingestions are essential in assessing the potential severity of poisoning and determining the need for antidotal therapy with N-acetylcysteine. Acetaminophen toxicity differs from many other poisonings in that there is delay of significant symptoms by 1 to 3 days after ingestion, whereas most other poisonings have definite symptoms within 6 hr of exposure.[27] This delay in onset makes it difficult to use signs, symptoms, and clinical diagnostic tests (such as serum transaminase, bilirubin, or INR) as an early means to assess the risk of acetaminophen toxicity.[9] A serum concentration of acetaminophen obtained at least 4 hr after an acute ingestion (Figure 5-1) can be used to assess whether a patient is at risk of developing acetaminophen hepatotoxicity.

The semilogarithmic plot of serum acetaminophen concentration vs. time (also called the Rumack-Matthew nomogram or acetaminophen nomogram) is also used to determine whether there is a need to administer N-acetylcysteine to reduce the risk of toxicity.[40] If the results are not expected to be available within 10 hr of ingestion, N-acetylcysteine is typically administered provisionally and then continued or discontinued based on the serum acetaminophen concentration. In situations when the specimen is sent to a reference laboratory, the results may take several days to be reported, and, consequently, the patient may receive the entire course of therapy that may last for 72 hr. Due to the widespread availability of acetaminophen, it is commonly ingested in suicide attempts. Several professional groups have advocated that all patients who are suspected of intentionally taking drugs should have a serum acetaminophen concentration determined as part of their evaluation in the ED.[17,20,28] In the case of acetaminophen poisoning, the serum concentration becomes a valuable determinant of recognition, therapy, and disposition.

A serum concentration can also guide the utilization or dosage determination of antidotes that are in short supply or are expensive, such as digoxin immune fragment antibody

MINICASE 6

A MOTHER CALLS A POISON CONTROL CENTER about her 16-year-old daughter, Kelly, who has ingested approximately 30 acetaminophen 500-mg tablets 1 hr ago. She thinks that her daughter was "trying to hurt herself." The pharmacist at the poison center refers the patient to the nearest hospital for evaluation due to the amount of acetaminophen and the intent of the ingestion. The mother is asked to bring any medicine to which Kelly may have had access. At the emergency department, Kelly vomits several times but has no other physical complaints or symptoms. A physical exam is unremarkable except for the vomiting. Baseline electrolytes, complete blood count, liver function tests, urine drug screen, and a pregnancy test are ordered. An intravenous line is placed and maintenance intravenous fluids are started. At 4 hr after the acetaminophen ingestion, a blood specimen is drawn to determine the serum acetaminophen concentration. Ninety minutes later, the result is reported as 234 μg/mL.

Question: Is this teenager at risk for acetaminophen hepatotoxicity? Should she be treated with N-acetylcysteine?

Discussion: When the serum acetaminophen concentration of 234 μg/mL is plotted on the acetaminophen nomogram at 4 hr, it is clearly above the treatment line. This indicates that Kelly is at risk for developing hepatotoxicity and that treatment with N-acetylcysteine should be initiated immediately. The dose of acetaminophen that Kelly ingested is also associated with a risk of developing hepatotoxicity, but patients with intentional overdoses (substance abuse or attempted suicide) do not always provide accurate histories. If the results of the acetaminophen assay would not be available within 2 hr of sampling or within 8–10 hr of ingestion, N-acetylcysteine therapy would be started provisionally. After learning the acetaminophen concentration, the decision to continue or stop therapy with N-acetylcysteine could be determined. Since most patients do not exhibit signs and symptoms of acute hepatic injury until 1–3 days after acute acetaminophen overdose, serum transaminase and bilirubin values would not be expected to be abnormal at the time of Kelly's assessment in the ED.

(Digibind and Digifab). Life-threatening acute or chronic digoxin may require the administration of digoxin immune fragment antibody to quickly reverse the toxic effects of digoxin. The dose of digoxin immune fragment antibody can be determined empirically, based on the amount ingested, or by a serum concentration obtained at least 6 hr after acute exposures.[41,42]

Number of vials of digoxin immune fragment antibody = serum concentration of digoxin (µg/mL) × 6 × patient weight (kg)/600.

Once the digoxin immune fragment antibody is administered, the serum concentration of digoxin precipitously rises and has no correlation to the degree of toxicity (Figure 5-2).[41] This sharp increase of digoxin reflects total digoxin (protein-bound and unbound) in the serum that has been redistributed from tissue sites. The digoxin bound to digoxin immune fragment antibody is not toxicologically active, and it is eventually excreted in the urine.

Unique Considerations

The timing of sample collection for poisoned or overdosed patients is variable due to the

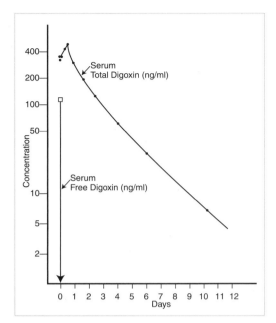

Figure 5-2. Serum digoxin concentrations changed dramatically after administration of digoxin immune fragment antibodies at time zero. Serum free digoxin was greater than 100 ng/mL at the time of administration and decreased to undectable amounts (<0.3 ng/mL) by 1 hr after antibody administration was complete. Serum total digoxin concentration (including that bound to the antibody) increased to >400 ng/mL during the first 12 hr and then fell rapidly. (Reprinted, with permission, from Reference 41.)

varying times of arrival at an ED after the exposure and to the delay in the recognition of poisoning[43] (unless it is obvious from the history or symptoms). Most specimens are collected at the time of admission to the ED except when specified times are important, such as acetaminophen or when adequate absorption has yet to occur (Table 5-8). This variability makes comparison of serum concentrations among patients difficult to clearly establish a relationship with the concentration and toxicity.

The pharmacokinetics of drugs and chemicals on overdose, sometimes termed *toxicokinetics*, can affect interpretation of a serum concentration.[9] Few studies have compared the pharmacokinetics of drugs in therapeutic and toxic doses since toxic doses cannot be administered to human volunteers and overdosed patients are too heterogeneous to make clear assessments.

TABLE 5-10

EFFECT OF OVERDOSAGE[a]	EXAMPLES
Slowed absorption due to formation of poorly soluble semisolid tablet masses in the gastrointestinal tract	Aspirin, lithium, phenytoin, sustained-release theophylline
Slowed absorption due to slowed gastrointestinal motility	Benztropine, nortriptyline
Slowed absorption due to toxin-induced hypoperfusion	Procainamide
Decreased serum protein binding	Lidocaine, salicylates, valproic acid
Increased volume of distribution associated with toxin-induced acidemia	Salicylates
Slowed elimination due to saturation of biotransformation pathways	Ethanol, phenytoin, salicylates, theophylline
Slowed elimination due to toxin-induced hypothermia (<35 °C)	Ethanol, propranolol
Prolonged toxicity due to formation of longer-acting metabolites	Carbamazepine, dapsone, glutethimide, meperidine

[a]*Compared to characteristics following therapeutic doses or resolution of toxicity.*
[b]*Reprinted, with permission, from Reference 9.*

Table 5-10. Influence of Toxicokinetic Changes in Poisoned and Overdosed Patients[b]

Nevertheless, there are several examples where the absorption, distribution, metabolism, and elimination of drugs are different on overdose (Table 5-10). It is difficult to apply pharmacokinetic parameters derived from therapeutic doses to situations when massive overdoses are involved.

Many patients who are poisoned or have overdosed are critically ill, and multiple samples of blood have been obtained for a variety of tests to monitor their condition. When the toxic agent is recognized late in the course of therapy or when serial determinations could be helpful in understanding some aspect of therapy or toxicity, scavenging aliquots of existing serum samples may be helpful for retrospective toxicological analysis. Laboratories often retain serum samples for several days in case a retest is needed so immediate consultation with the clinical laboratory technician is essential in order to save the specimen for testing. Another sample collection technique involves collecting a blood or urine specimen at presentation to the emergency department but not performing the assay. This approach, sometimes called *toxicology hold*, allows collection of specimen at a time when concentrations may be highest even if the need for the assay may not be clear.[13] The specimen can be refrigerated or frozen and assayed on request.

SPECIAL SITUATIONS

Other Biological Specimen

There is great interest in utilizing other biological specimen—such as hair, saliva, perspiration, and expired breath—for quantitative or qualitative analysis.[11,44] These are less invasive than venipuncture and provide unique markers of long-term exposure or use (Table 5-11). Once the technology has been fully validated and sampling techniques refined to minimize interference, there may be applications for point-of-care testing such as drug screens at the bedside and worksite or longitudinal evaluation of chronic use (e.g., cocaine and marijuana in hair samples).[45] To date, the Substance Abuse and Mental Health Services Administration has not accepted these alternative specimen for it regulatory requirements. Several point-of-care urine drug tests are available but have similar or inferior performance to immunoassays.[46] The most common application to date has been breath alcohol determination to assess driving impairment from ethanol use at the scene of an accident or arrest.[34]

Forensic and Legal Issues

In addition to clinical and regulatory applications for urine drug screens and serum drug concentrations, toxicological analysis has an important role in providing evidence for suspected cases of homicide, suicide, child abuse, drug-aided sexual assault (e.g., date rape), environmental contamination, malpractice, workers' compensation, insurance claims, and product liability litigation. Chemical exposure monitoring of workers or the work environment requires specialized approaches such as long-term, on-site monitoring by an industrial hygiene specialist. Toxicological tests are also important in establishing brain death in patients being considered for organ donation or to remove life support. It is important to establish that the apparent vegetative or unresponsive state is not due to drugs. Whenever legal action is anticipated, it is necessary to maintain a specimen chain of custody that can be documented as part of the evidence presentation.[13]

Postmortem analysis of biological specimen, such as gastric contents, organs, vitreous humor, bile, blood, and urine, can assist in the cause of death. These specimen are often collected at the time of autopsy which may be weeks after death. The study of the changes that occur in drug distribution and metabolism after death has been called *postmortem toxicology* or *necrokinetics*. In addition to diffusion of some drugs to or from tissues and blood after death, the effects of putrefaction, fluid shifts on drug concentrations, and chemical stability

	TYPE OF TEST	STRENGTHS	WEAKNESSES	DETECTION TIMES
TABLE 5-11	Urine	• Highest assurance of reliable results • Least expensive • Most flexibility in testing different drugs, including alcohol and nicotine • Most likely of all drug-testing methods to withstand legal challenge	• Specimen can be adulterated, substituted, or diluted • Limited window of detection • Test sometimes viewed as invasive or embarrassing • Biological hazard for specimen handling and shipping to lab	• Typically 1–5 days
	Hair	• Longer window of detection • Greater stability (does not deteriorate) • Can measure chronic drug use • Convenient shipping and storage (no need to refrigerate) • Collection procedure not considered invasive or embarrassing • More difficult to adulterate than urine • Detects alcohol/cocaine combination use	• More expensive • Test usually limited to basic 5-drug panel • Cannot detect alcohol use • Will not detect very recent drug use (1–7 days prior to test)	• Depends on the length of hair in the sample; hair grows about a half-inch per month, so a $1\frac{1}{2}$ inch specimen would show a 3-month history
	Oral fluids (saliva)	• Sample obtained under direct observation • Minimal risk of tampering • Noninvasive • Samples can be collected easily in virtually any environment • Can detect alcohol use • Reflects recent drug use	• Drugs and drug metabolites do not remain in oral fluids as long as they do in urine • Less efficient than other testing methods in detecting marijuana use	• Approximately 10–24 hr
	Sweat patch	• Noninvasive • Variable removal date (generally 1–7 days) • Quick application and removal • Longer window of detection than urine • No sample substitution possible	• Limited number of labs able to process results • People with skin eruptions, excessive hair, or cuts and abrasions cannot wear the patch • Passive exposure to drugs may contaminate patch and affect results	• Patch retains evidence of drug use for at least 7 days, and can detect even low levels of drugs 2–5 hr after last use

Table 5-11. Characteristics of Selected Specimens for Toxicological Analysis[44]

need to be considered. This is an evolving field of study, which has already demonstrated that postmortem drug concentrations from various biological specimens may not always be appropriately referenced to drug concentration results derived from living humans.[47–49]

Pediatrics

The toxicological testing of newborn babies, preschool-age poisoning victims, and adolescents involves several unique ethical, technical, and societal concerns. Intrauterine drug exposure can lead to medical complications of newborns and such abuse may be confirmed by drug screens. When mothers do not admit to prepartal drug use, the routine screening of a newborn's urine or meconium poses economic and practical challenges, such as difficulty in obtaining an adequate urine sample from a neonate and the preanalytical processing of meconium to make it suitable for analysis. Guidelines for newborn urine drug testing involve consideration of maternal and neonatal risk factors.[50]

The use of urine drug screens in the ED provide minimally useful information because the offending agent is typically known and attempts at concealment are infrequent.[51] However, a broad or focused drug screen may be helpful for cases of suspected child abuse by poisoning or when the history of the poisoning is unclear.[52]

Prerequisite drug testing of adolescents for participation in school activities and routine screening by school officials, concerned parents, and pediatricians, presents several ethical dilemmas. Parents and school officials want assurance that substance abuse is not occurring, but the confidentiality and consent of the adolescent should be recognized. The American Academy of Pediatrics[53] states that "involuntary, (mass, nonsuspicion-based, drug) testing is not appropriate in adolescents with decisional capacity—even with parental consent—and should be performed only if there is a strong medical or legal reason to do so." This policy statement is at odds with the desire of some parent groups[54] to perform such tests without the adolescent's consent and with court rulings upholding a school's ability to perform mass or random drug tests of its students.[44] Drug use in school-age children has been associated with a variety of risk taking behaviors, such as carrying a gun, engaging in unprotected sexual intercourse with multiple partners, and suffering injury from a physical fight.[55] These behaviors may indicate the need for monitoring drug abuse.

Sports and Drugs

Drugs have been used by amateur and professional athletes in hopes of enhancing athletic performance and by nonathletes to improve physical appearance. An estimated 5% of high school students have used androgenic anabolic steroids; of these students, 16–36% do not participate in sports but use steroids to change their appearance.[56–58] The types and variety of substances are typically different from those encountered in poisonings or substance abuse. Most workplace or clinical drug screens will not detect athletic performance enhancing drugs such as anabolic androgenic steroids, growth hormone, and erythroid-stimulating agents.[59] The international term for drug use in sports is *doping* and efforts to combat this practice are referred to as *doping control* or *antidoping*.[56,59]

Governing athletic organizations, such as the International Olympic Committee, the United States Olympic Committee, and the National Collegiate Athletic Association, have established policies and analytical procedures for testing athletes as well as lists of banned substances.[60] The technical and scientific challenges in detecting many of these substances are unique to this field.[59] The World Antidoping Agency has plans for all organized sports programs to standardize analytical tests, banned substances, and screening procedures. Using banned drugs can result in an unfair, artificial advantage for competitive athletes and physical injury or permanent disability from the drug's effects, such as those from anabolic steroids and ephedra.[57]

SUMMARY

Testing for substance abuse, poisonings, and overdose affects society at several levels. Knowledge of assay limitations, sampling procedures, interfering substances, patient factors, and regulatory requirements will aid in the interpretation of the value of the test and its clinical relevance. In this chapter, several approaches and applications are discussed, but other situations that involve potential toxins—such as environmental contamination, chemical terrorism,[61–64] and product safety testing—call for different approaches and pose unique challenges.

Sources of Information

Since test characteristics vary with the type of test, manufacturer, assay kit, setting, and application, information about a specific test is critical for proper utilization and interpretation. Good communication with laboratory technicians is an important first step in assuring proper testing. Laboratory technicians can provide guidance on sample collection, cutoff values, interfering substances, and other technical aspects. The package insert for immunoassays or other commercial assay kits is an important and specific guide to assay performance and known interfering substances with the specific assay. There are several textbooks that can be helpful in understanding techniques, values, and interfering substance and test availability.[65–67] Health care professionals in poison control centers (list available at www.aapcc.org or contact your local program at 1-800-222-1222 nationwide) can also provide useful information on laboratory tests particularly as they relate to poisonings. There is also a wealth of information in governmental publications of which many are available at Internet websites of governmental agencies such as the Substance Abuse and Mental Health Services Administration (www.samhsa.gov), Office of Drug Policy Control (www.whitehousedrugpolicy.gov), and the US Drug Enforcement Administration (www.dea.gov). These websites can also increase awareness of persistent or emerging drugs of abuse. QuickViews of eight common urine drug screens by immunoassay[11–15,18,25] include information on the signs and symptoms of these agents following abuse and overdose.[9,25,26,68]

Potential Roles of Pharmacists

A pharmacist's knowledge of drugs, pharmacokinetics, toxicology, and basic sciences can be helpful in the interpretation of toxicological tests in several settings. Pharmacists practicing in critical care units, emergency departments, substance abuse clinics, and hospital-based therapeutic drug monitoring programs often deal with patients suffering from substance abuse, poisoning, and overdose. Thus, interpretation of toxicological tests is an extremely important function. Pharmacists practicing in poison control centers are routinely consulted to interpret test results as they relate to acute or chronic poisonings, and some pharmacists assist medical review officers in their evaluation of workplace drug testing results. Those who have distinguished themselves with advanced practice and training in toxicology and therapeutic drug monitoring are often consulted as expert witnesses in cases involving the interpretation of toxicological tests. On a personal basis, pharmacists are also asked by family members, acquaintances, and patients about drug testing and the potential impact on their lives. It is often prudent to refer the person to the testing laboratory or physician who ordered the test in question when pertinent facts are not available or when they are unable to be properly assessed.

REFERENCES

1. Substance Abuse and Mental Health Services Administration. *Results from the 2001 National Household Survey on Drug Abuse: Volume I. Summary of National Findings.* Rockville, MD: Office of Applied Studies (NHSDA Series H-17, DHHS Publication No. SMA 02-3758); 2002. Available at: http://www.drugabusestatistics.samhsa.gov/oas/nhsda/2k1nhsda/PDF. Accessed January 24, 2003.
2. Office of National Drug Control Policy. *Drug Data Summary.* Washington, DC: Executive Office of the President; 2003. Available at: http://whitehousedrugpolicy.gov/pdf/drug_datasum.pdf. Accessed April 1, 2003.
3. Federal Bureau of Investigation. *Crime in the United States 2001: Uniform Crime Reports.* Washington, DC: U.S. Department of Justice; 2002. Available at: www.fbi.gov/Cius_01/01crime. Accessed March 31, 2003.
4. Litovitz TL, Klein-Schwartz W, Rodgers GC, et al. 2001 annual report of the American Association of Poison Control Centers toxic exposure surveillance system. *Am J Emerg Med.* 2002; 20:391–452.
5. Zhang Z, Huang LX, Brittingham AM. *Worker drug use and workplace policies and programs: results from the 1994 and 1997 national household survey on drug abuse.* Rockville, MD: Department of Health and Human Services, Substance Abuse and Mental Health Services Administration; 1999. Available at: http://www.samhsa.gov/oas/NHSDA/A-11/TOC.htm. Accessed January 24, 2003.
6. Johnston LD, O'Malley PM, Bachman JG. *Monitoring the future national results on adolescent drug use: overview of key findings, 2002.* (NIH Publication No. 03-5374). Bethesda, MD: National Institute on Drug Abuse; 2003. Available at: http://www.monitoringthefuture.org/pubs/monographs/overview2002.pdf. Accessed March 31, 2003.

7. Centers for Disease Control and Prevention. *Web-Based Injury Statistics Query and Reporting System (WISQARS) [Online]*. Atlanta, GA: National Center for Injury Prevention and Control, Centers for Disease Control and Prevention. Available at: www.cdc.gov/ncipc/wisqars. Accessed April 4, 2003.

8. Office of National Drug Control Policy. *Federal Drug Data Sources*. Washington, DC: Executive Office of the President. Available at: http://whitehousedrugpolicy.gov/drugfact/sources/html. Accessed March 31, 2003.

9. Chyka PA. Clinical toxicology. In: DiPiro JT, Talbert RL, Yee GC, et al, eds. *Pharmacotherapy: A Pathophysiologic Approach*. 5th ed. New York, NY: McGraw-Hill; 2002: 99–121.

10. Division of Workplace programs. *Drug Testing*. Rockville, MD: Substance Abuse and Mental Health Services Administration, Department of Health and Human Services. Available at: http://workplace.samhsa.gov/. Accessed October 19, 2002.

11. Anon. Tests for drugs of abuse. *Med Lett Drugs Ther*. 2002; 44:71–3.

12. Osterloh JD. Laboratory testing in emergency toxicology. In: Ford MD, Delaney KA, Ling LJ, et al, eds. *Clinical Toxicology*. Philadelphia, PA: W. B. Saunders; 2001: 51–60.

13. Rainey PM. Laboratory principles and techniques for evaluation of the poisoned or overdosed patient. In: Goldfrank LR, Flomenbaum NE, Lewin NA, et al, eds. *Goldfrank's Toxicologic Emergencies*. 7th ed. New York, NY: McGraw-Hill; 2002: 6993.

14. Rosenfeld W, Wingert WE. Scientific issues in drug testing and use of the laboratory. In: Schydlower M (ed). *Substance Abuse: A Guide for Health Professionals*. 2nd ed. Elk Grove, IL: American Academy of Pediatrics; 2002: 105–21.

15. Hammertt-Stabler CA, Pesce AJ, Cannon DJ. Urine drug screening in the medical setting. *Clinica Chimicia Acta*. 2002; 315:125–35.

16. Division of Workplace programs. *Federal Standards for Urine Drug Testing Cut-Off Concentrations*. Rockville, MD: Substance Abuse and Mental Health Services Administration, Department of Health and Human Services. Available at: http://workplace.samhsa.gov/DrugTesting/RegGuidance/UrineConcen.htm. Accessed March 28, 2003.

17. Wu AB, McKay C, Broussard LA, et al. National Academy of Clinical Biochemistry laboratory medicine practice guidelines: recommendations for the use of laboratory tests to support poisoned patients who present to the emergency department. *Clin Chem*. 2003; 49:357–79.

18. Phillips SD. Drug testing in the workplace. In: Ford MD, Delaney KA, Ling LJ, et al, eds. *Clinical Toxicology*. Philadelphia, PA: W. B. Saunders; 2001: 127–36.

19. Nice A, Leikin JB, Maturen A, et al. Toxidrome recognition to improve efficiency of emergency urine drug screens. *Ann Emerg Med*. 1988; 17:676–80.

20. American College of Emergency Physicians. Clinical policy for the initial approach to patients presenting with acute toxic ingestion or dermal or inhalation exposure. *Ann Emerg Med*. 1999; 33:735–61.

21. Carrigan TD, Field H, Illingworth RN, et al. Toxicological screening in trauma. *J Accid Emerg Med*. 2000; 17:33–7.

22. Substance Abuse and Mental Health Services Administration. *Medical Review Officer Manual for Federal Workplace Drug Testing Programs*. Rockville, MD: Department of Health and Human Services. Available at: http://workplace.samhsa.gov/DrugTesting/MedicalReviewOfficers/MROmannual.html. Accessed August 19, 2002

23. Office of Justice Programs. *Fact Sheet: Drug Testing and the Criminal Justice System*. Washington, DC: U.S. Department of Justice; 1992. Available at: http://www.ncjrs.org/pdffiles/dtest.pdf. Accessed October 22, 2002.

24. Wu AH. Urine adulteration before testing for drugs of abuse. In: Shaw LM, Kwong TC, Rosana TG, et al, eds. *The Clinical Toxicology Laboratory: Contemporary Practice of Poisoning Evaluation*. Washington, DC: American Association of Clinical Chemistry Press; 2001: 157–71.

25. Anon. Urine drug detection. In: Toll LL, Hurlbut KM, eds. *Poisindex*. Greenwood Village, CO: Thomson MICROMEDEX; vol 116. (Edition expires June 2003.)

26. Watson WA, Paloucek F. Managing acute drug toxicity. In: Koda-Kimble MA, Young LY, Kradjan WA, et al, eds. *Applied Therapeutics*. 7th ed. Philadelphia, PA: Lippincott Williams & Wilkins; 2001: 5-1 to 5-24.

27. Dart RC, Hurlbut KM, Kuffner EK, et al. *The 5-Minute Toxicology Consult*. Philadelphia, PA: Lippincott Williams & Wilkins; 2000.

28. National Poisons Information Service and Association of Clinical Biochemists. Laboratory analyses for poisoned patients: joint position paper. *Ann Clin Biochem*. 2002; 39:328–39.

29. Otten EJ, Prybysk M, Gesell LB. Ethanol. In: Ford MD, Delaney KA, Ling LJ, et al, eds. *Clinical Toxicology*. Philadelphia, PA: W. B. Saunders; 2001: 605–12.

30. Hammond KB, Rumack BH, Rodgerson DO. Blood ethanol: a report of unusually high levels in a living patient. *JAMA*. 1973; 226:63–4.

31. Van Heyningen C, Watson ID. Survival after very high blood alcohol concentrations (letter). *Ann Clin Biochem*. 2002; 39:416–17.

32. National Highway Traffic Safety Administration. *Setting Limits, Saving Lives: The Case for .08 BAC Laws*. Washington, DC: Department of Transportation; 2001. Available at www.nhtsa.gov/people/injury/alcohol. Accessed April 6, 2003.

33. Voas RB, Tippetts AS. *The Relationship of Alcohol Safety Laws to Drinking Drivers in Fatal Crashes*. Washington, DC: Department of Transportation, National Highway Traffic Safety Administration; 1999. Available at: http://www.nhtsa.dot.gov/people/injury/alcohol/limit.08/voas08/alcoholsafety.html. Accessed April 10, 2003.

34. Kwong TC. Point-of-care testing for alcohol. In: Shaw LM, Kwong TC, Rosana TG, et al, eds. *The Clinical Toxicology Laboratory: Contemporary Practice of Poisoning Evaluation*. Washington, DC: American Association of Clinical Chemistry Press; 2001: 190–6.

35. Orsay E, Doan-Wiggins L. Serum alcohol is not the same as blood alcohol concentration. *Ann Emerg Med*. 1995; 25:430–31.

36. Done AK. Salicylate intoxication: significance of measurements of salicylate in blood in cases of acute ingestion. *Pediatrics*. 1960; 26:800–7.

37. Dugandzic RM, Tierney MG, Dickinson GE, et al. Evaluation of the validity of the Done nomogram in the management of acute salicylate intoxication. *Ann Emerg Med*. 1989; 18:1186–90.

38. Gabow PA, Anderson RJ, Potts DE, et al. Acid-base disturbances in the salicylate-intoxicated adult. *Arch Intern Med*. 1978; 38:1481–4.

39. Sporer KA, Khayam-Bashi H. Acetaminophen and salicylate serum levels in patients with suicidal ingestion or altered mental status. *Am J Emerg Med*. 1996; 14:443–6.

40. Smilkstein MJ, Knapp GL, Kulig KW, et al. Efficacy of oral N-acetylcysteine in the treatment of acetaminophen overdose: analysis of the national multicenter study (1976 to 1985). *N Engl J Med*. 1988; 319:1557–62.

41. Zucker AR, Lacina SJ, DasGupta DS, et al. Fab fragments of digoxin-specific antibodies used to reverse ventricular fibrillation induced by digoxin ingestion in a child. *Pediatrics*. 1982; 70:468–71.

42. Antman EM, Wenger TL, Butler VP, et al. Treatment of 150 cases of life-threatening digitalis intoxication with digoxin-specific Fab antibody fragments: final report of a multicenter study. *Circulation*. 1990; 81:1744–52.

43. Bosse GM, Matyunas NJ. Delayed toxidromes. *J Emerg Med*. 1999; 17:679–90.

44. Office of National Drug Control Policy. *What You Need to Know About Drug Testing in Schools*. Washington, DC: Executive Office of the President; 2003. Available at: http://www.whitehousedrugpolicy.gov/pdf/drug_testing.pdf. Accessed March 28, 2003.

45. George S, Braithwaite RA. Use of on-site testing for drugs of abuse. *Clin Chem*. 2002; 48:1639–46.

46. Peace MR, Tarnai LD, Poklis A. Performance evaluation of four on-site drug-testing devices for detection of drugs of abuse in urine. *J Analyt Toxicol*. 2000; 589–94.

47. Leikin JB, Watson WA. Postmortem toxicology: what the dead can and cannot tell us. *J Toxicol Clin Toxicol*. 2003: 41:47–56.

48. Drummer OH, Gerostamoulos J. Postmortem drug analysis: analytical and toxicological aspects. *Therap Drug Monit*. 2002; 24:199–209.

49. Rao RB, Flomenbaum M. Postmortem toxicology. In: Goldfrank LR, Flomenbaum NE, Lewin NA, et al, eds. *Goldfrank's Toxicologic Emergencies*. 7th ed. New York, NY: McGraw-Hill; 2002: 1781–88.

50. Kwong TC, Ryan RM. Detection of intrauterine illicit drug exposure by newborn drug testing. *Clin Chem*. 1997; 43:235–42.

51. Belson MG, Simon HK, Sullivan K, et al. The utility of toxicologic analysis in children with suspected ingestions. *Pediatr Emerg Care*. 1999; 15:383–7.

52. Casavant MJ. Urine drug screening in adolescents. *Pediatr Clin N Am*. 2002; 49:317–27.

53. American Academy of Pediatrics. Testing for drugs of abuse in children and adolescents. *Pediatrics*. 1996; 98:305–7. Available at: http://www.aap.org/policy/01495.html. Accessed March 31, 2003.

54. Schwartz RH, Silber TJ, Heyman RB, et al. Urine testing for drugs of abuse. *Arch Pediatr Adolesc Med*. 2003; 157:158–61.

55. Grunbaum JA, Kann L, Kinchen SA, et al. Youth risk behavior surveillance—United States, 2001. In: *Surveillance Summaries*. MMWR 2002; 51(SS-4):1–66. Available at: http://www.cdc.gov/mmwr/PDF/ss/ss5104.pdf. Accessed July10, 2002.

56. Boyce EG. Use and effectiveness of performance-enhancing substances. *J Pharm Pract*. 2003: 16:22–36.

57. Chyka PA. Health risks of selected performance-enhancing drugs. *J Pharm Pract*. 2003: 16:37–44.

58. Prendergast HM, Bannen T, Erickson TB, et al. The toxic torch of the modern Olympic games. *Vet Human Toxicol*. 2003; 45:97–102.

59. Rollins DE. Drug testing in athletes at the 2002 Olympic Winter Games. *J Pharm Pract*. 2003: 16:15–21.

60. Anon. *Olympic Movement Anti-doping Code: Appendix A. Prohibited Classes of Substances and Prohibited Methods, 2003*. Lausanne, Switzerland: International Olympic Committee; 2003. Available at: http://multimedia.olympic.org/pdf/en_report_542.pdf. Accessed April 10, 2003.

61. Jortani S, Snyder JW, Valdes R Jr. The role of the clinical laboratory in managing chemical or biological terrorism. *Clin Chem*. 2000; 46:1883–93.

62. Krenzekok EP, ed. *Biological and Chemical Terrorism: A Pharmacy Preparedness Guide*. Bethesda, MD: American Society of Health-System Pharmacists; 2003.

63. McEvoy GK, ed. *AFHS DI Bioterrorism Resource Manual*. Bethesda, MD: American Society of Health-System Pharmacists; 2002.

64. Terriff C, Schwartz M, Lomaestro B. Bioterrorism: pivotal clinical issues. *Pharmacotherapy*. 2003; 23:274–90.

65. Hicks JM, Young DS, Rifai N. *DORA '00-02: Directory of Rare Analyses*. Washington, DC: American Association of Clinical Chemistry Press; 2000.

66. Baselt RC. *Disposition of Toxic Drugs and Chemicals in Man*. 6th ed. Foster City, CA: Biomedical Publications; 2002.

67. Shaw LM, Kwong TC, Rosana TG, et al, eds. *The Clinical Toxicology Laboratory: Contemporary Practice of Poisoning Evaluation*. Washington, DC: American Association of Clinical Chemistry Press; 2001.

68. National Institute on Drug Abuse. *InfoFacts*. Washington, DC: National Institutes of Health. Available at: http://www.nida.nih.gov/Infofax/Infofaxindex.html. Accessed April 3, 2003.

quickview – urine drug screen, amphetamines, and methamphetamine

PARAMETER	DESCRIPTION	COMMENTS
Critical value	Positive	Check for possible interferents; confirm result with confirmatory test such as GC-MS
Major causes of... **Positive results**	Following ingestion, intranasal application, inhalation, injection	Typical symptoms include CNS stimulation, euphoria, irritability, insomnia, tremors, seizures, paranoia, and aggressiveness; overdoses cause hypertension, tachycardia, stroke, arrhythmias, cardiovascular collapse, rhabdomyolysis, and hyperthermia
Associated signs and symptoms	None may be evident at time of specimen collection; may involve exposure to illicit substances; may involve exposure to medicines used for legitimate purposes or abuse	
After use, time to... **Negative result from light, sporadic use**	2–5 days; clearance is faster in acidic urine	Methylphenidate typically will not be detected
Negative result from chronic use	Up to 2 weeks	Mefenamic acid (Ponstel) may produce a false-negative result
Possible spurious positive results with immunoassays	Ephedrine, pseudoephedrine, ephedra (ma huang), phenylephrine, desoxyephedrine (Vicks Nasal Inhaler), selegiline, chlorpromazine, trazodone, bupropion, desipramine, amantadine, ranitidine, phenylpropanolamine, methylenedioxy-methamphetamine (MDMA), propylhexedrine, isometheptene (Midrin), labetalol, fenfluramine, phentermine, isoxsuprine, brompheniramine	False-positive result Consider patient's use of nonprescription drugs and dietary supplements; verify possible false positive with laboratory and assay package insert

quickview – urine drug screen, barbiturates

PARAMETER	DESCRIPTION	COMMENTS
Critical value	Positive	Check for possible interferents; confirm result with confirmatory test such as GC–MS
Major causes of... **Positive results**	Following ingestion; rarely injected or used as a suppository	Typical symptoms include sedation; overdoses cause coma, ataxia, nystagmus, depressed reflexes, hypotension, and respiratory depression; consider coingestion of ethanol; primidone is metabolized to phenobarbital
Associated signs and symptoms	None may be evident at time of specimen collection; may involve exposure to medicines used for legitimate purposes or abuse	
After use, time to... **Negative result from short-acting agents**	1–7 days	Depends on drug and extent and duration of use
Negative result from long-acting agents	1–3 weeks	Phenobarbital may be detected up to 4 weeks after stopping use
Possible spurious positive results with immunoassays		Verify possible false positive with laboratory and assay package insert

quickview – urine drug screen, benzodiazepines

PARAMETER	DESCRIPTION	COMMENTS
Critical value	Positive	Check for possible interferents; confirm result with confirmatory test such as GC-MS
Major causes of... **Positive results**	Following ingestion or injection	Benzodiazepines vary in cross-reactivity and detectability
Associated signs and symptoms	None may be evident at time of specimen collection; may involve exposure to medicines used for legitimate purposes or abuse; may involve exposure to illicit forms	Typical symptoms include drowsiness, ataxia, slurred speech, sedation; oral overdoses can cause tachycardia and coma with rare severe respiratory or cardiovascular depression; rapid IV use can cause severe respiratory depression; consider coingestion of ethanol
After use, time to... **Negative result**	Typically up to 2 weeks; up to 6 weeks with chronic use of some agents	Some benzodiazepines may persist for a longer period of time and some have an active metabolite that may or may not be detected; flunitrazepam may not be detected; not all benzodiazepines will be detected by all immunoassays
Possible spurious positive results with immunoassays		Verify possible false positive with laboratory and assay package insert

quickview – urine drug screen, benzoylecgonine (cocaine metabolite)

PARAMETER	DESCRIPTION	COMMENTS
Critical value	Positive	Check for possible interferents; confirm result with confirmatory test such as GC-MS
Major causes of... **Positive results**	Following snorting, inhalation, injection, topical application (vagina, penis) or rectal insertion; possible passive inhalation; ingestion	Typical symptoms include CNS stimulation that produces euphoric effects and hyperstimulation such as dilated pupils, increased temperature, tachycardia and hypertension; overdoses cause stroke, acute myocardial infarction, seizures, coma, respiratory depression, arrhythmias
Associated signs and symptoms	None may be evident at time of specimen collection with heavy or chronic use; may involve exposure to medicines used for legitimate purposes or abuse; may involve exposure to illicit forms	
After use, time to... **Negative result from light, sporadic use**	12–72 hr	Cross-reactivity with cocaethylene (metabolic product of concurrent cocaine and ethanol abuse) varies with the assay
Negative result from chronic use	Up to 1–3 weeks	
Possible spurious positive results with immunoassays	Topical anesthetics containing cocaine Coca leaf tea	False positive for drug abuse; false-positive result; false positives from -caine anesthetics (e.g., lidocaine, procaine, benzocaine) are unlikely; verify possible false positive with laboratory and assay package insert

quickview – urine drug screen, delta-9-tetrahydrocannabinol-9-carboxylic acid (marijuana metabolite)

PARAMETER	DESCRIPTION	COMMENTS
Critical value	Positive	Check for possible interferents; confirm result with confirmatory test such as GC-MS
Major causes of... **Positive results**	Following inhalation or ingestion; possible passive inhalation	May be caused by sodium phosphate used as drug screen adulterant; may be due to prescription for dronabinol
Associated signs and symptoms	None may be evident at time of specimen collection with heavy or chronic use; may involve exposure to illicit substances; may involve exposure to medicine used for legitimate purposes or abuse	Typical symptoms include delirium, conjunctivitis, food craving; other effects include problems with memory and learning, distorted perception, difficulty in thinking and problem solving, loss of coordination, sedation, and tachycardia
After use, time to... **Negative result from light, sporadic use**	7–10 days	May persist for a longer period of time with heavy, long-term use
Negative result from chronic use	6–8 weeks typically, up to 3 months possible	
Possible spurious positive results with immunoassays	Ibuprofen, naproxen, efavirenz, hemp seed, hemp oil	False-positive result
	Dronabinol	False-positive for abuse; verify possible false-positive with laboratory and assay package insert

quickview – urine drug screen, lysergic acid diethylamide (lsd)

PARAMETER	DESCRIPTION	COMMENTS
Critical value	Positive	Check for possible interferents; confirm result with confirmatory test such as GC-MS
Major causes of... **Positive results**	Following ingestion, placement in buccal cavity or ocular instillation	Not well-absorbed topically
Associated signs and symptoms	May involve exposure to illicit substances	Typical symptoms include unpredictable hallucinogenic effects; physical effects include mydriasis, elevated temperature, tachycardia, hypertension, sweating, loss of appetite, sleeplessness, dry mouth, and tremors; flashbacks months later are possible
After use, time to... **Negative result**	24–48 hr typically, up to 120 hr possible	
Possible spurious positive results with immunoassays		LSD is a schedule I drug with no legitimate routine medical use; verify possible false positive with laboratory and assay package insert

quickview – urine drug screen, opiates

PARAMETER	DESCRIPTION	COMMENTS
Critical value	Positive	Check for possible interferents; confirm result with confirmatory test such as GC-MS
Major causes of... **Positive results**	Following ingestion, injection, dermal application of drug containing patches, rectal insertion	Synthetic opioids (e.g., fentanyl, fentanyl derivatives, meperidine, methadone, pentazocine, propoxyphene, and tramadol) have minimal cross-reactivity and may not be detected
Associated signs and symptoms	None may be evident at time of specimen collection; may involve exposure to illicit substances; may involve exposure to medicines used for legitimate purposes or abuse; ingestion of large amounts of food products made with poppy seeds	Typical symptoms include CNS depression, drowsiness, miosis, constipation; overdoses cause coma, hypotension, respiratory depression, pulmonary edema, and seizures Heroin use is confirmed by the presence of 6-acetylmorphine (6-AM)
After use, time to... **Negative result**	2–3 days typically, up to 6 days with sustained-release formulations, up to 1 week with prolonged or heavy use	Mefenamic acid (Ponstel) may produce a false-negative result
Possible spurious positive results with immunoassays	Poppy seeds	False positive for drug abuse
	Rifampin, some fluoroquinolones, quinine	False-positive result; consider patient's legitimate use of opioid analgesics including long-term pain management and opioid withdrawal treatment with methadone, levo-alpha-acetylmethadol (ORLAAM), or buprenorphine (Subutex, Suboxone); verify possible false positive with laboratory and assay package insert

quickview – urine drug screen, phencyclidine (pcp)

PARAMETER	DESCRIPTION	COMMENTS
Critical value	Positive	Check for possible interferents; confirm result with confirmatory test such as GC-MS
Major causes of... **Positive results**	Following ingestion, inhalation, injection	Typical symptoms include hallucinations, schizophrenia-like behavior, hypertension, elevated temperature, diaphoresis, tachycardia; high doses cause nystagmus, ataxia, hypotension, bradycardia, depressed respirations, seizures, and coma
Associated signs and symptoms	None may be evident at time of specimen collection; may involve exposure to illicit substances; may involve exposure to medicines containing dextromethorphan or diphenhydramine used for legitimate purposes or abuse	
After use, time to... **Negative result from light, sporadic use**	2–10 days	May persist for a longer period of time with heavy, long-term use or massive overdose preceded by chronic use
Negative result from chronic use	Weeks or months	
Possible spurious positive results with immunoassays	Dextromethorphan, ketamine, diphenhydramine, sertraline	False positive result; verify possible false positive with laboratory and assay package insert

Chapter **6**

INTERPRETATION OF SERUM DRUG CONCENTRATIONS

Janis J. MacKichan

The pharmacist is a key member in the therapeutic drug monitoring process. This chapter is designed to review the indications for drug concentration monitoring and to discuss how drug concentrations obtained from the clinical laboratory, specialized reference laboratory, or physician's office should be interpreted. General considerations for interpretation will be described, as well as unique considerations for drugs that commonly undergo therapeutic drug monitoring. Future directions of therapeutic drug monitoring will also be discussed.

This chapter is not intended to provide an in-depth review of pharmacokinetic dosing methods; nevertheless, knowledge of certain basic pharmacokinetic terms and concepts is expected. The general phrase *drug concentration* will be used throughout the chapter unless specific references to serum, plasma, whole blood, saliva, or tears are more appropriate. The bibliography lists numerous texts about therapeutic drug monitoring and clinical pharmacokinetic principles with applications to clinical practice.

OBJECTIVES

After completing this chapter, the reader should be able to

1. Describe appropriate indications for drug concentration monitoring.
2. Describe characteristics of drugs that make them good candidates for drug concentration monitoring.
3. List and discuss the importance of information needed when requesting and reporting drug concentrations.
4. Discuss interpatient variation in a therapeutic range, including factors that may affect it.
5. Discuss the importance of documenting the time a sample is obtained relative to the last dose, as well as factors that can affect interpretation of a drug concentration, depending on when it was obtained.
6. Compare the types of specimens that may be obtained (serum, plasma, whole blood, and saliva), including reasons for choosing one over the other.
7. Describe the types of artifacts or interferences that may be caused by blood or saliva collection methods or by assay choice.
8. Compare linear to nonlinear pharmacokinetic behavior with respect to how drug concentration measurements are used to make dosage regimen adjustments.
9. Discuss the impact of altered serum binding, active metabolites, or stereoselective pharmacokinetics on the interpretation of drug concentration measurements.

THERAPEUTIC DRUG MONITORING

Therapeutic drug monitoring is broadly defined as the use of drug concentrations to optimize drug therapy for individual patients.[1] Prior to the use of drug concentrations to guide therapy, physicians adjusted drug doses based on their interpretation of clinical response. In many cases, drug doses were increased until obvious signs of toxicity were observed (e.g., nystagmus for phenytoin or tinnitus for salicylates). The idea that intensity and duration of pharmacologic response depended on serum concentration was first reported by Marshall[2] and then tested for the screening of antimalarials during World War II.[3] Koch-Weser, in a hallmark paper, described how steady-state serum levels of commonly used drugs can vary 10-fold among patients receiving the same dosage schedule.[4] He further described how serum concentrations predict intensity of therapeutic or toxic effects more accurately than dosage.

Starting in the 1960s, there was rapid improvement in analytical methods used for drug concentration measurements; extensive research correlating serum or plasma drug concentrations with clinical efficacy and toxicity quickly followed. Physicians, pharmacists, and laboratory technologists began forming specialized therapeutic drug monitoring or clinical pharmacokinetics services in hospitals starting in the 1970s. Today, with the emergence of immunoassays that require no specialized equipment, drug concentration measurements can be easily performed in physician offices.[5]

The drug concentration assays most widely available in hospital laboratories are for antiepileptics (carbamazepine, ethosuximide, primidone/phenobarbital, phenytoin, and valproic acid), cardiac drugs (digoxin, procainamide/N-acetylprocainamide, and quinidine), antibiotics (aminoglycosides and vancomycin), theophylline, and lithium. But there is new research showing correlations between drug concentration and response for additional groups of drugs such as the psychotropics, immunosuppressants, antimycobacterial, anticancer, and antiretroviral drugs. Drugs in these groups are currently monitored only in certain circumstances, in special treatment centers, or in research settings, but they may become more routinely monitored as the relationships between drug concentration and response become clearer.

The increased availability and convenience of drug assay methods has led to a number of concerns. Is therapeutic drug monitoring being done simply because it is available, rather than because it is clinical necessary? There are numerous reports of suboptimal therapeutic drug monitoring practices that contribute to inappropriate decision-making as well as wasted resources.[6–8] Questions are also being raised about whether therapeutic drug monitoring actually improves patient outcomes.[9] However, many clinicians claim that therapeutic drug monitoring is greatly underused and could, if appropriately used, further improve patient care as well save health care dollars.[10,11] Clearly, there is a need for more education of all health care professionals involved in the therapeutic drug monitoring process in order to make its use more appropriate and cost-effective. Such education efforts have been shown to effectively reduce the numbers of inappropriate serum drug concentration requests.[12]

Goal and Indications for Drug Concentration Monitoring

The primary goal of therapeutic drug monitoring is to maximize the benefit of a drug to a patient in the shortest possible time with minimal risk of toxicity. The number of hospitalizations or office visits used to adjust therapies or manage and diagnose adverse drug reactions may, therefore, be reduced, resulting in cost savings.

Drug concentration measurements should not be performed unless the result will affect some future action or decision. Monitoring should not be done simply because the opportunity presents itself; it should be used discriminatingly to answer clinically relevant questions and resolve or anticipate problems in drug therapy management.[13] The clinician should always ask, "Will this drug concentration value provide more information to me than sound clinical judgment alone?"[9] The following are examples of clinical situations and the clinical questions that drug concentration measurements might be able to answer:

- **Therapeutic confirmation:** A patient is on a regimen that appears to offer maximum benefit with acceptable side effects. *Question: What is the drug concentration associated with a therapeutic effect in this patient for future reference?*

- **Dosage optimization:** A patient has a condition in which clinical response is not easily measured, and has been initiated on a standard regimen of a drug. There is modest improvement and no symptoms of toxicity are evident. *Question: Can I increase the dose rate to further enhance effect? If so, by how much?*

- **Confirmation of suspected toxicity:** A patient is experiencing certain signs and symptoms that could be related to the drug. *Question: Are these signs and symptoms most likely related to a dose rate that is too high? Can I reduce the daily dose, and if so, by how much?*

- **Avoidance of inefficacy or toxicity:** A patient is initiated on a standard regimen of an antibiotic that is known to be poorly absorbed in a small percentage of patients. Sustained subtherapeutic concentrations of this drug can lead to drug-resistance. *Question: Will a higher daily dose be needed in this patient?* A patient has been satisfactorily treated on a dosage regimen of Drug A. The patient experiences a change in health or physiologic status or a second drug, suspected to interact with Drug A, is added. *Question: Will a dosage regimen adjustment be needed to avoid inefficacy or toxicity?*

- **Distinguishing noncompliance from treatment failure:** A patient has not responded to usual doses and noncompliance is a possibility. *Question: Is this a treatment failure or does the patient need counseling on compliance?*

Characteristics of Ideal Drugs For Therapeutic Drug Monitoring

Not all drugs are good candidates for therapeutic drug monitoring, no matter how appropriate the indication seems to be. Those for which drug concentration monitoring will be most useful have the following characteristics[14]:

- **Readily available assays:** Methods for drug concentration measurement must be available to the clinician at a cost to justify the information to be gained. Analytical methods for some drugs are routinely available in hospitals or in physician offices. Methods for newer drugs or drugs used in specialized treatment centers are not as widely available but, nevertheless, are essential for that patient population.

- **Lack of easily observable, safe, or desirable clinical endpoint:** Clinically, there is no immediate, easily monitored, and/or predictable clinical parameter to guide dosage titration. For example, waiting for arrhythmias or seizures to occur or resume may be an unsafe and undesirable approach to dosing antiarrhythmics and antiepileptics.

- **Dangerous toxicity or lack of effectiveness:** Toxicity or lack of effectiveness of the drug presents a danger to the patient. For example, serum drug concentrations of the antifungal drug, flucytosine, are not routinely monitored. However, specialized monitoring may be done to assure that levels are below 100 mg/L to avoid gastrointestinal side effects, blood dyscrasias, and hepatotoxicity. As another example, specialized monitoring of the protease inhibitors may be done to assure adequate levels since rapid emergence of antiviral resistance is observed with sustained exposure to subtherapeutic levels.

- **Unpredictable dose-response relationship:** There is an unpredictable dose-response relationship, such that a dose producing therapeutic benefit in one patient may cause toxicity in another patient. This would be true for drugs that have significant interpatient variation in pharmacokinetic parameters, drugs with nonlinear behavior, and drugs whose pharmacokinetic parameters are affected by concomitant administration of other drugs. For example, patients given the same daily dose of phenytoin can demonstrate a wide range of serum concentrations and responses.

- **Narrow therapeutic range:** The drug concentrations associated with therapeutic effect overlap considerably with the concentrations associated with toxic effects, such that the zone for therapeutic benefit without toxicity is very narrow. For example, the therapeutic range of phenytoin is widely accepted to be 10–20 mg/L for most patients; the upper limit of the range is only twice the lower limit.

- **Good correlation between drug concentration and efficacy or toxicity:** This criterion must apply if we are using drug concentrations to adjust the dosage regimen of a drug. For example, a patient showing unsatisfactory asthma control with a serum theophylline concentration of 5 mg/L is likely to show improved control with a doubling of the daily dose to attain a serum concentration of 10 mg/L.

Other than availability of an assay, it may not be necessary for a drug to fulfill all of the above characteristics for drug concentration monitoring to help guide clinical decision-making. Newer drugs that do not yet have clearly defined therapeutic ranges may only be monitored under special circumstances (e.g., to assure compliance). Other drugs may not have a clearly defined upper or lower limit to the therapeutic range but are monitored under special circumstances to assure efficacy or avoid toxicity. This goes back to the importance of the drug concentration for answering a specific clinical question: Will the information provided by this measurement help to improve the patient's drug therapy?

Information Needed for Planning and Evaluating Drug Concentrations

Drug concentrations should be interpreted in light of full information about the patient, including clinical status. Information about the timing of the sample relative to the last dose is especially critical and is one of the biggest factors making drug concentrations unusable or cost-ineffective.[6,15–17] Table 6-1 provides a list of the essential information needed for a drug concentration request. Laboratory request forms or computer entry forms must be designed to encourage entry of the most important information. All relevant information should be included on both the request form and the report form to facilitate accurate interpretation. Some hospital laboratories have minimized the number of inappropriate samples by refusing to run any samples that are not accompanied by critical information, such as the timing of the sample relative to the last dose.[6] The laboratory report form should also include the assay used; active metabolite concentration (if measured); and parameters reflecting the sensitivity, specificity and precision of the method.

Accuracy and completeness of the information provided on a laboratory request form is particularly important in light of the many problems that can occur during the therapeutic drug monitoring process. A drug concentration that seems to be illogical, given the information provided on the form, may be explained by a variety of factors as shown in Table 6-2.

Considerations for Appropriate Interpretation of Drug Concentrations

To appropriately interpret a drug concentration, it is important to have as many answers as possible to the following questions:

- **Therapeutic range:** What do the studies show to be the usual therapeutic range? How frequently will patients show response at a concentration below the lower limit of the usual range? How frequently will patients show toxicity at a level below the upper limit of the usual range? What are the usual signs and symptoms indicating toxicity?

- **Sample timing:** Was the sample drawn at a steady state? Was the sample drawn at a time during the dosing interval (if intermittent therapy) that reflects the intended indication for monitoring (a peak, a trough, or an average level)? During the dosing

TABLE 6-1

TYPE OF DATA	SPECIFIC DATA	WHY NECESSARY
Patient identification	Name, address, identification number, and physician name	All blood samples look alike and could easily be switched among patients without appropriate identification.
Patient demographics and characteristics	Age, gender, ethnicity, height, weight, and pregnancy	The therapeutic range for a given drug may depend on the specific indication being treated (e.g., digoxin for atrial arrhythmias versus heart failure). If there is no history of prior drug concentration measurements, information about concurrent disease states, physiologic status, and social habits may help with initial determination of population pharmacokinetic parameters, in order to determine if the resulting level is *expected* or not. Information about renal function and albumin is important if a total drug level is being measured for a drug normally highly bound to serum proteins. It is also important to know if any endogenous substances due to diseases will interfere with the assay. Electrolyte abnormalities may affect interpretation of a given concentration (e.g., digoxin).
History and physical examination	Condition being treated Organ involvement (renal, hepatic, cardiac, gastrointestinal, and endocrine) Fluid balance and nutritional status Labs (albumin, total protein, liver function enzymes, INR, bilirubin, serum creatinine or creatinine clearance, thyroid status, and electrolyte abnormalities) Smoking and alcohol history	
Specimen information	Time of collection Nature of specimen: blood, urine, or other body fluid Site of collection Order of sample, if part of a series Type of collection tube Time of receipt by laboratory	The time of collection relative to the dose is extremely important for proper interpretation. (Close to a trough? Closer to a peak?) Knowing the type of collection tube is important because of the many interferences that may occur. Important to know the collection site relative to the administration site, if intravenous route. If a series of samples is to be drawn, the labeled timing of the collection tubes can get mixed up.
Drug information	Name of drug to be assayed Current dosage regimen, including route Type of formulation (sustained-release, delayed-release, or prompt-release) Length of time on current regimen Time of last dose Concurrent drug therapy	It is important to know if the concentration was drawn at a steady state and when the level was drawn relative to the last dose. It is also important to know if there are any potential drug interferences with the assay to be used.
Drug concentration history	Dates and times of prior concentration measurements Response and drug regimen schedules associated with prior concentrations.	It is important to know what drug concentrations have been documented as effective or associated with toxicity. It is also important to know how drug concentrations have changed as a consequence of dosage regimen.
Purpose of assay and urgency of request	Therapeutic confirmation Suspected toxicity Anticipated inefficacy or toxicity due to change in physiologic/health status or drug-drug interaction Identification of drug failure Suspected overdose	This forces the clinician to have a specific clinical question in mind before ordering a sample. It also aids in the interpretation of results.

[a]Adapted, with permission, from Reference 14.
[b]Adapted, with permission, from Reference 18.

Table 6-1. Information Needed on Laboratory Request Form[a,b]

TABLE 6-2

CATEGORY OF FACTOR	SPECIFIC EXAMPLES
Related to drug administration or blood sampling logistics	• Wrong dose or infusion rate administered • Dose skipped or infusion held for a period of time • Dose given at time other than recorded; blood drawn as ordered • Dose given at right time; blood drawn at time other than recorded • Sample taken through an administration line which was improperly flushed prior to sample withdrawal • Sample taken from the wrong patient • Improper or prolonged storage prior to delivery to laboratory • Wrong collection tube/device used
Related to pharmacokinetics	• Sample is drawn prior to a steady state • Orders for digoxin samples are not clearly specified to be drawn at least 6 hr postdistribution • Samples are ordered for the wrong times relative to last dose to reflect specific needs (e.g., peaks and/or troughs) • Concentrations of active metabolites are not ordered when appropriate • Concentrations for total drug are ordered for a drug with unusual serum protein binding without recognition that the *usual* therapeutic range of total drug will not apply
Related to the laboratory	• The wrong drug is assayed • Critical active metabolites are not assayed • Interferences or artifacts caused by endogenous substances (bilirubin, lipids, and hemolysis) or concurrent drugs • Improper or prolonged storage prior to assay • Technical errors with the assay
Related to the patient	• Patient is not adherent with therapy

[a]Adapted, with permission, from Reference 18.
[b]Adapted, with permission, from Reference 20.

Table 6-2. Common Reasons Why Drug Concentration Results Do Not Make Sense[a,b]

interval, when is a peak level most likely to occur for the formulation administered? Does the formulation exhibit a lag-time for release or absorption, such that the lowest level will occur into the next dosing interval?

• **Specimen, collection method, and assay:** Was the collected specimen (serum, plasma, whole blood, and saliva) appropriate for the assay that was used? Was the blood collection method artifact-free or interference-free? Is saliva (or some other fluid) an appropriate noninvasive alternative to blood collection? Was the saliva collected according to a standardized protocol? Was the storage method appropriate based on studies of stability in the specimen used? Was the assay suitably sensitive and precise for concentrations being measured? Is there any reason to believe, based on the assay, that there might be interferences (over-reading, under-reading) from endogenous substances in the specimen, concurrent drugs, or metabolites?

• **Use of levels for dosage adjustment:** Does the drug display first-order (linear) pharmacokinetic behavior such that an increase in daily dose will produce a proportional increase in the drug concentration? Is the dosage adjustment method focused on attaining specific peaks and/or trough, or specific average levels?

- **Protein binding, active metabolites, and enantiomers:** How are total drug concentrations in serum interpreted in cases of altered serum protein binding? How are concentrations or contributions of active metabolite considered along with parent drug? Is the drug administered as a racemic mixture and if so, do the enantiomers differ in activity and pharmacokinetic behavior? Do certain physiologic or pathologic conditions affect a patient's response to the drug at a given concentration?

Each of these categories will be described in general below and, more specifically, for each drug or drug class in the Applications section.

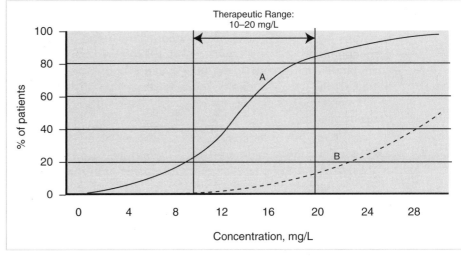

Figure 6-1. The therapeutic range for a hypothetical drug. Line A is the percentage of patients displaying a therapeutic effect; line B is the percentage of patients displaying toxicity.

THE THERAPEUTIC RANGE

A therapeutic range is best defined as a "range of drug concentrations within which the probability of the desired clinical response is relatively high and the probability of unacceptable toxicity is relatively low."[1] This means that the therapeutic range reported by a laboratory is actually a population-based average for which the majority of patients are expected to respond with acceptable side effects. Thus, there will always be some patients who exhibit therapeutic effect at drug concentrations below the lower limit, while others will experience unacceptable toxicity at levels below the upper limit. In essence, patients have their own unique therapeutic range.

Figure 6-1 illustrates how the probability of response and toxicity increases with drug concentration for a hypothetical drug and how a therapeutic range might be determined based on these relative probabilities. Figure 6-2 shows how patterns for response and toxicity can differ in two different patients receiving the same drug. If the hypothetical drug in question has an active metabolite that accumulates more than the parent drug in renal impairment, and if that metabolite contributes more to

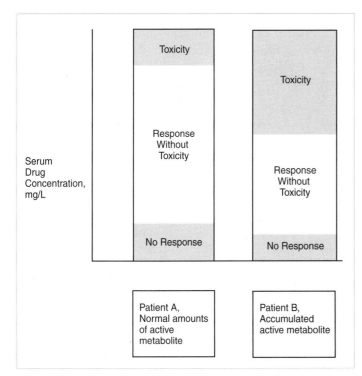

Figure 6-2. Representation showing how the therapeutic range of a hypothetical drug can differ in a patient with renal impairment because of accumulated active metabolite.

MINICASE 1

CHARLES W., A 65-YEAR-OLD-MALE asthmatic patient with a theophylline half-life of 8–9 hr, was started on an aminophylline infusion of 30 mg/hr at 8 p.m. on Monday. His doctor ordered a theophylline level for "Tuesday morning." The laboratory drew the blood Tuesday at 6 a.m. (a little more than one half-life later); a concentration of 7 mg/L was reported Tuesday afternoon at 3 p.m. The physician increased the rate of aminophylline infusion to 60 mg/hr because of poor clinical response and a relatively low theophylline concentration. (In the past, Charles W. required serum theophylline concentrations close to 13 mg/L to suppress his bronchospasm. His doctor assumed that doubling the infusion rate would double the serum theophylline concentration.)

At 3 p.m. on Wednesday, Charles W. complained of nausea, palpitations, and jitteriness; his heart rate was 110. The physician ordered a stat theophylline level; the laboratory called 2 hr later with a "critical value" of 27 mg/L, but the physician did not become informed until 11 p.m. Wednesday night. At this point, the physician decreased the rate to 40 mg/hr and ordered a level for Thursday morning. The laboratory drew blood at 6 a.m. Thursday (not quite one half-life later) and reported a concentration of 21.5 mg/L at 3 p.m. Thursday at which time the rate was decreased to the original 30 mg/hr. A level drawn 32 hr later was 12 mg/L.

Question: Why did the original rate of 30 mg/hr not yield a serum theophylline concentration of 12 mg/L as it did at the end of the case? What could have been done to avoid the bouncing concentrations and side effects?

Discussion: This type of "tail-chasing" scenario commonly occurs when the concept of steady state is not appreciated or applied. Given enough time after the initial infusion rate of 30 mg/hr (24 hr at the minimum, assuming a theophylline half-life of 8 hr), the serum theophylline level eventually would have reached 12 mg/L. The level obtained on Tuesday morning was approximately 60% of the eventual steady state level. By increasing the infusion rate based on a presteady state level, the physician caused toxicity in the patient and incurred unnecessary costs.

Minicase 1 is adapted from the second edition chapter titled "Interpretation of Serum Drug Concentrations," which was written by Scott L. Traub.

toxicity than to efficacy, then the therapeutic range in the patient with renal impairment will be narrower with lower concentrations. Concentration monitoring of the active metabolite would be especially important in that situation.

Drug concentration monitoring is often criticized by claims that therapeutic ranges are not sufficiently well-defined.[10,11] The lack of clearly-defined therapeutic ranges for older drugs is partially attributable to how these ranges were originally determined. Eadie describes the process that was typically used for determination of the therapeutic ranges of the antiepileptic drugs: "These ranges do not appear to have been determined by rigorous statistical procedures applied to large patient populations. Rather, workers seem to have set the lower limits for each drug at the concentration at which they perceived a reasonable (though usually unspecified) proportion of patients achieved seizure control, and the upper limit at the concentration above which overdosage-type adverse effects appear to trouble appreciable numbers of patients, the values then being rounded off to provide a pair of numbers, which are reasonably easy to remember."[13] In an ideal world, studies to define therapeutic ranges for drugs should use reliable methods for measurement of response and should be restricted to patients with the same diseases, age range, and concurrent medications.[1] In recent years, the Food and Drug Administration (FDA) has recognized the importance of determining concentration vs. response relationships early during clinical trials.[21]

What factors can affect a therapeutic range for a given patient? Anything that affects the pharmacodynamics of a drug, meaning the response at a given drug concentration, will affect the therapeutic range. These factors include

- **Indication:** Drugs that are used for more than one indication are likely to be interacting with different receptors. Thus, a different concentration vs. response profile might be expected depending on the disease being treated. For example, higher serum drug concentrations of digoxin are needed for treatment of atrial fibrillation as compared to congestive heart failure.

- **Active metabolites:** As shown in Figure 6-2, variable presence of an active metabolite can shift the therapeutic range for that individual patient up or down. These metabolites may behave in a manner similar to the parent drug or may interact with different receptors altogether. In either case, the relationship between parent drug concentration and response will be altered.

- **Concurrent drug treatment:** In a manner similar to active metabolites, the presence of other drugs that have similar pharmacodynamic activities will contribute to efficacy or toxicity but not to measurement of the drug concentration. The therapeutic range will be shifted.

- **Patient's age:** While there is not much information concerning developmental changes in pharmacodynamics, it is believed that the numbers and affinities of pharmacologic receptors change with progression of age from newborns to advanced age.[22] This would be expected to result in a shift of the therapeutic range.

- **Electrolyte status:** As an example, hypokalemia, hypomagnesemia, and hypercalcemia are all known to increase the cardiac effects of digitalis glycosides and enhance the potential for digoxin toxicity at a given serum concentration.[23]

- **Concurrent disease:** As an example, patients with underlying heart disease (coronary atherosclerotic heart disease, old myocardial infarction, or cor pulmonale) have increased sensitivity to digoxin.[23] There is also evidence that thyroid disease alters the usual response patterns of digoxin.[23]

- **Variable ratios of enantiomers:** Some drugs are administered as racemic mixtures of enantiomers, which may have different response/toxicity profiles as well as pharmacokinetic behaviors. Thus, a given level of the summed enantiomers (using an achiral assay method) will be associated with different levels of response or toxicity in patients with different proportions of the enantiomers. This has been extensively studied for disopyramide.[24]

- **Variable genotype:** There is growing evidence that response to certain drugs is genetically determined. In the future, patients may be genotyped before starting drug treatment in order to identify them as nonresponders, responders, or toxic responders.[25,26]

- **Variable serum protein binding:** Theoretically, only the unbound concentration of drug in blood is capable of establishing equilibrium with pharmacologic receptors, thus making it a better predictor of response than total drug concentration. Most drug concentrations in serum, plasma or blood, however, are measured as the summed concentration of bound and unbound drug. It is very likely that some of the patients who show toxicity within the conventional therapeutic range have abnormally low protein binding and high concentrations of unbound drug in blood.[27]

In summary, the therapeutic range reported by the laboratory is only an initial guide and is not a guarantee of desired clinical response in any individual patient. Every effort must be made to consider other signs of clinical response and toxicity in addition to the drug concentration measurement. Therapeutic ranges for the most commonly monitored drugs discussed in the Applications section of this chapter are reported in Table 6-3.

TABLE 6-3

	RECOMMENDED CONCENTRATIONS	RECOMMENDED TIMING	CONSIDERATIONS FOR INTERPRETATION: PROTEIN BINDING, ACTIVE METABOLITES, OTHER FACTORS
Analgesic/Anti-inflammatory			
Salicylate	100–250 mg/L	Trough or $C_{ss,avg}$. Steady state occurs after 1 week.	Salicylic acid binding to albumin is concentration-dependent. Unbound fractions increase in pregnancy and in patients with liver disease, nephrotic syndrome, and uremia. Lower total levels might be more appropriate in these patients with decreased serum binding.
Antiasthmatics			
Theophylline	Adult: 5–15 mg/L Neonate: 5–13 mg/L	Trough or $C_{ss,avg}$. Steady state occurs in 24 hr for an average adult nonsmoker.	Metabolite caffeine of minor significance in adults; may contribute to effect in neonates.
Caffeine	Neonate: 10–20 mg/L	Anytime during interval acceptable. Steady state not necessary.	
Antiepileptics			
Carbamazepine	4–12 mg/L	Trough or $C_{ss,avg}$. Steady state may require up to 2–3 weeks after initiation of full dose rate.	Lower total concentrations may be more appropriate in patients with decreased protein binding—liver disease, hypoalbuminemia, and hyperbilirubinemia.
Ethosuximide	40–100 mg/L	Anytime during interval. Steady state may require up to 12 days.	
Phenytoin	Adult: 10–20 mg/L Infant: 6–11 mg/L	Trough or $C_{ss,avg}$. Steady state may require up to 3 weeks.	Lower total phenytoin levels may be more appropriate in patients with decreased protein binding due to hypoalbuminemia (e.g., liver disease, nephrotic syndrome, pregnancy, cystic fibrosis, burns, trauma, malnutrition, AIDS, and advanced age), end stage renal disease, concurrent salicylic acid, or valproic acid.
Phenobarbital	15–40 mg/L	Anytime during interval. Steady state may require up to 3 weeks.	Phenobarbital, a metabolite of primidone, may be primary determinant of primidone effect; it must always be measured when primidone is administered.
Primidone	5–12 mg/L	Steady state may require up to 3 weeks.	
Valproic Acid	50–100 mg/L	Trough or $C_{ss,avg}$. Steady state may require up to 5 days.	Lower total valproic acid levels may be more appropriate in patients with hypoalbuminemia, (liver disease, cystic fibrosis, burns, trauma, malnutrition, and advanced age), hyperbilirubinemia, end-stage renal disease, and concurrent salicylic acid. Valproic acid shows interpatient variability in unbound fraction because of nonlinear protein binding; total concentrations will increase less than proportionately with increases in daily dose, while unbound concentrations will increase proportionately.
Antimicrobial Drugs			
Amikacin	Traditional Dosing Peaks: 20–30 mg/L Troughs: 1–8 mg/L	Traditional Dosing: steady state occurs after 3rd or 4th dose. Pulse dosing: per protocol.	
Gentamicin, Netilmicin, Tobramycin	Traditional Dosing Peaks: 6–10 mg/L Troughs: 0.5–2 mg/L	Traditional Dosing: steady state occurs after 3rd or 4th dose. Pulse dosing: per protocol.	

	RECOMMENDED CONCENTRATIONS	RECOMMENDED TIMING	CONSIDERATIONS FOR INTERPRETATION: PROTEIN BINDING, ACTIVE METABOLITES, OTHER FACTORS
Chloramphenicol	Adult: 10–20 mg/L Neonate: 7.5–14 mg/L	Peak. Steady state may require up to 24 hr.	
Vancomycin	Troughs: 5–10 mg/L	Trough, within 1 hr of next dose. Steady state may require up to 2–3 days in patients with normal renal function.	Desired trough levels may be higher in some institutions.
Cardiac Drugs			
Digoxin	0.5–2.0 µg/L	*NEVER* sooner than 6 hours after an oral dose. Steady state may require up to 7 days with normal renal function.	Digoxin toxicity more likely within therapeutic range in patients with hypokalemia, hypomagnesemia, hypercalcemia, underlying heart disease, and hypothyroidism. Patients with hyperthyroidism may be resistant at a given digoxin level.
Lidocaine	1.5–5 mg/L	Anytime during infusion once steady state is reached. Steady state may require up to 24 hr.	High lidocaine levels in postmyocardial infarction patients may not be associated with toxicity because of increased serum binding. Higher total levels may be acceptable in other conditions associated with increased binding—rheumatoid arthritis, cancer, morbid obesity, or any kind of physiologic trauma.
Procainamide/ N-acetyl-procainamide (NAPA)	Procainamide: 4–8 mg/L, up to 12 mg/L in some. NAPA: 5–30 mg/L	Trough, within 1 hr of next oral dose. Steady state may require up to 18 hr in normal function for steady state of both parent and NAPA.	NAPA levels will accumulate more than procainamide in patients with renal impairment; NAPA should always be measured along with procainamide in these patients. Levels of procainamide and NAPA should be separately compared to their own therapeutic ranges, rather than to a therapeutic range of summed concentrations.
Quinidine	2–5 mg/L	Trough, within 1 hr of next oral dose. Steady state may require up to 3 days.	Higher total levels may be acceptable in conditions associated with increased binding—myocardial infarction, cardiac surgery, atrial arrhythmias, heart failure, or any other kind of physiologic trauma.
Cytotoxic Drugs			
Methotrexate	0.01–0.1 µM (per protocol)	Per protocol for determination of leucovorin rescue regimen.	Decreased protein binding is observed in some situations, but implications for interpretation of total levels are unclear.
Immunosuppressives			
Cyclosporine	100–400 µg/L (whole blood, using specific assay)	Trough. Steady state may require up to 5 days.	Highly variable unbound fraction in blood. Higher total levels may be acceptable in patients with hypercholesterolemia or prior to acute rejection episodes (increased serum binding). Lower total levels might be acceptable in patients with decreased binding in serum (low cholesterol).
Psychotropics			
Amitriptyline	Amitriptyline + nortriptyline: 120–125 µg/L	12–14 hr after the bedtime dose for once-daily dosing. Steady state may require up to 11 days.	
Nortriptyline	50–150 µg/L		

	RECOMMENDED CONCENTRATIONS	**RECOMMENDED TIMING**	**CONSIDERATIONS FOR INTERPRETATION: PROTEIN BINDING, ACTIVE METABOLITES, OTHER FACTORS**
Imipramine	Imipramine + desipramine: 180–350 µg/L	12–14 hr after the bedtime dose for once-daily dosing. Steady state may require up to 6 days for steady state.	Unbound fractions are decreased in alcoholics and cardiac patients; higher total concentrations may be acceptable in patients suspected to have higher binding. Active metabolites (imipramine of desipramine and nortriptyline of amitriptyline) must always be determined in addition to the parent drug, as they contributed significantly to therapeutic effect.
Desipramine	115–250 µg/L		
Lithium	0.5–1.2 mEq/L	12 hr after the evening dose on BID or TID schedule. Steady state may require up to 1 week.	

Table 6-3. Data To Aid Interpretation of Concentrations of Drugs That Are Commonly Monitored

Sample Timing

Incorrect timing of sample collection is the most frequent source of error when therapeutic drug monitoring results do not agree with the clinical picture. Warner[17] reviewed five studies in which 70–86% of the samples obtained for therapeutic drug monitoring purposes were not usable. In most cases, this was the result of inappropriate sample timing, including lack of attention to the time required to reach a steady state. There are two primary considerations for sample timing: (1) how long to wait after initiation or adjustment of a dosage regimen, and (2) when to obtain the sample during a dosing interval.

At steady state. When a drug dosage regimen (a fixed dose given at a regular interval) is initiated, concentrations are initially low and gradually increase until a steady state is reached. Pharmacokinetically, *steady state* is defined as the condition in which the rate of drug entering the body is equal to the rate of its elimination. For the purpose of therapeutic drug monitoring, a steady state means that drug concentrations have leveled off at their highest and, when given as the same dose at a fixed interval, the concentration vs. time profiles are constant from interval to interval. This is illustrated in Figure 6-3 for a constant infusion and a chronic intermittent dosage regimen.

Drug concentration measurements should not be made until the drug is sufficiently close to a steady state, so that the maximum benefit of the drug is assured. The time required to

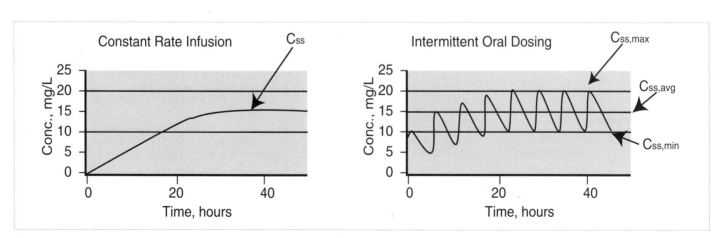

Figure 6-3. Concentration vs. time plots for a constant infusion and intermittent therapy after initiation of therapy, without a loading dose. The half-life for this hypothetical drug is 8 hr. Thus, 88% of the eventual average steady state concentration ($C_{ss,avg}$) is attained in 24 hr.

reach a steady state can be predicted if the drug's half-life is known. Eighty-eight percent of the ultimate steady state is reached after three half-lives; 94% after four half-lives; and 97% after five half-lives. This means the clinician should wait three half-lives at a minimum before obtaining a sample for monitoring purposes. The half-lives of drugs that are typically monitored are reported in the Applications section, and typical times to steady state are reported in Table 6-3.

Sometimes drugs are not given as a fixed dose at a fixed interval, or they may undergo diurnal variations in pharmacokinetic handling.[28,29] While the concentration vs. time profiles may differ from each other within a given day, the patterns from day-to-day will be the same if a steady state has been attained. In cases of irregular dosing or diurnal variations, it is important that drug concentration measurements on different visits be obtained at similar times of the day for comparative purposes.

An unusual situation is caused by autoinduction, as exemplified by carbamazepine. The half-life of carbamazepine is longer after the first dose but progressively shortens as the enzymes that metabolize carbamazepine are induced by exposure to itself.[30] The half-life of carbamazepine during chronic therapy cannot be used to predict the time required to reach a steady state. The actual time to reach a steady state is somewhere between the time based on the first-dose half-life and that based on the chronic-dosing half-life.

It is a common misconception that a steady state is reached faster when a loading dose is given. While a carefully chosen loading dose will provide desired target levels following that first dose, it will still require at least three half-lives to attain a true steady state. Whenever possible, it is best to allow more time for a steady state to be attained than less. This is also important because the average half-life for the population may not apply to a specific patient.

There are some exceptions to the rule of waiting until a steady state is reached before sampling. If there is suspected toxicity early during therapy, a drug concentration measurement is warranted and may necessitate immediate reduction of the dose rate. Dosing methods designed to predict maintenance dosage regimens use presteady state drug levels[31–35] and are useful when rapid individualization of the dosage regimen is needed.

Within the dosing interval. Figure 6-3 shows typical concentration vs. time profiles for a drug given by constant infusion and a drug given by oral intermittent dosing. Once a steady state is attained, drug concentrations during a constant infusion remain constant, and samples for drug concentration measurements can be obtained at anytime. When a drug is given intermittently, however, there is fluctuation in the drug concentration profile. The lowest concentration during the interval is known as the *steady state minimum concentration,* or the trough. The highest concentration is known as the *steady state maximum concentration,* or the peak. Also shown in Figure 6-3 is the *steady state average concentration* ($C_{ss,avg}$), which represents the time-averaged concentration during the dosage interval. An important principle of dosing for drugs that show first-order behavior is that the average concentration during the interval or day will change in direct proportion to the change in the daily dose. This is covered in more detail in the Use of Levels for Dosage Adjustment section

The degree of fluctuation within a dosing interval will depend on three factors: the half-life of the drug in that patient; how quickly the drug is absorbed (as reflected by the time at which a peak concentration occurs for that particular formulation); and the dosing interval. The least fluctuation (lowest peak:trough ratio) will occur for drugs with relatively long half-lives that are slowly absorbed or given as sustained-release formulations (prolonged peak time) and are given in divided doses (short dosing interval). However, drugs with relatively short half-lives that are quickly absorbed (or given as prompt-release products) and given only once daily will show the greatest amount of fluctuation within the interval.

TERESA R., A 37-YEAR-OLD FEMALE with chronic renal failure from long-term use of amphotericin B for a previous fungal infection, recently underwent a kidney transplant. She received an oral loading dose of cyclosporine followed by an oral maintenance regimen (100 mg every 12 hr), prednisone (1.5 mg/kg/day), and azathioprine (1 mg/kg/day). Eight days after the transplant, she developed urosepsis from *Escherichia coli* and was given gentamicin and piperacillin. She was hemodynamically stable, but 3 days later her kidney function declined (BUN from 25 to 50 mg/dL and urine output from 1000 to 400 mL per day). A gentamicin trough (2.5 mg/L) was only slightly above the target trough of 2 mg/L. A predose cyclosporine whole blood concentration was low at 110 µg/L using the monoclonal fluorescence polarization immunoassay (TDx®). Her kidney biopsy revealed signs of early rejection.

Teresa R. was taken off gentamicin and piperacillin and switched to ceftriaxone because it is cleared by nonrenal routes and not associated with nephrotoxicity. She was given boluses of methylprednisolone (15 mg/kg/day) for 2 days, and her oral cyclosporine was increased to 300 mg every 12 hr. Over the next 7 days, her renal function improved. At the end of that period, her predose cyclosporine concentration was 325 µg/L. Teresa R. was discharged and experienced no complications for a long time.

Question: What role did cyclosporine concentrations play here?

Discussion: Early rejection was suspected to be the cause of decreasing renal function rather than gentamicin toxicity, given the low gentamicin concentrations and only 3 days of therapy. Initial cyclosporine concentrations on the low end of the therapeutic range (100–400 µg/L) were consistent with this hypothesis and a biopsy confirmed it. Rejection was probably related to low cyclosporine concentrations, which generally need to be at the upper end of the therapeutic range early during therapy. An increase in the daily cyclosporine dose resulted in a proportional increase of the trough concentration into the range associated with long-term graft survival. If Teresa R.'s cyclosporine concentration had been greater than 400 µg/L and her biopsy showed no signs of rejection, cyclosporine nephrotoxicity would have been diagnosed and her cyclosporine dosage reduced.

Minicase 2 is adapted from the second edition chapter titled "Interpretation of Serum Drug Concentrations," which was written by Scott L. Traub.

The estimated degree of fluctuation (peak:trough ratio) for a given dosage regimen can be estimated by comparing the drug's half-life in a patient to the difference between the dosing interval and the estimated time required to reach a peak concentration.[36] The following guidelines may be used:

$\dfrac{\text{Interval} - \text{Peak Time}}{\text{Half-Life}}$	Peak:Trough Ratio
2.00	4.0
1.50	2.8
1.00	2.0
0.50	1.4
0.25	1.2

Using the information above, concentrations during the interval fluctuate very little (peaks are only 1.2 times troughs) if the difference between the dosing interval and peak time is one-quarter of the drug's half-life. In that case, it may be assumed that concentrations obtained anytime during the interval are almost equivalent; the peak, trough, and average concentrations are roughly equal.

The choice of timing for samples within the dosing interval should be based on the clinical question to be addressed. Troughs are usually recommended for therapeutic confirmation, especially if the therapeutic range was formulated based on trough levels as for most of the antiepileptic drugs.[13] Trough concentrations are also recommended if the indication for concentration monitoring is avoidance of inefficacy or distinguishing noncompliance from therapeutic failure. Trough concentrations should also be monitored if the patient tends to experience symptoms of inefficacy before the next dose (in which case a shortening of the dosing interval might be all that is needed). While it is logical to assume that the lowest concentration during the interval will occur immediately before the next dose, this is not always the case. Some products are formulated as delayed-release products (e.g., enteric-coated valproic acid) that are designed to be absorbed from the intestine rather than the stomach. As such, they may not begin to be absorbed for several hours after administration, and the level of drug from the previous dose continues to decline for several hours into the next interval. It is important to recognize that the predose level for those formulations is not the lowest level during the interval. (Figure 6-4)

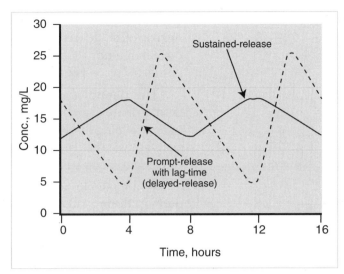

Figure 6-4. Concentration vs. time profiles for a prompt-release formulation that exhibits a lag-time in its release or absorption (delayed-release) as compared to a sustained-release formulation without lag-time. Note that the lowest concentration during the dosing interval for the delayed-release product occurs at a time that is typically expected for the peak to occur.

Peak concentrations are monitored less often for drugs given orally because the time at which peak concentrations occur is difficult to predict. If a peak concentration is indicated, the package insert should be consulted for peak times of individual products. Peak concentration monitoring would be appropriate if the patient complains of symptoms of toxicity at a time believed to correspond with a peak concentration. Peaks may also be used for intravenous drugs (aminoglycosides and chloramphenicol) because the time of the peak is known to correspond to the end of the infusion. For the aminoglycosides, the peak level is believed to be a predictor of efficacy, while for chloramphenicol the peak concentration predicts both efficacy and adverse effects.[37]

Sometimes the clinician wishes to get an idea of the average level of drug during the day or dosing interval. This is particularly useful when the level is to be used for a dosage adjustment. Pharmacokinetically, the average level equals the area-under-the-curve (AUC) during the dosing interval (requiring multiple samples) divided by the interval. (Note: The AUC during an interval or portion of an interval is used as the monitoring parameter in place of single drug concentration measurements for certain drugs, such as some immunosuppressant and cytotoxic drugs, because it provides a better indication of overall drug exposure.) However, determination of the AUC, or $C_{ss,avg}$, by multiple sampling is not cost-effective for the most commonly monitored drugs. The following are alternatives to estimating the $C_{ss,avg}$ without multiple samples:

- Look up the expected time to reach a peak concentration for the particular formulation and obtain a sample midway between that time and the end of the dosing interval.[20]
- Measure the trough level (as close to the time of administration of the next dose as possible) and use that along with the population value for the drug's volume of distribution (Vd) to estimate the peak level as follows:

$$Peak_{steady-state} = (Dose/Vd) + measured\ trough$$

Then take the simple average of the trough and the peak to get an estimate of the average steady-state level.

- If you have reason to believe that there is very little fluctuation during the dosing interval, then a sample drawn anytime during the interval will provide a reasonable reflection of the average concentration.

There are special and extremely important timing considerations for some drugs, such as digoxin. It must reach specific receptors, presumably in the myocardium, to exhibit its therapeutic effect, but this takes a number of hours after the dose is administered. Early after a digoxin dose, levels in serum are relatively high, but response is not yet evident because digoxin has not yet equilibrated at its site of action. Thus, only digoxin levels that are in the postdistribution phase should be monitored and compared to the reported therapeutic range.

The timing of samples for other drugs may be based on the requirements for certain dosing methods. This is true for the aminoglycosides and certain lithium dosing methods. Sample timing for drugs like methotrexate will be specified in protocols because concentrations are used to determine the need for rescue therapy with leucovorin to minimize methotrexate toxicity.

While samples for drug concentration measurements may be preferred at certain times during a dosing interval, visits to physician offices often do not coincide with desired times for blood draws. One is then faced with the matter of how to interpret a level that is drawn at a time that happens to be more convenient to the patient's appointment. The most critical pieces of information to obtain in this situation are (1) when the last drug dose was taken; (2) how compliant the patient has been; (3) timing of the sample relative to the last dose; and (4) when is the expected time of peak concentration. Some drugs are available as a wide variety of formulations (solutions, suspensions, prompt-release, and sustained- or extended-release solid dosage forms), and the package insert may be the best source of information for the expected peak time. Once again, drugs with relatively long half-lives given as sustained-release or slowly absorbed products in divided doses will have the flattest concentration vs. time profiles, and levels drawn anytime during the interval are going to be similar. However, prompt-release drugs with short half-lives given less frequently will show more fluctuation. Knowing the expected peak time for the formulation in question is especially important for drugs that show more fluctuation during that interval. In that case, one can at least judge if the reported concentration is closer to a peak, an average (if midway between the peak and trough), or a trough.

Specimens, Collection Methods, and Assays

Whole blood, plasma, and serum. Whole blood, plasma, serum, and ultrafiltrate of serum are commonly used specimens for drug concentration measurements. Unbound drug molecules in blood distribute themselves among red blood cells, binding proteins (albumin, alpha-1-acid glycoprotein (AAG), and lipoproteins) and plasma water based on how avidly they partition into red blood cells; the concentrations of binding proteins in blood; and the affinities of the binding proteins for the drug.[27]

Samples for plasma or whole blood analysis are collected in tubes that contain an anticoagulant. Plasma is created by centrifugation of the blood sample and collection of the upper layer containing plasma water, protein, unbound drug, and protein-bound drug. Samples for serum are collected in tubes without an anticoagulant and allowed to clot followed by centrifugation, while samples for unbound drug measurements, preferably serum, are ultrafiltered (as described below) to create serum water that contains only unbound drug. Concentrations of drug in ultrafiltrate of serum are always lower than the corresponding total (bound plus unbound) concentrations, especially for drugs that are highly bound to serum proteins. Because the only difference between plasma and serum is that the clotting factors have been consumed when serum is created, drug concentrations in plasma and serum are generally regarded to be equivalent. Concentrations of drug in whole blood are higher than the corresponding serum or plasma concentrations if the drug happens to concentrate within red blood cells.

The choice of serum, plasma or whole blood for a drug concentration measurement depends in part on the requirements of the assay to be used. Serum or plasma would be better if hemoglobin interferes with the assay. An assay with marginal sensitivity might be more useful if whole blood is used for a drug that concentrates in the red blood cell. Some of the newer physician office or desktop methods have the advantage of using capillary whole blood from fingersticks, thus obviating the need for centrifugation or other sample preparation steps.

The choice of blood collection method is extremely important. For plasma analyses, it is important to know if the particular anticoagulant interferes with the assay, affects the stability or protein binding of the drug, or even dilutes the sample.[38] There have been numerous reports that polymer-based gels, designed to form a barrier between serum and the clot during centrifugation, may also absorb drugs from the serum to varying extents. Technical improvements in these devices (know as *serum separator tubes*) have been made,[39] but, nevertheless, several groups have categorically recommended that separation gels not be used for blood collection unless rigorous testing has first been done.[40] Finally, there were a number of reports in the 1970s and 1980s of artifacts caused by contact of serum or plasma with rubber stoppers of evacuated blood collection tubes.[41,42] Tris-(2-butoxyethyl)phosphate (TBEP) in the rubber stoppers leached into the serum or plasma and displaced basic drugs from AAG, thus causing redistribution of unbound drug into the red blood cells. When the samples were centrifuged, the total plasma or serum drug concentration was decreased to varying extents. Although recent studies of reformulated stoppers for these tubes show no artifacts,[42] each laboratory must perform their own tests to assure that similar artifacts are not observed.

Specific recommendations for blood collection methods and collection tubes will be presented in the Applications sections that follow for each drug or drug category.

Alternatives to blood sampling. Saliva has been proposed as a noninvasive alternative to blood sampling, particularly for children, for a number of drugs.[43–45] Saliva is a natural ultrafiltrate of plasma and, thus, may provide a closer reflection of the therapeutically active unbound drug concentration in serum as compared to the total drug concentration.[46] Concentrations of drug in saliva are much lower than total concentrations in serum of highly bound drugs, and assay sensitivity should be considered if saliva samples are used for drug concentration monitoring.

Use of saliva drug concentration as a substitute for total or unbound drug concentration in serum or plasma requires that the saliva:plasma (S:P) drug concentration ratio be stable, at least within a patient. The S:P ratio, however, can be influenced by salivary flow rate, saliva pH, and contamination by residual drug in the mouth. With the exception of saliva pH, these factors can be controlled by careful selection of the collection method. The degree of a drug's ionization affects the extent to which it passively diffuses from blood into saliva. Blood pH is constant, but saliva pH varies widely during the day within a patient, and the S:P ratio may, therefore, change considerably during the day. Neutral drugs are not expected to show variable S:P ratios within patients,[46] while acids or bases with pKa values similar to blood pH are most likely to be sensitive to variations in saliva pH. Correction of the S:P ratio may be possible, however, if the saliva pH is measured.[47]

Whole saliva is most often collected, and it can be either *stimulated* or *unstimulated*. Stimulated saliva is preferred: it produces a larger volume, minimizes the pH gradient between saliva and blood, and provides more stable S:P ratios. Methods for stimulating whole saliva production include the chewing or rolling of inert materials (paraffin, wax, and glass marble) in the mouth or applying a small amount of citric acid to the tongue.[48] Novel methods have been proposed for collection of saliva for home monitoring purposes in children. One involves placing a gauze-wrapped cotton ball, with attached string, in the child's mouth for a period of time and squeezing saliva from the retrieved cotton using a plastic syringe.[49] Special devices that collect saliva from specific salivary glands are commercially available and offer the advantage of reduced viscosity and more reproducible results.[50] Regardless of the method used, contamination of saliva from residual drug in the mouth must be avoided by collecting saliva no earlier than 2–3 hr after a dose and rinsing the mouth with deionized water prior to collection. In some studies, an initial collection of saliva is discarded.

Lacrimal fluid has been proposed as an ideal medium for monitoring unbound drug, since it does not have the problem with pH changes.[51–53] Tears may be stimulated by exposing the eye to cigarette smoke or having the patient sniff formaldehyde fumes. In another method, tears are collected by hooking small strips of blotting paper over the lower lid of the eye for a few minutes.[52] The major limitation for assay of drug in tears is the sensitivity of the assay, since large volumes cannot be collected.

Storage. The following factors can affect drug concentrations in serum, serum ultrafiltrate, plasma, whole blood, and saliva: exposure to light, temperature, storage container, and presence of other drugs or endogenous substances. Specific information for each drug or drug category, if available, will be provided in the Applications sections.

Assays. Interpretation of any drug concentration measurement requires full knowledge of the strengths and limitations of the analytical method that was used. Laboratories should readily supply clinicians with all details of assay performance, including linearity, coefficients of variation at high and low concentrations, minimum detection limit, and potential interferences. While the laboratory must consistently conform to accepted standards for accuracy and reproducibility, requirements for assay sensitivity and specificity will depend on the intended use, the therapeutic range, the volume to be analyzed, and the nature of the specimen (serum/plasma, whole blood, serum ultrafiltrate, or saliva).

Knowledge of the sensitivity of a method (the ability to quantitate drug when drug is present) is helpful to interpret a laboratory report of *nondetectable*. If the method is highly sensitive, nondetectable may actually mean there is no drug in the sample. If the method is less sensitive, however, there could be drug in the sample but just not enough to register.[54] The minimum detection limit will be of greatest concern for drugs with lower therapeutic ranges (i.e., in the μg/L range) such as digoxin and the protease inhibitors. More sensitive assays are also required when there are small sample volumes, such as in neonates. Drug concentrations in saliva or in ultrafiltrates of serum may require more sensitive assays if the drugs are highly bound to serum proteins. In some cases, assays may be based on blood concentrations for drugs that concentrate in red blood cells in order to overcome limitations of sensitivity.[55]

Knowledge of the specificity (the ability to detect nothing when nothing is there) of a method is equally important. If the drug concentration report from the laboratory is higher than would be expected with no attendant toxicity, the clinician might suspect an interference with the assay. Substances that may interfere with assays include drug metabolites, other drugs, and endogenous substances (e.g., lipids, bilirubin, hemoglobin, or uremic byproducts that accumulate in renal impairment). As an example, endogenous digoxin-like immunoreactive substances accumulate in the serum of neonates, pregnant patients, and patients with liver or renal disease[56] and are reported to cause falsely elevated digoxin concentration readings. Some assays are purposely developed to be nonspecific for purposes of drug abuse screens. Examples are the immunoassays used for detection of *benzodiazepines*, *tricyclics*, or *barbiturates*.

Knowledge of the condition or appearance of the sample at the time of assay may be important. A sample with a milky appearance may indicate lipemia; one with a dark yellow to gold appearance may mean high bilirubin levels; one with a pinkish tinge may mean hemolysis. All of these conditions can result in either overreading (positive bias) or underreading (negative bias) of a drug concentration, depending on the analytical method. Drugs that are more concentrated in red blood cells than in serum will have artifactually high-serum concentration readings in a hemolyzed sample, while drugs that are less concentrated in the red blood cell will dilute the serum or plasma resulting in artifactually low readings.

High-performance liquid chromatography (HPLC) and gas-liquid chromatography (GLC) are still used in clinical laboratories and are considered in many cases to be the reference methods. Immunoassays have become the method of choice, however, because of ease of use, ability to automate, and rapid turnaround time. Of the immunoassays, the fluorescence polarization immunoassay (FPIA; TDx® System, Abbott Diagnostics) and the homogeneous enzyme-multiplied immunotechnique (EMIT®; Dade Behring) methods are the most commonly used. The immunologic methods are generally specific for the parent drug, but in some cases metabolites or other drug-like substances are recognized by the antibody. Certain drugs are not suitable for immunologic assays. Lithium, an electrolyte, is an example of this and must be analyzed using ion-selective electrode technology, atomic absorption spectroscopy, or flame emission photometry.

The increased interest in drug assay methods for use in ambulatory settings, such as physician offices, has led to the development of immunoassay systems purported to be fast, reliable, and cost-effective.[5,57–59] Most of these so-called desktop systems have the capacity to produce results within 1–5 min; some use whole blood. Prior to 1988, less than 10% of all clinical laboratories were required to meet quality standards. Growing concern about lack of quality control in settings such as physician offices led to adoption of the 1998 Clinical Laboratory Improvement Amendments (CLIA) in which three levels of testing complexity were defined: waived, moderately complex, and highly complex. All drug concentration measurement testing is currently classified either as moderate or high complexity, and laboratories that perform these assays must maintain a quality control program, participate in proficiency testing programs, and be periodically inspected.[5] These physician office methods vary in their reliability as compared to reference methods.[60–63]

Use of Levels for Dosage Adjustment

A chronic intermittent dosage regimen has three components: the dose rate, the dosing interval, and the dose. For the dosage regimen of 240 mg every 8 hr, the dose is 240 mg, the interval is 8 hr, and the dose rate can be expressed as 720 mg/day or 30 mg/hr. The dose rate is important because it determines the average concentration ($C_{ss,avg}$) during the day. The degree of fluctuation within a dosing interval is highly influenced by the dosing interval.

Dosage adjustments for linear behavior. If a drug is known to have first-order bioavailability and elimination behavior after therapeutic doses, one can use simple proportionality to make an adjustment in the daily dose:

- If average levels are being monitored or estimated, one can predict that the average, steady state drug concentration will increase in proportion to the increase in daily dose, regardless of any changes that were made in the dosing interval.
- If trough levels are monitored and the dosing interval will be held constant, the trough level will increase in proportion to the increase in daily dose.
- If trough levels are monitored for a drug that exhibits considerable fluctuation during the interval, and *both* the dose rate *and* dosing interval will be adjusted, the trough concentration will not be as easy to predict at a new steady state and is beyond the scope of this chapter. If the trough concentration can be used to estimate the $C_{ss,avg}$, as described above, the $C_{ss,avg}$ can be predicted with certainty to change in proportion to the change in daily dose.

Sampling after a dosage regimen adjustment, if appropriate, should not be done until a new steady state has been reached. For a drug with first-order behavior, this should take the same period of time (three half-lives at a minimum) that it did after initiation of therapy with this drug.

Dosage adjustments for drugs with nonlinear behavior. All drugs will show nonlinear elimination behavior if sufficiently high doses are given. Some drugs, however, show pronounced nonlinear (Michaelis-Menten) behavior following doses that produce therapeutic drug concentrations. This means that an increase in the dose rate of the drug will result in a greater-than-proportional increase in the drug concentration. Phenytoin is an example of a drug with this behavior. Theophylline, procainamide, and salicylate also show some degree of nonlinear behavior but only at the higher end of their therapeutic ranges (and not enough to require special dosing methods).

Methods have been described to permit predictions of the effect of dose rate increases for phenytoin[64] but are beyond the scope of this chapter. The most important rule to remember for dosage adjustments of drugs like phenytoin is to be conservative; small increases in the dose rate will produce unpredictably large increases in the serum drug concentration. It must also be remembered that the half-life of a drug like phenytoin will be progressively prolonged at higher dose rates. Increases in dose rate will require a longer period of time to reach a steady state as compared to when the drug was first initiated.

Population pharmacokinetic or Bayesian dosage adjustment methods, which involve the use of statistical probabilities, are preferred by many for individualization of therapy.[65] They are useful for drugs with both linear and nonlinear behavior.

Protein Binding, Active Metabolites, and Other Considerations

Altered serum binding. Total (unbound plus protein-bound) drug concentrations measured in blood, serum, or plasma are almost always used for therapeutic drug monitoring, despite the fact that unbound drug concentrations are more closely correlated to drug effect.[27] This is because it is easier to measure the total concentration and because the ratio of unbound to total drug concentration in serum is usually constant within and between individuals. For some drugs, however, the relationship between unbound and total drug concentration is extremely variable among patients, or it may be altered by disease or drug interactions. For drugs that undergo concentration-dependent serum binding, the relationship between unbound and total concentration varies *within* patients. In all of these situations, total drug concentration does not reflect the same level of activity as with normal binding and must be cautiously interpreted because the usual therapeutic range will not apply.

The direct measurement of unbound drug concentration would seem to be appropriate in these situations. Drugs for which total concentration monitoring is routinely performed (but for which unbound concentration monitoring has been proposed) include carbamazepine, disopyramide, lidocaine, phenytoin, quinidine, and valproic acid. Of these, correlations between unbound drug concentration and response have only been weakly established for carbamazepine and disopyramide[27] but more firmly established for phenytoin.[66]

Unbound drug concentration measurements involve an extra step prior to analysis—separation of the unbound from the bound drug. Equilibrium dialysis and ultracentrifugation may be used in a research setting, but ultrafiltration is the method of choice for a clinical laboratory.[27] Commercial systems for unbound drug concentration measurements involve centrifugation of serum in tubes containing a semipermeable membrane (e.g., Millipore Centrifree® UF device). The ultrafiltrate, containing unbound drug, is collected in small cup and assayed. The method used for analysis of the ultrafiltrate must be sufficiently sensitive since lower drug concentrations will be observed for highly bound drugs. Specificity of the assay may also be especially important. The ratio of metabolite to parent drug is likely to be greater in the ultrafiltrate since most metabolites are not as highly bound to protein as the parent. Thus, an immunoassay that shows acceptable specificity using total serum might show unacceptable specificity using ultrafiltrate.[67]

If unbound drug concentration measurements are unavailable, too costly, or considered impractical, the following alternative approaches to interpreting total drug concentrations in situations of altered serum protein binding may be used:

- **Use of equations to normalize the measured total concentration:** Sheiner and Tozer[68] were the first to propose equations that can be used to convert a measured total concentration of drug (phenytoin in this case) to what it would be if the patient had normal binding. Equations to normalize total phenytoin concentrations have been used for patients with hypoalbuminemia, impaired renal function, and concurrent valproic acid therapy.[36,69] Once the total level has been normalized, it may be compared to the conventional therapeutic range.

- **Normalize the measured total concentration using literature estimates of the abnormal unbound drug fraction:** An alternative method for normalizing the total concentration can be used if reasonable estimates of the abnormal and normal unbound reactions of the drug can be ascertained (i.e., from the literature). The normalized total concentration ($C_{normalized}$) can be estimated as

$$C_{normalized} = C_{measured} \times \frac{\text{Abnormal unbound fraction}}{\text{Normal unbound fraction}}$$

  where $C_{measured}$ is the measured total concentrations reported by the laboratory.

- **Predictive linear regression equations:** Some studies have reported the ability to predict unbound drug concentrations in the presence of displacing drugs if the total concentrations of both drugs are known. This has been done to predict unbound concentrations of phenytoin[70] and carbamazepine,[71] both in the presence of valproic acid. These unbound drug concentrations should be compared to corresponding therapeutic ranges of unbound drug, which can be estimated for any drug if the normal unbound fraction and the usual therapeutic range of total concentrations (TR) are known:

$$TR_u = TR \times \text{normal unbound fraction}$$

- **Use of saliva or tears as a substitute for unbound drug concentration:** This may be a reasonable alternative so long as studies have shown a strong correlation between unbound concentrations in serum and concentrations in saliva or lacrimal fluid. The concentration of drug in saliva or tears may not be equal to the concentration in serum ultrafiltrate. Therefore, the laboratory should have determined a reliable conversion factor for this. The calculated unbound concentration may then be compared to the estimated therapeutic range for unbound concentrations as described above.

Active metabolites. Interpretation of parent drug concentration alone, for drugs with active metabolites that are present to varying extents, is difficult at best. Active metabolites may contribute to therapeutic response, to toxicity, or to both. Since metabolites will likely have different pharmacokinetic characteristics, they will be affected differently than the parent drug under different physiologic and pathologic conditions.

For drugs like primidone (metabolized to phenobarbital) and procainamide (metabolized to N-acetylprocainamide), the laboratory will typically report both the parent and the metabolite as well as a therapeutic range for both. While a therapeutic range for the sum of procainamide and N-acetylprocainamide may be reported by some laboratories, this practice is discouraged since the parent and metabolites have different types of pharmacologic activities.

Enantiomeric pairs. Some drugs exist as an equal mixture (racemic mixture) of enantiomers, which are chemically identical but are mirror images of each other. Because they can interact differently with receptors, they may have very different pharmacodynamic and pharmacokinetic properties. The relative proportions of the enantiomers can differ widely among and within patients. Thus, a given concentration of the summed enantiomers (what is routinely measured using achiral methods) can represent very different activities.

Table 6-3 provides relevant information about protein binding, active metabolites, enantiomers, and other influences on serum concentration interpretation for drugs discussed in the Applications sections that follow.

APPLICATIONS

Analgesic/Anti-inflammatory Drugs

Salicylic Acid

Therapeutic range. The therapeutic range for the analgesic and antipyretic effects of salicylic acid is commonly reported as 20–100 mg/L.[72,73] Salicylate is more commonly monitored, however, for its anti-inflammatory effect: while the commonly reported therapeutic range is 100–250 mg/L,[72] effective concentrations may be as low as 70 mg/L and as high as 300 mg/L.[73] The concentrations associated with toxicity can overlap considerably with those associated with efficacy. Tinnitus, for example, may be experienced at concentrations as low as 200 mg/L. Indications for monitoring salicylate concentrations, other than suspected overdose or chronic salicylate abuse, include suspected toxicity; suspected noncompliance; change in renal function, mental status, acid-base balance or pulmonary status; and anticipated drug-drug interactions.

Sample timing. Salicylic acid undergoes nonlinear elimination, and, thus, the half-life progressively increases from 3 to 20 hr as drug accumulates to within the range of 100–300 mg/L.[74] Because of the progressive prolongation of half-life during initiation of therapy, samples for salicylate monitoring should not be obtained earlier than after 1 week of therapy.[75] The rate of salicylate absorption, while usually fast, is slowed during food intake or when enteric-coated formulations are administered.[75] Trough samples are generally advised for purposes of therapeutic drug monitoring, as they are the most reproducible.[75] Timing of the sample within the interval was not deemed critical in patients with juvenile rheumatoid arthritis who are dosed using an interval of 8 hr or less.[76]

Specimens, collection methods, and assays. Blood samples for determination of salicylate concentration should be collected in tubes without additives or in tubes containing heparin or EDTA.[72] Recent studies of certain evacuated serum separator tubes show they are also acceptable for blood collection for salicylate monitoring.[39,77] Saliva concentrations are extremely variable when compared to unbound salicylate concentrations, and the variability is not explained by pH alone.[45] Saliva is proposed to be a reasonable alternative to icteric serum, however, if a colorimetric method must be used.[72] Salicylate in serum may be stored refrigerated for up to 2 weeks.[72]

Colorimetric methods are used for salicylate determination as well as GLC, HPLC, and FPIA. The FPIA method performs exceptionally well and is recommended over colorimetric methods especially for icteric serum or plasma.[78,79]

Use of levels for dosage adjustment. Two of the metabolic pathways for salicylate are capacity-limited, such that increases in dose rate produce greater-than-proportional increases in unbound serum drug concentrations and response. Because there is also concentration-dependent serum protein binding, total concentrations may mask this nonlinear relationship between dose rate and unbound drug concentration. Droomgoole and Furst[73] provide an algorithm for adjustment of salicylate doses based on total serum salicylate levels.

Protein binding, active metabolites, and other considerations. The binding of salicylate to albumin is concentration-dependent. Specifically, it is approximately 90% bound at total concentrations of 100 mg/L and decreases to 76% bound at levels as high as 400mg/L.[73] The unbound fraction of salicylate is known to increase during pregnancy and in patients with nephrotic syndrome, liver disease, and uremia.[73] While salicylate would seem to be an ideal candidate for unbound concentration monitoring, a therapeutic range for unbound salicylate has not been established. Nevertheless, the clinician should be cautious that total concentrations within the usual therapeutic range may be associated with toxic responses in patients who are suspected to have abnormally low serum binding. No significant differences in the unbound percentage of salicylate in serum were observed among patients with juvenile rheumatoid arthritis, despite widely variable albumin concentrations, suggesting that total concentration monitoring is more appropriate in this group.[80]

Antiasthmatics

Theophylline

Therapeutic range. Many clinicians still use 10–20 mg/L as the accepted therapeutic range for theophylline for management of acute bronchospasm associated with asthma and chronic obstructive pulmonary disease. The 1997 NIH Expert Panel Report, *Guidelines for the Diagnosis and Management of Asthma,* stipulates, however, a more conservative range of 5–15 mg/L.[81] Most patients will respond at serum concentrations within this range, but levels up to 20 mg/L may be necessary in some patients.[81] There is an 85% probability of adverse effects with levels above 25 mg/L, and levels above 30–40mg/L can be associated with dangerous adverse events.[82] Adverse effects typically experienced by adults include nausea, vomiting, diarrhea, irritability, and insomnia at levels above 15 mg/L; supraventricular tachycardia, hypotension, and ventricular arrhythmias at levels above 40 mg/L; and seizures, brain damage, and even death at higher levels. It must also be noted that side effects such as nausea and vomiting, while common, do not occur in all patients and should never be considered prodromal to the occurrence of the more serious side effects.[36]

Theophylline is also indicated for treatment of neonatal apnea, although caffeine is usually preferred.[83] The therapeutic range in neonates is anywhere from 5–6 mg/L on the low end to 10–13 mg/L on the high end.[81,84–86] Adverse effects in neonates include lack of weight-gain, sleeplessness, irritability, diuresis, dehydration, hyperflexia, jitteriness, and serious cardiovascular and neurologic events.[82] Tachycardia has been reported in neonates with levels as low as 13 mg/L.[87]

In summary, there is considerable overlap of therapeutic and toxic effects within the usual therapeutic ranges reported for theophylline in neonates, children, and adults. Serum concentrations should, therefore, never be interpreted in the absence of information about the patient's clinical status. Indications for theophylline monitoring include therapeutic confirmation of effective levels after initiation of therapy or a dosage regimen adjustment, anticipated drug-drug interactions, change in smoking habits, and/or changes in health status that might affect the metabolism of theophylline.

Sample timing. The half-life of theophylline is greatly affected by age, disease, concurrent drugs, smoking, and any physiologic condition that affects its metabolism. The half-life of theophylline can range anywhere from 3 hr in children or adult smokers to greater than 50 hr in nonsmoking adults with severe heart failure or liver disease.[81] Steady state will be reached in 24 hr for the average patient with an elimination half-life of 8 hr[36] but will require much longer for patients with heart failure or liver disease (or for patients who are taking drugs known to inhibit theophylline metabolism). The time to steady state in neonates is reported to be approximately 6 days.[84]

The fluctuation of theophylline concentrations within a steady state dosing interval can be quite variable—depending not only on the frequency of administration, type of formulation (sustained- or prompt-release), and half-life—but also on whether or not the dose was taken with a meal.[82] There are many theophylline formulations available. Thus, it is important to consult the product information to determine the anticipated peak times. Peak times for prompt-release formulations are 1–2 hr;[36] peak times for sustained-release formulations occur later and are difficult to predict.

Trough concentrations of theophylline are most reproducible and should always be obtained if at all possible. Comparisons of trough levels from visit to visit will also be facilitated if samples are obtained at the same time of day on each visit. This is because of diurnal variations in the rate of theophylline absorption.[82]

Specimens, collection methods, and assays. Plasma or serum are used for most assays; whole blood may be used in some of the desktop systems.[82] There are no particular concerns about blood collection tubes. Prolonged storage in red-top evacuated tubes or serum separator tubes had no effect on theophylline concentrations in serum.[39]

Many studies suggest saliva theophylline concentrations to be reliable predictors of total or unbound theophylline concentrations in serum or plasma.[50,88,89] Both unstimulated and stimulated saliva were equally good predictors of theophylline concentrations in serum in one study.[88] Either citric acid or the chewing of Parafilm® may be used for stimulation of whole saliva production.[89] A study of an oral mucosal transudate collection device showed that once the S:P ratio was established for a given patient, saliva samples collected at home by the patient are reliable predictors of serum theophylline concentrations.[50]

While theophylline is often measured using HPLC, the most common assays in clinical laboratories are FPIA or EMIT®. The immunoassay methods offer acceptable sensitivity but may not be suitable for patients with renal failure who have accumulated theophylline metabolites.[90,91] A number of desktop systems designed for use in physician offices, including Vision® (Abbott), Seralyzer® (Ames), and AccuLevel® (Syntex), compare favorably with the FPIA and EMIT® methods.[82] Caffeine and theobromine interfere with theophylline measurements by some of the office methods[60]; the Vision® system shows no interferences by bilirubin and triglycerides, but hemolyzed samples give lower readings.[92]

Use of levels for dosage adjustment. Theophylline is usually assumed to undergo first-order elimination, but some of its metabolic pathways are nonlinear at concentrations at the higher end of the therapeutic range.[82] The clearance of theophylline decreases by 20% as daily doses are increased from 210 mg to 1260 mg.[82] While the magnitude of this nonlinear behavior does not require special methods for dosing, the clinician should expect somewhat greater-than-proportional increases in serum theophylline concentration with increases in dose rate, particularly as concentrations get into the upper end of the therapeutic range.

Protein binding, active metabolites, and other considerations. Theophylline is 35% bound to serum proteins in neonates and 40–50% bound to serum proteins in adults. Therefore, significant alterations in serum protein binding are unlikely.[82] Theophylline is metabolized to the active metabolite caffeine, which is of minor consequence in adults. Caffeine concentrations in the serum of neonates who are receiving theophylline, however, are approximately 30% of theophylline concentrations and therefore contribute to the effect of theophylline during treatment of neonatal apnea. This may account for the slightly lower therapeutic range of theophylline in neonates as compared to adults. There are many other metabolites of theophylline, none of which possess significant activity.

Caffeine

Therapeutic range. Caffeine is indicated for neonatal apnea (apnea of prematurity) and is recommended over theophylline because it can be given once daily and is considered to have a wider therapeutic range.[83] Concentrations as low as 5 mg/L may be effective, but most pediatric textbooks consider 10 mg/L to be the lower limit of the therapeutic range.[86,93] Most clinicians consider 20 mg/L to be the upper limit of the range, and serious toxicity is associated with serum concentrations above 50 mg/L. Signs of toxicity include jitteriness, vomiting, irritability, tremor of the extremities, tachypnea, and tonic-clonic movements. Serum concentration measurements of caffeine may only be indicated for neonates who do not respond as expected or if recurrence of apnea occurs after a favorable response.

Sample timing. The half-life of caffeine in preterm infants at birth is 65–103 hr.[93] Thus, a loading dose is always administered to attain effective levels as soon as possible. The long half-life means that caffeine concentrations will not fluctuate much during the interval, even when caffeine is administered once daily. Sampling in the postdistribution phase is recommended, but at least 2 hr postdose.

Baseline levels of caffeine must be obtained prior to the first caffeine dose in the following situations: (1) if the infant had been previously treated with theophylline, since caffeine is a metabolite of theophylline; and (2) if the infant was born to a mother who consumed caffeine prior to delivery. Reductions in the usual caffeine dose will be necessary if predose caffeine levels are present.

Specimens, collection methods, and assays. Because of the limited blood volume in neonates, it is generally recommended that blood samples of 75 μL or less be used.[86] Caffeine from blood samples is measured as either serum or plasma. Recommendations for collection tubes include evacuated tubes without additives or tubes containing EDTA. Refrigeration at 4 °C for at least 24 hr is acceptable.[93] Common assays for caffeine include HPLC, GLC, and immunoassay by EMIT®. The immunoassay method was demonstrated to be unaffected by hemolysis, hyperbilirubinemia, and lipemia.[94]

Saliva concentrations have been recommended as a noninvasive alternative to blood sampling, which would be particularly helpful in this population.[93,95] The reported S:P concentration ratio can vary depending on the methods used. Therefore, it is important that collection and assay methods be consistently used within a given institution. De Wildt et al.[93] developed a novel saliva collection method in which a cotton swab with attached gauze was placed in the mouth of the neonate 5–10 min after a drop of 1% citric acid solution had been placed in the cheek pouch. Saliva concentrations measured by HPLC predicted plasma concentrations reliably. Other collection methods (no stimulation or citric acid placed on the gauze) did not predict plasma concentrations as well.[93]

Use of levels for dosage adjustment. There is no data to suggest that caffeine undergoes nonlinear elimination. Thus, dosage adjustments by proportionality are acceptable. Dosage adjustments for caffeine are complicated by the fact that a true steady state is not reached for at least 4 days, so any adjustments should be conservative.

Protein binding, active metabolites, and enantiomers. Caffeine is only 31% bound to serum proteins[93] and has no active metabolites.

Antiepileptics

The antiepileptics that have clearly defined therapeutic ranges should be routinely monitored. Because they are used as prophylaxis for seizures that may not occur frequently, it is particularly important that effective serum concentrations of these drugs be assured early in therapy. Indications for monitoring antiepileptic drugs include[13,96] (1) documentation of an effective steady state concentration after initiation of therapy; (2) after dosage regimen adjustments; (3) after adding a drug that has potential for interaction; (4) changes in disease state or physiologic status that may affect the pharmacokinetics of the drug; (5) within hours of a seizure recurrence; (6) after an unexplained change in seizure frequency; (7) suspected dose-related drug toxicity; and (8) suspected noncompliance.

Carbamazepine

Therapeutic range. Carbamazepine is used to prevent partial seizures and generalized tonic-clonic seizures as well as bipolar disorder and trigeminal neuralgia.[30,81] Most studies indicate that serum concentrations between 4 and 12 mg/L are necessary for treatment of seizures and trigeminal neuralgia. Concentrations above 12 mg/L are most often associated with nausea and vomiting, unsteadiness, blurred vision, drowsiness, dizziness, and headaches in patients who are taking carbamazepine alone.[30] Patients taking other antiepileptic drugs such as primidone, phenobarbital, valproic acid or phenytoin may show these adverse effects at levels as low as 9 mg/L. Serious adverse reactions are seen at levels greater than 50 mg/L.[96]

Carbamazepine 10,11-epoxide is an active metabolite that can be present in concentrations that are 12–25% of carbamazepine but is not routinely monitored along with the parent drug. A suggested therapeutic range for this metabolite, used at some research centers, is 0.4–4 mg/L.[81]

In addition to the usual indications for monitoring, it is important to monitor carbamazepine concentrations if the patient is switched to another formulation (e.g., generic), since the bioavailability may be different.[96]

Sample timing. Because carbamazepine induces its own metabolism, it is recommended that initial dose rates of carbamazepine be relatively low and gradually increase over a 3–4 week period.[30] For maximal induction or deinduction to occur, 2–3 weeks may be required after the maximum dose rate has been attained. Thus, a total of 6–7 weeks may be required for a true steady state to be reached after initiation of therapy. After any dose rate changes or addition/discontinuation of enzyme-inducing or inhibiting drugs, 2–3 weeks will be required to reach a new steady state.[81]

A trough level is generally preferred if there is a choice. The absorption of conventional carbamazepine tablets from the gastrointestinal tract is relatively slow, reaching a peak between 4 and 8 hr after a dose.[97] Extended-release formulations are even more slowly absorbed. If carbamazepine is administered every 6 or 8 hr, serum levels during the dosing interval will remain fairly flat, and all levels will be fairly representative of a trough concentration. Less frequent dosing will result in more fluctuation in which case the time of the level relative to the last dose should be documented for appropriate interpretation. Use of the extended-release formulation of carbamazepine will minimize fluctuations caused by diurnal variations.[98] Nevertheless, it is recommended that samples on repeated visits always be obtained at the same time of the day for purposes of comparison.[96]

Specimens, collection methods, and assays. Either serum or plasma collected in EDTA-treated tubes are acceptable for total carbamazepine measurements. Oxalate and citrate were shown to cause significant negative interferences in the measurement of carbamazepine by EMIT® and a GLC method.[99] Recent studies of a new serum separator tube (SST II®, Becton-Dickinson) show that serum carbamazepine concentrations are stable for 24 hr at room temperature.[39] Saliva has been proposed as a convenient noninvasive alternative, especially for children and for home monitoring.[43,46,100] If saliva is used, a standardized protocol for obtaining the specimen must be approved by the laboratory. Both the chewing of Parafilm®[46] and stimulation by citric acid[101] have been used successfully. Saliva collected within 2 hr of oral administration may be contaminated by residual drug in the mouth.[30]

The most common assays for total carbamazepine include a wide variety of immunoassays, GLC, and HPLC.[97] Some of the immunoassays cross-react with the 10,11-epoxide metabolite.[102] This can be a particular problem if saliva is measured, as the ratio of epoxide to parent drug is higher in saliva.[101] The active carbamazepine 10,11-epoxide is generally not routinely measured separately, even though it has been shown to exhibit anticonvulsant activity. Assays for unbound carbamazepine, monitored rarely, are done by ultrafiltration followed by one of the other assay methods.[27] Severe hemolysis may result in inaccurate measurement by the immunologic methods in which case one of the chromatographic methods is suggested.[103]

Use of levels for dosage adjustment. Carbamazepine exhibits first-order behavior following therapeutic doses. Thus, increases in dose rate will result in a proportional increase in the average steady state level of carbamazepine. If the dose is adjusted without a change in the interval, a level drawn at the same time within the interval will increase in proportion to the increase in dose.

Protein binding, active metabolites, and enantiomers. In most patients, carbamazepine is 70 to 80% bound to serum proteins, including albumin and alpha-1-acid glycoprotein.[104] In some patients, however, unbound percentages as low as 10% have been reported.[81] Measurements of unbound carbamazepine concentrations are not generally recommended or necessary. Rather, total carbamazepine concentrations should be carefully interpreted in situations of suspected altered protein binding. Decreased binding might be anticipated in liver disease, hypoalbuminemia, or hyperbilirubinemia.[81] Increased binding might be expected in cases of physiologic trauma due to elevated alpha-1-acid glycoprotein concentrations, but this would be a rare occurrence. Valproic acid has been shown to displace carbamazepine from albumin; an equation was proposed to predict unbound carbamazepine concentrations in this situation.[71] Correlations between saliva and unbound carbamazepine concentrations are strong.[46] Thus, saliva sampling might be considered in situations of suspected alterations in carbamazepine binding.

Drug-drug interactions that are expected to result in a higher proportion of active 10,11-epoxide metabolite relative to the parent drug (e.g., concurrent phenytoin, phenobarbital, or valproic acid) may alter the activity associated with a given carbamazepine concentration. It is suggested that a lower therapeutic range of 4–8 mg/L be used when those drugs are given concurrently.[13]

Ethosuximide

Therapeutic range. Ethosuximide is the drug of choice for the management of absence seizures. The therapeutic range is generally considered to be 40–100 mg/L.[105] Eighty percent of patients will achieve partial control within that range, and 60% will be seizure-free. Some patients will require levels up to 150 mg/L.[81] Side effects are usually seen at concentrations above 70 mg/L and include drowsiness, fatigue, ataxia, and lethargy. Ethosuximide does not require as much monitoring as some of the other antiepileptics, but it is important to assure effective levels after initiation of therapy or a change in dosage regimen.

Sample timing. The half-life of ethosuximide is quite long—40–60 hr in adults and 25–35 hr in children.[97] Thus, it advised to wait as long as 1 week to 12 days before obtaining ethosuximide levels for monitoring purposes.[13,105] While it is generally advised that trough concentrations be obtained, levels drawn anytime during the dosing interval should be acceptable because there will be very little fluctuation if ethosuximide is given in divided doses. Peak concentrations of ethosuximide administered as a capsule are attained in less than 3 hr.[97]

Specimens, collection methods, and assays. Serum or plasma may be used for determination of ethosuximide concentrations. A variety of blood collection tubes have been tested, and none have interfered with measurement of ethosuximide.[42] Ethosuximide does not bind to serum proteins. Therefore, measurement of unbound levels is never necessary. Studies have shown saliva ethosuximide concentrations to be equal to serum or plasma concentrations, thus making saliva a convenient alternative, especially in children.[43,101]

Assays for ethosuximide include GLC, HPLC, and various immunoassays. Cross-reactivity by desmethylmethsuximide, the active metabolite of methsuximide, has been reported with both the EMIT® and TDx® assays.[97]

Use of levels for dosage adjustment. Ethosuximide is reported to display nonlinear elimination, but primarily at concentrations near the upper end of its therapeutic range. Somewhat greater-than-proportional increases in drug concentration with increases in doses can therefore be expected when higher dose rates are use.

Protein binding, active metabolites, and enantiomers. Ethosuximide is negligibly bound to serum proteins and its metabolites have insignificant activity. While ethosuximide is administered as a racemic mixture, the enantiomers have the same pharmacokinetic properties. Thus, measurement of the summed enantiomers is acceptable.[106]

Phenobarbital/Primidone

Primidone and phenobarbital are both used for management of generalized tonic-clonic and partial seizures. Phenobarbital is used for febrile convulsions and hypoxic ischemic seizures in neonates and infants. Primidone is used for treatment of essential tremor in the elderly.[96] Although primidone has activity of its own, most clinicians believe that phenobarbital—a metabolite of primidone—is predominantly responsible for primidone's therapeutic effects. These two drugs will, therefore, be considered together.

Therapeutic ranges. The therapeutic range of phenobarbital for treatment of tonic-clonic, febrile, and hypoxic ischemic seizures is generally regarded as 15–40 mg/L,[96] while concentrations as high as 70 mg/L may be required for refractory status epilepticus.[107] Eighty-four percent of patients are likely to respond with concentrations between 10 and 40 mg/L. Management of partial seizures seems to require higher phenobarbital concentrations than management of bilateral tonic-clonic seizures.[13] Concentrations of phenobarbital are always reported when primidone levels are ordered. The therapeutic range of primidone reported by most laboratories is 5–12 mg/L.[13,96] Fifteen to 20% of a primidone dose is metabolized to the active phenobarbital;[81] the side effects of primidone are mostly related to phenobarbital. Central nervous system side effects such as sedation and ataxia generally occur in chronically treated patients at phenobarbital levels between 35 and 80 mg/L. Stupor and coma have been reported at phenobarbital concentrations above 65 mg/L.[81,97,107]

Sample timing. The half-life of phenobarbital is the rate-limiting step for determining the time to reach steady state after primidone administration, and it is 5 days for neonates and between 3 and 5 days for adults.[107] Since phenobarbital or primidone dosage may be initiated gradually, steady state is not attained until 2–3 weeks after full dosage has been implemented. Because phenobarbital has such a long half-life, levels obtained anytime during the day would provide reasonable estimates of a trough concentration. Ideally, levels should be obtained from visit to visit at similar times of the day.[107]

Specimens, collection methods, and assays. Serum or plasma are acceptable for measurements of phenobarbital and primidone; whole blood is used for the desktop AccuLevel® assay of phenobarbital. Use of a new serum separator tube (SST II®, Becton-Dickinson) does not cause a problem with phenobarbital determinations.[39] The partitioning of phenobarbital into saliva is pH-sensitive. However, some studies have shown acceptable correlations with or without pH correction.[43] Saliva concentrations of primidone are particularly sensitive to saliva flow rate changes but show strong correlations with serum concentrations of primidone when standardized collection methods are used.[43] However, the clinical utility of just measuring primidone concentration in saliva is questionable.

Chromatographic methods (GLC, HPLC) may permit simultaneous determination of both primidone and phenobarbital, but immunoassays are most commonly used.[97] There is potential for cross-reactivity of the immunoassay methods with coadministered barbiturates.[97] The AccuLevel® assay for phenobarbital compares well with both EMIT® and TDx® methods, showing no interferences from endogenous substances or blood collection tube components.[108,109]

Use of levels for dosage adjustment. Phenobarbital and primidone exhibit first-order elimination behavior,[97,107] thus, a change in the dose rate of either drug will result in a proportional change in the average, steady state serum concentrations.

Protein binding, active metabolites, and enantiomers. Phenobarbital is approximately 50% bound to serum proteins (albumin) in adults; primidone is not bound to serum proteins.[96,110] Thus, total concentrations of both drugs are reliable indicators of the active, unbound concentrations of these drugs. While primidone has an active metabolite, phenylethylmalonamide (PEMA), the contribution to activity is unlikely to be significant.

Phenytoin

Therapeutic range. Phenytoin is used for all types of seizures except absence seizures and seizures caused by theophylline overdose.[96] It is also a Type 1b antiarrhythmic that is especially useful for digitalis-induced ventricular arrhythmias.[81] Studies have shown that serum or plasma concentrations of phenytoin between 10 and 20 mg/L will result in maximum protection from primary or secondary generalized tonic-clonic seizures in most adult patients with normal serum binding. Ten percent of patients with controlled seizures have phenytoin levels less than 3 mg/L, 50% have levels less than 7 mg/L, and 90% have levels less than 15 mg/L.[13] Levels at the lower end of the range are effective for bilateral seizures, while higher concentrations appear to be necessary for partial seizures.[13] The therapeutic range of total concentrations in infants is lower due to lower serum protein binding: 6–11 mg/L.[96] Concentration-related side effects include nystagmus, central nervous system depression (ataxia, inability to concentrate, confusion, and drowsiness), and changes in mental status, coma, or seizures at levels above 40 mg/L.[96,111] While mild side effects may be observed at concentrations as low as 5 mg/L,[111] there have been cases in which concentrations as high 50 mg/L have been required for effective treatment without negative consequences.[112]

Some clinicians have proposed that monitoring of phenytoin be limited to unbound concentrations, particularly in hospitalized patients.[66,113] The therapeutic range of unbound phenytoin levels is presumed to be 1–2 mg/L for laboratories that determine the unbound phenytoin fraction at 25 °C and 1.5–3 mg/L if done at 37 °C.[96]

Sample timing. The time required to attain a steady state after initiation of phenytoin therapy is difficult to predict due to phenytoin's nonlinear elimination behavior. While the $T_{50\%}$ is approximately 24 hr (considering the average population Vmax and Km values when levels are between 10 and 20 mg/L), there can be extreme variations in these population values. Half-lives between 6 and 60 hr have been reported in adults.[96] Thus, a steady state might not be attained for as long as 3 weeks. Some clinicians advise that samples be obtained prior to steady state (after 3–4 days) in order to make sure that levels are not climbing too rapidly.[111] Equations have been developed to predict the time required to reach a steady state once Km and Vmax values are known.[64] It is important to recognize that the time required to reach a steady state in a given patient will be longer each time the dose rate is further increased.

Most clinicians advise that predose phenytoin concentrations be monitored.[96] Phenytoin is quite slowly absorbed so that the concentration vs. time profile is fairly flat. This is especially true when oral phenytoin is administered 2 or 3 times per day. In this case, serum phenytoin drawn any time during the dosage interval is likely to be close to a trough concentration. The most fluctuation would be seen for the more quickly absorbed products (chewable tablets and suspension) in children (higher clearance of phenytoin) given once daily. In this case, it is particularly important to document the time of sample relative to the dose—to identify if the level is closer to a peak, a trough, or a $C_{ss,avg}$.

Specimens, collection methods, and assays. Serum or plasma are generally recommended for total phenytoin measurements. Blood collected for plasma should not be anticoagulated with citrate or oxalate because these anticoagulants are reported to cause negative interferences with measurements of phenytoin using the EMIT® method.[96,99] Anticoagulation with heparin is also of concern since activation of lipoprotein lipases may increase free fatty acid concentrations and displace phenytoin from albumin.[96] While serum separator tubes are generally not recommended,[96] recent studies of a new serum separator tube show that serum phenytoin concentrations are stable for 24 hr at room temperature using the SST II® (Becton-Dickinson) tubes.[39]

Saliva has been proposed as a viable alternative to monitoring plasma phenytoin concentrations, especially for children.[43,48,101] It has also been proposed as a useful specimen for monitoring unbound phenytoin concentrations, particularly in patients taking valproic acid concurrently.[43] Successful results in infants and children have been shown when saliva is stimulated using a small amount of citric acid on the tongue.[45] Since the S:P ratio is affected by salivary flow rate, it is particularly important that the saliva collection procedure be carefully standardized.[43]

Immunoassays are the most common methods for measurement of total phenytoin concentrations in serum or plasma.[64] The metabolites of phenytoin do not contribute to antiepileptic activity, but certain immunologic methods may measure accumulated phenytoin metabolites in patients with renal impairment. Immunoassays that use monoclonal antibodies or HPLC would be appropriate alternative methods for samples from patients with renal impairment.[67] Fosphenytoin, the phenytoin prodrug, interferes with both the EMIT® and TDx® methods. For this reason, serum for phenytoin monitoring should not be obtained earlier than 4 hr after administration at which time fosphenytoin has been maximally converted to phenytoin.[114] Assays for unbound phenytoin are usually done using ultrafiltered serum followed by one of the other assay methods.[67] The unbound phenytoin fraction is affected by temperature. Therefore, this variable must be controlled.[96] Hemolysis and lipemia do not interfere with phenytoin measurements using the TDx® FPIA method.[115]

Use of levels for dosage adjustment. Phenytoin exhibits pronounced nonlinear behavior following therapeutic doses. Thus, increases in dose rate will produce greater-than-proportional increases in the average serum concentration during the dosing interval. Several methods, described elsewhere,[64] use population and/or patient-specific Vmax and Km values to predict the most appropriate dose rate adjustment. The clinician must be aware that the size of phenytoin daily dose increases should typically not be greater than 30 or 60 mg using sodium phenytoin or 25 or 50 mg using the chewable tablets.

Protein binding, active metabolites, and enantiomers. The metabolites of phenytoin have insignificant activity. Phenytoin binds primarily to albumin in plasma and the normal unbound fraction of drug in plasma of adults is 0.1.[96,111] Lower serum binding of phenytoin is observed in neonates and infants and in patients with hypoalbuminemia, liver disease, nephrotic syndrome, pregnancy, cystic fibrosis, burns, trauma, malnourishment, AIDS, and advanced age. Concurrent drugs (valproic acid, salicylate, and other nonsteroidal anti-inflammatory drugs) are known to displace phenytoin.[81,116] Thus, a total level of phenytoin that is within the range of 10–20 mg/L in these patients might represent an unbound level that is higher than 1–2 mg/L (the therapeutic range of unbound levels). Total concentration of phenytoin in this situation can be misleading. Several approaches can be used in these situations: (1) an unbound phenytoin level can be ordered, if available; (2) the patient's unbound phenytoin level can be calculated by estimating the unbound fraction in the patient (using the literature) and multiplying that by the patient's measured phenytoin level (the resulting unbound level should then be compared to 1–2 mg/L); or (3) special equations may be used to convert the total phenytoin level to what it would be if the patient had normal serum protein binding.

The following equation was developed to normalize phenytoin (PHT) levels in patients with hypoalbuminemia and/or renal failure[81,111,117]:

$$\text{Normalized PHT level} = \frac{\text{Measured PHT level}}{(X \times \text{Albumin Concentration, Gm\%}) + 0.1}$$

The value "X" is 0.2 for patients with creatinine clearances equal to or above 25 mL/min and 0.1 for patients with end stage renal disease (creatinine clearances less than 10 mL/min). Total levels of phenytoin in patients with creatinine clearance values between 10 and 25 mL/min cannot be as accurately normalized; the clinical status of such patients should be carefully considered since total levels can be misleading. This equation for normalizing total phenytoin concentrations has been tested by groups of investigators in different groups of patients with mixed reviews; it is emphasized that it should only be used as a guide.

Valproic acid is known to increase the unbound fraction of phenytoin in serum.[118] It has also been variably reported to inhibit the metabolism of phenytoin. These two occurrences together could mean that a level within the range of 10–20 mg/L is associated with adverse effects and an unbound phenytoin level greater than 2 mg/L. If unbound phenytoin concentrations are not available, the following equation—modified from its original form[69,111]— may be useful to normalize the total phenytoin (PHT) level if the level of valproic acid (VPA) in that same sample has been measured:

Normalized PHT level = Measured PHT level + (0.01 × VPA level × Measured PHT level)

Other equations have been used for estimating the unbound phenytoin concentration in the presence of valproic acid.[119]

Valproic Acid

Therapeutic range. Valproic acid is used for management of absence seizures, in addition to partial and generalized tonic-clonic and myoclonic seizures. It is also used for bipolar disorder and prophylaxis against migraine headaches.[96] Most laboratories use 50–100 mg/L as the therapeutic range of total valproic acid concentrations. Some patients are effectively treated at lower levels, and others may require levels as high as 120 mg/L.[120] Levels at the upper end of the therapeutic range appear to be necessary for treatment of complex partial seizures.[120] The same therapeutic range is used for patients with migraines or bipolar disorder. The following concentration-related side effects may be seen: ataxia, sedation, lethargy, and fatigue at levels above 75 mg/L; tremor at levels above 100 mg/L; and stupor and coma at levels greater than 175 mg/L.[81] The therapeutic range of total valproic acid concentrations is confounded by the nonlinear serum protein binding of this drug, which might explain some of the variable response among and within patients at a given total serum concentration.[97]

Sample timing. The half-life of valproic acid ranges between 7 and 18 hr in children and adults and 17 and 40 hr in infants.[96] Thus, 3–5 days may be required to attain a steady state.[120] The pattern of change in valproic acid concentrations varies from interval to interval during the day because of considerable diurnal variation.[96,120] It is, therefore, recommended that samples always be obtained prior to the morning dose as this has been shown to be most consistent from day to day.[120] Considerable fluctuation within the interval will be seen with the immediate-release capsule and syrup, which are rapidly absorbed. The enteric-coated, delayed-release Depakote® tablet displays a shift-to-the-right with respect to its concentration vs. time profile, such that the lowest concentration during the interval may not be observed until 1–6 hr into the next dosing interval.[120] It is important to know, however, that concentrations during the interval following administration of the enteric-coated tablet will show considerable fluctuation. The extended-release and Sprinkle® capsules, if given in divided doses, provide less fluctuation in concentrations, and samples may be drawn at any time.

Specimens, collection methods, and assays. Serum or heparinized plasma are recommended; other anticoagulants may cross-react if immunoassay methods are used.[96,97,99] Concentrations of valproic acid in saliva are very low and do not correlate well with plasma concentrations.[43,48] Concentrations of valproic acid measured in tears collected using absorbent paper strips were shown to correlate well with unbound, valproic acid concentrations.[52]

Chromatographic methods (GLC, HPLC) are considered the most specific methods for determination of valproic acid concentrations. While EMIT® and TDx® are acceptable methods, there is some cross-reactivity with unsaturated metabolites.[97] Unbound valproic acid levels should be determined by ultrafiltration of fresh serum or serum that has been stored frozen; equilibrium dialysis is not recommended.[97] Unbound concentrations in ultrafiltrate have been measured by immunoassay or HPLC.[97,121]

Use of levels for dosage adjustment. The metabolism of unbound valproic acid is linear following therapeutic doses. Thus, unbound valproic acid levels will increase in proportion to increases in dose rate.[96,97] Because valproic acid shows nonlinear, saturable protein binding in serum over the therapeutic range, however, total concentrations will increase less than proportionally. This is important to keep in mind when interpreting total valproic acid levels.

Protein binding, active metabolites, and enantiomers. Valproic acid is 90–95% bound to albumin and lipoproteins in serum. The unbound fraction of valproic acid shows considerable interpatient variability. It is increased in conditions associated with hypoalbuminemia (e.g., liver disease, nephrotic syndrome, cystic fibrosis, burns, trauma, malnutrition, and advanced age)[81] and as a result of displacement by endogenous substances (e.g., bilirubin, free fatty acids, and uremic substances in end stage renal disease) and by other drugs (e.g., salicylate and other nonsteroidal anti-inflammatory drugs).[81,122] The increase in the unbound fraction of valproic acid during labor is believed to be the result of displacement by higher concentrations of free fatty acids.[123] Valproic acid also shows intrapatient variability in the unbound fraction due to nonlinear binding. The unbound fraction of valproic acid is fairly constant at lower concentrations but progressively increases as total concentrations rise above 75 mg/L.[96] Thus, total concentrations do not reflect unbound concentrations at the upper end of the therapeutic range. A therapeutic range for unbound valproic acid concentrations can only be approximated; assuming unbound fractions of 0.05–0.1 and a therapeutic range of total valproic acid concentrations of 50–100 mg/L, an unbound therapeutic range of 2.5–10 mg/L can be deduced.

Other Antiepileptic Drugs

Several of the newer antiepileptic drugs do not have characteristics that make them suitable candidates for serum concentration monitoring.[124] Gabapentin has a fairly wide therapeutic index, and, like oxcarbazepine, does not show much variability among patients in pharmacokinetics. Vigabatrin serum levels do not correlate with clinical effect because of its unusual mechanism of action—irreversible binding to an enzyme. Lamotrigine, felbamate, tiagabine, topiramate, and zonisamide, however, have characteristics that might make concentration monitoring helpful for guiding therapy. Severe adverse reactions observed in the postmarketing period have resulted in severe restrictions of felbamate use. Therefore, it will not be discussed here.

MINICASE 3

DANIEL I., A 45-YEAR-OLD MALE, had been taking sodium phenytoin 330 mg at bedtime for 12 years for control of tonic-clonic seizures that first occurred after head trauma in a motor vehicle accident. He was started on omeprazole 10 days ago for esophageal reflux refractory to famotidine 40 mg/day. In the past year, his only other medications were nontherapeutic multivitamins and occasional ibuprofen for tendonitis.

Today, his wife called the doctor's office because Daniel I. had become increasingly confused, lethargic, and dizzy over the past 3–4 days and complained today of visual disturbances (diplopia). His reflux had improved greatly. On examination, nystagmus on lateral gaze was present. A phenytoin concentration drawn 14 hr after his last dose was 36 mg/L; he was told to stop taking the phenytoin for the next three nights. He was also told to stop taking omeprazole and was placed back on famotidine 40 mg twice a day with antacids prn. Daniel I. restarted his phenytoin at 300 mg/day after 3 days, and after 14 more days, a serum phenytoin concentration measured from a sample drawn 12 hr after his last dose was 14 mg/L. He was seizure free.

Question: What was the probable cause of the patient's elevated phenytoin concentration? What signs and symptoms were related to phenytoin toxicity?

Discussion: The probable cause of Daniel I.'s elevated concentration was the addition of omeprazole, which inhibits the enzymes involved in phenytoin's metabolism. A reversal of elevated concentrations and symptoms after withdrawal of omeprazole confirms the interaction. The sign of toxicity here is nystagmus; the symptoms are confusion, lethargy, dizziness, and double vision. Their appearance is expected at an average concentration of 36 mg/L.

Altered serum binding of phenytoin would not explain any of the findings in this patient. First, decreased serum binding alone would *decrease* the total serum phenytoin concentration, not increase it. Second, altered serum binding in the absence of altered metabolism would not affect the unbound concentration of phenytoin, and, hence, the pharmacologic effect. Folic acid, which may be in the multivitamins, cannot explain the elevated phenytoin concentrations either. Folic acid in sufficiently high doses has the potential to increase the clearance of phenytoin, thus lowering total levels of phenytoin. Besides, Daniel I. has been taking these vitamins for at least the last year. While cimetidine is known to increase phenytoin concentrations, famotidine does not.

The blood samples that were drawn for phenytoin that were drawn for phenytoin measurements were both approximately midway between the time of peak concentration and the time of the next dose. Thus, these levels are fairly representative of average levels during the dosing interval. The first level (36 mg/L) was probably not at steady state and could have risen further had the physician not told the patient to stop taking the phenytoin. The second level, obtained 17 days after restarting the phenytoin, most likely reflected a steady state. Even if the half-life of phenytoin was as long as 60 hr in this patient, 88% of the steady state would have been reached in 1 week. The extra week gave time for the omeprazole to wash out and for the enzymes to resume their usual activity.

Minicase 3 is adapted from the second edition chapter titled "Interpretation of Serum Drug Concentrations," which was written by Scott L. Traub.

Lamotrigine. The considerable pharmacokinetic variability among patients taking lamotrigine, due in part to significant drug-drug interactions, makes it a good candidate for therapeutic drug monitoring.[124,125] The therapeutic range of lamotrigine was originally defined as 1–4 mg/L, but more recently 3–14 mg/L has been proposed.[126] Some patients may tolerate concentrations above 20 mg/L.[127] It has been suggested that concomitant therapy with other antiepileptics may alter the response to lamotrigine or its side effect profile at a given lamotrigine serum concentration.[125] The half-life of lamotrigine can range from between 15–60 hr. Thus, one should wait at least 1 week before obtaining samples after initiating or adjusting lamotrigine therapy.[124,125] This drug exhibits linear pharmacokinetics. Therefore, dose-rate adjustments will result in proportionate changes in average serum concentrations. Because it is only 55% bound to serum proteins, measurements of unbound lamotrigine levels in serum are not necessary. Saliva concentrations of lamotrigine may be a useful alternative to blood sampling.[128] There are HPLC assays currently available for lamotrigine.[126] Routine lamotrigine monitoring is generally not recommended, but serum concentrations might be helpful to determine if lack of response is related to unusually low levels or noncompliance.[126]

Tiagabine. Tiagabine shows pronounced interpatient pharmacokinetic variability. Trough levels greater than 40 mg/L are associated with improved seizure control, but there is wide variation in response at any given total concentration.[124] This could, in part, be due to variable serum binding (96% bound in serum on average). Valproic acid, salicylate, and naproxen have been shown to displace tiagabine from serum proteins.[124] Tiagabine half-life ranges from 4–13 hr and may be even shorter in the presence of enzyme inducing drugs.[125] Tiagabine shows linear elimination behavior following therapeutic doses. Studies to clarify the therapeutic range or utility of total concentration monitoring are clearly needed.

Topiramate. Topiramate levels are particularly influenced by interactions with other drugs, with levels as much as 2-fold lower when enzyme-inducing drugs are administered concurrently.[129] The half-life ranges from 12–30 hr, and it has linear elimination behavior.[124, 125] Topiramate is negligibly bound to serum proteins but shows saturable binding to red blood cells, thus suggesting that whole blood might be a preferable specimen for monitoring.[125] Effective serum levels are generally reported to be between 3.4 and 5.2 mg/L with further improvement seen at levels above 10 mg/L.[124] No active metabolites have been identified.[124] An FPIA assay method has been developed.[124,125]

Zonisamide. The pharmacokinetics of zonisamide are variable among patients and also highly influenced by interactions with other drugs.[124] Zonisamide is approximately 50% bound to serum proteins, and, like topiramate, shows saturable binding to red blood cells, suggesting that whole blood monitoring might be preferable.[125] The half-life is 50–70 hr but may be as short as 25 hr when enzyme inducers are coadministered. There are some reports suggesting nonlinear behavior at higher doses. The plasma concentration range associated with response is 7–40 mg/L; cognitive dysfunction is reported at levels above 30 mg/L.[125] No active metabolites have been identified.[124] Both HPLC and immunoassays are available.

Antimicrobials

Aminoglycosides

Therapeutic ranges. Amikacin, gentamicin, netilmicin, and tobramycin are administered intravenously to treat infections of Gram-negative organisms that are resistant to less toxic antibiotics.[37] They are bactericidal, and, thus, their efficacy is highly related to peak concentration after an infusion.[130] They also exhibit a postantibiotic effect in which bacterial killing continues even after the serum concentration is below the minimum inhibitory concentration (MIC).[81] The concentration-dependent killing and postantibiotic effects of the aminoglycosides explain why extended-interval (pulse) dosing of the aminoglycosides is shown to be safe and effective in many patients. Nephrotoxicity and ototoxicity are the most frequently reported adverse effects of the aminoglycoside antibiotics. Ototoxicity seems to be associated with a prolonged course of treatment (for greater than 7–10 days) with peaks above 12–14 mg/L for gentamicin, netilmicin, and tobramycin and 35–40 mg/L for amikacin.[81] Patients with trough levels above 2–3 mg/L (gentamicin, netilmicin, and tobramycin) or 10 mg/L (amikacin) for sustained periods of time are predisposed to increased risk of nephrotoxicity.[81]

Therapeutic ranges for peaks and troughs are reported for the aminoglycosides and pertain only to traditional dosing approaches. For gentamicin, netilmicin, and tobramycin, peaks between 6 and 10 mg/L and troughs between 0.5 and 2 mg/L are recommended.[131] The approximately 4-fold higher minimum inhibitory concentration (MIC) for amikacin explains why peaks between 20 and 30 mg/L and troughs between 1 and 8 mg/L are recommended.[131] There is no therapeutic range when the pulse-dosing method is used; doses are given to attain peaks that are approximately 10 times the MIC, and troughs are intended to be nondetectable within 4 hr of administration of the next dose.[130,132] A serum level drawn sometime after infusion of the dose is used only for adjustment of the dosing interval, not to check for efficacy or toxicity.

There has been some concern over the years that aminoglycosides are overmonitored. Uncomplicated patients with normal renal function, who do not have life-threatening infections and will be treated for less than 5 days, may not need to have serum aminoglycoside levels measured.[132] At the other extreme, dosage individualization using serum levels of aminoglycosides are absolutely necessary in patients with serious infections who are on prolonged treatment courses, especially if unusual pharmacokinetic parameters are expected (e.g., renal impairment, burns, cystic fibrosis, extremes of age, sepsis, and pregnancy) and if risk of toxicity is high (such as in patients taking concomitant loop diuretics or nephrotoxic drugs [e.g., amphotericin, cyclosporine, or vancomycin]).[131,132]

Sample timing. For pulse dosing in patients with normal renal function, a steady state is never reached since each dose is washed out prior to the next dose. The method developed by Nicolau et al. (the so-called Hartford method) requires that a single blood sample be obtained between 6 and 14 hr after the end of the first infusion.[133] This sample is referred to as a *random sample*, but the time of the collection must be documented. The level is used with a nomogram in order to determine if a different dosing interval should be used.[37,133] Levels that are too high, according to this nomogram, will indicate that the drug is not being cleared as well as originally predicted, suggesting the need for a longer interval. For traditional dosing, it is important to wait until a steady state is reached before obtaining blood samples. The half-lives of the aminoglycosides are 1.5–3 hr for adults with normal renal function but as long as 72 hr in patients with severe renal impairment.[81] Since the dosing interval for aminoglycosides is usually adjusted to be 2–3 times the drug's half-life, then a conservative rule of thumb is that steady state is reached after the third or fourth dose.[37,81,132] Some patients may have blood samples drawn immediately after the first dose ("off the load") in order to determine their pharmacokinetic parameters for purposes of dosage regimen individualization. These would most likely be patients who are anticipated to have unpredictable pharmacokinetic parameters, and who require immediate effective treatment because of life-threatening infections.

Two blood samples are sufficient for purposes of individualizing traditional aminoglycoside therapy, and will provide reasonable estimates of aminoglycoside pharmacokinetic parameters.[36] It is crucial that the times of the sample collections be accurately recorded.[37,130] The two samples should be spaced sufficiently apart from each other so that an accurate determination of the log-linear slope can be made, in order to determine the elimination rate constant. One sample (sometimes referred to as the *measured peak*) should be drawn no earlier than 30–60 min after the end of drug infusion. A second sample may be drawn any time later, but is usually drawn within 30 min of the start of infusion of the next dose (assumed to be the trough).[37,130,132] If it is expected that the trough level will be close to the limit of the assay sensitivity, the second sample may be drawn earlier.[36] Once the elimination rate constant has been calculated using these two levels, the true peak and true trough can be calculated and their values compared to desired target peaks and troughs.

Specimens, collection methods, and assays. Serum or EDTA-treated plasma is recommended. Blood collection tubes using gel barriers are acceptable for serum.[134,135] Heparin has been shown to interfere with some assays and is not recommended unless the laboratory has ruled out any problems.[37] A recent study showed that gentamicin concentrations in citric acid-stimulated saliva of pediatric patients were good predictors of trough plasma gentamicin concentrations, but only when pulse dosing was used (24-hr dosing interval).[136] It was suggested gentamicin may require a long period of time to fully equilibrate between plasma and saliva, thus explaining the lack of correlations when divided doses were used.[136]

Aminoglycoside concentrations in cerebrospinal fluid are between 10% and 50% of serum concentrations; no therapeutic ranges for cerebrospinal fluid concentrations have been established.[37]

Serum or plasma should either be assayed within 2 hr of collection, or frozen at 0–5 °C.[37] This is particularly important for samples that contain B-lactam antibiotics such as carbenicillin, mezlocillin or ticarcillin. The B-lactam antibiotics, commonly administered with aminoglycosides, physically bind aminoglycoside antibiotics in blood resulting in their inactivation.[37,81,130] In vivo, this means the aminoglycoside is cleared more rapidly than usual. The primary concern, however, is continued inactivation of the aminoglycoside that can occur after a blood sample has been collected. A serum concentration that is 7 mg/L at the time of collection might become 6 mg/L after a period of time at room temperature. Use of the artifactually low serum concentration would lead to errors in determination of the aminoglycoside pharmacokinetic parameters. If immediate assay is not possible, the serum or plasma sample should be immediately frozen.

Use of levels for dosage adjustment. The pulse dosing method was developed to take advantage of the concentration-related killing and postantibiotic effects of the aminoglycosides. A mg/kg dose is administered in order to attain a peak concentration that is approximately 10 times the MIC. Then a sample is obtained between 6 and 14 hr after the end of the infusion and compared to a nomogram, which indicates the appropriate dosing interval—usually 24, 36, or 48 hr.[133] The pulse dosing method is not routinely recommended for certain patients, including those with endocarditis, renal failure, meningitis, osteomyelitis, or burns and patients who are pregnant.[132] However, studies are ongoing to show safety and efficacy in more subpopulations of patients. The results of clinical trials do not consistently show a reduction in nephrotoxicity, and it has been proposed that pulse doses be lowered to provide daily areas-under-the-curve similar to those measured following traditional daily doses.[130,137]

Serum concentrations of aminoglycosides obtained during traditional dosing are used to determine an individual patient's pharmacokinetic parameters, as well as the true peak and true trough in order to compare these to desired target levels. Equations that account for time of drug infusion are used to determine an appropriate dosing interval and dose.[131,138] Other dosage adjustment methods include nomograms[131] and population pharmacokinetic (Bayesian) methods.[138]

Protein binding, active metabolites, and enantiomers. The aminoglycosides are less than 10% bound to serum proteins,[131] and unbound concentrations will always reflect total concentrations in serum. The metabolites of the aminoglycosides are inactive.

Chloramphenicol

Therapeutic range. Chloramphenicol is a broad spectrum antibiotic reserved for treatment of serious infections, including treatment of meningitis caused by ampicillin-resistant *Haemophilus influenzae* type b.[37,139] The therapeutic range for peak levels is generally considered to be 10–20 mg/L. A dose-related reversible type of bone marrow depression may occur and is associated with sustained peak serum levels above 25 mg/L. Irreversible aplastic anemia occurs rarely and is not believed to be related to the serum concentration of chloramphenicol. A somewhat lower therapeutic range may be used for neonates (7.5–14 mg/L)[86] because of the lower serum binding of chloramphenicol in this group—32% vs. 53% in adults.[139] Toxic reactions, including fatalities, have occurred in premature infants and newborns who have had sustained chloramphenicol serum levels above 40–50 mg/L.[37,139] These reactions, known as the "Gray syndrome," are likely caused by the immature conjugation and renal clearance pathways in these patients.

Chloramphenicol should be monitored closely in patients to guide dosing and avoid toxicity in patients with liver or renal disease or in whom drug-drug interactions are anticipated.[37] One study in children, ages 1–66 months, showed progressive decreases in chloramphenicol levels during treatment, suggesting that this group should be frequently monitored.[140] It is important that baseline blood counts and hepatic and renal function tests be done before initiation of therapy and repeated during treatment.

Sample timing. The half-life of chloramphenicol is 2–5 hr in adults; steady state is usually assumed to occur within 12–24 hr.[139] The half-life in neonates and infants may range from 8 to 22 hr.[141] Thus, a steady state should not be assumed in these groups for at least 3 days.

Because both efficacy and toxicity to chloramphenicol are related to peak levels, it is necessary to anticipate when the peak level will occur. Chloramphenicol is available orally as either chloramphenicol base or the chloramphenicol palmitate, which is hydrolyzed to active chloramphenicol in the intestine. Chloramphenicol succinate is the only available intravenous product and is hydrolyzed to chloramphenicol by esterases in the liver, kidneys, and lungs. The peak times for chloramphenicol, therefore, depend not only on the rate of absorption or infusion but also on the rate of hydrolysis in the case of these prodrugs.[139] Times associated with peak serum concentrations of chloramphenicol are approximately 1 hr for the orally administered base, 1.5–3 hr for the orally administered palmitate suspension, and between 0.5 and 1 hr after the end of a 30-min succinate infusion.[37] Times of peak chloramphenicol levels following intravenous infusion of the succinate to infants are highly affected by infusion rate, injection site, volume of fluid in the tubing, and type of infusion system.[142] It is important that specific guidelines be established at individual institutions to best estimate the times at which peak chloramphenicol levels will occur.

Specimens, collection methods, and assays. Both serum and plasma are acceptable for analysis of chloramphenicol. Gel barrier serum separator tubes have not caused a problem with chloramphenicol.[37] There is some suggestion that serum or plasma should be protected from light.[37] Also, in vitro hydrolysis of the succinate has been reported, and samples are not stable when stored at –20 °C for longer than 1 week.[143] The most commonly used assays for chloramphenicol are HPLC and immunoassay (EMIT®). The immunoassay method has the necessary sensitivity and specificity but does not permit measurements of palmitate or succinate concentrations.[144] HPLC is sufficiently sensitive and may also permit simultaneous determination of both prodrug and active drug. This ability to determine concentrations of prodrug would only be useful for explaining the reason for a particular chloramphenicol level. For example, low concentrations of chloramphenicol along with high concentrations of the succinate would indicate limited capacity for hydrolysis of the prodrug.[139]

Cerebrospinal fluid concentrations of chloramphenicol are sometimes measured (in which case the assay must assure the necessary sensitivity). Concentrations in cerebrospinal fluid need to be above the MIC of the organism, usually between 1 and 6 mg/L.[37] Saliva concentrations of chloramphenicol are not reliable predictors of serum chloramphenicol concentrations.[145]

Use of levels for dosage adjustment. Chloramphenicol has linear elimination characteristics. Therefore, serum chloramphenicol concentrations should change in proportion to the change in daily dose.

Protein binding, active metabolites, and enantiomers. Chloramphenicol is 53–60% bound in the serum of adults, with lower binding in neonates (32%) and adults with cirrhosis (42%).[139] Unbound chloramphenicol concentrations in neonates who have total concentrations between 7.5 and 14 mg/L are similar to unbound concentrations in adults who have total levels between 10 and 20 mg/L.[86] None of the metabolites of chloramphenicol show significant activity, and, therefore, do not need to be considered when interpreting chloramphenicol serum concentrations.

Vancomycin

Therapeutic range. Vancomycin, a glycopeptide antibiotic with a narrow spectrum of activity, is used intravenously to treat gram-positive cocci and bacilli resistant to other antibiotics.[37,81] Emergence of vancomycin-resistant enterococci has led to the need to restrict its use. The major toxicities associated with vancomycin are nephrotoxicity and ototoxicity (likely aggravated by concurrent administration of other nephro- and ototoxic drugs). Another adverse effect known as *red man syndrome* (intense flushing, tachycardia, and hypotension) is usually associated with infusion rates faster than 20 mg/min.

While many institutions monitor both peaks and troughs of vancomycin, this practice has been questioned. Unlike the aminoglycosides, vancomycin is bactericidal, and maintaining levels above the MIC during the dosing interval is what is important. It is usually assumed that trough concentrations for vancomycin should be between 5 and 10 mg/L. While some have advocated higher troughs,[36,146] most agree that the risk of nephrotoxicity is greater with sustained troughs above 10 mg/L.[37,130,147] While it is sometimes recommended that peak concentrations must be kept below 50 mg/L to avoid ototoxicity, this recommendation is based on only two cases.[130] It is more likely that ototoxicity is the result of both peaks and troughs being too high (an excessively high total vancomycin exposure).[130] Some pharmacokinetic dosing methods are, therefore, based on targeting peak vancomycin serum concentrations between 30 and 40 mg/L.[36]

Vancomycin is routinely monitored in all patients in some hospitals, but many question the need for this in uncomplicated patients with normal renal function.[37,130] Indications for monitoring include decreased or changing renal function, especially in patients receiving other nephrotoxic or ototoxic drugs; patients expected to have unusual pharmacokinetics (burns, malignancies, and intravenous drug abusers); patients on therapy for longer than 10 days; patients showing poor response; and patients with unusually high MICs.[37,147,148]

Sample timing. The half-life of vancomycin is 7–9 hr in adults with normal renal function but can be as long as 120–140 hr in patients with renal failure. Vancomycin half-life is approximately 7 hr in full-term infants, 2–3 hr in children, and 12 hr in patients older than 65. Half-lives in obese patients are 3–4 hr and 4 hr in burn patients.[81,147] Samples should be obtained as troughs, within 0.5–1 hr of the start of the next infusion. Winter proposed a simple method whereby the peak vancomycin concentration can be estimated using a single trough level, thus obviating the need to draw two levels if pharmacokinetic dosing is to be performed.[36]

Specimens, collection methods, and assays. Serum or plasma, using EDTA-treated tubes, may be used. Heparinized tubes should be avoided based on reports of instability of vancomycin in the presence of heparin. There are no reports or problems using serum separator tubes.[37]

Immunoassays (EMIT® and FPIA) are the most common assays used for routine measurements of serum or plasma vancomycin concentration measurements. HPLC may also be used. Serum vancomycin concentrations in patients with renal failure will likely be overestimated if the Abbott TDx® FPIA method is used. This is because of cross-reactivity of the polyclonal antibody with vancomycin crystalline degradation product, which accumulates in renal failure patients.[149] The EMIT® method and a modified FPIA method (Abbott, AxSYM®), both using monoclonal antibodies, do not significant overestimate vancomycin serum concentrations in these patients.[150] Serum vancomycin concentrations determined by the Abbott TDx® method are reported to be falsely low in patients with hyperbilirubinemia.[151]

Use of levels for dosage adjustment. Vancomycin elimination is linear, and an increase in the dose (without a change in the dosing interval) can be expected to provide a proportional change in the trough (and peak) serum concentration. More sophisticated prediction methods are required, however, if the dosing interval is adjusted with or without a change in dose.

Many methods have been proposed for vancomycin dosage regimen adjustment.[36,81,152] A relatively simple method proposed by Winter[36] permits the use of a single trough level (drawn within 1 hr of the start of the next infusion) along with an assumption of the population distribution volume to predict the necessary pharmacokinetic parameters needed for individualization. Once those parameters are determined, the aminoglycoside individualization equations can be used to target desired peak and trough vancomycin concentrations.

Protein binding, active metabolites, and enantiomers. Vancomycin is 30–55% bound to serum proteins in adults with normal renal function. The binding is lower (19%) in patients with end stage renal disease.[152] With binding this low, total concentrations of vancomycin will always provide reliable indications of the unbound concentrations in serum. Vancomycin metabolites are inactive, and, thus, do not contribute to effect or toxicity.

Amphotericin B

While amphotericin B continues to be considered the drug of choice for most systemic fungal infections, serum concentration monitoring is not recommended.[153] The nephrotoxic effects of amphotericin B do not appear to be related to serum concentration, and the range of concentrations associated with beneficial effect is, likewise, unclear.[153]

Flucytosine

Therapeutic range. Flucytosine is a synthetic antifungal agent that is often used in combination with amphotericin B for treatment of systemic fungal infections.[154] It is also used increasingly in combination with the azole antifungal agents and is part of a new therapeutic approach in the treatment of certain tumors, such as colorectal carcinoma.[155] Most clinicians agree that peak serum concentrations of flucytosine should be kept below 100 mg/L to avoid dose-related hepatotoxicity, bone marrow depression, and gastrointestinal disturbances.[130,155,156] Some clinicians also advise that trough concentrations of flucytosine be kept between 25 and 50 mg/L (or kept above 25 mg/L) in order to avoid rapid formation of resistance.[130,154,155] If a constant infusion is used, steady state serum concentrations of 50 mg/L should be targeted.[130] The hepatotoxicity and bone marrow suppression are both usually reversible with discontinuation. Indications for monitoring flucytosine include avoidance of toxicity—particularly in patients with impaired renal function or who are receiving concomitant amphotericin B—and avoidance of resistance due to sustained low levels.[130,154–156]

Sample timing. The half-life of flucytosine is approximately 3–4 hr in patients with normal renal function;[155] it is usually advised to wait 24 hr before a steady state is assumed.[156] The half-life can be as long as 85 hr in patients with renal failure[154] in which case steady state would not be reached for approximately 10 days. Peak concentrations should be obtained 1–2 hr after an oral dose[130,154,155] or 30 min after the end of an infusion.[153] The peak time occurs later after an oral dose of flucytosine in patients with poor renal function[155] because of either slowed absorption or a shift in peak time related to the drug's longer half-life. Trough concentrations, if indicated, should be drawn within 30 min of the next dose.

Specimens, collection methods, and assays. Serum is the most common specimen reported for analysis. There do not appear to be special precautions for blood collection devices. The most common assays include microbiological, GLC, HPLC, and an automated enzymatic method.[154,156,157] The enzymatic method compares well to HPLC but shows some degree of nonspecificity with icteric and lipemic samples.[157]

Use of levels for dosage adjustment. Because there are no reports of nonlinear elimination behavior, a given increase in dose rate or infusion rate should produce a proportional increase in serum flucytosine concentration.

Protein binding, active metabolites, and enantiomers. Flucytosine does not exist as enantiomers, has no active metabolites, and is minimally bound to serum proteins.

Fluconazole, Itraconazole, Ketoconazole

Therapeutic ranges. Firm relationships between serum concentration, effect, and toxicity have not been established for any of the azole antifungal drugs, which limit the routine therapeutic monitoring of these drugs. Serum concentrations of the azoles have been measured and documented following successful therapy, but serum concentrations associated with toxicity have not been determined. For itraconazole, serum concentrations above 0.25 mg/L of the parent drug are associated with chronic therapy.[158] Combined levels of itraconazole and its active hydroxy metabolite of 1 mg/L or higher are also recommended.[130] Serum concentrations of ketoconazole between 1.5 and 6 mg/L, and fluconazole between 30 and 90 mg/L have been associated with chronic therapy.[153,156]

The primary reason for monitoring the azole antifungal drugs is to assure efficacy. Itraconazole levels are known to be relatively low in patients with AIDS or acute leukemia, most likely due to malabsorption and concurrent administration of enzyme inducing drugs.[159] For this reason, some consider the serum concentration monitoring of itraconazole to be essential in patients with life-threatening fungal infections.[153] Ketoconazole is recommended for monitoring only in patients with treatment failure or relapse, or if drug-drug interactions or malabsorption are suspected.[153,156] Fluconazole is the least likely to require monitoring, as its absorption is predictable and it is less affected by drug-drug interactions.[153]

Sample timing. The half-life of itraconazole ranges between 20 and 60 hr. Thus, steady state will not be attained for 1–2 weeks after initiation of therapy or adjustment of the dosage regimen.[156,159] A steady state can be expected for fluconazole in 5–7 days and for ketoconazole after 48 hr.[156] Since the purpose of monitoring the azoles is to assure that minimum levels of drug are present, trough levels should be obtained when possible.

Specimens, collection methods, and assays. Serum is the most common specimen reported for analysis of the azole drugs. There do not appear to be any reported problems associated with blood collection methods. The most common assays for the azoles include microbiological, GLC, and HPLC.[153,156,159] Because itraconazole has an active metabolite that may be present at concentrations that are 2–3 times higher than the parent drug,[158] concentration readings using microbiologic assays will be higher than those reported using the chromatographic methods.[159] An HPLC method that measures both the parent and hydroxylated metabolite is preferred for itraconazole. Although concentrations of fluconazole in stimulated saliva were highly correlated with concentrations in plasma, accuracy of plasma concentration prediction was not adequate.[160]

Use of levels for dosage adjustment. Although azole levels are not used for purpose of dosage adjustment, ketoconazole and fluconazole exhibit first-order elimination behavior, and increases in dose rate or infusion rate can be expected to produce proportional increases in drug concentrations.[153] Itraconazole is reported to have nonlinear elimination behavior, such that greater-than-proportional increases in serum drug concentration should be expected.[130,159]

Protein binding, active metabolites, and enantiomers. Itraconazole and ketoconazole are 98–99% bound to serum proteins, primarily albumin, while fluconazole is only 11–12% bound.[159] It is possible that some of the inability to correlate total serum concentrations with response and toxicity is complicated by variable serum protein binding among patients. Itraconazole concentrations in the presence of variable quantities of the active may also complicate the correlation of itraconazole serum concentrations with effect and toxicity.[158]

Antimycobacterials

The optimal use of therapeutic drug monitoring for mycobacterial infections is currently under study. Drugs that are FDA-approved and considered first line as part of an initial four-drug regimen are isoniazid, rifampin, pyrazinamide, and either ethambutol or streptomycin. Of these, isoniazid and rifampin are the most important based on their relatively high potency and favorable side-effect profiles. Second line agents that are more toxic must be used if drug resistance emerges and include ethionamide, cycloserine, capreomycin, para-aminosalicylic acid, and dapsone.[161]

It is essential that adequate levels of these antimycobacterial drugs be present in serum for effective treatment. This does not always occur, even in patients in whom compliance has been documented.[161] Lower-than-expected levels of antimycobacterial drugs have been reported in patients with HIV infections and in some cases is associated with malabsorption.[162] There is also considerable potential for drug-drug interactions among the antimycobacterial drugs, given the effects of rifampin, isoniazid, and the fluoroquinolones in either inducing or inhibiting cytochrome P450 isozymes.[163] Drugs used to treat HIV patients may also contribute to this drug-drug interaction quagmire.

A study in non-HIV infected tuberculosis patients who were not responding to treatment as expected showed that 29–68% of them had serum antimycobacterial drug levels below target ranges.[164] In another study, a small percentage of nonresponding patients all showed suboptimal levels of rifampin.[165] After dosage adjustments were made, all patients responded to treatment. The authors recommended that low serum rifampin levels be suspected in patients who do not respond after 3 months of supervised drug administration, or earlier in patients with HIV infection, malnutrition, known gastrointestinal or malabsorptive disease, or hepatic or renal disease.

Specialized laboratories have been developed that offer sensitive and specific assays for serum concentrations for the most commonly used antimycobacterial drugs.[161] As more specific information about the efficacy of therapeutic drug monitoring of these drugs becomes available, more laboratories and services of this type will likely be available.[166]

Antiretrovirals

Therapeutic ranges. There is growing evidence that favors serum concentration monitoring of drugs used in the treatment of HIV-1 infection, in particular the protease inhibitors (PIs) and the nonnucleoside reverse-transcriptase inhibitors (NNRTIs). These drugs, particularly the PIs, show marked interpatient variability in their pharmacokinetics, and retrospective studies show strong relationships between drug concentrations and virologic response.[167] In addition, suboptimal levels of the antiretroviral drugs are associated with acquired drug resistance and virologic failure.[168] A substudy of the randomized, prospective clinical trial, ATHENA, showed that patients who underwent drug concentration monitoring for the antiretroviral drugs had a significantly higher likelihood of virological response as compared to those who did not undergo monitoring.[167] National treatment guidelines from the Netherlands and United Kingdom have already incorporated therapeutic drug monitoring as the standard of practice in the treatment of HIV-1 infection.[167]

Minimum effective concentrations have been determined for the most common PIs based on in vitro determinations of drug concentrations (corrected for serum binding) required for 50% or 90% inhibition of replication in the patient's virus isolate (IC_{50} or IC_{90}). Attention has turned more recently, however, to the use of a new parameter that may be a better predictor of response. The inhibitory quotient (IQ) is the ratio of the patient's trough plasma concentration to the IC_{50} or IC_{90}.[167] A high IQ would indicate more drug is present in the patient than is needed for virologic response, while a low IQ would indicate inadequate drug levels or a resistant virus. Recent studies show virologic response may be better related to IQ than to trough levels alone.[167] Future studies may focus on the definition of therapeutic ranges of IQ rather than minimum concentrations.

The most common PIs are amprenavir, indinavir, lopinavir, nelfinavir, ritonavir, and saquinavir; the most commonly used NNRTIs are efavirenz and nevirapine. Some clinicians advocate the monitoring of these drugs in all patients on initiation of therapy to assure adequate levels; others reserve use for selected situations including patients with renal or liver disease, pregnancy, children, patients at risk for drug interactions, and suspected toxicity.[167,169]

Sample timing. Half-lives of the NNRTIs average 25–50 hr,[170] and steady state will be reached after a week in most patients. However, a steady state will be reached within 2 days for the PIs, which have half-lives ranging from 2–12 hr.[170] Predose samples are recommended as the minimum effective concentrations and the inhibitory quotients are based on the lowest drug concentration during the dosing interval. There may be logistic problems with this timing, however, in cases when the drug is administered once daily in the evening. Some drugs, such as nelfinavir, exhibit a lag in their absorption, such that the lowest concentration actually occurs about an hour after administration of the next dose.

Specimen, collection methods, and assays. Serum or plasma has been used as the specimen for analysis. It is important that the possible influence of gel barrier or serum separator tubes be determined by the laboratory prior to use. Given the high binding of these drugs to alpha-1-acid glycoprotein, tubes with stoppers possibly formulated with TBEP must be avoided. Nevirapine concentrations in citric-acid simulated saliva strongly correlated with concentrations in plasma and plasma ultrafiltrate.[171] Indinavir concentrations in saliva also show promise as noninvasive alternatives to plasma concentrations.[172] Concentration monitoring in saliva for the other antiretroviral drugs is not likely to be as promising because they are highly protein bound (>90%), and assay sensitivity would be limiting.

HPLC is most commonly used to determine serum concentrations of the antiretroviral drugs. A recently developed assay is able to simultaneously determine concentrations of six PIs and two NNRTIs in a single run using ultraviolet absorption detection.[173]

Use of levels for dosage adjustment. Dosage adjustments of the antiretroviral drugs, for the most part, should result in proportional changes in the trough serum drug concentration, provided the dosing interval is not altered. Reports showing serum drug concentrations to be unpredictable after dosage adjustments in some patients suggest that noncompliance with antiretroviral regimens is a major concern.[167] Serum concentrations of amprenavir, lopinavir, nelfinavir, and saquinavir may be difficult to maintain above their minimum effective concentrations because of rapid clearances and large first-pass effects. Rather than increasing their dose rate, ritonavir, a potent inhibitor of CYP3A4-mediated metabolism in the gut wall and liver, may be coadministered as a *pharmacoenhancer*. This results in decreased gastrointestinal enzyme catabolism of the PI, higher trough levels, and, in most cases, prolonged elimination half-lives.[174]

Protein binding, active metabolites, and enantiomers. The serum protein binding of efavirenz and indinavir is 50–60%, while the protein binding of the other antiretrovirals is greater than 90%.[170] Alpha-1-acid glycoprotein and albumin are the primary binding proteins for these drugs in serum.[167] As would be expected, there is considerable variability in the unbound fraction of these drugs in serum. In addition, alpha-1-acid glycoprotein concentrations are elevated in patients with HIV-1 infection and can return to normal with treatment. Thus, the same total level of the drug would be expected to reflect a lower level of response early in treatment as compared to later. Clearly, total concentrations of the PIs and NNRTIs should be cautiously interpreted if unusual serum binding is anticipated, but no clear guidelines are yet available.[167] Only nelfinavir has a metabolite that is known to be active.[167] While studies indicate the measurement of the metabolite is probably not crucial, there is likely to be considerable variability among and within patients in the presence of this metabolite.

Cardiac Drugs

Digoxin

Therapeutic ranges. There has been a dramatic reduction in digoxin toxicity since the advent of therapeutic drug monitoring for digoxin.[56] Digoxin's inotropic effect is the basis for its use for treatment of congestive heart failure, while its negative chronotropic effects form the basis for treatment of atrial arrhythmias such as atrial fibrillation, atrial flutter, and paroxysmal atrial tachycardia. The commonly reported therapeutic range is 0.5–2.0 µg/L in adults[56,175] and 1–2.6 µg/L in neonates.[86] The lower end of the range (0.5–1 µg/L) is generally used for treatment of heart failure, with levels up to 1.5 µg/L possibly leading to additional benefit.[81] Higher serum digoxin concentrations are required for treatment of atrial arrhythmias (0.8–1.5 µg/L), with additional benefit gained in some patients with levels up to 2 µg/L.[81]

Fifty percent of patients with serum digoxin concentrations above 2.5 µg/L show some form of digoxin toxicity.[81] Symptoms of toxicity include muscle weakness; gastrointestinal complaints (anorexia, nausea, vomiting, abdominal pain, and constipation); CNS effects (headache, insomnia, confusion, vertigo, and changes in color vision); and serious cardiovascular effects (second or third degree AV block, bradycardia, premature ventricular contractions, and ventricular tachycardia).[81,175] In fact, many of the cardiac arrhythmias observed with high digoxin concentrations resemble the clinical condition being treated, hence the need to monitor serum digoxin concentrations to distinguish toxicity from inadequate therapy.

There are several physiologic or pathologic conditions that can shift the therapeutic range of digoxin. Its toxicity may be more likely within the therapeutic range if the patient has hypokalemia, hypomagnesemia, hypercalcemia, or underlying heart disease (e.g., coronary atherosclerotic heart disease or an old myocardial infarction).[23,56] Patients with hyperthyroidism are believed to be more resistant to digoxin.[23]

The primary indications for digoxin monitoring include (1) suspected digoxin toxicity in order to determine the appropriate amount of antidote (digoxin-immune Fab fragments; Digibind®) needed; (2) suspected poisoning from ingestion of plants or herbal medications that contain structurally similar glycosides, (3) impaired renal function to adjust the dose rate; and (4) suspected interactions with drugs such as antibiotics, cholestyramine, kaolin-pectin, amiodarone, quinidine, verapamil, cyclosporine, spironolactone, and St. John's wort.[23,36]

Sample timing. The average digoxin half-life in adults with normal renal function is approximately 2 days; at least 7 days are recommended to attain a steady state.[36,175] In the case of treatment of digoxin overdose with digoxin-immune Fab fragments (a fragment of an antibody that is very specific for digoxin), blood samples for serum digoxin measurements should not be obtained sooner than 10 days after administration of the fragments.[56,175] Since most immunoassays measure both the free and Fab-bound digoxin, premature sampling would lead to artifactually high digoxin concentration readings.

Samples drawn during the absorption and distribution phases after administration of digoxin cannot be appropriately interpreted by comparison to the usual therapeutic range. Digoxin levels in blood do not reflect the more important levels in myocardial tissue until at least 6 hr after the dose (some say at least 8 hr).[36,175] Blood samples should, therefore, be drawn anytime between 6 hr after the dose and right before the next dose (Figure 6-5).

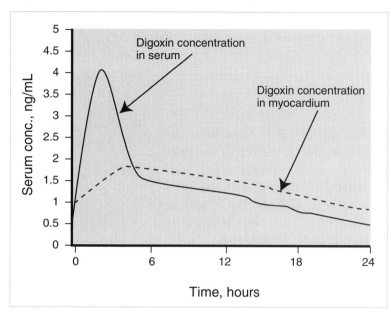

Figure 6-5. Simulated plot showing concentrations of digoxin in serum (ng/mL) and concentrations in *myocardial tissue* (units not provided) after a dose of digoxin at steady state. Tissue concentrations do not parallel concentrations in serum until at least 6 hr after the dose.

Inappropriate timing of samples for digoxin determinations is a major problem in hospitals. One study showed that 55% of the samples submitted to the laboratory for digoxin analysis lacked clinical value because of inappropriate timing.[176] In another study, standardization of digoxin administration times for 1700 and blood sample times for 0700 resulted in a dramatic reduction in inappropriately timed samples.[177] Another recommendation is that the laboratory immediately contact the clinician if digoxin levels are above 3.5 µg/L.[175] If it is confirmed that the sample was drawn too early after the dose, another sample should be requested. Alternatively, the laboratory should collect sample timing information as part of the laboratory request form and refuse to assay any samples that are inappropriately timed.

Specimens, collection methods, and assays. Serum or plasma, anticoagulated with heparin or EDTA, may be used. In general, serum separator tubes should be avoided. Serum is recommended if ultrafiltration is to be done for purposes of determining unbound concentrations of digoxin in patients treated with Fab fragments (Digibind®). Samples are stable for 24 hr at 2–8 °C and 1–2 weeks at –20 °C.[175] Saliva concentrations of digoxin have been measured in a number of studies, but none show a sufficiently strong correlation with either total or unbound levels in serum. Part of the poor correlation was proposed to be related to active secretion of digoxin into saliva or interferences from endogenous digoxin-like immunoreactive substances (DLIS).[136]

Digoxin serum concentrations are measured almost exclusively using commercial immunoassay methods.[56,175] The digoxin antibodies used in these immunoassays cross-react to varying extents with digoxin metabolites, endogenous DLIS, and other drugs and their metabolites (spironolactone and its active metabolite canrenone, digitoxin, and digitoxin metabolites). In fact, immunoassays for digoxin may cross-react with structurally similar substances in Chinese medicines (e.g., dried venom of Chinese toad) or plants (oleander) and, therefore, may be used to detect the presence of these substances, which cause digoxin-like toxicity.[175] It is important to note that these interferences can result in overreading or underreading of digoxin. One study comparing nine different commercial immunoassay methods showed that three of the nine methods underreported potentially toxic digoxin concentrations because of negative interferences caused by spironolactone and canrenone.[63] Potentially interfering digoxin metabolites will accumulate in renal impairment; DLIS are predominant in the blood of patients with renal and liver disease, those who are pregnant, and in neonates.[56] The high potential for interferences reinforces the importance of monitoring signs and symptoms in addition to serum levels.

One major cause of interference with digoxin serum concentration determinations by immunoassay is the presence of Fab fragments (Digibind®) used as an antidote to digoxin toxicity. The digoxin antibodies from the immunoassay cause this interference by competing with the Fab fragments for digoxin in the same samples. In patients with renal failure, this source of interference persists for more than 10 days after administration of the antidote. Ultrafiltration of the serum sample removes the digoxin-bound Fab fragments and permits a fairly reliable measurement of the unbound digoxin concentration.[178] Newer assays have been developed to directly measure unbound digoxin in the presence of Digibind® without ultrafiltration.[179]

Use of levels for dosage adjustment. Dose rate adjustments of digoxin based on serum digoxin concentrations are straightforward. Because of linear elimination behavior, a given increase in the daily digoxin dose will produce a proportional increase in the serum concentration at that time during the dosing interval. Again, it is extremely important that a serum level used for dose rate adjustment be obtained no earlier than 6–8 hr after the last dose.

Protein binding, active metabolites, and enantiomers. Digoxin is only 20–30% bound to serum proteins.[23] Therefore, total concentrations in serum will reflect the pharmacologically active unbound concentration. The biologic activity of digoxin metabolites is modest compared to the parent drug, and variable presence of metabolites should not affect the interpretation of a digoxin serum concentration.

Lidocaine

Therapeutic range. Lidocaine is a Type 1B antiarrhythmic used as second line therapy for treatment for ventricular tachycardia and fibrillation. It is also used for management of chronic pain syndromes of neurogenic origin.[56,81] The therapeutic range used for these indications is 1.5–5 mg/L with concentrations greater than 6 mg/L considered to be toxic.[81,175] Minor side effects—drowsiness, dizziness, euphoria, and paresthesias—may be observed at serum concentrations above 3 mg/L. More serious side effects observed at concentrations above 6 mg/L include muscle twitching, confusion, agitation, and psychoses, while cardiovascular depression, AV block, hypotension, seizures, and coma may be observed at concentrations above 8 mg/L.[81,175]

Lidocaine is not monitored as commonly as some of the other cardiac drugs because its effect (abolishment of the ECG-monitored arrhythmia) is easy to directly observe. Indications should be restricted to situations in which the expected response is not evident (inefficacy or toxicity) or when decreased hepatic clearance is suspected or anticipated: liver disease, congestive heart failure, advanced age, and/or concurrent propranolol or cimetidine.[56,175]

Sample timing. The half-life of lidocaine ranges from 1.5 hr to as long as 5 hr in patients with liver disease.[81] Thus, steady state may not be attained for 18–24 hr even if a loading dose is administered. Because lidocaine is administered as a continuous infusion, there are no fluctuations in levels, and blood for lidocaine serum concentration determinations can be drawn anytime at steady state.

Specimens, collection methods, and assays. Blood collected in serum separator tubes and tubes using TBEP-containing rubber stoppers have resulted in artifactually low lidocaine levels. A new formulation of the Becton-Dickinson serum separator tube, SST II®, has been shown to be acceptable, however, with complete recovery of lidocaine from serum stored for as long as 7 days.[39] Plasma is also acceptable as a specimen if heparin or EDTA are used as the anticoagulants.[175] Lidocaine is stable in serum or plasma stored 24 hr at 2–8 °C or 1–2 weeks at –20 °C.[175]

Immunoassays for determination of lidocaine are commercially available and show little cross-reactivity with lidocaine metabolites.[56] They do not permit separate determination of the primary active metabolite, monoethylglycinexylidide (MEGX), which has 80–90% of the activity of lidocaine.[175] Chromatographic methods (HPLC and GLC) are preferred if monitoring of the active metabolite is deemed necessary.

Use of levels for dosage adjustment. Adjustments of lidocaine infusion rate should result in a proportional increase in lidocaine serum concentration.

Protein binding, active metabolites, and enantiomers. The unbound percentage of lidocaine is normally 30% but can range from 10–40% due to variations in alpha-1-acid glycoprotein concentrations. Alpha-1-acid glycoprotein concentrations are decreased in patients with nephrotic syndrome and increased in conditions of physiologic trauma, after surgery, and in patients with rheumatoid arthritis, cancer, and morbid obesity.[175] Thus, higher total concentrations may be considered therapeutic for patients with higher alpha-1-acid glycoprotein concentrations.

Alpha-1-acid glycoprotein concentrations are also increased after a myocardial infarction, resulting in a lower unbound lidocaine fraction during prolonged infusions of lidocaine in these patients.[180] The combination of higher total levels of lidocaine during prolonged infusions (believed to be due to competition between lidocaine and its accumulated metabolites[181]) and a lower unbound fraction mean that unbound lidocaine concentrations during prolonged infusions are probably therapeutic. It is important to be aware that total lidocaine levels at the higher end of the therapeutic range may not present a danger of toxicity in patients receiving prolonged infusions of lidocaine after a myocardial infarction.

The monoethylglycinexylidide metabolite of lidocaine (MEGX) has 80–90% of the antiarrhythmic potency of lidocaine, and its concentration accumulates in renal failure. Since the MEGX metabolite is not as highly bound as lidocaine, ratios of unbound MEGX to lidocaine can be high, especially in patients with renal impairment. Estimated unbound MEGX:lidocaine ratios were 0.68 in a group of patients following a myocardial infarction.[182] Thus, MEGX may contribute to the pharmacologic effects of lidocaine in a substantial number of patients.[182] While there is anecdotal evidence that MEGX and the glycinexylidide metabolite of lidocaine (GX) contribute to the toxicity of lidocaine, no definitive evidence exists.[182]

Procainamide

Therapeutic range. Procainamide is used orally for long-term suppression of ventricular arrhythmias and long-term prevention of chronic supraventricular tachycardia, atrial fibrillation, and atrial flutter.[81] It may also be used intravenously for life-threatening ventricular arrhythmias, among other indications.[183] The therapeutic range of procainamide is complicated by the presence of an active metabolite, *N*-acetylprocainamide (NAPA), which has different electrophysiologic properties. Procainamide is a Type 1A antiarrhythmic, while NAPA is a Type III antiarrhythmic.[56,81,175] The enzyme that acetylates procainamide is bimodally distributed, such that patients are either slow or fast acetylators. In addition, NAPA is more dependent on the kidneys for elimination than is procainamide, and its levels accumulate more than procainamide for a given level of renal impairment.[175,180] Thus, the ratio of NAPA to procainamide in serum can be quite variable, necessitating the use of separate therapeutic ranges for the parent and metabolite.

Most patients respond when serum procainamide concentrations are between 4 and 8 mg/L; some receive additional benefit with levels up to 12 mg/L.[183] There have been reports of patients requiring levels between 15 and 20 mg/L without adverse effects.[36,183] Serum concentrations of NAPA associated with efficacy are reported to be as low as 5 mg/L and as high as 30 mg/L. Most clinicians consider toxic NAPA levels to be above 30–40 mg/L.[175,183] Some clinicians feel that NAPA does not need to be monitored except in patients with renal impairment.[183] Most laboratories, however, automatically measure both procainamide and NAPA concentrations in the same sample. The practice of summing the two concentrations and comparing to a therapeutic range for summed procainamide and NAPA (often reported as 10–30 mg/L) is to be discouraged.[81,175] To do this validly, the molar units of the two chemicals would need to be used.[56] More importantly, however, is the fact that procainamide and

NAPA have completely different electrophysiologic behaviors. The best practice is to independently compare each chemical to its own reference range.[56,81,175]

Side effects to procainamide and NAPA are similar. Anorexia, nausea, vomiting, diarrhea, weakness, and hypotension may be seen with procainamide levels above 8 mg/L, while levels above 12 mg/L may be associated with more serious adverse effects: heart block, ventricular conduction disturbances, new ventricular arrhythmias, and even cardiac arrest.[81] A syndrome known as *torsades de pointes* may also be seen after procainamide administration,[81] although this is more commonly seen after quinidine or disopyramide administration.

Indications for procainamide and NAPA serum level monitoring include recurrence of arrhythmias that were previously controlled, suspected toxicity or overdose, anticipated pharmacokinetic alterations caused by drug-drug interactions (including amiodarone, cimetidine, ofloxacin, and trimethoprim), and disease state changes (renal failure or congestive heart failure, in particular).[81,175,180,183]

Sample timing. The half-life of procainamide in adults without renal impairment or congestive heart failure ranges from 2.5 hr (fast acetylator) to 5 hr (slow acetylator).[81,175] The half-life of NAPA is longer, averaging 6 hr in patients with normal renal function, and up to 40 hr in patients with renal impairment.[81,183] Thus, a steady state of both chemicals is not observed until at least 18 hr in patients with good renal function or as long as 5 days in renal impairment. Most clinicians agree that serum procainamide and NAPA levels should be obtained as a trough, within 1 hr of administration of the next dose.[81,175,183] For extended-release products that are administered at a dosing interval of 6 hr or less, levels will not fluctuate much and could be obtained at any time to reflect an average steady state level.[183] It is recommended, however, that the sampling time within the interval be consistent from visit to visit. For intervals greater than 6 hr, a trough is preferred. It must be noted that delayed absorption may occur with some procainamide products,[175] such that the predose level may not represent the lowest level within the dosing interval.

Specimens, collection methods, and assays. Serum or plasma, anticoagulated with heparin, EDTA, or oxalate, may be used.[175] Recovery of procainamide and NAPA are not affected by use of serum separator tubes, but the influence of any special blood collection devices should always be confirmed by individual laboratories.[175] Serum and plasma are stable for 24 hr at 2–8 °C, and for 1–2 weeks at –20 °C.[175] Saliva levels of procainamide and NAPA have been shown to correlate strongly with plasma levels and are proposed as acceptable, noninvasive alternatives to blood sampling.[184]

The most commonly used commercial, automated assays for procainamide and NAPA are FPIA (TDx®) and EMIT®. These methods require separate determinations of procainamide and NAPA on the same serum sample. Samples that are hemolyzed, lipemic, or icteric may affect the reading of these immunoassay methods.[175] Chromatographic methods (HPLC and GLC) allow the simultaneous measurement of procainamide and NAPA and are not subject to interferences from hemoglobin, lipids, or bilirubin.[175]

Use of levels for dosage adjustment. The 24% lower clearance of procainamide at higher dose rates has been attributed to nonlinear hepatic clearance.[185] The clinician should be aware that increases in dose rate may produce somewhat greater-than-proportional increases in serum procainamide concentration in some patients, particularly those with serum levels at the upper end of the therapeutic range.

Protein binding, active metabolites, and enantiomers. Procainamide is only 10–20% bound to serum proteins.[56,175] Thus, total procainamide and NAPA levels always reflect the pharmacologically active unbound concentrations of these drugs.

Quinidine

Therapeutic range. Quinidine is used to chemically convert atrial fibrillation or flutter to normal sinus rhythm and to manage supraventricular or ventricular arrhythmias.[81,175,186] Parenteral quinidine gluconate is also indicated for the treatment of patients with life-threatening *plasmodium falciparum* malaria. It is considered a second-line therapy by many clinicians because of its side effect profile.[81] The therapeutic range for quinidine in serum is most commonly reported as 2–5 mg/L[175] with toxic levels seen most commonly above 6 mg/L.[81,186] Common side effects are gastrointestinal in nature (anorexia, nausea, and diarrhea) and more serious side effects include cinchonism (blurred vision, lightheadedness, tremor, giddiness, and tinnitus), hypotension, and ventricular arrhythmias.[81,175] Torsades de pointes is more likely to occur at concentrations at the lower end of the therapeutic range, thus complicating the interpretation of quinidine concentrations.[56]

Indications for monitoring of quinidine concentrations include therapeutic confirmation; suspected toxicity; recurrence of arrhythmias after initial suppression; suspected drug-drug interactions or other conditions known to alter quinidine pharmacokinetics; suspected noncompliance; and changes in administered formulation.[81,175,186]

Sample timing. The half-life of quinidine is reported to range from 4–8 hr in adults and up to 10 hr in patients with liver disease. Steady state should be attained within 2 or 3 days, and most clinicians agree that samples should be drawn as a trough within 1 hr of the next dose.[56,81,175]

Specimens, collection methods, and assays. Serum or plasma may be used. Plasma should be collected in EDTA-treated tubes. Serum separator tubes should generally be avoided.[175] Quinidine in serum or plasma is stable for 1–2 weeks at –20 °C.[175]

Quinidine in serum or plasma is most frequently assayed using immunoassay (EMIT® or TDx®), but HPLC may also be used. Dihydroquinidine (an impurity in quinidine dosage forms), quinine, and the quinidine metabolite, 3-hydroxyquinidine, may all interfere to varying extents with immunoassay methods.[175] Moderate (20%) cross-reactivity with the 3-hydroxy metabolite is seen with the FPIA (TDx®) method.[56]

Use of levels for dosage adjustment. Quinidine displays linear elimination behavior for most patients; a change in daily quinidine dose will cause a proportional change in the average steady state serum quinidine concentration. Nonlinear elimination may be evident in some patients, due either to saturable first-pass metabolism or saturable renal tubular secretion.[186] Thus, a greater-than-proportional increase in average quinidine concentration with increase in daily quinidine dose may be evident in some patients.

Protein binding, active metabolites, and enantiomers. Quinidine is a weak base that is normally between 70% and 80% bound to albumin and alpha-1-acid glycoprotein in serum of healthy patients.[175] These protein levels are known to increase in trauma, myocardial infarction, cardiac surgery, atrial fibrillation/flutter, and congestive heart failure, and the percentage binding of quinidine can increase to as high as 92% in these patients.[81] The unbound fraction of quinidine was shown to be decreased in patients with atrial fibrillation or atrial flutter,[187] and unbound quinidine concentration was shown to correlate better with ECG interval changes than total quinidine.[188] All of this suggests that total serum concentrations of quinidine must be cautiously interpreted in patients with suspected elevations in alpha-1-acid glycoprotein concentrations. A total quinidine level that is above 5 mg/L could be therapeutic with respect to unbound quinidine concentration.

An impurity, dihydroquinidine, may be present in amounts that are between 10% and 15% of the labeled amount of quinidine and is believed to have similar electrophysiologic properties as quinidine.[175] The 3-hydroxyquinidine metabolite has activity that is less than the parent (anywhere between 20% and 80% have been reported) and is not as highly bound to serum proteins.[180] Although not reported, this leads one to wonder about possible accumulation of these substances in renal failure patients with a resultant shift in the quinidine therapeutic range.

Other Cardiac Drugs

Amiodarone. Amiodarone is classified as a Type III antiarrhythmic and is restricted for treatment of life-threatening recurrent ventricular arrhythmias that do not respond to adequate doses of other antiarrhythmics. The primary metabolite, desethylamiodarone, has similar electrophysiologic properties as amiodarone[56] and accumulates to levels similar to or higher than the parent drug, especially in renal failure patients. The concentration vs. effect relationship for amiodarone is poorly defined; some say that serum concentrations between 0.5 and 2.5 mg/L are associated with effectiveness with minimal toxicity.[56] The occurrence of toxicity, however, appears to be more reliably related to the total amount of drug administered rather than serum concentration. Laboratories that measure serum amiodarone concentrations report only the parent drug, despite high levels of the active metabolite. In general, therapeutic drug monitoring of amiodarone is of limited benefit because activity of the drug is mostly associated with concentrations in the tissue.[56] Serum concentrations might be most useful in cases of suspected noncompliance.

Disopyramide. Disopyramide is used to treat established ventricular arrhythmias. Because it is proarrhythmic and a powerful negative inotrope, its use is restricted to selected patients.[175] Disopyramide has several characteristics that confound the use of serum disopyramide concentration monitoring. It is administered as a racemic mixture, and only the S(+) enantiomer is believed to significantly contribute to the drug's antiarrhythmic effect.[24] Both enantiomers demonstrate concentration-dependent binding, such that increases in dose rate produce proportional increases in unbound (pharmacologically active) enantiomer but less-than-proportional increases in total summed enantiomer concentration.[24,56,175] The primary metabolite of disopyramide, mono-N-dealkyldisopyramide, has 50% of the antiarrhythmic activity of the parent but 2–4 times the anticholinergic activity, which is responsible for many of the side effects.[175] The metabolite accumulates more than disopyramide in renal failure patients. Despite all of these confounding factors, most laboratories monitor summed enantiomer levels of total parent drug only (no metabolite) and, in most cases, rely on a therapeutic range between 2 and 5 mg/L with levels greater than 7 mg/L considered toxic.[175] The use of serum disopyramide concentrations as a guide to dosage adjustments is, understandably, on the decline. Indications that might be appropriate include suspected toxicity or noncompliance and drug-drug interactions or diseases that are anticipated to affect the pharmacokinetics of the enantiomers.[175]

Flecainide. Flecainide, classified as a Type 1C antiarrhythmic, is indicated for prevention of paroxysmal atrial fibrillation/flutter or paroxysmal supraventricular tachycardias. Like the other Type 1C antiarrhythmics, it is proarrhythmic and, therefore, should not be used in patients with a recent history of myocardial infarction or AV block.[175] Flecainide is administered as a racemic mixture, but unlike disopyramide, there is little difference in the pharmacologic effects of these enantiomers.[56] The commonly used therapeutic range, based on the flecainide acetate salt, is 200–1000 µg/L; the range based on the flecainide base is 175–870 µg/L.[56,175] Toxicity is likely observed at acetate concentrations greater than 1600 µg/L.[56] Although this is a fairly wide therapeutic range, the pharmacokinetics of flecainide are quite variable among patients, suggesting that serum concentration monitoring might be helpful. Indications for monitoring may include patients who have a recent myocardial infarction, impaired renal function, or in whom drug-drug interactions are suspected.[175] The serum binding of flecainide is low (32–58%) so that total flecainide concentrations provide a reliable reflection of the active, unbound concentration. Flecainide is assayed by FPIA or HPLC.[175]

Mexiletine. Mexiletine is structurally similar to lidocaine but has the advantage that it can be given orally. It is used for prevention of ventricular arrhythmias and may also be used for treatment of chronic pain syndromes.[56] It is given as a racemic mixture—with the S(+) enantiomer showing greater activity than the R(−) enantiomers—and is only 50–60% bound to serum proteins. Mexiletine is usually assayed by achiral methods (GLC or HPLC); no studies have yet been done to relate effect to individual enantiomers.[56] The therapeutic range for the summed total enantiomers is most commonly reported to be 0.5–2.0 mg/L.[56,180] Toxicity may occur, however, at concentrations within the range of effective concentrations.[180] Mild side effects may be seen between 0.8 and 3 mg/L, and severe side effects between 1 and 4.4 mg/L.[180] Because the extent of mexiletine absorption can be significantly affected by changes in the rate of gastric emptying, patients receiving narcotics and those who have had a recent myocardial infarction might benefit from serum concentration monitoring.[180] Higher serum levels of mexiletine may be seen in patients with liver disease and patients with congestive heart failure.[189]

Cytotoxic Drugs

While cytotoxic drugs have characteristics that make them ideal candidates for therapeutic drug monitoring (narrow therapeutic indices and variable pharmacokinetics) they have many more characteristics that make therapeutic drug monitoring difficult or unsuitable.[190,191] They lack a simple, immediate indication of pharmacologic effect in order to aid definition of a therapeutic range (the ultimate outcome of *cure* could be years). They are given in combination with other cytotoxic drugs, such that concentration vs. effect relationships for any single drug are difficult to isolate. They are used to treat cancer, which is a highly heterogeneous group of diseases, each possibly having its own concentration vs. effect relationships. Finally, many of these drugs require tedious assay techniques. In summary, cytotoxic drugs are not routinely monitored because they are in need of more clearly defined therapeutic ranges. If ranges are established, they are usually more helpful to avoid toxicity than to define zones for efficacy.

Methotrexate

Therapeutic range. Methotrexate is the only antimetabolite drug for which serum concentrations are routinely monitored.[190] It acts by blocking the conversion of intracellular folate to reduced folate cofactors necessary for cell replication. While cancer cells are more susceptible to the toxic effects of methotrexate, healthy host cells are also affected by prolonged exposure to methotrexate. It is for this reason that leucovorin, a folate analogue that prevents further cell damage, is administered following high-dose methotrexate treatments.[190] Measurements of serum methotrexate concentrations at critical times following high-dose methotrexate regimens are imperative to guide the amount and duration of leucovorin rescue treatments, thus preventing methotrexate toxicity. Institution of protocols for methotrexate serum concentration monitoring for this purpose has resulted in dramatic reductions in high-dose methotrexate-related toxicity and mortality.[192]

While it is known that methotrexate levels must be sufficiently high in order to prevent relapse of the malignancy,[192] the specific range of levels defining efficacy has been difficult to define. However, the relationship between methotrexate levels and toxicity has been much more clearly defined. Depending on the protocol, methotrexate levels that remain above 0.01–0.1 μM for longer than 48 hr are associated with a high risk of cytotoxicity.[36,193] Prolonged levels of methotrexate can lead to nephrotoxicity, myelosuppression, gastrointestinal mucositis, and liver cirrhosis.[190,192]

Serum concentration monitoring is not generally indicated when relatively low doses of methotrexate are given for chronic diseases such as rheumatoid arthritis, asthma, psoriasis, and maintenance for certain cancers.[193]

Sample timing. The timing of samples for determination of methotrexate concentrations is highly dependent on the administration schedule. As one example of such a protocol, a methotrexate dose may be administered by infusion over 24 hr followed by a regimen of leucovorin doses starting 36 hr after the start of methotrexate infusion. Guidelines would be given for additional or larger leucovorin doses depending on the methotrexate levels in samples drawn 48 or 72 hr after the start of the methotrexate infusion. It is important that methotrexate levels continue to be monitored until they are below the critical levels (usually between 0.01 and 0.1 µM).[36,190]

Specimen, collection methods, and assays. Serum or plasma concentrations are generally used. Saliva concentrations correlate poorly with total and unbound methotrexate concentrations, precluding the clinical use of saliva as a noninvasive alternative for blood samples.[194] Rapid reporting of methotrexate levels is important, and the immunoassay methods are preferred for determination of methotrexate levels. All immunoassays have different specificities and sensitivity limits and none stand out as clearly superior.[192] The most widely used method, FPIA, offers a sensitivity limit as low as 0.05 µM, and minimal (1.5%) cross-reactivity with the major metabolite, 7-hydroxymethotrexate.[192] Chromatographic methods such as HPLC must be used if quantitation of methotrexate metabolites is desired, most likely for research purposes.

Use of levels for dosage adjustment. Methotrexate and leucovorin doses are based on protocols.

Protein binding, active metabolites, and enantiomers. Methotrexate binding to albumin in serum ranges from 20–57%.[190] While studies have shown the unbound fraction of methotrexate to be increased by concomitant administration of NSAIDs, salicylate, sulfonamides, and probenecid, the implications for interpretation of methotrexate levels are probably not important.[193] The methotrexate metabolite, 7-hydroxymethotrexate, has only 1/100th the activity of methotrexate but may cause nephrotoxicity due to precipitation in the renal tubules.[192]

Other Cytotoxic Drugs

Crom and Evans[192] provide an excellent summary of cytotoxic drugs and the types of measurements that have been used to predict their toxicity and/or response. Correlations between response or toxicity and areas under the serum concentration vs. time curves (AUC) for total drug have been shown for busulfan, fluorouracil, hexamethylene, bisacetamide, and vincristine.[192,195,196] Unbound AUC values for etoposide and teniposide, which demonstrate concentration-dependent binding, correlate more strongly with toxicity than corresponding total plasma AUC values.[197] Systemic drug clearance has been predictive of response/toxicity for amsacrine, fluorouracil, methotrexate, and teniposide.[192,198] Steady state average serum concentrations or concentrations at designated postdose times have also been predictive of response/toxicity for cisplatin, etoposide, and methotrexate.[192] Finally, concentrations of cytosine-arabinoside metabolite in leukemic blasts and concentrations of mercaptopurine metabolite in red blood cells have been predictive of response or toxicity for these drugs. Correlations between systemic exposure and response/toxicity for cyclophosphamide, carmustine, and thiotepa have also been reported.[199]

Other than methotrexate, none of the assays for these drugs (often done by HPLC) is available commercially as an immunoassay. While most studies up to this point have focused on use of cytotoxic drug concentration measurements to minimize toxicity, future studies will be increasingly focused on use of drug concentrations to maximize efficacy.

Immunosuppressants

Cyclosporine

Therapeutic range. Cyclosporine is a potent cyclic polypeptide used for prevention of graft-vs.-host disease in bone marrow transplant graft rejection in solid organ (kidneys, liver, heart, lungs, and pancreas) transplant recipients. It is also used for the management of psoriasis, rheumatoid arthritis, and other autoimmune diseases. The therapeutic range of cyclosporine is highly dependent on the specimen (whole blood or serum/plasma) and assay. Most transplant centers use whole blood with one of the more specific assays—HPLC or immunoassays that use monoclonal antibodies (monoclonal radioimmunoassay or monoclonal fluorescence polarization immunoassay).[81,200] The commonly cited therapeutic range for whole blood using one of these specific methods is 100–400 µg/L.[81] Therapeutic ranges are lower if serum or plasma is used and higher if a less specific assay is used, such as an immunoassay based on polyclonal antibodies. The therapeutic range also depends on the specific organ transplantation procedure, as well as the stage of treatment after surgery (higher concentrations during induction and lower concentrations during maintenance to minimize side effects).[55,81,201–203] Thus, it is important that the therapeutic range guidelines established by each center be used. While most centers still use trough levels to adjust cyclosporine doses, there is renewed interest in targeting areas under the blood concentration vs. time curve instead. Studies that have investigated the use of single cyclosporine concentrations measured 2 hr after the dose, as a surrogate for the AUC value, suggest a better clinical outcome as compared to the use of single trough levels.[200,204]

Cyclosporine has a narrow therapeutic index and extremely variable pharmacokinetics among and within patients. The implications of ineffective therapy and adverse reactions are serious. Thus, it is imperative that cyclosporine concentrations be monitored in all patients starting immediately after transplant surgery.[81,202] The primary side effects associated with high cyclosporine blood concentrations are nephrotoxicity, neurotoxicity, hypertension, hyperlipidemia, hirsuitism, and gingival hyperplasia.[55,81,202] Blood cyclosporine concentrations should also be monitored when there are signs of rejection, adverse reactions, or suspected noncompliance.[55,202]

Sample timing. Monitoring is often done immediately after surgery before a steady state is reached. Initially, levels may be obtained daily or every other day, then every 3–5 days, then monthly. Changes in dose rate or initiation or discontinuation of potential enzyme inducers or inhibitors will require resampling once a new steady state is reached. The half-life of cyclosporine ranges from 6 to 27 hr. Thus, 3–5 days is generally adequate in most patients for attainment of a new steady state. Most centers continue to sample predose (trough) cyclosporine levels, while some are using 2-hr postdose levels, which appear to more closely predict total exposure to cyclosporine as measured by AUC.[200,204] Multiple samples to determine the AUC is generally unnecessary.

Specimens, collection methods, and assays. Blood concentrations of cyclosporin are 2–5 times the concentration in serum because of extensive partitioning into red blood cells. Whole blood is the preferred specimen and should be collected in tubes with EDTA.[55] Samples are stable for 7 days in plastic tubes at 4 °C.[205] Capillary blood by skin puncture is also acceptable.[55] While the popular monoclonal immunoassays offer improved specificity over the older polyclonal versions, they continue to measure varying amounts of cross-reactive metabolites.[55,200] The reference method of HPLC offers optimal specificity but takes longer; it might be considered in selected cases where significant interferences from metabolites are suspected.

Use of levels for dosage adjustment. In most cases, simple proportionality may be used for dosage adjustments. Trough or 2-hr postdose levels will change in proportion to the change in dose rate.

Protein binding, active metabolites, and enantiomers. Cyclosporine is 90–95% bound to albumin and lipoproteins in blood.[203] Unbound fractions in blood vary widely among patients and are weakly correlated to lipoprotein concentrations in blood.[203] For example, lower unbound fractions of cyclosporine have been reported in patients with hypercholesterolemia.[55] Lindholm and Henricsson reported a significant drop in the unbound fraction of cyclosporine in plasma immediately prior to acute rejection episodes.[206] An association between low cholesterol levels (and presumably high unbound fractions of cyclosporine) and increased incidence of neurotoxicity has also been reported.[55] These studies suggest that efforts to maintain all patients within a certain range of total concentrations may be misleading. Routine monitoring of unbound cyclosporine levels is not yet feasible, given the many technical difficulties with this measurement. Instead, the clinician should cautiously interpret total levels of cyclosporine in situations where altered protein binding of cyclosporine has been reported.

Other Immunosuppressants

Tacrolimus. Tacrolimus is a macrolide antibiotic with immunosuppressant activity and is generally used in combination with other immunosuppressant drugs. Like cyclosporine, whole blood is the preferred specimen. Trough blood concentrations of tacrolimus as high as 20 µg/L are targeted during initial treatment and gradually decrease to between 5 and 10 µg/L during maintenance therapy, often after 12 months.[55] Toxicities to tacrolimus are very similar to those with cyclosporine, including nephrotoxicity and neurotoxicity.[202] The unpredictable and variable extent of tacrolimus bioavailability (9–43%) contribute to the need for monitoring of this drug.[202] Monitoring should always be done after changes in dose rate or initiation/discontinuation of enzyme inducing or inhibiting agents.[36] The half-life of tacrolimus ranges from 4–41 hr, and a new steady state will be attained after approximately 5 days.[55] While trough concentrations are still the method of choice for monitoring,[204] a second level might be needed if Bayesian approaches to dosage individualization are used.[207] The majority of centers use immunoassay methods, either a microparticle enzyme immunoassay (MEIA) or EMIT®, which show some cross-reactivity with tacrolimus metabolites. More specific methods, such as HPLC, may be required in patients with liver disease who are anticipated to have high levels of metabolites.[55] Bilirubin and alkaline phosphatase do not interfere with measurements of tacrolimus using MEIA, but abnormally high hematocrit levels caused underreading of tacrolimus.[208] Tacrolimus appears to exhibit linear elimination behavior. Thus, an increase in the daily dose is expected to result in a proportional increase in the steady state trough level. Tacrolimus is 75–99% bound to plasma proteins (albumin and alpha-1-glycoprotein).[55] While there is no information at this point that unbound tacrolimus concentrations correlate better with response or toxicity,[202] it is prudent to be cautious with interpretation of total tacrolimus concentrations in patients with suspected alterations in protein binding.

Mycophenolic acid. Mycophenolate mofetil, the prodrug of mycophenolic acid, is often used in combination with cyclosporine or tacrolimus with or without corticosteroids.[55] While troughs of mycophenolic acid may be monitored (levels between 2.5 and 4 mg/L are targeted with good success[204]), AUC values appear to be better predictors of efficacy.[209] Reliable measurements of AUC require at least three samples to be drawn (trough, 30 min, and 120 min postdose) with a desired target AUC range of 30–60 mg × hr/L.[209] The half-life of mycophenolic acid is approximately 17 hr. Thus, a new steady state will be attained approximately 3 days after a dose rate change or the addition/discontinuation of drugs that affect the metabolism of mycophenolic acid. In contrast to cyclosporine, tacrolimus, and sirolimus, plasma anticoagulated with EDTA is the preferred specimen for mycophenolic acid concentration measurements.[55] The acyl glucuronide metabolite of mycophenolic acid is active, but its clinical significance for the interpretation of mycophenolic acid levels is not yet clear. This metabolite cross-reacts with immunoassay using the EMIT® method, giving higher readings as compared to HPLC.[55] Mycophenolic acid is 97% bound to plasma proteins, and the unbound fraction is greatly influenced by changes in albumin concentration, displacement by metabolites, renal failure, and hyperbilirubinemia.[200] Several groups of investigators suggest that unbound mycophenolic acid concentrations should be monitored when altered binding is suspected.[55,209–211] There is evidence that unbound mycophenolic acid concentration may be a better predictor of adverse effects.[210]

Sirolimus. Sirolimus is a macrolide antibiotic with potent immunosuppressant activity. When used in combination with cyclosporine or tacrolimus, trough blood concentrations of 4–12 µg/L are generally targeted.[204] It has a relatively long half-life (60–82 hr),[55,200] and a new steady state will not be attained in many patients until at least 10 days after dose rate adjustments or the addition/discontinuation of interacting drugs. At present, trough concentrations are used for monitoring as they correlate well with AUC.[200] Whole blood is the preferred specimen and should be collected using EDTA as the anticoagulant.[212] Samples are not stable at temperatures above 35 °C but may be stored at room temperature for up to 24 hr, between 2 and 8 °C for up to 7 days, and at 20 °C for up to 3 months.[212] An MEIA method is under development, but it overestimates sirolimus concentrations measured by HPLC because of cross-reactivities with sirolimus metabolites.[55]

Psychotropics

Amitriptyline, Nortriptyline, Imipramine, Desipramine

Therapeutic ranges. Three of the tricyclic antidepressants (TCAs) are recommended for therapeutic drug monitoring by the American Psychiatric Association: imipramine, desipramine, and nortriptyline.[213] Desipramine and nortriptyline, while drugs in their own right, are also active metabolites of imipramine and amitriptyline, respectively. Thus, amitriptyline is included as a fourth tricyclic antidepressant for serum concentration monitoring. Therapeutic ranges for these drugs have been fairly well-established.

When imipramine is administered, combined serum concentrations of imipramine and desipramine that are considered therapeutic but not toxic are between 180 and 350 µg/L.[36,213,214] Combined levels above 1000 µg/L are extremely serious.[214] When desipramine is administered, levels between 115 and 250 µg/L are frequently associated with therapeutic effect.[213,214] When amitriptyline is administered, combined serum concentrations of amitriptyline and nortriptyline should be between 120 and 250 µg/L.[36,213] Combined levels above 450 µg/L are not likely to produce additional response, and toxicity is likely. The therapeutic range of nortriptyline is the most firmly established of these four drugs; target serum concentrations after nortriptyline administration are between 50 and 150 µg/L.[36,213,215]

Potential cardiotoxicity is the major reason to monitor the TCAs. However, the most common side effects are anticholinergic in nature—dry mouth, constipation, urinary retention, and blurred vision.[213] Toxicities seen at higher concentrations include cardiac conduction disturbances (with prolonged QRS interval evident on EKG), seizures, and coma.[213] For all of the TCAs, these toxic effects occur at serum concentrations that are approximately 5 times those needed for antidepressant efficacy.[11]

Some clinicians advocate routine monitoring of TCAs in all patients once a steady state has been attained in order to adjust the maintenance regimen (so that desired target concentrations are attained). Since it would take 3 or more weeks beyond the final dose rate adjustment to fully assess clinical response, this would shorten the overall dosage titration period as compared to a trial and error dose rate adjustment method.[36] A dosage individualization method, using serum nortriptyline levels drawn following the first dose, was used for this purpose and resulted in patients being discharged 6 days earlier and returning to work 55 days earlier as compared to a control group.[33] Response rates to TCAs are reported to increase from 30–40% to as high as 80% by use of serum TCA concentration monitoring.[216] Other indications for monitoring include (1) suspected noncompliance or inadequate response; (2) suspected toxicity; and (3) suspected unusual or altered pharmacokinetics (children, elderly, and drug interactions).

Sample timing. While the half-lives of amitriptyline and nortriptyline range from 9 to 56 hr with a steady state attained within 4–11 days in most patients,[215] the half-lives of imipramine and desipramine range from 6–28 hr with a steady state attained in 6 days.[214,215] As a general rule, the clinician should wait at least a week before drawing any blood samples for serum concentration monitoring. Peak serum concentrations within the dosing interval following oral administration of the TCAs occur between 2 and 8 hr.[217] Trough levels are more reproducible but inconvenient since patients usually take the drug once-daily at bedtime. Therefore, a standardized sampling time is commonly used—12 to 14 hr after the bedtime dose.[36,215] Since this sample is taken midway through the dosing interval, it provides a fairly good approximation of the average steady state level of TCA. If the TCA happens to be given in divided doses, a 4- to 6-hr postdose sample time is recommended.[213,215]

Specimens, collection methods, and assays. Serum or plasma collected using EDTA as the anticoagulant is preferred. There is some suggestion that heparin lowers the concentrations of TCAs,[213] and there were numerous reports in the literature about TCAs having spuriously low serum levels due to displacement from alpha-1-acid glycoprotein by TBEP in the rubber stopper. Although the stopper has since been reformulated, it is a good idea to avoid blood collection materials that have not been tested by the laboratory, as well as special serum separator tubes with gel barriers.[213] Serum or plasma should be immediately separated from red blood cells to avoid the possibility of hemolysis.[213] Serum or plasma can be stored for 24 hr at room temperature, for 4 weeks at 4 °C, or for more than 1 year at –20 °C.

Chromatographic and immunoassay methods are most commonly used for measurements of serum TCA concentrations with immunoassay being most common.[214,215] Of the two available immunoassay methods, only the EMIT® system uses a monoclonal antibody to determine individual concentrations of these four TCAs. The FPIA method (TDx®) measures for the presence of all tricyclic drugs (*total tricyclics*) using a less specific polyclonal antibody and is, therefore, useful for toxicology screenings.[213] False positives may result from such screenings, however, if carbamazepine is present.[218] One limitation of the EMIT® method is that the tertiary amines (imipramine, amitriptyline, and others) cross-react with one another, while the secondary amines (desipramine and nortriptyline) also cross-react with one another.[213] This becomes a problem if the patient is receiving more than one TCA or is being switched from one to another.

Use of levels for dosage adjustment. Some mild nonlinearity has been described for desipramine, in which case, increases in the daily dose will be expected to produce somewhat greater-than-proportional increases in the standardized 12-hr sample. The other TCAs, however, exhibit proportionality. A method proposed by Browne et al.[33] for the dosing of nortriptyline involves the use of a serum level drawn following a first dose to predict an appropriate maintenance dosage regimen. This method, very similar to methods used for initiation of lithium therapy, is not commonly used but has demonstrated great promise in speeding up the dose-titration period.

Protein binding, active metabolites, and assays. The TCAs in general are highly bound to serum proteins, including albumin, alpha-1-acid glycoprotein, and lipoproteins.[217] The binding of TCAs is increased in cardiac patients, alcoholic patients, and others who have elevated alpha-1-acid glycoprotein concentrations.[217] The unbound percentage of imipramine varies from 4 to 41% among patients.[217] Based on this, one would expect unbound TCA serum concentrations to be much better predictors of response than total concentrations, particularly in populations suspected to have unusually high or low serum binding. Until now, studies that have attempted to examine this have not been able to clarify relationships between response and total serum concentrations based on variable protein binding. Assays for accurate and direct measurement of unbound TCA concentrations in serum need to be sufficiently sensitive for these kinds of studies.

The TCAs are extensively metabolized and undergo significant first-pass metabolism. While the primary active metabolites have been identified and are separately measured, other active metabolites can accumulate in some circumstances and affect the response at a given parent drug concentration. In one study, levels of conjugated and unconjugated hydroxylated metabolites of the TCAs were markedly elevated in patients with renal failure and believed to contribute to the hypersensitivity of these patients to TCA side effects.[219]

Lithium

Therapeutic range. Lithium is a monovalent ion used for the treatment of manic-depressive illness and the manic phase of affective disorders. The concentration units for lithium are expressed as mEq/L, which is the same as mmol/L. While the overall therapeutic range for treatment of manic depression is stipulated as 0.5–1.2 mEq/L in the American Psychiatric Association practice guidelines,[213] there appear to be two distinct ranges used in practice, depending on the stage of therapy. For acute management of manic depressive episodes, 0.8–1 mEq/L are desired, going up to 1.2 mEq/L if necessary.[36,81] For maintenance treatment, 0.6 to 0.8 mEq/L is usually recommended.[36,81] Serum concentrations above 1.5 mEq/L are associated with fine tremors of the extremities, gastrointestinal disturbances, muscle weakness, fatigue, polyuria and polydipsia. Concentrations above 2.5 mEq/L are associated with coarse tremors, confusion, delirium, slurred speech, and vomiting. Concentrations above 2.5–3.5 are life-threatening and potentially lethal: seizures, coma, and death.[213,215,220] It is important to point out that the values for the therapeutic ranges are based on samples obtained at a specific time during the day—just before the morning dose and at least 12 hr after the evening dose for patients taking a BID or TID regimen.[36,221]

Most clinicians require that every patient taking lithium be regularly monitored,[81] which is very cost effective considering the potential avoidance of toxicity.[215] Specific indications for lithium concentration monitoring include evaluation of noncompliance; suspicion of toxicity; confirmation of the level associated with efficacy; and any situation in which altered pharmacokinetics of the drug is anticipated (drug-drug interactions, pregnancy, children, geriatric patients, and fluid and electrolyte imbalance). Despite the strong indication for lithium monitoring in all patients, 37% of lithium users on Medicaid did not have serum drug concentrations monitored.[222]

Sample timing. The half-life of lithium ranges from 18–24 hr, and steady state will be reached within a week of therapy.[36] However, 4–6 weeks of treatment may be required after that before the full response to the drug can be assessed.[81,220] When initiating lithium therapy, it is recommended that serum levels be measured every 2–3 days (before a steady state is reached) to assure that levels do not exceed 1.2 mEq/L during that time.[81,220] Because of the extreme variability of serum lithium levels during the absorption and distribution periods, the current standard of practice is to draw all samples for lithium serum concentration determination 12 hr after the evening dose, regardless of whether a BID or TID schedule is used. For example, the time for blood sampling for a patient on a 0900/1500/2100 schedule would be right before the 0900 dose.[81] Because of this standardized sampling time, you do not see patients taking lithium on a once daily basis.[220]

Specimens, collection methods, and assays. While plasma is acceptable, it must be collected using sodium heparin as the anticoagulant, not lithium heparin. Serum is the preferred specimen, therefore, just to avoid any possible confusion.[215] The serum sample should be rejected if there is any evidence of hemolysis since release of high concentrations of lithium from the red blood cells will artifactually raise the serum concentration.[213] To minimize the chance of hemolysis, serum should be separated from the red blood cells within 1 hr of collection.[215] Other than one exception, involving an interference from a silica clot activator,[223] blood collection tubes generally have not introduced any artifacts for lithium assays. Lithium in serum or plasma is stable at room temperature or refrigeration temperature for extended periods of time.[213]

Lithium erythrocyte concentration has been proposed to correlate better with response and toxicity since it represents intracellular lithium.[36,213] This method, however, has never been routinely adopted for monitoring. Saliva concentrations of lithium have been proposed as noninvasive substitutes for serum or plasma lithium concentrations. However, the S:P ratio is quite variable, even within some patients. The average S:P ratio ranges from two to four and is affected by many variables. If the S:P ratio is shown to be stable for an individual patient over time, saliva monitoring might prove to be useful for some patients.[221,224] Based on an audit of clinical laboratories in Europe and the United Kingdom, flame emission photometry and atomic absorption spectroscopy are still the most commonly used methods for lithium quantitation and offer excellent precision, accuracy, and few interferences.[225] Ion-selective electrode (ISE) methods are more rapid and less costly but may have problems with interferences. Carbamazepine, quinidine, procainamide, *N*-acetylprocainamide, lidocaine, and valproic acid can all produce biases in lithium measurements by ISE.[213] High calcium levels may also produce a positive bias with some ISE methods.[213] A new colorimetric dry slide-based serum lithium assay is concluded to offer an acceptable alternative to currently available methods for monitoring lithium.[226]

Use of levels for dosage adjustment. Lithium exhibits linear elimination behavior and proportionality can be assumed when dosage adjustments are made. The assumption of linearity is the basis for several dosing methods that are used for initiating lithium therapy in patients. The Cooper method[34] involves drawing a sample for lithium analysis 24 hr after a first dose of 600 mg. The resulting level, believed to provide a reflection of the drug's half-life, is used with a nomogram that indicates the optimal maintenance regimen. The Perry method[35] requires that two levels be drawn during the postabsorption- postdistribution phase after a first dose of lithium. These two levels are used to determine the first-order elimination rate constant, which can then be used to determine the expected extent of lithium accumulation in the patient. The maintenance regimen required to attain a desired target lithium concentration in that patient can then be determined. Population-pharmacokinetic dosing-initiation methods (Bayesian) can also be used.[81]

Protein binding, active metabolites, and enantiomers. Lithium is not bound to serum proteins, nor is it metabolized.

Other Psychotropics

Other Antidepressants. Assays have been developed to document the serum concentrations observed following administration of other cyclic antidepressants (bupropion, clomipramine, and doxepin), as well as the selective serotonin reuptake inhibitors.[11,227–229] While working ranges have been established, there does not appear to be any compelling reason for routine monitoring of these drugs given their relatively wide therapeutic indices and favorable side effect profiles. Because 50% of patients do not achieve optimal relief from symptoms of depression, some clinicians advocate the use of serum concentration monitoring in patients who do not initially respond to identify noncompliance or to identify unusually low serum concentrations.[11,213]

Antipsychotics. The existence of optimal therapeutic ranges for most antipsychotic drugs remains controversial.[216,230] There is some evidence for therapeutic ranges for haloperidol and clozapine; ranges for other drugs are primarily based on average serum concentrations observed during chronic therapy.[215,216,231] However, therapeutic drug monitoring would seem appropriate based on the pronounced interindividual differences in pharmacokinetics of these drugs, problems with noncompliance, and significant drug-drug interactions in these patients. It also seems reasonable that initiation of therapy guided by serum concentration monitoring could significantly shorten the dose-titration period since there is a delayed onset of clinical response. One difficulty in establishing clear therapeutic range guidelines is that chronicity of illness and duration of antipsychotic drug exposure can shift the therapeutic range; separate therapeutic ranges may need to be developed depending on duration of illness.[231]

FUTURE OF TDM

Drug assays are rapidly improving with regard to specificity, sensitivity, speed, and convenience. Methods that separate drug enantiomers may help to elucidate therapeutic ranges for compounds administered as racemic mixtures.[232] Capillary electrophoresis-based assays will be increasingly used in clinical laboratories because of their low cost, specificity, utility for small sample volumes, and speed.[233] Methods for measurement of drugs in hair samples are being proposed for assessment of long-term drug compliance.[234] Implanted amperometric biosensors, currently used for glucose monitoring, may be useful for continuous monitoring of drug concentrations.[235] Subcutaneous microdialysis probes may also be useful for continuous drug monitoring, particularly since they monitor pharmacologically active unbound drug concentrations.[236] Desktop assay methods, currently used in private physician offices, group practices, clinics, and emergency rooms, could eventually be used in community pharmacies in the future.[237]

The therapeutic drug monitoring of the near future may also involve genotyping of patients before they receive certain drugs in order to identify those subsets of patients who will be *nonresponders* or *toxic responders*. Such genotype testing would not require special sample timing, might be possible using noninvasive methods (e.g., hair, saliva, and buccal swabs), and would only need to be done once as the result would apply over a lifetime. This type of testing will help patients to receive the best drug for the indication and rapid individualization of drug dosage to achieve desired target concentrations.[25,26,238] This will likely result in increased demand for rapid and reliable genotyping tests from clinical laboratories currently involved in routine therapeutic drug monitoring.

There is a movement to change the terminology and practice of therapeutic drug monitoring to something called *target concentration strategy* or *target concentration intervention*.[239] Critics of the therapeutic drug monitoring terminology claim that it suggests a passive process that is only concerned with after-the-fact monitoring to assure that levels are within an ill-defined range without proper regard to evaluation of the response to the drug in an individual patient.[22,239] Target concentration intervention is essentially a new name for a process used by clinical pharmacokinetics services for years and involves the following steps: (1) choosing a target concentration (usually within the commonly accepted therapeutic range) for a patient; (2) initiating therapy to attain that target concentration using best-guess population pharmacokinetic parameters; (3) fully evaluating response at the resulting steady state concentration; and (4) adjusting the regimen as needed using pharmacokinetic parameters that have been further refined by use of the drug concentration measurement(s).

Methods to improve the therapeutic drug monitoring process itself are needed. Every effort should be made to focus on patients who are most likely to benefit from therapeutic drug monitoring, and minimize time and money spent on monitoring that provides no value.[9] The biggest problems with the process continue to be lack of education, communication, and documentation.[6,17] Approaches to changing physician behavior with regard to appropriate sampling and interpretation include educational sessions; formation of formal therapeutic drug monitoring services; multidisciplinary quality improvement efforts; and computerization of requests for drug concentration measurement samples.[240] Pharmacists will continue to have a pivotal role in the education of physicians and others involved in the therapeutic drug monitoring process. Future studies that evaluate the effect of therapeutic drug monitoring on patient outcomes will likely use quality management approaches.[241]

REFERENCES

1. Evans WE. General principles of applied pharmacokinetics. In: Evans WE, Schentag JJ, Jusko WJ, eds. *Applied Pharmacokinetics: Principles of Therapeutic Drug Monitoring*. 3rd ed. Vancouver, WA: Applied Therapeutics; 1992: 1.1–1.8.

2. Marshall EK. Experimental basis of chemotherapy in the treatment of bacterial infections. *Bull N Y Acad Med*. 1940; 16:722–31.

3. Shannon JA. The study of antimalarials and antimalarial activity in the human malarias. *Harvey Lect*. 1946; 41:43–89.

4. Koch-Weser J. Drug therapy. Serum drug concentrations as therapeutic guides. *N Engl J Med*. 1972; 287:227–31.

5. Oles KS. Therapeutic drug monitoring analysis systems for the physician office laboratory: a review of the literature. *DICP*. 1990; 24:1070–7.

6. Carroll DJ, Austin GE, Stajich GV, et al. Effect of education on the appropriateness of serum drug concentration determination. *Ther Drug Monit*. 1992; 14:81–4.

7. Mason GD, Winter ME. Appropriateness of sampling times for therapeutic drug monitoring. *Am J Hosp Pharm*. 1984; 41:1796–801.

8. Travers EM. Misuse of therapeutic drug monitoring: an analysis of causes and methods for improvement. *Clin Lab Med*. 1987; 7:453–72.

9. Ensom MH, Davis GA, Cropp CD, et al. Clinical pharmacokinetics in the 21st century. Does the evidence support definitive outcomes? *Clin Pharmacokinet*. 1998; 34:265–79.

10. Walson PD. Therapeutic drug monitoring in special populations. *Clin Chem*. 1998; 44:415–9.

11. Burke MJ, Preskorn SH. Therapeutic drug monitoring of antidepressants: cost implications and relevance to clinical practice. *Clin Pharmacokinet*. 1999; 37:147–65.

12. Bates DW. Improving the use of therapeutic drug monitoring. *Ther Drug Monit*. 1998; 20:550–5.

13. Eadie MJ. Therapeutic drug monitoring—antiepileptic drugs. *Br J Clin Pharmacol*. 2001; 52(suppl 1):S11–S20.

14. Robinson JD, Taylor W.J. Interpretation of serum drug concentrations. In: Taylor WJ, Caviness MHD, eds. *A Textbook for the Application of Therapeutic Drug Monitoring*. Irving, TX: Abbott Laboratories, Diagnostics Division; 1986: 31–45.

15. D'Angio RG, Stevenson JG, Lively BT, et al. Therapeutic drug monitoring: improved performance through educational intervention. *Ther Drug Monit*. 1990; 12:173–81.

16. Sieradzan R, Fuller AV. A multidisciplinary approach to enhance documentation of antibiotic serum sampling. *Hosp Pharm*. 1995; 30:872–7.

17. Warner A. Setting standards of practice in therapeutic drug monitoring and clinical toxicology: a North American view. *Ther Drug Monit*. 2000; 22:93–7.

18. Traub SL. Interpretation of serum drug concentrations. In: Traub SL, ed. *Basic Skills in Interpreting Laboratory Data*. 2nd ed. Bethesda, MD: American Society of Health-System Pharmacists; 1996: 61–92.

19. Miller JJ, Straub RW Jr, Valdes R Jr. Digoxin immunoassay with cross-reactivity of digoxin metabolites proportional to their biological activity. *Clin Chem*. 1994; 40:1898–903.

20. Murphy JE. Introduction. In: Murphy JE, ed. *Clinical Pharmacokinetics Pocket Reference*. 2nd ed. Bethesda, MD: American Society of Health-System Pharmacists; 2001: xxxv–xlvii.

21. Bowers LD. Analytical goals in therapeutic drug monitoring. *Clin Chem*. 1998; 44:375–80.

22. Reed MD, Blumer JL. Therapeutic drug monitoring in the pediatric intensive care unit. *Pediatr Clin North Am*. 1994; 41:1227–43.

23. Reuning RH, Geraets, DR, Rocci, ML, et al. In: Evans WE, Schentag JJ, Jusko WJ, eds. *Applied Pharmacokinetics: Principles of Therapeutic Drug Monitoring*. 3rd ed. Vancouver, WA: Applied Therapeutics; 1992: 20.1–20.48.

24. Lima JJ, Wenzke SC, Boudoulas H, et al. Antiarrhythmic activity and unbound concentrations of disopyramide enantiomers in patients. *Ther Drug Monit*. 1990; 12:23–8.

25. Ensom MH, Chang TK, Patel P. Pharmacogenetics: the therapeutic drug monitoring of the future? *Clin Pharmacokinet*. 2001; 40:783–802.

26. McLeod HL, Evans WE. Pharmacogenomics: Unlocking the human genome for better drug therapy. *Annu Rev Pharmacol Toxicol*. 2001; 41:101–21.

27. MacKichan JJ. Influence of protein binding and use of unbound (free) drug concentrations. In: Evans WE, Schentag JJ, Jusko WJ, eds. *Applied Pharmacokinetics: Principles of Therapeutic Drug Monitoring*. 3rd ed. Vancouver, WA: Applied Therapeutics; 1992: 5.1–5.48.

28. Bruguerolle B. Chronopharmacokinetics. Current status. *Clin Pharmacokinet*. 1998; 35:83–94.

29. Reinberg A, Smolensky MH. Circadian changes of drug disposition in man. *Clin Pharmacokinet*. 1982; 7:401–20.

30. MacKichan JJ, Kutt H. Carbamazepine. In: Taylor WJ, Finn AL, eds. *Individualizing Drug Therapy: Practical Applications of Drug Monitoring*. Vol. 2. New York, NY: Gross, Townsend, Frank, Inc.; 1981:1–25.

31. Rodvold KA, Paloucek FP, Zell M. Accuracy of 11 methods for predicting theophylline dose. *Clin Pharm.*1986; 5:403–8.

32. Slattery JT, Gibaldi M, Koup JR. Prediction of maintenance dose required to attain a desired drug concentration at steady-state from a single determination of concentration after an initial dose. *Clin Pharmacokinet.* 1980; 5:377–85.

33. Browne JL, Perry PJ, Alexander B, et al. Pharmacokinetic protocol for predicting plasma nortriptyline levels. *J Clin Psychopharmacol.* 1983; 3:351–6.

34. Cooper TB, Simpson GM. The 24-hr lithium level as a prognosticator of dosage requirements: a 2-year follow-up study. *Am J Psychiatry.* 1976; 133:440–3.

35. Perry PJ, Alexander B, Dunner FJ, et al. Pharmacokinetic protocol for predicting serum lithium levels. *J Clin Psychopharmacol.* 1982; 2:114–8.

36. Winter ME. *Basic Clinical Pharmacokinetics.* 4th ed. Baltimore, MD: Lippincott Williams & Wilkins; 2004.

37. Hammett-Stabler C, Johns T. Laboratory guidelines for monitoring of antimicrobial drugs. *Clin Chem.* 1998; 44:1129–40.

38. Uges DR. Plasma or serum in therapeutic drug monitoring and clinical toxicology.*Pharm Weekbl Sci.* 1988; 10:185–8.

39. Bush V, Blennerhasset J, Wells A, et al. Stability of therapeutic drugs in serum collected in vacutainer serum separator tubes containing a new gel (SST II). *Ther Drug Monit.* 2001; 23:259–62.

40. Kaplan LA. Standards of laboratory practice: guidelines for the maintaining of a modern therapeutic drug monitoring service. *Clin Chem.* 1998; 44:1072.

41. Devine JE. Drug-protein binding interferences caused by the plasticizer TBEP. *Clin Biochem.* 1984; 17:345–7.

42. Janknegt R, Lohman JJ, Hooymans PM, et al. Do evacuated blood collection tubes interfere with therapeutic drug monitoring? *Pharm Weekbl Sci.* 1983; 5:287–90.

43. Liu H, Delgado MR. Therapeutic drug concentration monitoring using saliva samples. Focus on anticonvulsants. *Clin Pharmacokinet.* 1999; 36:453–70.

44. Bailey B, Klein J, Koren G. Noninvasive methods for drug measurement in pediatrics. *Pediatr Clin North Am.* 1997; 44:15–26.

45. Gorodischer R, Koren G. Salivary excretion of drugs in children: theoretical and practical issues in therapeutic drug monitoring. *Dev Pharmacol Ther.* 1992; 19:161–77.

46. MacKichan JJ, Duffner PK, Cohen ME. Salivary concentrations and plasma protein binding of carbamazepine and carbamazepine 10,11-epoxide in epileptic patients. *Br J Clin Pharmacol.* 1981; 12:31–7.

47. Nishihara K, Uchino K, Saitoh Y, et al. Estimation of plasma unbound phenobarbital concentration by using mixed saliva. *Epilepsia.* 1979; 20:37–45.

48. Gorodischer R, Burtin P, Verjee Z, et al. Is saliva suitable for therapeutic monitoring of anticonvulsants in children: an evaluation in the routine clinical setting. *Ther Drug Monit.* 1997; 19:637–42.

49. Chee KY, Lee D, Byron D, et al. A simple collection method for saliva in children: potential for home monitoring of carbamazepine therapy. *Br J Clin Pharmacol.* 1993; 35:311–3.

50. Holden WE, Bartos F, Theime T, et al. Theophylline in oral mucosal transudate. A practical method for monitoring outpatient therapy. *Am Rev Respir Dis.* 1993; 147:739–43.

51. Barre J, Didey F, Delion F, et al. Problems in therapeutic drug monitoring: free drug level monitoring. *Ther Drug Monit.*1988; 10:133–43.

52. Nakajima M, Yamato S, Shimada K, et al. Assessment of drug concentrations in tears in therapeutic drug monitoring: I. Determination of valproic acid in tears by gas chromatography/mass spectrometry with EC/NCI mode. *Ther Drug Monit.* 2000; 22:716–22.

53. Monaco F, Piredda S, Mutani R, et al. The free fraction of valproic acid in tears, saliva, and cerebrospinal fluid. *Epilepsia.*1982; 23:23–6.

54. Friedman H, Greenblatt DJ. Rational therapeutic drug monitoring. *JAMA.* 1986; 256:2227–33.

55. Wong SH. Therapeutic drug monitoring for immunosuppressants. *Clin Chim Acta.* 2001; 313:241–53.

56. Campbell TJ, Williams KM. Therapeutic drug monitoring: antiarrhythmic drugs. *Br J Clin Pharmacol.* 2001; 52(suppl 1):S21–S34.

57. Nierenberg DW. Measuring drug levels in the office: rationale, possible advantages, and potential problems. *Med Clin North Am.* 1987; 71:653–64.

58. Blecka LJ, Jackson GJ. Immunoassays in therapeutic drug monitoring. *Clin Lab Med.* 1987; 7:357–70.

59. Taylor AT. Office therapeutic drug monitoring. *Prim Care.* 1986; 13:743–60.

60. Cook JD, Platoff GE, Koch TR, et al. Accuracy and precision of methods for theophylline measurement in physicians' offices. *Clin Chem.* 1990; 36:780–3.

61. Wallinder H, Gustafsson LL, Angback K, et al. Assay of theophylline: in vivo and in vitro evaluation of dry chemistry and immunoassay vs. high-performance liquid chromatography. *Ther Drug Monit.* 1991; 13:233–9.

62. Iosefsohn M, Soldin SJ, Hicks JM. A dry-strip immunometric assay for digoxin on the Ames Seralyzer. *Ther Drug Monit.*1990; 12:201–5.

63. Steimer W, Muller C, Eber B. Digoxin assays: frequent, substantial, and potentially dangerous interference by spironolactone, canrenone, and other steroids. *Clin Chem.* 2002; 48:507–16.

64. Tozer TN, Winter ME. Phenytoin. In: Evans WE, Schentag JJ, Jusko WJ, eds. *Applied Pharmacokinetics: Principles of Therapeutic Drug Monitoring.* 3rd ed. Vancouver, WA: Applied Therapeutics; 1992: 25.1–25.44.

65. Jelliffe RW, Schumitzky A, Van Guilder M, et al. Individualizing drug dosage regimens: roles of population pharmacokinetic and dynamic models, Bayesian fitting, and adaptive control. *Ther Drug Monit.* 1993; 15:380–93.

66. Burt M, Anderson DC, Kloss J, et al. Evidence-based implementation of free phenytoin therapeutic drug monitoring. *Clin Chem*. 2000; 46:1132–5.

67. Roberts WL, Annesley TM, De BK, et al. Performance characteristics of four free phenytoin immunoassays. *Ther Drug Monit*. 2001; 23:148–54.

68. Sheiner LB, Tozer TN, Winter ME. Clinical pharmacokinetics: the use of plasma concentrations of drugs. In: Melmon KL, Morelli HF, eds. *Clinical Pharmacology: Basic Principles in Therapeutics*. New York, NY: MacMillan; 1978: 71–109.

69. Kerrick JM, Wolff DL, Graves NM. Predicting unbound phenytoin concentrations in patients receiving valproic acid: a comparison of two prediction methods. *Ann Pharmacother*. 1995; 29:470–4.

70. Haidukewych D, Rodin EA, Zielinski JJ. Derivation and evaluation of an equation for prediction of free phenytoin concentration in patients comedicated with valproic acid. *Ther Drug Monit*. 1989; 11:134–9.

71. Haidukewych D, Zielinski JJ, Rodin EA. Derivation and evaluation of an equation for prediction of free carbamazepine concentrations in patients comedicated with valproic acid. *Ther Drug Monit*. 1989; 11:528–32.

72. White S, Wong SH. Standards of laboratory practice: analgesic drug monitoring. National Academy of Clinical Biochemistry. *Clin Chem*. 1998; 44:1110–23.

73. Dromgoole SH, Furst DE. Salicylates. In: Evans WE, Schentag JJ, Jusko WJ, eds. *Applied Pharmacokinetics: Principles of Therapeutic Drug Monitoring*. 3rd ed. Vancouver, WA: Applied Therapeutics; 1992: 32.1–32.34.

74. Levy G. Pharmacokinetics of salicylate in man. *Drug Metab Rev*. 1979; 9:3–19.

75. Levy G, Tsuchiya T. Salicylate accumulation kinetics in man. *N Engl J Med*. 1972; 287:430–2.

76. Pachman LM, Olufs R, Procknal JA, et al. Pharmacokinetic monitoring of salicylate therapy in children with juvenile rheumatoid arthritis. *Arthritis Rheum*. 1979; 22:826–31.

77. Dasgupta A, Yared MA, Wells A. Time-dependent absorption of therapeutic drugs by the gel of the Greiner Vacuette blood collection tube. *Ther Drug Monit*. 2000; 22:427–31.

78. Berkovitch M, Uziel Y, Greenberg R, et al. False-high blood salicylate levels in neonates with hyperbilirubinemia. *Ther Drug Monit*. 2000; 22:757–61.

79. Karnes HT, Beightol LA. Evaluation of fluorescence polarization immunoassay for quantitation of serum salicylates. *Ther Drug Monit*. 1985; 7:351–4.

80. Poe TE, Mutchie KD, Saunders GH, et al. Total and free salicylate concentrations in juvenile rheumatoid arthritis. *J Rheumatol*. 1980; 7:717–23.

81. Bauer LA. *Applied Clinical Pharmacokinetics*. New York, NY: McGraw-Hill; 2001.

82. Edwards DJ, Zarowitz BJ, Slaughter RL. Theophylline. In: Evans ME, Schentag JJ, Jusko WJ, eds. *Applied Pharmacokinetics: Principles of Therapeutic Drug Monitoring*. 3rd ed. Vancouver, WA: Applied Therapeutics, Inc.; 1992: 13.1–13.38.

83. Scanlon JE, Chin KC, Morgan ME, et al. Caffeine or theophylline for neonatal apnoea? *Arch Dis Child*. 1992; 67:425–8.

84. Darsey EH. Theophylline. In: Murphy JE, ed. *Clinical Pharmacokinetics Pocket Reference*. 2nd ed. Bethesda, MD: American Society of Health-System Pharmacists; 2001: 345–60.

85. Pesce AJ, Rashkin M, Kotagal U. Standards of laboratory practice: theophylline and caffeine monitoring. National Academy of Clinical Biochemistry. *Clin Chem*. 1998; 44:1124–8.

86. Koren G. Therapeutic drug monitoring principles in the neonate. National Academy of Clinical Biochemistry. *Clin Chem*. 1997; 43:222–7.

87. Aranda JV, Chemtob S, Laudignon N, et al. Pharmacologic effects of theophylline in the newborn. *J Allergy Clin Immunol*. 1986; 78:773–80.

88. Blanchard J, Harvey S, Morgan WJ. Relationship between serum and saliva theophylline levels in patients with cystic fibrosis. *Ther Drug Monit*. 1992; 14:48–54.

89. Kirk JK, Dupuis RE, Miles MV, Gaddy GD, Miranda-Massari JR, Williams DM. Salivary theophylline monitoring: reassessment and clinical considerations. *Ther Drug Monit*. 1994; 16:58–66.

90. Patel JA, Clayton LT, LeBel CP, et al. Abnormal theophylline levels in plasma by fluorescence polarization immunoassay in patients with renal disease. *Ther Drug Monit*. 1984; 6:458–60.

91. Jenny RW, Jackson KY. Two types of error found with the Seralyzer ARIS assay of theophylline. *Clin Chem*. 1986; 32:2122–3.

92. Chan KM, Koenig J, Walton KG, et al. The theophylline method of the Abbott "Vision" analyzer evaluated. *Clin Chem*.1987; 33:130–2.

93. de Wildt SN, Kerkvliet KT, Wezenberg MG, et al. Use of saliva in therapeutic drug monitoring of caffeine in preterm infants. *Ther Drug Monit*. 2001; 23:250–4.

94. Aranda JV, Beharry K, Rex J, et al. Caffeine enzyme immunoassay in neonatal and pediatric drug monitoring. *Ther Drug Monit*. 1987; 9:97–103.

95. Lee TC, Charles BG, Steer PA, et al. Saliva as a valid alternative to serum in monitoring intravenous caffeine treatment for apnea of prematurity. *Ther Drug Monit*. 1996; 18:288–93.

96. Warner A, Privitera M, Bates D. Standards of laboratory practice: antiepileptic drug monitoring. National Academy of Clinical Biochemistry. *Clin Chem*. 1998; 44:1085–95.

97. Levy RH, Anderson GD. Carbamazepine, valproic acid, phenobarbital, and ethosuximide. In: Evans WE, Schentag JJ, Jusko WE, eds. *Applied Pharmacokinetics: Principles of Therapeutic Drug Monitoring*. 3rd ed. Vancouver, WA: Applied Therapeutics; 1992: 26.1–26.29.

98. Bonneton J, Iliadis A, Genton P, et al. Steady state pharmacokinetics of conventional vs. controlled-release carbamazepine in patients with epilepsy. *Epilepsy Res*. 1993; 14:257–63.

99. Godolphin W, Trepanier J, Farrell K. Serum and plasma for total and free anticonvulsant drug analyses: effects on EMIT assays and ultrafiltration devices. *Ther Drug Monit.* 1983; 5:319–23.

100. Rosenthal E, Hoffer E, Ben-Aryeh H, et al. Use of saliva in home monitoring of carbamazepine levels. *Epilepsia.* 1995; 36:72–4.

101. Drobitch RK, Svensson CK. Therapeutic drug monitoring in saliva. An update. *Clin Pharmacokinet.* 1992; 23:365–79.

102. Contin M, Riva R, Albani F, et al. Determination of total and free plasma carbamazepine concentrations by enzyme multiplied immunoassay: interference with the 10,11-epoxide metabolite. *Ther Drug Monit.* 1985; 7:46–50.

103. Lacher DA, Valdes R Jr, Savory J. Enzyme immunoassay of carbamazepine with a centrifugal analyzer. *Clin Chem.* 1979; 25:295–8.

104. MacKichan JJ, Zola EM. Determinants of carbamazepine and carbamazepine 10,11-epoxide binding to serum protein, albumin and alpha 1-acid glycoprotein. *Br J Clin Pharmacol.* 1984; 18:487–93.

105. Garnett WR. Ethosuximide. In: Murphy JE, ed. *Clinical Pharmacokinetics Pocket Reference.* 2nd ed. Bethesda, MD: American Society of Health-System Pharmacists; 2001: 155–63.

106. Villen T, Bertilsson L, Sjoqvist F. Nonstereoselective disposition of ethosuximide in humans. *Ther Drug Monit.* 1990; 12:514–6.

107. Anderson DM, Tallian KB. Phenobarbital. In: Murphy JE, ed. *Clinical Pharmacokinetics Pocket Reference.* 2nd ed. Bethesda, MD: American Society of Health-System Pharmacists; 2001: 271–84.

108. Fairchild L, Wong E, Li TM, et al. Phenobarbital monitoring in whole blood with a quantitative noninstrumented test. *Ther Drug Monit.* 1991; 13:425–7.

109. Nielsen IM, Gram L, Dam M. Comparison of AccuLevel and TDx: evaluation of on-site monitoring of antiepileptic drugs. *Epilepsia.* 1992; 33:558–63.

110. Eadie MJ. Therapeutic drug monitoring—antiepileptic drugs. *Br J Clin Pharmacol.* 1998; 46:185–93.

111. Winter ME. Phenytoin and fosphenytoin. In: Murphy JE, ed. *Clinical Pharmacokinetics Pocket Reference.* 2nd ed. Bethesda, MD: American Society of Health-System Pharmacists; 2001: 285–303.

112. Kozer E, Parvez S, Minassian BA, et al. How high can we go with phenytoin? *Ther Drug Monit.* 2002; 24:386–9.

113. Banh HL, Burton ME, Sperling MR. Interpatient and intrapatient variability in phenytoin protein binding. *Ther Drug Monit.* 2002; 24:379–85.

114. Kugler AR, Annesley TM, Nordblom GD, et al. Cross-reactivity of fosphenytoin in two human plasma phenytoin immunoassays. *Clin Chem.* 1998; 44:1474–80.

115. Oeltgen PR, Shank WA Jr, Blouin RA, et al. Clinical evaluation of the Abbott TDx fluorescence polarization immunoassay analyzer. *Ther Drug Monit.* 1984; 6:360–7.

116. Toler SM, Wilkerson MA, Porter WH, et al. Severe phenytoin intoxication as a result of altered protein binding in AIDS. *DICP.* 1990; 24:698–700.

117. Anderson GD, Pak C, Doane KW, et al. Revised Winter-Tozer equation for normalized phenytoin concentrations in trauma and elderly patients with hypoalbuminemia. *Ann Pharmacother.* 1997; 31:279–84.

118. MacKichan JJ. Protein binding drug displacement interactions fact or fiction? *Clin Pharmacokinet.* 1989; 16:65–73.

119. May TW, Rambeck B, Jurges U, et al. Comparison of total and free phenytoin serum concentrations measured by high-performance liquid chromatography and standard TDx assay: implications for the prediction of free phenytoin serum concentrations. *Ther Drug Monit.* 1998; 20:619–23.

120. Gidal BE, Graves NM. Valproic acid. In: Murphy JE, ed. *Clinical Pharmacokinetics Pocket Reference.* 2nd ed. Bethesda, MD: American Society of Health-System Pharmacists; 2001: 361–73.

121. Liu H, Montoya JL, Forman LJ, et al. Determination of free valproic acid: evaluation of the Centrifree system and comparison between high-performance liquid chromatography and enzyme immunoassay. *Ther Drug Monit.* 1992; 14:513–21.

122. Dasgupta A, Volk A. Displacement of valproic acid and carbamazepine from protein binding in normal and uremic sera by tolmetin, ibuprofen, and naproxen: presence of inhibitor in uremic serum that blocks valproic acid-naproxen interactions. *Ther Drug Monit.* 1996; 18:284–7.

123. Bardy AH, Hiilesmaa VK, Teramo K, et al. Protein binding of antiepileptic drugs during pregnancy, labor, and puerperium. *Ther Drug Monit.* 1990; 12:40–6.

124. Tomson T, Johannessen SI. Therapeutic monitoring of the new antiepileptic drugs. *Eur J Clin Pharmacol.* 2000; 55:697–705.

125. Perucca E. Is there a role for therapeutic drug monitoring of new anticonvulsants? *Clin Pharmacokinet.* 2000; 38:191–204.

126. Chong E, Dupuis LL. Therapeutic drug monitoring of lamotrigine. *Ann Pharmacother.* 2002; 36:917–20.

127. Perucca E, Dulac O, Shorvon S, et al. Harnessing the clinical potential of antiepileptic drug therapy: dosage optimization. *CNS Drugs.* 2001; 15:609–21.

128. Tsiropoulos I, Kristensen O, Klitgaard NA. Saliva and serum concentration of lamotrigine in patients with epilepsy. *Ther Drug Monit.* 2000; 22:517–21.

129. Contin M, Riva R, Albani F, et al. Topiramate therapeutic monitoring in patients with epilepsy: effect of concomitant antiepileptic drugs. *Ther Drug Monit.* 2002; 24:332–7.

130. Begg EJ, Barclay ML, Kirkpatrick CM. The therapeutic monitoring of antimicrobial agents. *Br J Clin Pharmacol.* 2001; 52(suppl 1):S35–S43.

131. Zaske DE. Aminoglycosides In: Evans WE, Schentag JJ, Jusko WJ, eds. *Applied Pharmacokinetics: Principles of Therapeutic Drug Monitoring.* 3rd ed. Vancouver, WA: Applied Therapeutics; 1992: 14.1–14.47.

132. Murphy JE. Aminoglycosides. In: Murphy JE, ed. *Clinical Pharmacokinetics Pocket Reference.* 2nd ed. Bethesda, MD: American Society of Health-System Pharmacists; 2001: 23–59.

133. Nicolau DP, Freeman CD, Belliveau PP, et al. Experience with once-daily aminoglycoside program administered to 2,184 adult patients. *Antimicrob Agents Chemother.* 1995; 39:650–5.

134. Landt M, Smith CH, Hortin GL. Evaluation of evacuated blood-collection tubes: effects of three types of polymeric separators on therapeutic drug-monitoring specimens. *Clin Chem.* 1993; 39:1712–7.

135. Koch TR, Platoff G. Suitability of collection tubes with separator gels for therapeutic drug monitoring. *Ther Drug Monit.* 1990; 12:277–80.

136. Berkovitch M, Bistritzer T, Aladjem M, et al. Clinical relevance of therapeutic drug monitoring of digoxin and gentamicin in the saliva of children. *Ther Drug Monit.* 1998; 20:253–6.

137. Barclay ML, Kirkpatrick CM, Begg EJ. Once daily aminoglycoside therapy. Is it less toxic than multiple daily doses and how should it be monitored? *Clin Pharmacokinet.* 1999; 36:89–98.

138. Tod MM, Padoin C, Petitjean O. Individualizing aminoglycoside dosage regimens after therapeutic drug monitoring: simple or complex pharmacokinetic methods? *Clin Pharmacokinet.* 2001; 40:803–14.

139. Nahata MC. Chloramphenicol. In: Evans WE, Schentag JJ, Jusko WJ, eds. *Applied Pharmacokinetics: Principles of Therapeutic Drug Monitoring.* 3rd ed. Vancouver, WA: Applied Therapeutics; 1992: 16.1–16.24.

140. Coakley JC, Hudson I, Shann F, et al. A review of therapeutic monitoring of chloramphenicol in patients with Haemophilus influenzae meningitis. *J Paediatr Child Health.* 1992; 28:249–53.

141. Soldin OP, Soldin SJ. Review: therapeutic drug monitoring in pediatrics. *Ther Drug Monit.* 2002; 24:1–8.

142. Nahata MC. Intravenous infusion conditions. Implications for pharmacokinetic monitoring. *Clin Pharmacokinet.* 1993; 24:221–9.

143. Nahata MC, Powell DA. Bioavailability and clearance of chloramphenicol after intravenous chloramphenicol succinate. *Clin Pharmacol Ther.* 1981; 30:368–72.

144. Schwartz JG, Casto DT, Ayo S, et al. A commercial enzyme immunoassay method (EMIT) compared with liquid chromatography and bioassay methods for measurement of chloramphenicol. *Clin Chem.* 1988; 34:1872–5.

145. Koup JR, Lau AH, Brodsky B, et al. Relationship between serum and saliva chloramphenicol concentrations. *Antimicrob Agents Chemother.* 1979; 15:658–61.

146. Zimmermann AE, Katona BG, Plaisance KI. Association of vancomycin serum concentrations with outcomes in patients with gram-positive bacteremia. *Pharmacotherapy.* 1995; 15:85–91.

147. Frye RF, Matzke GR. Vancomycin. In: Murphy JE, ed. *Clinical Pharmacokinetics Pocket Reference.* 2nd ed. Bethesda, MD: American Society of Health-System Pharmacists; 2001: 375–87.

148. Pou L, Rosell M, Lopez R, et al. Changes in vancomycin pharmacokinetics during treatment. *Ther Drug Monit.* 1996; 18:149–53.

149. Somerville AL, Wright DH, Rotschafer JC. Implications of vancomycin degradation products on therapeutic drug monitoring in patients with end-stage renal disease. *Pharmacotherapy.* 1999; 19:702–7.

150. Trujillo TN, Sowinski KM, Venezia RA, et al. Vancomycin assay performance in patients with acute renal failure. *Intensive Care Med.* 1999; 25:1291–6.

151. Wood FL, Earl JW, Nath C, et al. Falsely low vancomycin results using the Abbott TDx. *Ann Clin Biochem.* 2000; 37(part 3):411–3.

152. Matzke GR. Vancoymcin. In: Evans WE, Schentag JJ, Jusko WJ, eds. *Applied Pharmacokinetics: Principles of Therapeutic Drug Monitoring.* 3rd ed. Vancouver, WA: Applied Therapeutics; 1992:15.1–15.31.

153. British Society for Antimicrobial Chemotherapy Working Part. Laboratory monitoring of antifungal chemotherapy. *Lancet.* 1991; 337:1577–80.

154. Petersen D, Demertzis S, Freund M, et al. Individualization of 5-fluorocytosine therapy. *Chemotherapy.* 1994; 40:149–56.

155. Vermes A, Guchelaar HJ, Dankert J. Flucytosine: a review of its pharmacology, clinical indications, pharmacokinetics, toxicity and drug interactions. *J Antimicrob Chemother.* 2000; 46:171–9.

156. Summers KK, Hardin TC, Gore SJ, et al. Therapeutic drug monitoring of systemic antifungal therapy. *J Antimicrob Chemother.* 1997; 40:753–64.

157. Huang CM, Kroll MH, Ruddel M, et al. An enzymatic method for 5-fluorocytosine. *Clin Chem.* 1988; 34:59–62.

158. Al-Rawithi S, Hussein R, Al-Moshen I, et al. Expedient microdetermination of itraconazole and hydroxyitraconazole in plasma by high-performance liquid chromatography with fluorescence detection. *Ther Drug Monit.* 2001; 23:445–8.

159. Haria M, Bryson HM, Goa KL. Itraconazole. A reappraisal of its pharmacological properties and therapeutic use in the management of superficial fungal infections. *Drugs.* 1996; 51:585–620.

160. Koks CH, Crommentuyn KM, Hoetelmans RM, et al. Can fluconazole concentrations in saliva be used for therapeutic drug monitoring? *Ther Drug Monit.* 2001; 23:449–53.

161. Peloquin CA. Using therapeutic drug monitoring to dose the antimycobacterial drugs. *Clin Chest Med.* 1997; 18:79–87.

162. Sahai J, Gallicano K, Swick L, et al. Reduced plasma concentrations of antituberculosis drugs in patients with HIV infection. *Ann Intern Med.* 1997; 127:289–93.

163. Yew W. Clinically significant interactions with drugs used in the treatment of tuberculosis. *Drug Saf.* 2002; 25:111–33.

164. Kimerling ME, Phillips P, Patterson P, et al. Low serum antimycobacterial drug levels in non-HIV-infected tuberculosis patients. *Chest.* 1998; 113:1178–83.

165. Mehta JB, Shantaveerapa H, Byrd RP Jr, et al. Utility of rifampin blood levels in the treatment and follow-up of active pulmonary tuberculosis in patients who were slow to respond to routine directly observed therapy. *Chest.* 2001; 120:1520–4.

166. Yew WW. Therapeutic drug monitoring in antituberculosis chemotherapy: clinical perspectives. *Clin Chim Acta.* 2001; 313:31–6.

167. Van Heeswijk RP. Critical issues in therapeutic drug monitoring of antiretroviral drugs. *Ther Drug Monit.*–2002; 24:323–31.

168. Back DJ, Khoo SH, Gibbons SE, Merry C. The role of therapeutic drug monitoring in treatment of HIV infection. *Br J Clin Pharmacol.* 2001; 52(suppl 1):S89–S96.

169. Khoo SH, Gibbons SE, Back DJ. Therapeutic drug monitoring as a tool in treating HIV infection. *Aids.* 2001; 15(suppl 5):S171–S181.

170. Dasgupta A, Okhuysen PC. Pharmacokinetic and other drug interactions in patients with AIDS. *Ther Drug Monit.* 2001; 23:591–605.

171. van Heeswijk RP, Veldkamp AI, Mulder JW, et al. Saliva as an alternative body fluid for therapeutic drug monitoring of the nonnucleoside reverse transcription inhibitor nevirapine. *Ther Drug Monit.* 2001; 23:255–8.

172. Wintergerst U, Kurowski M, Rolinski B, et al. Use of saliva specimens for monitoring indinavir therapy in human immunodeficiency virus-infected patients. *Antimicrob Agents Chemother.* 2000; 44:2572–4.

173. Titier K, Lagrange F, Pehourcq F, et al. High-performance liquid chromatographic method for the simultaneous determination of the six HIV-protease inhibitors and two nonnucleoside reverse transcriptase inhibitors in human plasma. *Ther Drug Monit.* 2002; 24:417–24.

174. Moyle GJ, Back D. Principles and practice of HIV-protease inhibitor pharmacoenhancement. *HIV Med.* 2001; 2:105–13.

175. Valdes R Jr, Jortani SA, Gheorghiade M. Standards of laboratory practice: cardiac drug monitoring. National Academy of Clinical Biochemistry. *Clin Chem.* 1998; 44:1096–109.

176. Bernard DW, Bowman RL, Grimm FA, et al. Nighttime dosing assures postdistribution sampling for therapeutic drug monitoring of digoxin. *Clin Chem.* 1996; 42:45–9.

177. Matzuk MM, Shlomchik M, Shaw LM. Making digoxin therapeutic drug monitoring more effective. *Ther Drug Monit.* 1991; 13:215–9.

178. Ujhelyi MR, Green PJ, Cummings DM, et al. Determination of free serum digoxin concentrations in digoxin toxic patients after administration of digoxin Fab antibodies. *Ther Drug Monit.* 1992; 14:147–54.

179. Ocal IT, Green TR. Serum digoxin in the presence of digibind: determination of digoxin by the Abbott AxSYM and Baxter Stratus II immunoassays by direct analysis without pretreatment of serum samples. *Clin Chem.* 1998; 44:1947–50.

180. Brown JE, Shand DG. Therapeutic drug monitoring of antiarrhythmic agents. *Clin Pharmacokinet.* 1982; 7:125–48.

181. Bauer LA, Brown T, Gibaldi M, et al. Influence of long-term infusions on lidocaine kinetics. *Clin Pharmacol Ther.* 1982; 31:433–7.

182. Pieper JA, Johnson KE. Lidocaine. In: Evans WE, Schentag JJ, Jusko WJ, eds. *Applied Pharmacokinetics: Principles of Therapeutic Drug Monitoring.* 3rd ed. Vancouver, WA: Applied Therapeutics; 1992: 21.1–21.37.

183. Pieper JA. Procainamide. In: Murphy JE, ed. *Clinical Pharmacokinetics Pocket Reference.* 2nd ed. Bethesda, MD: American Society of Health-System Pharmacists; 2001: 205–28.

184. Koike Y, Mineshita S, Uchiyama Y, et al. Monitoring of procainamide and N-acetyl-procainamide concentration in saliva after oral administration of procainamide. *Am J Ther.* 1996; 3:708–14.

185. Coyle JD, Lima, J.J. Procainamide. In: Evans WE, Schentag JJ, Jusko WJ, eds. *Applied Pharmacokinetics: Principles of Therapeutic Drug Monitoring.* 3rd ed. Vancouver, WA: Applied Therapeutics; 1992: 22.1–22.33.

186. Nolan PE, Evans CM. Quinidine. In: Murphy JE, ed. *Clinical Pharmacokinetics Pocket Reference.* 2nd ed. Bethesda, MD: American Society of Health-System Pharmacists; 2001:319–43.

187. McCollam PL, Crouch MA, Watson JE. Altered protein binding of quinidine in patients with atrial fibrillation and flutter. *Pharmacotherapy.* 1997; 17:753–9.

188. Ochs HR, Grube E, Greenblatt DJ, et al. Intravenous quinidine: pharmacokinetic properties and effects on left ventricular performance in humans. *Am Heart J.* 1980; 99:468–75.

189. Bauman J. Mexilitine. In: Taylor W, Caviness MHD, eds. *A Textbook for Clinical Application of Therapeutic Drug Monitoring.* Irving, TX: Abbott Laboratories, Diagnostics Division; 1986: 125–31.

190. Lennard L. Therapeutic drug monitoring of cytotoxic drugs. *Br J Clin Pharmacol.* 2001; 52(suppl 1):S75–S87.

191. Hon YY, Evans WE. Making TDM work to optimize cancer chemotherapy: a multidisciplinary team approach. *Clin Chem.* 1998; 44:388–400.

192. Crom WR, Evans WE. Methotrexate. In: Evans WE, Schentag JJ, Jusko WJ, eds. *Applied Pharmacokinetics: Principles of Therapeutic Drug Monitoring.* 3rd ed. Vancouver, WA: Applied Therapeutics; 1992: 29.1–29.42.

193. Teresi ME, McCormick JN. Methotrexate. In: Murphy JE, ed. *Clinical Pharmacokinetics Pocket Reference.* 2nd ed. Bethesda, MD: American Society of Health-System Pharmacists; 2001: 247–69.

194. Press J, Berkovitch M, Laxer R, et al. Evaluation of therapeutic drug monitoring of methotrexate in saliva of children with rheumatic diseases. *Ther Drug Monit.* 1995; 17:247–50.

195. McCune JS, Gibbs JP, Slattery JT. Plasma concentration monitoring of busulfan: does it improve clinical outcome? *Clin Pharmacokinet.* 2000; 39:155–65.

196. Tabak A, Hoffer E, Rowe JM, et al. Monitoring of busulfan area under the curve: estimation by a single measurement. *Ther Drug Monit.* 2001; 23:526–8.

197. Sparreboom A, Nooter K, Loos WJ, et al. The (ir)relevance of plasma protein binding of anticancer drugs. *Neth J Me*. 2001; 59:196–207.

198. Gusella M, Ferrazzi E, Ferrari M, et al. New limited sampling strategy for determining 5-Fluorouracil area under the concentration-time curve after rapid intravenous bolus. *Ther Drug Monit*. 2002; 24:425–31.

199. Petros WP, Colvin OM. Metabolic jeopardy with high-dose cyclophosphamide?—not so fast. *Clin Cancer Res*. 1999; 5:723–4.

200. Holt DW, Armstrong VW, Griesmacher A, et al. International Federation of Clinical Chemistry/International Association of Therapeutic Drug Monitoring and Clinical Toxicology working group on immunosuppressive drug monitoring. *Ther Drug Monit*. 2002; 24:59–67.

201. Oellerich M, Armstrong VW, Kahan B, et al. Lake Louise Consensus Conference on cyclosporin monitoring in organ transplantation: report of the consensus panel. *Ther Drug Monit*. 1995; 17:642–54.

202. Karlix J, Walker J. Antirejection agents. In: Murphy JE, ed. *Clinical Pharmacokinetics Pocket Reference*. 2nd ed. Bethesda, MD: American Society of Health-System Pharmacists; 2001: 79–96.

203. Yee GC, Salomon, DDR. Cyclosporine. In: Evans ME, Schentag JJ, Jusko WJ, eds. *Applied Pharmacokinetics: Principles of Therapeutic Drug Monitoring*. 3rd ed. Vancouver, WA: Applied Therapeutics; 1992: 28.1–28.40.

204. Johnston A, Holt DW. Immunosuppressant drugs—the role of therapeutic drug monitoring. *Br J Clin Pharmacol*. 2001; 52(suppl 1):S61–S73.

205. Faynor SM, Robinson R. Suitability of plastic collection tubes for cyclosporine measurements. *Clin Chem*. 1998; 44:2220–1.

206. Lindholm A, Henricsson S. Intra- and interindividual variability in the free fraction of cyclosporine in plasma in recipients of renal transplants. *Ther Drug Monit*.1989; 11:623–30.

207. Macchi-Andanson M, Charpiat B, Jelliffe RW, et al. Failure of traditional trough levels to predict tacrolimus concentrations. *Ther Drug Monit*. 2001; 23:129–33.

208. Kuzuya T, Ogura Y, Motegi Y, et al. Interference of hematocrit in the tacrolimus II microparticle enzyme immunoassay. *Ther Drug Monit*. 2002; 24:507–11.

209. Shaw LM, Pawinski T, Korecka M, et al. Monitoring of mycophenolic acid in clinical transplantation. *Ther Drug Monit*. 2002; 24:68–73.

210. Weber LT, Shipkova M, Armstrong VW, et al. The pharmacokinetic-pharmacodynamic relationship for total and free mycophenolic Acid in pediatric renal transplant recipients: a report of the German study group on mycophenolate mofetil therapy. *J Am Soc Nephrol*. 2002; 13:759–68.

211. Ensom MH, Partovi N, Decarie D, et al. Pharmacokinetics and protein binding of mycophenolic acid in stable lung transplant recipients. *Ther Drug Monit*. 2002; 24:310–4.

212. Yatscoff RW, Boeckx R, Holt DW, et al. Consensus guidelines for therapeutic drug monitoring of rapamycin: report of the consensus panel. *Ther Drug Monit*. 1995; 17:676–80.

213. Linder MW, Keck PE Jr. Standards of laboratory practice: antidepressant drug monitoring. National Academy of Clinical Biochemistry. *Clin Chem*. 1998; 44:1073–84.

214. DeVane CL. Cyclic antidepressants. In: Murphy JE, ed. *Clinical Pharmacokinetics Pocket Reference*. 2nd ed. Bethesda, MD: American Society of Health-System Pharmacists; 2001: 119–42.

215. Mitchell PB. Therapeutic drug monitoring of psychotropic medications. *Br J Clin Pharmacol*. 2001; 52(suppl 1):S45–S54.

216. Eilers R. Therapeutic drug monitoring for the treatment of psychiatric disorders. Clinical use and cost effectiveness. *Clin Pharmacokinet*. 1995; 29:442–50.

217. DeVane CL, Jarecke, C.R. Cyclic antidepressants. In: Evans WE, Schentag JJ, Jusko WJ, eds. *Applied Pharmacokinetics: Principles of Therapeutic Drug Monitoring*. 3rd ed. Vancouver, WA: Applied Therapeutics; 1992: 33.1–33.47.

218. Chattergoon DS, Verjee Z, Anderson M, et al. Carbamazepine interference with an immune assay for tricyclic antidepressants in plasma. *J Toxicol Clin Toxicol*. 1998; 36:109–3.

219. Lieberman JA, Cooper TB, Suckow RF, et al. Tricyclic antidepressant and metabolite levels in chronic renal failure. *Clin Pharmacol Ther*. 1985; 37:301–7.

220. Carson SW, Roberts SH. Lithium. In: Murphy JE, ed. *Clinical Pharmacokinetics Pocket Reference*. 2nd ed. Bethesda, MD: American Society of Health-System Pharmacists; 2001: 229–45.

221. Carson SW. Lithium. In: Evans WE, Schentag JJ, Jusko WJ, eds. *Applied Pharmacokinetics: Principles of Therapeutic Drug Monitoring*. 3rd ed. Vancouver, WA: Applied Therapeutics; 1992: 34.1–34.26.

222. Marcus SC, Olfson M, Pincus HA, Zarin DA, Kupfer DJ. Therapeutic drug monitoring of mood stabilizers in Medicaid patients with bipolar disorder. *Am J Psychiatry* 1999; 156:1014-8.

223. Sampson M, Ruddel M, Albright S, et al. Positive interference in lithium determinations from clot activator in collection container. *Clin Chem*. 1997; 43:675–9.

224. Perry R, Campbell M, Grega DM, et al. Saliva lithium levels in children: their use in monitoring serum lithium levels and lithium side effects. *J Clin Psychopharmacol*. 1984; 4:199–202.

225. Thomson AH, Watson ID, Wilson JF, et al. An audit of therapeutic drug monitoring service provision by laboratories participating in an external quality assessment scheme. *Ther Drug Monit*. 1998; 20:248–52.

226. Frezzotti A, Margarucci AM, Coppa G, et al. An evaluation of the Ektachem serum lithium method and comparison with flame emission spectrometry. *Scand J Clin Lab Invest*. 1996; 56:591–6.

227. Burke MD. Principles of therapeutic drug monitoring. *Postgrad Med*. 1981; 70:57–63.

228. Leucht S, Steimer W, Kreuz S, et al. Doxepin plasma concentrations: is there really a therapeutic range? *J Clin Psychopharmacol*. 2001; 21:432–9.

229. DeVane CL. Metabolism and pharmacokinetics of selective serotonin reuptake inhibitors. *Cell Mol Neurobiol*. 1999; 19:443–66.

230. Javaid JI. Clinical pharmacokinetics of antipsychotics. *J Clin Pharmacol*. 1994; 34:286–95.

231. Preskorn SH, Burke MJ, Fast GA. Therapeutic drug monitoring. Principles and practice. *Psychiatr Clin North Am*. 1993; 16:611–45.

232. Williams ML, Wainer IW. Role of chiral chromatography in therapeutic drug monitoring and in clinical and forensic toxicology. *Ther Drug Monit*. 2002; 24:290–6.

233. Thormann W, Theurillat R, Wind M, et al. Therapeutic drug monitoring of antiepileptics by capillary electrophoresis. Characterization of assays via analysis of quality control sera containing 14 analytes. *J Chromatogr A*. 2001; 924:429–37.

234. Williams J, Patsalos PN, Mei Z, et al. Relation between dosage of carbamazepine and concentration in hair and plasma samples from a compliant inpatient epileptic population. *Ther Drug Monit*. 2001; 23:15–20.

235. Wang J. Amperometric biosensors for clinical and therapeutic drug monitoring: a review. *J Pharm Biomed Anal*. 1999; 19:47–53.

236. Stahle L, Alm C, Ekquist B, et al. Monitoring free extracellular valproic acid by microdialysis in epileptic patients. *Ther Drug Monit*. 1996; 18:14–8.

237. Campbell M. Community-based therapeutic drug monitoring. Useful development or unnecessary distraction? *Clin Pharmacokinet*. 1995; 28:271–4.

238. Innocenti F, Ratain MJ. Update on pharmacogenetics in cancer chemotherapy. *Eur J Cancer*. 2002; 38:639–44.

239. Holford NH. Target concentration intervention: beyond Y2K. *Br J Clin Pharmacol*. 2001; 52(suppl 1):S55–S59.

240. Bates DW, Soldin SJ, Rainey PM, et al. Strategies for physician education in therapeutic drug monitoring. *Clin Chem*. 1998; 44:401–7.

241. Schumacher GE, Barr JT. Total testing process applied to therapeutic drug monitoring: impact on patients' outcomes and economics. *Clin Chem*. 1998; 44:370–4.

BIBLIOGRAPHY

Bauer LA. *Applied Clinical Pharmacokinetics*. New York, NY: McGraw-Hill; 2001.

Burton ME, Shaw LM, Schentag JJ, Evans WE, eds. *Pharmacokinetics and Pharmacodynamics: Principles of Therapeutic Drug Monitoring*. 4th ed., in press. Baltimore, MD: Lippincott Williams & Wilkins; 2004.

Murphy JE, ed. *Clinical Pharmacokinetics Pocket Reference*. 2nd ed. Bethesda, MD: American Society of Health-System Pharmacists; 2001.

Tayor WJ, Caviness MHD, eds. *A Textbook for the Application of Therapeutic Drug Monitoring*. Irving, TX: Abbot Laboratories, Diagnostics Division; 1986.

Winter ME. *Basic Clinical Pharmacokinetics*. 4th ed. Baltimore, MD: Lippincott Williams & Wilkins; 2004.

Chapter **7**

ELECTROLYTES, OTHER MINERALS, AND TRACE ELEMENTS

Alan Lau and Lingtak-Neander Chan

Determination of serum electrolyte concentrations is among the most commonly used laboratory tests by clinicians for assessment of medical conditions and disease states. The use of various nutrition management modalities has increased the need for checking serum concentrations of electrolytes and trace elements. The purpose of this chapter is to present the physiological basis of the need to determine serum concentrations of common electrolytes, minerals, and trace elements. The appropriate interpretation of these laboratory values and the clinical significance are addressed.

This chapter is particularly relevant to clinicians involved in nutritional support, since the optimal use of parenteral and enteral nutritional regimens requires the monitoring of serum electrolyte, mineral, and trace element concentrations. In addition, clinicians in many other practice settings, including those in critical care, cardiology, and nephrology, often make important therapeutic decisions based on serum electrolyte and mineral values; their patients often have multiple-organ failure, resulting in various acute and chronic disturbances.

Commonly, the first three tests (sodium, potassium, and chloride) addressed in this chapter are considered electrolytes. However, other minerals, such as magnesium, calcium, and phosphate, are often measured as a part of the serum chemistry panel. Calcium and phosphate metabolism are frequently discussed in the context of the endocrine system because of their influence by vitamin D and parathyroid hormone. Serum carbon dioxide content, often measured in conjunction with electrolytes, is discussed in Chapter 9 because of its significance for the evaluation of acid-base disorders. Listed in Table 7-1, a background for the materials in this chapter, are the normal daily dietary intakes of electrolytes, minerals, and trace elements.

Although the serum concentrations of trace elements are not routinely measured in most settings, patients on chronic enteral and parenteral nutrition therapy may require assessment of the serum concentrations of these elements, as malnutrition and critical illnesses can alter the homeostasis of trace elements and often lead to their deficiencies. Furthermore, clinicians should appreciate the interplay among electrolytes and trace elements and evaluate all laboratory values in the appropriate context rather than considering each as a separate, independent entity.

TABLE 7-1

NUTRIENT	NORMAL DAILY DIETARY INTAKE
Sodium	Highly variable; average 5.6–7.2 g (243–355 mEq)
Potassium	50–100 mEq
Chloride	Varies with potassium and sodium intakes
Magnesium	300–400 mg
Calcium	~1000 mg
Phosphate	700–800 g
Copper	2–5 mg
Zinc	4–14 mg
Manganese	3–4 mg
Chromium	50–100 µg

Table 7-1. Normal Dietary Intake of Electrolytes, Other Minerals, and Trace Elements

OBJECTIVES

After completing this chapter, the reader should be able to

1. Describe the homeostatic mechanisms involved in plasma sodium and water balance and distinguish between hyponatremia and hypernatremia.
2. Describe the physiology of intracellular and extracellular potassium equilibrium and the signs and symptoms of hypokalemia and hyperkalemia.
3. List common causes of serum chloride abnormalities.
4. List common conditions resulting in serum magnesium abnormalities and describe signs and symptoms of hypomagnesemia and hypermagnesemia.
5. Describe the relationship among the metabolism of calcium, phosphate, parathyroid hormone (PTH), and vitamin D.
6. List common conditions resulting in serum calcium abnormalities and describe signs and symptoms of hypocalcemia and hypercalcemia.
7. List common conditions resulting in serum copper, zinc, manganese, and chromium abnormalities and describe the signs and symptoms associated with them.
8. In the context of a clinical case description, including history and physical examination, interpret the results of laboratory tests used to assess sodium, potassium, chloride, calcium, phosphate, magnesium, copper, zinc, manganese, and chromium.

ELECTROLYTES

The traditional units, International System (SI) units as well as their conversion factors for electrolytes, minerals, and trace elements discussed in this chapter, are listed in Table 7-2.

Sodium

Normal range: 136–145 mEq/L
or 136–145 mmol/L

Sodium is the most abundant cation in the extracellular fluid. It is the major contributor to serum osmolality, which is important in regulating water movement between the extracellular (i.e., intravascular and interstitial) and intracellular compartments. Thus, discussion of serum sodium must include a discussion of body water.[1] Sodium disorders are often associated with body water imbalance. If total body water changes without an accompanied change in total body solute, plasma osmolality will be affected and may result in hyponatremia. Once the physiology of sodium and water is mastered, abnormalities in serum sodium are easy to understand.

TABLE 7-2

NUTRIENT	TRADITIONAL UNITS	CONVERSION FACTORS TO SI UNITS	SI UNITS
Sodium	mEq/L	1	mmol/L
Potassium	mEq/L	1	mmol/L
Chloride	mEq/L	1	mmol/L
Magnesium	mEq/L	0.5	mmol/L
Calcium	mg/dL	0.25	mmol/L
Phosphate	mg/dL	0.3229	mmol/L
Copper	µg/dL	0.1574	µmol/L
Zinc	µg/dL	0.1530	µmol/L
Manganese	µg/L	18.2	µmol/L
Chromium	µg/L	18.3	nmol/L

Table 7-2. Conversion Factors to SI Units

Physiology

The principal role of sodium is the regulation of serum osmolality as well as fluid balance. Sodium is also needed for maintaining the appropriate transmembrane electric potential for neuromuscular functioning.[2] Figure 7-1 summarizes the physiology of water and sodium. In general, calculation or measurement of serum osmolality is especially helpful in the presence of hyponatremia. Normal serum osmolality is usually between 280–295 mOsm/kg H_2O. The presence of a significant amount of any other extracellular solutes (e.g., sodium, toxins, and organic solvents) will lead to an increase of serum osmolality.

The regulation of body water and plasma volume can directly or indirectly affect serum sodium concentration. The kidneys are the primary organs responsible for the regulation of body sodium and water. The glomeruli receive and filter about 180 L of water and 600 g (nearly 26,000 mEq) of sodium per day. On average, less than 2 L of water and between 0.1–40 g of sodium are excreted in the urine, depending on the body fluid status. Generally speaking, 100% of the plasma sodium is filtered by the glomeruli, but less than 1% is excreted in the

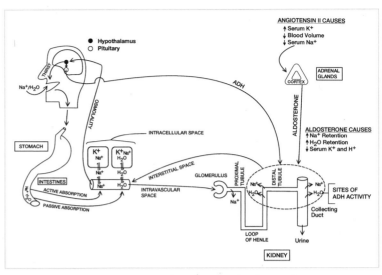

Figure 7-1. Homeostatic mechanisms involved in sodium, potassium, and water balance.

urine under normal circumstances. The proximal tubule and the loop of Henle each account for approximately 45% of sodium reabsorption.[3] In the presence of a change in effective circulating volume, baroreceptors and osmoreceptors are triggered to result in appropriate hemodynamic and volume changes. Baroreceptors are located in the carotid sinus, aortic arch, cardiac atria, hypothalamus, and the juxtaglomerular apparatus in the kidney. Osmoreceptors are present primarily in the hypothalamus. The three major mediators involved include antidiuretic hormone (ADH), renin-angiotensin-aldosterone system, and atrial natriuretic factor (ANF). The resulting renal effects include alteration of glomerular filtration rate and sodium reabsorption/excretion.

Antidiuretic hormone (vasopressin). Antidiuretic hormone (ADH), also known as arginine vasopressin, is a nonpeptide hormone that plays a key role in the regulation of water balance and osmolality. Thus, it has a pivotal effect on serum sodium concentration. It is secreted by the magnocellular neurons in the supraoptic and paraventricular nuclei of the hypothalamus, where both osmoreceptors and baroreceptors are present to detect any change of volume status in the body. Its release is stimulated by (1) hypovolemia (detected by baroreceptors), (2) thirst, (3) increased serum osmolality, and (4) angiotensin II. The plasma half-life of ADH is 10–20 min, and it is rapidly cleared by the liver, kidneys, and a plasma enzyme called *vasopressinase*.

ADH decreases urine output by increasing the permeability of the collecting tubules to increase the net reabsorption of water, resulting in concentrated urine. Circulating serum ADH binds to type 2 vasopressin (V2) receptors in the collecting tubule, which in turn stimulates the formation of a water channel, known as *aquaporin-2*. Aquaporin-2 facilitates the reabsorption of water from the lumen back into the renal blood supply, causing a decrease in diuresis. However, if serum sodium is high but blood volume is normal, the baroreceptors override the release of ADH, thus preventing volume overload (i.e., hypervolemia).[3]

In patients with syndrome of inappropriate ADH secretion (SIADH), an abnormally high quantity of ADH is present. This condition results in increased water reabsorption leading to a low serum sodium concentration (dilutional effect). Urine osmolality and urine electrolyte concentrations are increased due to the decreased urinary excretion of free water. Conversely, *central diabetes insipidus* occurs when an inadequate amount of ADH is synthesized or released.

In some situations, the kidneys fail to respond to normal or high quantities of circulating ADH. This condition is called *nephrogenic diabetes insipidus*. In central or nephrogenic diabetes insipidus (Chapter 13), little water reabsorption occurs, resulting in a large urine output of low urine osmolality. However, thirst usually causes these individuals to consume the quantity of water needed to replenish their diminished blood volume.[3] Otherwise, the excessive urine output will result in dehydration. (Chapter 8 offers an in depth discussion of the effects of other diseases on urine composition.)

Drugs can also increase ADH release, which is a common cause of SIADH. Drugs that are known to cause SIADH include chlorpropamide, tolbutamide, cyclophosphamide, carbamazepine, opiate derivatives, clofibrate, oxytocin, vincristine, phenothiazines, and some tricyclic antidepressants. Because of their ability to increase ADH release, some of these drugs are used in the treatment of diabetes insipidus.

Renin-angiotensin-aldosterone system. Renin is a glycoprotein that catalyzes the conversion of angiotensinogen to angiotensin I, which is further converted to angiotensin II primarily in the lungs. However, angiotensin II can also be formed locally in the kidneys. Angiotensin II causes significant vasoconstriction, which is important in maintaining optimal perfusion pressure to end organs when plasma volume has decreased. But more importantly, angiotensin II induces the release of aldosterone, ADH, and, to a much less extent, cortisol.

Aldosterone is a potent mineralocorticoid. It affects the distal tubular reabsorption of sodium rather than water.[4] This hormone is released from the adrenal cortex. Besides angiotensin II, various dietary and neurohormonal factors including low serum sodium, high serum potassium, and low blood volume can also stimulate its release. Aldosterone increases the urinary secretion of potassium from the distal tubules in exchange for sodium reabsorption.

Aldosterone has a profound effect on serum potassium, and its effect on serum sodium is relatively minor. As serum sodium increases, so does water reabsorption following the osmotic gradient.[3] Renal arteriolar blood pressure (BP) then increases, which increases the glomerular filtration rate (GFR). Ultimately, more water and sodium pass through the distal tubules, overriding the initial effect of aldosterone.[3,4]

Atrial natriuretic factor. Atrial natriuretic factor (ANF), also known as atrial natriuretic peptide, is a vasodilatory hormone synthesized and primarily released by the right atrium. It is secreted in response to plasma volume expansion, as a result of increased atrial stretch. ANF inhibits the juxtaglomerular apparatus, zona glomerulosa cells of the adrenal gland, and the hypothalamus-posterior pituitary. As a result, a global down regulation of renin, aldosterone, and ADH, respectively, is achieved. ANF directly induces glomerular hyperfiltration and reduces sodium reabsorption in the collecting tubule. A net increase in sodium excretion is achieved. Therefore, ANF can decrease serum and total body sodium.

Finally, the homeostatic mechanism for water and sodium also involves the equilibrium among intravascular, interstitial, and intracellular spaces.[3] The net movement of water goes from an area of low osmolality to one of high osmolality. This effect can be readily observed in patients with a low serum osmolality due to either a low serum sodium concentration or high serum water. In these patients, water moves toward the higher osmolality in the interstitial space to equalize the osmolar gap.[3] In the presence of high hydrostatic and oncotic pressure gaps across capillary walls, the net effect is excessive interstitial water accumulation and edema formation.[3,4]

Sodium moves among cells, interstitial spaces, and intravascular spaces. It may be easiest to interpret serum sodium values by conceptualizing the amount of sodium ion in the blood as fixed and the volume of water as variable. In this way, interpretation focuses on determining the causes of excessive or diminished serum water. Serum sodium is reported per liter of plasma water; as such, this value reflects not only sodium but also water. Consequently, when interpreting abnormal sodium values, the practitioner must determine if the problem is due to a sodium and/or water imbalance.

Hyponatremia

Hyponatremia is defined as a serum sodium concentration less than 136 mEq/L (<136 mmol/L). Serum sodium reflects total body water rather than total body sodium; hyponatremia may occur in the presence of low, normal, or high total body sodium. Therefore, natremic status cannot be assessed without regard to the fluid and water status of the patient. Clinicians must consider the patient's physical findings and medical history. More importantly, the patient's renal function, hydration status, and fluid intake and output should be assessed and closely monitored. The most common causes of hyponatremia can be broken down into two types: sodium depletion in excess of total body water loss and dilutional hyponatremia (i.e., water intake greater than water output, implying impaired water excretion). Dilutional hyponatremia can be further categorized into five subtypes: (1) primary dilutional hyponatremia (e.g., SIADH and renal failure); (2) neuroendocrine (e.g., adrenal insufficiency and myxedema); (3) psychiatric disorder (e.g., psychogenic polydipsia); (4) osmotic hyponatremia (e.g., severe hyperglycemia), and (5) thiazide diuretics-induced.

Most patients with hyponatremia remain asymptomatic until serum sodium is less than 120 mEq/L. Infusion of hypertonic saline is usually not necessary unless serum sodium concentration is less than 120 mEq/L or altered mental status is present. As with most electrolyte disorders, the chronicity of the imbalance is a major determinant of the severity of signs and symptoms. For example, hyponatremia in patients with congestive heart failure (CHF) secondary to volume overload and decreased renal perfusion is less likely to be symptomatic than a patient who is hyponatremic due to rapid infusion of a hypotonic solution. The most commonly reported symptoms associated with hyponatremia are altered mental status and mental confusion (Table 7-3). If serum sodium continues to fall, cerebral edema can worsen and intracranial pressure will continue to rise. More severe symptoms such as seizure, coma, and, subsequently, death may result.[3–6]

TABLE 7-3

SIGNS	SYMPTOMS
Abnormal sensorium	Agitation
Cheyne-Stokes respiration	Anorexia
Depressed deep-tendon reflexes	Apathy
Hypothermia	Disorientation
Seizures	Lethargy
Muscle cramps
Nausea

Table 7-3. Signs and Symptoms of Hyponatremia

Hyponatremia associated with decreased total body sodium. Hyponatremia associated with low total body sodium reflects a reduction in total body water, with an even larger reduction in total body sodium. This condition is primarily caused by depletion of extracellular fluid volume, which stimulates ADH release to increase renal water reabsorption even at the expense of hypo-osmolality. Some common causes include vomiting; diarrhea; intravascular fluid losses due to burns, peritonitis, and pancreatitis; hypoaldosteronism (Addison's disease); and certain forms of renal failure (e.g., salt-wasting nephropathy).[3] This type of hyponatremia may also occur in patients treated too aggressively with diuretics who receive sodium-free solutions (e.g., dextrose 5% in water) as replacement fluid.

Low serum sodium can also result when a large quantity of an osmotically active substance enters the bloodstream.[3] Physiologically, water follows the osmotic active substances and the osmotic gradient, resulting in a dilutional hyponatremia. This situation can occur with mannitol infusions and hyperglycemia. In hyperglycemia, the high serum glucose concentration results in high serum osmolarity, thus creating an osmolar gap between the plasma compartment and the extracellular fluid. This gap leads to a shift of water into the intravascular space, diluting the serum sodium concentration and results in hyponatremia.[3,5]

Additionally, the hyperglycemia leads to an osmotic diuresis. Hence, dilutional hyponatremia occurs as long as the rate of water moving from the cells into the blood is greater than the volume of water excreted through the urine. As cellular water diminishes and diuresis continues, plasma sodium may increase progressively.[3,5]

Patients with hyponatremia associated with low total body sodium often exhibit signs and symptoms of dehydration. These manifestations include thirst, dry mucous membranes, weight loss, sunken eyes, diminished urine output, and diminished skin turgor.[3]

Hyponatremia associated with normal total body sodium. Also called euvolemic or dilutional hyponatremia, this condition refers to impaired water excretion without any alteration in sodium excretion. Etiologies include any mechanism that enhances ADH secretion or potentiates its action at the collecting tubules. This condition can occur during states of glucocorticoid deficiency, severe hypothyroidism, administration of water to a patient with impaired water excretion capacity, and SIADH.[3,5]

As the name implies, SIADH is a disorder in which continued ADH secretion occurs despite low serum osmolality. Secretion may be drug induced. Therefore, the clinician should consider potential causative agents. These agents generally can be divided into two categories (Table 7-4):

1. Drugs that act centrally to cause ADH release.
2. Drugs that have ADH-like action or potentiate ADH's effect at the collecting tubules.

In addition to drugs, a number of disease states and medical conditions also precipitate SIADH. Some tumors, such as lung cancer, pancreatic carcinoma, thymoma, and lymphoma, may produce ADH ectopically. In contrast, head trauma, subarachnoid hemorrhage (SAH), hydrocephalus, Guillain-Barré syndrome, pulmonary aspergillosis, and occasionally tuberculosis may increase hypothalamic ADH production. Patients with SIADH have a high urine osmolality (i.e., concentrated urine, usually >200 mOsm/kg H_2O) and urine sodium excretion (usually >20 mEq/L); normal renal, adrenal, and thyroid function; and no evidence of volume abnormalities.[3,5]

Hyponatremia associated with increased total body sodium. This condition, the most common form of hyponatremia, implies an increase in total body sodium with a larger increase in total body water. Hyponatremia is frequently observed in edematous states such as CHF, cirrhosis, nephrotic syndrome, and chronic renal failure. In these conditions, water and sodium excretion from the kidneys is impaired. Edema is one hallmark sign of hyponatremia with increased total body sodium.[3,5]

TABLE 7-4

DRUGS THAT INCREASE ADH SECRETION

Carbamazepine

Chlorpropamide

Clofibrate

Cyclophosphamide

Diuretics

Narcotics

Nicotine

Vincristine

DRUGS THAT HAVE ADH-LIKE ACTION OR POTENTIATE ADH RENAL EFFECT

Acetaminophen

ADH analogs

Chlorpropamide

Cyclophosphamide

Diuretics

Nonsteroidal anti-inflammatory drugs (NSAIDs)

Table 7-4. Drugs Associated with Dilutional Hyponatremia

Fractional Excretion of Sodium (FE$_{Na}$)

Normal range: 1–2%

When a serum sodium value is abnormal, the clinician should identify possible etiologies by determining whether the abnormality is associated with low, normal, or high total body sodium. A urine sample (preferably from a 24-hr urine collection) is needed to determine renal handling of sodium. Then FE$_{Na}$, the measure of the percentage of filtered sodium excreted in the urine (Chapter 8), must be calculated:

$$FE_{Na} (\%) = \frac{\text{Urine Na / Serum Na}}{\text{UCr / SCr}} \times 100\%$$

Values greater than 2% indicate that the kidneys are excreting a higher than normal fraction of the filtered sodium, implying renal tubular damage. Conversely, FE$_{Na}$ values less than 1% indicate renal sodium retention suggesting prerenal causes of renal dysfunction (e.g., hypovolemia and cardiac failure). Since acute diuretic therapy can increase the FE$_{Na}$ to 20% or more, urine samples should be obtained at least 24 hr after diuretics have been discontinued.[3] Minicase 1 demonstrates how to calculate FE$_{Na}$:

MINICASE 1

ALICE W., A 74-YEAR-OLD WHITE FEMALE, had a history of coronary artery disease, CHF, and insulin-dependent diabetes mellitus (IDDM). She was brought to the emergency department by her daughter, who complained about her mother's increasing disorientation over the past week. Medications at the time of admission were benazepril 10 mg oral daily, digoxin 0.125 mg oral daily, furosemide 40 mg oral twice a day, nitroglycerin patch 0.2 mg/hr, diphenhydramine 25 mg every bedtime, NPH plus regular insulin subcutaneously twice a day, and acetaminophen 650 mg prn. She last took these medications the morning before admission. Alice W. also drank many cans of diet cola every day.

A review of systems revealed lethargy and apathism with no apparent distress. Vital signs showed a sitting BP of 110/75 (standing BP not measured), a regular heart rate of 96, and a rapid and shallow respiratory rate of 36. Alice W.'s physical examination was pertinent for bilaterally depressed deep-tendon reflexes. Her laboratory findings were unremarkable, except for a serum sodium of 120 mEq/L (136–145 mEq/L) and a serum glucose of 185 mg/dL (70–110 mg/dL). A urine collection was started on admission to the hospital. Her 24-hr collection showed: urine volume, 2280 mL (<2000 mL); SCr, 1.0 mg/dL (0.7–1.5 mg/dL); urine creatinine, 32 mg/dL; and urine sodium, 12 mEq/L.

Question: What subjective and objective data for Alice W. are consistent with a diagnosis of hyponatremia? What are the potential etiologies of hyponatremia in this patient?

Discussion: Aside from her low serum sodium concentration, Alice W. is exhibiting symptoms of hyponatremia (e.g., lethargy, apathy, and rapid and shallow breathing [Cheyne-Stokes respiration]) and diminished deep-tendon reflexes. A clinician must determine volume status when assessing a patient with sodium abnormality. However, Alice W. currently does not exhibit any signs or symptoms of dehydration or fluid overload. To identify possible etiologies, a determination must be made as to whether the hyponatremia is associated with low, normal, or high total body sodium. Since Alice W. last took her diuretic yesterday morning, her 24-hr urine collection may be used for calculating FE$_{Na}$:

$$0.3\% = \frac{12 \text{ mEq/L}}{120 \text{ mEq/L}} \div \frac{32 \text{ mg/dL}}{1.0 \text{ mg/dL}} \times 100$$

Therefore, Alice W. is trying to preserve sodium in the presence of her hyponatremia, which implies a deficit in total body water with a larger deficit in total body sodium. This condition may be due to aggressive furosemide treatment, with replacement of her lost body fluid with a low sodium or sodium-free solution (e.g., dextrose 5% in water or free water).

Blood Urea Nitrogen (BUN): Serum Creatinine (SCr) Ratio

Normal range: <20:1

The BUN: SCr ratio can also provide helpful information in regard to the bodily fluid status and help assess sodium status. When this ratio is higher than 20, dehydration is usually present. As extracellular fluid volume is diminished, the kidneys increase their reabsorption of urea but not creatinine. Therefore, BUN increases by a larger magnitude than the SCr concentration in dehydrated individuals, leading to a rise in the BUN: SCr ratio. (Chapter 8 offers a more in-depth discussion.)

Hypernatremia

Hypernatremia is defined as a serum sodium concentration greater than 145 mEq/L (>145 mmol/L). It is less common than hyponatremia. High serum sodium concentrations are most common in patients with either an impaired thirst mechanism (e.g., neurohypophyseal lesion—common after strokes) or an inability to replace water depleted through normal insensible losses (i.e., uncontrollable water loss through respiration or skin) or from renal or GI losses. All hypernatremic states increase serum osmolality. Like hyponatremia, hypernatremia may occur in the presence of high, normal, or low total body sodium content.[3,4,6]

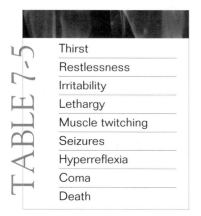

TABLE 7-5
Thirst
Restlessness
Irritability
Lethargy
Muscle twitching
Seizures
Hyperreflexia
Coma
Death

Table 7-5. Signs and Symptoms of Hypernatremia

The clinical manifestations of hypernatremia primarily involve the neurological system (Table 7-5). These manifestations are the consequence of cellular dehydration, particularly in the brain. In adults, acute elevation in serum sodium above 160 mEq/L (>160 mmol/L) is associated with 75% mortality. Unfortunately, neurological sequelae are common even in survivors. Elevated urine specific gravity, indicating concentrated urine, is uniformly observed. Hematocrit values may not be useful because changes in total body water also can affect erythrocyte water.[3-6] In order to assess the etiology of hypernatremia, it is important to determine (1) urine production; (2) sodium intake; and (3) renal solute concentrating ability, which reflects ADH activity.

Hypernatremia associated with low total body sodium. Hypernatremia with low total body sodium results when both sodium and water losses occur, but water is lost to a greater extent.[3] The thirst mechanism generally increases water intake, but this adjustment is not always possible (e.g., institutionalized elderly patients). This condition may also be iatrogenic when hypotonic fluid losses (e.g., profuse sweating and diarrhea) are replaced with an inadequate quantity of water and salt. In these circumstances, fluid losses should be replaced with dextrose 5% in water or sodium chloride 0.45%.[3,5]

These patients have high urine osmolalities (>800 mOsm/L, roughly equivalent to a specific gravity of 1.023) and low urine sodium concentrations (<10 mEq/L), indicating that the renal concentrating mechanisms are intact. Patients often exhibit orthostatic hypotension, flat neck veins, tachycardia, poor skin turgor, and dry mucous membranes. In addition, the BUN: SCr ratio may be greater than 20, indicating dehydration.[3,5]

Hypernatremia associated with normal total body sodium. Also called euvolemic hypernatremia, this condition refers to a general water loss without sodium loss.[3] Because of water redistribution between the intracellular and extracellular fluid, no volume contraction is usually evident unless water loss is substantial (Minicase 2). Etiologies include increased insensible water loss (e.g., fever, extensive burns, and mechanical ventilation) and central and nephrogenic diabetes insipidus. The clinician should be aware of drugs that may cause nephrogenic diabetes insipidus (Table 7-6).[3,5] (Chapter 12 covers diabetes insipidus in more detail.)

MINICASE 2

TODD M., A 21-YEAR-OLD MALE, was admitted to the neurosurgical service for a complete hypophysectomy to reduce an expanding pituitary tumor affecting his optic nerve. He was otherwise in good health and on no chronic medication. His postoperative medications included morphine (administered in a patient-controlled analgesia pump) and cefazolin 1 g every 8 hr.

Within 3 hr after surgery, Todd M.'s urine output reached 4.5 L. His physical exam was unremarkable, and his vital signs were stable. Clinical laboratory tests included serum sodium 152 mEq/L (136–145 mEq/L), potassium 3.8 mEq/L (3.5–5.0 mEq/L), chloride 102 mEq/L (96–106 mEq/L), carbon dioxide content 24 mEq/L (24–30 mEq/L), glucose 98 mg/dL (70–110 mg/dL), serum phosphate 2.9 mg/dL (2.6–4.5 mg/dL), BUN 9 mg/dL (8–20 mg/dL), and SCr 0.9 mg/dL (0.7–1.5 mg/dL). Urine specific gravity was 1.003 (1.010–1.020). On day 2, his urine volume reached 14 L, and he complained of excessive thirst.

Question: What subjective and objective data for Todd M. are consistent with a diagnosis of hypernatremia? What are the potential etiologies of hypernatremia in this patient?

Discussion: Aside from his serum sodium concentration and excessive thirst, Todd M. is not exhibiting any sign or symptom specific to hypernatremia. Usually, the first step in identifying possible etiologies is determining whether the hypernatremia is associated with low, normal, or high total body sodium (i.e., calculating FE_{Na} and measuring urine osmolality and specific gravity). However, Todd M.'s urine specific gravity may be used as a surrogate marker since FE_{Na} and urine osmolality were not measured.

Because this problem is acute, potential causes must be considered so that appropriate interventions can be made. Given the rapid onset of polyuria shortly after Todd M.'s complete hypophysectomy, a lack of circulating ADH probably caused his sodium-water imbalance. Todd M.'s hypernatremia is associated with a normal total body sodium (also called euvolemic hypernatremia) since ADH affects only the excretion of water. If his urine had been tested, his urine osmolality probably would be low, indicating production of dilute urine. This supposition is indirectly supported by his low urine specific gravity. His condition, therefore, is probably due to a general water loss without sodium loss. Since this abnormality was detected early, Todd M.'s only clinical manifestations were polyuria and polydipsia.

IV fluid replacement with dextrose 5% is adequate for correcting his hypernatremia. However, vasopressin (ADH) or its analog will be needed for long-term therapy.

Hypernatremia associated with high total body sodium. This form of hypernatremia is the least common, since sodium homeostasis is maintained indirectly through the control of water, and defects in the system usually affect total body water more than total body sodium.[3] This form of hypernatremia is usually due to exogenous administration of high sodium-containing solutions such as

- Resuscitative efforts using hypertonic sodium bicarbonate.
- Inadvertent intravenous (IV) infusion of hypertonic saline (i.e., solutions >0.9% sodium chloride).
- Inadvertent dialysis against high sodium-containing solution.
- Sea water, near drowning.

Primary hyperaldosteronism and Cushing's disease also may cause this form of hypernatremia. Large quantities of sodium can be found in the urine of these patients. Signs and symptoms include diminished skin turgor and elevated plasma proteins.[3,5]

Potassium

Normal range: 3.5–5.0 mEq/L or 3.5–5.0 mmol/L

Potassium is the primary cation in the intracellular space, with an average intracellular fluid concentration of about 140 mEq/L (140 mmol/L). The major physiological role of potassium is in the regulation of muscle and nerve excitability. It

TABLE 7-6

Acetohexamide
Amphotericin B
Angiographic dyes
Cisplatin
Colchicine
Demeclocycline
Foscarnet
Gentamicin
Glyburide
Lithium
Loop diuretics
Methicillin
Methoxyflurane
Norepinephrine
Osmotic diuretics
Propoxyphene
Thiazide diuretics
Tolazamide
Vinblastine

Table 7-6. Drugs that Can Cause Nephrogenic Diabetes Insipidus

may also play important roles in the control of intracellular volume (similar to the ability of sodium in controlling extracellular volume), protein synthesis, enzymatic reactions, and carbohydrate metabolism.[7,8]

Physiology

The most important aspect of potassium physiology is its effect on muscle and nervous tissue excitability.[2] During periods of potassium imbalance, the cardiovascular system is of principal concern. Similar to other muscle tissues, the function of cardiac muscle cells depends on their ability to change their resting-state electrical potentials when exposed to the proper stimulus, resulting in muscle contraction and nerve conduction.[7,8]

One important aspect of potassium homeostasis is its distribution equilibrium. In a 70-kg man, the total body potassium content is about 4000 mEq. Of that amount, only 60 mEq is located in the extracellular fluid with the remainder residing within cells. The average daily Western diet contains 50–100 mEq of potassium, which is completely and passively absorbed in the upper gastrointestinal tract. To enter cells, potassium must first pass through the extracellular compartment. If the serum potassium concentrations rise above 6 mEq/L (>6 mmol/L), symptomatic hyperkalemia may occur. Abnormalities in potassium homeostasis may be related to disturbances in insulin, aldosterone, acid-base balance, renal function, or gastrointestinal and skin losses. These conditions can be modulated by various pathological states as well as pharmacotherapy. Although potassium may affect different bodily functions, its effect on the cardiac muscle is the most important due to the potential life-threatening effect of arrhythmias, caused by either high or low serum potassium concentrations.[4,6–10]

Renal homeostasis. When the serum potassium concentration is high, the body has two different mechanisms to restore potassium balance. One quick way is to shift the plasma potassium into the cells, while the other slower mechanism is renal elimination.[10] The kidneys are the primary organs involved in the control and elimination of potassium. Potassium is freely filtered at the glomeruli and almost completely reabsorbed before the filtrate reaches the distal tubules. However, an amount equal to about 10% of the filtered potassium is then secreted into the urine at the distal and collecting tubules. Virtually all the potassium recovered in urine is, therefore, delivered via tubular secretion rather than glomerular filtration.[7]

In the distal tubule, potassium is being secreted into the tubule while sodium is reabsorbed. There are several mechanisms that can modulate the activity of this sodium-potassium exchange. Aldosterone plays an important role since it increases potassium secretion into the urine[10] (Figures 7-1 and 7-2). The hormone is secreted by the adrenal glands in response to high serum potassium concentrations. The delivery of large quantities of sodium and fluid to the distal tubules may also cause potassium secretion and its subsequent elimination, as seen in diuretic-induced hypokalemia.[11] As the delivery of sodium and fluid is decreased, potassium secretion declines.

The presence of anions in the distal tubules, which are relatively permeable to reabsorption, can increase renal potassium loss because the negatively charged anions attract positively charged potassium ions. This mechanism is responsible for hypokalemia caused by renal tubular acidosis and the administration of high doses of a penicillin (e.g., carbenicillin).[10] Potassium secretion is also influenced by the potassium concentration in distal tubular cells.

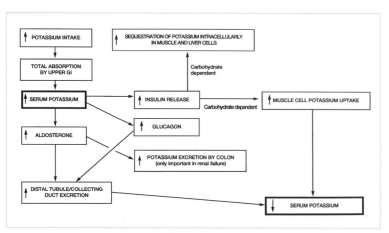

Figure 7-2. The homeostatic sequence of events in the body to maintain serum potassium within a narrow concentration range.

When the intracellular potassium concentration rises, as with dehydration, potassium secretion into the urine increases.

In addition to the mechanisms addressed above, there are several additional points that we should consider regarding maintenance of potassium homeostasis:

1. Although the kidneys are the primary route of elimination, potassium secretion into the colon becomes important in patients with advanced renal failure.[10]
2. Unlike sodium, the kidneys are not fully able to arrest potassium's secretion into the urine. During hypokalemia, the urinary potassium concentration may be as low as 5 mEq/L, but potassium excretion does not completely cease.

The modulation of renal potassium excretion by these mechanisms may take hours to cause significant changes in serum potassium concentration, even when drastic, acute changes have taken place. Extrarenal mechanisms, therefore, often play very important roles in keeping the serum potassium concentration within the narrow acceptable range.

Arterial pH homeostasis. Another potentially relevant factor influencing renal potassium secretion is arterial pH. When arterial pH increases due to metabolic—but not respiratory—alkalosis, there is a compensatory shift of hydrogen ions out of the cells and into the extracellular fluid (bloodstream).[7] To maintain the electropotential gradient, potassium moves intracellularly. Although there is no immediate change in the amount of total body potassium, this movement of ions increases the cellular potassium content, primarily in muscle tissues.

The shift in potassium and hydrogen ions may also be found in the renal distal tubular cells. During alkalosis, renal potassium secretion into the urine is increased. During the early phase of metabolic alkalosis, serum potassium concentration is reduced due to intracellular shift without a change in total body amount. Later on, the serum potassium concentration declines through increased renal loss, resulting in reduced body store.

Metabolic acidosis has the opposite effect. Decreased arterial pH results in an extracellular shift of potassium as a result of intracellular shift of hydrogen ions, causing an elevated serum potassium concentration.[7] Since the intracellular potassium content of the distal tubular cell is decreased, secretion of potassium in the urine is diminished. Chronically, however, the potassium loss gradually increases in the urine due to unknown mechanisms.

When a severe metabolic acid-base abnormality exists, the serum potassium concentration should be corrected to reflect the change in transcellular shifting (redistribution) of potassium. For every 0.1 U reduction in arterial pH less than 7.4, roughly 0.6 mEq/L (range: 0.2–1.7 mEq/L) should be added to the serum potassium value:

$$K_{corr} = ([7.4 - pH]/0.1 \times 0.6 \text{ mEq/L}) + K_{uncorr}$$

where K_{corr} is the corrected serum potassium concentration and K_{uncorr} is the uncorrected or measured serum potassium concentration (Minicase 3).[7]

Although total body potassium does not change abruptly in alkalemia or acidemia, arrhythmias can occur if the serum potassium concentration changes drastically. Even a small percentage change in intracellular potassium can produce a clinically significant change in extracellular concentrations.

Acute homeostasis. Figure 7-2 summarizes the acute homeostatic mechanism involved in potassium distribution. In hyperkalemia, along with the release of aldosterone, increased glucagon and insulin release also contribute to reducing the serum potassium concentration. Glucagon stimulates potassium secretion into the distal tubules and collecting ducts, while insulin helps to drive potassium intracellularly. This insulin-potassium interaction is completely independent of transcellular glucose transport. Although insulin is not a major controlling factor in potassium homeostasis, it is useful in the emergency treatment of hyperkalemia.[7,12]

ANDREW D., A 65-YEAR-OLD, 150-LB MALE, was admitted to University Hospital for surgical management of acute urinary retention due to long-standing bladder outlet obstruction. His past medical history was significant for hypertension and diet-controlled Type II diabetes mellitus. His medications included propranolol 120 mg oral twice a day, furosemide 80 mg oral twice a day, and enalapril 10 mg oral every morning.

A review of Andrew D.'s systems was unremarkable, except for his inability to urinate. Vital signs included respiratory rate 25, pulse 60 and regular, and BP 190/98–190/102 mm Hg. Positive physical findings included an audible S_4 heart sound and decreased deep-tendon reflexes bilaterally. The only other abnormal clinical finding was an indurated, fixed prostate gland. Abnormal clinical laboratory tests included serum potassium 5.6 mEq/L (3.5–5.0 mEq/L), serum carbon dioxide 16 mEq/L (24–30 mEq/L), glucose 237 mg/dL (70–110 mg/dL), phosphate 6.4 mg/dL (2.6–4.5 mg/dL), BUN 56 mg/dL (8–20 mg/dL), and SCr 3.3 mg/dL (0.7–1.5 mg/dL). A presurgery arterial blood gas showed pH 7.30 (7.36–7.44), partial pressure of carbon dioxide (pCO_2) 17 mm Hg (36–44 mm Hg), and partial pressure of oxygen (pO_2) 99 mm Hg (80–100 mm Hg).

Due to postsurgical complications, Andrew D. was placed on a daily peripheral vein hyperalimentation solution containing dextrose 5%, amino acids 3%, sodium chloride 50 mEq, potassium chloride 30 mEq, potassium phosphate 40 mEq (based on potassium), calcium gluconate 4.6 mEq, magnesium sulfate 16.2 mEq, and multivitamin supplements 10 mL. Over the next several days, Andrew D. complained of muscle weakness, and his urine output dropped to 20 mL/hr. His pulse was 40 and irregular, and his BP was 130/65 mm Hg. His electrocardiogram (ECG) showed flat P waves, tall T waves, and widened QRS intervals. A repeat serum chemistry revealed a serum potassium concentration of 7.1 mEq/L (3.5–5.0 mEq/L).

Question: What subjective and objective data for Andrew D. are consistent with a diagnosis of hyperkalemia? What are the potential etiologies of hyperkalemia in this patient?

Discussion: Aside from his high serum potassium concentration, Andrew D. is exhibiting signs and symptoms of hyperkalemia (e.g., muscle weakness, rhythm disturbances, worsening of bradycardia, and reduced BP).

Andrew D. has several predisposing factors that may have contributed to his hyperkalemia. First, he has mild metabolic acidosis. This condition resulted in an extracellular shifting of potassium, causing an elevated serum potassium concentration. Although clinically insignificant, his serum potassium value may be corrected for his acidosis to reflect his extracellular potassium status more accurately. The serum potassium value must be corrected as follows:

$$K_{corr} = ([7.4 - pH]/0.1 \times 0.6 \text{ mEq/L}) + K_{uncorr}$$
$$K_{corr} = ([7.4 - 7.3]/0.1 \times 0.6 \text{ mEq/L}) + 7.1 = 7.7 \text{ mEq/L}$$

This correction implies that if acidemia is corrected, serum potassium will increase by 0.6 mEq/L without any addition of potassium to the body. This equation becomes more significant during severe metabolic acid-base disorders.

Second, although the potassium balance usually is not disturbed until the GFR falls to less than 10 mL/min, Andrew D.'s renal impairment contributed to his hyperkalemia. His creatinine clearance is about 22 mL/min. Since angiotensin-converting enzyme inhibitors decrease urine potassium excretion by inhibiting the renin-angiotensin-aldosterone system, enalapril also may have contributed to this patient's hyperkalemia (decreased output). Although β_2-adrenergic receptors potentiate the movement of potassium from extracellular fluid to the intracellular fluid compartment, propranolol (a β_1- and β_2-adrenergic receptor inhibitor) does not appear to have a clinically significant effect on serum potassium concentrations.

Finally, the potassium content of Andrew D.'s hyperalimentation solution is 70 mEq. Although this value is consistent with the average Western diet (50–100 mEq), this quantity may be inappropriately high (increased intake) given his renal impairment.

Pharmacological stimulation of β_2-adrenergic receptors may also affect the transcellular equilibrium of potassium. It leads to the movement of potassium from extracellular fluid to the intracellular fluid compartment. β_2-adrenergic agonist (e.g., albuterol) can, therefore, be used to treat certain hyperkalemic patients.[7-9]

Hypokalemia

Hypokalemia is defined as a serum potassium concentration less than 3.5 mEq/L (<3.5 mmol/L). It may indicate true or apparent potassium deficit, although the signs and symptoms are indistinguishable.[10] To interpret the significance of low potassium values, the clinician should determine whether hypokalemia is due to intracellular shifting of potassium (apparent deficit) or increased loss from the body (true deficit) (Table 7-7).

Intracellular shifting occurs as a result of metabolic alkalosis or after administration of insulin, dextrose, or ß$_2$-adrenergic agonists.[9,13] Parenteral nutrition solutions can drive potassium into cells due to their high glucose, insulin, and amino acid content. Potassium, as an intracellular cation, is taken up during the formation of new cells. Increased loss of potassium can occur in the kidneys or gastrointestinal tract. There may be decreased potassium reabsorption in the proximal tubules or increased secretion in the distal tubules and collecting ducts.[10]

Amphotericin B. Proximal tubular damage can occur with amphotericin B therapy, resulting in renal tubular acidosis. Reabsorption of potassium, magnesium, and bicarbonate may all be affected, leading to hypokalemia, hypomagnesemia, and metabolic acidosis.[7,13] Concurrent deficiency in magnesium may affect the ability to restore potassium balance. Magnesium maintains the sodium-potassium adenosine triphosphate (ATP) pump activity and facilitates renal preservation of potassium. A hypokalemic patient who is also hypomagnesemic may not, therefore, respond to potassium replacement therapy unless the magnesium balance is restored.[7,8,12]

Diuretics. The most common class of drugs associated with renal potassium wasting is diuretics. Although their mechanisms of natriuretic action differ, diuretic-induced hypokalemia is primarily caused by increased secretion of potassium at the distal sites in the nephron in response to an increased load of exchangeable sodium. Diuretics increase the distal urinary flow by inhibiting sodium reabsorption. This increased delivery of fluid and sodium in the distal segment of the nephron results in an increase in sodium reabsorption at that site. To maintain a neutral electropotential gradient in the lumen, potassium is excreted as sodium is reabsorbed. Therefore, any inhibition of sodium absorption by diuretics proximal to or at the distal tubules can increase potassium loss. Renal potassium excretion is further enhanced when nonabsorbable anions are present in the urine.

Use of loop diuretics (e.g., furosemide) and thiazides (e.g., hydrochlorothiazide) may both result in hypokalemia. However, low doses of thiazide (≤50 mg/day of hydrochlorothiazide) may exert an antihypertensive effect without having a high risk of developing severe hypokalemia. In fact, the seventh report of the Joint National Committee on Detection, Evaluation and Treatment of High Blood Pressure (JNC-7) recommended thiazide-type diuretics for hypertension treatment in most patients.[14] In order to minimize the risk for developing hypokalemia and other electrolyte imbalances, low doses of thiazides (e.g., 12.5–25 mg of hydrochlorothiazide or chlorthalidone) should now be used instead of the high doses (e.g., 100 mg/day) that were used previously. Serum potassium concentrations should be monitored regularly to avoid the increased risk for cardiovascular events secondary to hypokalemia and other electrolyte imbalance. In addition, elderly patients with ischemic heart disease and patients receiving digoxin are more susceptible to the adverse consequences of hypokalemia.[15-17]

TABLE 7-7

APPARENT DEFICIT —INTRACELLULAR SHIFTING OF POTASSIUM
Alkalosis
ß$_2$-adrenergic stimulation
Insulin
TRUE DEFICIT
Decreased intake
"Tea and toast" diet
Alcoholism
Indigence
Potassium-free IV fluids
Anorexia nervosa
Bulimia
Increased output
Extrarenal
Vomiting
Diarrhea
Laxative abuse
Intestinal fistulas
Renal
Corticosteroids
Amphotericin B
Diuretics
Hyperaldosteronism
Cushing's syndrome
Licorice abuse

Table 7-7. Etiologies of Hypokalemia

Spironolactone, triamterene, and amiloride are not expected to cause potassium loss due to their mode of action. In fact, they cause retention of potassium due to their effects on aldosterone-dependent (spironolactone) and aldosterone-independent (triamterene and amiloride) exchange sites in the collecting tubules. These agents are also magnesium sparing.[11,18]

Other causes. Conditions that cause hyperaldosteronism, either primary (e.g., adrenal tumor) or secondary to other causes (e.g., renovascular hypertension), can produce hypokalemia.[13] Cushing's syndrome leads to increased circulation of mineralocorticoids such as aldosterone. Corticosteroids with strong mineralocorticoid activity (e.g., cortisone) also can cause hypokalemia.[10]

GI loss of potassium can be important. Aldosterone influences not only renal potassium handling but also that of the intestines.[10] A decrease in extracellular volume increases aldosterone secretion, resulting in renal and colonic potassium wasting. Diarrheal fluid can contain 20–120 mEq/L (20–120 mmol/L) of potassium; consequently, profuse diarrhea can rapidly result in potassium imbalance. In contrast, vomitus contains only 0–32 mEq/L (0–32 mmol/L) of potassium, and loss secondary to vomiting is unlikely to be significant. However, with severe vomiting, the resultant metabolic alkalosis may lead to hypokalemia due to intracellular shifting of potassium. Finally, patients receiving potassium-free parenteral fluids can become hypokalemic if not monitored properly.[7,10]

Clinical diagnosis. Signs and symptoms of hypokalemia involve many physiological systems. However, abnormalities in the cardiovascular system may result in serious consequences (i.e., disturbances in cardiac rhythm). Hypokalemia-induced arrhythmias are of particular concern in patients receiving digoxin. Both digitalis glycosides and hypokalemia inhibit the sodium-potassium ATP pump in the cardiac cells. Together, they can deplete intracellular potassium, which may result in fatal arrhythmias. The signs and symptoms of hypokalemia are listed in Table 7-8. Skeletal muscle weakness is often seen; severe depletion may lead to decreased reflexes and paralysis. Death can occur from respiratory muscle paralysis.[7,9,19]

Hyperkalemia

Hyperkalemia is defined as a serum potassium concentration greater than 5.0 mEq/L (>5.0 mmol/L). As with hypokalemia, hyperkalemia may indicate a true or apparent potassium imbalance, although the signs and symptoms are indistinguishable.[10] To interpret a high serum potassium value, the clinician should determine whether hyperkalemia is due to apparent excess caused by extracellular shifting of potassium or true potassium excess in the body caused by increased intake with diminished excretion (Table 7-9).[4,6,9,11]

Causes. Since renal excretion is the major route of potassium elimination, renal failure is the most common cause of hyperkalemia. However, potassium handling by the nephrons is well-preserved until the GFR falls to less than 10% of normal. Many patients with renal impairment can, therefore, maintain a near normal, serum potassium concentration. They are still prone to developing hyperkalemia if excessive potassium is consumed and when renal function deteriorates.[9,12]

Increased potassium intake rarely causes any problem without significant renal impairment. In subjects with normal renal function, increased potassium intake will lead to in-

TABLE 7-8

CARDIOVASCULAR
Decrease in T-wave amplitude
Development of U waves
Hypotension
Increased risk of digoxin toxicity
PR prolongation (with severe hypokalemia)
Rhythm disturbances
ST segment depression
QRS widening (with severe hypokalemia)

METABOLIC/ENDOCRINE (MOSTLY SERVE AS COMPENSATORY MECHANISMS)
Decreased aldosterone release
Decreased insulin release
Decreased renal responsiveness to ADH

NEUROMUSCULAR
Areflexia (with severe hypokalemia)
Cramps
Loss of smooth muscle function (ileus and urinary retention with severe hypokalemia)
Weakness

RENAL
Inability to concentrate urine
Nephropathy

Table 7-8. Signs, Symptoms, and Other Effects of Hypokalemia

creased renal excretion and redistribution to the intracellular space through the action of aldosterone and insulin, respectively. Interference with either mechanism may result in hyperkalemia. Decreased aldosterone secretion can occur with Addison's disease or other defects affecting the hormone's adrenal output.[7,12]

Use of potassium-sparing diuretics is a common cause of hyperkalemia, especially in patients with renal function impairment. Concurrent use of potassium supplements (including potassium-rich salt substitutes) will also increase the risk. Pathological changes affecting the proximal or distal renal tubules can also lead to hyperkalemia.[7,12]

Similar to hypokalemia, hyperkalemia can result from transcellular shifting of potassium. In the presence of severe metabolic acidosis, potassium shifts from the intracellular to the extracellular space, which may result in a clinically significant increase in the serum potassium concentration.[10]

Clinical diagnosis. The cardiovascular manifestations of hyperkalemia are of major concern. They include cardiac rhythm disturbances, bradycardia, hypotension, and, in severe cases, cardiac arrest. At times, muscle weakness may occur before these cardiac signs and symptoms. To appreciate the potent effect of potassium on the heart, one has to realize that potassium is the principal component of cardioplegic solutions commonly used to arrest the rhythm of the heart during cardiac surgeries.[7,9,12]

Causes of spurious laboratory results. There are several conditions that will result in fictitious hyperkalemia in which the high serum concentration reported is not expected to have any significant clinical sequelae. Erythrocytes, like other cells, have high potassium content. When there is substantial hemolysis in the specimen collection tube, the red cells will release potassium in quantities large enough to produce misleading results. Hemolysis may occur when a very small needle is used for blood draw, the tourniquet is too tight, or when the specimen stands too long or is mishandled. By looking at the color of the serum after the specimen is centrifuged, one can determine if significant hemolysis is present. The normally clear serum becomes red as red blood cells are broken down. When a high serum potassium concentration is reported in a patient without pertinent signs and symptoms, the test needs to be repeated to rule out hemolysis.[6,7,10]

A similar phenomenon can occur when the specimen is allowed to clot (when non-heparinized tubes are used) because platelets and white cells are also rich in potassium. In patients with leukemia or thrombocytosis, the potassium concentration should be obtained from plasma rather than serum samples. However, the normal plasma potassium concentration is 0.3–0.4 mEq/L lower than serum values.

TABLE 7-9

APPARENT EXCESS—EXTRACELLULAR SHIFTING OF POTASSIUM
Metabolic acidosis
TRUE EXCESS
Increased intake
Endogenous
Hemolysis
Rhabdomyolysis
Muscle crush injuries
Burns
Exogenous
Salt substitutes
Drugs (e.g., penicillin potassium)
Decreased output
Chronic or acute renal failure
Drugs
Potassium-sparing diuretics
Angiotensin-converting enzyme inhibitors
NSAIDs
β_2-adrenergic antagonists
Heparin
Trimethoprim
Deficiency of adrenal steroids
Addison's disease

Table 7-9. Etiologies of Hyperkalemia

Chloride

Normal range: 96–106 mEq/L or 96–106 mmol/L

Physiology

Chloride is the most abundant extracellular anion. However, its intracellular concentration is small (about 4 mEq/L). Chloride is passively absorbed from the upper small intestine. In the distal ileum and large intestine, its absorption is coupled with bicarbonate ion secretion. Chloride is primarily regulated by the renal proximal tubules, where it is exchanged for bicarbonate ions. Throughout the rest of the nephron, chloride passively follows sodium and water.

Chloride is influenced by the extracellular fluid balance and acid-base balance.[19,20] Although homeostatic mechanisms do not directly regulate chloride, they indirectly regulate it through changes in sodium and bicarbonate. The role of chloride is primarily passive. It balances out positive charges in the extracellular fluid and, by passively following sodium, helps to maintain extracellular osmolality. Finally, chloride fills in electronegative voids created by bicarbonate ion depletion.

Hypochloremia and Hyperchloremia

Serum chloride values are used as confirmatory tests to identify fluid balance and acid-base abnormalities.[21] Like sodium, a change in the serum chloride concentration does not necessarily reflect a change in total body content. Rather, it indicates an alteration in fluid status and/or acid-base balance. One of the most common causes of hyperchloremia in hospitalized patients is from saline infusion. Chloride has the added feature of being influenced by bicarbonate. Therefore, it would be expected to decrease to the same proportion as sodium when serum is diluted with fluid and to increase to the same proportion as sodium during dehydration. However, when a patient is on acid-suppressive therapy (e.g., cimetidine or omeprazole), has had nasogastric suction, or is profusely vomiting, a greater loss of chloride than sodium can occur because gastric fluid contains 1.5–3 times more chloride than sodium. Gastric outlet obstruction, protracted vomiting in alcoholism, and self-induced vomiting can also lead to hypochloremia.

Drug and parenteral nutrition causes. Even though drugs can influence serum chloride concentrations, they rarely do so directly. For example, although loop diuretics (e.g., furosemide) and thiazide diuretics (e.g., hydrochlorothiazide) inhibit chloride uptake at the loop of Henle and distal nephron, respectively,[18] the hypochloremia that may result is due to the concurrent loss of sodium and contraction alkalosis.[21] Since chloride passively follows sodium, salt and water retention can transiently raise serum chloride concentrations. This effect occurs with corticosteroids, guanethidine, and NSAIDs such as ibuprofen. Also, parenteral nutrition solutions with a chloride:sodium ratio greater than 1 are associated with an increased risk of hyperchloremia. Acetate or phosphate salts used in place of chloride salts (e.g., potassium chloride) reduce this risk. Acetazolamide also can cause hyperchloremia.

Acid-base status and other causes. The acid-base balance is partly regulated by renal production and excretion of bicarbonate ions. The proximal tubules are the primary regulators of bicarbonate. These cells exchange bicarbonate with chloride to maintain the intracellular electropotential gradient. The clinician must understand that the renal excretion of chloride increases during metabolic alkalosis, resulting in a reduced serum chloride concentration.

The opposite situation also may be true—metabolic or respiratory acidosis results in an elevated serum chloride concentration. Hyperchloremic metabolic acidosis is not common but may occur when the kidneys are unable to conserve bicarbonate, as in interstitial renal disease (e.g., obstruction, pyelonephritis, and analgesic nephropathy), GI bicarbonate loss (e.g., cholera and staphylococcal infections of the intestines), and acetazolamide-induced carbonic anhydrase inhibition. Falsely elevated chloride rarely occurs from bromide toxicity due to a lack of distinction between these two halogens by the laboratory's chemical analyzer.

(Since the signs and symptoms associated with hyperchloremia and hypochloremia are related to fluid status or the acid-base balance and underlying causes, rather than to chloride itself, the reader is referred to discussions in Chapter 9.)

OTHER MINERALS

Magnesium

Normal range: 1.5–2.2 mEq/L or 0.75–1.1 mmol/L

Physiology

Magnesium has a widespread physiological role in neuromuscular functions and maintaining enzymatic functions. Magnesium acts as a cofactor for phosphorylation of adenosine triphosphates (ATP) from adenosine diphosphates (ADP). Magnesium is also vital for binding macromolecules to organelles (messenger ribonucleic acid, RNA, to ribosomes).

Magnesium's bodily regulation is not well-understood. The average 70-kg adult body contains 2000 mEq of magnesium with the following distribution:

- 50–60% in bone (about 30% is slowly exchangeable with extracellular fluid).
- 30–40% in intracellular fluid.
- 1–2% in extracellular fluid (for plasma magnesium, about 60% is free; approximately 15% is complexed to anions, especially bicarbonate; and 25% is bound to protein, primarily albumin).

The average daily magnesium intake is 20–40 mEq/day. Approximately 30% of ingested magnesium is absorbed from the jejunum and ileum by passive diffusion and an active process that is coupled to calcium absorption. Because of this coupling system, low magnesium intake can facilitate calcium absorption from the intestines. There is evidence to suggest that 1,25 dihydroxy-calcitriol also regulates magnesium absorption across the intestinal lumen. Primarily the kidneys excrete magnesium, where unbound serum magnesium is freely filtered at the glomerulus. All but about 3–5% of filtered magnesium is normally reabsorbed (~100mg/day). In other words, 97% of the filtered magnesium is reabsorbed under normal circumstances. Reabsorption is primarily through the ascending limb of the Loop of Henle (50–60%). About 30% is reabsorbed in the proximal tubule and 7% from the distal tubule. This explains why loop diuretics have a more profound effect on renal magnesium wasting. The drive of magnesium reabsorption is mediated by the charge difference generated by the sodium-potassium-chloride cotransport system in the lumen. Urinary magnesium accounts for one-third of the total daily magnesium output. The other two-thirds are in the gastrointestinal tract (e.g., stool).

The regulation of magnesium is primarily driven by magnesium concentration present in the plasma. Changes in plasma magnesium concentrations cause potent effects on its renal reabsorption and stool losses. These effects are seen in 3–5 days and may persist for a long time. Hormonal regulation of magnesium seems to be much less critical for its homeostasis.

Factors affecting calcium homeostasis also affect magnesium homeostasis.[22] A decline in serum magnesium concentration stimulates the release of PTH, which increases serum magnesium by increasing both its release from bone stores and its renal reabsorption. Hyperaldosteronism causes increased magnesium renal excretion. Insulin by itself does not alter serum magnesium concentration. But in hyperglycemic state, insulin causes a rapid intracellular uptake of glucose. This process causes an increase in the phosphorylation by sodium-potassium ATPase on the cell membrane, which subsequently decreases serum magnesium concentration that is used as a cofactor. Excretion of magnesium is influenced by serum calcium and phosphate concentrations. Magnesium movement generally follows that of phosphate (i.e., if phosphate declines, magnesium also declines) and is the opposite of calcium.[21,22] Other factors that increase magnesium reabsorption include acute metabolism acidosis, hyperthyroidism, and chronic ethanol use.

Hypomagnesemia

Hypomagnesemia is defined as a serum magnesium concentration less than 1.5 mEq/L (<0.75 mmol/L). The common causes of hypomagnesemia include renal wasting, chronic alcohol use, diabetes mellitus, protein-calorie malnutrition, refeeding syndrome, and postparathyroidectomy. Since serum magnesium deficiency can be offset by magnesium release from bone, muscle, and heart stores, serum values may not be a useful indicator of cellular depletion and complications (e.g., arrhythmias). However, low serum magnesium usually indicates low cellular magnesium as long as the patient has a normal extracellular fluid volume.[22,23]

Causes. Magnesium deficiency is more common than magnesium excess. Depletion usually results from excessive loss from the GI tract or kidneys (e.g., use of loop diuretics). Magnesium depletion is not commonly the result of decreased intake because the kidneys can cease magnesium elimination in 4–7 days to conserve the ion. However, with chronic alcohol consumption, deficiency can occur from a combination of poor intake, poor GI absorption (e.g., vomiting or diarrhea), and increased renal elimination. Depletion can also occur from poor intestinal absorption (e.g., small-bowel resection). Diarrhea can be a source of magnesium loss because diarrhea stools may contain as much as 14 mEq/L (7 mmol/L) of magnesium.

Urinary magnesium loss may result from diuresis or tubular defects, such as the diuretic phase of acute tubular necrosis. Some patients with hypoparathyroidism may exhibit low magnesium serum concentrations from renal loss and, possibly, decreased intestinal absorption. Other conditions associated with magnesium deficiency include hyperthyroidism, primary aldosteronism, diabetic ketoacidosis, and pancreatitis. Magnesium deficiency in these states may be particularly dangerous because they often are associated with potassium and calcium deficiencies. Although loop diuretics lead to significant magnesium depletion, thiazide diuretics do not cause hypomagnesemia, especially at lower doses (≤50 mg/day). Furthermore, potassium-sparing diuretics (spironolactone, triamterene, and amiloride) are also magnesium sparing and have some limited clinical role in diuretic-induced hypokalemia and hypomagnesemia.[22,24]

Clinical diagnosis. Magnesium depletion is usually associated with neuromuscular symptoms such as weakness, muscle fasciculation with tremor, tetany, and increased reflexes.[22] They occur because the release of acetylcholine to motor endplates is affected by the presence or absence of magnesium. Motor endplate sensitivity to acetylcholine is also affected. When serum magnesium decreases, acetylcholine release increases, resulting in increased muscle excitation.

Magnesium also affects the central nervous system (CNS). Magnesium depletion can cause personality changes, disorientation, convulsions, psychosis, stupor, and coma.[22,25] Severe hypomagnesemia may result in hypocalcemia due to intracellular cationic shifts. Many symptoms of magnesium deficiency are due to decreased calcium.

Perhaps the most important effects of magnesium imbalance are on the heart. Decreased magnesium in cardiac cells may manifest as a prolonged QT interval (increased risk of arrhythmias, especially torsades de pointes).[25] Moderately decreased concentrations can cause ECG abnormalities similar to those observed with hypokalemia. In addition, vasodilatation may occur by a direct effect on blood vessels and ganglionic blockade.

A 24–hr urine magnesium excretion test may be helpful in determining the magnitude of total body magnesium deficiency. If the value is normal, the patient is not considered deficient as long as serum magnesium is also normal. The diagnosis of total body magnesium deficiency is established if the serum magnesium concentration is normal but the 24-hr urinary magnesium excretion is low. Magnesium replacement therapy is indicated.

MINICASE 3 DESCRIBED THE CASE OF ANDREW D., a 65-year-old male with hyperkalemia, metabolic acidosis, and renal impairment. His hyperalimentation solution contained an inappropriately high amount of potassium for his condition. When the potassium content was reduced to 30 mEq, his signs and symptoms of hyperkalemia resolved. However, Andrew D. developed severe pneumonia and required intubation and mechanical ventilation. To reduce gastric pH and the likelihood of stress ulcers, he received 30 mL of aluminum-magnesium hydroxide antacid every 2 hr through his nasogastric tube.

Three days after his intubation, Andrew D. developed bradycardia again and appeared drowsy. His bedside neurological exam revealed bilaterally depressed deep-tendon reflexes. Andrew D.'s vital signs included respiratory rate 26, pulse 45 and regular, and BP 145/78 mm Hg. Abnormal clinical laboratory tests included serum potassium 5.3 mEq/L (3.5–5.0 mEq/L), serum carbon dioxide content 17 mEq/L (24–30 mEq/L), phosphate 6.9 mg/dL (2.6–4.5 mg/dL), BUN 60 mg/dL (8–20 mg/dL), SCr 3.5 mg/dL (0.7–1.5 mg/dL), and magnesium 7.2 mEq/L (1.5–2.2 mEq/L).

Question: What subjective and objective data for Andrew D. are consistent with a diagnosis of hypermagnesemia? What are the potential etiologies of hypermagnesemia in this patient?

Discussion: Aside from his high serum magnesium concentration, Andrew D. is exhibiting signs and symptoms of hypermagnesemia, including drowsiness, bradycardia, and depressed deep-tendon reflexes. Hypermagnesemia commonly is associated with severe renal impairment; however, it may be due to increased magnesium intake and decreased magnesium output. Although magnesium balance usually is not disturbed until the GFR falls below 10 mL/min, Andrew D.'s renal impairment is a contributing factor. Another factor is the daily magnesium dose that he receives from his hyperalimentation solution and the antacid (increased intake).

Hypermagnesemia

Hypermagnesemia is defined as a serum magnesium concentration greater than 2.7 mEq/L (>1.3 mmol/L).

Causes. Besides magnesium overload (e.g., over-replacement of magnesium, treatment for preeclampsia, and antacid/laxative overuse), the only other cause of hypermagnesemia is renal dysfunction. The magnesium content of antacids and laxatives should be considered when a patient has renal disease (Minicase 4). Rapid infusions of IV solutions containing large amounts of magnesium, such as those given for myocardial infarction, preeclampsia, and status asthmaticus, may lead to hypermagnesemia.

Clinical diagnosis. Plasma magnesium concentrations below 5 mEq/L (<2.5 mmol/L) rarely cause serious symptoms. Relatively no specific symptoms such as muscle weakness decrease in deep tendon reflex and fatigue may be present. As magnesium concentration rises above 5 mEq/L, more serious symptoms such as lethargy, mental confusion, and hypotension may be observed (Table 7-10).[22,24,27] In severe hypermagnesemia (>7.5 mEq/L), life-threatening symptoms, including coma, paralysis, or cardiac arrest, can be observed and urgent therapy is indicated.

Treatment for severe or symptomatic hypermagnesemia may include intravenous calcium gluconate 1–2 g over 30 min to reverse neuromuscular and cardiovascular blockade of magnesium. Increased elimination magnesium can be achieved by forced diuresis with intravenous saline hydration and a loop diuretic agent. Hemodialysis should be reserved as a last resort.

TABLE 7-10		
	2–5 mEq/L	Bradycardia, flushing, sweating, sensation of warmth, nausea, vomiting. Decreased serum calcium and decreased clotting mechanisms
	6 mEq/L	Drowsiness and decreased deep-tendon reflexes
	10–15 mEq/L	Flaccid paralysis and increased PR and QRS intervals
	>15 mEq/L	Respiratory distress and asystole

Table 7-10. Signs and Symptoms of Hypermagnesemia

Calcium

Normal range: 8.5–10.8 mg/dL or 2.1–2.7 mmol/L for adults

Physiology

Calcium plays an important role in the propagation of neuromuscular activity, regulation of endocrine functions (e.g., pancreatic insulin release and gastric hydrogen secretion), blood coagulation including platelet aggregation, and bone and tooth metabolism.[2,28]

The serum calcium concentration is closely regulated by a complex interaction among PTH, serum phosphate, vitamin D system, and target organ (Figure 7-3). About one-third of the ingested calcium is actively absorbed from the proximal area of the small intestine, facilitated by 1,25-dihydroxycholecalciferol (1,25-DHCC or calcitriol, the most active form of vitamin D). Passive intestinal absorption is negligible with intake of less than 2 g/day. The average daily calcium intake is 2–2.5 g/day.

The normal adult body contains about 1000 g of calcium, with only 0.5% found in the extracellular fluid; 99.5% is integrated into bones. The tissue concentration of calcium is, therefore, small. Since bone is constantly remodeled by osteoblasts and osteoclasts, a small quantity of bone calcium is in equilibrium with the extracellular fluid. Extracellular calcium exists in three forms:

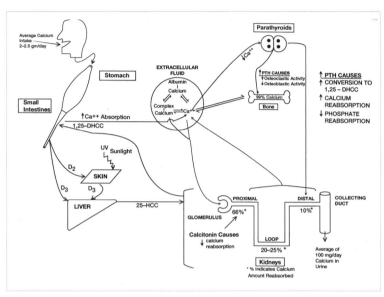

Figure 7-3. Calcium physiology: relationship with vitamin D, calcitonin, PTH, and albumin.

1. Complexed to bicarbonate, citrates, and phosphates (6%).
2. Protein bound, mostly to albumin (40%).
3. Ionized or free fraction (54%).

The equilibrium among these three forms determines the homeostasis of calcium.

Intracellular calcium. Imbalance of body calcium will lead to disturbances in muscle contraction and nerve action.[28] Within the cells, calcium maintains a low concentration. The calcium that is attracted into the negatively charged cell is either actively pumped out or sequestered by mitochondria or the endoplasmic reticulum. This difference in intracellular concentration allows calcium to be used for transmembrane signaling. In response to stimuli, calcium is either allowed to enter a cell or released from internal cellular stores where it interacts with specific intracellular proteins to regulate cellular functions or metabolic processes.[2,26,27] Calcium enters cells through one of the three types of calcium channels that have been identified: T (transient or fast), N (neuronal), and L (long lasting or slow). Subsets of these channels may exist. Calcium channel-blockers likely affect the L channels.[29]

In muscle, calcium is released from the intracellular sarcoplasmic reticulum. The released calcium binds to troponin and stops troponin from inhibiting the interaction of actin and myosin. This interaction results in muscle contraction. Muscle relaxation occurs when calcium is pumped back into the sarcoplasmic reticulum. In cardiac tissue, calcium becomes important during phase 2 of the action potential. During this phase, fast entry of sodium stops and calcium entry through slow channels begins (Figure 7-4), resulting in contraction. During repolarization, calcium is actively pumped out of the cell.[2]

Calcium channel-blocking drugs (e.g., nifedipine, diltiazem, and verapamil) inhibit the movement of calcium into muscle cells, thus decreasing the strength of contraction. The areas most sensitive to these effects appear to be the sinoatrial and atrioventricular nodes and vascular smooth muscles (which explains the hypotensive effects of nifedipine).

Extracellular calcium. Complex-bound calcium usually accounts for less than 1 mg/dL (<0.25 mmol/L) of blood calcium. The complex usually is formed with bicarbonate, citrate, or phosphate. In patients with chronic renal failure, calcium may also be bound with sulfate because the anion is retained. Phosphate plays an important role in calcium homeostasis. Under normal physiological conditions, the product of calcium concentration times phosphate concentration (the so-called calcium-phosphate product) is relatively constant: an increase in one ion necessitates a corresponding decline in the other. In addition, many homeostatic mechanisms that control calcium also regulate phosphate. This relationship is particularly important in renal failure; the decreased phosphate excretion may ultimately lead, through a complex mechanism, to hypocalcemia, especially if the hyperphosphatemia is untreated.[30,31]

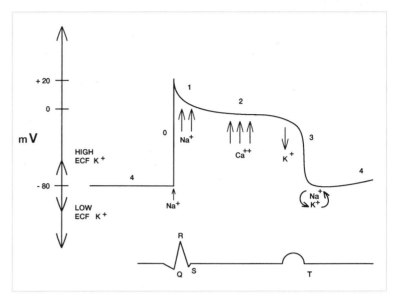

Figure 7-4. Cardiac intracellular potential and its relationship to the ECG.

Calcium is bound primarily to serum albumin (80%) and globulins (20%). Protein-bound calcium is in equilibrium with ionized calcium, which is affected by the serum anion concentration and blood pH. This equilibrium is important since ionized calcium is the physiologically active moiety. Alkalosis increases protein binding of calcium, resulting in a lower free fraction, whereas acidosis has the opposite effect. In patients with respiratory or metabolic alkalosis, the signs and symptoms of hypocalcemia may become more pronounced due to increased binding. Conversely, signs and symptoms of hypercalcemia become more apparent in patients with metabolic or respiratory acidosis. Therefore, total serum calcium concentration, which is commonly reported by clinical laboratories, is less important than the quantity of ionized calcium available. In fact, it is the free fraction that is closely regulated by the different homeostatic mechanisms.

Clinically, the most important determinant of ionized calcium concentration is the amount of serum proteins (primarily albumin) available for binding. The normal serum calcium range is 8.5–10.8 mg/dL (2.1–2.7 mmol/L) for a patient with a serum albumin of approximately 4 g/dL (40 g/L). Since less of the calcium will be protein bound in hypoalbuminemic patients, this "normal" range must be corrected based on the serum albumin concentration to reflect the additional quantity of free (active) calcium when less protein is available for binding. The following formula may be used:

$$Ca_{corr} = ([4.0 - albumin] \times 0.8 \text{ mg/dL}) + Ca_{uncorr}$$

where Ca_{corr} is the corrected serum calcium concentration, and Ca_{uncorr} is the uncorrected serum calcium concentration. For example, a clinician may be asked to write parenteral nutrition orders for an emaciated cancer patient. The serum albumin is 1.9 g/dL (19 g/L), and the serum calcium is 7.7 mg/dL (1.9 mmol/L) (calcium concentration is commonly reported as total calcium—not free or ionized fraction—unless specifically requested). At first glance, one might consider the calcium to be low. But with the reduced serum albumin concentration, more ionized calcium is available to cells.

$$Ca_{corr} = ([4.0 - 1.9] \times 0.8) + 7.7 = 9.4 \text{ mg/dL (2.34 mmol/L)}$$

The corrected serum calcium concentration is, thus, within the normal range. In severe hypoalbuminemia, as seen in nutritionally deprived patients, an apparently low total serum calcium may in fact be sufficient or even excessive. If such a patient were given IV albumin, the free fraction of calcium would acutely decline. The measured total calcium concentration will need to be corrected for the new albumin concentration.

Although this serum calcium correction method may be useful, the clinician must be aware of its potential for inaccuracy. The correction factor of 0.8 represents an average value and is not specific for the patient being cared for. If an accurate free concentration is needed, a direct measurement of serum ionized calcium concentrations may be conducted by most clinical laboratories (normal range: 4.6–5.2 mg/dL or 1.15–1.38 mmol/L).

Other less important factors can influence the calcium-protein equilibrium. While sodium may affect binding and, with severe hyponatremia, increased calcium-protein binding may be found, severe hypernatremia may reduce binding. In addition, hypothermia may decrease calcium binding.

Influence of vitamin D system. Small amount of calcium is excreted daily into the GI tract through saliva, bile, and pancreatic and intestinal secretions. However, the primary route of elimination is filtration by the kidneys. Calcium is freely filtered at the glomeruli, where approximately 65% is reabsorbed at the proximal tubules under partial control of calcitonin and 1,25-DHCC. Roughly 25% is reabsorbed in the loop of Henle, and another 10% is reabsorbed at the distal tubules under the influence of PTH.

Vitamin D is important for:

- Intestinal absorption of calcium.
- PTH-induced mobilization of calcium from bone.
- Calcium reabsorption in the proximal renal tubules.

Vitamin D must undergo several conversion steps before the active form, calcitriol or 1,25-DHCC, is formed. Vitamin D is absorbed by the intestines in two forms, vitamin D_2 (7-dehydrocholesterol) and vitamin D_3 (cholecalciferol). Vitamin D_2 is converted into vitamin D_3 in the skin by the sun's ultraviolet radiation. One of the causes of childhood hypocalcemia, rickets, is caused by reduced exposure to sunlight, resulting in diminished production of vitamin D_3.

Liver enzymes hydroxylate vitamin D_3 to calcifediol or 25-hydroxycholecalciferol (25-HCC), which is then hydroxylated by the kidneys to form the active 1,25-DHCC. This last conversion step is regulated by PTH. When PTH is increased during hypocalcemia, renal production of 1,25-DHCC increases, resulting in increased intestinal absorption of calcium. 1,25-DHCC may in turn regulate PTH synthesis and secretion.[30,32]

Influence of calcitonin. Calcitonin is a hormone secreted by specialized C cells of the thyroid gland in response to high level of circulating ionized calcium. Calcitonin inhibits osteoclastic activity, thereby inhibiting bone resorption. It also decreases calcium reabsorption in the renal proximal tubules to result in increased renal calcium clearance.[28] There are different forms of calcitonin available for the treatment of acute hypercalcemia.

Influence of parathyroid hormone. PTH is the most important hormone involved in calcium homeostasis. It is secreted by the parathyroid glands, which are embedded in the thyroid, in direct response to low circulating ionized calcium. PTH closely regulates, and is regulated by, the vitamin D system in maintaining the serum ionized calcium concentration within a narrow range. Generally, PTH increases the serum calcium concentration and stimulates renal conversion of 25-HCC to 1,25-DHCC, which enhances calcium absorption from the intestines. Conversely, 1,25-DHCC is a potent suppressor of PTH synthesis via a direct mechanism that is independent of the serum calcium concentration.[28,31] The normal reference range for serum PTH concentrations is 10–60 pg/mL.

Tubular reabsorption of calcium and phosphate at the distal nephron is controlled by PTH; it increases renal reabsorption of calcium and decreases the reabsorption of phosphate, resulting in lower serum phosphate and higher serum calcium concentrations. Perhaps the most important effect of PTH is on the bone. In the presence of PTH, osteoblastic activity is diminished and the bone-resorption processes of osteoclasts are increased. These effects increase serum ionized calcium, which feeds back to the parathyroid glands to decrease PTH output.[30]

The suppressive effect of 1,25-DHCC (calcitriol) on PTH secretion is used clinically in patients with chronic renal failure who have excessively high serum PTH concentrations due to secondary hyperparathyroidism. PTH is a known

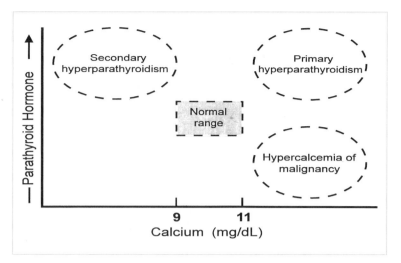

Figure 7-5. Interpretation of serum PTH concentrations with concomitant serum calcium concentrations.

uremic toxin, and its presence in supraphysiological concentrations has numerous adverse effects (e.g., suppressed erythropoiesis by the bone marrow and increased osteoclastic resorption of bones with replacement by fibrous tissue).[33] Figure 7-5 depicts the relationship between serum PTH and serum calcium concentrations.

Abnormalities. True abnormal serum concentrations of calcium may result from an abnormality in any of the previously mentioned mechanisms, including

- Altered intestinal absorption.[8,30,31,34]
- Altered number or activity of osteoclast and osteoblast cells in bone.[8,30,31,34]
- Changes in renal reabsorption of calcium.[8,30,31,34]
- Calcium or phosphate IV infusions.

Patients with chronic renal failure have increased serum phosphate and decreased serum calcium concentrations as a result of the following factors that interact via a complex mechanism: decreased phosphate clearance by the kidneys, decreased renal production of 1,25-DHCC, and skeletal resistance to the calcemic action of PTH. This interaction is further complicated by the metabolic acidosis of renal failure, which can increase bone resorption to result in decreased bone integrity. This complex process is counteracted by administering calcitriol, phosphate binders, and calcium supplements to keep serum calcium and phosphate concentrations near normal and to prevent secondary hyperparathyroidism.[31,36]

Hypocalcemia

Hypocalcemia indicates a total serum calcium concentration of less than 8.5 mg/dL (<2.1 mmol/L). The most common cause of hypocalcemia is low serum proteins. As discussed previously, the ionized calcium concentration may indeed be acceptable, and the patient should remain asymptomatic and often no treatment is required.

The most common causes of true reduction in total serum calcium are disorders of vitamin D metabolism and PTH production (Table 7-11). Osteomalacia (in adults) and rickets (in children) can be caused by a lack of dietary calcium or vitamin D, diminished synthesis of vitamin D_3 from insufficient sunlight exposure,

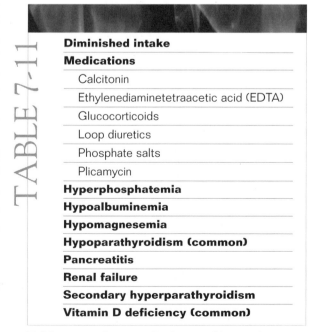

TABLE 7-11
Diminished intake
Medications
Calcitonin
Ethylenediaminetetraacetic acid (EDTA)
Glucocorticoids
Loop diuretics
Phosphate salts
Plicamycin
Hyperphosphatemia
Hypoalbuminemia
Hypomagnesemia
Hypoparathyroidism (common)
Pancreatitis
Renal failure
Secondary hyperparathyroidism
Vitamin D deficiency (common)

Table 7-11. Common Etiologies of Hypocalcemia

or resistance by the intestinal wall to the action of vitamin D. The reduction in serum calcium leads to secondary hyperparathyroidism, which increases bone resorption. With long-standing disease, bones lose their structural integrity and become more susceptible to fracture. The diminished serum calcium concentration, if significant, may result in tetany.

Diminished intake. Although uncommon, diminished intake of calcium is an important cause of hypocalcemia, especially in patients receiving long-term total parental nutrition solutions.[37,38]

Medications. Excessive use of certain drugs to lower serum calcium by either increasing bone deposition or decreasing renal reabsorption of calcium may lead to hypocalcemia. These drugs include plicamycin, calcitonin, glucocorticoids, loop diuretics, etidronate, pamidronate, and alendronate.

IV bicarbonate administration and hyperventilation can cause systemic alkalosis, resulting in a decrease in ionized serum calcium. This decrease is usually important only in patients who already have low serum calcium concentrations. Other drugs that may cause hypocalcemia include phenytoin, phenobarbital, aluminum-containing antacids, cis-platinum, theophylline, sodium fluoride, and magnesium sulfate.

Another cause is rapid IV administration of phosphate salts (a common ingredient in total parental nutrition solutions), especially at high doses. Phosphate can bind calcium and form an insoluble product. This product can deposit into soft tissues, causing metastatic calcification or hardening of normally pliable tissues.[37,38] Soft-tissue deposition of the calcium-phosphate complex (e.g., in lungs and blood vessels) occurs when the serum solubility product of calcium times phosphate exceeds 70. The risk of deposition is higher in patients with alkalosis. Other than the intravenous route, a large amount of phosphate may be absorbed from the GI tract with the use of certain enema and laxative preparations (e.g., Fleet's enema).[33]

Hypoparathyroidism effects. Hypoparathyroidism can reduce serum calcium concentrations. The most common cause of hypoparathyroidism is thyroidectomy, when the parathyroids are removed along with the thyroid glands. Since PTH is the major hormone regulating calcium balance, its absence significantly reduces serum calcium.[38]

Hyperparathyroidism effects. Hypocalcemia is commonly seen in patients with secondary hyperparathyroidism resulting from chronic renal failure (see Figure 7-5). The mechanism is complex and involves elevated serum phosphate concentrations and reduced activation of vitamin D. PTH acts on the bone to increase calcium and phosphate resorption. Since renal phosphate elimination is reduced because of the renal failure, serum phosphate concentration remains high and depresses serum calcium level. Because of the high phosphate concentrations in the intestinal wall, dietary calcium is bound and absorption is impaired while phosphate absorption continues.

Metabolic acidosis, which is common in chronic renal failure, further enhances bone resorption. With prolonged severe hyperparathyroidism, excessive osteoclastic resorption of bones continues to result in replacement of bone material by fibrous tissues. This condition is termed *osteitis fibrosa cystica*.[31,34,35] Such diminution of bone density may result in pathological fractures. Although the serum calcium concentrations are low, patients may not show symptoms of hypocalcemia because the accompanying acidosis helps to maintain a proper balance of ionized serum calcium through the reduction in protein binding.

Magnesium effects. Similar to potassium, calcium balance depends strongly on magnesium homeostasis. Therefore, if a hypocalcemic patient is also hypomagnesemic, as a result of loop diuretic therapy, calcium replacement therapy may not be effective unless magnesium balance is restored.

Clinical diagnosis. As with any electrolyte disorder, the severity of the clinical manifestations of hypocalcemia depends on the acuteness of onset. Hypocalcemia can at times be a medical emergency with symptoms primarily in the neuromuscular system.[37,38] They include fatigue, depression, memory loss, hallucinations, and, in severe cases, seizures and tetany. The early signs of hypocalcemia are finger numbness, tingling and burning of extremities, and paresthesia. Mental instability and confusion may be seen in some patients as the primary manifestation.

Tetany is the hallmark of severe hypocalcemia. The mechanism of muscle fasciculation of tetany is the loss of the inhibitory effect of ionized calcium on muscle proteins. In extreme cases, this loss leads to increased neuromuscular excitability that can progress to laryngospasm and tonic-clonic seizures. Chvostek's and Trousseau's signs are hallmarks of hypocalcemia. Chvostek's sign is a unilateral spasm induced by a slight tap over the facial nerve. Trousseau's sign is a carpal spasm elicited when the upper arm is compressed by a blood pressure cuff.[31,38,40]

As hypocalcemia worsens, the cardiovascular system may be affected, as evidenced by myocardial failure, cardiac arrhythmias, and hypotension.[37,38] Special attention should be given to serum calcium concentrations in patients receiving diuretics, corticosteroids, digoxin, vitamin preparations, antacids, lithium, and parenteral nutrition and in patients with renal disease.

Hypercalcemia

Hypercalcemia indicates a total serum calcium concentration greater than 10.8 mg/dL (>2.7 mmol/L).

Causes. The most common causes of hypercalcemia are malignancy and primary hyperparathyroidism (see Figure 7-5). Malignancies can increase serum calcium by several mechanisms. Osteolytic metastases can arise from breast, lung, thyroid, kidney, or bladder cancer. These tumor cells invade bone and produce substances that directly dissolve bone matrix and mineral content. Some malignancies, such as multiple myeloma, can produce factors that stimulate osteoclast proliferation and activity. Another mechanism is the ectopic production of PTH or PTH-like substances by tumor cells, resulting in a pseudohyperparathyroid state.[39,41]

In primary hyperparathyroidism, inappropriate secretion of PTH from the parathyroid gland, usually due to adenoma, increases serum calcium concentrations. The other major cause of hypercalcemia in hyperparathyroidism is the increased renal conversion of 25-HCC to active 1,25-DHCC. As the serum calcium concentration rises, the renal ability to reabsorb calcium may be exceeded, leading to increased urinary calcium concentration and the subsequent formation of calcium-phosphate and calcium-oxalate renal stones. Typically, this condition results from parathyroid adenomas but may also be caused by primary cell hyperplasia, primary chief-cell hyperplasia, or other carcinomas.[31,41]

Approximately 2% of patients treated with thiazide diuretics may develop hypercalcemia. Patients at risk are those with hyperparathyroidism. The mechanism appears to be multifactorial and includes enhanced renal reabsorption of calcium and decreased plasma volume.

The milk-alkali syndrome (Burnett's syndrome), rarely observed today, is another drug-related cause of hypercalcemia.[33] This syndrome occurs from a chronic high intake of milk or calcium products combined with an absorbable antacid (e.g., calcium carbonate, sodium bicarbonate, or magnesium hydroxide). This syndrome was more common in the past when milk or cream was used to treat gastric ulcers and before the advent of nonabsorbable antacids. Renal failure can occur as a result of calcium deposition in soft tissues.[33,42]

Hypercalcemia can also result from[28,40,41,43]:

- Excessive administration of IV calcium salts.
- Calcium supplements.
- Chronic immobilization.
- Paget's disease.
- Sarcoidosis.
- Hyperthyroidism.
- Acute adrenal insufficiency.
- Some respiratory diseases.
- Lithium-induced renal calcium reabsorption.
- Excessive vitamin D, vitamin A, or thyroid hormone, which increases intestinal absorption.
- Tamoxifen.
- Androgenic hormones.
- Estrogen.
- Progesterone.

Clinical diagnosis. Similar to hypocalcemia and other electrolyte disorders, the severity of the clinical manifestations of hypercalcemia depends on the acuteness of onset. Hypercalcemia can be a medical emergency, especially when serum concentrations rise above 14 mg/dL (>3.5 mmol/L). Symptoms associated with this condition often consist of vague GI complaints such as nausea, vomiting, abdominal pain, dyspepsia, and anorexia. More severe GI complications include peptic ulcer disease, possibly due to increased gastrin release, and acute pancreatitis.[43,44]

Severe hypercalcemic symptoms primarily involve the neuromuscular system (e.g., lethargy, obtundation, psychosis, cerebellar ataxia, and, in severe cases, coma and death). However, EKG changes and spontaneous ventricular arrhythmias may also be seen. It may also enhance the inotropic effects of digoxin, increasing the likelihood of cardiac arrhythmias.[35–38]

Renal function may be affected by hypercalcemia through the ability of calcium to inhibit the adenyl cyclase–cyclic adenosine monophosphate system that mediates the ADH effects on the collecting ducts. This inhibition results in diminished conservation of water by the kidneys. The renal effect is further compounded by diminished solute transport in the loop of Henle, leading to polyuria, nocturia and polydipsia.[28] Other chronic renal manifestations include nephrolithiasis, nephrocalcinosis, chronic interstitial nephritis, and renal tubular acidosis.

In addition, hypercalcemia can cause vasoconstriction of the renal vasculature, resulting in a decrease in renal blood flow and GFR. If hypercalcemia is allowed to progress, oliguric acute renal failure may ensue.[28] With an increased calcium-phosphate product (>70), soft-tissue calcification with the calcium-phosphate complex may occur.

The signs and symptoms described above are mostly seen in patients with severe hypercalcemia. With serum concentrations less than 13 mg/dL (3.2 mmol/L), most patients should be asymptomatic.

Causes of spurious laboratory results. False hypercalcemia can occur if the tourniquet is left in place too long when the blood specimen is drawn. This results from increased plasma-protein pooling in the phlebotomized arm. Falsely elevated calcium should be suspected if serum albumin is greater than 5 g/dL (>50 g/L). Table 7-12 contains the normal range values for tests related to calcium metabolism.

TABLE 7-12

Calcium (free)	4.6–5.2 mg/dL
Calcium (total)	8.5–10.5 mg/dL
1,25-DHCC	16–42 pg/mL
Phosphate	2.6–4.5 mg/dL
PTH	10–60 pg/mL
Urine calcium	0–300 mg/day
Urine hydroxyproline	10–50 mg/day (adults)
Urine phosphate	average: 1 g/day

Table 7-12. Normal Ranges for Tests Related to Calcium Metabolism

Phosphate

Normal range: 2.6–4.5 mg/dL or 0.84–1.45 mmol/L for adults

Many factors that influence serum calcium concentrations also affect serum phosphate, either directly or indirectly. Laboratory values for calcium and phosphate should, therefore, be interpreted together. Since phosphate exists as several organic and inorganic moieties in the body, some clinical laboratories simply report the phosphate value as phosphorus.

Physiology

Phosphate is a major intracellular anion with several functions. It is important for intracellular metabolism of proteins, fats, and carbohydrates and is a major component in phospholipid membranes, RNAs, nicotinamide diphosphate (an enzyme cofactor), cyclic adenine and guanine nucleotides (second messengers), and phosphoproteins. Another important function of phosphate is in the formation of high-energy bonds for the production of ATP, which is a source of energy for many cellular reactions. Phosphate is a component of 2,3-diphosphoglycerate (2,3-DPG), which regulates the release of oxygen from hemoglobin (Hgb) to tissues. In addition, phosphate has a regulatory role in the glycolysis and hydroxylation of cholecalciferol. It is also an important acid-base buffer.[35,40]

A balanced diet for adults usually contains about 800–1500 mg/day of phosphate. About two-thirds is actively absorbed from the small intestine. Some of the phosphate is absorbed passively with calcium and some is absorbed under the influence of 1,25-DHCC, which also increases the intestinal absorption of calcium. However, phosphate is the first of the two to be absorbed.[40]

Diminished phosphate absorption occurs when large quantities of calcium or aluminum are present in the intestines due to formation of insoluble phosphate compounds. The large quantities of calcium and aluminum may result from the consumption of antacids. In fact, for patients with chronic renal failure who have high serum phosphate concentrations, calcium- and aluminum-containing antacids are given with meals as phosphate binders to reduce intestinal phosphate absorption.[45]

Phosphate is widely distributed in the body throughout the

- Plasma.
- Extracellular fluid.
- Cell membrane structures.
- Intracellular fluid.
- Collagen.
- Bone.

Bone holds 85% of the body's phosphate. About 90% of plasma phosphate is filtered at the glomeruli, and the majority is actively reabsorbed at the proximal tubule. Some reabsorption also takes place in the loop of Henle, distal tubules, and possibly the collecting ducts.[31] The amount of phosphate excreted renally is, therefore, the amount filtered minus the amount reabsorbed. Increased urinary phosphate excretion can result from an increase in plasma volume and the action of PTH, which can block phosphate reabsorption throughout the nephron. In contrast, vitamin D_3 and its metabolites can directly stimulate proximal tubular phosphate reabsorption. In all, 90% of eliminated phosphate is excreted renally while the remainder is secreted into the intestines.[31,35,46] Renal handling of phosphate, especially the proximal tubules, therefore, plays an important role in maintaining the homeostatic balance of phosphate. Renal phosphate transport is active, saturable, and pH and sodium ion dependent. However, most changes in serum phosphate result from changes in either the GFR or the rate of tubular reabsorption.[2,31,35]

Serum phosphate and calcium concentrations as well as PTH and vitamin D levels are intimately related with each other. Serum phosphate indirectly controls PTH secretion via a negative feedback mechanism. With a decrease in the serum phosphate concentration, the conversion of vitamin D_3 to 1,25-DHCC increases (which increases serum concentrations of both phosphate and calcium). Both the intestinal absorption and renal reabsorption of phosphate is increased. The concomitant increase in serum calcium then directly decreases PTH secretion. This decrease in serum PTH concentration permits further increase in renal phosphate reabsorption.[30,31]

A true phosphate imbalance may be due to an abnormality in any of the previously discussed mechanisms and hormones for maintaining calcium and phosphate homeostasis. These abnormalities may include altered intestinal absorption, altered number or activity of osteoclast and osteoblast cells in bone, changes in renal reabsorption of calcium and phosphate, and IV infusions of calcium or phosphate salts.[35,40]

Hypophosphatemia

Hypophosphatemia indicates a serum phosphate concentration of less than 2.6 mg/dL (<0.84 mmol/L). Whereas hyperphosphatemia primarily occurs in renal failure, hypophosphatemia can occur as a result of renal dysfunction as well as other conditions. There following three clinical conditions are common causes of decreased serum phosphate concentrations:

1. Increased renal excretion.[40,47,48]
2. Intracellular shifting.
3. Decreased phosphate or vitamin D intake.[41,47,48]

To identify the etiology of hypophosphatemia, the serum and urine phosphate concentrations ought to be considered simultaneously. Low urine and serum phosphates indicate either a diminished phosphate intake or excessive use of phosphate-binding antacids. An increased urine phosphate suggests either hyperparathyroidism or renal tubular dysfunction. If the increased urine phosphate is accompanied by elevated serum calcium, the presence of primary hyperparathyroidism or decreased vitamin D metabolism must be considered.

Common causes. Hypophosphatemia is usually due to decreased renal reabsorption or increased GFR, shift of phosphate from extracellular to intracellular fluid, alcoholism, or malnutrition. Phosphate is required in total parenteral nutrition solutions to promote muscle growth and fat replacement and to replenish hepatic glycogen storage in malnourished patients. The infusion of concentrated glucose solution increases insulin secretion from the pancreas, which facilitates glucose and phosphate cell entry. Phosphate is used to form phosphorylated hexose intermediates during cellular utilization of glucose. An inadequate phosphate content in these nutrition fluids can decrease anabolism, glycolysis, ATP, and 2,3-DPG production.[48]

Infusion of concentrated glucose solutions, especially when accompanied by insulin, can produce hypophosphatemia by shifting phosphate intracellularly. This condition, known as refeeding syndrome, can occur when an inadequate amount of phosphate is given with the parenteral nutrition solutions; large amounts of phosphate are taken up by the newly produced cells during anabolism.

Hypophosphatemia can also occur during hyperkalemia treatment with insulin and dextrose. In addition, aluminum- and calcium-containing antacids, as well as magnesium hydroxide, are potent binders of intestinal phosphate.[45] Overuse of these agents can severely reduce serum phosphate concentrations in patients with normal renal function. Moreover, calcitonin, glucagon, and ß-adrenergic stimulants can decrease serum phosphate concentrations. Thiazide and loop diuretics can increase renal phosphate excretion. However, this effect is often insignificant clinically in otherwise healthy individuals.

Other conditions known to cause hypophosphatemia include nutritional recovery after starvation, treatment of diabetic ketoacidosis, decreased absorption or increased intestinal loss, alcohol withdrawal, diuretic phase of acute tubular necrosis, and prolonged respiratory alkalosis. To compensate for respiratory alkalosis, carbon dioxide shifts from intracellular to extracellular fluid. This shift increases the intracellular fluid pH, which activates glycolysis and intracellular phosphate trapping. Metabolic acidosis, in contrast, produces a minimal change in serum phosphate.

Uncommon causes. Burn patients often retain a great amount of sodium and water. During wound healing diuresis often ensues, which results in substantial loss of phosphate. Since anabolism also occurs during recovery, hypophosphatemia may be inevitable without proper replacement. Moderate reductions in serum phosphate can occur from prolonged nasogastric suctioning, gastrectomy, small bowel or pancreatic disease resulting in malabsorption, and impaired renal phosphate reabsorption of phosphate in patients with multiple myeloma, Fanconi syndrome, heavy-metal poisoning, amyloidosis, and nephrotic syndrome.[47,48]

Severe hypophosphatemia. Severe phosphate depletion (<1 mg/dL or <0.32 mmol/L) can occur during diabetic ketoacidosis. The resultant acidosis mobilizes bone, promotes intracellular organic substrate metabolism, and releases phosphate into the extracellular fluid. The glycosuria and ketonuria caused by diabetic ketoacidosis results in an osmotic diuresis that increases the urinary clearance of phosphate. The combined effects of these events may produce a normal serum phosphate concentration with severe intracellular deficiency. When the diabetic ketoacidosis is corrected with insulin, phosphate accompanies glucose to move intracellularly. Serum phosphate is usually reduced within 24 hr of treatment. As the acidosis is being corrected, there is further intracellular shifting of phosphate to result in profound hypophosphatemia. The accompanying volume repletion may exacerbate the problem further.

Clinical diagnosis. Patients with moderate reductions in serum phosphate (2–2.5 mg/dL or 0.64–0.81 mmol/L) are often asymptomatic. Neurological irritability may occur as the serum phosphate concentration drops below 2 mg/dL (<0.64 mmol/L). Severe hypophosphatemia is often associated with muscle weakness, rhabdomyolysis, paresthesia, hemolysis, platelet dysfunction, and cardiac and respiratory failure.

CNS effects often include encephalopathy, confusion, obtundation, seizures, and, ultimately, coma. The mechanism for these effects may involve decreased glucose utilization by the brain, decreased brain cell ATP, or cerebral hypoxia from increased oxygen-Hgb affinity, secondary to diminished erythrocyte 2,3-DPG content. This decreased content results in decreased glycolysis, which leads to decreased 2,3-DPG and ATP production. The decreased contents of 2,3-DPG and ATP result in an increased affinity of Hgb for oxygen, eventually leading to decreased tissue oxygenation. The ensuing cerebral hypoxia may explain the persistent coma often seen in patients with diabetic ketoacidosis. Hemolysis may occur but is rarely seen at serum phosphate concentrations greater than 0.5 mg/dL (>0.16 mmol/L).

Hyperphosphatemia

Hyperphosphatemia indicates a serum phosphate concentration greater than 4.5 mg/dL (>1.45 mmol/L). There are three basic causes for elevated serum phosphate concentration:

1. Decreased renal phosphate excretion.
2. Shift of phosphate from intracellular to extracellular fluid.
3. Increased intake of vitamin D or phosphate products (orally, rectally, or IV).

Elevated phosphate concentration may also result from reduced PTH secretion, increased body catabolism, and some malignant conditions (e.g., leukemias and lymphomas).[4,47,48]

Causes. The most common cause of hyperphosphatemia is renal dysfunction, which usually occurs as the GFR falls below 25 mL/min. Chronic renal failure can result in secondary hyperparathyroidism, which can further reduce renal phosphate clearance. The increase in serum phosphate concentration increases the risk for deposition of insoluble calcium-phosphate complex in soft tissues (i.e., metastatic calcification). This deposition reduces the serum concentration of ionized calcium and leads to increased PTH production and release. Sustained period of high PTH level leads to excessive bone resorption, which will severely weaken its structural integrity.[36,40]

Hyperphosphatemia can be caused by a shift of phosphate from intracellular to extracellular fluid. This shift of phosphate can occur in massive cell break down as a result of chemotherapy for leukemia or lymphoma, rhabdomyolysis, and during septic shock. In addition, hyperthyroidism can elevate serum phosphate by increasing bone resorption and PTH suppression and also by directly increasing renal tubular phosphate reabsorption.

Clinical diagnosis. Signs and symptoms of hyperphosphatemia commonly result from the accompanying hypocalcemia and hyperparathyroidism (see Hypocalcemia section). Renal function may diminish if hyperphosphatemia is left untreated. If renal failure occurs, phosphate clearance is further reduced to cause even greater increases in the serum phosphate concentration and further decline in the serum calcium concentration (Minicase 5).[36,40,45]

MINICASE 5

PAUL M., A 65-YEAR-OLD MAN, had a 1-week history of nausea, vomiting, and general malaise. His appetite had severely decreased over the past 2 months. He had a long-standing history of uncontrolled hypertension and diabetes mellitus as well as diabetic nephropathy, retinopathy, and neuropathy.

Paul M.'s current medications included levothyroxine 0.1 mg oral daily, metoclopramide 10 mg oral 3 times a day, and regular insulin subcutaneously twice a day. His physical examination revealed a BP of 160/99 mm Hg, diabetic retinopathic changes with laser scars bilaterally, and diminished sensation bilaterally below the knees.

Paul M.'s laboratory values were as follows: serum sodium 146 mEq/L (136–145 mEq/L), potassium 4.7 mEq/L (3.5–5.0 mEq/L), chloride 104 mEq/L (96–106 mEq/L), serum carbon dioxide content 15 mEq/L (24–30 mEq/L), SCr 7.9 mg/dL (0.7–1.5 mg/dL), BUN 92 mg/dL (8–20 mg/dL), and a random blood glucose of 181 mg/dL (70–110 mg/dL). On detection of his renal failure, additional laboratory tests were obtained: calcium 7.5 mg/dL (8.5–10.8 mg/dL), phosphate 9.1 mg/dL (2.6–4.5 mg/dL), total serum protein 5.2 g/dL (5.5–9.0 g/dL), albumin 3 g/dL (3.5–5 g/dL), and uric acid 8.9 mg/dL (3.4–7.0 mg/dL).

Paul M. was started on a daily peripheral hyperalimentation solution containing dextrose 5%, amino acids 3%, sodium chloride 50 mEq, potassium chloride 10 mEq, potassium phosphate 30 mEq (based on potassium), calcium gluconate 4.6 mEq, magnesium sulfate 8.1 mEq, and multivitamin supplements 10 mL. Over the next several days, he complained of finger numbness, tingling, and burning of extremities. Paul M. also experienced increasing confusion and fatigue. A neurological examination was positive for both Chvostek's and Trousseau's signs. Repeated laboratory tests showed substantial changes in serum calcium (6.1 mg/dL) and phosphate (10.4 mg/dL). The patient's intact serum PTH was 280 pg/mL (10–60 pg/mL).

Question: What subjective and objective data for Paul M. are consistent with a diagnosis of calcium and phosphate abnormalities? What are the potential etiologies of calcium-phosphate disorder in this patient?

Discussion: Paul M. has three laboratory abnormalities relating specifically to calcium-phosphate metabolism: (1) hypocalcemia, (2) hyperphosphatemia, and (3) severe hyperparathyroidism. He is exhibiting classic signs and symptoms of hypocalcemia, such as finger numbness, tingling, burning of extremities, confusion, fatigue, and positive Chvostek's and Trousseau's signs.

Chronic renal failure, as seen in Paul M., commonly is associated with hypocalcemia, hyperphosphatemia, hyperparathyroidism, and vitamin D deficiency. These calcium-phosphate abnormalities frequently lead to the secondary complication of renal osteodystrophy. As stated previously, no single mechanism is responsible for these abnormalities.

At earlier stages of his renal disease, Paul M.'s kidneys probably were retaining phosphate. As his serum phosphate concentration rose, his ionized calcium concentration fell and stimulated PTH release. This release led to secondary hyperparathyroidism. High concentrations of PTH reduced this patient's renal tubular reabsorption of phosphate and increased its excretion. Both his serum phosphate and calcium concentrations then returned to normal as a result of hyperparathyroidism (Figure 3).

As Paul M.'s renal disease worsened (GFR fell below 30 mL/min), his renal tubules ceased to respond adequately to his high serum PTH concentrations. Hyperphosphatemia developed. In response to the hypocalcemia that followed, calcium was mobilized from the bone by a PTH-mediated mechanism. However, this compensatory response obviously was not adequate since hypocalcemia and hyperphosphatemia persisted.

Although concentrations were not measured, this persistent hyperphosphatemia probably contributed to the diminished renal conversion of 25-HCC to its biologically active metabolite 1,25-DHCC. As a result, the gut absorption of dietary calcium was diminished. Vitamin D deficiency also contributed to hypocalcemia and mobilization of calcium from bone. The metabolic acidosis of renal failure potentially present in Paul M. also may contribute to a negative calcium balance in the bone.

Paul M. was relatively asymptomatic up to this point, primarily because these laboratory abnormalities developed chronically and were, therefore, better tolerated. When nausea and vomiting developed and his appetite decreased, his oral calcium intake probably was substantially reduced. This reduction potentially enhanced his malaise. During this period of malnutrition, the patient's serum albumin concentration also diminished, which further contributed to his hypocalcemia.

Since calcium is reported as total calcium and not as the free or ionized fraction, Paul M.'s total serum calcium concentration must be corrected for his serum albumin value. For every 1 g/dL reduction in serum albumin less than 4 g/dL, 0.8 mg/dL should be added to his serum calcium concentration. Therefore, when corrected for his serum albumin concentration of 3 g/dL, Paul M.'s first serum calcium value of 7.5 mg/dL is equivalent to a total concentration of 8.3 mg/dL. Likewise, his second serum calcium value of 6.1 mg/dL is equivalent to a total concentration of 6.9 mg/dL.

During hospitalization, the calcium content of Paul M.'s hyperalimentation solution was apparently not adequate for correcting or sustaining his serum calcium concentration. Therefore, the worsening of his hypocalcemia augmented his hyperparathyroidism and increased his serum phosphate concentration.

Causes of Spurious Laboratory Results

Hemolysis can occur during phlebotomy, which may lead to a falsely elevated serum phosphate concentration. If the serum is not separated soon after phlebotomy, phosphate may be falsely decreased as it is taken up by the cellular components of blood.

Similar to what may occur to specimens for potassium concentration determination, when the blood is allowed to clot with the use of nonheparinized tubes, phosphate may leach out of the platelets to result in falsely elevated concentration. In patients with thrombocytosis, phosphate concentrations should, therefore, be obtained from plasma rather than serum samples.

Serum phosphate may vary by 1–2 mg/dL (0.32–0.64 mmol/L) after meals. Meals rich in carbohydrates can reduce serum phosphate, and meals high in phosphate, such as diary products, can increase serum phosphate. When accurate assessment of the phosphate concentration is necessary, the blood specimens should be obtained from the patient after fasting.

TRACE ELEMENTS

Copper

Normal range: 65–155 µg/dL (10–24.6 µmol/L) for serum copper

18–40mg/dL for ceruloplasmin

0.47 ± 0.06 mg/g for erythrocyte superoxide dismutase (SOD)

Physiology

The relationship between copper homeostasis and human diseases dated backed to 1912 shortly after Wilson's disease was described. In the early 1930s, a relationship between copper deficiency and anemia was suspected, although the hypothesis was not well-accepted and proven at that time. Subsequently, the physiological functions of copper were better understood and its link to pathogenesis was better appreciated in the 1970s. An official dietary copper recommendation and adequate daily dietary intake was introduced the first time in 1979.

Copper plays an integral part in the synthesis and functions of many circulating proteins and enzymes. In addition, copper is an essential factor for the formation of connective tissues, such as the cross-linking of collagen and elastin. Copper also shares similar physiological functions with iron.[49] In the central nervous system, copper is required for the formation or maintenance of myelin and other phospholipids. Cuproenzymes (copper-dependent enzymes) are crucial in the metabolism of catecholamines. For example, the functions of dopamine hydroxylase and monoamine oxidase are impaired by copper deficiency. Copper also affects the function of tyrosinase function in melanin synthesis, which is responsible for the pigmentation of skin, hair, and eyes. Deficiency of tyrosinase results in albinism. Other physiological functions of copper include thermal regulation, glucose metabolism, blood clotting (e.g., factor V function), and protection of cells against oxidative damage.[50,51]

The normal adult daily intake of copper, from both animal and plant sources, is 2–3 mg. Plant copper is in the inorganic (free ionic) form, while meat (animal) copper is in the form of cuproproteins (copper-protein complex). Inorganic copper is absorbed in the upper portion of the GI tract (stomach and proximal duodenum) under acidic conditions. Cuproprotein copper is absorbed below the pancreatic duct after digestion. The absorption of copper from the GI tract is saturable. The oral bioavailability of copper ranges from 15–97% and shows a negative correlation with the amount of copper present in the diet.

Once absorbed, copper is bound to a mucosal copper-binding protein called *metallothionein* (a sulfur-rich, metal-binding protein present in intestinal mucosa). From this protein, copper is slowly released into the circulation, where it is absorbed by the liver and other tissues.[50] Animal data suggest that the liver serves as the ultimate depot for copper storage.

Copper absorption may be reduced by a high intake of zinc (>20 mg/day), ascorbic acid, and dietary fiber. Zinc may induce the synthesis of intestinal metallothionein and form a barrier to copper ion absorption.[50,51]

The normal adult body contains 75–150 mg of copper, which is significantly lower compared with other trace elements such as zinc and iron. Approximately one-third of the total body copper is found in the liver and brain at high tissue concentrations.[52] Another one-third is located in the muscles at low tissue concentrations. The rest is found in the heart, spleen, kidneys, and blood (erythrocytes and neutrophils).[50,52]

In the plasma, copper is highly bound (~95%) to an α_2-glycoprotein to form ceruloplasmin (also known as ferroxidase I), a blue copper protein.[49] This protein contains 6–7 copper atoms per molecule. The fraction of plasma copper associated with ceruloplasmin seems to be relatively constant for the same individual. But a significant inter-individual variation is present. The remainder of the plasma copper is bound to albumin and amino acids or is free.[50,52] Copper is eliminated mainly by biliary excretion (average 25 µg/kg/day), with only 0.5–3% of daily intake found in the urine.[50]

Ceruloplasmin is considered the most reliable indicator of copper status because of its large and relatively stable binding capacity with plasma copper. Therefore, when evaluating copper status in the body, ceruloplasmin concentration should be assessed together with plasma copper concentration.

Hypocupremia

Copper deficiency is relatively uncommon in humans.[51] Hypocupremia usually occurs in infants with chronic diarrhea or malabsorption syndrome or low-birth-weight infants fed with milk (rather than formulas).[49,51,53] Premature infants, who typically have low copper stores, are at a higher risk for developing copper deficiency under these circumstances.[50]

Copper deficiency can also occur in patients receiving long-term parenteral nutrition parenteral nutrition. Certain malabsorption syndromes (e.g., celiac disease and ulcerative colitis), protein-wasting enteropathies, and nephrotic syndrome may also cause copper deficiency. However, symptomatic deficiency is rare.[49,53] A vegetarian diet may also be a risk factor because (1) some major food sources of copper are meat, and (2) plant sources have a high-fiber content that may interfere with copper absorption.[49]

Prolonged hypocupremia leads to a syndrome of neutropenia and iron-deficiency anemia correctable with copper.[53] The anemia is normocytic or microcytic and hypochromic. It is due mainly to poor iron absorption and ineffective heme incorporation of iron.[45,52] Copper deficiency can affect any system or organ whose enzymes require copper for proper functioning. As such, copper deficiency may lead to abnormal glucose tolerance, arrhythmias, hypercholesterolemia, atherosclerosis, depressed immune function, defective connective tissue formation, demineralization of bones, and pathological fractures.[51]

There are two well-known genetic defects associated with impaired copper metabolism in humans. Menkes' syndrome (also called kinky- or steely-hair syndrome) is an X-linked disorder that occurs in 1 out of every 50,000 to 100,000 live births. This disease leads to defective copper absorption, and the patients are usually deceased by the age of 3. Patients with Menkes' syndrome have reduced copper concentrations in the blood, liver, and brain.[49,51] These patients (mostly children) suffer from slow growth and retardation, defective keratinization and pigmentation of hair, hypothermia, and degenerative changes in the aortic elastin and neurons. Progressive nerve degeneration in the brain results in intellectual deterioration, hypotonia, and seizures. However, anemia and neutropenia, hallmark symptoms of nutritional copper deficiency, are not found in Menkes' diseases. Administration of parenteral copper increases serum copper and ceruloplasmin concentrations, but it seems to have no effect in slowing disease progression.

Wilson's disease is an autosomal recessive disease of copper storage. Its occurrence is uncertain but is believed to be less frequent than Menkes' disease. Wilson's disease appears to be associated with altered copper catabolism and excretion of ceruloplasmin copper into the bile. It is associated with elevated urinary copper loss and low plasma ceruloplasmin and copper concentrations. However, copper deposition occurs in the liver, brain, and cornea. If untreated, significant copper accumulation in these organs will eventually lead to irreversible damage such as cirrhosis and neurological impairment. Interestingly, treatment with dietary adjustment of copper intake does not seem to be effective. Chelation therapy using D-penicillamine is much more effective in preventing copper deposition. Oral zinc supplementation has also been used to decrease excessive copper accumulation.

Hypercupremia

Copper excess is not common in humans and usually occurs with a deliberate attempt to ingest large quantities of copper. The exact amount of copper that results in toxicity is unknown. Acute or long-term ingestions of greater than 15 mg of elemental copper may lead to symptomatic copper poisoning.[52] It has also been reported that drinking water with 2–3 mg/L of copper is associated with hepatotoxicity in infants. Like other metallic poisonings, acute copper poisoning leads to nausea, vomiting, intestinal cramps, and diarrhea.[52] Larger ingestions lead to shock, hepatic necrosis, intravascular hemolysis, renal impairment, coma, and death.[53] Patients with primary biliary cirrhosis and biliary atresia tend to have very high intrahepatic copper concentration.[49,50,53] In addition, since copper has an important role in the neurological system, it has been suggested that copper-induced free radical-induced neurodegeneration may be a contributive factor for Alzheimer's disease. There is no known treatment for hypercupremia.

Zinc

Normal range: 70–130 μg/dL or 10.7–19.9 μmol/L

Physiology

Next to iron, zinc is the most abundant trace element in the body. It is an essential nutrient that is a constituent of, or a cofactor to, many enzymes. These metalloenzymes participate in the metabolism of carbohydrates, proteins, lipids, and nucleic acids.[50] As such, zinc influences[50,53]

- Tissue growth and repair.
- Cell membrane stabilization.
- Bone collagenase activity and collagen turnover.
- Immune response, especially T cell mediated response.
- Sensory control of food intake.
- Spermatogenesis and gonadal maturation.
- Normal testicular function.

The normal adult body contains 1.5–2.5 g of zinc.[51] Beside supplementation with zinc capsules, dietary intake is only source of zinc for humans. Food sources of zinc include meat products, oysters, and legumes.[50] Food zinc is largely bound to proteins and released below the common duct for absorption by the ileum. Ionic zinc found in zinc supplements is absorbed in the duodenum due to a lower pH in that region.[50] Body zinc stores control, to some extent, the percentage of zinc that is absorbed from food and mineral supplements. Foods rich in calcium, dietary fiber, or phytate may interfere with zinc absorption, as can folic acid supplements.[50]

After absorption, zinc is transported from the small intestine to the portal circulation where it binds to proteins such as albumin, transferrin, and globulins.[50] Circulating zinc is bound mostly to serum proteins; two-thirds are loosely bound to albumin and prealbumin while one-third is bound tightly to α_2-macroglobulin.[53] Only 2–3% (3 mg) of zinc is either in free ionic form or bound to amino acids.[50]

Zinc distributes to many organs. Tissues high in zinc include the liver, pancreas, spleen, lungs, eyes (retina, iris, cornea, and lens), prostate, skeletal muscle, and bone. Because of their mass, skeletal muscle (60–62%) and bone (20–28%) have the highest zinc contents of body tissues.[50] Only 2–4% of total body zinc is contained in the liver. In blood, 85% is in erythrocytes, although each leukocyte contains 25 times the zinc content of an erythrocyte.[51]

Although plasma zinc concentration can be measured, it is a poor indicator of total body zinc status. Since 98% of total body zinc is present in tissues and end organs, plasma zinc concentration tends to be maintained by continuous shifting from intracellular sources. Additionally, metabolic stress, such as infection, acute myocardial infarction, and critical illnesses increase intracellular shifting of zinc to the liver and lower serum zinc concentrations, even when total body zinc is normal. Conversely, serum zinc concentrations may be normal during starvation or wasting syndromes due to release of zinc from tissues and cells.[50] Therefore, serum/plasma zinc concentration alone has little clinical meaning. It has been suggested that the rate of zinc turnover in the plasma provides better assessment of the body zinc status. This may be achieved by measuring 24–hr zinc loss in body fluids (e.g., urine and stool). However, this approach is rarely practical for critically ill patients as renal failure is often present. Alternatively, some investigators have suggested determining zinc turnover and mobilization by adjusting plasma zinc concentration with serum α_2-macroglobulin and albumin concentrations.[56,57] Others suggest monitoring the functional indices of zinc—such as erythrocyte alkaline phosphatase, serum superoxide dismutase, and lymphocyte 5' nucleotidase—to evaluate bodily zinc status. However, the clinical validity of these test require further investigation.

Zinc undergoes substantial enteropancreatic recirculation and is excreted primarily in pancreatic and intestinal secretions. Zinc is also lost dermally through sweat, hair and nail growth, and skin shedding. Except in certain disease states, only 2% of zinc is lost in the urine.[50]

Hypozincemia

In Western countries, zinc deficiency is rare from inadequate intake. Persons with serum zinc concentrations below 70 μg/dL (<10.7 μmol/L) are at an increased risk for developing symptomatic zinc deficiency. Given the caveats of measuring serum zinc concentrations in certain disease states, response to zinc supplements may be the only way of diagnosing this deficiency. In many chronic diseases, it is unclear whether zinc deficiency is clinical or subclinical due to reduced protein binding.[53] Conditions leading to deficiency may be divided into five classes (Table 7-13)[50,53]:

1. Low intake.
2. Decreased absorption.
3. Increased utilization.
4. Increased loss.
5. Unknown causes.

The most likely candidates for zinc deficiency are infants; rapidly growing adolescents; menstruating, lactating, or pregnant women; persons with low meat intake; institutionalized patients;

TABLE 7-13

LOW INTAKE
Anorexia
Nutritional deficiencies
Alcoholism
Chronic renal failure
Premature infants
Some vegetarian diets
Therapy with hyperalimentation solutions
DECREASED ABSORPTION
Acrodermatitis enteropathica
Malabsorption syndromes
INCREASED UTILIZATION
Adolescence
Lactation
Menstruation
Pregnancy
INCREASED LOSS
Alcoholism
β-Thalassemia
Cirrhosis
Diabetes mellitus
Diarrhea
Diuretic therapy
Enterocutaneous fistula drainage
Exercise (long term, strenuous)
Glucagon
Loss of enteropancreatic recycling
Nephrotic syndrome
Protein-losing enteropathies
Sickle cell anemia
Therapy with hyperalimentation solutions
UNKNOWN CAUSES
Arthritis and other inflammatory diseases
Down syndrome

Table 7-13. Etiologies of Zinc Deficiency

SIGNS

Acrodermatitis enteropathica

Anemia

Anergy to skin test antigens

Complicated pregnancy

    Excess bleeding

    Maternal infection

    Premature or stillborn birth

    Spontaneous abortion

    Toxemia

Decreased basal metabolic rate

Decreased circulating thyroxine (T_4) concentration

Decreased lymphocyte count and function

Effect on fetus, infant, or child

    Congenital defects of skeleton, lungs, and CNS

    Fetal disturbances

    Growth retardation

    Hypogonadism

Impaired neutrophil function

Impairment and delaying of platelet aggregation

Increased susceptibility to dental caries

Increased susceptibility to infections

Mental disturbance

Pica

Poor wound healing

Short stature in children

Skeletal deformities

SYMPTOMS

Acne and recurrent furunculosis

Ataxia

Decreased appetite

Defective night vision

Hypogeusia

Hyposmia

Impotence

Mouth ulcers

Table 7-14. Signs and Symptoms of Zinc Deficiency

and patients on zinc-deficient parenteral nutrition solutions.[53] Acrodermatitis enteropathica is an autosomal, recessive disorder involving zinc malabsorption that occurs in infants of Italian, Armenian, and Iranian heritage. It is characterized by severe dermatitis, chronic diarrhea, emotional disturbances, and growth retardation.[50] Examples of malabsorption syndromes that may lead to zinc deficiency include Crohn's disease, ulcerative colitis, celiac sprue (gluten enteropathy), and short-bowel syndrome.

Excessive zinc may be lost in the urine (hyperzincuria), as occurs in alcoholism, ß-thalassemia, diabetes mellitus, diuretic therapy, nephrotic syndrome, sickle cell anemia, and therapy with parenteral nutrition. Severe or prolonged diarrhea (e.g., inflammatory bowel diseases and graft vs. host disease) may lead to significant zinc loss in the stool. Excessive zinc may be lost through cutaneous route in burn patients and athletes who routinely perform strenuous exercises.[50,53] Patients with end-stage liver disease frequently have depleted zinc storage due to decreased functional hepatic cell mass.

Because zinc is involved in a diverse group of enzymes, its deficiency manifests in numerous organs and physiological systems (Table 7-14).[50] Dysgeusia (lack of taste) and hyposmia (diminished smell acuity) are common. Pica is a pathological craving for specific food or nonfood substances (e.g., geophagia). Chronic zinc deficiency, as occurs in acrodermatitis enteropathica, leads to growth retardation, anemia, hypogonadism, hepatosplenomegaly, and impaired wound healing. Additional signs and symptoms of acrodermatitis enteropathica include diarrhea; vomiting; alopecia; skin lesions in oral, anal, and genital areas; paronychia; nail deformity; emotional lability; photophobia; blepharitis; conjunctivitis; and corneal opacities.[50,53]

Hyperzincemia

Zinc is one of the least toxic trace elements.[53] Clinical manifestations of excess zinc occur with chronic, high doses of a zinc supplement. However, patients with Wilson's disease who commonly take high doses of zinc rarely show signs of toxicity. This situation may be due to stabilization of serum zinc concentrations during high-dose administration.[50] As much as 12 g of zinc sulfate (>2700 mg of elemental zinc) taken over 2 days has caused drowsiness, lethargy, and increases in serum lipase and amylase concentrations. Nausea, vomiting, and diarrhea also may occur.[50]

Serum zinc concentrations must be measured using nonhemolyzed samples. Erythrocytes and leukocytes, like many other cells, are rich in zinc. When they are allowed to hemolyze in the tube (e.g., too small a needle is used to draw the sample, tourniquet is too tight, or specimen stands too long or is mishandled), these cells release zinc into the specimen in quantities large enough to produce misleading results. This phenomenon can also occur when the specimen is allowed to clot (with nonheparinized tubes).[50]

Manganese

Normal range: clinically relevant plasma concentration not validated

Physiology

Manganese is an essential trace element that serves as a cofactor for numerous diverse enzymes involved in carbohydrate, protein, and lipid metabolism; protection of cells from free radicals; steroid biosynthesis; and metabolism of biogenic amines.[54] Interestingly, manganese deficiency does not affect the functions of most of these enzymes, presumably because magnesium may substitute for manganese in most instances.[53] In animals, manganese is required for normal bone growth, lipid metabolism, reproduction, and CNS regulation.[51]

Manganese has an important role in the normal function of the brain, primarily through its effect on biogenic amine metabolism. This effect may be responsible for the relationship between brain concentration of manganese and catecholamine.[54]

The manganese content of the adult body is 10–20 mg. Manganese homeostasis is regulated through the control of its absorption and excretion.[54] Plants are the primary source of food manganese since animal tissues have low contents.[54] Manganese is absorbed from the small intestine by a mechanism similar to that of iron.[51] However, only 3–4% of the ingested manganese is absorbed. Dietary iron and phytate may affect manganese absorption.[49]

Human and animal tissues have low manganese content.[54] Tissues relatively high in manganese are the bone, liver, pancreas, and pituitary gland.[49,54] Most circulating manganese is loosely bound to the β_1-globulin transmanganin, a transport protein similar to transferrin.[51,53] In situations of overexposure, excess manganese accumulates in the liver and brain, causing severe neuromuscular signs and symptoms.[49]

Manganese is excreted primarily in biliary and pancreatic juices. In manganese overload, other GI routes of elimination may also be used. Little manganese is lost in urine.[53,54]

Manganese Deficiency

Due to its relative abundance in plant sources, manganese deficiency is rare among the general population.[49] Deficiency normally occurs after several months of deliberate manganese omission from the diet.[53,54] Little information is available regarding serum manganese concentrations and disease states in humans.[53]

Information from the signs and symptoms of manganese deficiency comes from experimental subjects who intentionally followed low-manganese diets for many months. Their signs and symptoms included weight loss, slow hair and nail growth, color change in hair and beard, transient dermatitis, hypocholesterolemia, and hypotriglyceridemia.[54]

Adults and children with convulsive disorders have lower mean serum manganese concentrations than normal subjects, although a cause-and-effect relationship has not been established. However, serum manganese concentrations correlate with seizure frequency.[54] Animals deficient in manganese show defective growth, skeletal malformation, ataxia, reproductive abnormalities, and disturbances in lipid metabolism.[49,53]

Manganese Excess

Manganese is one of the least toxic trace elements.[53] Its excess primarily occurs through inhalation of manganese compounds (e.g., manganese mines).[54] Since excess drug accumulates in the liver and brain, severe neuromuscular manifestations occur. They include encephalopathy and profound neurological disturbances mimicking Parkinson's disease.[49,53,54] These manifestations are not surprising since metabolism of biogenic amines is altered in both manganese excess and Parkinson's disease. Other signs and symptoms include anorexia, apathy, headache, impotence, and speech disturbances.[53] Inhalation of manganese products may lead to manganese pneumonitis.[54]

Chromium

Normal range: clinical implication unknown

Physiology

The main physiological role of chromium is as a cofactor for insulin.[55] In its organic form, chromium potentiates the action of endogenous and exogenous insulin, presumably by augmenting its adherence to cell membranes.[49] The organic form is in the dinicotinic acid-glutathione complex or glucose tolerance factor (GTF).[51] Chromium is the metal portion of GTF; with insulin, GTF affects the metabolism of glucose, cholesterol, and triglycerides.[53] Therefore, chromium is important for glucose tolerance, glycogen synthesis, amino acid transport, and protein synthesis. Chromium is also involved in the activation of several enzymes.[51]

The adult body contains an average of 5 mg of chromium.[53] Food sources of chromium include brewer's yeast, spices, vegetable oils, unrefined sugar, liver, kidneys, beer, meat, dairy products, and wheat germ.[50,51] GTF is present in the diet and can be synthesized from inorganic trivalent chromium (Cr^{+3}) available in food and dietary supplements.[50] Chromium is absorbed via a common pathway with zinc; its degree of absorption is inversely related to dietary intake, varying from 0.5 to 2%.[49,50] Absorption of Cr^{+3} from GTF is 10–25%, but the absorption is only 1% for inorganic chromium.[51]

Chromium circulates as free Cr^{3+}, bound to transferrin and other proteins, and as the GTF complex.[50,53] GTF is the biologically active moiety and is more important than total serum chromium concentration.[53] Trivalent chromium accumulates in the hair, kidneys, skeleton, liver, spleen, lungs, testes, and large intestine. GTF concentrates in insulin-responsive tissues such as the liver.[50,51]

The metabolism of chromium is not well-understood for several reasons[51]:

- Low concentrations in tissues.
- Difficulty in analyzing chromium in biological fluids and tissue samples.
- Presence of different chromium forms in food.

Homeostasis is controlled by release of chromium from GTF and by dietary absorption.[50] The kidneys are the main route of elimination.[53] The urinary excretion of chromium is constant despite variability in the fraction absorbed. However, excretion increases after glucose or insulin administration.[50,53] Insulin, or a stimulus for insulin release, can mobilize chromium from its stores. This increased release in chromium then is lost in the urine. Therefore, circulating insulin controls the daily loss and requirement of chromium.[55]

Chromium Deficiency

It is important to stress that body chromium status cannot be reliably assessed.[50] Serum or plasma chromium may not be in equilibrium with other pools. As with other trace elements, the risk for developing deficiency may be increased in patients receiving prescribed nourishment low in chromium content (e.g., parenteral nutrition solutions).[55] Marginal deficiencies or defects in utilization of chromium may be present in the elderly, patients with diabetes, or patients with atherosclerotic coronary artery disease.[50] The hepatic stores of chromium decrease 10-fold in the elderly, suggesting a predisposition to deficiency. Since chromium is involved in lipid and cholesterol metabolism, its deficiency is a suspected risk factor for the development of atherosclerosis.[50,55]

Urinary losses of chromium due to hyperglycemia, coupled with marginal intake, predispose to deficiency that worsens glucose tolerance metabolism.[55] This mechanism is suspected for chromium deficiency in patients with Type II diabetes mellitus.[50,55] Finally, multiparous women are at a higher risk than nulliparous women for becoming chromium deficient because, over time, chromium intake may not be adequate to meet fetal needs and maintain a mother's stores.[55]

The manifestation of chromium deficiency may involve insulin resistance and disturbance in glucose metabolism. Such abnormalities may be divided into three stages:

1. Glucose intolerance occurs but is masked by a compensatory increase in insulin release.
2. Impaired glucose tolerance and disturbance in lipid metabolism are clinically evident.
3. Marked insulin resistance and manifestations of diabetes' unresponsiveness to insulin are evident.[55]

However, there is no conclusive report supporting the benefit of chromium supplementation in patients with diabetes or in those who with impaired glucose metabolism.

Chromium deficiency may lead to hypercholesterolemia and, as a result, serve as a risk factor for development of atherosclerotic disease.[50] Low chromium tissue concentrations have been associated with cardiovascular disease, although a cause-and-effect relationship has not been established. Likewise, a negative correlation has been established between cardiovascular morbidity and mortality and chromium intake.[55]

Chromium Excess

Chromium has very low toxicity. As such, information is lacking about the clinical significance of a high body chromium content.

SUMMARY

Hyponatremia and hypernatremia may be associated with high, normal, or low total body sodium. Hyponatremia may be due to abnormal accumulation of water in the intravascular space (dilutional hyponatremia), a decline in both extracellular water and sodium, or a reduction in total body sodium with the water balance remaining normal. Hypernatremia is most common in patients with either an impaired thirst mechanism (e.g., neurohypophyseal lesion) or an inability to replace water depleted through normal insensible losses or from renal or GI losses. Signs and symptoms of a sodium and water imbalance mostly involve the neurological system. The most common symptom of hyponatremia is confusion. However, if sodium continues to fall, seizure, coma, and death may result. Thirst is a major symptom of hypernatremia; an elevated urine specific gravity, indicating concentrated urine, is uniformly observed.

Hypokalemia and hyperkalemia may indicate either a true or an apparent (due to transcellular shifting) potassium imbalance. Hypokalemia can occur due to excessive loss from the kidneys (diuretics) or GI tract (vomiting). The most serious manifestation involves the cardiovascular system (i.e., cardiac arrhythmias). Renal impairment, usually in the presence of high intake, commonly causes hyperkalemia. Like hypokalemia, the most serious clinical manifestations of hyperkalemia involve the cardiovascular system.

A serum chloride concentration serves as a confirmatory test to identify fluid balance and acid-base abnormalities. Hypochloremia may be diuretic induced and is due to the concurrent loss of sodium and contraction alkalosis. Hyperchloremia may occur with parenteral nutrition solutions with a chloride:sodium ratio greater than 1. Signs and symptoms associated with these conditions are related to the fluid status or acid-base balance and underlying causes rather than to chloride itself.

Hypomagnesemia usually results from excessive loss from the GI tract (e.g., nasogastric suction, biliary loss, or fecal fistula) or from the kidneys (e.g., diuresis). Magnesium depletion is usually associated with neuromuscular symptoms such as weakness, muscle fasciculation with tremor, tetany, and increased reflexes. Increased magnesium intake in the presence of renal dysfunction commonly causes hypermagnesemia. Neuromuscular signs and symptoms opposite those caused by hypomagnesemia are observed.

The most common causes of true hypocalcemia are disorders of vitamin D metabolism and PTH production. In acute settings, hypocalcemia can be a medical emergency and lead to cardiac arrhythmias and tetany. Symptoms primarily involve the neuromuscular system.

The most common causes of hypercalcemia are malignancy and primary hyperparathyroidism. In acute settings, hypercalcemia can be a medical emergency and lead to cardiac arrhythmias. Symptoms often consist of vague GI complaints such as nausea, vomiting, abdominal pain, anorexia, constipation, and diarrhea.

The most common causes of hypophosphatemia are decreased intake and increased renal loss. Although mild hypophosphatemia is usually asymptomatic, severe depletion (<1 mg/dL or <0.32 mmol/L) is typically associated with muscle weakness, rhabdomyolysis, paresthesia, hemolysis, platelet dysfunction, and cardiac and respiratory failure. The most common cause of hyperphosphatemia is renal dysfunction, usually occurring as the GFR falls below 25 mL/min. Signs and symptoms of this condition are due primarily to the hypocalcemia and hyperparathyroidism that often ensue.

Hypocupremia is uncommon in humans but can occur in infants, especially those born prematurely, those who have chronic diarrhea or a malabsorption syndrome, or those whose diet consists mostly of milk. Prolonged hypocupremia leads to a syndrome of neutropenia and iron-deficiency anemia correctable with copper.

Copper excess is not common in humans and usually occurs with a deliberate attempt to ingest large quantities. Like other metallic poisonings, acute copper poisoning leads to nausea and vomiting, intestinal cramps, and diarrhea.

Likely candidates for zinc deficiency are infants; rapidly growing adolescents; menstruating, lactating, or pregnant women; persons with low meat intake; institutionalized patients; and patients on parenteral nutrition solutions. Because zinc is involved with a diverse group of enzymes, its deficiency manifests in numerous organs and physiological systems. Zinc excess occurs with chronic, high doses of a zinc supplement. Signs and symptoms include nausea, vomiting, diarrhea, drowsiness, lethargy, and increases in serum lipase and amylase concentrations.

Manganese deficiency normally occurs after several months of deliberate omission from the diet. Signs and symptoms include weight loss, slow hair and nail growth, color change in hair and beard, transient dermatitis, hypocholesterolemia, and hypotriglyceridemia. Manganese excess primarily occurs through inhalation of manganese compounds (e.g., manganese mines). Due to excess accumulation, severe neuromuscular manifestations occur, including encephalopathy and profound neurological disturbances mimicking Parkinson's disease. Inhalation of manganese products may lead to manganese pneumonitis.

The risk for developing chromium deficiency increases in patients receiving prescribed nourishment low in chromium content (e.g., parenteral nutrition solutions). The main manifestations of deficiency involve insulin resistance and disturbance in glucose metabolism.

REFERENCES

1. Sterns RH, Spital A, Clark EC. Disorders of water balance. In: Kokko JP, Tannen RL, eds. *Fluids and Electrolytes*. 3rd ed. Philadelphia, PA: W. B. Saunders; 1996: 63–109.
2. Guyton AC, Hall JE. *Textbook of Medical Physiology*. 10th ed. Philadelphia, PA: W. B. Saunders; 2001.
3. Berl T, Schrier RW. Disorders of water metabolism. In: Schrier RW, ed. *Renal and Electrolyte Disorders*. 6th ed. Philadelphia, PA: Lippincott Williams & Wilkins; 2003: 1–63.
4. Rose BD. *Clinical Physiology of Acid-Base and Electrolyte Disorders*. 5th ed. New York, NY: McGraw-Hill; 2001.
5. Briggs JP, Singh IIJ, Sawaya BE, et al. Disorders of salt balance. In: Kokko JP, Tannen RL, eds. *Fluids and Electrolytes*. 3rd ed. Philadelphia, PA: W. B. Saunders; 1996: 3–62.
6. Halperin ML, Goldstein MB, eds. *Fluid, Electrolyte, and Acid-Base Physiology: A Problem-Based Approach*. 2nd ed. Philadelphia, PA: W. B. Saunders; 1994.
7. Zull DN. Disorders of potassium metabolism. *Emerg Med Clin North Am*. 1989; 7:771–94.
8. Oh MS, Carroll HJ. Electrolyte and acid-base disorders. In: Chernow B, ed. *The Pharmacologic Approach to the Critically Ill Patient*. 3rd ed. Baltimore, MD: Williams & Wilkins; 1994: 957–68.
9. Peterson LN, Levi M. Disorders of potassium metabolism. In: Schrier RW, ed. *Renal and Electrolyte Disorders*. 6th ed. Philadelphia, PA: Lippincott Williams & Wilkins; 2003: 171–215.
10. Tannen RL. Potassium disorders. In: Kokko JP, Tannen RL, eds. *Fluids and Electrolytes*. 3rd ed. W. B. Saunders; 1996: 111–99.
11. Rose BD. Diuretics. *Kidney Int*. 1991; 39:336–52.
12. Williams ME. Endocrine crises. Hyperkalemia. *Crit Care Clin*. 1991; 7:155–74.
13. Freedman BI, Burkart JM. Endocrine crises: hypokalemia. *Crit Care Clin*. 1991; 7:143–53.
14. The seventh report of the Joint National Committee on Prevention, Detection, Evaluation, and Treatment of High Blood Pressure: The JNC 7 Report. *JAMA*. 2003; 289:2560–72.
15. Siegel D, Hulley SB, Black DM, et al. Diuretics, serum and intracellular electrolyte levels, and ventricular arrhythmias in hypertensive men. *JAMA*. 1992; 267:1083–9.
16. Moser M. Current hypertension management: separating fact from fiction. *Cleve Clin J Med*. 1993; 60:27–37.
17. Papademetriou V, Burris JF, Notargiacomo A, et al. Thiazide therapy is not a cause of arrhythmia in patients with systemic hypertension. *Arch Intern Med*. 1988; 148:1272–6.
18. Ellison DH. Diuretic drugs and the treatment of edema: from clinic to bench and back again. *Am J Kidney Dis*. 1994; 23:623–43.
19. Shapiro JI, Kaehny WD. Pathogenesis and management of metabolic acidosis and alkalosis. In: Schrier RW, ed. *Renal and Electrolyte Disorders*. 6th ed. Philadelphia, PA: Lippincott Williams & Wilkins; 2003: 115–153.
20. Kaehny WD. Pathogenesis and management of respiratory and mixed acid-base disorders. In: Schrier RW, ed. *Renal and Electrolyte Disorders*. 6th ed. Philadelphia, PA: Lippincott Williams & Wilkins; 2003: 154–70.
21. Koch SM, Taylor RW. Chloride ion in intensive care medicine. *Crit Care Med*. 1992; 20:227–40.
22. Alfrey AC. Normal and abnormal magnesium metabolism. In: Schrier RW, ed. *Renal and Electrolyte Disorders*. 6th ed. Philadelphia, PA: Lippincott Williams & Wilkins; 2003: 278–302.
23. Salem M, Munoz R, Chernow B. Hypomagnesemia in critical illness: a common and clinically important problem. *Crit Care Clin*. 1991; 7:225–52.
24. Rude RK. Magnesium disorders. In: Kokko JP, Tannen RL, eds. *Fluids and Electrolytes*. 3rd ed. Philadelphia, PA: W. B. Saunders; 1996: 421–45.
25. Ghamdi SM, Cameron EC, Sutton RA. Magnesium deficiency: pathophysiologic and clinical overview. *Am J Kidney Dis*. 1994; 24:737–52.
26. Berkelhammer C, Bear RA. A clinical approach to common electrolyte problems: hypomagnesemia. *Can Med Assoc J*. 1985; 132:360–8.
27. Van-Hook JW. Endocrine crises: hypermagnesemia. *Crit Care Clin*. 1991; 7:215–23.
28. Kumar R. Calcium disorders. In: Kokko JP, Tannen RL, eds. *Fluids and Electrolytes*. 3rd ed. Philadelphia, PA: W. B. W. B. Saunders; 1996: 391–419.
29. Zelis R, Moore R. Recent insights into the calcium channels. *Circulation*. 1989; 80(suppl IV):14–6.
30. Brown AJ, Dusso AS, Slatopolsky E. Vitamin D analogues for secondary hyperparathyroidism. *Nephrol Dial Transplant*. 2002; 17(suppl)10:10–9.

31. Hruska KA, Slatopolsky E. Disorders of phosphorus, calcium, and magnesium metabolism. In: Schrier RW, Gottschalk CW, eds. *Diseases of the Kidney.* 7th ed. Philadelphia, PA: Lippincott Williams & Wilkins; 2001: 2607–60.

32. Slatopolsky E, Lopez-Hilker S, Delmez J, et al. The parathyroid-calcitriol axis in health and chronic renal failure. *Kidney Int.* 1990; 29(suppl):S41–7.

33. Hudson JQ, Johnson CA. Chronic renal failure. In: Young LY, Koda-Kimble MA, eds. *Applied Therapeutics: The Clinical Use of Drugs.* 7th ed. Philadelphia, PA: Lippincott Williams & Wilkins; 2001: 30.1–30.38.

34. Malluche HH, Mawad H, Koszewski NJ. Update on vitamin D and its newer analogues: actions and rationale for treatment in chronic renal failure. *Kidney Int.* 2002; 62(2):367–74.

35. Zaloga GP, Chernow B. Divalent ions: calcium, magnesium, and phosphorus. In: Chernow B, ed. *The Pharmacologic Approach to the Critically Ill Patient.* 3rd ed. Baltimore, MD: Williams & Wilkins; 1994: 777–804.

36. Ritz E, Matthias S, Seidel A, et al. Disturbed calcium metabolism in renal failure—pathogenesis and therapeutic strategies. *Kidney Int.* 1992; 42(suppl 38):S37–42.

37. Zaloga GP. Hypocalcemic crisis. *Crit Care Clin.* 1991; 7: 191–200.

38. Zaloga GP. Hypocalcemia in critically ill patients. *Crit Care Med.* 1992; 20: 251–62.

39. Mundy GR. Hypercalcemia of malignancy. *Kidney Int.* 1987; 31:142–55.

40. Popovtzer MM. Disorders of calcium, phosphorus, vitamin D, and parathyroid hormone activity. In: Schrier RW, ed. *Renal and Electrolyte Disorders.* 6th ed. Philadelphia, PA: Lippincott Williams & Wilkins; 2003: 216–77.

41. Hall TG, Schaiff RA. Update on the medical treatment of hypercalcemia of malignancy. *Clin Pharm.* 1993; 12:117–25.

42. Randall RE, Straus MB, McNeely WF, et al. The milk-alkali syndrome. *Arch Intern Med.* 1961; 107:63–81.

43. Bilezikian JP. Management of acute hypercalcemia. *N Engl J Med.* 1992; 326:1196–1203.

44. Davis KD, Attie MF. Management of severe hypercalcemia. *Crit Care Clin.* 1991; 7:175–90.

45. Delmez JA, Slatopolsky E. Hyperphosphatemia: its consequences and treatment in patients with chronic renal disease. *Am J Kidney Dis.* 1992; 19:303–17.

46. Dennis VW. Phosphate disorders. In: Kokko JP, Tannen RL, eds. *Fluids and Electrolytes.* 3rd ed. Philadelphia, PA W. B. Saunders; 1996: 359–90.

47. Peppers MP, Geheb M, Desai T. Endocrine crises: hypophosphatemia and hyperphosphatemia. *Crit Care Clin.* 1991; 7:201–14.

48. Halevy J, Bulvik S. Severe hypophosphatemia in hospitalized patients. *Arch Intern Med.* 1988; 148:153–5.

49. Williams SR, ed. *Nutrition and Diet Therapy.* St. Louis, MO: C. V. Mosby; 1993.

50. Flodin N, ed. *Pharmacology of Micronutrients.* New York, NY: Alan R. Liss; 1988.

51. Robinson CH, Lawler MR, Chenoweth WL, et al., eds. *Normal and Therapeutic Nutrition.* 7th ed. New York, NY: Macmillan; 1990.

52. Grant JP, Ross LH. Parenteral nutrition. In: Chernow B, ed. *The Pharmacologic Approach to the Critically Ill Patient.* 3rd ed. Baltimore, MD: Williams & Wilkins; 1994: 1009–33.

53. Lindeman RD. Minerals in medical practice. In: Halpern SL, ed. *Quick Reference to Clinical Nutrition.* 2nd ed. Philadelphia, PA: J. B. Lippincott; 1987: 295–323.

54. Hurley LS. Clinical and experimental aspect of manganese in nutrition. In: Prasad AR, ed. *Clinical, Biochemical, and Nutritional Aspects of Trace Elements.* 1st ed. New York, NY: Alan R. Liss; 1982: 369–78.

55. Mertz W. Clinical and public health significance of chromium. In: Prasad AS, ed. *Clinical, Biochemical, and Nutritional Aspects of Trace Elements.* 1st ed. New York, NY: Alan R. Liss; 1982: 315–23.

56. De Haan KE, De Goeij JJ, Van Den Hamer CJ, et al. Changes in zinc metabolism after burns: observations, explanations, clinical implications. *J Trace Elem Electrolytes Health Dis.* 1992; 6:195–201.

57. Foote JW, Delves HT. Albumin bound and α_2-macroglobumin blund zinc concentrations in the sera of healthy adults. *J Clin Pathol.* 1984; 37:1050–4.

PARAMETER	DESCRIPTION	COMMENTS
Common reference ranges	136–145 mEq/L (136–145 mmol/L)	Measure of water status
Adults	130–140 mEq/L (130–140 mmol/L)	Premature
Pediatrics	135–145 mEq/L (135–145 mmol/L)	Older
Critical value	>160 or <120 mEq/L (>160 or <120 mmol/L)	Acute changes more dangerous than chronic abnormalities
Natural substance?	Yes	Most abundant cation in extracellular fluid
Inherent activity?	Yes	Maintenance of transmembrane electric potential
Location Storage Secretion/excretion	Mostly in extracellular fluid Filtered by kidneys, mostly reabsorbed; some secretion in distal nephron	Closely related to water homeostasis
Major causes of... **High results**	Multiple (discussed in text)	Can occur with low, normal, or high total body sodium
Associated signs and symptoms	Mostly neurological	Table 7-5
Low results	Multiple (discussed in text)	Can occur with low, normal, or high total body sodium
Associated signs and symptoms	Mostly neurological	Table 7-3, 7-4
After insult, time to... **Initial elevation or positive result**	Hours to years, depending on chronicity	The faster the change, the more dangerous the consequences
Peak values	Hours to years, depending on chronicity	
Normalization	Days, if renal function is normal	Faster with appropriate treatment
Drugs often monitored with test	Diuretics, angiotensin-converting enzyme inhibitors (ACE) inhibitors, ADH analogs	Any drug that affects water homeostasis
Causes of spurious results	None	

PARAMETER	DESCRIPTION	COMMENTS
Common reference ranges **Adults and pediatrics**	3.5–5.0 mEq/L (3.5–5.0 mmol/L)	Age: >10 days old
Critical value	>7 or <2.5 mEq/L (>7 or <2.5 mmol/L)	Acute changes more dangerous than chronic abnormalities
Natural substance?	Yes	Most abundant cation; 98% in intracellular fluid
Inherent activity?	Yes	Control of muscle and nervous tissue excitability, acid–base balance, intra-cellular fluid balance
Location Storage Secretion/excretion	98% in intracellular fluid Mostly secreted by distal nephron	Some via GI tract secretion
Major causes of... **High results**	Renal failure (GFR <10 mL/min)	Usually with increased intake
Associated signs and symptoms	Mostly cardiac	ECG changes, bradycardia, hypotension, cardiac arrest

Continued

Continued

PARAMETER	DESCRIPTION	COMMENTS
Low results	Decreased intake or increased loss	Usually combination of the two
Associated signs and symptoms	Involves many physiological systems	Table 7-8
After insult, time to...		
Initial elevation or positive result	Hours to years, depending on chronicity	The faster the change, the more dangerous the consequences
Peak values	Hours to years, depending on chronicity	
Normalization	Days, if renal function is normal	Faster with appropriate treatment
Drugs often monitored with test	Diuretic, ACE inhibitors, amphotericin B, *cis*-platinum	Potassium-containing preparations if renal failure present
Causes of spurious results	Hemolyzed samples (falsely elevated)	High potassium content in erythrocytes

PARAMETER	DESCRIPTION	COMMENTS
Common reference ranges		
Adults and pediatrics	96–106 mEq/L (96–106 mmol/L)	
Critical value		Depends on underlying disorder
Natural substance?	Yes	
Inherent activity?	Yes	Primary anion in extracellular fluid and gastric juice, cardiac function, acid-base balance
Location		
Storage	Extracellular fluid	Most abundant extracellular anion
Secretion/excretion	Passively follows sodium and water	Also influenced by acid-base balance
Major causes of...		
High results	Dehydration Acidemia	
Associated signs and symptoms	Associated with underlying disorder	
Low results	Nasogastric suction Vomiting Serum dilution Alkalemia	
Associated signs and symptoms	Associated with underlying disorder	
After insult, time to...		
Initial elevation or positive result	Hours to years, depending on chronicity	The faster the change, the more dangerous the consequences
Peak values	Hours to years, depending on chronicity	
Normalization	Days, if renal function is normal	Faster with appropriate treatment of underlying disorder
Drugs often monitored with test	Same as with sodium	
Causes of spurious results	Bromides; iodides (falsely elevated)	

PARAMETER	DESCRIPTION	COMMENTS
Common reference ranges **Adults and pediatrics**	1.5–2.2 mEq/L (0.75–1.1 mmol/L)	
Critical value	>5 or <1 mEq/L (>2.5 or <0.5 mmol/L)	Acute changes more dangerous than chronic abnormalities
Natural substance?	Yes	
Inherent activity?	Yes	Enzyme cofactor, thermoregulation, muscle contraction, nerve conduction, calcium and potassium homeostasis
Location **Storage**	50% bone, 45% intracellular fluid, 5% extracellular fluid	
Secretion/excretion	Filtration by kidneys	3–5% reabsorbed
Major causes of... **High results**	Renal failure	Usually in presence of increased intake
Associated signs and symptoms	Neuromuscular manifestations	Table 7-10
Low results	Excessive loss from GI tract or kidneys Decreased intake	Alcoholism and diuretics
Associated signs and symptoms	Neuromuscular and cardiovascular manifestations including weakness, muscle fasciculations, tremor, tetany, increased reflexes, and ECG abnormalities	More severe with acute changes
After insult, time to... **Initial elevation or positive result**	Hours to years, depending on chronicity	The faster the change, the more dangerous the consequences
Peak values	Hours to years, depending on chronicity	
Normalization	Days, if renal function is normal	Faster with appropriate treatment
Drugs often monitored with test	Diuretics and magnesium-containing antacids	
Causes of spurious results	Hemolyzed samples (falsely elevated)	

PARAMETER	DESCRIPTION	COMMENTS
Common reference ranges **Adults**	8.5–10.8 mg/dL (2.1–2.7 mmol/L)	Approximately half is bound to serum proteins; only ionized (free) calcium is physiologically active
Pediatrics	8–10.5 mg/dL (2–2.6 mmol/L)	
Critical value	>14 or <7 mg/dL (>3.5 or <1.8 mmol/L)	Also depends on serum albumin and pH values
Natural substance?	Yes	
Inherent activity?	Yes	Preservation of cellular membranes, propagation of neuromuscular activity, regulation of endocrine functions, blood coagulation, bone metabolism, phosphate homeostasis

Continued

Continued

PARAMETER	DESCRIPTION	COMMENTS
Location Storage	99.5% in bone and teeth	Very closely regulated
Secretion/excretion	Filtration by kidneys	Small amounts excreted into GI tract from saliva, bile, and pancreatic and intestinal secretions
Major causes of... High results	Malignancy Hyperparathyroidism	Also thiazide diuretics, lithium, vitamin D, and calcium supplements
Associated signs and symptoms	Vague GI complaints and neurological, cardiovascular, and renal signs	More severe with acute onset
Low results	Vitamin D deficiency Hypoparathyroidism Hyperphosphatemia Pancreatitis Loop diuretics Calcitonin Renal failure Hypoalbuminemia	Hypocalcemia due to hypoalbuminemia is asymptomatic (ionized calcium concentration unaffected)
Associated signs and symptoms	Primarily neuromuscular (e.g., fatigue, depression, memory loss, hallucinations, seizures, tetany)	More severe with acute onset
After insult, time to... Initial elevation or positive result	Hours to years, depending on chronicity	The faster the change, the more dangerous the consequences
Peak values	Hours to years, depending on chronicity	
Normalization	Days, if renal function is normal	Faster with appropriate treatment
Drugs often monitored with	Loop diuretics, calcitonin, vitamin D, calcium supplements, phosphate binders	
Causes of spurious results	Hypoalbuminemia	Ionized calcium concentration usually unaffected

PARAMETER	DESCRIPTION	COMMENTS
Common reference ranges Adults Pediatrics	2.6–4.5 mg/dL (0.84–1.45 mmol/L) 4–7.1 mg/dL (1.3–2.3 mmol/L)	
Critical value	>8 or <1 mg/dL (>2.6 or <0.3 mmol/L)	Acute changes more dangerous than chronic abnormalities
Natural substance?	Yes	Most abundant intracellular anion
Inherent activity?	Yes	Bone and tooth integrity, cellular membrane integrity, phospholipid synthesis, acid-base balance, calcium homeostasis, enzyme activation, formation of high-energy bonds
Location Storage	Extracellular fluid, cell membrane structure, intracellular fluid, collagen, bone	85% in bone
Secretion/excretion	Filtration by kidneys	Mostly reabsorbed

Continued

Continued

PARAMETER	DESCRIPTION	COMMENTS
Major causes of...		
High results	Decreased renal excretion Extracellular shifting Increased intake of phosphate or vitamin D	Renal failure the most common cause
Associated signs and symptoms	Due primarily to hypocalcemia and hyperparathyroidism	QuickView for calcium (hypocalcemia)
Low results	Increased renal excretion Intracellular shifting Decreased intake of phosphate or vitamin D	Also can occur in renal failure
Associated signs and symptoms	Bone pain, weakness, malaise, hypocalcemia, cardiac failure, respiratory failure	Usually due to diminished intracellula ATP and erythrocyte 2,3-DPG concentrations
After insult, time to...		
Initial elevation or positive result	Usually over months to years	
Peak values	Usually over months to years	
Normalization	Over days with renal transplantation	
Drugs often monitored with test	Calcium-containing antacids, vitamin D, phosphate binders	
Causes of spurious results	Hemolyzed samples (falsely elevated) and methotrexate (falsely elevated)	

PARAMETER	DESCRIPTION	COMMENTS
Common reference ranges		
Adults	75–150 µg/dL (11.8–23.6 µmol/L)	
Pediatrics	20–70 µg/dL (3.1–11 µmol/L)	0–6 months
	90–190 µg/dL (14.2–29.9 µmol/L)	6 years
	80–160 µg/dL (12.6–25.2 µmol/L)	12 years
Critical value	Not applicable	
Natural substance?	Yes	
Inherent activity?	Yes	Companion to iron, enzyme cofactor, Hgb synthesis, collagen and elastin synthesis, metabolism of many neu-rotransmitters, energy generation, regulation of plasma lipid levels, cell protection against oxidative damage
Location		
Storage	One-third in liver and brain; one-third in muscles; the rest in heart, spleen, kidneys, and blood (erythrocytes and neutrophils)	95% of circulating copper is protein bound as ceruloplasmin
Secretion/excretion	Mainly by biliary excretion; only 0.5–3% of daily intake found in urine	
Major causes of...		
High results	Deliberate ingestion of large amounts (>15 mg of elemental copper) Wilson's disease	Uncommon in humans

Continued

Continued

PARAMETER	DESCRIPTION	COMMENTS
Associated signs and symptoms	Nausea, vomiting, intestinal cramps, diarrhea	Larger ingestions lead to shock, hepatic necrosis, intravascular hemolysis, renal impairment, coma, and death
Low results	Infants with chronic diarrhea Malabsorption syndromes Decreased intake over months Menkes' syndrome	
Associated signs and symptoms	Neutropenia, iron-deficiency anemia, abnormal glucose tolerance, arrhythmias, hypercholesterolemia, atherosclerosis, depressed immune function, defective connective tissue formation, demineralization of bones	Can affect any system or organ whose enzymes require copper for proper functioning
Drugs often monitored with test	Copper supplements and hyperalimentation solutions	Serum copper concentrations not routinely monitored

PARAMETER	DESCRIPTION	COMMENTS
Common reference ranges **Adults and pediatrics**	70–130 µg/dL (10.7–19.9 µmol/L)	Increased risk for developing symptomatic zinc deficiency
Critical value	<70 µg/dL (<10.7 µmol/L)	
Natural substance?	Yes	
Inherent activity?	Yes	Enzyme constituent and cofactor; carbohydrate, protein, lipid, and nucleic acid metabolism; tissue growth; tissue repair; cell membrane stabilization; bone collagenase activity and collagen turnover; immune response; food intake control; spermatogenesis and gonadal maturation; normal testicular function
Location **Storage**	Liver, pancreas, spleen, lungs, eyes (retina, iris, cornea, lens), prostate, skeletal muscle, bone, erythrocytes, neutrophils	60–62% in skeletal muscle, 20–28% in bone 2–4% in liver
Secretion/excretion	Primarily in pancreatic and intestinal secretions; also lost dermally through sweat, hair and nail growth, and skin shedding	Except in certain disease states, only 2% lost in urine
Major causes of... **High results**	Large intake	Uncommon in humans
Associated signs and symptoms	Drowsiness, lethargy, nausea, vomiting, diarrhea, increases in serum lipase and amylase concentrations	
Low results	Low intake (infants) Decreased absorption (acrodermatitis enteropathica) Increased utilization (rapidly growing adolescents and menstruating, lactating, or pregnant women) Increased loss (hyperzincuria)	Rare from inadequate dietary intake
Associated signs and symptoms	Manifests in numerous organs and physiological systems	Table 7-14

Continued

Continued

PARAMETER	DESCRIPTION	COMMENTS
Drugs often monitored with test	Zinc supplements and hyperalimentation solutions	Serum zinc concentrations not routinely monitored
Causes of spurious results	Hemolyzed samples; 24-hr intrapatient variability	High zinc content in erythrocytes and neutrophils

PARAMETER	DESCRIPTION	COMMENTS
Common reference ranges		
Adults	2–3 µg/L (36–55 µmol/L)	
Pediatrics	2.4–9.6 µg/L (44–175 µmol/L)	Newborn
	0.8–2.1 µg/L (15–38 µmol/L)	2–18 years
Critical value	Not applicable	
Natural substance?	Yes	
Inherent activity?	Yes	Enzyme cofactor; carbohydrate, protein, and lipid metabolism; protection of cells from free radicals; steroid biosynthesis; metabolism of biogenic amines; normal brain function
		Magnesium may substitute for manganese in most instances
Location		
Storage	Bone, liver, pancreas, pituitary gland	Circulating manganese loosely bound to transmanganin
Secretion/excretion	Primarily in biliary and pancreatic juices; little lost in urine	Other GI routes also may be used in manganese overload
Major causes of...		
High results	Primarily through inhalation of manganese compounds, such as in manganese mines	One of least toxic trace elements
Associated signs and symptoms	Encephalopathy and profound neurological disturbances mimicking Parkinson's disease	Accumulates in liver and brain
Low results	After several months of deliberate omission from diet	Rare from inadequate dietary intake
Associated signs and symptoms	Weight loss, slow hair and nail growth, hair color change, transient dermatitis, hypocholesterolemia, hypotriglyceridemia	Seen mostly in experimental subjects
Drugs often monitored with test	Manganese supplements and hyperalimentation solutions	Serum manganese concentration not routinely monitored

PARAMETER	DESCRIPTION	COMMENTS
Common reference ranges		
Adults	1–5 µg/L (18–92 nmol/L)	Analysis of chromium in biological fluids and tissues is difficult
Pediatrics	Unknown	Analysis of chromium in biological fluids and tissues is difficult
Critical value	Unknown	
Natural substance?	Yes	
Inherent activity?	Yes	Cofactor for insulin and metabolism of glucose, cholesterol, and triglycerides
Location		
Storage	Hair, kidneys, skeleton, liver, spleen, lungs, testes, large intestines	Chromium circulates as free Cr^{3+}, bound to transferrin and other proteins, and as organic complex
Secretion/excretion	Excretion in urine	Circulating insulin controls daily loss
Major causes of...		
Low results	Decreased intake	
Associated signs and symptoms	Glucose intolerance; hyperinsulinemia; hypercholesterolemia; possibly, cardiovascular disease	Mainly due to its role as insulin cofactor
Drugs often monitored with test	Chromium supplement and hyperalimentation solution	Serum chromium concentration not routinely monitored

Chapter **8**

THE KIDNEYS

Thomas J. Comstock and Kandace V. Whitley

Through the excretion of water and solutes, the kidneys are responsible in large part for maintaining homeostasis within the body. They also function in the activation and synthesis of many substances that affect blood pressure, mineral metabolism, and red cell production. The purpose of this chapter is to provide insight to the interpretation of laboratory tests in the assessment of kidney function, as well as insight to the interpretation of a urinalysis.

OBJECTIVES

After completing this chapter, the reader should be able to

1. Describe the normal physiology of the kidneys.
2. Differentiate the renal handling of urea and creatinine.
3. Describe clinical situations where blood urea nitrogen (BUN) and/or serum creatinine (SCr) is elevated.
4. Cite clinical situations where BUN and SCr are and are not reliable indicators of renal function and explain why.
5. Determine creatinine clearance (CrCl) given a patient's 24-hr urine creatinine (UCr) excretion and SCr.
6. Estimate CrCl given a patient's height, weight, sex, age, and SCr and identify limitations of the methods for estimation of kidney function.
7. Discuss the various components assessed by macroscopic and microscopic urine analyses.
8. Assess the utility of urine protein measurements as an indicator of kidney disease.
9. Describe situations where urinary electrolyte determinations and the fractional excretion of sodium (FE_{Na}) test are useful diagnostically and therapeutically.
10. Describe the uses as well as the limitations of urine urea nitrogen in monitoring nutritional status.

RENAL PHYSIOLOGY

The functional unit of the kidneys is the nephron (Figure 8-1), and each of the two kidneys contains about 1 million nephrons. The major components of the nephron include the glomerulus, proximal tubule, loop of Henle, distal tubule, and collecting duct. Blood is delivered to the glomerulus, the filtering portion of the nephron, via the afferent arteriole. Acting as microfilters, the pores of glomerular capillaries allow substances with a molecular weight of up to 40,000 daltons to pass through them. Plasma proteins, such as albumin (mw 65 kd) and red blood cells do not normally pass through the glomerulus. Most drugs are small enough to be freely filtered at the glomerulus, with the exception of large proteins and drugs bound to plasma proteins.

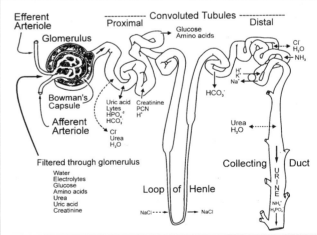

Figure 8-1. The nephron. Arrows pointing toward the nephron represent substances entering from the peritubular blood or interstitial space. Arrows heading away represent reabsorption. Solid arrows represent an active (energy-requiring) process, and dashed arrows represent a passive process. PCN = penicillin.

The proximal tubule avidly reabsorbs large quantities of water along with glucose, amino acids, uric acid, sodium, chloride, bicarbonate, and other electrolytes. Sodium, chloride, and water are further reabsorbed in the loop of Henle. The distal tubule controls the amounts of sodium, potassium, bicarbonate, phosphate, and hydrogen that ultimately are excreted, and the collecting duct regulates the amount of water in the urine as a result of the effect of antidiuretic hormone (ADH), which facilitates water reabsorption.[1]

As shown in Figure 8-1, substances can enter the nephron from the peritubular blood (secretion) or interstitial space. Substances also are reabsorbed from the tubule back into the systemic circulation via the peritubular vasculature. Tubular secretion occurs via two primary pathways in the proximal tubule: the organic acid transport (OAT) system and the organic cation transport (OCT) system. While each system is somewhat specific for anions and cations, respectively, some drugs are excreted by both pathways, such as probenecid. Creatinine, an endogenous product of muscle metabolism and a common marker to assess kidney function, enters the tubule primarily by filtration through the glomerulus. However, a small amount of creatinine is also secreted by the OCT system into the proximal tubule.

Blood flow to the kidneys is determined, in large part, by cardiac output with about 20% or 1.2 L/min directed to the kidneys. Renal plasma flow is directly related to renal blood flow by taking the patient's hematocrit into consideration as follows:

$$RPF = RBF \times (1 - Hct) \tag{1}$$

where RPF = renal plasma flow; RBF = renal blood flow; and Hct = hematocrit. The normal value for renal plasma flow is about 625 mL/min. Of the plasma that reaches the glomerulus, about 20% is filtered and enters the proximal tubule, resulting in a glomerular filtration rate (GFR) of about 125 mL/min. The GFR is often used as a measure of the degree of kidney function in a patient. The kidneys filter about 180 L of fluid each day; of this amount, they excrete only 1.5 L as urine. Thus, more than 99% of the glomerular filtrate is absorbed back into the bloodstream. Many solutes that are not reabsorbed are concentrated in the urine, and include endogenous substances such as creatinine, and exogenous compounds such as some drugs. Although beta-lactam antibiotics (e.g., penicillins and cephalosporins) are filtered through the glomerulus, a large percentage enters the nephron via tubular secretion. If a renally eliminated drug or substance is filtered (but not secreted) from the blood into the tubule (and not reabsorbed once in the tubule), its renal clearance is equal to the GFR, such as for aminoglycoside antibiotics.[1]

TESTS TO ESTIMATE GLOMERULAR FILTRATION RATE

Tests that estimate the GFR use endogenous markers such as creatinine and exogenous markers such as inulin, iothalamate, and radioactive substances (e.g., ethylenediamine tetra-acetic acid [^{51}Cr-EDTA], diethylenetriamine pentaacetic acid [^{99m}Tc-DTPA], and ^{131}I-iothalamate). Tests for creatinine clearance generally correlate with the GFR as measured using the more specific exogenous markers, with inulin clearance considered the "gold standard."

Clinicians should determine whether the actual GFR (inulin clearance) or a surrogate clearance (of any substance except inulin) would give the most useful or accurate information, depending on the intended use. For example, although the GFR as measured by inulin clearance is the most accurate measure of GFR, creatinine clearance (CrCl) may yield better results for pharmacokinetic dosing of drugs, since most kinetic studies use CrCl as the measure of kidney function to estimate drug clearance and develop dosing strategies. CrCl can also be estimated through nomograms based on the serum creatinine value and limited patient demographic data. While these methods are widely used to assess kidney function, it is important to be aware of their limitations. The blood urea nitrogen concentration (urea) has also been used as a marker of kidney function. It is freely filtered at the glomerulus and does not undergo tubular secretion, but it is reabsorbed along with water, thereby providing an accurate measure of renal function. During conditions of dehydration, there is increased reabsorption of water from the proximal tubule, and urea reabsorption is increased. The result is an increased serum urea concentration (BUN), which may falsely suggest impaired kidney function. The serum creatinine is a more accurate indicator of kidney function under these conditions as it does not undergo reabsorption.

Inulin and Related Marker Substances

Inulin is a fructose polysaccharide, an inert carbohydrate, with a molecular weight of 5200 daltons, which is not bound to plasma proteins. It is freely filtered through the glomerulus and is not metabolized, secreted, or reabsorbed. As a result of these characteristics, the renal clearance of inulin can be used as a measure of a patient's GFR:

$$CL_{renal, inulin} = \text{rate of inulin excretion}/C_{p,inulin} \tag{2}$$

$$\text{Rate of excretion} = \text{rate of filtration} + \text{rate of secretion} - \text{rate of reabsorption} \tag{3}$$

$$\text{where } C_{p,inulin} = \text{plasma inulin concentration}$$

$$\text{For inulin, rate of secretion} = 0 \text{ and rate of reabsorption} = 0;$$

$$\text{Rate of filtration} = GFR \times C_p \times f_{up} \tag{4}$$

$$\text{where } f_{up} = \text{fraction unbound in plasma, and } f_{up,inulin} = 1.0;$$

$$\text{therefore, } CL_{renal,inulin} = GFR \times C_{p,inulin}/C_{p,inulin} = GFR \tag{5}$$

The inulin clearance test consists of administering an intravenous dose of inulin to achieve a desired plasma concentration, followed by a maintenance intravenous infusion to sustain the concentration. Plasma and urine inulin concentrations are measured along with the urine flow rate to calculate the renal inulin clearance.[2]

$$CL_{renal, inulin} = \frac{UFR \times C_{u,inulin}}{C_{p,inulin}} \tag{6}$$

where UFR = urine flow rate; $C_{u,inulin}$ = urine inulin concentration; $C_{p,inulin}$ = plasma inulin concentration. Since inulin is eliminated entirely by the kidneys, it is also possible to measure kidney function without the collection of urine. Following IV bolus administration, plasma concentrations decline in a first-order manner, and total body clearance is calculated as dose/area under the plasma concentration-time curve ($\emptyset \rightarrow$ infinity). This clearance value will estimate GFR since inulin is eliminated only by glomerular filtration. While this procedure is practical for patients with normal kidney function due to the rapid elimination of inulin from the plasma, patients with reduced kidney function will have a prolonged elimination phase due to the reduced renal clearance of inulin, which limits the practical application of this approach, especially in the clinical research setting.

Although the inulin clearance test has ideal pharmacokinetics and is not radioactive, it is mainly used as a research tool because it is invasive and requires specialized analytical methods. Moreover, pharmacokinetic studies in patients with renal dysfunction usually relate drug clearance to CrCl as opposed to the true GFR. Therefore, dosage adjustments should generally be based on CrCl.

Other procedures that measure the GFR include the clearance of iothalamate, ^{51}Cr-EDTA, ^{99m}Tc-DTPA, or ^{131}I-iothalamate. Although some authorities feel that these tests are more suitable for clinical use than inulin is, they still require the injection of a foreign substance (some radioactive) into the patient as well as repeated blood sampling and/or timed urine collections. Therefore, these methods are not widely accepted clinically and they are not discussed further in this chapter. Alternatively, measurement of the two endogenous substances, urea (BUN) and serum creatinine (SCr), is widely used in clinical practice.

Urea (Blood Urea Nitrogen)

Normal range: 8–20 mg/dL or 2.9–7.1 mmol/L

Blood urea nitrogen (BUN) is actually the concentration of nitrogen (as urea) in the *serum* and not in RBCs (blood) as the name implies. Although the renal clearance of urea can be measured, it does not meet the requirements for an ideal GFR marker (i.e., a substance that is not bound to plasma proteins, filtered but not secreted from the blood into the tubule, and not reabsorbed once in the tubule). Its serum concentration depends on urea production (which occurs in the liver) and tubular reabsorption in addition to glomerular filtration. Therefore, clinicians must consider factors other than filtration when interpreting changes in BUN.

When viewed with other laboratory and clinical data, BUN can be used to assess or monitor hydration, renal function, protein tolerance, and catabolism in numerous clinical settings (Table 8-1). Also, it is used to predict the risk of uremic syndrome in patients with severe renal failure. Concentrations above 100 mg/dL (35.7 mmol/L) are associated with this risk.

Elevated BUN

Urea production is increased by

- A high-protein diet (including amino acid infusions).
- Upper gastrointestinal (GI) bleeding (blood is digested as dietary protein).
- Administration of corticosteroids, tetracyclines, or any other drug with antianabolic effects.

Usually, about 50% of the filtered urea is reabsorbed, but this amount is inversely related to the rate of urine flow in the tubules. In other words, the slower the urine flows, the more time the urea has to leave the tubule and re-enter surrounding capillaries (reabsorption). Urea reabsorption tends to change in parallel with sodium, chloride, and water reabsorption. Since severely dehydrated patients avidly reabsorb sodium, chloride, and water, larger amounts of urea are also absorbed.

Urine flow, in turn, is affected by fluid balance and blood pressure (BP). For example, dehydrated patients have low urine flow and develop high concentrations of urea nitrogen in the blood. Likewise, a patient with a pathologically low BP develops diminished urine flow secondary to decreased renal blood flow with a subsequently diminished GFR. Congestive heart failure and reduced renal blood flow, despite increased intra-

TABLE 8-1

PRERENAL CAUSES

Decreased renal perfusion: dehydration, blood loss, shock, severe heart failure

Increased protein breakdown or antianabolism (increased urea production): gastrointestinal bleed, crush injury, burn, fever, corticosteroids, tetracyclines, excessive amino acid or protein intake

INTRARENAL (INTRINSIC) CAUSES

Acute renal failure: nephrotoxic drugs, severe hypertension, glomerulonephritis, tubular necrosis

Chronic renal dysfunction: pyelonephritis, diabetes, glomerulonephritis, renal tubular disease, amyloidosis, arteriosclerosis, collagen vascular disease, polycystic kidney, chronic analgesic overuse

POSTRENAL CAUSES

Obstruction of ureter, bladder neck, or urethra

Table 8-1. Common Causes of True BUN Elevations (Azotemia)

vascular volume, is a common cause of elevated BUN. Causes of abnormally high BUN (also called azotemia) are listed in Table 8-1.

Chloral hydrate may interfere with some assays and cause *falsely* high BUN values. Fortunately, SCr and BUN are routinely measured together in most laboratories because of predetermined automatic analyzer setups.[3] Simultaneous assays that assess the same organ may help to identify interferences when results are discordant.

Decreased BUN

In and of itself, a low BUN does not have pathophysiological consequences. BUN may be truly low in patients who are malnourished or have profound liver damage (due to inability to synthesize urea). Intravascular fluid overload may initially dilute BUN (causing low concentrations), but many causes of extravascular volume overload, which are associated with third spacing of fluids into tissues (e.g., congestive heart failure, renal failure, and nephritic syndrome) result in increased BUN.

Chloramphenicol and streptomycin interference with some assays may also cause BUN to appear low. Likewise, assays based on urease reactions may yield falsely low BUN values (depressed up to 25%) if blood is collected in tubes containing sodium fluoride (gray-top tube), sometimes used for glucose preservation.[3]

Creatinine

Analytical Methods

The measurement of creatinine to assess the urinary excretion rate was first suggested by Folin in 1904.[4] His assay quantified creatinine by forming creatinine picrate in an alkaline environment. The picrate salt appears as varying intensities of an orange-red color. Many laboratories still use a modification (Jaffe) of this assay but read the color more accurately (±2%) with spectrophotometry. This assay is only fairly specific because noncreatinine chromogens are measured as creatinine (see Causes of False Serum Creatinine Results section).

Some laboratories now use an automated enzymatic method to determine true creatinine—it does not measure noncreatinine chromogens.[5] These practitioners argue that CrCl measured using a true creatinine assay correlates better with those determined using inulin.[6] However, this automated assay is time-consuming and disrupts the counterbalancing of creatinine secretion (discussed later) when the GFR is estimated from CrCl. Laboratories using true creatinine assays should report a lower normal range (0.4–1.0 mg/dL or 35–88 µmol/L).

Serum Creatinine

Normal range: 0.7–1.5 mg/dL or 62–133 µmol/L for adults; 0.2–0.7 mg/dL or 18–62 µmol/L for young children

Creatinine and its precursor creatine are nonprotein, nitrogenous biochemicals of the blood. After synthesis in the liver, creatine diffuses into the bloodstream. Creatine then is taken up by muscle cells, where some of it is stored in a high-energy form, creatine phosphate. Creatine phosphate acts as a readily available source of phosphorus for regeneration of adenosine triphosphate (ATP) and is required for transforming chemical energy to muscle action.

Creatinine is a spontaneous decomposition product of creatine and creatine phosphate. The daily production of creatinine is about 2% of total body creatine, which remains constant if muscle mass is not significantly changed. In normal patients at steady state, the rate of creatinine production equals its excretion. Therefore, creatinine concentrations in the serum (SCr) vary little from day to day in patients with healthy kidneys.

For children with *normal* renal function, the expected SCr can be estimated in milligrams per deciliter by multiplying the child's height in inches by 0.01.[7] For International

System (SI) units (micromoles per liter), the equation becomes height in centimeters times 0.35. These formulas are not surprising since the relationship between height and muscle mass is known. Although only rough estimates are obtained, they may be useful for children who cannot or will not tolerate venipuncture. Extensive reference range tables have been generated for infants and children.[8]

After an acute insult to nephrons, the amount of time needed to reach a new steady-state SCr depends on the half-life of creatinine at that time. Interpretation based on a pre-steady-state SCr concentration (if rising) leads to overestimation of the GFR. The half-life of creatinine in a 70-kg person with a CrCl of 120 mL/min is 3.5 hr. The typical maximal daily increase in SCr is 1–2 mg/dL (88–177 µmol/L). Higher rates (especially without decreased urine output) suggest an assay interference. Some evidence (albeit controversial), however, indicates that SCr may increase faster than 2 mg/dL/day (177 µmol/L/day) in rhabdomyolysis-induced renal failure.[9]

The time required to reach 95% of steady state in patients with 50, 25, and 10% of normal kidney function (120 mL/min) is about 1, 2, and 4 days, respectively. Therefore, if renal function suddenly declines to 10% of normal, SCr would not fully reflect the functional disability until 4 days later.

Causes of true changes in serum creatinine. A rise in SCr almost always indicates worsening renal function. Diseases and nephrotoxins that adversely affect the kidney's ability to filter and excrete metabolic end-products (e.g., creatinine) and drugs (e.g., digoxin and aminoglycoside antibiotics) disrupt the steady state, causing these chemicals to accumulate in the blood.

In addition, drugs such as cimetidine, triamterene, amiloride, spironolactone, trimethoprim,[10] probenecid, aspirin,[11] and pyrimethamine[12] inhibit tubular secretion of creatinine. Although they may cause true increases in SCr, these increases are not from a decreased GFR.[13] Patients on these drugs may have suppressed urinary excretion of creatinine. Therefore, their renal function, as estimated by CrCl, may be incorrectly assessed to be worse than it really is. Some investigators have exploited this property and used cimetidine to improve the accuracy of CrCl as an estimate of the true GFR (cimetidine inhibits tubular secretion of creatinine).[14,15] Whereas cimetidine successfully blocks the tubular secretion of creatinine, ranitidine has no effect on CrCl.[16] This lack of effect is also expected for the other H_2-receptor antagonists due to their low molar plasma concentrations compared with cimetidine. Administered as a single oral dose of 800 mg, cimetidine effectively blocks the tubular secretion of creatinine such that the resulting CrCl measured during a 3-hr urine collection is a more accurate assessment of GFR.[17] This is important for the assessment of kidney function in patients with progressive kidney disease so that the efficacy of treatment can be appropriately assessed.

Unlike BUN, SCr is not influenced much by usual changes in diet or urine flow. A large intake of roasted meats, however, may temporarily increase SCr due to the presence of creatinine in the meal.[18] Likewise, there is a strong relationship between the amount of protein in the diet and creatinine *excretion* but not SCr.[19]

Since SCr is a byproduct of muscle metabolism, severely decreased muscle mass (cachexia) or activity may be reflected by low SCr. Thus, patients with spinal cord injuries and muscle inactivity have decreased creatinine production.[20] For similar reasons, patients who have been in a coma or on neuromuscular blocking agents for a prolonged time tend to have decreased creatinine excretion rates with normal or low SCr. Conversely, very muscular patients occasionally have slightly elevated SCr with elevated creatinine excretion and normal CrCl and GFR. As expected, vigorous exercise may temporarily increase SCr (by an average of 0.5 mg/dL or 44 µmol/L), but normal exercise does not.[21]

Clinicians should rightfully surmise, therefore, that as long as no abnormalities exist in muscle mass and there has been no recent meat ingestion, an increased SCr almost always reflects a decreased GFR. The converse is not always true; a normal SCr does not necessarily imply a normal GFR. As part of the aging process, both muscle mass and renal function diminish. Therefore, SCr remains in the normal range because as the kidneys become less capable of filtering and excreting creatinine, they also are presented with decreasing amounts. Thus, practitioners should not rely solely on SCr as an index of renal function. They should also obtain or estimate CrCl.

Besides aging, some pathophysiological changes can affect the relationship between SCr and CrCl. For example, renal dysfunction is underestimated on the basis of SCr alone in cirrhotic patients.[22] Their low SCr is, in part, due to a decreased hepatic synthesis of creatine, the precursor of creatinine. In cirrhotic patients, it is prudent to perform a measured CrCl (see Calculating Creatinine Clearance from a Timed Urine Collection section). If the patient also has hyperbilirubinemia, assay interference by elevated bilirubin also may contribute to the low SCr.

Causes of false serum creatinine results. Unusually large amounts of noncreatinine chromogens (e.g., uric acid, glucose, fructose, acetone, acetoacetate, pyruvic acid, and ascorbic acid) in the serum, as measured by the Jaffe (alkaline picrate) assay, commonly lead to falsely increased SCr concentrations.[23] For example, an increase in glucose of 100 mg/dL (5.6 mmol/L) is likely to elevate SCr falsely by 0.5 mg/dL (44 µmol/L) in some assays. Likewise, serum ketones high enough to spill into the urine may falsely increase SCr[24,25] and UCr. This false effect is important because diabetic patients are prone to nephropathy and are likely to undergo unnecessary evaluation for renal failure when presenting with ketoacidosis. Like ketones, acetoacetate may be elevated enough to cause falsely elevated SCr after a 48-hr fast or in diabetic ketoacidosis.

With some automated analyzers, turbid or chylous samples (occurring in patients with hyperlipidemias) may produce erratic results. Patients receiving intravenous (IV) fat emulsions may have this potential under certain circumstances. Fortunately, when astute technologists observe turbidity, they remove chylomicrons to circumvent the interference.

Another endogenous substance, bilirubin, may falsely lower results (by 0.4–0.8 mg/dL or 35–70 µmol/L) if concentrations are greater than 10 mg/dL (171 µmol/L) with both the alkaline picrate and enzymatic assays.[26] Patients with bilirubin this high are easily identified because of their jaundice.

Unlike most other interferents noted above, flucytosine affects only the enzymatic assays.[27] This interference is especially important because patients may concomitantly receive two antifungal agents, flucytosine and the nephrotoxic agent amphotericin B. An increase in SCr may be attributed to amphotericin B-induced nephrotoxicity when it is actually from assay interference. Not all interference observations are false positives. Dopamine and dobutamine have been reported to cause a false decrease in the measured SCr when using the enzymatic method (Ektachem) by as much as 10–100%.[28]

Potential interferences with common SCr assays are listed in Table 8-2—most of the substances cause concentration-dependent alterations. Therefore, drawing blood samples (for SCr) far apart from anticipated peak concentrations of the listed substances should minimize interferences.

Concomitant BUN and Serum Creatinine

Simultaneous BUN and SCr determinations can furnish valuable information to aid in the interpretation of these values. This is particularly true for acute renal impairment. In acute renal failure with suspected dehydration, BUN and SCr are elevated. However, the BUN:SCr ratio is often 20:1 or higher (SI: 0.08:1 or higher). This observation is due to the differences

TABLE 8-2

SUBSTANCE	INTERFERENCE[b] WITH	
	JAFFE ASSAY	ENZYMATIC ASSAY
Acetoacetic acid		
Acetone		
Ascorbic acid (high doses)		
Bilirubin (>10 mg/dL)[c]		
Cefoxitin		
Cephalothin		
Dopamine		
Flucytosine		
Fructose		
Glucose (>250 mg/dL)		
Ketones		
Levodopa		
Lidocaine[d]		
Lipid emulsions		
Methyldopa		

[a] Compiled from References 3 and 29–37. These substances may also interfere with measurement of UCr if excreted in the urine mostly unmetabolized.
[b] __= false elevation of results; __= false suppression of results; __= no significant effect.
[c] SI: 171 µmol/L total bilirubin.
[d] Interferes with the EKTA enzymatic assay.

Table 8-2. Drugs and Other Substances that May Interfere Chemically with SCr Assays[a]

in the renal handling of urea and creatinine. Recall that urea is reabsorbed with water, and under conditions of dehydration and/or decreased renal perfusion, water reabsorption is increased as is urea. The effect is an increased BUN due to decreased renal urea excretion. Since creatinine is not reabsorbed, it is not affected by increased water reabsorption, although decreased renal perfusion may decrease glomerular filtration if prolonged, leading to an increased serum creatinine. In this case, the BUN would be increased to a greater degree, still leading to a BUN:SCr >20:1.

When acute changes in kidney function are observed, BUN:SCr ratios greater than 20:1 suggest prerenal causes of acute renal impairment (Table 8-1) whereas ratios from 10:1 to 20:1 (SI: from 0.04:1 to 0.08:1) suggest intrinsic kidney damage. However, as previously noted, both types may occur simultaneously, confounding typical interpretations. Furthermore, a ratio greater than 20:1 is not clinically important if both SCr and BUN are within normal limits (e.g., SCr = 0.8 mg/dL and BUN = 20 mg/dL).

Creatinine Clearance

Normal range: 90–140 mL/min/1.73 m²

From a practical clinical perspective, determination of CrCl provides the best approximation of the GFR. Creatinine is close to the ideal natural substance for this estimation because it is eliminated almost entirely by glomerular filtration. For individuals with normal kidney function, tubular secretion accounts for about 10% of the creatinine excreted in the urine, so it overestimates GFR. As kidney function declines, the percent of creatinine secretion increases significantly, to the point that it equals the filtration rate at GFR values of approximately 20 mL/min.[6] Creatinine may also be eliminated by gut flora, an important mechanism primarily in patients with chronic kidney disease.[41,42]

Despite the small degree of tubular secretion during normal kidney function, CrCl accurately estimates the GFR because substances that contribute to the color of the common Jaffe assay reaction (noncreatinine chromogens) in the serum are read as creatinine throughout the range of normal to mildly decreased GFRs. The noncreatinine chromogens (e.g., uric acid, glucose, fructose, acetone, pyruvic acid, acetoacetate, and ascorbic acid) affect the serum assay much more than the measurement of creatinine in urine. The overestimation of SCr increases the denominator of the clearance equation. The impact of overestimation is canceled out by the comparable effect (in the opposite direction) of creatinine elimination by secretion, which increases the numerator.

MINICASE 1

J. C., A 43-YEAR-OLD FEMALE, with a long history of Crohn's disease (regional enteritis), was admitted to Community Hospital with an exacerbation described as bloody, pusy, diarrhea; abdominal pain; anorexia; weight loss (5 lb); and weakness. All had worsened over the past 2 weeks.

A physical examination revealed an emaciated (5-ft 9-in; 40 kg; BSA of 1.3 m²) but mildly Cushingoid woman with moderate abdominal distress and dehydration, tachycardia (heart rate of 100), oral temperature of 101.5 °F (38.6 °C), BP of 100/50 mm Hg, macerated anal area, pallor, and mild finger clubbing. J. C. had been taking prednisone, 10 mg/day, for the past year and until now had experienced no serious flare-ups of her disease. On admission, prednisone was replaced with IV methylprednisolone 40 mg twice a day.

Laboratory included

- Sodium, 130 mEq/L (136–145 mEq/L).
- Potassium, 3.2 mEq/L (3.5–5.0 mEq/L).
- Chloride, 96 mEq/L (96–106 mEq/L).
- Carbon dioxide, 20 mEq/L (24–30 mEq/L).
- Glucose, 185 mg/dL (70–110 mg/dL).
- Phosphorus, 2.5 mg/dL (2.6–4.5 mg/dL).
- Hemoglobin (Hgb), 9 g/dL (12–16 g/dL).
- White blood cell (WBC) count, 15,000 cells/mm³ (4800–10,800 cells/mm³) with 80% neutrophils.
- BUN, 33 mg/dL (8–20 mg/dL).
- SCr, 0.8 mg/dL (0.7–1.5 mg/dL).

Over the next 3 days, J. C. received fluid and electrolyte replacement and 2 U of packed RBCs. On day 3, her test results were

- Sodium, 140 mEq/L.
- Potassium, 3.6 mEq/L.
- Chloride, 102 mEq/L.
- Carbon dioxide, 25 mEq/L.
- Glucose, 130 mg/dL.
- Phosphorus, 3.5 mg/dL.
- Hgb, 9.5 g/dL.
- WBC count, 18,000 cells/mm³ with 85% neutrophils.
- BUN, 25 mg/dL.
- SCr, 0.6 mg/dL.

On day 4, because J. C.'s Hgb did not improve much—her oral nutritional intake was inadequate and bowel rest was desired—she was given another 2 U of blood and started on total parenteral nutrition (TPN). TPN was composed of appropriate vitamins and minerals, amino acids 3 g/kg/day, and 30 nonprotein kcal/kg/day including fat emulsion 500 mL every day. Because she was still febrile (spiking temperatures to 103 °F or 39.4 °C) with leukocytosis (WBC count of 16,000 cells/mm³) and abdominal rigidity, an intra-abdominal infection was suspected. Therefore, cefoxitin 2 g every 6 hr was started.

By day 6, J. C. defervesced and her Hgb was 11 g/dL. However, her BUN was 40 mg/dL and her SCr was 2.2 mg/dL (serum was not turbid). Her urinalysis was normal with no ketones, glucose, muddy brown (granular) casts, or tubular epithelial cells; her serum glucose was 150 mg/dL. J. C.'s urine output was difficult to determine because of loss during diarrhea.

Because her SCr was elevated, a 24-hr urine collection for creatinine was started 6 hr later after insertion of a Foley catheter. J. C. was also switched to cefotetan 2 g every 12 hr. At the same time, a repeat BUN and SCr were 39 and 0.8 mg/dL, respectively. On the next day, the 24-hr UCr was 700 mg in a volume of 1900 mL and SCr was 0.7 mg/dL.

Question: What type of renal dysfunction was J. C. experiencing? What were the likely causes of her elevated BUN and SCr? How often should BUN and SCr be determined?

Discussion: This case is rather complex because many factors might affect SCr and BUN at various times. One fairly certain interpretation is that, on day 6, cefoxitin caused the SCr to be falsely elevated to 2.2 mg/dL. The argument for this conclusion is strong because

1. SCr would rarely decline by 1.4 mg/dL in only 6–12 hr in patients not being hemodialyzed.

2. Other SCr measurements were all around 0.7–0.8 mg/dL.

3. Cefoxitin interference with common creatinine assays is well-documented.[32,33,38]

Because J. C.'s SCr was elevated to 2.2 mg/dL and because renal hypoperfusion (BP of 100/50 mm Hg) might have led to kidney damage and her urine output was unknown, a CrCl test was done to try to clarify SCr. Her CrCl was 93 mL/min/1.73 m², which would be expected if her renal function were normal. The clinician should keep in mind, however, that renal function, as determined by CrCl, may be overestimated in malnourished patients[39] like J. C.

Although it did not seem to happen with J. C., the measurement of UCr would also be falsely elevated if the cefoxitin washout period was inadequate and this antibiotic was still in her urine. In this case, the measured CrCl would be exaggerated. More evidence of normal renal function was that catheter-collected urine showed good output (1900 mL; almost 2 mL/kg/hr) and urinalysis revealed no significant casts (discussed later).

There are several possible reasons why J. C.'s BUN values were elevated. On admission, dehydration could have hemoconcentrated the BUN. In fact, after rehydration, her BUN decreased to 25 mg/dL. Although her SCr also declined (albeit slightly), if hemoconcentration contributed to the initial azotemia, at first glance one would expect other serum constituents to *decline*. The opposite occurred. There is no paradox, however, since J. C. probably received many of these substances parenterally during the first 3 days.

Severe dehydration may have also increased her BUN secondary to diminished renal blood flow (prerenal cause). A BUN:SCr ratio of greater than 20:1 is consistent with prerenal azotemia. J. C.'s ratio was 40:1. The patient's relatively low SCr, which may have been a reflection of little muscle mass, increased this ratio *artificially*. Finally, the fact that J. C. was on chronic steroids may have contributed to her elevated BUN.

On day 6, J. C.'s BUN was 40 mg/dL despite rehydration. A SCr of 2.2 mg/dL and a BUN:SCr ratio of 10:1–20:1 are consistent with acute renal failure, and it is not uncommon for prerenal problems to lead to acute renal failure.[40] Fortunately, as mentioned, her SCr was spuriously elevated.

On day 6, three causes of the high BUN are possible:

1. J. C.'s steroid dose had been increased substantially. As mentioned, steroids can lead to an elevated BUN by their antianabolic properties (a byproduct of increased gluconeogenesis from cellular proteins).

2. J. C. was receiving excessive amino acids and relatively inadequate calories. Although increasing BUN from parenteral nutrition usually occurs only with diminished renal function, it can occur in this scenario.

3. Stress from exacerbation of Crohn's disease and her infection may also have contributed to J. C.'s elevated BUN values due to increased protein catabolism.

There is no consensus about the optimal frequency for determining SCr or CrCl. With this patient, the BUN and SCr tests were ordered whenever the clinician needed to assess therapy, renal function, or state of hydration. A CrCl was ordered only after other results appeared discrepant.

In patients in the initial phases of acute renal failure, SCr tests are done almost every day; in chronic renal failure, every 4–6 months usually suffices. While patients are on drugs such as aminoglycosides, determinations are customarily conducted every 3 days. The frequency of taking SCr levels depends on the disease or drug being monitored as well as the patient's history. In general, CrCl is tested only if renal function cannot be reliably assessed by SCr and BUN alone.

At low GFRs, however, creatinine secretion overtakes the balancing effects of measuring noncreatinine chromogens, causing an overestimation of GFRs by as much as 50%.[6,23]

Interpreting Creatinine Clearance Values with Other Renal Parameters

As alluded to previously, the most common clinical uses for CrCl and SCr include

- Assessing kidney function in patients with acute or chronic renal failure.
- Monitoring the effects of drug therapy on slowing the progression of kidney disease.
- Monitoring patients on nephrotoxic drugs.
- Determining dosage adjustments for renally eliminated drugs.

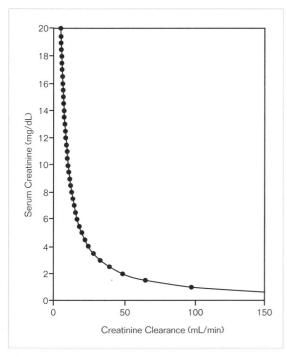

Figure 8-2. This plot represents the inverse relationship between SCr and CrCl. Below 50 mL/min, there is a greater increase of SCr compared to CrCl vales greater than 50 mL/min. The simulation is based on a patient with a urine creatinine excretion rate of 1400 mg/day.

Because the relationship between SCr and CrCl is inverse and geometric as opposed to linear (Figure 8-2), significant declines in CrCl may occur before SCr rises above the normal range. For example, as CrCl slows, SCr rises very little until more than 50% of the nephrons have become nonfunctional. Therefore, SCr alone is not a sensitive indicator of early kidney dysfunction.

Calculating Creatinine Clearance from a Timed Urine Collection

Although shorter collection periods (3–8 hr) appear to be adequate and often more reliable,[43] CrCl is routinely calculated using a 12- or 24-hr UCr excretion result and SCr. Creatinine excretion is normally 20–28 mg/kg/24 hr in men and 15–21 mg/kg/24 hr in women. In children, normal excretion (milligrams per kilogram per 24 hr) should be approximately 15 + (0.5 × age), where age is in years.

Because its excretion remains relatively consistent within these ranges, UCr is often used as a check for complete urine collection when creatinine or other substances (e.g., amylase, urea, protein, hormones, and catecholamines) are being measured. In adults, some clinicians discount a urine sample if it contains less than 10 mg of creatinine/kg/24 hr; they assume that the collection was incomplete. However, 8.5 mg/kg/day might be a better cutoff, especially in critically ill elderly patients.[44] UCr assays are affected by most of the same substances that affect SCr. To interfere significantly, however, the substance must appear in the urine in concentrations at least equal to those found in the blood.

Endogenous CrCl is calculated with the following formula:

$$CrCl = ([UCr \times V]/[SCr \times t]) \times 1.73/BSA \qquad (7)$$

where CrCl is the creatinine clearance in mL/min/1.73 m^2; UCr = urine creatinine concentration; V = volume of urine produced during the collection interval; SCr = serum creatinine concentration; t = time of the collection interval, and BSA = body surface area (m^2). BSA can be estimated using the standard method of Dubois and Dubois[45]:

$$BSA \ (m^2) = 0.20247 \times height(m)^{0.725} \times weight(kg)^{0.425} \qquad (8)$$

BSA also can be estimated using the following equation from Mosteller[46]:

$$BSA \ (m^2) = ([height(cm) \times weight(kg)]/3600)^{1/2} \qquad (9)$$
$$e.g., BSA = SQRT \ ([cm*kg]/3600)$$

Adjustment of CrCl to a standard BSA (1.73 m^2) allows direct comparison with normal CrCl ranges since such tables are in units of milliliters per minute per 1.73 m^2. The CrCl value adjusted for BSA is the number of milliliters cleared per minute for each 1.73 m^2 of the patient's BSA. Therefore, such adjustment in a large person (>1.73 m^2) reduces the original nonadjusted clearance value since the assumption is that clearance would be lower if the patient were smaller. In practice, it is only important to adjust CrCl for BSA in patients who are much smaller (e.g., children) or larger (e.g., tall weightlifters) than 1.73 m².

Estimating Creatinine Clearance without Urine Collection

A 24-hr urine collection for CrCl determination is labor intensive, expensive, time-consuming, and cumbersome. The most common problem is that all excreted urine is not collected. In addition, therapy or other diagnostic studies may have to be delayed until after the collection period. Therefore, clinicians have sought methods for estimation of CrCl. Although results from estimations have long been considered not as accurate as test results from measuring UCr, they can be obtained quickly and easily, and in most cases, exceed the reliability of urine methods due to the difficulty of obtaining a complete collection. Several different methods have been developed over the past 30 years or more, and the following summarizes the ones important for clinical practice today.

The National Kidney Foundation has recently developed sets of evidence-based clinical practice guidelines referred to collectively as the Kidney Disease Quality Outcomes Initiative (K/DOQI).[47] The guidelines cover the topics of hemodialysis and peritoneal dialysis adequacy, vascular access, anemia, nutrition, and the most recent, chronic kidney disease (CKD). The CKD guidelines focus on evaluation, classification, and stratification for the purpose of identifying patients at risk and initiating therapies to prevent or minimize further progression of disease. Two approaches for the estimation of kidney function in adults are highlighted in the report as acceptable methods. The first is the well-recognized Cockcroft-Gault equation, which estimates CrCl using the following equation[48]:

$$\text{CrCl (mL/min)} = ([140 - \text{age}] \times \text{weight[kg]}/[\text{SCr} \times 72]) \times 0.85 \text{ (if female)} \qquad (10)$$

This equation is based on linear regression of the 24-hr urine creatinine excretion as a function of age in 249 men with stable kidney function. It was derived from the regression line, $\text{PCr} = 28 - (0.2 \times \text{age})$, where PCr = creatinine production, mg/kg/d, and the standard equation for calculating renal clearance. In unusually small or large individuals, Equation 10 should be adjusted for BSA by multiplying the result by 1.73/patient's BSA. This adjustment generates results in milliliters per minute per 1.73 m². Some clinicians, however, prefer to adjust the milliliters-per-minute value to a 72-kg person (as opposed to BSA). The formula then is simplified to:

$$\text{CrCl (mL/min/72 kg)} = [(140 - \text{age})/\text{SCr}] \times 0.85 \text{ (if female)} \qquad (11)$$

where SCr is in milligrams per deciliter and age is in years.

The more recently developed method is based on data collected during the Modification of Diet in Renal Disease (MDRD) study.[47,49] Based on patient demographic data and a true measure of GFR, using ^{125}I-iothalamate, the investigators developed the following relationship:

$$\text{GFR (mL/min/1.73 m}^2) = 170 \times (\text{SCr})^{-0.999} \times (\text{age})^{-0.176} \times (\text{BUN})^{-0.170} \times (\text{Alb})^{+0.318} \qquad (12)$$
$$\times (0.762 \text{ if female}) \times (1.180 \text{ if African American})$$

Analysis of various forms of the equation yielded several with similar predictive performance, and the following, referred to as the *abbreviated MDRD*, has broader appeal as it is independent of the BUN and albumin concentrations.[47,50]

$$\text{GFR (mL/min/1.73 m}^2) = 186 \times (\text{SCr})^{-1.154} \times (\text{age})^{-0.203} \times (0.742 \text{ if female}) \qquad (13)$$
$$\times (1.210 \text{ if African American})$$

An important difference between the MDRD methods and the Cockcroft-Gault is that the latter is based on GFR, and the former is based on CrCl. The clinical effect of this difference has not been assessed prospectively as related to dosage regimen design based on kidney function, since most clinical studies evaluating drug elimination in patients with kidney disease have been based on CrCl. The MDRD method does serve as a new tool to assess kidney function and the impact of interventions to slow the progression of disease. The method is recommended by K/DOQI as the preferred approach to assess kidney function in adults, and clinical laboratories are encouraged to report the estimated GFR along with the SCr as it is a more useful measure of kidney function. Limitations in the interpretation of the GFR will apply to those conditions discussed above where the SCr may not be a reliable measurement of the true steady-state value.

For children, the K/DOQI Guidelines recommend the Schwartz[51] and Counahan-Barratt[52] formulae as acceptable methods for estimation of GFR. Difference in the constants for the two equations has been suggested to be due to different assays for measurement of SCr.

$$\text{Schwartz: } CrCl \text{ (mL/min)} = 0.55 \times \text{length(cm)}/SCr\text{(mg/dL)} \qquad (14)$$

$$\text{Counahan-Barratt: (mL/min/1.73m}^2) = 0.43 \times \text{length(cm)}/SCr\text{(mg/dL)} \qquad (15)$$

None of these methods is valid in a patient being hemodialyzed since dialysis contributes to creatinine elimination.

For patients with unstable kidney function, the above methods are not appropriate for the assessment of kidney function, as a steady-state SCr is required. With SCr changing, two values are necessary to assess the rate of change. Here, the Jelliffe and Jelliffe approach is useful. For this method (modified from Reference 53) refer to the following Steps 1–6:

1. *Estimate patient's ideal body mass (IBM) from height in inches:*

$$IBM \text{ (lb)} = 130 + 3 \text{ (height} - 60) \text{ in males} \qquad (16)$$

$$IBM \text{ (lb)} = 120 + 3 \text{ (height} - 60) \text{ in females} \qquad (17)$$

For example, a 70-in-tall woman has an ideal body mass of 150 lb. If the patient's actual weight is less than the estimated ideal body mass, the actual weight should be used. Pounds are converted to kilograms (divided by 2.2) for Step 2.

2. *Estimate steady-state (unadjusted) UCr:*

$$UCr = IBM \text{ } (29.3 - [0.20 \times \text{age]}) \text{ in males} \qquad (18)$$

$$UCr = IBM \text{ } (25.3 - [0.18 \times \text{age]}) \text{ in females} \qquad (19)$$

where UCr is in milligrams per 24 hr, ideal body mass is in kilograms, and age is in years.

3. *Correct UCr for nonrenal elimination using a correction factor (CF):*

$$CF = 1.035 - 0.034(SCr) \qquad (20)$$

An average SCr can be used if more than one has been run. Then,

$$UCr' = UCr \times CF \qquad (21)$$

where UCr´ is creatinine excretion corrected for nonrenal (mostly GI) elimination. Step 3 can be omitted unless SCr is greater than 2.5 mg/dL; at that point, it begins to affect UCr´ more drastically.

4. *Estimate daily accumulation (or loss) of creatinine* (Cr˜):

$$Cr˜ = \frac{4\,(IBM)(SCr_2 - SCr_1)}{T} \tag{22}$$

where SCr_2 is the current SCr and SCr_1 is the SCr T days ago. If there has been no upward or downward trend in SCr (i.e., it is stable), creatinine approaches zero and this adjustment is not needed.

5. *Adjust UCr for daily accumulation or loss:*

$$UCr_\Delta = UCr´ - Cr˜ \tag{23}$$

where UCr_D is the estimated UCr excretion adjusted for nonrenal elimination and *changing* renal function.

6. *Calculate CrCl:*

$$CrCl \ (mL/min/1.73 \ m^2) = \frac{UCr_\Delta \times 0.12}{SCr \times BSA} \tag{24}$$

The question of which SCr to use is controversial. If one suspects that CrCl will continue to fall or rise, the most recent value, SCr_2, probably should be used. Otherwise, the average of SCr_2 and SCr_1 should be used.

URINALYSIS

Urinalysis is another tool that clinicians can use to search for or evaluate renal and nonrenal problems (e.g., endocrine, metabolic, and genetic). A routine urinalysis, as the name implies, is done as a screening test during many hospital admissions and initial physician visits. It is also performed periodically in patients in nursing homes and other settings. Since many different methods are used to assess the components of a urinalysis, only the common ones are discussed here.

Accurate interpretations can be made only if urine is properly collected as well as handled. Techniques are mainly standardized and aim to avoid contamination (the urine should be sterile) by normal flora of external mucous membranes of the vagina or uncircumcised penis or by microorganisms on the hands. Therefore, these areas are cleansed and physically kept away from the urine flow. During menses or heavy vaginal secretions, a fresh tampon should be inserted before cleansing. Midstream urine alone (1 cup) is customarily used as the specimen. However, first-voided (2-cup) and even 3-cup urines may provide information about the prostate in males.

Once voided, the urine should be brought to the laboratory as soon as possible to prevent its deterioration. If the sample is not refrigerated, bacteria multiply; they use glucose (if any) as a food source. Glucose concentrations fall and ketones may evaporate with prolonged standing. Another problem is that formed elements (Microscopic Analysis section) begin decomposing within 2 hr. With excessive exposure to light, bilirubin and urobilinogen are oxidized. Unlike other substances, however, protein is hardly affected by prolonged standing.[54]

After the urine sample is collected, it may undergo three types of testing: macroscopic, microscopic, and chemical.

Macroscopic Analysis (General Appearance)

The color of normal urine varies greatly—from totally clear to dark yellow or amber—depending on the concentration of solutes. Color comes primarily from the pigments urochrome and urobilin. Fresh normal urine is not cloudy or hazy, but urine may become cloudy if urates (in an acid environment) or phosphates (in an alkaline environment) crystallize or precipitate out of solution. These salts become less soluble as the urine cools from body temperature.

Turbidity may also occur when large numbers of RBCs or WBCs are present. An unusual amount of foam may be from protein or bile acids. Table 8-3 lists causes of different urine colors. Drugs that cause or exacerbate any of the medical problems listed in Table 8-3 can also be considered indirect causes of discolored urine.

Microscopic Analysis (Formed Elements)

Microscopic analysis typically involves

1. Centrifuging the urine at 2000 revolutions per minute for 5 min.
2. Pouring off all "loose" supernatant.
3. Mixing the sediment with the residual supernatant.
4. Examining the resulting suspension under 400–455 × magnification (also described as high-power field).

This segment of the urinalysis is the most time-consuming and costly. Therefore, many authorities have suggested that dipstick chemical screening (described later) be used to determine whether the urine sediment should be examined microscopically.[56] Some practitioners found that when the urine was negative for protein, blood, and leukocytes, omitting microscopy missed potentially significant findings in only 1.5–3% of specimens. Whether microscopic analysis is done routinely or selectively, one should look for the three "Cs"—cells, casts, and crystals.

Cells

Theoretically, no cells should be seen during microscopic examination of urine. In practice, however, an occasional cell or two is found. These cells include microorganisms, RBCs, WBCs, and tubular epithelial cells.

TABLE 8-3

COLOR	CAUSE	POSSIBLE UNDERLYING ETIOLOGIES
Red to orange	Myoglobin	Crush injuries, electric shock, seizures, cocaine-induced muscle damage
	Hemoglobin	Hemolysis (malaria, drugs, strenuous exercise)
	Porphyrins	Porphyria, lead poisoning, liver disease
	Drugs/chemicals	Drugs/chemicals causing above diseases. As dyes: rifampin, phenazopyridine, danthron,[b] emodin,[c] daunorubicin, doxorubicin, phenolphthalein,[b] phenothiazines, senna,[b] chlorzoxazone
	Food	Beets, rhubarb, blackberries, cold drink dyes, carrots
Blue to green	Biliverdin	Oxidation of bilirubin (poorly preserved specimen)[d]
	Bacteria	Pseudomonas or Proteus in urinary tract infections (rare), particularly in urine drainage bags
	Drugs/chemicals	As dyes: amitriptyline, azuresin, methylene blue, Clorets® abuse, Clinitest® ingestion, mitoxantrone, triamterene, resorcinol
Brown to black	Myoglobin	Crush injuries, electric shock, seizures, cocaine-induced muscle damage
	Bile pigments	Hemolysis, bleed into tissues, liver disease
	Melanin	Melanoma (prolonged exposure to air)[d]
	Methemoglobin	Methemoglobinemia from drugs, dyes, etc.
	Porphyrins	Porphyria and sickle cell crisis
	Drugs/chemicals	As dyes: cascara,[b] chloroquine, clofazimine, emodin,[b] senna,[b] chemicals ferrous salts, methocarbamol, metronidazole, nitrofurantoin, sulfonamides

[a] Adapted from References 3, 54, and 55 and various anecdotal reports.
[b] In acidic urine.
[c] In basic (alkaline) urine.
[d] After prolonged standing or exposure to air.

Table 8-3. Causes of Various Urine Coloring[a]

Microorganisms (normal range: zero to trace). Although urine is sterile normally, fungi, bacteria, and other single-cell organisms can be seen in patients with a urinary tract infection or colonization. Even if ordered, some laboratories do not perform urine cultures unless there is significant bacteriuria. *Significant bacteriuria* may be defined as an initial positive dipstick screen for leukocyte esterase and/or nitrites (Chemical Analysis section). Likewise, some laboratories do not process cultures further (e.g., identification, quantification, and susceptibility) if more than one or two different bacterial species is seen on initial plating.

Additionally, some labs do not perform susceptibility testing if more than one organism (some more than two) is isolated or if less than 100,000 (some use 50,000 as the cutoff) colony-forming units (cfu) per milliliter per organism are measured with a midstream, clean-catch sample. The common cutoff for urine obtained through a catheter is less than 10,000. The rationale is that the chance of isolating pathogens is low with low colony counts. In the case of multiple bacteria, contamination by vaginal, rectal, hand, or other flora is assumed.

Most laboratories use unspun urine for microbiological screening. However, investigators using *centrifuged*, stained sediment found the highest sensitivity (98%) and specificity (89%) when the criterion for significant bacteriuria was one or more bacteria per oil-immersion field.[57] Microscopic findings were compared with the "gold standard," quantitative urine culture, where the isolate is deemed to be a pathogen if seen in quantities of 100,000 cfu or more per milliliter. Unfortunately, studies on this topic are difficult to compare because of slight differences in technical methods and varying ideas about what constitutes significant bacteriuria.

Red blood cells (normal range: one to three per high-power field). A few RBCs occasionally are found in a healthy patient's urine, particularly after exertion, trauma, or fever. If persistent, however, even small numbers may reflect urinary tract pathology. RBCs are seen in glomerulonephritis, infection (pyelonephritis), renal infarction or papillary necrosis, tumors, stones, and coagulopathies. In some of these disorders, hematuria may turn the urine pink or red (gross hematuria).

If the specimen is not collected properly, vaginal blood may contaminate the urine. Many squamous epithelial cells also appear in this case, suggesting that the erythrocytes did not originate from the urinary tract but probably from the vaginal walls.

White blood cells (normal range: zero to two per high-power field). Potentially significant pyuria has been defined as three or more WBCs per high-power field of centrifuged urine sediment. Alone, this finding is not specific for a particular disease and may even occur in the absence of pathology. Pyuria is usually associated with a bacterial urinary tract infection. However, inflammation in the tract also may lead to this finding.

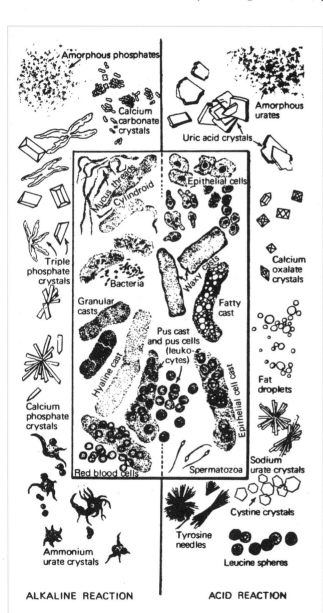

Figure 8-3. Possible microscopic (100–200x) findings (mostly abnormal) in urine sediment. Elements on the left are more likely to be seen in alkaline urine; those on the right are more likely in acid urine. (Reproduced, with permission, from Krupp MA, Sweet NJ, Jawetz E, et al. *Physician's Handbook.* 19th ed. Norwalk, CT: Lange Medical Publications; 1979.)

Urethritis provides an interesting example of how integration of pyuria with other urinalysis findings can provide diagnostic information. In women complaining of dysuria, pus in the urine without microscopic bacteria is highly suggestive of chlamydial urethritis. Negative tests for hematuria and proteinuria strengthen this diagnosis.

Tubular epithelial cells (normal range: zero or one per high-power field). One epithelial cell per high-power field is often found in normal subjects. Cells originating from the renal tubules are small, round, and mononuclear. Their quantity increases dramatically when the tubules are damaged (e.g., acute tubular necrosis) or heavy proteinuria occurs (nephrotic syndrome).

Numerous flat, irregular, vaginal epithelial cells with small nuclei suggest contamination.

Casts

Casts are cylindrical masses of glycoproteins (e.g., Tamm-Horsfall mucoprotein) that form in the tubules. As shown in Figure 8-3, casts have relatively smooth and regular margins (as opposed to clumps of cells) because they conform to the shape of the tubular lumen. To oversimplify, their production is similar to the pouring of wax into a tubular mold to make (usually short) candles.

Under certain conditions, casts are released into the urine (called *cylinduria*). Even normal urine can contain a few clear casts. These formed elements are fragile and dissolve more quickly in warm, alkaline urine. Types include hyaline, cellular, granular, waxy, and broad; their causes are listed in Table 8-4.

Hyaline casts. Being clear, hyaline casts are difficult to observe under a microscope. They are seen with exercise, fever, and proteinuria. They are not indicative of intrinsic renal disease, but of a small volume of concentrated urine or a prerenal problem, such as CHF or dehydration.

Cellular casts. In contrast to hyaline casts, cellular casts are seen with intrinsic renal disease. They form when leukocytes, RBCs, or renal tubular epithelial cells become entrapped in the gelatinous matrix forming in the tubule. Their clinical significance is the same as that of the cells themselves; unlike free cells, however, cells in casts originate from within the kidneys. In other words, WBC casts suggest *intrarenal* inflammation and/or upper urinary tract infection, usually pyelonephritis. Epithelial cell casts indicate definite tubular destruction, while RBC casts are seen in glomerulonephritis or ischemic injury to the kidneys.

Granular and waxy casts. Granular and waxy casts are older, degenerated forms of the other types. Granular (also called muddy brown) casts are most typical of acute tubular necrosis and, therefore, are seen in renal damage secondary to ischemic or toxic insults (e.g., shock, sepsis, liver failure with increased bilirubin, aminoglycoside toxicity, and contrast media toxicity). Since waxy casts occur in many diseases, they do not offer much diagnostic information.

TABLE 8-4

CAST	CAUSE
Red cell	Acute glomerulonephritis, renal infarct, subacute bacterial endocarditis, Goodpasture's syndrome, lupus nephritis, vasculitis
White cell	Acute pyelonephritis or interstitial nephritis
Epithelial cell	Toxicity from salicylates and heavy metals, tubular necrosis, cytomegalovirus infection
Hyaline	Prerenal azotemia (from CHF, dehydration, etc.) or strenuous exercise
Granular	Acute tubular necrosis; less often in severe pyelonephritis and glomerulonephritis
Waxy	Renal failure or severe tubular atrophy
Broad	May be any of above types, but larger width reflects diameter of their origin (collecting ducts); seen in acute and chronic renal failure

*Adapted from Reference 54.

Table 8-4. Causes of Various Types of Casts in Urine[a]

P. D., A 78-YEAR-OLD, 5-FT 5-IN, 125-LB FEMALE, was admitted to the hospital 2 days ago for pneumonia in her left lower lobe and postprandial epigastric pain. She had a history of chronic obstructive pulmonary disease requiring oral steroids 2 or 3 times a year and many previous admissions for pneumonia. She had developed worsening shortness of breath and fever over the past few days.

P. D. also had a history of chronic renal failure secondary to diabetes and hypertension. Her SCr had typically been about 3 mg/dL and her BUN about 50 mg/dL. A stain of sputum revealed many Gram-negative rods, and cultures grew *Pseudomonas aeruginosa* susceptible only to ceftazidime and imipenem. Her SCr concentrations on the previous 2 days were 3.2 and 3.0 mg/dL, and her BUNs were 50 and 55 mg/dL. Her urine output averaged 1200 mL/day with an intake of about 1800 mL during the past 2 days. A hemocult test (for blood in stools) was positive on two occasions.

P. D. was empirically started on ceftriaxone on admission. However, the pharmacist wanted to change her antibiotic to imipenem (the attending physician usually used 500 mg every 6 hr for this type of infection) and start nizatidine. Both drugs need dosage adjustment in patients with renal dysfunction.

Question: How should P. D.'s renal function be estimated? How should her drug dosages be adjusted?

Discussion: Because P. D.'s SCr values did not change significantly from her usual poor baseline, her CrCl can be estimated using the Cockcroft-Gault[48] method, Equation 10. With a SCr of 3.0 mg/dL, the equation gives an estimate of 13.8 mL/min. Equation 8 yields a BSA of 1.61 m². To adjust the CrCl for BSA, 13.8 is multiplied by 1.73/BSA to get a CrCl of 14.8 mL/min/1.73 m². This adjustment affects the CrCl insignificantly because P. D. did not have a very large or small body size.

Because of possible active gastrointestinal bleeding, the nizatidine dose is usually 150 mg twice a day. However, at a CrCl of 20–50 mL/min, the manufacturer recommends a dose of 150 mg every day; at a CrCl of less than 20 mL, 150 mg every other day is suggested. Because P. D.'s CrCl was stable at about 15 mL/min, nizatidine should be started at 150 mg every other day but changed to every day if epigastric pain or bleeding persists.

In patients with normal renal function, imipenem 500 mg is often given every 6 hr; occasionally, doses as high as 1000 mg every 8 hr are given for this type of infection. The manufacturer suggests using 500 mg every 6 hr if the CrCl is 31–70 mL/min, 500 mg every 8 hr if it is 21–30 mL/min, and 500 mg every 12 hr if it is 6–20 mL/min. Since P. D.'s CrCl was 15 mL/min, she should be given 500 mg every 12 hr.

Crystals

Crystalluria, if differentiated by type, can help to identify patients with certain local and systemic diseases. Urate crystals are found in acid urine and dissolve on warming; phosphate crystals form in alkaline urine and dissolve with acidification. The former occur in patients with uric acid uropathy; the latter occur in patients with urinary infections caused by urea-splitting bacteria (e.g., *Proteus*) and in patients with persistently alkaline urine for other reasons. Both crystals also may be found in normal urine.

CHEMICAL ANALYSIS (SEMIQUANTITATIVE TESTS)

For this discussion, biochemical analysis of urine includes protein; pH; specific gravity; bilirubin, bile, and urobilinogen; blood and hemoglobin; leukocyte esterase; nitrite; and glucose and ketones. All of these semiquantitative tests can be performed quickly using modern dipsticks containing one or more reagent-impregnated pads. When using these strips, the clinician must carefully apply the urine to the pads as instructed and wait the designated time before comparing pad colors to the color chart. Possible results associated with various colors are displayed in Table 8-5.

TABLE 8-5

TEST	RESULTS						
Leukocyte esterase	Negative	Trace	Small +	Moderate ++	Large +++		
Nitrite	Negative	Positive					
Urobilinogen	Normal 0.2 mg/dL	Normal 1 mg/dL	2 mg/dL	4 mg/dL	8 mg/dL		
Protein	Negative	Trace	30 mg/dL +	100 mg/dL ++	300 mg/dL +++	³2000 mg/dL ++++	
PH	5	6	6.5	7	7.5	8	8.5
Blood (Hgb)	Negative	Nonhemolyzed Trace	Hemolyzed Trace	Small +	Moderate ++	Large +++	
Specific gravity	1.000	1.005	1.010	1.015	1.020	1.025	1.030
Ketones	Negative	Trace 5mg/dL	Small 15mg/dL	Moderate 40mg/dL	Large 80mg/dL	Large 160mg/dL	
Bilirubin	Negative	Small +	Moderate ++	Large +++			
Glucose	Negative	1/10 g/dL (trace) 100mg/dL	1/4 g/dL 250 mg/dL	1/2 g/dL 500 mg/dL	1 g/dL 1000 mg/dL	³2 g/dL ³2000 mg/dL	

ᵃ Multistix 10 SG, Bayer.

Table 8-5. Examples of Tests Available and Possible Results from Multitest Urine Dipstickᵃ

Protein

Normal range: zero to trace or <200 mg/g UCr

The more common causes of proteinuria are listed in Table 8-6. Even the persistent presence of as little as 150 mg of protein in the urine per day is abnormal. Most protein that passes into the urine is either albumin or globulins.

Abnormal permeability of the glomerular-limiting membrane, prototypically seen in nephrotic syndrome, allows large quantities of albumin to enter the urine. Even trace amounts in patients with noninsulin-dependent diabetes (type II) are associated with increased mortality.[58] Large quantities of globulins (e.g., Bence-Jones proteins) in the urine suggest multiple myeloma. Furthermore, small to moderate amounts of protein may be seen in the urine of patients with dysfunctioning renal tubules since they cannot reabsorb the small amounts of proteins that are normally filtered.

The National Kidney Foundation Kidney Disease Outcome Quality Initiative (K/DOQI) Clinical Practice Guidelines for Chronic Kidney Disease[47] recommend monitoring guidelines for urinary protein and albumin in patients to detect kidney disease. For patients not at increased risk of kidney disease (i.e., no diabetes, no hypertension), the standard dipstick for urine protein is the initial screen. If ≥1+, the patient should be further evaluated with a spot total protein/creatinine ratio. If greater than 200 mg/g, then the pa-

TABLE 8-6

Little proteinuria (<0.5 g/day)
Hemoglobinuria (hemolysis)
High BP
Lower urinary tract infection
Fever
Renal tubular damage
Exercise

Moderate proteinuria (0.5–3 g/day)
CHF (severe)
Chronic glomerulonephritis
Acute glomerulonephritis (sometimes major)
Diabetic nephropathy
Pyelonephritis
Multiple myeloma
Preeclampsia of pregnancy

Major proteinuria (>3 g/day)
Amyloid disorders
Chronic glomerulonephritis (severe)
Diabetic nephropathy (severe)
Lipoid nephrosis
Lupus nephritis
Focal glomerulosclerosis (AIDS or heroin abuse)

Table 8-6. Causes of Proteins in Urine

tient should undergo diagnostic evaluation for kidney disease. For those patients already at increased risk, the initial screen should be performed with an albumin-specific dipstick. If positive, then further quantitative evaluation should be performed using a spot albumin/creatinine ratio. If ≥30 mg/g, then a diagnostic evaluation should be performed. Routine screening for urinary albumin is not indicated in patients not at increased risk. Due to difficulties with overnight and 24-hr collections, K/DOQI recommends spot urine testing. The protein (or albumin)-to-creatinine ratio accounts for urine volume effects on protein concentration and standardizes the protein or albumin excretion to creatinine excretion.

The color indicator test strips used to detect and measure protein in the urine contain a buffer mixed with a dye (usually tetrabromphenol blue). In the absence of albumin, the buffer holds the pH at 3, maintaining a yellow color. If present, albumin reduces the activity coefficient of hydrogen ions (the pH rises), producing a blue color. However, urine containing globulins, including 50% of Bence-Jones proteins, is misread as negative. Improper interpretation also may result if the buffer is neutralized by very alkaline urine or is washed off by excessive urine ("drenching"). A newer semiquantitative test uses tablets impregnated with reagents similar to those in the strips. This test, for professional use only, detects albumin concentrations as low as 4 mg/dL.

The more traditional acetic acid and sulfosalicylic acid methods, being less specific, detect globulins and Bence-Jones proteins as well as albumin. These methods are based on the denaturing of protein to produce turbidity. Although they are sensitive to more proteins, they are not specific for proteins. For example, penicillins, especially those administered in large doses (e.g., penicillin G and nafcillin), caused false positives with the acid methods in some studies. Discordantly, one study suggested that beta-lactam antibiotics, including penicillin G, ampicillin, methicillin, and cefazolin, do not interfere with the acid tests for urine protein.[59]

Information regarding interferences with specific tests for detecting proteinuria is included in Table 8-7. When the dipstick method shows negative proteinuria in a patient suspected with this problem (cloudy or foamy urine), the sulfosalicylic or acetic acid method should be used to confirm the result. Conversely, when drug interference is suspected with an acid assay, the dipstick test should be used.

TABLE 8-7

TYPE OF TEST	PROTEINS DETECTED	FALSE POSITIVES	FALSE NEGATIVES
Reagent strip (dipstick)	Albumin (5–10 mg/dL)	Skin disinfectants Sodium bicarbonate Acetazolamide	Very dilute urine High salt concentration
Heat and acetic acid	Albumin (5–10 mg/dL) Globulins Bence Jones	Phosphates and urates Tolbutamide, sulfonamides, penicillins (high dose), tolmetin	Highly buffered alkaline urine
Sulfosalicylic acid	Albumin (0.25 mg/dL) Globulins Bence Jones Glycoproteins	Same as for heat and acetic acid, plus cephalothin and chlorpromazine	Highly buffered alkaline urine

ᵃ Adapted from Reference 54.

Table 8-7. Interferences with Tests for Protein in Urineᵃ

pH

Normal range: 4.5–8.0

Sulfuric acid, resulting from the metabolism of sulfur-containing amino acids, is the primary acid generated by the daily ingestion of food. Normally, the kidneys can eliminate the acid load by excreting acid itself and sodium hydroxide ions. In fact, healthy persons can acidify the urine to pH 4.5, although the average pH is around 6. Any pH close to the reference range can be interpreted as normal as long as it reflects the kidneys' attempts at regulating blood pH. Conversely, a pH within the reference range may be considered abnormal if it is the opposite of what normal homeostasis should produce.

In general, acidic (vs. neutral) urine deters bacterial colonization. Alkaline urine may be seen with either

- Urinary tract infections caused by urea-splitting bacteria such as *Proteus mirabilis* (via ammonia production).
- Tubular defects causing decreased net tubular hydrogen ion secretion, as in renal tubular acidosis.

By their intended or unintended pharmacological actions, drugs also can cause true pH changes; they do not interfere with the reagents used to estimate urine pH. Drugs that induce diseases associated with pH changes are indirect causes. These and other causes of acidic and alkaline urine are listed in Table 8-8. Persistent pHs greater than 7.0 are associated with calcium carbonate, calcium phosphate, and magnesium–ammonium phosphate stones; pHs below 5.5 are associated with cystine and uric acid stones.

pH is usually estimated (in 0.5 increments) by use of test strips containing methyl red and bromthymol blue indicators. These strips undergo a series of color changes from orange to blue over a pH range of 5.0–8.5. In addition, pH can be precisely measured with electronic pH meters.

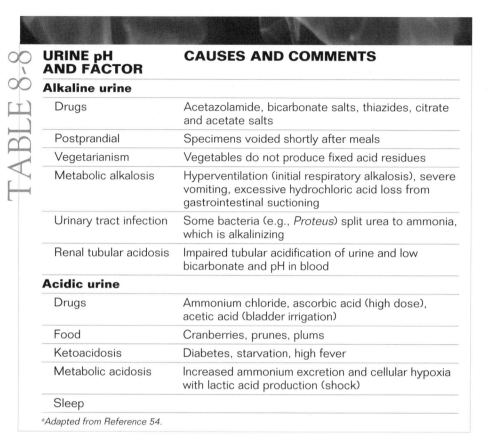

TABLE 8-8

URINE pH AND FACTOR	CAUSES AND COMMENTS
Alkaline urine	
Drugs	Acetazolamide, bicarbonate salts, thiazides, citrate and acetate salts
Postprandial	Specimens voided shortly after meals
Vegetarianism	Vegetables do not produce fixed acid residues
Metabolic alkalosis	Hyperventilation (initial respiratory alkalosis), severe vomiting, excessive hydrochloric acid loss from gastrointestinal suctioning
Urinary tract infection	Some bacteria (e.g., *Proteus*) split urea to ammonia, which is alkalinizing
Renal tubular acidosis	Impaired tubular acidification of urine and low bicarbonate and pH in blood
Acidic urine	
Drugs	Ammonium chloride, ascorbic acid (high dose), acetic acid (bladder irrigation)
Food	Cranberries, prunes, plums
Ketoacidosis	Diabetes, starvation, high fever
Metabolic acidosis	Increased ammonium excretion and cellular hypoxia with lactic acid production (shock)
Sleep	

[a]Adapted from Reference 54.

Table 8-8. Factors Affecting Urine pH[a]

Specific Gravity

Normal range: 1.010–1.025

The kidneys are responsible for maintaining the blood's osmolality within a narrow range (285–300 mOsm/kg). To do so, however, the kidneys must vary the osmolality of the urine over a wider range. Although osmolality is the best measure of the kidneys' concentrating ability, determining osmolality is difficult. Fortunately, it correlates well with specific gravity when the urine contains normal constituents. Because specific gravity is related to the weight (and not the number) of particles in solution, particles with a weight different from that of sodium chloride (the solute usually in the highest concentration there) can widen the disparity.

Sodium is normally the main contributor to the specific gravity of urine. Nevertheless, other endogenous substances (e.g., glucose, urea, and protein) also can affect it. If the urine contains protein or glucose, the specific gravity is greater at a fixed osmolality than in normal urine. In diabetics, for example, each increase of 270 mg/dL glucose raises the specific gravity by 0.001. This increase would not usually confound matters until the urine reached 2 g/dL, which would account for about 0.010 of the specific gravity (a 50–100% rise from baseline).

Proteinuria affects the specific gravity even less; heavy proteinuria (0.4 g/dL) raises it by only 0.001. On the other hand, if the urine contains unusual amounts of urea (a less dense molecule), the specific gravity could be lowered and then interpreted as a sign of the kidneys having lower than actual concentrating ability.

Exogenous substances (e.g., drugs) that concentrate in the urine can increase the specific gravity. For example, after a radiologic study of the kidneys, the iodinated contrast material that appears in the urine may raise the specific gravity to 1.040. Dextran also may cause increases in this parameter. Furthermore, penicillins that are administered in large quantities can increase the urine's specific gravity according to the following formula:

$$\text{true SG} = \text{lab SG} - \left[6 \times \frac{0.8 \times \text{carbenicillin (g/day)}}{\text{24-hr urine volume (mL)}} \right] \tag{25}$$

where SG is specific gravity.[60] For penicillin G, 4.7 would be used instead of 6. Dehydrated patients typically concentrate urine to a specific gravity of 1.020–1.030. A specific gravity greater than 1.030 is likely to be caused by drugs such as carbenicillin.

Several diseases usually affect specific gravity. In chronic renal failure, the kidneys first lose their ability to concentrate and then their ability to produce dilute urine. When about 80% of the nephron mass is destroyed, the specific gravity hovers around 1.010, the specific gravity of plasma. The urine of patients with diabetes insipidus has low values (<1.005), whereas high values are found in patients with inappropriate secretion of antidiuretic hormone (ADH). In general, *urinary* specific gravity should be considered abnormal if it is the opposite (high vs. low and vice versa) of what normal physiology should produce based on the concurrent *plasma* specific gravity.

Specific gravity is routinely measured with a urinometer or refractometer. The urinometer is akin to a graduated buoy; it requires sufficient urine volume to float freely. The reading is adjusted according to the urine temperature. The refractometer uses the refractive index as a basis and needs only a few milliliters of urine and no temperature adjustment.

Bilirubin, Bile, and Urobilinogen

Normal range: zero to trace

A dark yellow or brown color generally suggests bilirubin in the urine. Most test strips and some tablets (Ictotest) rely on bilirubin's reaction with a diazotized organic dye to yield a distinct color. Patients on phenazopyridine and some phenothiazines may have false-positive results. Truly positive results are found in patients with liver disease (jaundice) or internal bleeding.

Urobilinogen (formed by bacterial conversion of conjugated bilirubin in the intestine) increases in the urine when the turnover of heme pigments is abnormally rapid, as in hemolytic anemia, CHF with liver congestion, cirrhosis, viral hepatitis, and drug-induced hepatotoxicity. Elevated urobilinogen may be premonitory of early hepatocellular injury, such as hepatitis, because it is affected before serum bilirubin. Alkaline urine is also associated with increased urobilinogen concentrations due to enhanced renal elimination.

Urobilinogen may decrease (if previously elevated) in patients started on antibiotics (e.g., neomycin, chloramphenicol, and tetracycline) that reduce the intestinal flora producing this substance. Urobilinogen is usually absent in total biliary obstruction, since the substance cannot be formed. Increased urobilinogen in the absence of bile in the urine suggests a hemolytic process. Finally, both substances degrade in specimens exposed for prolonged periods to bright fluorescent light or room temperature.

Blood and Hemoglobin

Normal range: zero to trace

Lysed RBCs and, therefore, hemoglobin may be present in the urine when the urinary tract is damaged. In addition, after intravascular hemolysis and saturation of serum haptoglobin, free hemoglobin may spill into the urine. This hemoglobinuria occurs within a few hours of severe hemolysis and lasts less than a day. Hemolysis may occur with hereditary diseases (e.g., sickle cell anemia, spherocytosis, and glucose-6-phosphate dehydrogenase deficiency) or paroxysmal nocturnal hemoglobinuria and may be induced by many drugs.

Hemoglobin acts as a peroxidase and catalyzes the oxidation of o-toluidine by peroxide, producing a blue color. When urine is tested for occult blood with common dipsticks, povidone-iodine can cause positive readings in the absence of hemoglobin. Since this antiseptic is often used to prepare the urethral meatus before urine collection for cultures and the same urine also may be used for hemoglobin testing, this fact is clinically relevant.

Because of its structural similarity with hemoglobin, myoglobin in the urine (which may appear after muscle trauma, infarction, or infection) also leads to a positive test despite the absence of hematuria. Conversely, high doses of vitamin C may cause a false negative by inhibiting the reaction rate.

Leukocyte Esterase

Normal range: zero to trace

Many dipsticks can detect leukocyte esterase and give a semiquantitative estimate of pyuria. WBC esterases differ enough from esterases of serum, urine, and kidney tissue to yield reliable results. Specificity and sensitivity are around 96% and 85%, respectively.

Some clinicians think that reading the strip at 5 min (as opposed to the indicated 2 min) decreases false negatives. In fact, the sensitivity of the WBC esterase test (based on more than three WBCs per high-power field in sediment of spun urine) approaches 100% if the strip is read after 5 min. As is often the case, however, increased sensitivity is at the expense of specificity. In one study, the false-positive rate increased from 4.5 to 22% with the 5-min read time.[56] Based on these findings, the WBC pad on the strip should be read at 1–2 min and, if negative, again at 5 min. If the test is positive only at the second reading, a significant—but low—number of WBCs are probably in the urine.

One example of how this test may be applied in an office or clinic involves a woman suspected of having a lower urinary tract infection (dysuria, frequency, and urgency). If she has significant pyuria (2+ or greater leukocyte esterase), she could be started immediately on empiric therapy. In the absence of pyuria, however, therapy could be withheld pending full urinalysis and culture results.[61]

Vitamin C and phenazopyridine interfere with the leukocyte esterase test. Phenazopyridine causes either false-negative or unreadable results.[62]

Nitrite

Normal range: none

Nitrite may be present in the urine as a result of Gram-negative bacterial metabolism of dietary nitrates to nitrites. In this assay, an aromatic amine reacts with any nitrite to produce a colored azo dye. If bacteria that are incapable of this metabolism are causing the infection (Gram-positive bacteria), the test falsely indicates that no bacteria are present. Recent antibacterial therapy and high doses of ascorbic acid also may cause false-negative results.

A positive nitrite test usually corresponds with a positive leukocyte esterase test. However, a positive WBC test may occur with inflammation, whereas the nitrite test pad is only positive when bacteria are present.

Glucose and Ketones

Normal range: none

Glucose in the urine is suggestive of diabetes mellitus. Ketones in the urine are also suggestive of diabetes mellitus, especially when glucose is present. Aspirin has been reported to cause a false-negative ketone test, whereas levodopa and phenazopyridine may cause false-positive ketone results.

URINARY ELECTROLYTES AND SODIUM (%FE$_{NA}$) TEST

Like most laboratory tests, urinary electrolytes are rarely definitive for any diagnosis. They can confirm suspicions of a particular medical problem from the history, physical examination, and other laboratory data. They also can assist in determining whether the kidneys are retaining these electrolytes. Along with the results of a urinalysis and serum electrolytes, urinary electrolyte tests allow the practitioner to rule possible diseases in or out of the differential diagnosis.

Because normal values have not been firmly established, these tests can be properly interpreted only in the context of the clinical situation and dietary intake. In general, however, because the kidneys play a major role in maintaining the balance of these electrolytes, any concentration in the urine is *normal* if it favors a normal fluid and serum electrolyte status. A related test, the %FE$_{Na}$, can assist with common diagnostic dilemmas involving the kidneys' ability to regulate electrolytes.

Urinary Sodium, Potassium, and Chloride

The electrolyte that is most commonly measured in the urine is sodium. Occasionally, it is also useful to measure potassium and chloride. Interpretation of urinary sodium, potassium, and chloride is summarized

TABLE 8-9

MEDICAL PROBLEM	ELECTROLYTE VALUE	LIKELY DIAGNOSIS
	Sodium	
Volume depletion	0–10 mEq/L	Extrarenal sodium loss
	>10 mEq/L	Renal sodium wasting or adrenal insufficiency
Acute oliguria	0–10 mEq/L	Prerenal azotemia
	>30 mEq/L	Acute tubular necrosis, except contrast-media-induced failure
Hyponatremia	0–10 mEq/L	Volume depletion or edematous diseases
	Greater than diet intake	Inappropriate ADH secretion or adrenal insufficiency
	Potassium	
Hypokalemia	0–10 mEq/L	Nonrenal potassium loss
	>10 mEq/L	Renal potassium loss
	Chloride	
Metabolic alkalosis	0–10 mEq/L	Chloride-responsive alkalosis
	Same as diet intake	Chloride-resistant alkalosis

[a] Adapted from References 63 and 64.
[b] Random samples, assuming no drug therapy that will influence excretion. See exceptions in text.

Table 8-9. Interpretation of Urinary Sodium, Potassium, and Chloride[a,b]

in Table 8-9. For these electrolytes, there is no conversion to SI units since milliequivalents per liter is equivalent to millimoles per liter.

Sodium

Normal range: varies widely

The major diagnostic use of random urinary sodium concentrations is in patients with simultaneous volume depletion, acute oliguria, and hyponatremia.[63] In the volume-depleted patient, urinary sodium may help to determine the underlying cause of the sodium loss. When the amount of sodium in the urine is negligible, volume depletion is probably caused by GI or other nonrenal sodium or fluid losses. On the other hand, the presence of sodium suggests renal or adrenal insufficiency if a drug-induced etiology and osmotic diuresis can be excluded.

The underlying cause of a sudden stoppage (anuria) or sharp drop in urine output (acute oliguria) must be quickly assessed. Most often, it is related to either prerenal azotemia or acute tubular necrosis. Patients with pure prerenal oliguria should have markedly diminished urinary sodium concentrations (<5–10 mEq/L). Conversely, in acute tubular necrosis, the values are commonly greater than 30–40 mEq/L. Exceptions are patients with burns, cirrhosis (hepatorenal syndrome), and contrast-media-induced renal failure.[64] An FE_{Na} determination or microscopic examination of the urine (showing granular casts) may firm up a diagnosis of acute tubular necrosis.

Hyponatremia associated with urinary sodium excretion that equals or exceeds dietary intake is often seen with inappropriate ADH secretion (increased water reabsorption) or adrenal insufficiency (decreased sodium reabsorption). Low serum sodium with very low urinary sodium (regardless of diet) is consistent with enhanced tubular reabsorption. Expansion of extracellular volume or development (or worsening) of edematous diseases (e.g., CHF, cirrhosis, and nephrotic syndrome) is the usual underlying cause. This is due to the combination of a reduced effective arterial blood volume, reduced renal perfusion, and increased renal reabsorption of sodium; hyponatremia occurs as the result of the nonosmotic release of ADH in an attempt to expand the blood volume and increase renal perfusion. Furthermore, patients receiving therapeutic doses of heparin for more than a few days may not retain sodium properly because of impaired aldosterone activity.

In addition, clinicians responsible for monitoring drug therapy have another use for this test: assessing a patient's compliance with a diuretic regimen. Compliant patients should have moderate to high concentrations (>10–20 mEq/L) of sodium in their urine.

Potassium

Normal range: varies widely

For patients with unexplained hypokalemia, urinary potassium may provide useful information. Concentrations greater than 10 mEq/L in a hypokalemic patient usually mean that the kidneys are responsible for the loss. This scenario may occur with potassium-wasting diuretics, high-dose sodium penicillin therapy (e.g., disodium ticarcillin and sodium penicillin), metabolic acidosis or alkalosis, and a few intrinsic renal disorders. Concomitant hypokalemia and low urinary potassium (<10 mEq/L) suggest GI loss (including chronic laxative abuse) as the cause of low serum potassium.

Chloride

Normal range: varies

If metabolic alkalosis is persistent, urinary chloride determination may be of value. Since this disorder is commonly from GI losses of hydrochloric acid or is diuretic induced, urinary chloride levels are not needed.

Usually, urinary sodium and chloride concentrations parallel each other: if sodium is high, chloride is high and vice versa. The direction of change, however, may diverge if the need for urinary electroneutrality is overpowering. For example, if there is heavy excretion of cations other than sodium (K^+, NH_4^+, Ca^{++}, and H^+), more chloride than sodium would have to be excreted. Therefore, in a dehydrated patient, where typically both urinary sodium and chloride are low, this situation would lead to the appearance of only low urine sodium. For similar reasons, the opposite divergence (only a low urinary chloride) may be seen in the dehydrated patient who is excreting large amounts of anions other than chloride (bicarbonate; high-dose penicillins such as ticarcillin and piperacillin [PCN-COO⁻]).

Elevated urinary chloride without elevated urinary sodium generally occurs when the kidneys respond to metabolic acidosis and attempt to eliminate excess acid as ammonium chloride. Therefore, the urinary anion gap, calculated as $(U_{Na} + U_K) - U_{Cl}$, becomes negative. This calculation can be used to distinguish the normal anion gap acidosis caused by diarrhea (or other GI alkali loss) from that caused by distal renal tubular acidosis. In both disorders, serum potassium is usually low. In patients with renal tubular acidosis, however, urinary pH is always greater than 5.3.

Usually, excretion of urinary hydrogen ions during diarrhea acidifies the urine. However, hypokalemia leads to enhanced ammonia synthesis by the proximal tubular cells. Despite acidemia, the excess urinary ammonia (NH_3) accepts a hydrogen ion to become ammonium (NH_4^+), which increases the urine pH in some patients with diarrhea. The ammonium picks up chlorine ions and is excreted in the urine, creating a negative urinary anion gap. Hence, the urinary anion gap should be negative in the patient with diarrhea, regardless of the urine pH.

In contrast, although hypokalemia may result in enhanced proximal tubular ammonia synthesis in *distal* renal tubular acidosis, the inability to secrete hydrogen ions into the collecting tubule in this condition limits ammonium chloride formation and excretion. Therefore, the urinary anion gap is positive in distal renal tubular acidosis.

%FE$_{Na}$ Test

In distinguishing prerenal from intrarenal causes (e.g., acute tubular necrosis) of sudden oliguria or azotemia, the %FE$_{Na}$ test has a diagnostic discrimination far better (96–100%) than urinary sodium determinations. The better discrimination is because the overlap with urinary sodium is great, the ranges for prerenal and intrarenal diseases are 5–40 and 10–80 mEq/L, respectively.[64,65]

Only a "spot" or random (vs. 12–24-hr) urine collection is required, along with a concomitant serum sample. The laboratory should measure sodium and creatinine in the urine and serum. The calculation is

$$\%FE_{Na} = \frac{U_{Na}}{S_{Na}} \div \frac{UCr}{SCr} \times 100 \qquad (26)$$

where U_{Na} and S_{Na} are urine and serum sodium in milliequivalents per liter or millimoles per liter, and UCr and SCr are in milligrams per deciliter or micromoles per liter.

In a normal subject with a GFR of 120 mL/min and a daily sodium excretion of 120 mEq, %FE$_{Na}$ is 0.5%. If the result is between 0.5 and 1%, the cause of the oliguria is probably prerenal (e.g., dehydration, volume depletion, or CHF). If %FE$_{Na}$ is >1–2%, the patient probably has acute tubular necrosis.[65] Table 8-10 lists %FE$_{Na}$ values in various disorders.

In a few situations, however, %FE$_{Na}$ may not conform to the usual patterns. It may be 1% or less despite the absence of prerenal azotemia (i.e., in the presence of nonoliguric acute renal failure) in patients with diseases causing sodium-avid states (e.g., ascites of liver disease,

CHF, hepatorenal syndrome, nephrotic syndrome, and burns).[67] Moreover, with acute tubular necrosis caused by radiocontrast media, $\%FE_{Na}$ is often less than 1%.[68]

URINE UREA NITROGEN AND NITROGEN BALANCE

Urine urea nitrogen is used primarily to determine the nitrogen balance in patients receiving extraordinary nutritional support (e.g., parenteral nutrition). Urine usually is collected for 24 hr, and the amount of nitrogen in urea is measured by various assays. The typical amounts found in practice are 5–25 g/day. The total nitrogen content of the urine is actually sought, and nitrogen within urea is a surrogate measure. Although clinicians assume that the urea nitrogen accounts for 80–90% of the total nitrogen content, the percentage is variable and decreases in certain diseases (e.g., liver disease).[69]

Low (<1%)	High (>1%)
Prerenal azotemia	Acute tubular necrosis
Acute glomerulonephritis	Urinary obstruction
Hepatorenal syndrome	Chronic uremia
Renal transplant rejection	Diuretics

[a] See exceptions in text.

Table 8-10. $\%FE_{Na}$ Test Results in Various Conditions[66,a]

Not all assays produce the same result on the same specimen. Some laboratories use instruments that convert urea to ammonia and then quantitate nitrogen from ammonia (no correction for pre-existing ammonia in the specimen). This technique generates results that are 5–10% higher than assays that do not convert urea.[70] Chloramphenicol and sulfonamides may cause falsely low results due to assay interference with most commercially available kits.

Estimating Total Nitrogen Elimination

The formula,

$$\text{total nitrogen loss (g)} = (UUN \times 1.25) + 2 \tag{27}$$

where UUN is urine urea nitrogen, is often used to estimate total *body* nitrogen losses (in grams). Then this amount is compared to the amount of nitrogen intake in the form of amino acids for estimation of the nitrogen balance. The 1.25 adjusts the urine urea nitrogen to the total nitrogen content; it is assumed that only 80% of the total nitrogen content is in the form of urea (most of the rest is in ammonia). The 2 in this formula represents the amount of nitrogen (in grams) lost via nonrenal routes, primarily the stool. Some investigators, however, have proposed that urine urea nitrogen plus an actual measurement of urinary ammonia more accurately approximates the urine's total nitrogen content.[71]

Estimating Nitrogen Balance

A positive nitrogen balance (more nitrogen in than out) is an important therapeutic goal for malnourished patients receiving parenteral and enteral nutrition. Clinicians should strive for at least a nitrogen equilibrium (in equals out).

The amount of amino acids (same as proteins) taken in by a patient can be converted to the approximate amount of incoming nitrogen (in grams) by dividing amino acids by 6.25, since 16% (1/6.25) of the average amino acid's weight is from nitrogen atoms. The amount of nitrogen going out is represented by Equation 27 or (UUN × 1.25) + 2. Therefore, a positive nitrogen balance is represented by

$$(\text{amino acid intake}/6.25) - (1.25\ UUN + 2) > 0 \tag{28}$$

where amino acid intake and urine urea nitrogen are in grams over 24 hr. In malnourished patients, a balance of zero is not adequate. Clinicians typically strive for an excess of at least 4 g of incoming nitrogen per day. Drugs (steroids) and diseases that cause the BUN to rise due to catabolic or antianabolic activity also can cause the urine urea nitrogen to rise.

SUMMARY

The kidneys play a major role in the regulation of fluids, electrolytes, and the acid-base balance. Kidney function is affected by the cardiovascular, pulmonary, endocrine, and central nervous systems. Therefore, abnormalities in these systems may be reflected in renal or urine tests. The urinalysis is useful as a mirror for organ systems that generate substances (e.g., blood/biliary system and urobilinogen) ultimately eliminated in the urine. A urinalysis allows indirect examination without invasive procedures.

A rise in BUN without a simultaneous rise in SCr is not specific for intrinsic renal disease. However, concomitant elevations in BUN and SCr almost always reflect intrinsic kidney damage. The GFR should be estimated based on the patient's SCr and demographic characteristics using the MDRD equation, as it is a more reliable index of kidney function than SCr alone. Monitoring the urine albumin excretion is useful as a measure of response to therapy for progressive kidney disease. Clinicians responsible for pharmacotherapy in patients with kidney disease rely heavily on these tests.

Urine urea nitrogen, the amount of urea nitrogen excreted in the urine per time period (usually 24 hr), is used almost exclusively for determining a patient's nitrogen balance. A positive nitrogen balance in a malnourished patient who is being fed intravenously or orally (especially if it occurs with a nonfluid weight gain) suggests that the patient is generating new muscular and circulating proteins.

REFERENCES

1. Vander AJ, Navar LG, eds. *Renal Physiology*. 6th ed. New York, NY: McGraw-Hill; 2002.
2. Levey AS. Use of glomerular filtration rate measurements to assess the progression of renal disease. *Semin Nephrol.* 1989; 9:370–79.
3. Young DS. *Effects of Drugs on Clinical Laboratory Tests*. 3rd ed. Washington, DC: American Association for Clinical Chemistry Press; 1990.
4. Kasiske BL, Keane WF. Laboratory assessment of renal disease: clearance, urinalysis, and renal biopsy. In: Brenner BM, ed. *Brenner & Rector's The Kidney*. 6th ed. Philadelphia, PA: W. B. Saunders; 2000.
5. Fossati P, Prencipe L, Berti G. Enzymatic creatinine assay: a new colorimetric method based on hydrogen peroxide measurement. *Clin Chem.* 1983; 29:1494–6.
6. Bauer JH, Brook CS, Byrch RN. Clinical appraisal of creatinine clearance as a measurement of glomerular filtration rate. *Am J Kidney Dis.* 1982; 2:337–46.
7. Rubin MI, Barratt TM, eds. *Pediatric Nephrology*. Baltimore, MD: Williams & Wilkins; 1975: 21.
8. Savory DJ. Reference ranges for serum creatinine in infants, children and adolescents. *Ann Clin Biochem.* 1990; 27:99–101.
9. Oh MS. Does serum creatinine rise faster in rhabdomyolysis? *Nephron.* 1993; 63:255–7.
10. Muther RS. Drug interference with renal function tests. *Am J Kidney Dis.* 1983; 3:118–20.
11. Bennett WM, Porter GA. Aspirin and renal function (letter). *N Engl J Med.* 1977; 296:1168.
12. Opravil M, Keusch G, Lüthy R. Pyrimethamine inhibits renal secretion of creatinine. *Antimicrob Agents Chemother.* 1993; 37:1056–60.
13. Perrone R, Madias N, Levey A. Serum creatinine as an index of renal function: new insights into old concepts. *Clin Chem.* 1992; 38:1933–53.
14. Hilbrands LB, Artz MA, Wetzels JF, et al. Cimetidine improves the reliability of creatinine as a marker of glomerular filtration. *Kidney Int.* 1991; 40:1171–6.
15. Hellerstein S, Alon U, Blowey D, et al. Use of serum creatinine concentration for estimation of glomerular filtration rate. *Am J Dis Child.* 1993; 147:719–20.
16. van den Berg JG, Koopman MG, Arisz L. Ranitidine has no influence on tubular creatinine secretion. *Nephron.* 1996; 74:705–8.
17. Zaltzman JS, Whiteside C, Cattran D, et al. Accurate measurement of impaired glomerular filtration using single-dose oral cimetidine. *Am J Kidney Dis.* 1996; 27:504–11.
18. Mayersohn M, Conrad KA, Achari R. The influence of a cooked meat meal on creatinine plasma concentration and creatinine clearance. *Br J Clin Pharmacol.* 1983; 15:227–30.
19. Lew SQ, Bosch JP. Effect of diet on creatinine clearance and excretion in young and elderly healthy subjects and in patients with renal disease. *J Am Soc Nephrol.* 1991; 2:856–65.
20. Kaji D, Strauss I, Kahn T. Serum creatinine in patients with spinal cord injury. *Mt Sinai J Med.* 1990; 57:160–4.
21. Rama R, Ibáñez J, Pagés T, et al. Plasma and red cell magnesium levels and plasma creatinine after a 100 km race. *Rev Esp Fisiol.* 1993; 49:43–8.

22. Caregaro L, Menon F, Angeli P, et al. Limitations of serum creatinine level and creatinine clearance as filtration markers in cirrhosis. *Arch Intern Med.* 1994; 154:201–5.

23. Kampmann JP, Hansen JM. Glomerular filtration rate and creatinine clearance. *Br J Clin Pharmacol.* 1981; 12:7–14.

24. Lebel RR, Gutmann FD, Mazumdar DC, et al. Creatinine determination in ketosis (letter). *N Engl J Med.* 1984; 310:1671.

25. Watts GF, Pillay D. Effects of ketones and glucose on the estimation of urinary creatinine: implications for microalbuminuria screening. *Diabetic Med.* 1990; 7:263–5.

26. Delanghe JR, Louagie HK, De Buyzere ML, et al. Glomerular filtration rate and creatinine production in adult icteric patients. *Clin Chim Acta.* 1994; 224:33–44.

27. Mitchell EK. Flucytosine and false elevation of serum creatinine level. *Ann Intern Med.* 1984; 101:278.

28. Daly TM, Kempe KC, Scott MG, et al. "Bouncing" creatinine levels (letter). *New Engl J Med.* 1996; 334:1749–50.

29. Blass KG, Ng DS. Reactivity of acetoacetate with alkaline picrate: an interference of the Jaffe reaction. *Clin Biochem.* 1988; 21:39–47.

30. Kenny D. A study of interferences in routine methods for creatinine measurement. *Scand J Clin Lab Invest.* 1993; 212(53 suppl):43–7.

31. Halstead AC, Nanji AA. Artifactual lowering of serum creatinine levels in the presence of hyperbilirubinemia (letter). *JAMA.* 1984; 251:38–9.

32. Piveral K, Miller SC, Baird DR, et al. Apparently raised serum creatinine levels due to cephalosporins (letter). *JAMA.* 1986; 255:323–4.

33. Nanji AA, Poon R, Hinberg I. Interference by cephalosporins with creatinine measurement by desk-top analyzers. *Eur J Clin Pharmacol.* 1987; 33:427–9.

34. Weber JA, van Zanten AP. Interferences in current methods for measurements of creatinine. *Clin Chem.* 1991; 37:695–700.

35. Santeiro ML, Thompson DF, Sagraves R. Flucytosine interference with serum creatinine determinations. *Drug Intell Clin Pharm.* 1988; 22:879–80.

36. Viraraghavan S, Blass KG. Effect of glucose on alkaline picrate: a Jaffe interference. *J Clin Chem Clin Biochem.* 1990; 28:95–105.

37. Nanji AA, Whitlow KJ. Spurious increase in serum creatinine associated with intravenous methyldopa therapy. *Drug Intell Clin Pharm.* 1984; 18:896–7.

38. Ducharme MP, Smythe M, Strohs G. Drug-induced alterations in serum creatinine concentrations. *Ann Pharmacother.* 1993; 27:622–33.

39. Lau AH, Berk SI, Prosser T, et al. Estimation of creatinine clearance in malnourished patients. *Clin Pharm.* 1988; 7:62–5.

40. Badr KF, Ichikawa I. Prerenal failure: a deleterious shift from renal compensation to decompensation. *N Engl J Med.* 1988; 319:623–9.

41. Jones JD, Burnett PC. Creatinine metabolism in humans with decreased renal function: creatinine deficit. *Clin Chem.* 1974; 20:1204–12.

42. Mitch WE, Mackenzie W. A proposed mechanism for reduced creatinine excretion in severe chronic renal failure. *Nephron.* 1978; 21:248–54.

43. Lemann J, Bidani AK, Bain RP, et al. Use of the serum creatinine to estimate glomerular filtration rate in health and early diabetic nephropathy. *Am J Kidney Dis.* 1990; 16:236–43.

44. Pesola GR, Akhavan I, Carlon GC. Urinary creatinine excretion in the ICU: low excretion does not mean inadequate collection. *Am J Crit Care.* 1993; 2:462–6.

45. Dubois D, Dubois EF. Clinical calorimetry: X. formula to estimate the approximate surface area if height and weight be known. *Arch Intern Med.* 1916; 17:863–71.

46. Mosteller RD. Simplified calculation of body-surface area. *N Engl J Med.* 1987; 317:1098.

47. NKF K/DOQI Advisory Board. Clinical practice guidelines for chronic kidney disease: evaluation, classification, and stratification. *Am J Kidney Dis.* 2002; 39(2 suppl):S1–246.

48. Cockcroft DW, Gault MH. Prediction of creatinine clearance from serum creatinine. *Nephron.* 1976; 16:31–41.

49. Levey AS, Bosch JP, Lewis JB, et al. A more accurate method to estimate glomerular filtration rate from serum creatinine. A new prediction equation. Modification of diet in renal disease study group. *Ann Intern Med.* 1999; 130:461–70.

50. Levey AS, Greene T, Kusek JW, et al. A simplified equation to predict glomerular filtration rate from serum creatinine (abstract). *J Am Soc Nephrol.* 2000; 11:A0828.

51. Schwartz GJ, Feld LG, Langford DJ. A simple estimate of glomerular filtration rate in full-term infants during the first year of life. *J Pediatr.* 1984; 104:849–54.

52. Counahan R, Chantler C, Ghazali S et al. Estimation of glomerular filtration rate from plasma creatinine concentration in children. *Arch Dis Child.* 1976; 51:875–8.

53. Jelliffe RW, Jelliffe SM. A computer program for estimation of creatinine clearance from unstable serum creatinine concentration. *Math Biosci.* 1972; 14:17–24.

54. Widmann FK. *Clinical Interpretation of Laboratory Tests.* 9th ed. Philadelphia, PA: F. A. Davis; 1983.

55. Wallach J. *Interpretation of Diagnostic Tests.* 3rd ed. Boston, MA: Little, Brown; 1982: 537–9.

56. Shaw ST Jr, Poon SY, Wong ET. Routine urinalysis: is the dipstick enough? *JAMA.* 1985; 253:1596–600.

57. Jenkins RD, Fenn JP, Matsen JM. Review of urine microscopy for bacteriuria. *JAMA.* 1986; 255:3397–403.

58. Mogensen CE. Microalbuminemia predicts clinical proteinuria and early mortality in maturity-onset diabetes. *N Engl J Med.* 1984; 310:356–60.

59. Yosselson-Superstine S, Sinai Y. Drug interference with urine protein determination. *J Clin Chem Clin Biochem.* 1986; 24:103–6.

60. Zwelling LA, Balow JE. Hypersthenuria in high-dose carbenicillin therapy. *Ann Intern Med.* 1978; 89:225–6.

61. Komaroff AL. Urinalysis and urine culture in women with dysuria. *Ann Intern Med.* 1986; 104:212–8.

62. Kerr JE, Magee-Nolan C, Schuster BL. Interference with phenazopyridine with the leukocyte esterase dipstick. *JAMA.* 1986; 256:38–9.

63. Harrington JT, Cohen JJ. Measurement of urinary electrolytes: indications and limitations. *N Engl J Med.* 1975; 293:1241–3.

64. Sherman RA, Eisinger RP. The use and misuse of urinary sodium and chloride measurements. *JAMA.* 1982; 247:3121–4.

65. Espinel CH. The FE_{Na} test: use in the differential diagnosis of acute renal failure. *JAMA.* 1976; 236:579–81.

66. Espinel CH. Diagnosis of acute and chronic renal failure. *Clin Lab Med.* 1993; 13:89–102.

67. Diamond JR, Yoburn DC. Nonoliguric acute renal failure associated with a low fractional excretion of sodium. *Ann Intern Med.* 1982; 96:597–600.

68. Fang LS, Sirota RA, Ebert TH, et al. Low fractional excretion of sodium with contrast media-induced acute renal failure. *Arch Intern Med.* 1980; 140:531–3.

69. Loder PB, Kee AJ, Horsburgh R, et al. Validity of urinary urea nitrogen as a measure of total urinary nitrogen in adult patients requiring parenteral nutrition. *Crit Care Med.* 1989; 17:309–12.

70. Boehm KA, Helms RA, Storm MC. Assessing the validity of adjusted urinary urea nitrogen as an estimate of total urinary nitrogen in three pediatric populations. *J Parenter Enter Nutr.* 1994; 18:172–6.

71. Burge JC, Choban P, McKnight T, et al. Urinary ammonia plus urinary urea nitrogen as an estimate of total urinary nitrogen in patients receiving parenteral nutrition support. *J Parenter Enter Nutr.* 1993; 17:529–31.

Chapter **9**

ARTERIAL BLOOD GASES AND ACID-BASE BALANCE

Thomas G. Hall

Maintenance of normal pH in the body is required for normal organ function. Cellular metabolism continually produces acidic substances that must be excreted to prevent acid accumulation. The lungs, kidneys, and a complex system of buffers allow the body to maintain acid-base homeostasis. Arterial blood gases (ABGs) include the pH, arterial partial pressures of oxygen (PaO_2) and carbon dioxide ($PaCO_2$), and the bicarbonate (HCO_3^-) concentration. By evaluating the ABGs, the clinician can assess a patient's acid-base status. The serum anion gap and lactate concentrations provide additional information to classify and evaluate the most likely causes of acid-base disorders.

This chapter reviews acid-base physiology and control, discusses laboratory tests used to assess acid-base status, and provides a method to evaluate potential causes of acid-base disorders. This chapter also reviews the use of ABGs to evaluate the oxygenation and ventilation functions of the lungs.

OBJECTIVES

After completing this chapter, the reader should be able to

1. Discuss the normal physiology of acid-base balance.
2. Describe the role of the kidneys in maintaining acid-base balance.
3. Describe the role of the lungs in gas exchange and maintaining acid-base balance.
4. Explain the functions of carbon dioxide, bicarbonate, and carbonic acid as the body's principal buffer system.
5. List the four simple acid-base disorders, their important causes, and accompanying laboratory test results.
6. Evaluate a patient's acid-base status and identify common causes, given the clinical presentation and laboratory data.
7. In a case study, use the results of ABGs and serum bicarbonate concentration to assess acid-base disorders, ventilation, and oxygenation.
8. In a case study, use the results of the anion gap and serum lactate concentration to evaluate acid-base disorders.

ACID-BASE PHYSIOLOGY

The pH of arterial blood is normally maintained within the narrow range of 7.36–7.44.[1,2] Values of arterial pH 7.35 and lower are termed *acidemia*, and values of arterial pH 7.45 and higher are termed *alkalemia*. A disorder that lowers pH is an *acidosis*, and a disorder that raises pH is an *alkalosis*. The distinction between these terms is often blurred. However, recognition of these concepts is critical to a thorough understanding of acid-base physiology. The arterial pH may be normal in mixed acid-base disorders (e.g., respiratory acidosis plus metabolic alkalosis) or only mildly altered even in significant acid-base disorders due to compensatory mechanisms.

Generally, the lungs and kidneys maintain acid-base homeostasis. Acid-base disorders are categorized according to the primary abnormality; the underlying biochemical event that disturbs the pH. The lungs excrete carbon dioxide (CO_2), which is the primary volatile acid in the body. When carbon dioxide elevation is the primary abnormality, the disorder is termed *respiratory acidosis*; a deficit of carbon dioxide is termed *respiratory alkalosis*. The kidneys regulate blood concentrations of bicarbonate (HCO_3^-). When the primary abnormality is a deficit of bicarbonate the disorder is termed *metabolic acidosis*; an excess of bicarbonate is termed *metabolic alkalosis*. Laboratory assessment of acid-base status is usually performed on samples of arterial blood, which accurately reflect acid-base status in the body under most conditions.

Acid-Base Balance

Metabolism of glucose, fats, and protein as energy sources result in the daily production of 15,000 mmol of carbon dioxide, which acts as an acid in the body, and 50–100 mEq of nonvolatile acids (e.g., sulfuric acid).[3] This continual load of acidic substances must be buffered initially to prevent acute acidosis. After being buffered, these acids must be excreted to prevent exceeding the body's buffer capacity. Carbon dioxide is excreted by the lungs and the nonvolatile acids are excreted by the kidneys.

The principal buffer in the body is the carbonic acid/bicarbonate system. Other buffers, including proteins, phosphate, and hemoglobin (Hgb), also contribute to maintenance of normal pH. However, the carbonic acid/bicarbonate system is particularly important in understanding acid-base physiology for two reasons:

1. The key components of this system, CO_2 as the acid and HCO_3^- as the base, are routinely measured in clinical laboratories. These parameters are used to estimate the overall acid-base status of the body. Because all buffer systems exist in equilibrium in the body, any change in acid-base status is reflected equally in each system. Thus, even though other buffers are important, accurate assessment of acid-base status may be made using only one system.
2. The lungs and kidneys closely regulate the concentrations of CO_2 and HCO_3^-, allowing rapid and precise control over acid-base equilibrium. Pathology in these organs often is associated with acid-base disorders.

Carbonic Acid/Bicarbonate Buffer System

Carbonic acid (H_2CO_3), a weak acid, and its conjugate base, bicarbonate (HCO_3^-), exist in equilibrium with hydrogen ions (H^+):

$$HCO_3^- + H^+ \rightleftarrows H_2CO_3$$

If hydrogen ions are added to the body or released as a result of cellular metabolism, the H^+ concentration rises and is reflected by a fall in pH. However, a large portion of the hydrogen ions combines with bicarbonate to form carbonic acid, lessening the effect on pH. The effect of the acid is buffered, and the pH remains at or near normal.

In aqueous solutions, carbonic acid reversibly dehydrates to form water and carbon dioxide. This reaction is catalyzed in the body by the enzyme carbonic anhydrase (CA), which is present in many tissues:

$$\overset{\text{CA}}{HCO_3^- + H^+ \rightleftarrows H_2CO_3 \rightleftarrows CO_2 + H_2O}$$

Nearly all carbonic acid in the body exists as carbon dioxide gas. Therefore, carbon dioxide is the acid form of the carbonic acid/bicarbonate buffer system. When hydrogen ions are released, the concentration of bicarbonate falls, and the concentration of carbon dioxide gas rises as the acid is buffered.

The Henderson-Hasselbalch equation for the carbonic acid/bicarbonate buffer system describes the mathematical relationship among pH, bicarbonate concentration in milliequivalents per liter, and partial pressure of carbon dioxide (pCO_2, a measure of the concentration of carbon dioxide gas in fluid) in millimeters of mercury:

$$pH = 6.1 + \log \left(\frac{HCO_3^-}{0.03 \times pCO_2} \right)$$

This equation demonstrates an important point: the *ratio* of the bicarbonate and carbon dioxide concentrations, not the absolute values, determines pH. The concentration of bicarbonate or carbon dioxide can change dramatically, but if the other value changes proportionately in the same direction, pH remains unchanged.

For arterial blood, the most commonly sampled medium, the normal ratio of bicarbonate (in milliequivalents per liter) to $PaCO_2$ (in millimeters of mercury) is 0.6:1. This ratio results in a pH of 7.40 when the bicarbonate concentration is normal (24 mEq/L ± 2 or 24 mmol/L ± 2) and the $PaCO_2$ is normal (40 mm Hg ± 4 or 5.3 kPa ± 0.5). It is impossible to predict the pH accurately or to assess a patient's acid-base status from either the bicarbonate concentration or $PaCO_2$ alone. If both are known, however, the pH can be calculated from this equation. In fact, when clinical laboratories evaluate ABGs, only the pH and $PaCO_2$ are measured. The bicarbonate concentration is then calculated from this equation.

Role of Kidneys and Lungs

The kidneys regulate the concentration of bicarbonate in extracellular fluid, and the lungs regulate the $PaCO_2$. An understanding of the functions of these organs is necessary to evaluate ABGs and acid-base status.

Kidneys

The principal role of the kidneys in maintaining acid-base homeostasis is to regulate the concentration of bicarbonate in the blood. Since bicarbonate is readily filtered at the glomerulus, the kidneys reabsorb filtered bicarbonate to prevent depletion. Approximately 90% of this reabsorption takes place in the proximal tubule and is catalyzed by carbonic anhydrase (Figure 9-1). Filtered bicarbonate combines with hydrogen ions secreted by the tubule cell to form carbonic acid. The enzyme carbonic anhydrase, located in the brush border of the tubule, catalyzes conversion of carbonic acid to carbon dioxide. The uncharged CO_2 readily crosses the cell membrane and passively diffuses into the renal tubule cell. Inside the cell, carbonic acid and bicarbonate are reformed, also catalyzed by carbonic anhydrase. The bicarbonate is reabsorbed into capillary blood. The net result of this process is reabsorption of sodium and bicarbonate. Drugs that inhibit carbonic anhydrase (e.g., acetazolamide) can cause metabolic acidosis by inhibiting this process, causing excessive quantities of bicarbonate to be lost in the urine.

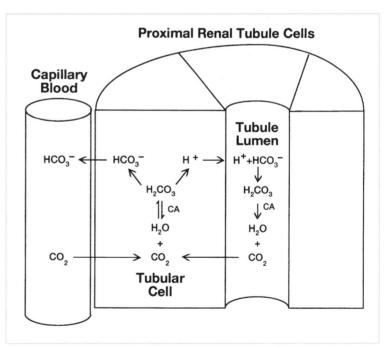

Figure 9-1. Reabsorption of bicarbonate from the proximal renal tubule cell.

The other major role of the kidneys, as discussed previously, is to excrete the 50–100 mEq/day of nonvolatile acids that are produced by the body. This process occurs primarily in the distal tubule and also requires carbonic anhydrase. The hydrogen ions that are secreted into the tubule lumen are buffered by phosphates and ammonia, so the urine pH is usually acidic but typically not less than 4.50.

Lungs

The principal role of the lungs in maintaining acid-base balance is to regulate the $PaCO_2$. After blood returns from the tissues to the right side of the heart, it is pumped through the pulmonary artery to the lungs. In the capillaries, carbon dioxide readily diffuses from the blood into the alveoli of the lungs and is excreted in exhaled air.

The rate of carbon dioxide excretion is directly proportional to the rate of air passing into and out of the lungs. Under resting conditions, normal individuals take 14–18 breaths/min. The amount of air in each breath, known as the *tidal volume*, is about 500 mL. Ventilation can be increased by increasing either the rate of respiration or the tidal volume.

Chemoreceptors in the arteries and the medulla in the brain are capable of rapidly increasing or decreasing ventilation in response to changes in pH and the arterial partial pressures of oxygen (PaO_2) and carbon dioxide ($PaCO_2$). This ability allows rapid response to changes in acid-base status and is a reason that the carbonic acid/bicarbonate buffer system is physiologically important. An elevated $PaCO_2$ is usually associated with hypoventilation, and a low $PaCO_2$ is usually associated with hyperventilation.

The other major function of the lungs is to oxygenate the blood. Inspired oxygen diffuses from the alveoli into capillary blood and is bound to Hgb in red blood cells. The oxygen is carried throughout the body via the arterial system and is released to tissues for utilization. Oxygen in arterial blood is present in three forms:

1. Oxygen gas (measured as PaO_2).
2. Dissolved oxygen.
3. Oxygen bound to Hgb (oxy-Hgb).

However, over 90% of the total arterial oxygen content is as oxy-Hgb. As the oxygenated blood passes through the capillaries, dissolved and gaseous oxygen are taken up by tissues, and additional oxygen rapidly dissociates from Hgb and becomes available for tissue uptake.

ARTERIAL BLOOD GASES

ABG evaluations include measurements of the arterial pH, PaO_2, and $PaCO_2$. The bicarbonate concentration is calculated from the pH and $PaCO_2$ using the equations listed previously. Proper evaluation of ABG results requires specific knowledge about each test.

pH

Normal range: 7.36–7.44

The pH of arterial blood is the first value to consider when using the ABGs to assess a patient's acid-base status. As stated previously, pH values of 7.35 and lower represent acidemia, and pH values of 7.45 and higher represent alkalemia. When a patient's acid-base status is evaluated, the patient must first be classified as having normal pH, acidemia, or alkalemia. It is important to recognize that a normal pH does not exclude the possibility of an acid-base disorder. Mixed acid-base disorders may result in a normal pH.

Critical values of pH are difficult to specify. Frequently, other manifestations of the underlying disorder producing the acid-base disturbance will dictate the urgency with which treatment must be offered. In general, pH values <7.20 or >7.60 represent levels that may require therapy to reverse the specific detrimental effects of the pH value.[4]

Spurious values of pH are most commonly due to inadvertent sampling of venous, rather than arterial blood. The pH of venous blood is slightly more acidic than arterial blood.

Arterial Partial Pressure of Carbon Dioxide

Normal range: 36–44 mm Hg or 4.8–5.9 kPa

Evaluation of the $PaCO_2$ (commonly seen on lab reports as pCO_2) provides information about the adequacy of lung function in excreting carbon dioxide, the acid form of the carbonic acid/bicarbonate buffer system. Because carbon dioxide is a small, uncharged molecule, it diffuses readily from pulmonary capillary blood into the alveoli in normal lungs. Therefore, an elevated $PaCO_2$ usually implies inadequate ventilation.

It is the pH, not the absolute value of $PaCO_2$ that determines the criticality of the patient's situation. Like the pH, spurious values for $PaCO_2$ are usually due to inadvertent venous sampling, which has a higher carbon dioxide content.

Arterial Partial Pressure of Oxygen

Normal range: 80–100 mm Hg or 10.7–13.3 kPa

Evaluation of the PaO_2 (commonly seen on lab reports as pO_2) provides information about the level of oxygenation of arterial blood. If effective circulation is achieved, a normal PaO_2 generally means that oxygen delivery to tissues is adequate. PaO_2 is commonly reduced in conjunction with an elevated $PaCO_2$ in states associated with hypoventilation. In fact, the PaO_2 is more likely to be diminished because carbon dioxide is much more freely diffusible across the pulmonary capillary and alveolar membranes. Therefore, diseases that impair gas exchange in the lungs can produce hypoxemia, which stimulates increased ventilation. Hyperventilation may fail to correct the hypoxemia but may produce a normal or low $PaCO_2$.

Figure 9-2 shows the sigmoid relationship between the percentage of available oxygen-binding sites on Hgb that are occupied and the PaO_2. The Hgb saturation remains above 90% as long as the PaO_2 is above 60 mm Hg (8 kPa). Since most oxygen in arterial blood is present as oxy-Hgb, oxygen delivery to tissues generally remains adequate even though the PaO_2 drops to as low as 60 mm Hg. However, PaO_2 values less than 60 mm Hg are associated with rapid falls in Hgb saturation and dramatic decreases in oxygen delivery to tissues.

This relationship is important to remember because ABGs measure PaO_2. Even though PaO_2 values between 60 mm Hg (8 kPa) and normal (80–100 mm Hg or 10.7–13.3 kPa) suggest a disease process, oxygen therapy may not be urgently needed since Hgb saturation is still above 90%. However, PaO_2 values less than 60 mm Hg indicate a more significant reduction in Hgb saturation and impaired tissue oxygen delivery. This impairment may require rapid supplemental oxygen therapy. The atmosphere contains 21% oxygen, and increasing this concentration with supplemental oxygen therapy frequently reverses hypoxemia. Oxygen is administered by increasing the fraction of inspired oxygen (FiO_2) to 24–100%.

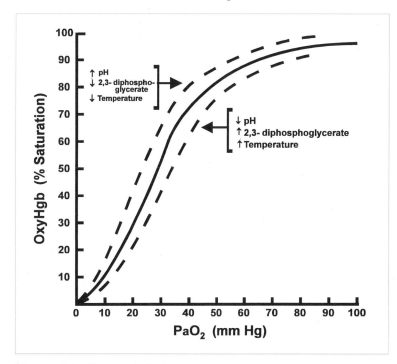

Figure 9-2. Oxygen–Hgb dissociation curve.

Spuriously low values of PaO_2 are seen with inadvertent venous blood samples or when the arterial blood sample is not stored in ice before the test is run. If kept at room temperature, cellular metabolism results in significant oxygen consumption, lowering the PaO_2 value. Conversely, air bubbles in the syringe may result in oxygen diffusion into the sample, spuriously raising the PaO_2 value.

Several conditions can alter oxygen–Hgb dissociation. Acidosis, fever, and increased concentrations of 2,3-diphosphoglycerate (2,3-DPG) shift the curve in Figure 9-2 to the right, making oxygen more readily available for delivery to tissues. Alkalosis and decreased 2,3-DPG concentrations shift the curve to the left, increasing oxygen binding to Hgb and potentially reducing oxygen delivery to tissues.

Serum Bicarbonate

Normal range: 24–30 mEq/L or 24–30 mmol/L

Once the $PaCO_2$ and pH are measured, the bicarbonate concentration is calculated and reported with the ABG results. Either the bicarbonate from the ABG determination or the total carbon dioxide content of serum (discussed below) can be used to assess acid-base disorders.

OTHER TESTS TO ASSESS ACID-BASE BALANCE AND OXYGENATION

Total Carbon Dioxide (Serum Bicarbonate)

Normal range: 24–30 mEq/L or 24–30 mmol/L

The total carbon dioxide concentration is determined by acidifying serum to convert all of the bicarbonate present to carbon dioxide. The total carbon dioxide content is then determined. However, since 95% of total serum carbon dioxide consists of converted bicarbonate, this value is actually a measure of the bicarbonate concentration. Therefore, the term *serum bicarbonate* is often used to describe the results of this test, even though clinical laboratories may report the test as the total carbon dioxide content. Although the name *total carbon dioxide* implies that it is a measure of acid, it is important to recognize that this test represents bicarbonate, the base form of the carbonic acid/bicarbonate buffer system. Like the $PaCO_2$ test, the urgency of need for response to abnormal total carbon dioxide values is determined by the pH. Some laboratories also report the bicarbonate or base deficit, which is the difference between the measured value and normal.

Anion Gap

Normal range: 3–11 mEq/L or 3–11 mmol/L

The anion gap is a calculated value that is helpful in categorizing and evaluating possible causes of metabolic acidosis.[5] For the body to remain electrically neutral, the numbers of all positively and negatively charged ions must be equal. However, clinical laboratories do not routinely measure all ions. Many positively charged ions (e.g., sodium, potassium, calcium, and magnesium) are measured. Sodium (Na^+) typically accounts for the majority of cations in extracellular fluids. Some anions (e.g., chloride, bicarbonate, and phosphate) are routinely measured, but others (e.g., sulfate, lactate, and pyruvate) are not. Serum proteins are also sources of negative charges that are difficult to quantify.

The number of *unmeasured* anions normally exceeds the number of *unmeasured* cations. When this difference is increased above the upper limit of normal, it often reflects an increase in negatively charged, weak acids. The presence of an increased anion gap in conjunction with metabolic acidosis provides the clinician with useful information about possible causes of acidosis. By convention, the anion gap is calculated using sodium to approximate the measured cations, and chloride (Cl⁻) and bicarbonate to approximate the measured anions:

$$\text{anion gap} = Na^+ - (Cl^- + HCO_3^-)$$

In conditions that cause metabolic acidosis either by production of hydrochloric acid (HCl) or by excessive loss of bicarbonate, which the kidneys primarily replace with chloride, the anion gap remains normal. The normal anion gap exists in these disorders because chloride anions replace bicarbonate, and both values are included in the calculation of the anion gap. These conditions are termed *hyperchloremic* or *normal anion gap* metabolic acidosis.

In other conditions, organic acids are formed that dissociate into unmeasured anions. In diabetic ketoacidosis, lipid catabolism produces the ketone bodies b-hydroxybutyrate and acetoacetate. In methanol intoxication methanol is metabolized to formic acid, which dissociates to produce formate and hydrogen ions. The anions b-hydroxybutyrate, acetoacetate, and formate are not measured in routine electrolyte panels or included in the calculation of the anion gap. They produce acidemia, a decrease in serum bicarbonate as this buffer is consumed, and an increase in the calculated anion gap. These conditions are examples of *elevated anion gap* metabolic acidosis. The presence of an elevated anion gap in any patient is highly suggestive of a metabolic acidosis.

The normal value for the anion gap has been reduced within the last several years because of changes in clinical chemistry methodologies for measuring chloride ions.[6] This shift has resulted in an increase in the normal range for chloride and a subsequent decrease in the normal value of the anion gap. Prior to this change, the normal anion gap was 8–12 mEq/L (8–12 mmol/L). The normal value at most institutions is now 3–11 mEq/L (3–11 mmol/L). However, this range may vary due to the variability in normal ranges of the values used to calculate anion gap. Clinicians should verify the normal range for anion gap at their institutions.

Various factors can alter the anion gap, making interpretation more difficult.[7] In particular, hypoalbuminemia, hyperlipidemia, lithium intoxication, and multiple myeloma decrease the anion gap. Albumin is one principal source of unmeasured anions, so hypoalbuminemia decreases unmeasured anions and the anion gap. Hyperlipidemia reduces the anion gap both by occupying space in the plasma volume and by interfering with the laboratory assay for chloride. Lithium is a positively charged ion not included in the anion gap calculation. In cases of intoxication, it can decrease the anion gap. Multiple myeloma produces positively charged proteins and reduces the anion gap by increasing unmeasured cations.

The anion gap can also be altered by many electrolyte abnormalities. In particular, abnormalities involving ions not included in the calculation of the anion gap (e.g., potassium and calcium) can affect the anion gap. Therefore, the anion gap must always be interpreted cautiously.

Serum Lactate

Normal ranges: 0.5–1.5 mEq/L or 0.5–1.5 mmol/L (venous) and 0.5–2.0 mEq/L or 0.5–2.0 mmol/L (arterial)

Lactate is a byproduct of the anaerobic metabolism of glucose as an energy source.[8] Metabolism of glucose yields pyruvate, which can be converted to lactate in a reaction catalyzed by lactate dehydrogenase (LDH) (Figure 9-3). Lactate is transported to the liver and converted back to pyruvate.

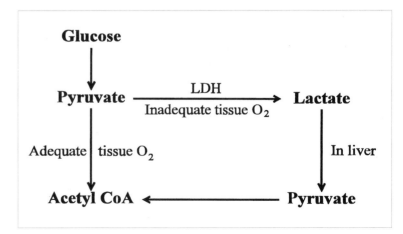

Figure 9-3. Lactate metabolism.

When tissues are normally oxygenated, pyruvate is converted to acetyl coenzyme A (acetyl CoA) and is utilized as an energy source via aerobic metabolism. In patients with inadequate tissue perfusion (e.g., septic shock) or increased tissue metabolic rates (e.g., status epilepticus), anaerobic metabolism predominates. Anaerobic metabolism increases the conversion of pyruvate to lactate, increasing lactate concentrations. When inadequate tissue perfusion is present, lactate is not transported to the liver, further increasing lactate concentrations. If these processes are severe or not reversed, lactic acidosis (a type of metabolic acidosis) can occur. Drugs or other conditions that impair lactate or pyruvate metabolism can also produce elevated lactate concentrations. Lactate levels above 5 mEq/L are usually associated with critical illness and require urgent treatment.

Venous Partial Pressure of Oxygen

Normal range: ≥70 mm Hg or ≥9.3 kPa

It has been recognized for many years that in critically ill patients or during cardiopulmonary resuscitation, venous blood gases may provide a more accurate measure of the adequacy of tissue oxygenation than arterial blood gases.[9] In particular, the venous partial pressure of oxygen has been suggested as a test that better reflects tissue oxygenation. This is because the amount of oxygen remaining in venous blood after passing through the tissues reflects both oxygen delivery (DO_2) and oxygen consumption (VO_2). When venous partial pressure of oxygen is measured in pulmonary arterial blood, which reflects mixed venous blood from all tissues in the body, it is termed *mixed venous oxygen* (SvO_2). The normal value for SvO_2 is ≥70 mm Hg. Values below this indicate that tissues are extracting an unusually large fraction of the delivered oxygen, and that increasing oxygen delivery or reducing tissue metabolic activity may be indicated. Studies evaluating the role of SvO_2 as a guide to treatment in critically ill patients are inconclusive. However, SvO_2 may be monitored in selected critically ill patients.

Oxygen Saturation by Pulse Oximetry

Normal range: >95%

As an alternative to PaO_2 values obtained with ABGs, measuring the oxygen-Hgb saturation with pulse oximetry can also assess the level of oxygenation.[10] Pulse oximetry is based on the principle that oxy-Hgb molecules absorb different amounts of light than nonoxygenated Hgb. In pulse oximetry a probe is placed on the finger or earlobe. Light of specific wavelength is transmitted through the tissues, and the light intensity is measured on the opposite side of the tissue. The amount of light absorption is proportional to the relative amounts of oxy-Hgb and Hgb present in arterial blood. The instrument calculates oxygen saturation from this ratio. This method is commonly used when frequent, noninvasive monitoring of oxygenation is needed (e.g., for patients receiving intravenous midazolam or opiates to provide moderate sedation for invasive procedures). Pulse oximetry provides a continuous estimate of oxygen saturation without the need for frequent arterial blood sampling. It is important to remember that the PaO_2 can fall dramatically, and the oxygen saturation will stay above 90%. Significant impairment of oxygenation may occur with minimal change in oxygen saturation. The results of pulse oximetry must be interpreted with this understanding.

Several factors can interfere with the accuracy of pulse oximetry. Presence of large amounts of carboxyhemoglobin (CO-Hgb), seen in heavy smokers and in carbon monoxide poisoning, falsely increases the estimated oxygen saturation. Hyperbilirubinemia also produces CO-Hgb and can falsely increase the oxygen saturation measured by pulse oximetry. Methemoglobinemia, often produced due to exposure to oxidizing substances, can produce false elevations or decreases in pulse oximetry measurements. Methylene blue produces significant decreases in the estimated oxygen saturation as measured by pulse oximetry. Physical factors such as excessive motion, skin pigmentation, and nail polish can affect the pulse oximetry measurement, and, finally, hypoperfusion or use of potent vasoconstrictors can interfere with the pulse oximetry reading.

BASIC PRINCIPLES IN ACID-BASE ASSESSMENT

Table 9-1 summarizes the expected laboratory results in the four simple acid-base disorders. For each disorder, the primary laboratory abnormality is accompanied by a compensatory change. For example, the primary abnormality in metabolic acidosis is a fall in serum bicarbonate, and the compensatory change is a fall in $PaCO_2$. These compensatory changes reflect the body's attempts to return the bicarbonate/carbon dioxide ratio and pH closer to the normal range.

DISORDER	pH	PRIMARY ALTERATION	COMPENSATORY ALTERATION	NORMAL LEVEL OF COMPENSATION[b]
Metabolic acidosis	↓	↓↓↓ HCO_3^-	↓↓ $PaCO_2$	↓ $PaCO_2$ = 1.2 x ↓ HCO_3^-
Metabolic alkalosis	↑	↑↑↑ HCO_3^-	↑↑ $PaCO_2$	↑ $PaCO_2$ = 0.6 x ↑ HCO_3^-
Respiratory acidosis (acute)	↓↓	↑↑↑ $PaCO_2$	↑ HCO_3^-	↑ HCO_3^- = 0.1 x ↑ $PaCO_2$
Respiratory acidosis (chronic)	↓	↑↑↑ $PaCO_2$	↑↑ HCO_3^-	↑ HCO_3^- = 0.4 x ↑ $PaCO_2$
Respiratory alkalosis (acute)	↑↑	↓↓↓ $PaCO_2$	↓ HCO_3^-	↓ HCO_3^- = 0.2 x ↓ $PaCO_2$
Respiratory alkalosis (chronic)	↑	↓↓↓ $PaCO_2$	↓↓ HCO_3^-	↓ HCO_3^- = 0.4 x ↓ $PaCO_2$

[a]Arrows signify direction and relative magnitude of change from normal values of $PaCO_2$ (40 mm Hg) and HCO_3^- (24 mEq/L).
[b]Normal compensation can vary by approximately ±10% from calculated values.

TABLE 9-1

Table 9-1. Laboratory Results in Simple Acid-Base Disorders[a]

An important principle in interpreting these laboratory tests is to recognize that the body never overcompensates and rarely completely compensates for an acid-base disorder. The only exception is chronic respiratory alkalosis in which the kidneys can completely compensate. Therefore, the pH and direction of change of the $PaCO_2$ and serum bicarbonate generally can be used to classify simple acid-base disorders.

Although respiratory compensation for metabolic acid-base disorders occurs within minutes to hours because the lungs can alter carbon dioxide excretion rapidly, renal compensation for respiratory disorders is slower. Acute respiratory acidosis and alkalosis are associated with minimal compensation (Table 9-1). Tissue buffers (e.g., protein and Hgb) are responsible for this compensation. Renal compensation, accomplished by altering the bicarbonate excretion, requires 6–12 hr to be initiated and is not complete for 3–5 days.

When assessing a patient's acid-base status, one should always evaluate the pH first. Once the patient is categorized as being acidemic, alkalemic, or normal, evaluation of the $PaCO_2$ and serum bicarbonate allows categorization of the acid-base disorder. In simple disorders, either the $PaCO_2$ or the serum bicarbonate is abnormal. If compensation has occurred, the other test (serum bicarbonate or $PaCO_2$) is also altered in the same direction. The direction of change in pH, $PaCO_2$, and serum bicarbonate is usually consistent with only one form of simple acid-base disorder.

The formulas listed in Table 9-1 for normal levels of compensation are estimates only; variability exists in the normal response. Generally, compensatory changes within 10% of the values predicted in Table 9-1 are consistent with normal compensation. Changes higher than 10% from predicted values should prompt consideration of a mixed acid-base disorder, such as metabolic alkalosis plus respiratory acidosis or metabolic acidosis plus respiratory alkalosis. Changes lower than 10% from predicted values may also suggest a mixed disorder, such as a combined metabolic and respiratory acidosis or metabolic and respiratory alkalosis. In patients with metabolic acidosis, comparing the decrease in serum bicarbonate with the increase in the anion gap is useful. If the anion gap is elevated but not to the same degree that the bicarbonate has fallen, a combination of anion gap and hyperchloremic metabolic acidosis, caused by two underlying disorders, may be present.

In the case of renal compensation for respiratory acid-base disorders, values intermediate between acute and chronic compensation may indicate either that a mixed disorder is present or that adequate time for compensation has not elapsed. Information from the patient's history and physical examination, including temporal relationships, must be assessed to help evaluate the laboratory data. The minicases and discussions that follow build on this overview to demonstrate evaluation of patients with acid-base disorders.

Metabolic Acidosis

Patients with metabolic acidosis display an arterial pH less than 7.36 (acidemia) and a low serum bicarbonate concentration, determined either with ABGs or as the total carbon dioxide concentration on the serum chemistry panel. Under most circumstances, the body compensates by hyperventilating to increase carbon dioxide excretion, resulting in a low $PaCO_2$ value (Table 9-1).

Common causes of metabolic acidosis are listed in Table 9-2. Once metabolic acidosis is diagnosed, the next step in patient assessment is calculation of the anion gap. This step helps to determine the cause of the acidosis. As shown in Table 9-2, some causes of metabolic acidosis typically produce an increased anion gap, while others produce a normal gap. With a normal anion gap, the serum chloride is elevated, producing a hyperchloremic metabolic acidosis.

Several drugs can cause metabolic acidosis and are listed in Table 9-2. Several of the nucleoside reverse-transcriptase inhibitors used to treat human immunodeficiency virus (HIV) infection have been reported to cause lactic acidosis.[11] Propofol has been reported to cause lactic acidosis, primarily in critically ill pediatric patients, when used for sedation.[12,13] Prolonged, high dose infusion of intravenous lorazepam, which contains propylene glycol, has also been reported to cause lactic acidosis in critically ill patients.[14]

Metabolic Alkalosis

An elevated pH with an elevated serum bicarbonate concentration confirms the presence of metabolic alkalosis. Although some respiratory compensation occurs as a result of hypoventilation and carbon dioxide retention, compensation is relatively minor in metabolic

TABLE 9-2

ELEVATED ANION GAP	NORMAL ANION GAP (HYPERCHLOREMIC)
Renal failure	**Renal tubular acidosis**
Ketoacidosis	**Diarrhea**
Diabetes mellitus	**Drugs/toxins**
Starvation	Carbonic anhydrase inhibitors (e.g., acetazolamide)
Ethanol	Amphotericin B
Lactic acidosis	Lithium carbonate
Shock—septic, cardiogenic, hypovolemic	Lead
Severe hypoxemia	Ammonium chloride
Carbon monoxide poisoning	Arginine hydrochloride
Tonic-clonic seizures	Topiramate
Liver disease	
Drugs	
Metformin	
Propofol (primarily in children)	
Nucleoside reverse-transcriptase inhibitors	
Intravenous lorazepam (due to vehicle)	
Nitroprusside (cyanide accumulation)	
Intoxications	
Methanol	
Ethylene glycol	
Salicylates	

Table 9-2. Common Causes of Metabolic Acidosis[1–3,5,11–18]

MINICASE 1

A 27-YEAR-OLD FEMALE, M. M., was brought to the emergency department in a somnolent state. Her roommate stated that M. M. was diabetic and took insulin shots several times a day. The patient complained the previous evening of a headache and fatigue. Her vital signs included heart rate (HR) 120/min with blood pressure (BP) 110/60 mm Hg supine, HR 140/min with BP 80/40 mm Hg sitting, respiration rate 28/min with deep respirations, and temperature 99.5 °F (37.5 °C). Mucous membranes were dry, and tenting of the skin was present.

M. M. responded to stimuli only by opening her eyes and mumbling; she was unable to answer questions or follow commands. Deep tendon reflexes were mildly hyporeactive. Lung, cardiac, and abdominal exams were normal. Laboratory data included sodium 132 mEq/L (136–145 mEq/L), potassium 4.8 mEq/L (3.5–5.0 mEq/L), chloride 102 mEq/L (96–106 mEq/L), total carbon dioxide 10 mEq/L (24–30 mEq/L), serum creatinine (SCr) 1.4 mg/dL (0.7–1.5 mg/dL), glucose 600 mg/dL (70–110 mg/dL), and white blood cell (WBC) count 10,000 cells/mm³ (4800–10,800 cells/mm³). ABGs on room air were pH 7.23 (7.36–7.44), $PaCO_2$ 22 mm Hg (36–44 mm Hg), PaO_2 100 mm Hg (80–100 mm Hg), and serum bicarbonate 9 mEq/L (24–30 mEq/L).

Question:: What acid-base disorder does M. M. exhibit? What is her anion gap? What is the cause of her acid-base disorder? How are the physical exam findings consistent with this acid-base disorder?

Discussion: M. M.'s pH of 7.23 is clearly in the acidemic range. Further evaluation of the ABGs reveals a markedly low bicarbonate value, suggesting metabolic acidosis. The low $PaCO_2$ value, representing respiratory compensation, confirms this assessment. The level of respiratory compensation is consistent with the expected degree of compensation described in Table 9-1. The bicarbonate value has fallen by approximately 15 mEq/L from a normal value of 24, and the $PaCO_2$ has been reduced by 18 (1.2 x 15 mEq/L, as predicted in Table 9-1) to 22 mm Hg from the normal of 40 mm Hg. These values suggest that M. M. has only metabolic acidosis and not a mixed acid-base disorder.

The importance of compensation for acid-base disorders can be appreciated by calculating the expected pH in M. M. if respiratory compensation had not occurred. If the $PaCO_2$ had stayed at 40 mm Hg with a serum bicarbonate of 9 mEq/L, the pH would be 6.98 (Henderson-Hasselbalch equation).

M. M.'s anion gap of 20 mEq/L (132 – [102 + 10]) is elevated, allowing classification of the disorder as a metabolic acidosis with elevated anion gap. The most likely cause is diabetic ketoacidosis (Table 9-2), as suggested by her medical history and the elevated glucose concentration. Ketoacidosis produces an elevated anion gap due to the production of the ketone bodies, b-hydroxybutyrate and acetoacetate, byproducts of fat metabolism. The presence of rapid, deep respirations (Kussmaul) indicates the hyperventilation response to the acidosis and represents the body's attempt to reduce the carbon dioxide concentration to maintain a more normal pH in the presence of diminished bicarbonate.

---

alkalosis. The most common causes of metabolic alkalosis (Table 9-3) are

- Loss of gastric acid as a result of persistent vomiting or nasogastric suction.

- Loss of intravascular volume and chloride ion as a result of diuretic use.

Metabolic alkalosis due to loss of gastric acid may be prevented by administration of proton pump inhibitors (e.g., omeprazole) or histamine-2 antagonists (e.g., famotidine), which block gastric acid secretion.

Metabolic alkalosis also occurs in hospitalized patients as a result of improper anion balance in parenteral nutrition solutions or over treatment of metabolic acidosis with bicarbonate. In parenteral nutrition solutions, anions are typically provided as acetate and chloride. Because acetate is metabolized to bicarbonate, excessive acetate and inadequate chloride administration can produce metabolic alkalosis. In patients with metabolic acidosis due to circulatory failure, administration of sodium bicarbonate initially returns the pH toward normal. However, after restoration of adequate circulation, excessive bicarbonate and meta-

TABLE 9-3

Loss of gastric acid
Vomiting
Nasogastric suction

Mineralocorticoid excess
Hyperaldosteronism
Exogenous mineralocorticoids

Hypokalemia

Alkali administration
Oral
Parenteral nutrition with excessive acetate
Excessive administration of bicarbonate in metabolic acidosis

Diuretic therapy
Loop diuretics (e.g., furosemide)
Thiazide diuretics (e.g., hydrochlorothiazide)

Table 9-3. Common Causes of Metabolic Alkalosis[1–3]

MINICASE 2

A 45-YEAR-OLD MALE, J. C., was admitted to the general surgery service because of a constant, gnawing abdominal pain lasting 3 days. The pain was present in the left, upper abdominal quadrant and extended to his back. He came to the hospital when the pain got so severe that he was no longer able to eat or drink.

J. C. had a history of mild hypertension treated with hydrochlorothiazide 25 mg PO/day. He smoked one pack of cigarettes per day and admitted to consuming two or three martinis with lunch and dinner each day.

J. C.'s vital signs included HR 120/min with BP 120/70 mm Hg supine, HR 132/min with BP 100/60 mm Hg sitting, respiration rate 16/min, and temperature 98.6 °F (37 °C). His physical exam was remarkable only for dry mucous membranes and marked left, upper-quadrant abdominal tenderness with guarding. Bowel sounds were present but hypoactive, and rebound tenderness was absent.

J. C. was diagnosed with acute pancreatitis and was ordered to receive nothing by mouth. Intermittent nasogastric suction was initiated. At that time, laboratory data included sodium 135 mEq/L (136–145 mEq/L), potassium 4.0 mEq/L (3.5–5.0 mEq/L), chloride 98 mEq/L (96–106 mEq/L), total carbon dioxide 32 mEq/L (24–30 mEq/L), SCr 1.4 mg/dL (0.7–1.5 mg/dL), glucose 140 mg/dL (70–110 mg/dL), calcium 9.0 g/dL (8.5–10.8 mEq/L), albumin 4.0 g/dL (3.5–5 g/dL), amylase 1100 IU/L, and lipase 840 IU/L. J. C. was given IV fluids and morphine 4–10 mg intramuscularly every 4 hr as needed for pain.

Thirty-six hours later, his pain had improved slightly and his BP was normal, but he complained of generalized weakness. His ABGs were pH 7.53 (7.36–7.44), $PaCO_2$ 47 mm Hg (36–44 mm Hg), PaO_2 100 mm Hg (80–100 mm Hg), and serum bicarbonate 38 mEq/L (24–30 mEq/L).

Question: What acid-base disorder is present? What is the cause? What acid-base disorder was present on admission, and what was the cause?

Discussion: The elevated pH of 7.53 confirms the presence of an alkalemia. The possible causes are respiratory alkalosis, which would present with a low $PaCO_2$, and metabolic alkalosis, which would present with an elevated serum bicarbonate concentration. In J. C., the elevated serum bicarbonate of 38 mEq/L and slightly elevated $PaCO_2$ in compensation are consistent with the diagnosis of metabolic alkalosis.

His degree of hypoventilation and carbon dioxide retention is consistent with the expected degree of respiratory compensation predicted in Table 9-1. The serum bicarbonate is elevated by 14 mEq/L from the normal value of 24 mEq/L. The expected respiratory compensation for this serum bicarbonate concentration (Table 9-1) is approximately 8 mm Hg (0.6 x 14 mEq/L increase in bicarbonate), and the $PaCO_2$ is elevated by 7 mm Hg (from approximate normal of 40 mm Hg). Therefore, J. C. appears to have a simple compensated metabolic alkalosis. The most likely cause is the nasogastric suction, which results in removal of hydrogen ions from the stomach (Table 9-3).

Although definitive classification of J. C.'s acid-base status on admission is not possible since his ABGs were not done, he probably had a mild metabolic alkalosis at that time as well. The increase in bicarbonate, history of diuretic use, and evidence of intravascular volume depletion (i.e., orthostatic hypotension, dry mucous membranes, and reduced oral intake) are consistent with this conclusion.

TABLE 9-4

CNS Disorders
   Cerebral vascular accident
   Tumor
   Sleep apnea
   Drugs (e.g., opioids and sedative/hypnotics)

Lung disorders
   Airway obstruction
   Asthma
   Chronic obstructive pulmonary disease (e.g., chronic bronchitis)
   Pulmonary edema

Neuromuscular disorders
   Myasthenia gravis
   Guillain-Barré syndrome
   Hypokalemia
   Hypophosphatemia
   Neuromuscular blocking drugs

Table 9-4. Common Causes of Respiratory Acidosis[1–3,19]

bolic alkalosis may be present until the kidneys return the bicarbonate concentration to normal.

Respiratory Acidosis

Respiratory acidosis is usually synonymous with hypoventilation.[19] This condition can be a result of numerous causes (Table 9-4) in three general categories:

1. Impaired central nervous system (CNS) respiratory drive.
2. Impaired gas exchange in the lungs.
3. Impaired neuromuscular function affecting the diaphragm and/or chest wall.

Laboratory results consistent with respiratory acidosis are a low pH with an elevated $PaCO_2$, indicating inadequate excretion of carbon dioxide. Because the kidneys require 6–12 hr to initiate and 3–5 days to complete compensation, acute respiratory acidosis is associated with much greater alterations in pH than chronic respiratory acidosis. For example, a typical patient with an acute rise in $PaCO_2$ to 60 mm Hg (8 kPa) will have a pH of 7.26 with a serum bicarbonate of 26 mEq/L (26 mmol/L; Table 9-1 and Henderson-Hasselbalch equation). If the same patient's $PaCO_2$ remains at 60 mm Hg for 3–5 days when full renal compensation occurs, the serum bicarbonate will rise to 32 mEq/L (32 mmol/L). This returns the arterial pH to a nearly normal value of 7.35. While acute respiratory acidosis associated with hypoxemia may be life threatening, chronic compensated respiratory acidosis often requires no therapeutic intervention.

MINICASE 3

A 63-YEAR-OLD MALE, T. K., arrived at the Family Practice Clinic for a routine follow-up. He had a history of hypertension, coronary artery disease, and chronic bronchitis but had experienced no episodes of chest pain for the last month. T. K. had a chronic cough productive of approximately 2 cups of white-yellow sputum per day and shortness of breath after walking one block. These symptoms were unchanged over the past 3 months. His medications were enalapril 10 mg oral 2 times a day, simvastatin 40 mg oral daily, enteric-coated aspirin 325 mg oral daily, ipratropium bromide inhaler two puffs 4 times a day, albuterol inhaler two puffs as needed for shortness of breath, and nitroglycerin 0.4 mg sublingually as needed for chest pain.

T. K.'s vital signs included HR 90/min, BP 130/85 mm Hg, respiration rate 28/min, and temperature 98.6 °F (37 °C). His physical exam revealed rales and rhonchi throughout both lung fields. His laboratory data included sodium 134 mEq/L (136–145 mEq/L), potassium 3.6 mEq/L (3.5–5.0 mEq/L), chloride 92 mEq/L (96–106 mEq/L), total carbon dioxide 34 mEq/L (24–30 mEq/L), SCr 1.2 mg/dL (0.7–1.5 mg/dL), and glucose 160 mg/dL (70–110 mg/dL). ABGs on room air were pH 7.35 (7.36–7.44), $PaCO_2$ 60 mm Hg (36–44 mm Hg), PaO_2 65 mm Hg (80–100 mm Hg), and serum bicarbonate 32 mEq/L (24–30 mEq/L).

Question: What acid-base disorder does this patient have and what is the cause? Is this disorder acute or chronic?

Discussion: Inspection of the ABGs reveals that T. K. is acidemic, with a slightly low pH of 7.35. If he had a metabolic acidosis, his serum bicarbonate would be expected to be low. Instead, both the serum bicarbonate and the $PaCO_2$ are elevated. These values are consistent with a compensated respiratory acidosis. Patients with chronic bronchitis commonly exhibit chronic respiratory acidosis due to impaired ventilation (Table 9-4).[18] The body compensates by avidly reabsorbing bicarbonate to return the bicarbonate/carbon dioxide ratio and pH nearer to normal. The degree of renal compensation, as well as the history of chronic, stable symptoms, is consistent with a chronic disorder (Table 9-1). The anion gap is normal at 8 mEq/L (134 – [92 + 34]), as expected in patients with respiratory acidosis.

Respiratory Alkalosis

Increased ventilation results in increased carbon dioxide excretion (low $PaCO_2$), elevated pH, and respiratory alkalosis. Typically, the symptoms of respiratory alkalosis are mild and consist of dizziness, lightheadedness, and paresthesias. Acute respiratory alkalosis, commonly produced by the anxiety–hyperventilation syndrome, is usually a benign disorder and reverses either spontaneously or as a result of rebreathing expired air. Mild chronic respiratory alkalosis is also usually a benign disorder, but in some situations it may have more serious consequences.[20]

Common causes of respiratory alkalosis are listed in Table 9-5.

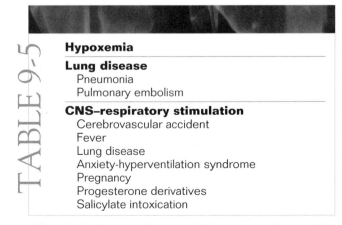

Hypoxemia
Lung disease
Pneumonia
Pulmonary embolism
CNS–respiratory stimulation
Cerebrovascular accident
Fever
Lung disease
Anxiety-hyperventilation syndrome
Pregnancy
Progesterone derivatives
Salicylate intoxication

Table 9-5. Common Causes of Respiratory Alkalosis[1–3,20]

MINICASE 4

A 24-YEAR-OLD MALE, B. H., was brought to the emergency department from the obstetrical floor for evaluation of syncope. He was assisting his wife in Lamaze breathing techniques when he fainted. His laboratory data included sodium 140 mEq/L (136–145 mEq/L), potassium 3.8 mEq/L (3.5–5.0 mEq/L), chloride 102 mEq/L (96–106 mEq/L), serum bicarbonate 24 mEq/L (24–30 mEq/L), SCr 0.8 mg/dL (0.7–1.5 mg/dL), and glucose 140 mg/dL (70–110 mg/dL). B. H.'s ABGs were pH 7.60 (7.36–7.44), $PaCO_2$ 25 mm Hg (36–44 mm Hg), PaO_2 120 mm Hg (80–100 mm Hg), and serum bicarbonate 24 mEq/L (24–30 mEq/L).

Question: What acid-base disorder does this patient exhibit?

Discussion: B. H.'s arterial pH is in the alkalemic range. Since the serum bicarbonate concentration is not elevated, this condition is not likely to be metabolic alkalosis. However, his $PaCO_2$ is low—consistent with respiratory alkalosis. The most likely cause is hyperventilation (Table 9-5). Because the alkalosis developed acutely, the kidneys did not have adequate time to compensate, and his pH rose enough to cause syncope.

MINICASE 5

A 24-YEAR-OLD-FEMALE, P. M., was brought to the emergency department after her roommate found her unconscious in their apartment. The roommate reports that P. M. has been despondent for the past 3 months after breaking up with her boyfriend and after being fired from her job. During ambulance transfer, P. M. vomited, and the emesis contained several white tablet fragments.

The roommate reports that P. M. takes only oral contraceptives, and there are no other prescription medications in the apartment. She does state that there are over-the-counter bottles of acetaminophen, ibuprofen, aspirin, and cough and cold products in the apartment.

P. M.'s vital signs included HR 100/min with BP 120/70 mm, respiration rate 30/min, and temperature 101 °F. (38.3 °C) Her physical exam was remarkable only for dry mucous membranes. Bowel sounds were present but hypoactive, and rebound tenderness was absent. She was noted to be somnolent and responded to questions only with moans.

Laboratory data included sodium 136 mEq/L (136–145 mEq/L), potassium 3.2 mEq/L (3.5–5.0 mEq/L), chloride 98 mEq/L (96–106 mEq/L), total carbon dioxide 15 mEq/L (24–30 mEq/L), SCr 1.0 mg/dL (0.7–1.5 mg/dL), and glucose 120 mg/dL (70–110 mg/dL). Her ABGs were pH 7.36 (7.36–7.44), $PaCO_2$ 28 mm Hg (36–44 mm Hg), PaO_2 100 mm Hg (80–100 mm Hg), and serum bicarbonate 15 mEq/L (24–30 mEq/L).

Question: What acid-base disorder is present? What is the most likely cause?

Discussion: Inspection of the pH reveals that the arterial pH is normal. However, both the $PaCO_2$ and serum bicarbonate are low. This combination of tests suggests that a mixed acid-base disorder may be present and emphasizes the need to fully evaluate the ABG results. The $PaCO_2$ is approximately 12 mm Hg below the normal value, which is consistent with respiratory alkalosis. The expected degree of renal compensation for this degree of decline in $PaCO_2$ is 2–5 mEq/L, depending on the time available for compensation to have occurred. This would result in a serum bicarbonate level of 19–22 mEq/L. The serum bicarbonate level is lower than would be expected in renal compensation, and the anion gap is elevated, so the patient must also have metabolic acidosis. The patient is displaying a mixed acid-base disorder, respiratory alkalosis combined with elevated anion gap metabolic acidosis. This combination of acid-base disorders is often seen in patients with salicylate toxicity. This is because of the direct respiratory stimulant effects of salicylate, displayed in P. M. by her tachypnea, and because salicylate also impairs oxidative metabolism, producing an anion gap metabolic acidosis.

SUMMARY

This chapter reviews acid-base physiology and disorders and presents a method of evaluating a patient's acid-base status. The lungs regulate the concentration of carbon dioxide, the acid form of the carbonic acid/bicarbonate buffer system. The kidneys regulate the concentration of bicarbonate.

Evaluation of ABGs requires identification of whether the patient is acidemic, alkalemic, or has a normal pH. Once this determination is made, the disorder can be categorized into a metabolic or respiratory type by examining both the $PaCO_2$ and serum bicarbonate. Assessment of the degree of compensation and comparison with expected levels of compensation, along with an evaluation of other patient information, allows detection of mixed acid-base disorders.

These basic skills enable the clinician to assess a patient's acid-base status quickly and effectively.

REFERENCES

1. Narins RG, Emmett M. Simple and mixed acid-base disorders: a practical approach. *Medicine*. 1980; 59:161–87.
2. McMullin ST, Hall TG, Kleiman-Wexler RL. Acid-base disorders. In: Koda-Kimble MA, Young LY, eds. *Applied Therapeutics: The Clinical Use of Drugs*. 7th ed. Philadelphia, PA: Lippincott Williams & Wilkins; 2001: 9.1–9.15.
3. Rose BD, Post TW. *Clinical Physiology of Acid-Base and Electrolyte Disorders*. 5th ed. New York, NY: McGraw-Hill; 2001.
4. Adrogué HJ, Madias NE. Management of life-threatening acid-base disorders. *N Engl J Med* 1998; 338:26–34, 107–11.
5. Goodkin DA, Gollapudi GK, Narins RG. The role of the anion gap in detecting and managing mixed metabolic acid-base disorders. *Clin Endocrinol Metab*. 1984; 13:333–49.
6. Winter SD, Pearson JR, Gabow PA, et al. The fall of the serum anion gap. *Arch Intern Med*. 1990; 150:311–3.
7. Salem MM, Mujais SK. Gaps in the anion gap. *Arch Intern Med*. 1992; 152:1625–9.
8. Mizrock BA. Lactic acidosis in critical illness. *Crit Care Med*. 1992; 20:80–93.
9. Weil MH, Rackow EC, Trevino R, et al. Difference in acid-base state between venous and arterial blood during cardiopulmonary resuscitation. *N Engl J Med*. 1986; 315:153–6.
10. Sinex JE. Pulse oximetry: principles and limitations. *Am J Emerg Med*. 1999; 17:59–67.
11. Carr A, Miller J, Law M, et al. A syndrome of lipoatrophy, lactic acidemia and liver dysfunction associated with HIV nucleoside analogue therapy: contribution to protease inhibitor-related lipodystrophy syndrome. *AIDS*. 2000; 14:F25–32.
12. Parke TJ, Stevens JE, Rice AS, et al. Metabolic acidosis and fatal myocardial failure after propofol infusion in children: five case reports. *Brit Med J*. 1992; 305:613–6.
13. Perrier ND, Baerga-Varela Y, Murray MJ. Death related to propofol use in an adult patient. *Crit Care Med*. 2000; 28:3071–3.
14. Reynolds HN, Teiken P, Regan M, et al. Hyperlactatemia, increased osmolar gap, and renal dysfunction during continuous lorazepam infusion. *Crit Care Med*. 2000; 28:1631–4.
15. Humphrey SH, Nash DA. Lactic acidosis complicating sodium nitroprusside therapy. *Ann Intern Med*. 1978; 88:58–9.
16. Kay TD, Hogan PG, McLeod SE, et al. Severe irreversible proximal renal tubular acidosis and azotaemia secondary to cidofovir. *Nephron*. 2000; 86:348–9.
17. Vittecoq D, Dumitrescu L, Beaufils H, et al. Fanconi syndrome associated with cidofovir therapy (letter). *Antimicrob Ag Chemother*. 1997; 41:1846.
18. Takeoka M, Holmes GL, Thiele E, et al. Topiramate and metabolic acidosis in pediatric epilepsy. *Epilepsia*. 2001;42:387–92.
19. Weinberger SE, Schwartzstein RM, Weiss JW. Hypercapnia. *N Engl J Med*. 1989; 321:1223–31.
20. Laffey JG, Kavanagh BP. Hypocapnia. *N Engl J Med*. 2002; 347:43–53.

Chapter **10**

PULMONARY FUNCTION AND RELATED TESTS

Gary Milavetz and Mary Teresi

Pulmonary function tests (PFTs) provide objective and quantifiable measures of lung function and are useful in the diagnosis, evaluation, and monitoring of respiratory disease. In addition, PFTs can assess response or effectiveness of therapy and detect pulmonary side effects of medications. Spirometry, a test that measures the movement of air into and out of the lungs during various breathing maneuvers, is the most frequently used PFT. Other tests of lung function include plethysmography, carbon monoxide diffusion capacity, exercise testing, and bronchoprovocation challenge tests. Arterial blood gases (ABGs) also are useful to assess lung function. Interpretation of ABGs is discussed elsewhere.

Diagnosis and monitoring of many pulmonary diseases, including diseases of gas exchange, often requires measurement of the flow or volume of air inspired and expired by the patient. Appropriate pharmacotherapeutic agents can be chosen and evaluated by using PFTs. Clinicians frequently review changes in these tests to monitor therapy for patients with asthma, cystic fibrosis (CF), emphysema, and other respiratory diseases, as well as to monitor lung function after thoracic radiation or lung transplantation. This chapter discusses the mechanics and interpretation of PFTs.

OBJECTIVES

After completing this chapter, the reader should be able to

1. Identify common PFTs and list their use and limitations.
    a. Spirometry
    b. Plethysmography
    c. Carbon monoxide diffusion capacity
    d. Airway reactivity tests
    e. Specialized tests
        i. Infant pulmonary function testing
        ii. Sputum inflammatory markers
2. Describe how PFTs are performed and discuss factors affecting the validity of the results.
3. Interpret commonly used PFTs, given clinical and other laboratory data.
4. Discuss how PFTs are used in the diagnosis of pulmonary diseases.
5. Discuss how PFTs are used in the monitoring of drug therapy.

ANATOMY AND PHYSIOLOGY OF LUNGS

The purpose of the lungs is to take oxygen from the atmosphere and exchange it for carbon dioxide in the blood. The movement of air in and out of the lungs is called *ventilation*; the movement of blood through the lungs is termed *perfusion*.

Air enters the body through the mouth and nose and travels through the pharynx to the trachea. The trachea splits into the left and right main stem bronchi, and these bronchi deliver inspired air to the respective lungs. The left and right lungs are in the pleural cavity of the thorax. These two spongy, conical structures are the primary organs of respiration.

The right lung has three lobes while the left lung has only two lobes, thus leaving space for the heart. The thoracic cavity is separated from the abdominal cavity by the diaphragm. The diaphragm—a thin sheet of dome-shaped muscle—contracts and relaxes during breathing. The lungs are contained within the rib cage but rest on the diaphragm. Between the ribs are two sets of intercostal muscles. These muscles attach to each upper and lower rib.

During inhalation, the intercostal muscles and the diaphragm contract, enlarging the thoracic cavity. This action generates a negative intrathoracic pressure, allowing air to rush in through the nose and mouth down into the pharynx, trachea, and lungs. During exhalation, these muscles relax and a positive intrathoracic pressure causes air to be pushed out of the lungs. Normal expiration is a passive process that results from the natural recoil of the expanded lungs. However, in people with rapid or labored breathing, the accessory muscles and abdominal muscles often contract to help force air out of the lungs more quickly and completely. Within the lungs, the main bronchi continue to split successively into smaller bronchi, bronchioles, terminal bronchioles, and finally alveoli. In the alveoli, carbon dioxide is exchanged for oxygen across a thin membrane separating capillary blood from inspired air.

The ability of the lungs to expand and contract to inhale and exhale air is affected by the compliance (degree of stiffness) of the lung tissue. Processes that result in scarring of lung tissue (bronchiectasis) can decrease compliance, thus affecting the flow and volume of air moved by the lungs. The degree of ease in which air can pass through the airways is known as *resistance*. The number, length, and diameter of the airways determine resistance. A patient with a high degree of resistance may not be able to take a full breath in or to exhale fully (some air may become trapped in the lungs).

To have an adequate exchange of the gases, there must be a matching of ventilation (V) and perfusion (Q). An average V:Q ratio, determined by dividing alveolar ventilation (4 L/min) by cardiac output (5 L/min), is 0.8. A mismatch may result from a cardiovascular anomaly (e.g., pulmonary embolus) that shunts blood away from normal alveoli. Ventilation in this area of the lung is "wasted," and the V:Q ratio approaches infinity. The converse occurs when there is normal perfusion to alveoli that have collapsed ("dead" space).

For the respiration process to be complete, *diffusion* must occur in the alveoli. By the diffusion mechanism, gases in the alveoli equilibrate from areas of high concentration to areas of low concentration. Hemoglobin (Hgb) releases carbon dioxide and adsorbs oxygen through the alveolar walls. If these walls thicken, diffusion is hampered. Membrane thickening may result from an acute or chronic inflammatory process such as acute pulmonary edema from congestive heart failure or pneumonia, chronic tuberculosis, silicosis, and other fibrotic conditions. V:Q mismatching also can decrease the pulmonary diffusing capacity.

The various PFTs can measure airflow in or out of the lungs, indicate how much air is in the lung parenchyma, and provide information on ventilation and perfusion, gas diffusion, or specific changes in airway tone or reactivity.

TABLE 10-1

TYPE	PATHOPHYSIOLOGY	EXAMPLE
Outflow obstruction	Reversible	Asthma
	Irreversible	Emphysema
Restrictive ventilation	Parenchymal infiltration	Pulmonary hemosiderosis and sarcoid
	Loss of lung volume	Pneumothorax, pneumonectomy, pleural effusions
	Extrathoracic compression	Kyphosis, morbid obesity, ascites, chest wall deformities
Mixed outflow obstruction and restrictive ventilation	All of the above	Chronic obstructive pulmonary disease
Diffusion capacity	Pulmonary fibrosis	Interstitial fibrosis

Table 10-1. Types of Pulmonary Disease

CLINICAL USE OF PULMONARY FUNCTION TESTING

PFTs are useful in many clinical situations. They aid in the diagnostic differentiation of various pulmonary diseases. For example, with obstructive lung diseases (e.g., asthma or chronic bronchitis), the underlying pathophysiology is a reversible or irreversible obstruction to airflow in the airways. In restrictive diseases (e.g., kyphosis or sarcoid), the lungs are restricted in the amount of air they can contain. Obstructive diseases usually decrease the flow of air, but not its volume. On the other hand, restrictive diseases usually decrease the volume of air but not its flow (Table 10-1).

In addition, serial PFTs allow tracking of the progression of pulmonary diseases and the need for or response to various treatments. They also help to establish a baseline of respiratory function prior to surgical, medical, or radiation therapy. Subsequent serial measurements then aid in the detection and tracking of changes in lung function caused by these therapies. Similarly, serial PFTs can be used to evaluate the risk of lung damage from exposure to environmental or occupational hazards.

In brief, PFTs are performed to

- Evaluate respiratory symptoms.
- Screen for respiratory disease.
- Assess disease severity.
- Preoperatively determine the risk of thoracic or upper abdominal surgery.
- Monitor the progression of lung disease.
- Evaluate the response to therapy.
- Assess the risk of pulmonary exposure to environmental toxins.
- Monitor drug or radiation pulmonary toxicity.

Table 10-2 summarizes the selected uses of PFTs.

PROCEDURES AND EQUIPMENT

Spirometry

Spirometry is a test that measures various aspects of breathing and lung function. Like most medical tests, spirometry has seen changes over the years in equipment, computer support, and recommendations for standardization. In an effort to maximize the usefulness of spirometry results, the American Thoracic Society (ATS) developed[2] and updated[3,4] recommendations for the standardization of spirometry. These recommendations are intended to decrease the variability of spirometry testing by improving the performance of the test. The recommendations cover equipment, quality control, training and education of people conducting the test, and training of patients performing the test. The recommendations also provide criteria for acceptability and reproducibility of the patient's spirometry efforts and guidelines on interpreting the spirometry test results.

Spirometry is performed by having a person breathe into a tube (mouth piece) connected to a machine (spirometer) that measures the amount and flow of inhaled and/or exhaled air. The physical forces of the airflow and the total amount of air inhaled and/or exhaled are converted by transducers to electrical signals and displayed on a computer screen. Manufacturers should be able to provide documentation that their spirometer meets or exceeds ATS recommendations for accuracy and precision for all PFT parameters measured over the entire volume range of the instrument. This is particularly important as portable, hand-held spirometers are becoming available for use at home or smaller healthcare centers.[5] Some spirometers require that the patient inhale before inserting the mouthpiece and forcefully exhaling (open-

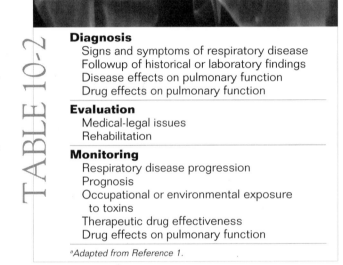

TABLE 10-2

Diagnosis
Signs and symptoms of respiratory disease
Followup of historical or laboratory findings
Disease effects on pulmonary function
Drug effects on pulmonary function

Evaluation
Medical-legal issues
Rehabilitation

Monitoring
Respiratory disease progression
Prognosis
Occupational or environmental exposure
  to toxins
Therapeutic drug effectiveness
Drug effects on pulmonary function

Adapted from Reference 1.

Table 10-2. Selected Uses of PFTs[a]

circuit system). Other spirometers require that the mouthpiece be inserted and several normal breaths be taken before the airflow is measured (closed-circuit system).

Prior to performing spirometry, the appropriate technique should be explained and demonstrated to the patient. Spirometry results are highly dependent on the patient's inhalation and exhalation, so the importance of completely filling and emptying the lungs of air during the test should be emphasized. Since the patient must respond to commands and have reasonably mature motor control and coordination, children younger than about 5 years generally cannot meet ATS reproducibility criteria for this test.

During spirometry nose clips should be worn to minimize air loss through the nose. Patients may sit or stand, but the position must be indicated on the report and should be kept constant as results can vary between the two positions.[6] The patient should not lean or slump and any restrictive clothing (such as ties or tight belts) should be loosened or removed.

For "forced" efforts, which measure forced vital capacity (FVC), forced expiratory volume in one second (FEV_1), peak expiratory flow rate (PEFR), and forced expiratory flow at 25–75% of vital capacity (FEF_{25-75}) (described in detail below), the patient takes a full deep breath in and then blasts the air out as quickly and forcefully as possible. During this maneuver, airflow and the total amount of air expired can be simultaneously measured and *flow-volume curve* and *volume-time curve* can be generated on the PFT screen or test result printout (Figure 10-1). The effort should last for 6 sec or until the volume-time curve plateaus (unless dealing with someone with very restrictive disease or a child).

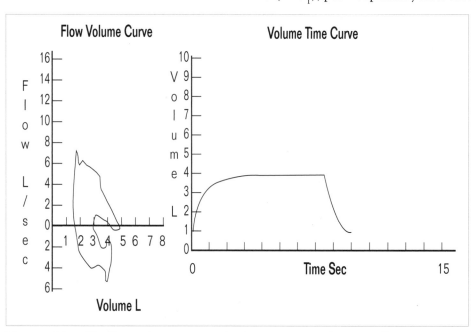

Figure 10-1. The flow-volume curve and volume-time curve from an effort meeting ATS acceptability criteria. The flow-volume curve has a deep inspiratory effort with a sharp complete expiratory flow. The volume-time curve demonstrates both a plateau and an exhalation time of greater than 6 sec.

Because the results of spirometry depend on the patient's effort, ATS recommends that at least three acceptable efforts be obtained with a goal of having the two highest measurements of FVC and FEV_1 vary by less than 0.2 L.[4] Acceptability criteria include

- Satisfactory start of test (no excessive hesitation or false start).
- No coughing during the first second of the effort.
- No early termination of the effort.
- No interruption in airflow (e.g., glottic closure).
- No evidence of a leak (mouth not tightly sealed around mouthpiece).
- No evidence of an obstructed mouthpiece (tongue, false teeth).

Some spirometry parameters, vital capacity (VC), total lung capacity (TLC), residual volume (RV), expiratory reserve volume (ERV), inspiratory reserve volume (IRV), and slow vital capacity (SVC), are measured after a normal, relaxed, complete breath out followed by a full inhalation and a full exhalation. Airflow should be at a relatively constant rate. The acceptability criteria listed above also apply to this maneuver.

After the data is generated, the patient's spirometry results are generally compared to the predicted values for people of similar age, height, and gender. Race also may affect the predicted values, but this factor is not included in all programs.

Body Plethysmography

For body plethysmography, the patient is seated in a large, closed box. Inside, a mouthpiece contains a pressure transducer. It senses the intrathoracic pressure generated when the patient rapidly and forcefully puffs against the closed mouthpiece. These data are then placed into Boyle's law:

$$\frac{P_1 \times V_1}{T_1} = \frac{P_2 \times V_2}{T_2}$$

where

P_1 = pressure inside the box where the patient is seated (atmospheric pressure)

V_1 = volume of the box

P_2 = intrathoracic pressure generated by the patient

V_2 = calculated volume of the patient's thoracic cavity

Because temperature (T_1 and T_2) is constant throughout testing, it is not included in the calculations.

After these data are generated, the patient's plethysmography results are usually compared to references from a presumed normal population. This comparison necessitates the generation of predicted values for that patient if he or she were completely normal and healthy. Through complex mathematical formulas, sitting and standing height, weight, age, gender, race, barometric pressure, and altitude are factored in to give predicted values for the pulmonary functions being assessed.[7]

Instead of a patient's results being compared with set "normal values," the results are described either as a percentage of predicted values or with standard deviations (SDs) from the mean of a physically matched healthy population of the same age. With few exceptions, either comparison is acceptable; some pulmonary function laboratories report both values. However, standard deviation comparisons should not be used with PFTs that are not normally distributed in the population, such as residual volume.

PULMONARY FUNCTION TESTS

PFTs measure lung volumes, lung flow, and diffusion capacity as well as airway reactivity, compliance, resistance, and conductance.

Lung Volume Tests

Lung volume tests routinely measure the

- Tidal volume (TV).
- Inspiratory capacity (IC).
- Inspiratory reserve volume (IRV).
- Expiratory reserve volume (ERV).
- Forced vital capacity (FVC).
- Slow vital capacity (SVC).
- Residual volume (RV).
- Functional residual capacity (FRC).
- Total lung capacity (TLC).

Lung volume tests indicate the amount of gas contained in the lungs at the various stages of inflation.[8] RV, FRC, and TLC may be obtained by several methods, including (1) body plethysmography with application of Boyle's law or (2) gas dilution. The different methods can have small but real effects on the values reported. Gas dilution methods only measure ventilated areas, whereas body plethysmography measures both ventilated and nonventilated areas. Therefore, body plethysmography values may be larger in patients with nonventilated or poorly ventilated lung areas.[8]

Tidal Volume, Inspiratory Capacity, and Inspiratory and Expiratory Reserve Volumes

The tidal volume (TV) is the amount of air inhaled and exhaled at rest. It is usually a very small proportion of the lung volume (~500–750 mL) and is infrequently used as a measure of respiratory disease.

The volume measured from the point of the TV where inhalation normally begins to maximal inspiration is known as the IC.

The volume measured from the "top" of the TV (i.e., initial point of normal exhalation) to maximal inspiration is known as the IRV. During exhalation, the volume from the "bottom" of the TV (i.e., initial point of normal inhalation) to maximal expiration is referred to as the ERV.

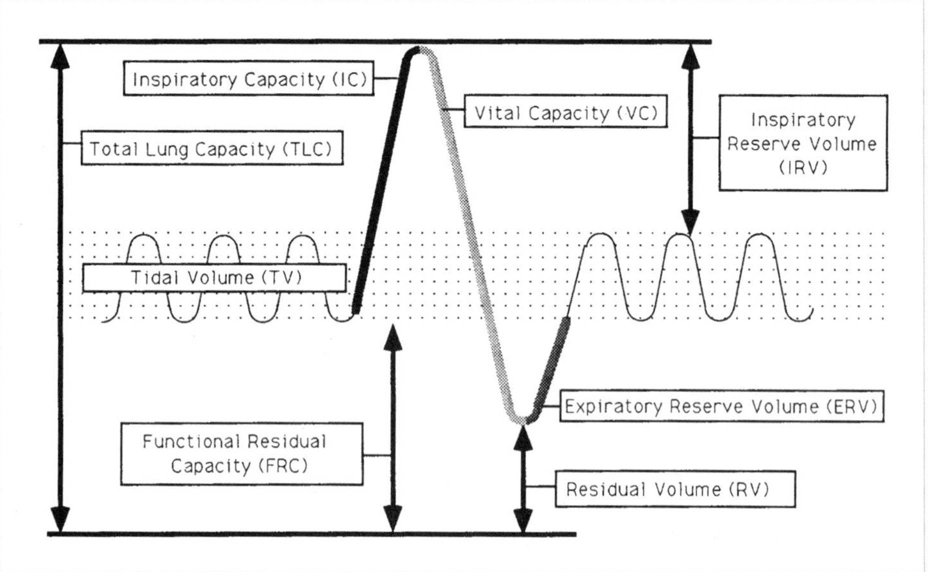

These four volumes, depicted graphically in Figure 10-2, are measured by spirometry.

Figure 10-2. Lung volumes and capacities—a schematic representation of various lung compartments based on a typical spirogram. (Graphic artwork by Michele Betterton.)

Forced Vital Capacity and Slow Vital Capacity

The forced vital capacity (FVC) is the total volume of air exhaled as hard and as fast as possible after a maximal inhalation. When the full inhalation-exhalation procedure is repeated slowly—instead of forcefully and rapidly—it is called the *slow vital capacity* (SVC). This value is the maximum amount of air exhaled after a full and complete inhalation.

In patients with normal airway function, FVC and SVC are usually similar. Therefore, they are shown together in Figure 10-2 as vital capacity. In patients with diseases, such as chronic obstructive pulmonary disease (COPD), results often show temporal divergence. During the initial stages of the disease, the FVC decreases before the SVC. The SVC remains normal because interluminal thoracic pressures are not elevated during the maneuver. Because of the forcefulness of the airflow, however, the FVC shows evidence of air trapping and airway collapse much earlier in the disease process.

Residual Volume

Following full exhalation to the expiratory reserve volume (ERV), the amount of air left in the lungs is called the *residual volume* (RV). This air volume, not measurable by spirometric methods, is usually obtained by body plethysmography. The RV typically approximates 1 L. Without the RV, the lungs would collapse like deflated balloons. In diseases characterized by obstructions that trap air in the lungs (e.g., asthma), the RV increases; the patient is less able to mobilize air trapped behind these obstructions.

Functional Residual Capacity

The functional residual capacity (FRC) is the summation of the ERV and RV. It is the volume of gas remaining in the lungs at the end of the TV. It also may be defined as a balance point between chest wall forces that increase volume and lung parenchymal forces that decrease volume.

An increased FRC represents hyperinflation of the lungs and usually indicates airway obstruction. The FRC may be decreased in diseases that affect many alveoli (e.g., pneumonia) or by restrictive changes, especially those due to fibrotic pulmonary tissue changes.

Total Lung Capacity

The *total lung capacity* (TLC) is the summation of the RV and the vital capacity. It is the total amount of gas contained in the lungs. The TLC also may be referred to as *thoracic gas volume*.

Lung Flow Tests

Lung flow tests routinely assess the

- Forced expiratory volume (FEV).
  - FEV_1
- Peak expiratory flow rate (PEFR).
- Forced expiratory flow (FEF).
  - FEF_{25-75}

These values and a flow-volume curve (discussed in Flow-Volume Curves section) are obtained by spirometry. The flow-volume loop is a graphic representation of inspiration and expiration (Figure 10-3).

Forced Expiratory Volume

The full, forced inhalation-exhalation procedure was already described as the FVC. Changes in this measurement from baseline reflect the degree of current airway obstruction. During this maneuver, the computer can

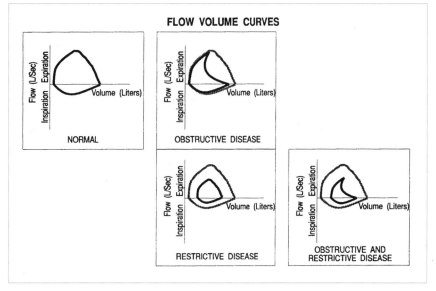

Figure 10-3. Flow-volume loops seen with common obstructive and restrictive pulmonary diseases. (Graphic artwork by Michele Betterton.)

discern the amount of air exhaled at specific time intervals of the FVC. By convention, $FEV_{0.5}$, FEV_1, FEV_3, and FEV_6 are the amounts of air exhaled after 0.5, 1, 3, and 6 sec, respectively. Of these measurements, FEV_1 has the most clinical relevance, primarily as an indicator of large airway function. Only air contained in the large airways (oropharnyx, trachea, main stem bronchi, and early, large bronchi) can be mobilized for exhalation in this short time.

The normal range for FEV_1 is 0.75–5.5 L. This range is large because of the physical variables among patients, as discussed previously. Usually, a patient's value is described either as a percentage of a predicted value or as a standard deviation from the mean of a physically matched population of the same age.

A value greater than 80% of the predicted normal value or within ±2 SD is considered normal. However, someone with an FEV_1 of 110% of predicted normal value at a baseline visit and an FEV_1 of 90% of predicted normal value at a follow-up visit is demonstrating a significant reduction in lung function even though both values are above 80% of the normal predicted value. Values less than or equal to 80% or below 2 SD are abnormal and related to airway obstruction. Normal values are often seen in patients with reversible airway obstruction when their disease is not "active." However, during acute exacerbation, their FEV_1 values may be markedly decreased.

In both obstructive and restrictive diseases, the FEV_1 usually shows a reduction in flow. The magnitude of change in FEV_1 can indicate the severity of the obstructive airway disease. Degrees of severity may be reported as mild (61–80% of predicted), moderate (41–60%), and severe (≤40%).

The ratio of FEV_1 to the FVC is another way to estimate the presence and amount of obstruction in the airways. This ratio indicates the amount of air mobilized in 1 sec as a percentage of the total amount of movable air. Normal, healthy individuals can exhale approximately 50% of their FVC in the first 0.5 sec, about 80% in 1 sec, and about 98% in 3 sec.

Patients with obstructive disease usually show a decreased ratio, and the actual percentage reduction varies with the severity of obstruction. Generally, this ratio is normal (or high) in patients with restrictive diseases, because both the FVC and FEV_1 are similarly reduced from normal in these disorders. The effects of pulmonary disease on some common PFTs are presented in Table 10-3.

TABLE 10-3

DISEASE	VITAL CAPACITY	RV	FEV_1: FVC
Chronic obstructive (chronic bronchitis and emphysema)	Normal or decreased	Normal or increased	Decreased
Reversible obstructive (asthma)	Normal or decreased	Increased	Decreased
Restrictive (extrapulmonary and intrapulmonary)	Decreased	Decreased	Normal
Combined obstructive and restrictive	Decreased	Decreased	Decreased

Table 10-3. Effects of Pulmonary Disease on PFTs

Peak Expiratory Flow Rate

The peak expiratory flow rate (PEFR), or peak flow, occurs within the first milliseconds of expiratory flow and is a measure of the maximum airflow rate. It can be measured during spirometry along with FVC, FEV_1 and FEF_{25-75}. However, due to the availability of simple hand-held devices (peak flow meters), PEFR can easily be measured at a patient's home or bedside and is widely used as an indicator of large airway obstruction.

Because the National Asthma Education Program (NAEP) strongly recommends using peak flow based home monitoring plans for asthma patients,[8] the most recent ATS guidelines include recommendations for home peak flow meters. Peak flow meters must measure PEFR within an accuracy of ±10% of reading or ±20 L, whichever is greater, with PEFRs between 60–400 L/min for children and from 100–850 L/min for adults. Because PEFR meters are not calibrated, the package insert should provide the average life span of the instrument as well as cleaning and maintenance instructions.[4] The more recent National Asthma Education and Prevention Program (NAEPP) report found that the literature did not clearly demonstrate that a PEFR home monitoring plan was better than a home symptom monitoring plan in improving outcomes of asthma.[9] However, the report still recommends use of home PEFR for patients with moderate to severe asthma.

Like FEV_1, the PEFR has a wide normal range. Healthy men achieve values of 400–800 L/min; healthy women achieve values of 200–600 L/min. A comparison of the current reading with a patient's best values is most useful. At the time of worsened obstruction, the patient's values are markedly decreased from the best values. Values of 50–100 L/min (or less if the flow meter is capable of lower readings) indicate severe, acute obstruction.

Usually, the peak flow is reduced in obstructive diseases but is normal in restrictive diseases. A decreased peak flow also may indicate a mechanical obstruction (e.g., foreign body aspiration).

Forced Expiratory Flow

Forced expiratory flow (FEF) measures airflow rate during forced expiration. While FEV measures the volume of air during expiration, FEF measures the rate of air movement. The FEF from 25–75% of vital capacity is known as FEF_{25-75}. This test specifically measures the flow rate of air in the medium and small airways (bronchioles and terminal bronchioles). Because asthma affects these airways the most, FEF_{25-75} is a good indicator of small airway obstruction.

Flow rates decrease in obstructive disease but remain normal in restrictive disease (see Table 10-3). FEF_{25-75} also gradually decreases with age. The flow from 75–100% of vital capacity is called *alveolar airflow*. This parameter may markedly diminish as airways collapse with increased intrathoracic pressure. Such pressure occurs in severe acute asthma when large obstructions are present in terminal bronchioles.

Diffusion Capacity Tests

Tests of gas exchange measure the ability of gases to cross (diffuse) the alveolar-capillary membrane and are useful in assessing interstitial lung disease.[10] Typically, these tests measure the per minute transfer of a gas, usually carbon monoxide, from the alveoli to the blood. The diffusion capacity may be lessened following losses in the surface area of the alveoli or thickening of the alveolar-capillary membrane. Thickening may be due to fibrotic changes.

These test results can be confounded by a loss of diffusion capacity due to poor ventilation, which may be related to closed or partially closed airways (as with atelectasis, pneumonia, or airway obstruction) or to a ventilation-perfusion mismatch (as with pulmonary emboli or cor pulmonale). The diffusion capacity of the lungs to carbon monoxide (DL_{CO}) can be measured by either a single-breath or steady-state test.

In the single-breath test, the patient deeply inhales—to vital capacity—a mixture of 0.3%, carbon monoxide, 10% helium, and air. After holding the breath for 10 sec, the patient exhales fully; the concentrations of carbon monoxide and helium are measured during the end of expiration (i.e., alveolar flow). These concentrations are compared to the inspired concentrations to determine the amount diffusing across the alveolar membrane. The mean value for carbon monoxide is about 25–30 mL/min/mm Hg.

In the steady-state test, the patient breathes a 0.1–0.2% concentration of carbon monoxide for 5–6 min. In the final 2 min, the expired gases are collected and an arterial blood gas (ABG) is obtained. The exhaled gas is measured for total volume and concentrations of carbon monoxide, carbon dioxide, and oxygen. The ABG is analyzed for carbon dioxide. These values are used to calculate the amount of gas transferred across the alveolar membrane per unit of time, usually a minute. The usual mean value may be slightly less with the steady-state method than the single-breath method. Furthermore, females typically have slightly lower values than males, probably due in part to slightly smaller lung volumes.

These tests of diffusion capacity are useful for assessing pulmonary fibrotic changes. Diffusion capacity is decreased in diseases that cause alveolar fibrotic changes. Changes may be idiopathic, such as those seen with sarcoid or environmental or occupational disease (asbestosis), or be induced by drugs (e.g., nitrofurantoin, amiodarone, and bleomycin).[11,12] Anything that alters Hgb, decreases the red cell Hgb concentration (see Chapter 14), or changes diffusion across the red cell membrane may alter the DL_{CO}. The DL_{CO} also reflects the pulmonary capillary blood volume. An increase in this volume (pulmonary edema or asthma) increases the DL_{CO}.

Flow-Volume Curves

Figure 10-3 shows several flow-volume curves where the expiratory flow is plotted against the exhaled volume.[13] As explained earlier, these curves are graphic representations of inspiration and expiration. The shape of the curve indicates both the type of disease and the severity of obstruction.

Obstructive changes result in decreased airflows at lower lung volumes, revealing a characteristic concave appearance. In obstructive cases, the loop size is similar to that of a healthy individual unless there is severe, acute obstruction. Flow-volume curves are often used with other PFTs. Minicase 5 demonstrates other PFT values that may occur in a patient with acute obstruction producing a concave flow-volume curve.

Restrictive changes result in a shape similar to that of a healthy individual, but the size is considerably smaller. The flow-volume loop also reveals mixed obstructive and restrictive disease by a combination of the two patterns.

Airway Reactivity Tests

Bronchodilator (Reversibility) Studies

One of many criteria used in the diagnostic work-up of reversible airway disease is spirometry with reversibility. The patient is asked to perform spirometry immediately before and 15 to 30 min after the administration of an inhaled short-acting β_2-adrenergic agonist. An improvement of FEV_1 by at least 12% indicates a significant reversible component to the lung disease. Bronchodilator studies are also used to assess a patient's response to these medi-

---

MINICASE 1

ED W., A 22-YEAR-OLD MALE with a 14-year history of asthma, reported increasing symptoms of coughing, wheezing, shortness of breath, and chest tightness over the past 12 hr. He came to the clinic for an evaluation of this acute exacerbation of his disease. His only treatment was two puffs of an epinephrine metered-dose inhaler (Primatene Mist), which he used every 1–2 hr with good response.

After a brief history and physical examination, pre- and postbronchodilator spirometry was performed using two puffs of isoproterenol from a metered-dose inhaler. Auscultation revealed breath sounds only on forced expiration.

The spirometry revealed the following results:

PFT	Predicted	Prebronchodilator Measured	% Predicted	SD	Postbronchodilator Measured	SD	% Change
FVC (L)	3.63	3.23	89	-0.70	3.22	-0.73	0
FEV₁ (L)	3.24	2.24	69	-2.33	2.87	-0.77	28
FEV₁:FVC (%)	89	69	–		89	–	29

Question: What would be a better treatment for Ed W.?

Discussion: Isoproterenol is used because of its rapid onset, strong β_2-activity, and short duration of effect. The PFTs are obtained within 5 min of the isoproterenol dose. The predicted values are obtained from formulas that take into account the patient's age, gender, and height.

Although values greater than 80% of predicted are considered normal, a preferable way to evaluate PFTs is to compare the results to the population as a whole. In this manner, standard deviation is used to compare individual results to the general population. Most PFTs are normally distributed, so any value falling within ±2 SD is considered normal.

Ed W. is bronchodilator responsive, as evidenced by the reversal to normal of his FEV_1 and FEV_1: FVC values. These values are interpreted as normal because the standard deviation returns to within ±2 of the predicted percentage. Since Ed W.'s FVC is normal prebronchodilator, it cannot by definition return to normal. Auscultation of an asthmatic usually finds breath sounds on expiration. Some patients may not experience these breath sounds on expiration but exhibit them on forced expiration. In either case, this finding indicates small airway obstructions.

Because of his responsiveness, Ed W.'s therapy should include inhaled β_2-selective agonists for his acute exacerbation. Therefore, Ed W. should use an albuterol-metered dose inhaler instead of his epinephrine inhaler.

MINICASE 2

SANDRA S., A 44-YEAR-OLD FEMALE with kyphosis (abnormal spinal curvature), had routine PFTs assessed during an annual physical examination. On initial review, her PFTs appeared abnormally decreased. Nevertheless, the patient had no complaints of respiratory symptoms now or in the past. Furthermore, her spinal curvature and general health had not changed.

Sandra S.'s PFTs revealed the following results:

PFT	Predicted	Prebronchodilator Measured	% Predicted	SD	Postbronchodilator Measured	SD	% Change
FVC (L)	3.68	0.81	22	-3.73	0.91	-3.57	12
FEV$_1$ (L)	3.05	0.79	26	-5.12	1.05	-4.96	15
FEV$_1$:FVC (%)	83	98	–	–	95	–	–
RV:TLC (%)	30	–	–	–	29	–	–

Question: Why is the FEV$_1$:FVC ratio useful in this case?

Discussion: This case is an example of restrictive lung disease. Because Sandra S.'s thoracic cavity is small and deformed compared to that of a normal, healthy person of similar size and age, her PFTs appear abnormally decreased. Therefore, it is imperative to assess the FEV$_1$:FVC ratio, which is within normal limits. This result indicates that Sandra S.'s airways function normally, even though she has less than normal expansion of her lung tissue. Further indication of restrictive rather than obstructive lung function is the normal RV:TLC ratio. She has an extrapulmonary cause for her decreased thoracic volume. An example of an important intrapulmonary cause for decreased thoracic volume includes neoplasm. Anything that limits (restricts) the lung's ability to expand can alter PFTs.

cations.[14] A significant improvement in FEV$_1$ would indicate that the patient may benefit from maintenance bronchodilator therapy, such as a long-acting ß$_2$-adrenergic agonist (salmeterol or formoterol) or theophylline in combination with an inhaled steroid. Without a positive response, further bronchodilator therapy is unlikely to elicit meaningful improvement. Patients with emphysema, however, frequently show a decreased flow pattern with little PFT response to bronchodilators but still feel better after using them. The various types of results seen with these tests are illustrated in the minicases.

Some clinicians use anticholinergics (e.g., ipratropium or atropine) as bronchodilators instead of a ß$_2$-adrenergic agonist, particularly for patients with COPD (e.g., chronic bronchitis or emphysema). The reversibility procedure is the same. Anticholinergics have demonstrated efficacy in treating COPD both as intervention (acute treatment) and maintenance therapy. Efficacy is lacking in the treatment of asthma. Other medications besides ß$_2$-adrenergic agonists, such as corticosteroids and anticholinergics, may still be necessary in controlling these respiratory diseases.

Bronchoprovocation Challenge Testing

Bronchial provocation testing (BPT) measures the reactivity of the airways to known concentrations of agents that induce airway narrowing. These tests are often referred to as "challenges," as the airways are challenged with increasing doses of a provoking agent until a desired drop in lung function occurs. Agents used to provoke the lung include inhaled methacholine,[15] histamine,[16] adenosine,[17] and specific allergens.[18] ATS has published guidelines for methacholine and exercise challenge testing to enhance the safety, accuracy, and validity of the tests.[19]

BPT begins by measuring baseline spirometry parameters to ensure it is safe to conduct the test. BPT should not be performed if the FEV$_1$ is less than 60% of predicted.[19] Most BPTs

THE FATHER OF AN 8-YEAR-OLD GIRL with chronic asthma called the clinic pharmacy to ask if his daughter, Frances P., should begin a short course of high-dose oral corticosteroids for her increased asthmatic symptoms. Frances P. was well until 18 hr ago when she experienced increased coughing, wheezing, and chest tightness.

Frances P. used a peak flow meter twice a day, recording the best of three efforts each time. Usually, her peak flow was approximately 250 L/min. On this day, before use of her albuterol metered-dose inhaler, her peak flow was 120 L/min. After her inhaled bronchodilator, it was 170 L/min. Although Frances P.'s symptoms improved after the albuterol, they did not completely resolve.

Question: Should corticosteroids be used in this patient? If so, should the delivery method be oral or inhaled?

Discussion: Peak flow meters are useful objective indicators of large airway function. In this case, the patient assesses her peak flow twice daily for reference. Usually, patients record the best of several efforts.

On this day, Frances P. used the meter before and after her inhaled bronchodilator to indicate whether her airway obstructions adequately responded to albuterol. Because her peak flow improved but did not return to normal, her symptoms are not fully bronchodilator responsive. Some clinicians administer a short course of high-dose oral corticosteroids at this point. Oral corticosteroids are the appropriate choice for acute exacerbation of asthma. Inhaled corticosteroids are used for maintenance therapy of chronic asthma.

---

then begin with nebulization of a solution of phosphate buffered saline. This both serves as a placebo to assess the airway effect of nebulization and establishes baseline airway function from which the amount of pulmonary function to be reduced is calculated. Then an extremely low concentration of the selected bronchoconstrictor agent is nebulized followed by spirometry at 30 and 90 min from the end of the nebulization. Additional spirometry efforts may be done to meet or exceed ATS criteria. Optimally, the FEV_1 values should be within 0.10 L of each other.[19] The patient inhales gradually increasing concentrations of the bronchoconstrictor at specific time intervals (usually 5 min) until a predesignated amount of airway restriction is attained. This is usually defined as a reduction in FEV_1 by at least 20% from the saline control. The challenge data is then summarized into a single number, the $PC_{20}FEV_1$ (mg/mL). This refers to the provocation concentration of the bronchoconstricting agent that would produce a 20% reduction in FEV_1.

For methacholine, a $PC_{20}FEV_1$ of <1.0 mg/mL indicates moderate to severe bronchial hyperresponsiveness (BHR), 1.0–4.0 mg/mL as mild BHR, 4.0–16 mg/mL as borderline BHR and >16 mg/mL as normal bronchial responsiveness. During a BPT, patients may experience transient respiratory symptoms such as cough, shortness of breath, wheezing, and chest tightness. An inhaled, short acting β_2-adrenergic agonist or anticholinergic agent may be administered to alleviate symptoms and quicken the return of the FEV_1 to the baseline value. Because BPTs can elicit severe, life-threatening bronchospasm, they should only be performed by trained personnel with medications to treat severe bronchospasm on-hand in the testing area.

BPTs are used to aid in the diagnosis of asthma, when the more common tests (symptom history, spirometry with reversibility) cannot confirm or reject the diagnosis, to evaluate the effects of drug therapy on airway hyperreactivity, and for research. This technique is frequently used to assess the effect of bronchodilating and anti-inflammatory drugs on the airways. Using this technique, the magnitude and duration of different drugs' effects on the airways may be compared.[15,17,18]

MINICASE 4

GREG A., A 13-YEAR-OLD BOY, came to a clinic complaining of increased coughing, wheezing, and chest tightness for 3 days. He had a 9-year history of asthma. His asthma usually was controlled with two puffs of a cromolyn metered-dose inhaler 4 times a day and two puffs of an albuterol metered-dose inhaler when needed for acute symptoms. Greg A. was currently using his albuterol 4 or 5 times a day with an incomplete response. He has had a viral upper respiratory infection for about 1 week. Chest auscultation revealed breath sounds on expiration. A chest x-ray was not obtained, nor were arterial blood gases (ABGs).

PFTs revealed the following results:

PFT	Prebronchodilator				Postbronchodilator		
	Predicted	Measured	% Predicted	SD	Measured	SD	% Change
FVC (L)	2.92	1.26	43	-7.39	1.15	-8.25	-9
FEV_1 (L)	2.49	0.54	22	-12.15	0.56	-11.85	4
FEV_1:FVC (%)	85	43	–	–	49	–	–
FEF_{25-75} (L/sec)	2.86	0.20	7	-10.02	0.25	-9.09	25

Because of the viral upper respiratory infection (subsequent increase in respiratory symptoms with increasing albuterol use) and PFT results indicating no bronchodilator response, Greg A. was placed on a short course of high-dose oral prednisone, 40 mg twice a day, until completely symptom free for 24 hr. He was told to call the clinic if he was not symptom free in 10 days. The PFTs were considered bronchodilator unresponsive because the postbronchodilator values did not normalize to within ±2 SD of the mean for that population. Greg A. called the clinic on day 11 and indicated that he had improved considerably but was not completely clear. His inhaled β_2-agonist use had decreased to 1 or 2 times a day with the clearing of his symptoms. He was told to continue prednisone, 40 mg twice a day, for an additional 3 days and then to return to the clinic for follow-up PFTs.

On day 14, Greg A.'s PFTs revealed the following results:

PFT	Prebronchodilator				Postbronchodilator		
	Predicted	Measured	% Predicted	SD	Measured	SD	% Change
FVC (L)	2.92	2.93	100	0.01	3.00	0.22	2
FEV_1 (L)	2.49	2.40	96	-0.29	2.72	0.70	13
FEV_1:FVC (%)	85	82	–	–	91	–	–
FEF_{25-75} (L/sec)	2.86	2.32	73	-0.84	2.25	0.84	89

Question: Should this patient's chronic maintenance therapy be altered?

Discussion: After 14 days of prednisone, the patient's asthma is back in control. The PFTs have returned to the predicted values; Greg A's coughing, wheezing, and chest tightness are resolved. Moreover, his chest is clear to auscultation.

The remaining reduced FEF_{25-75} indicates residual obstructions in the patient's small airways. They would eventually be cleared up if the prednisone was continued. The oral steroid is stopped, and Greg A. started on inhaled fluticasone 110 µg/puff, two puffs twice a day, as maintenance therapy. Because of the relatively short duration of the prednisone therapy and the beginning of inhaled fluticasone, tapering of prednisone is not necessary.

This presentation is common for patients with viral induced asthma. They have a "cold" that lasts 10–14 days and exacerbates their asthma. The exacerbation starts with increasing asthma symptoms that may, but usually do not, respond to β-agonists. A short course of high-dose oral prednisone brings the asthma back into control.

Exercise Challenge Testing

Exercise- or exertion induced bronchospasm (EIB) occurs in the majority of patients with asthma. The etiology of EIB is thought to be related to the cooling and drying of the airways caused by the rapid breathing during exercise. Exercise challenge testing is used to confirm or rule out EIB and to evaluate the effectiveness of medications used to treat or prevent EIB.

Exercise tests are usually done with a motor driven treadmill (with adjustable speed and grade) or a electromagnetically braked cycle ergometer. Heart rate should be monitored throughout the test. Nose clips should be worn and the room air should be dry and cool, to promote water loss from the airways during the exercise test. In most patients, symptoms are effectively blocked by use of an inhaled bronchodilator immediately prior to beginning exercise or other exertion causing the problem. After obtaining baseline spirometry, the exercise test is started at a low speed that is gradually increased over 2–4 min until the heart rate is 80–90% of the predicted maximum or the work rate is at 100%. The duration of the exercise is age and tolerance dependent. Children <12 years of age generally take 6 min while older children and adults take 8 min to complete the test. After the exercise is completed, the patient does serial spirometry at 5-min intervals for 20–30 min. FEV_1 is the primary outcome variable. A 10% or more decrease in FEV_1 from baseline is generally accepted as an abnormal response, though some clinicians feel a 15% decrease is more diagnostic of EIB.[19]

Specialized Tests

Infant Pulmonary Function Testing

With advances in respiratory technology, use of infant pulmonary function testing is re-emerging as a possible tool for investigating the development of the lungs, the progression of lung disease, and the response to pulmonary treatment interventions. The equipment costs around $100,000 and requires specialized training. As the equipment, procedures, measurements, and interpretation of results are becoming more standardized, the role of this test in diagnosing, monitoring, and treating lung disease in infants should become clearer.[20–22]

Inflammatory Markers

Airway inflammation is involved in a number of airway diseases. The ability to easily measure markers or indicators of this inflammatory process would improve our understanding of airway disease and its treatment.

Bronchial alveolar lavage. Bronchial alveolar lavage (BAL) is a direct measurement of the cells or proteins found in pulmonary secretions. Samples are attained during bronchoscopy. This procedure is the direct visualization of the lumen of the airways, and it can be accomplished with either a flexible bronchoscope or a rigid device. Generally, a flexible device is smaller and more maneuverable and, hence, easier for the patient to tolerate during the procedure. Flexible bronchoscopy may be performed while the patient is consciously sedated, whereas general anesthesia is required for a rigid bronchoscopy procedure.

The advantage of the larger rigid bronchoscope is that it allows removal of a small foreign body through its lumen. When either device is used and there is a desire to understand what is in the pulmonary secretions of the patient, a small amount of fluid, usually a buffered, warmed and sterile normal saline, is flushed into the airways and then drawn back out and sent to a laboratory for analysis. The microscopic analysis usually looks for cellular components and proteins found in the airways although it may be specific for other markers. Common cellular analysis items include numbers and types of eosinophils, neutrophils, lymphocytes, mast cells, and macrophages while protein matter include histamine and subcellular components. The invasiveness of this method limits its use, especially for monitoring changes in lung inflammation over short period of times.

KENT N., A 46-YEAR-OLD MALE, presented to a respiratory clinic for evaluation of his persistent cough and shortness of breath. His respiratory symptoms had been consistent, neither increasing nor decreasing for several months. They had progressively worsened over the past 15–20 years. Currently, Kent N. produced a teaspoonful to a tablespoonful of sputum each 24 hr. He had no history of fever, sore throat, or rhinitis but had been smoking at least one pack of cigarettes each day for 30 years.

A brief physical exam revealed a thin adult male with breath sounds on inspiration and expiration during auscultation. His pulse was 76 beats/min with regular rate and rhythm and no murmurs heard. His blood pressure was 134/78 mm Hg, and his temperature was 98.9 °F (37.2 °C). A chest radiograph revealed increased bronchiolar markings and slight hyperinflation with barrel chest. ABGs were not obtained.

PFTs revealed the following results (postbronchodilator values were obtained after two puffs of isoproterenol from a metered-dose inhaler):

PFT	Predicted	Prebronchodilator			Postbronchodilator		
		Measured	% Predicted	SD	Measured	SD	% Change
VC (L)	4.60	1.41	31	-8.10	1.94	-5.94	38
FEV_1 (L)	3.80	0.61	16	-12.5	0.71	-11.47	16
FEV_1:FVC (%)	83	43	–	–	37	NA[a]	NA[a]
FEF_{25-75} (L/sec)	4.03	0.21	5	-9.29	0.21	-9.29	0
SVC (L)	4.60	–	–	–	2.15	-5.22	NA[a]
TLC (L)	6.94	–	–	–	5.99	NA[a]	NA[a]
RV (L)	2.33	–	–	–	3.83	NA[a]	NA[a]
RV:TLC (%)	34	–	–	–	64	NA[a]	NA[a]

[a]NA = not applicable.

Question: What factors suggest a diagnosis of COPD?

Discussion: The poor prebronchodilator PFT results and the lack of a postbronchodilator response support the diagnosis of COPD. Kent N.'s poor baseline PFTs indicate that he is markedly obstructed. Furthermore, his lack of response to a strong ß-agonist indicates that the obstructions in his lungs are not caused primarily (if at all) by bronchospasms. The obstructions could be caused by inflammation and airway damage.

The breath sounds present during both inspiration and expiration also are compatible with a diagnosis of COPD. Breath sounds on expiration are compatible with the diagnosis of asthma, while breath sounds on inspiration are usually associated with stridor. Breath sounds occur when air rushes over and through the partial obstructions in the airways.

The chest x-ray also is compatible with long-term pulmonary changes associated with COPD. Over a long period, airway linings thicken with mucous and cellular debris. These obstructions occlude the distal airways and increase the density of pulmonary tissue to x-rays. With long-term obstructions, a patient "retains" air, increasing the RV and subsequent RV:TLC ratio. These changes result in hyperinflation on the x-ray. In addition, the patient's chest increases in thickness and becomes more rounded (barrel chested).

Although ABGs could be obtained, these tests are rarely cost effective and useful in the evaluation of a stable COPD patient. The obvious cause of Kent N.'s disease is his cigarette smoking.

Induced Sputum.[23] In the past, sputum samples were thought to be difficult to obtain and often unreliable. Patients were asked to cough a sample of sputum into a collection cup. However, many patients could not produce enough sputum for analysis, and often the sample contained more spit than sputum. With the introduction of newer methods of inducing sputum production and processing the resultant sample, sputum indices are being evaluated for diagnosing and tracking the progression of disease as well as for comparing response to various therapies. Induced sputum generally gives a higher recovery of viable cells and produces better slides for cell differential and counting than sputum samples obtained from the patient just trying to cough up sputum. From the sputum sample, total cell counts, cytokines, chemokines, adhesion molecules, and other inflammatory mediators can be measured. To induce sputum, patients inhale nebulized hypertonic saline. Patients are generally pretreated with a short-acting β_2-adrenergic agonist to prevent airway bronchospasm from the hypertonic saline. Sputum samples should be kept in ice and processed as soon as possible.

Nasal and exhaled nitric oxide. Measurement of nasal and exhaled concentrations of nitric oxide (NO) is being evaluated as a possible noninvasive test of airway inflammation. Although multiple studies have been published, the lack of standardization in the equipment, methodologies, and measurement technique in various disease states has limited the application of NO to the clinical setting. To aid the advancement of this test, ATS published recommendations for standardizing the test procedures.[24]

Compliance

The elasticity of the lungs and/or thorax is measured by pulmonary compliance. Compliance is the change in volume divided by the change in pressure. Pulmonary compliance varies with the amount of air contained in the lungs. Therefore, compliance is often normalized relative to the FRC (the ratio of compliance to the FRC). This ratio is also helpful in comparing patients with normal lung function to those with disease. Pressure is related to the effort needed to expand the lungs. As the pulmonary tissue nears its maximal elastic stretch, greater pressure is needed to stretch farther.

Decreased compliance is observed in patients with decreased volume secondary to pulmonary fibrosis, edema, atelectasis, and some pneumonias. Decreased compliance is also seen when the pressure needed to expand the lungs is increased, as with the loss of surfactant (e.g., hyaline membrane disease and adult respiratory distress syndrome). Pulmonary compliance increases in conditions where less pressure is needed to inflate the lungs. Because of progressive tissue destruction and reduced tissue elasticity, patients with emphysema demonstrate increased pulmonary compliance.

Resistance and Conductance

When the change in pressure is divided by the change in flow, the result is *airway resistance*. This value may be useful in differentiating obstructive from restrictive pulmonary disease or from normal pulmonary function. In obstructive diseases, resistance related to blockage of airflow increases. The magnitude of this increase is related to the amount and severity of the obstruction, and, because of airway narrowing, resistance may increase during acute asthma attacks. Increases also may be seen in emphysema and bronchitis due to obstructive changes. Decreased resistance is rarely clinically meaningful.

Some clinicians prefer to speak in terms of conductance rather than resistance. Conductance is the inverse of resistance. To compare resistance or conductance from one time or patient to another, the value is divided by the lung volume when the measurement was made. These new normalized values are referred to as the *specific airway resistance* or *specific airway conductance*.

MINICASE 6

PATRICK E., A 14-YEAR-OLD BOY with CF, was admitted to a hospital for pulmonary exacerbation. He was diagnosed at age 3 after having poor growth and weight gain and a long history of respiratory symptoms. Since the diagnosis, he had required one or two hospitalizations each year to reverse his decreasing pulmonary functions and worsening symptoms. Typically, his hospital treatment included intensive antibiotic therapy and chest physiotherapy.

Before therapy was started and serially every other day during this admission, PFTs were obtained with the following results:

PFT	Predicted	Measured on Admission		Measured on 12th Day		Best Ever Measurements	
		Pre[a]	Post[a]	Pre	Post	Pre	Post
FVC (L)	3.61	2.85	2.78	3.86	3.85	3.92	3.92
FEV$_1$ (L)	3.18	1.82	1.90	2.72	2.75	2.81	2.91
FEF$_{25-75}$ (L/sec)	4.32	1.04	1.22	1.81	1.95	2.07	2.33
SVC (L)	3.61	–	3.57	–	3.60	3.63	3.75
RV (L)	1.37	–	1.62	–	1.62	1.49	1.41
RV:TLC (%)	29	–	31	–	31	30	30

[a]Pre and Post indicate before and after inhaled bronchodilator administration, respectively.

Question: Why monitor "best ever" values in a patient with CF?

Discussion: Patrick E.'s PFTs improved until they reached the maximum possible. Since CF is a chronic, progressive disease, he probably cannot attain the predicted values. The predicted values are based on normal healthy patients, not people with a chronic progressive pulmonary disease. Therefore, Patrick E.'s "best ever" results become the goals of therapy. The listed tests are usually monitored in CF patients because they represent large airway function (FEV$_1$), small airway function (FEF$_{25-75}$), trapped air (RV and RV:TLC ratio), and general lung function (FVC and SVC).

SUMMARY

This chapter discusses the importance of pulmonary function testing as it relates to the diagnosis, treatment, and monitoring of respiratory disease states. After a review of the anatomy and physiology of the lungs, the mechanics of obtaining PFTs were emphasized. By understanding these mechanics, a clinician can better understand the interpretation of PFTs, and findings from different PFTs can help differentiate between diagnoses and therapeutic recommendations. Most PFT results need to be interpreted within the context of the other findings from the medical history and from other laboratory or clinical test results.

Common tests of airflows and lung volumes are primarily used to characterize airway functions and diseases. These measurements may indicate the need for specific pharmacotherapeutic interventions. For example, clinicians recommending a peak flow meter for home monitoring of severe asthma will find the information obtained useful when considering appropriate therapeutic interventions.

Other tests, such as diffusion capacity, indicate the ability of a gas to diffuse through lung tissues and the general thickness of the membranes lining the alveoli. Specialized tests, such as bronchoprovocational and bronchodilator studies, are used to guide treatment choices. Clearly, the PFTs are an important tool to aid the clinician in decision making.

REFERENCES

1. Crapo RO. Pulmonary function testing. *N Engl J Med.* 1994; 331:25–30.
2. American Thoracic Society. Standardization of spirometry. *Am Rev Respir Dis.* 1979; 119:831–8.
3. American Thoracic Society. Standardization of spirometry: 1987 update. *Am Rev Respir Dis.* 1987; 136:1286–96.
4. American Thoracic Society. Standardization of spirometry: 1994 update. *Am J Respir Crit Care Med.* 1995; 152:1107–36.
5. Bastian-Lee Y, Ghavasse R, Richter H, et al. Assessment of a low-cost home monitoring spirometer for children. *Pediatr Pulmonol.* 2002; 33:388–94.
6. Townsend MC. Spirometric forced expiratory volumes measured in the standing versus sitting position. *Am Rev Respir Dis.* 1984; 103:123–4.
7. Clausen JL. Prediction of normal pulmonary function testing. *Clin Chest Med.* 1989; 10:135–43.
8. National Asthma Education Program. *Expert Panel Report: Guidelines for the Diagnosis and Management of Asthma.* NIH publication 91 3042. Bethesda, MD: Department of Health and Human Services; 1991.
9. National Asthma Education and Prevention Program. Expert panel report: guidelines for the diagnosis and management of asthma update on selected topics, 2002. *J Allergy Clin Immunol.* 2002; 110(suppl, 5):S141–S219.
10. Ruppel G. *Manual of Pulmonary Function Testing.* 2nd ed. St. Louis, MO: C. V. Mosby; 1979:65–76.
11. Cooper JA, White DA, Matthay RA. Drug-induced pulmonary disease. Part 1: cytotoxic drugs. *Am Rev Respir Dis.* 1986; 133:321–40.
12. Cooper JA, White DA, Matthay RA. Drug-induced pulmonary disease. Part 2: noncytotoxic drugs. *Am Rev Respir Dis.* 1986; 133:488–505.
13. Gardner RM, Crapo RO, Nelson SB. Spirometry and flow-volume curves. *Clin Chest Med.* 1989; 10:145–54.
14. Iafrate RP, Massey KL, Hendeles L. Current concepts in clinical therapeutics: asthma. *Clin Pharm.* 1986; 5:206–27.
15. Ahrens RC, Hendeles L, Clarke WR, et al. Therapeutic equivalence of Spiros dry powder inhaler and Ventolin metered-dose inhaler. A bioassay using methacholine. *Am J Respir Crit Care Med.* 1999; 160:1238–43.
16. Cockroft DW, Killian DN, Mellon JJ, et al. Bronchial reactivity to inhaled histamine: a method and clinical survey. *Clin Allergy.* 1977; 7:235–43.
17. Taylor DA, Jensen MW, Kannar V, et al. A dose-dependent effect of the novel inhaled corticosteroids ciclesonide on airway responsiveness to adenosine-5'-monophosphate in asthmatic patients. *Am J Respir Crit Care Med.* 1999; 160:237–43.
18. Swystun VA, Bhagat R, Kalra S, et al. Comparison of 3 different doses of budesonide and placebo on the early asthmatic response to inhaled allergen. *J Allergy Clin Immunol.* 1998; 102:363–67.
19. American Thoracic Society. Guidelines for methacholine and exercise challenge testing: 1999. *Am J Respir Crit Care Med.* 1999; 161:309–29.
20. Series—Standard for Infant Respiratory Function Testing. ERS/ATS Task Force: tidal breath analysis for infant pulmonary function testing. *Eur Respir J.* 2002; 16:1180–92.
21. Series—Standard for Infant Respiratory Function Testing. ERS/ATS Task Force: specifications for equipment used for infant pulmonary function testing. *Eur Respir J.* 2002; 16:731–40.
22. Series—Standard for Infant Respiratory Function Testing. ERS/ATS Task Force: specifications for signal processing and data handling used for infant pulmonary function testing. *Eur Respir J.* 2002; 16:1016–22.
23. Efthimiadis A, Pizzichini E, Pizzichini MM, et al. *Sputum Examination for Indices of Airway Inflammation: Laboratory Procedures.* Astra DracoAB. Lund, Sweden: Canadian Thoracic Society; 1997.
24. American Thoracic Society. Recommendations for standardized procedures for the online and offline measurement of exhaled lower respiratory nitric oxide and nasal nitric oxide in adults and children: 1999. *Am J Respir Crit Care Med.* 1999; 160:2104–17.

Chapter **11**

THE HEART AND MYOCARDIAL INFARCTION

Wafa Y. Dahdal

The heart has two basic properties: electrical and mechanical. The two work in harmony to propel blood, delivering oxygen and nutrients to all body tissues. The pumping action is accomplished by means of striated muscles, which largely compose the myocardium. A number of diseases disrupt the mechanical function of the heart including the acute coronary syndromes (ACSs). Management of ACS and its complications contribute greatly to the overall health of and cost incurred by the society.

Laboratory tests are essential for the diagnosis and prognosis of patients with ACS. Accurate and expeditious assessment guides individualized treatment to optimize a patients' short- and long-term outcomes. Conversely, rapid exclusion of the diagnosis permits early discharge from the coronary care unit or hospital. Laboratory tests used in evaluating the patient with possible ACS are discussed in this chapter, and a number of other diagnostic tests are briefly described.

OBJECTIVES

After completing this chapter, the reader should be able to

- Describe the normal physiology of the heart.
- Explain the roles of the different biochemical markers in the diagnosis of ACS.
- Describe the electrocardiogram changes reflected by myocardial ischemia and infarction.
- Given a patient's history, clinical presentation, cardiac biochemical markers, and ECG findings, assess the presence and severity of ACS.
- Describe the role of pharmacologic agents in noninvasive imaging studies.
- Describe other diagnostic procedures used for the evaluation of ischemic heart disease (IHD) and ACS.

CARDIAC PHYSIOLOGY

Normal Function

The heart consists of two pumping structures, the right and the left. Each is composed of an upper chamber, the atrium, and a lower chamber, the ventricle. The atrium serves as a passive portal to the ventricle and is a weak pump that helps move blood into the ventricle. The atrium is responsible for 20–30% of ventricular filling. The right and left ventricles supply the primary force that propels blood through the pulmonary and peripheral circulation, respectively (Figure 11-1).

The functional unit of the heart is comprised of a network of noncontractile cells that form the conduction system responsible for originating and conducting action potentials from the atria to the ventricles, which leads to the excitation and contraction of the striated muscles responsible for the pumping of the blood to the other organs.

The normal adult human heart contracts rhythmically at approximately 70 beats/min. Each cardiac cycle is divided into a systolic and diastolic phase. During each cycle, blood

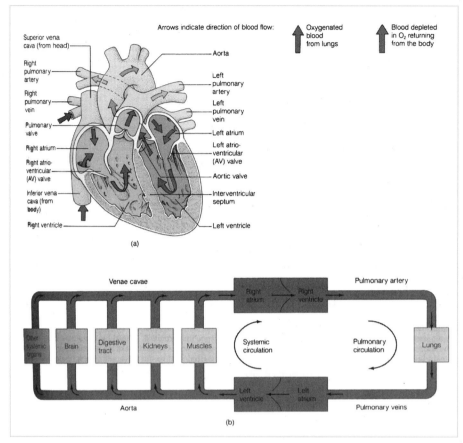

Figure 11-1. Blood flow through and pump action of the heart. (a) Blood flow through the heart. (b) Dual pump action of the heart. (Reproduced, with permission, from Sherwood L. *Human Physiology: From Cells to Systems* (Non-InfoTrac Version). 4th ed. Brooks/Cole; 2001.)

from the systemic circulation is returned to the heart via the veins, and the blood empties from the superior and inferior vena cava into the right atrium. During the diastolic phase, blood passively fills the right ventricle through the tricuspid valve with an active filling phase by atrial contraction just prior to end-diastole. Blood is then pumped from the right ventricle through the pulmonary artery to the lungs where carbon dioxide is removed and the blood is oxygenated. From the lungs, blood returns to the heart via the pulmonary veins and empties into the left atrium. Again, during diastole, blood empties from the left atrium through the mitral valve into the main pumping chamber, the left ventricle, which propels blood into the peripheral circulation via the aorta (Figure 11-1). At rest, the normal heart pumps approximately 4–6 L of blood per minute. Maintaining normal cardiac output is dependent on the heart rate and stroke volume. The *stroke volume*, defined as the volume of blood ejected during systole, is determined by intrinsic and extrinsic factors including myocardial contractility, preload, and afterload.

The coronary arteries, the arteries supplying the heart muscle, branch from the aorta just beyond the aortic valve and are filled with blood mostly during diastole. The major coronary arteries are depicted in Figure 11-2. In the face of increased myocardial metabolic needs, the heart is able to increase coronary blood flow by vasodilation to meet the myocardial oxygen demand.

Dysfunction

Decreased cardiac output compromises tissue perfusion and, depending on the severity and duration, may lead to significant acute and chronic complications. A number of cardiac dis-

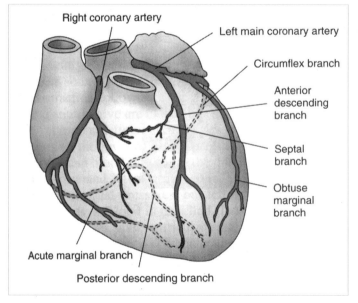

Figure 11-2. Coronary arteries and their principal branches in humans. (Reproduced, with permission, from Kusumoto F. Cardiovascular disorders: heart disease. In: McPhee SJ, Lingappa VR, Ganong WF, et al. *Pathophysiology of Disease: An Introduction to Clinical Medicine.* 3rd ed. McGraw-Hill; 2000.)

eases lead to decreased cardiac output including hypertensive heart diseases, systolic or diastolic heart failure, valvular diseases, congenital heart diseases, diseases of the myocardium, conduction abnormalities, and myocardial infarction (MI). The rest of this chapter focuses on the diagnosis and assessment of acute MI (AMI) within the new classification of the acute coronary syndromes (ACSs).

Patients with acute symptoms of myocardial ischemia may be experiencing one of three ACSs. These are unstable angina (UA), non-ST-segment elevation MI (NSTEMI), or ST-segment elevation MI (STEMI) (Figure 11-3).

UA may be caused by one or a combination of five different mechanisms: ·

1. A nonocclusive thrombus formation on a preexisting atherosclerotic plaque.
2. Dynamic obstruction of the coronary flow caused by coronary spasm or vasoconstriction.
3. Progressive mechanical obstruction and narrowing of the coronary lumen.
4. Inflammation and/or infection (e.g., *Chlamydia pneumoniae*, *Helicobacter pylori*, cytomegalovirus, or herpes simplex virus).
5. Secondary conditions causing increased myocardial oxygen demand or impaired oxygen supply (e.g., thyrotoxicosis, anemia).[1]

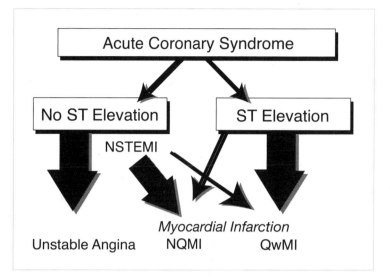

Figure 11-3. Nomenclature of ACSs. Patients with ischemic discomfort may present with or without ST-segment elevation on the ECG. The majority of patients with ST-segment elevation (large arrow) ultimately develop a Q-wave AMI (QwMI), whereas a minority (small arrow) develop a non-Q-wave AMI (NQMI). Patients who present without ST-segment elevation are experiencing either UA or an NSTEMI. The distinction between these two diagnoses is ultimately made based on the presence or absence of a cardiac marker detected in the blood. Most patients with NSTEMI do not evolve a Q wave on the 12-lead ECG and, subsequently, are referred to as having sustained a non-Q-wave MI (NQMI); only a minority of NSTEMI patients develop a Q wave and are later diagnosed as having Q-wave MI. Not shown is Prinzmetal's angina, which presents with transient chest pain and ST-segment elevation but rarely MI. The spectrum of clinical conditions that range from US to non-Q-wave AMI and Q-wave AMI is referred to as ACSs. (Reproduced, with permission, from Reference 6.)

The most common cause for ACSs is atherosclerotic plaque rupture and subsequent obstruction of the coronary lumen by fibrin, platelet aggregates, and red blood cells leading to myocardial necrosis. When a coronary artery is occluded, the location, extent, and duration of occlusion determine the progression and severity of infarction resulting in UA, NSTEMI, or STEMI.

Complication of AMI includes cardiogenic shock, congestive heart failure, ventricular and atrial arrhythmias, ventricular rupture or septal defect, cardiac tamponade, pericarditis, papillary muscle infarction, mitral regurgitation, and embolism. Initial assessment of the patient presenting with ACS may be complicated by the presence and severity of the above complications.

LABORATORY TESTS TO EVALUATE ACUTE CORONARY SYNDROMES

Three criteria for the diagnosis of AMI were identified by the World Health Organization and, subsequently, modified by the Joint European Society of Cardiology/American College of Cardiology Committee to include clinical presentation, electrocardiography, and elevated biochemical markers of myocardial necrosis.[2,3]

Clinical presentation does not distinguish among UA, NSTEMI, and STEMI. The electrocardiogram (ECG) differentiates between NSTEMI and STEMI. Cardiac-specific biochemical markers help differentiate between UA and MI. The release of detectable quantities of biochemical markers in the peripheral circulation indicates severe myocardial injury and is more consistent with AMI than UA. Markers are detected in the peripheral circulation within a few hours after the initial insult in NSTEMI and STEMI, but not UA. In the era of reperfusion therapy, diagnosing ACS accurately and without delay is crucial for risk stratification and appropriate, life-saving treatment implementation. This section describes the laboratory tests used in the diagnosis of ACS. Special emphasis is placed on the new biochemical markers. Other noncardiac specific tests are presented briefly.

MARKER	MW (D)	RANGE OF TIME TO INITIAL ELEVATION (hr)	MEAN TIME TO PEAK ELEVATIONS (nonthrombolysis)	TIME TO RETURN TO NORMAL RANGE	MOST COMMON SAMPLING SCHEDULE
cTnl	23,500	3–12	24 hr	5–10 days	Once at least 12 hr after CP
cTnT	33,000	3–12	12 hr–2 days	5–14 days	Once at least 12 hr after CP
CK-MB	86,000	3–12	24 hr	2–3 days	Every 12 hr × 3[a]
Myoglobin	17,800	1–4	6–7 hr	24 hr	Frequent; 1–2 hr after CP
LDH	135,000	10	24–48 hr	10–14 days	Once at least 24 hr after CP

[a]Increased sensitivity can be achieved with sampling every 6 or 8 hr. (Adapted, with permission, from Reference 4.)

Table 11-1. Biochemical Markers Used in the Diagnosis of AMI

Biochemical Cardiac Markers

Infarction of myocardial cells disrupts membrane, integrity-leaking intracellular macromolecules into the peripheral circulation where they are detected. The criteria of an ideal biochemical marker for the diagnosis of acute coronary syndromes include[4]

1. High specificity: present in high concentrations in the myocardial tissues and absent from nonmyocardial tissue.
2. High sensitivity: detects minor injury to the myocardium.
3. Release and clearance kinetics provide expedient and practical diagnosis:
   a. Rapidly released into the blood after injury to facilitate early diagnosis.
   b. Persists for sufficient time to provide convenient diagnostic time window.
4. Measured level of the marker is in direct proportional relationship with the extent of myocardial injury.
5. Assay technique is commercially available and is easy, inexpensive, and rapid.

Currently, no known marker meets every one of the above criteria. However, the cardiac-specific troponins have a number of attractive features and have gained acceptance as the biochemical markers of choice in the evaluation of patients with ACS.[3,5,6]

Cardiac-Specific Troponin I, Diagnostic Level: <1.5 ng/mL

Cardiac-Specific Troponin T, Diagnostic Level: <0.1 ng/mL

Troponin is a protein complex consisting of three subunits: troponin C (TnC), troponin I (TnI), and troponin T (TnT). The three subunits are located along thin filaments of myofibrils, and they regulate Ca^{+2}-mediated interaction of actin and myosin necessary for the contraction of striated muscles. TnC binds Ca^{+2}, TnI inhibits actomyosin ATPase, and TnT attaches to tropomyosin on the thin filaments. The TnC expressed by cells in cardiac and skeletal muscle is identical. On the contrary, TnI and TnT expressed by cardiac cells are encoded by distinct genes different from those in skeletal cells. Distinct amino acid sequences between the two isoforms allow for specific antibody development without cross-reactivity. Monoclonal antibody-based immunoassays have been developed to detect cardiac-specific TnI (cTnI) and cardiac-specific TnT (cTnT). Quantitative and qualitative assays are commercially available.

Cardiac-specific TnI and cTnT are highly specific and sensitive for myocardial infarction.[7-9] Following myocardial injury, serum cTnI and cTnT begin to rise above the upper reference limit within 3–12 hr, peak in 24 hr (cTnI) or 12 hr–2 days (cTnT), and returns to normal in 5–10 days (cTnI) or 5–14 days (cTnT) (Table 11-1). The initial rise of troponin is due to the release of cytoplasmic troponin whereas the later rise is due to the release of complexed troponin from disintegrating myofilaments (Figure 11-4).[10] Troponins are most beneficial in identifying AMI 6 hr or more after symptom onset. Patients with normal serum levels at presentation should be reassessed between 6–12 hr after onset of symptoms if clinical index of suspicion is high.[6] Levels typically increase more than 20 times above the reference limit. The prolonged time course of elevation of cTnI and cTnT is useful for the late diagnosis of AMI (Figure 11-5).

Two cutoff limits for interpreting levels of troponin have been identified: (1) upper reference limit defined as the 97.5th percentile of the values measured in normal controls, and (2) acute-myocardial-infarction decision limit defined as a level of troponin measurement consistent with AMI, as defined by the World

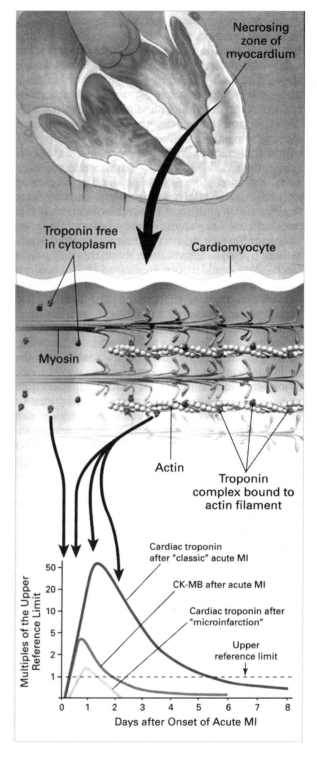

Figure 11-4. Release of cardiac troponins in acute myocardial infarction. The zone of necrosing myocardium is shown at the top of the figure, followed in the middle portion of the figure by a diagram of a cardiomyocyte that is in the process of releasing biomarkers. Most troponin exists as a tripartite complex of C, I, and T components that are bound to actin filaments, although a small amount of troponin is free in the cytoplasm. After disruption of the sarcolemmal membrane of the cardiomyocyte, the cytoplasmic pool of troponin is released first (left-most arrow in bottom portion of figure), followed by a more protracted release from the disintegrating myofilaments that may continue for several days (three-headed arrow). Cardiac troponin levels rise to about 20–50 times the upper reference limit (the 99th percentile of values in a reference control group) in patients who have a classic acute myocardial infarction (MI) and sustain sufficient myocardial necrosis to result in abnormally elevated levels of the MB fraction of creatine kinase (CK-MB). Clinicians can now diagnose episodes of microinfarction by sensitive assays that detect cardiac troponin elevations above the upper reference limit, even though CK-MB levels may still in the normal reference range. (Reproduced, with permission, from Reference 10.)

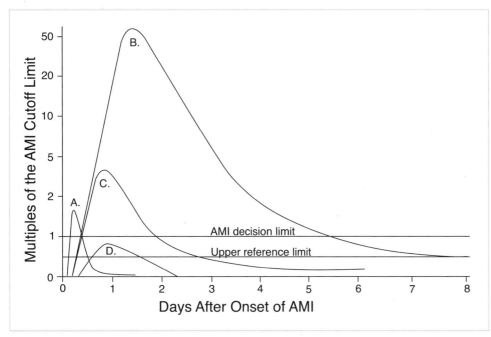

Figure 11-5. Plot of the appearance of cardiac markers in blood vs. time after onset of symptoms. Peak A, early release of myoglobin or CK-MB isoforms after AMI; Peak B, cardiac troponin after AMI; Peak C, CK-MB after AMI; Peak D, cardiac troponins after unstable angina. Data are plotted on a relative scale where 1.0 is set at the AMI cutoff concentration. (Reproduced, with permission, from Reference 5.)

Health Organization and on the basis of the creatine kinase isoenzyme MB (CK-MB). Later, a standardized upper reference limit was defined as an abnormally increased level of cTnI and cTnT exceeding that of 99% of a reference control group.[3]

Several analytical factors should be considered with troponin assays. The first-generation troponin T ELISA was limited by lack of specificity to cardiac troponin and long turnaround time (90 min at 20 °C and 45 min at 37 °C). Second-generation troponin T ELISA was improved by changing the antibody detected to the cardiac-specific antibody M11.7, resulting in enhanced specificity.[11] The currently available third-generation assay (Elecsys, Roche Diagnostics) uses recombinant human cardiac troponin T as standard material enabling reproducibility and standardization of cTnT assays with a normal cutoff concentration of 0.1 μg/L and a turnaround time of 9–12 min.[12] Qualitative assays are also available.

In contrast to cTnT, cTnI assays lack the standardization between multiple commercially available assays developed by different manufacturers. A number of factors complicate the standardization of the assays including (1) cTnI released from disintegrating myocytes may be free cTnI, complexed with cTnC, or a combination of the two forms as well as free-cTnI degradation products; (2) the different forms undergo oxidation, phosphorylation, and proteolysis after release form cells; and (3) the differences in the matrices used and the commutability from an artificial matrix to a physiologic one.[13] Different specificities of the antibodies used for detecting free and complexed cTnI may lead to variations in the cutoff concentration or abnormal levels of cTnI in the available immunoassays. Considerable variation (up to 20-fold) in cTnI levels may be observed when measured by different methods causing ambiguity in clinical interpretation.[14–16] Standardization of the different immunoassays is underway.[13,17] Until then, when interpreting results of cTnI, clinicians should employ the upper reference limit and AMI diagnostic cutoff values for the particular assay used in each institution's laboratory. Table 11-2 provides an example of one institutions' interpretive data for cardiac troponin I.

Because cTnI or cTnT is not detected in the peripheral circulation of healthy individuals, and the high sensitivity of the available assays, *micro-*

TABLE 11-2

RESULTS	INTERPRETATION
≤0.6 ng/mL	May be expected in apparently healthy individuals.
<1.5 ng/mL	May be associated with myocardial damage but have limited specificity within the analytical error of the test.
≥1.5 ng/mL	Consistent with myocardial damage. Any condition resulting in myocardial cell damage may elevate troponin I results. Myocardial infarction is typically accompanied by a rise and fall in troponin I results.

[a]1.5 ng/mL diagnostic cutoff was established for ACS:180 cTnI assay resulting in 94.6% sensitivity and 98.8% specificity.

Table 11-2. An Example of Interpretive Data for Cardiac Troponin I[a]

infarction of myocytes may be detected (see Figure 11-4). Significant prognostic information may be inferred from troponin levels. In a study of patients presenting to the emergency department with chest pain, negative qualitative bedside testing of cTnI and cTnT was associated with low risk for death or myocardial infarction within 30 days (event rates of 0.3 and 1.1, respectively).[18] Other large, clinical trials have documented that elevated troponin levels are strong, independent predictors of mortality and serious adverse outcome 30–42 days after ACSs.[19,20] The findings lead to the hypothesis that elevated troponins may be a marker of severe occlusion of the affected coronary arteries and unstable, ruptured plaques. The risk of 30-day cardiac death or myocardial infarction in patients presenting with angina at rest within 48 hr is estimated to be 15–20% in troponin-positive patients vs. <2% in troponin-negative patients. Further subclassification of these patients based on troponin findings may prove to be valuable for risk stratification and appropriate management.[21]

A number of conditions may cause detectable serum levels of troponins (Table 11-3). The utilization of cardiac troponins in patients with renal dysfunction has been controversial. Most data indicate that cTnI is highly specific, but it should be considered as a useful but an imperfect marker in patients with renal insufficiency and end-stage renal disease.[22] Recently it was found that cTnT predicted a 30-day composite end-point of death or myocardial infarction in patients with ACS regardless of their level of creatinine clearance.[23]

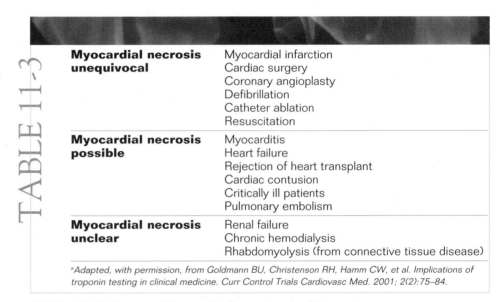

TABLE 11-3		
Myocardial necrosis unequivocal	Myocardial infarction Cardiac surgery Coronary angioplasty Defibrillation Catheter ablation Resuscitation	
Myocardial necrosis possible	Myocarditis Heart failure Rejection of heart transplant Cardiac contusion Critically ill patients Pulmonary embolism	
Myocardial necrosis unclear	Renal failure Chronic hemodialysis Rhabdomyolysis (from connective tissue disease)	

[a]Adapted, with permission, from Goldmann BU, Christenson RH, Hamm CW, et al. Implications of troponin testing in clinical medicine. Curr Control Trials Cardiovasc Med. 2001; 2(2):75–84.

Table 11-3. Causes of Detectable Serum Levels of Troponins[a]

In high-risk patients with non-ST-segment elevation ACS undergoing percutaneous coronary intervention (PCI), cTnI re-elevation, defined as a postprocedural elevation >1 times admission levels, was associated with a significant increase in in-hospital and 6-months mortality.[24] Another study showed elevated cTnI after successful PCI to be an independent predictor of 12-months mortality in patients with chronic renal insufficiency (serum creatinine ≥1.8 mg/dL, not on dialysis). Patients with cTnI >3 times normal values were particularly at higher risk.[25]

Creatine Kinase

Normal range: males, 40–200 IU/L or 667–3334 nmol sec/L
females, 35–150 IU/L or 583–2501 nmol sec/L

Creatine kinase (CK) is an enzyme that stimulates the transfer of high-energy phosphate groups. CK is found in skeletal muscle, myocardium, and the brain. Circulating serum CK is directly related to the individual's muscle mass.

Serum CK concentrations rise sharply 4–8 hr after the onset of chest pain associated with AMI, peak in 24 hr, and return to normal in 3–4 days. Maximum concentrations of CK may reach 5–7 times the normal values. Serial CK measurements following AMI provide excellent sensitivity (98%) but poor specificity (67%). Other causes for increased serum CK concentrations include any musculoskeletal injury or diseases, intramuscular (IM) injections, and a number of medications (Table 11-4).

TABLE 11-4

SKELETAL MUSCLE CAUSES	CARDIAC CAUSES
Dermatomyositis	Myocarditis
Polymyositis	Pericarditis
Muscular dystrophy	AMI
Myxedema	
Malignant hyperpyrexia	
Vigorous exercise	
Malignant hyperthermia syndrome	
Rhabdomyolysis	
Delerium tremens	
Seizures	
Trauma	

MEDICATIONS	OTHER CAUSES
3-hydroxy-3-methylglutaryl coenzyme A reductase inhibitors	Hypothyroidism
	Renal failure
Amphotericin B	Cerebrovascular accident
Clofibrate	Pulmonary embolism
Ethanol (binge drinking)	Severe hypokalemia
Lithium	
Halothane	
Succinylcholine	
Barbiturate poisoning	
Large doses of aminocaproic acid	
Intramuscular injections	

Table 11-4. Causes of Elevated CK Levels

Creatine Kinase Isoenzymes

Normal range: CK-MB <12 IU/L or <3–6% of total CK

The enzyme CK is a dimer of two B monomers (CK-BB), two M monomers (CK-MM), or a hybrid of the two (CK-MB). The three isoenzymes are found in different sources: CK-BB, found in the brain, lungs, and intestinal tract; CK-MM, found primarily in skeletal and cardiac muscle; and CK-MB, found predominantly in the myocardium but also in skeletal muscle. Fractionation of total CK into three isoenzymes increases the diagnostic specificity of the test for AMI.

The CK-MB isoenzyme is most specific for myocardial tissue and has been used for the diagnosis of AMI. Serum CK-MB concentrations begin to rise 3–12 hr after the onset of symptoms, peak in 24 hr, and return to baseline in 2–3 days. Other causes for elevated CK-MB levels include trauma, skeletal muscle injury, or surgical procedures involving the small intestine, tongue, diaphragm, uterus, or prostate.[26]

Electrophoresis separation followed by fluorometric analysis of isoenzyme bands is used to determine the actual CK-MB concentration in international units per liter (IU/L). The range cutoff for the upper limit of normal when the actual CK-MB concentration is determined is 5–25 IU/L. Alternatively, CK-MB as a percentage of the total CK concentration is determined by dividing the CK-MB concentration by the total CK concentration. The cutoff for the upper limit of normal for this value is usually 3–6%. The diagnosis of AMI is strongly suggested when CK-MB as a percentage of total CK was greater than 5% or when the actual CK-MB concentration was greater than 10 IU/L.

Laboratory artifacts may cause false-positive elevations of CK-MB. When using column chromatography assays, false-positive results may be caused by carryover of elevated CK-MM isoenzyme into fractions that normally contain CK-MB. In addition, variant isoenzymes that migrate as a band between CK-MM and CK-MB on electrophoresis may be interpreted as CK-MB on quantitative assays. These variants are usually due to immunoglobulin G complexed to CK-BB or to a mitochondrial source of CK, which differs slightly from cytoplasmic CK. An uncommon problem of qualitative electrophoretic assays is nonspecific fluorescence from other proteins (especially albumin), which may exhibit migration similar to that of other fractions.

Most laboratories currently use the newer CK-MB immunoassay using direct chemiluminometric technology. The assay measures the immunological activity of CK-MB using two monoclonal antibodies and reports the concentration in mass units (ng/mL) or SI units (nmol/L). The conversion formula is 1.0 ng/mL = 0.0125 nmol/L. These new monoclonal antibody immunoassay methodologies are highly sensitive and specific. Furthermore, they do not show the interferences common to earlier immunoassay or traditional electrophoretic and chromatographic methods.

When interpreting serum CK-MB levels, the timing of blood specimen collections in relation to the onset of symptoms must be assessed. Lack of absolute cardiac specificity (skeletal muscle, healthy persons) limits CK-MB interpretation. Other causes for elevated CK-MB levels are listed in Table 11-5 and are usually not associated with the typical rise and fall in serum levels as seen in AMI. To differentiate between cardiac and noncardiac sources of CK-MB elevation, the relative index (RI), or the ratio of CK-MB to total CK concentrations, can be used and is calculated using the following equation:

$$RI = \frac{\text{Measured CK-MB (ng/mL)}}{\text{Total CK Activity (IU/L)}} \times 100$$

This index is useful for samples with abnormally elevated total CK to differentiate MB released from cardiac vs. skeletal muscle. An index greater than 2 is suggestive of myocardial necrosis.

TABLE 11-5

FALSE ELEVATIONS	MYOCARDIAL DAMAGE
Isoenzyme variant	Myocardial infarction
Nonspecific fluorescence	Myocardial puncture/trauma
Spillover of CK-MM	Myocarditis
	Pericarditis

PERIPHERAL SOURCE OF CK-MB	SYSTEMIC DISEASES WITH CARDIAC INVOLVEMENT
Athletic activity (e.g. marathons)	Hyperthermia
Cesarean section	Hypothermia
Surgery (gastrointestinal, prostate)	Muscular dystrophy
Myositis	Reye's syndrome
Rhabdomyolysis	
Tumors	

MISCELLANEOUS	
Hypothyroidism	
Renal failure	
Subarachnoid hemorrhage	

aAdapted, with permission, from Lee TH, Goldman L. Serum enzyme assays in the diagnosis of acute myocardial infarction. Ann Intern Med. 1986; 105(2):221–33.

Table 11-5. Causes of Elevated CK-MB Levels[a]

CK-MB Isoforms

Once CK-MB, also known as the $CK\text{-}MB_2$ isoform while in the myocardial tissue, is released into the circulation following an AMI, it undergoes metabolism by lysine carboxypeptidase producing the more negatively charged isoform $CK\text{-}MB_1$. In healthy individuals, the two isoforms are in equilibrium and the normal levels are 0.5–1 IU/L. One study showed that elevated $CK\text{-}MB_2$ levels of >1.0 IU/L and increased ratio of $CK\text{-}MB_2$ to $CK\text{-}MB_1$ of ≥1.5 has a sensitivity of AMI diagnosis in the emergency department of 59% when measured at 2–4 hr and 92% at 4–6 hr of symptoms.[27] Another study showed that CK-MB isoforms were most sensitive and specific (91% and 89%) when measured 6 hr after onset of chest pain in patients with myocardial infarction presenting to the emergency department.[28] Similar to CK-MB, the isoforms lack absolute cardiac specificity. In addition, assays are not widely available for clinical use. The role of CK-MB isoforms among other biochemical markers remains to be defined.[29]

Myoglobin

Myoglobin is a low-molecular-weight heme protein found in cardiac and skeletal muscle. This protein is one of two preferred markers for the early detection of AMI and automated immunoassays are commercially available. Serum levels are detected within 1–4 hr and peak 6–7 hr after the onset of symptoms. The early rise of myoglobin levels after onset of symptoms makes it the most appropriate and convenient test for early detection of AMI. Myoglobin is cleared rapidly by renal glomerular filtration and levels return to reference value 24 hr following AMI. The fast rise and fall of myoglobin levels make it an appropriate marker to detect reinfarction if occurring 24 hr after the initial insult. In addition, in patients presenting with AMI receiving thrombolytic therapy, elevated baseline or 12–hr myoglobin levels predict 30-day mortality and may be useful in triaging patients following reperfusion.[30,31]

Myoglobin is highly sensitive to myocardial ischemia and is most useful in ruling out AMI. Lack of specificity to cardiac muscle limits the interpretation of myoglobin levels. Differential conditions leading to false-positive results include skeletal muscle injury of any cause, trauma, and renal failure.

MINICASE 1

JAMES S., A 65-YEAR-OLD CAUCASIAN MAN, presented to the emergency department complaining of chest pain that started 2 hr ago. The pain is characterized as substernal pressure associated with slight shortness of breath and was not relieved by one sublingual nitroglycerin tablet. His past medical history includes hypertension, diabetes, and a history of myocardial infarction 3 years ago. He smokes one pack of cigarettes every other day.

On physical examination, James S. had a blood pressure of 134/90 mmHg and a pulse of 81 bpm. Heart and lung examinations were normal. Initial ECG showed a 1-mm depression in leads II, III, and aVF and 0.5-mm depression in leads V_5 and V_6. Biochemical markers tested are as follows:

	CK-MB (<5.0 ng/mL)	TROPONIN I (<1.5 ng/mL)
At presentation	2.0	0.05
6 hr later	2.5	1.8

Question: What is the most likely assessment of James S.' presentation?

Discussion: On presentation, the ECG findings are consistent with inferolateral ST-segment depression, which is consistent with ischemia and unstable angina. Biochemical markers, however, are not elevated at baseline. Based on the ECG and the marker findings, James S. may be diagnosed as having unstable angina (UA).

The assumption that James S. has UA based on normal markers may be erroneous since his symptoms started 2 hr ago and the release kinetics of both CK-MB and troponin I are such that the levels begin to rise between 3–12 hr after onset of AMI. A second set of markers should be drawn and the levels should be assessed between 6–12 hr after onset of symptoms since the clinical presentation is highly suspicious. The second set of biochemical markers drawn 6 hr later was mildly positive for myocardial infarction (elevated troponin I). Thus, James S. is experiencing a non-ST-segment elevation myocardial infarction (NSTEMI) rather than UA.

Lactate Dehydrogenase

Normal range: 100–210 IU/L or 1667–3501 nmol sec/L

Lactate dehydrogenase (LDH) is an enzyme that catalyzes the reversible formation of lactate from pyruvate. Following AMI, serum LDH rises in 24–48 hr, peaks at 2–3 days, and returns to normal in 8–14 days after the onset of chest pain. The major limitation to LDH is the lack of specificity as it is found in numerous organs and tissues including the heart, liver, lungs, kidneys, skeletal muscle, red blood cells, and lymphocytes. Electrophoresis fractionation of LDH to its five major isoenzymes (LDH_1–LDH_5) better distinguishes the site of origin, but these tests are not specific for AMI. The heart contains mainly LDH_1 and to a lesser extent LDH_2. In the past, elevation of LDH_1 or a ratio of LDH_1:LDH_2 greater than one was used in the differential diagnosis of AMI. Since the development of more cardiac-specific markers, LDH and LDH isoenzymes are no longer recommended for the evaluation of the patient with ACS.[5]

Aspartate Aminotransferase

Normal range: males, 0–37 IU/L or 0–617 nmol sec/L
females, 0–31 IU/L or 0–517 nmol sec/L

Aspartate aminotransferase (AST) is an enzyme involved in amino acid synthesis. AST is widely distributed in the liver, heart, skeletal muscle, red blood cells, kidneys, and pancreas. Serum levels of AST rise within 12 hr of AMI, peak in 24–48 hr, and return to baseline in 3–4 days. Poor specificity of AST for myocardial cell damage led to its replacement by more cardiac-specific markers.

Recommendations for Measurement of Biochemical Markers

The time of the patient's presentation in relation to the onset of AMI should always be considered when interpreting laboratory results. The release and clearance kinetics of the different biochemical markers in relation to the time of presentation from initial onset of symptoms dictate the appropriate biomarker to accurately diagnose ACS. Early-rising biochemical markers (myoglobin or CK-MB isoforms) are most appropriate for patients presenting within 6 hr of onset of symptoms. Troponins are better markers for patients presenting 6 hr or later after AMI. A combination of an early marker with troponins is an acceptable practice and is adopted by most laboratories.[5]

Risk stratification based on cardiac biochemical markers indicative of myocardial necrosis impacts on patient outcomes and management decisions. The extent of myocardial necrosis is an important determinant of the risk of death. Troponins are more sensitive to the presence of myocardial damage than myoglobin and creatine kinase. Specific cTnI and cTnT have emerged as the preferred cardiac biochemical markers for the evaluation of patients with ACS.[5,6]

Troponins, CK-MB, and myoglobin may be used as indicators of reperfusion in patients undergoing successful recanalization of the infarct-related artery. Also, biochemical markers may be used to predict successful reperfusion therapy by thrombolytic therapy or percutaneous transluminal coronary angioplasty (PCTA). Successful reperfusion causes a *washout phenomenon* where a bolus amount of the markers is released, which is associated with a higher and earlier peak and faster clearance from the circulation. At least two blood samples are collected (just before and at 90 min after initiation of therapy).

In patients undergoing surgical procedures, troponins are most useful in the assessment of perioperative myocardial infarction. Because other biochemical markers lack cardiac specificity, they may be elevated secondary to the operation rather than AMI.

The availability of rapid, convenient assay—especially in the emergency departments—enhances timely and cost-effective assessment and disposition of patients. Point-of-care tests are available for troponins, CK-MB, and myoglobin.

Other Biochemical Markers

Other biochemical markers that may prove of value in the assessment of patients with ACS include markers of coagulation cascade activity and of acute phase inflammation. Fibrinopeptide and fibrinogen are markers of increased coagulation activity and appear to be associated with increased risk and a poor clinical outcome in patients with UA.[32,33] Similarly, elevated levels of C-reactive protein, serum amyloid A, or interleukin-6, which are acute phase inflammation markers, have been shown to predict an increased risk of adverse outcomes of ACS patients.[34–38]

Miscellaneous Laboratory Tests

A number of noncardiac specific laboratory abnormalities may be manifested in patients with AMI. These include nonspecific elevation of serum glucose, white blood cells, and erythrocyte sedimentation rate, and alterations in lipid profile findings. Recognition of these abnormalities as secondary to AMI precludes misinterpretation or misdiagnosis of other disorders.

Serum Glucose

Normal range: 70–110 mg/dL or 3.9–6.1 mmol/L when fasting

Following AMI, patients may present with elevations of serum glucose, apparently related to stress, and may persist for several weeks. The elevation may be found in diabetic as well as nondiabetic patients. Measurement of glycosylated hemoglobin may help to differentiate hyperglycemia caused by the stress of diabetic AMI.[39,40]

White Blood Cells

Normal range: 4.8–10.8 × 10³ cells/mm³ or 4.8–10.8 × 10⁹ cells/L for adults

White blood cell count may be increased in patients presenting with AMI in response to myocardial tissue necrosis or secondary to increased adrenal glucocorticoid secretion due to stress. Polymorphonuclear leukocytosis of 10,000–20,000 cells/mm³ (10–20×10^9 cells/L) may be seen 12–24 hr after onset of symptoms and may last for 1–2 weeks depending on extent of tissue necrosis. Fever may accompany leukocytosis.

Erythrocyte Sedimentation Rate

Normal range: males, 1–15 mm/hr
females, 1–20 mm/hr

Erythrocyte sedimentation rate (ESR) is an acute phase reactant that increases in patients with AMI. ESR usually peaks on day 4 or 5 and may remain elevated for 3–4 weeks post-AMI.

Lipid Panel

Total cholesterol and low-density lipoprotein may be decreased when measured 48–72 hr post-MI and may persist for 6–8 weeks afterward.

ELECTROCARDIOGRAPHY

Electrocardiography is the recording of the electrical activity of the heart on an electrocardiogram (ECG).

Normal Conduction System and Electrocardiogram Recording

The conduction system is composed of specialized, noncontractile cells that serve to originate and conduct action potentials in the appropriate sequence and at an appropriate rate from the atria to the ventricles. At rest, the cardiac cells are more negatively charged intracellularly than extracellularly, or polarized, with a voltage difference of 60–90 mV. When excited, ionic currents across cell membranes lead to charge shifting where the interior of the cells become more positive or depolarized, and an action potential is generated. Calcium influx leads to the excitation-contraction coupling of the cells. Subsequently, the action potential is propagated and the cells return to normal resting state (repolarization). Depolarization is the electrical phenomena that leads to myocardial contraction, and repolarization is the electrical phenomena that leads to myocardial relaxation. The ECG provides a pictorial presentation of the depolarization and repolarization of atrial and ventricular cells that can be assessed by reviewing a number of waves and intervals.

Normally, an electrical impulse originates in the sinoatrial (SA) node and is propagated through Bachmann's bundle and internodal tracts, the atrioventricular (AV) node, His bundle, the left and right bundle branches, and the Purkinje fibers resulting in one cardiac cycle. Each cardiac cycle is presented on ECG by the P wave reflecting atrial depolarization, the QRS complex reflecting ventricular depolarization, and the T wave reflecting ventricular repolarization (Figure 11-6). By placing multiple leads on the patient, the electrical impulses of the heart are recorded from different views. The standard ECG is composed of twelve leads: six limb leads (I, II, III, AVR, AVL, and AVF) and six chest leads (V_1–V_6). Different leads provide specific information on different aspects of heart chambers and coronary arteries.

Electrocardiographic Findings in Acute Coronary Syndrome

In patients with ACS, the ECG is an essential diagnostic tool providing immediate and invaluable data vital for the expeditious diagnosis, prognosis, and management. A 12-lead ECG should be obtained within 10 min of presentation to the emergency department if ACS is suspected. Careful reading of the ECG by an experienced clinician provides information on the (1) presence of myocardial ischemia, injury, or infarction, (2) location of the infarction, and (3) the site of occlusion in the coronary artery involved.

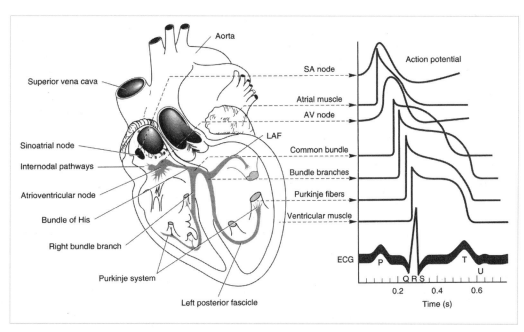

Figure 11-6. Conducting system of the heart. Typical transmembrane action potentials for the SA and AV nodes, other parts of the conduction system, and the atrial and ventricular muscles are shown along with the correlation to the extracellularly recorded electrical activity (i.e., the electrocardiogram [ECG]). The action potentials and ECG are plotted on the same time axis but with different zero points on the vertical scale. The PR interval is measured form the beginning of the P wave to the beginning of the QRS. (LAF, left anterior fascicle.) (Reproduced, with permission, from Kusumoto F. Cardiovascular disorders: heart disease. In: McPhee SJ, Lingappa VR, Ganong WF, et al. *Pathophysiology of Disease: An Introduction to Clinical Medicine.* 3rd ed. McGraw-Hill; 2000.)

The classic ECG pattern of myocardial infarction is reflected by three changes: (1) T-wave inversion, (2) ST-segment elevation, or (3) appearance of Q waves. The leads in which ECG changes occur reflect the anatomic site of the infarction (Table 11-6). T-wave inversions or ST-segment depression suggest acute ischemia whereas ST-segment elevation or Q waves suggest acute infarction. ST-segment elevation is the earliest sign of myocardial infarction and occurs within hours of onset of symptoms. As the infarction evolves, changes to the QRS complex include loss of R-wave height and the development of pathologic Q waves defined by a width of ≥1 mm and a depth of >25% of the QRS complex height. Q waves may appear within 1–2 hr of onset of symptoms, often 12 hr, and, occasionally, up to 24 hr.[41] Figure 11-7 depicts ECG evolution during acute STEMI (Q-wave) and NSTEMI (non-Q-wave) myocardial infarction.

ECG changes indicative of established MI and myocardial ischemia that may progress to MI, as defined by the Joint European Society of Cardiology/American College of Cardiology Committee, are summarized in Table 11-7.[3]

In addition to diagnosing ACS, ECG findings provide prognostic information. Patients presenting with angina at rest with transient ST-segment changes >0.05 mV, new or presumed

TABLE 11-6

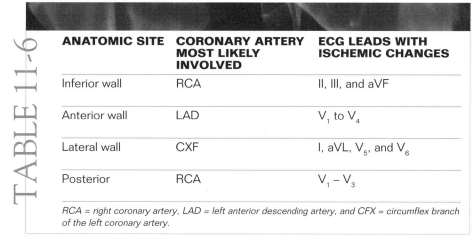

ANATOMIC SITE	CORONARY ARTERY MOST LIKELY INVOLVED	ECG LEADS WITH ISCHEMIC CHANGES
Inferior wall	RCA	II, III, and aVF
Anterior wall	LAD	V_1 to V_4
Lateral wall	CXF	I, aVL, V_5, and V_6
Posterior	RCA	$V_1 – V_3$

RCA = right coronary artery, LAD = left anterior descending artery, and CFX = circumflex branch of the left coronary artery.

Table 11-6. Localization of Left Ventricular Myocardial Infarction by Anatomical Relationships of Leads

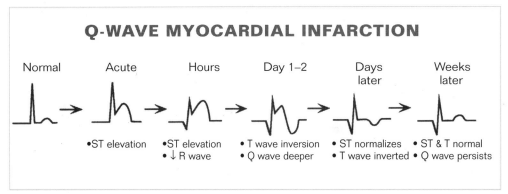

Q-WAVE MYOCARDIAL INFARCTION

Normal	Acute	Hours	Day 1–2	Days later	Weeks later
	• ST elevation	• ST elevation • ↓ R wave	• T wave inversion • Q wave deeper	• ST normalizes • T wave inverted	• ST & T normal • Q wave persists

Figure 11-7. ECG evolution during (a) acute Q-wave myocardial infarction and (b) non-Q-wave myocardial infarction. (Reproduced, with permission, from Sabatine MS, O'Gara PT, Lilly LS. Acute Myocardial Infarction. In: Lilly LS. *Pathophysiology of Heart Disease.* 2nd ed. Williams and Wilkins; 1998.)

bundle-branch block, or sustained ventricular tachycardia are at high risk of short-term death or nonfatal MI.[6]

IMAGING STUDIES

A number of imaging modalities contribute to the diagnosis and assessment of ACS, including chest roentgenography, echocardiography, cardiac catheterization, perfusion imaging, computed tomography, magnetic resonance imaging, and positron-emission tomography. For patients presenting with ACS, these tests may be used when clinical presentation, biochemical markers, and ECG are nondiagnostic with high clinical suspicion.

Chest Roentgenogram

Chest radiography taken at the initial presentation of patients with ACS provides early estimation of the size of the left heart chambers. In addition, presence and degree of pulmonary congestion indicates elevated left-ventricular end-diastolic pressure, which may result from sizeable infarction of the left ventricle.

Echocardiography

Echocardiography is based on sound transmitted to and through the heart. Different tissues present different acoustical impedance (resistance to transmitting sound). Transthoracic echocardiography (TTE) involves sound waves from a transducer positioned on the anterior chest directed across cardiac tissues. The sound is reflected back in different frequencies and images of cardiac anatomy are displayed on an oscilloscope or an electronic monitor.

Two-dimensional echocardiography records multiple views providing cross-sectional images of the heart and great coronary arteries. Clinical uses include anatomic assessment of the heart and coronary arteries and functional assessment of cardiac chambers and valves. Contrast agents may be injected to visualize blood flow. M-mode, or motion-mode, records the motion of individual structures. Doppler echocardiography uses sound or frequency ultrasound to record the velocity and direction of blood and wall motion; it is based on the principle of bouncing ultrasound waves off of a moving object (e.g., red blood cells). This method permits the assessment of valvular and wall motion abnormalities.

TABLE 11-7

ESTABLISHED MI

Any Q wave in leads V_1 through V_3, Q wave ≥30 ms (0.03 sec) in leads I, II, aVL, V_4, V_5, or V_6. (The Q wave changes must be present in any two contiguous leads, and be ≥1 mm in depth.)

MYOCARDIAL ISCHEMIA THAT MAY PROGRESS TO MI

1. Patients with ST-segment elevation
   New or presumed new ST-segment elevation at the J point in two or more contiguous leads with the cutoff points ≥0.2 mV in leads V_1, V_2, or V_3 and ≥0.1 mV in other leads (contiguity in the frontal plane is defined by the lead sequence aVL, inverted aVR, II, aVF, III).

2. Patients without ST-segment elevation[a]
   a. ST-segment depression
   b. T wave abnormalities only

[a]*New or presumed new ST-segment depression or T wave abnormalities, or both, should be observed in two or more contiguous leads. Also, new or presumed new symmetric inversion of T waves ≥1 mm should be present in at least two contiguous leads. (Adapted, with permission, from Reference 3.)*

Table 11-7. ECG Changes Indicative of Established MI and Myocardial Ischemia that may Progress to MI

TTE may have an important role in assessing patients with ACS presenting with apparent large infarct and hemodynamic instability. Information provided includes wall motion abnormalities to assess the extent of the infarct or the level of function of the remaining myocardium, recognition of complications such as postinfarction ventricular septal defect, and presence of left ventricular thrombi.[42] In addition, TTE can be combined with exercise and pharmacologic stress testing to assess stress-induced structural or functional abnormalities (e.g., wall motion abnormality associated with ischemia) in patients with ischemic heart disease.

Transesophageal echocardiography (TEE) involves mounting the transducer at the end of a flexible endoscope and passing it through the esophagus to position it closer to the heart. TEE provides higher resolution of the posterior cardiac structures making it ideal for viewing the atria, cardiac valves, and aorta. Clinical indications include detection of atrial thrombi, mitral valve vegetations, or thoracic aortic dissection. TEE has no role in the diagnosis or assessment of patients with ACS.

Cardiac Catheterization

Cardiac catheterization involves the introduction of a catheter through the femoral or brachial artery, which is advanced to the heart chambers or great vessels guided by fluoroscopy. Measurements collected include intracardiac pressures, hemodynamic data, and blood flow in the heart chambers and coronary arteries.

PRESENTING DIAGNOSIS	RECOMMENDATION
Asymptomatic or class I angina	Patients who do not have treated diabetes with asymptomatic ischemia or mild angina with one or more significant lesions in one or two coronary arteries suitable for PCI with a high likelihood of success and a low risk of morbidity and mortality. The vessels to be dilated must subtend a large area of viable myocardium.
Moderate or severe symptoms (angina class II to IV, UA or NSTEMI) with single- or multivessel coronary disease on medical therapy	Patients with one or more significant lesions in one or more mocoronary arteries suitable for PCI with a high likelihood of success and low risk of morbidity or mortality. The vessel(s) to be dilated must subtend a moderate or large area of viable myocardium and have high risk.
Acute transmural MI patients as an alternative to thrombolysis	1. As an alternative to thrombolytic therapy in patients with AMI and ST-segment elevation or new or presumed new left bundle branch block who can undergo angioplasty of the infarct artery ≤2 hr from the onset of ischemic symptoms or >2 hr if symptoms persist, if performed in a timely fashion by individuals skilled in the procedure and supported by experienced personnel in an appropriate laboratory environment. 2. In patients who are within 36 hr of an acute ST elevation/Q wave or new left bundle branch block myocardial infarction who develop cardiogenic shock, are <75 years of age, and revascularization can be performed within 18 hr of the onset of shock by individuals skilled in the procedure and supported by experienced personnel in an appropriate laboratory environment.
After thrombolysis	Objective evidence for recurrent infarction or ischemia (rescue PCI).
During subsequent hospital management after acute therapy for AMI including primary PCI	1. Spontaneous or provocable myocardial ischemia during recovery from infarction. 2. Persistent hemodynamic instability.

[a]Adapted, with permission, from Reference 43.

Table 11-8. Conditions for Which There is Evidence for and/or General Agreement that Percutaneous Coronary Intervention (PCI) is Useful and Effective[a]

TABLE 11-8

MINICASE 2

WILLIAM N., A 44-YEAR-OLD MALE with no previous cardiac history, was seen by a local physician 1 day after first feeling palpitations. His physician noted a tachycardic pulse with a heart rate of about 130 beats/min. William N. was sent to the local emergency department where an ECG revealed atrial fibrillation with a ventricular rate of 200 beats/min. Adenosine 6 mg was given, resulting in transient slowing of the rate to 150 beats/min. Intravenous (IV) verapamil produced no change in either heart rate or rhythm but did drop the patient's blood pressure (BP).

Synchronized direct current cardioversion was then attempted, resulting in ventricular fibrillation. William N. was then resuscitated for approximately 90 min until normal sinus rhythm returned. He received 10 direct current cardioversions, vasopressin, and amiodarone.

William N. was then transferred by emergency aircare to a university hospital and admitted to the cardiovascular intensive care unit (ICU). At admission, his ECG showed a short PR interval and a wide QRS with slurred upstroke (D wave) consistent with the Wolff-Parkinson-White syndrome. His laboratory results on admission were normal, except for an elevated leukocyte count of 23,800 cells/mm^3 (4800–10,800 cells/mm^3), serum creatinine (SCr) of 2.1 mg/dL (0.7–1.5 mg/dL), calcium of 8.2 mg/dL (8.5–10.8 mg/dL), phosphate of 6.3 mg/dL (2.6–4.5 mg/dL), uric acid of 9.9 mg/dL (3.4–7.0 mg/dL), and AST of 511 IU/L (0–37 IU/L). His glucose drawn on admission was 294 mg/dL (70–110 mg/dL). Over the ensuing 5 days, his cardiac enzymes were as follows:

HOSPITAL Day	Time	CK (40–200 IU/L)	CK-MB INDEX (0–1.9 %)
1	1525	1843	2.6
	2250	5062	1.1
2	0627	6273	0.6
	1244	6876	0.4
	1809	7030	–
3	0611	7768	–
4	0448	5478	–
5	0714	2813	0.1
6	0755	1051	0.1
7	0710	408	0.1

Question: What is the appropriate explanation for the above laboratory values?

Discussion: In this case, the patient presented with an arrhythmia and received multiple direct current cardioversions and prolonged chest compression. He had no symptoms of AMI and no ECG changes indicative of ischemia. The CK enzymes increased to extremely high concentrations, but only the first was positive for significant MB (positive CK-MB index). This finding was not interpreted as AMI since it was the only abnormal CK-MB and probably reflected a small amount of myocardial injury due to repeated cardioversions.

The CK enzyme concentrations were increased for a prolonged period—much longer than would be expected in a usual AMI. This finding probably reflected prolonged release from traumatized tissues and slowed elimination as a result of acute renal failure (SCr peaked at 2.1 mg/dL) that developed secondary to hypotension and reduced renal perfusion during resuscitation. Both phosphate and uric acid were elevated because of developing renal failure. The leukocyte count was elevated secondary to the stressful event and possible aspiration during resuscitation. The AST elevation most likely represented hepatic injury secondary to reduced hepatic perfusion during the code.

Coronary Angiography

Coronary angiography, also referred to as angiocardiography or coronary arteriography, utilizes contrast media that is injected into the coronary arteries. X-ray exposures are examined to assess the location and severity of coronary atherosclerotic lesions. Therapeutic interventions may be performed during the catheterization including percutaneous transluminal coronary angioplasty (PTCA) and stent placement. Table 11-8 summarizes the conditions for which there is evidence for and/or general agreement that percutaneous coronary intervention is useful and effective.[43] Brachytherapy and drug-eluting (sirolimus and paclitaxel) stents are being studied to reduce in-stent restenosis.

Left Ventriculography

Left ventriculography is the injection of contrast media into the left ventricle to assess its structure and function. Wall motion abnormalities and left ventricular ejection fraction are evaluated during this procedure.

Nuclear Imaging

Nuclear imaging involves the injection of tracer amounts of radioactive elements that concentrate in certain areas of the heart. A gamma camera is then rotated around the patient, and multiple planar images are taken to detect the radioactive emissions and form an image of the deployment of the tracer in the different regions of the heart. Single-photon emission computed tomography (SPECT) is the most common imaging technique.

Nuclear imaging is used to assess blood flow through the heart and myocardial perfusion, locate and assess severity of myocardial ischemia and infarction, and evaluate myocardial metabolism.

Myocardial Perfusion Imaging

Thallium-201 (^{201}Tl) became available in 1974 and was the conventional radiopharmaceutical agent used until the early 1990s, at which time technetium-99m (^{99m}Tc)-labeled compounds such as ^{99m}Tc-sestamibi and ^{99m}Tc-tetrofosmin were introduced for visualization of myocardial perfusion. The imaging agents measure the relative distribution of myocardial blood flow between normal and stenotic coronary arteries.

^{201}Tl, a potassium analog is taken up by healthy functioning tissue in a manner similar to potassium. ^{201}Tl is taken up at reduced rates by ischemic myocardial tissue and is not distributed to or taken up by regions of myocardial infarction. Imaging with ^{201}Tl for detection of infarction is accomplished with the patient at rest and is optimal within 6 hr of symptom onset. ^{201}Tl is injected intravenously and imaging is initiated 10–20 min after injection; imaging is repeated 2–4 hr later to determine whether redistribution occurred. The diagnosis of AMI must be inferred by a lack of regional myocardial uptake of the radiotracer. ^{201}Tl imaging for a perfusion defect has a sensitivity of about 90% if applied within the first 24 hr after symptom onset and falls sharply thereafter.

^{99m}Tc is an infarct-avid agent. It concentrates in necrotic myocardial tissue, presumably because it enters myocardial cells and selectively binds to calcium and calcium complexes. Abnormal intracellular uptake of calcium is a feature of irreversible cell death and begins as early as 12 hr after AMI and may persist for 2 weeks. ^{99m}Tc scans may be positive as early as 4 hr after the onset of AMI symptoms. The peak sensitivity for the scan is between 48–72 hr, but generally remains positive for up to 1 week post AMI. When obtained within 24–72 hr after onset of infarction, the scan has a diagnostic sensitivity of 90–95% in patients with Q-wave AMI, or 38–92% in patients with non-Q-wave AMI. ^{99m}Tc imaging has moderate specificity, with an overall range of 60–80%.

^{201}Tl perfusion imaging is widely utilized in patients with atypical chest pain following a nondiagnostic (symptoms or findings consistent with coronary artery disease are not evident during test) or false-positive stress testing to determine if coronary artery atherosclerosis is the cause of symptoms. In addition, since redistribution is a marker of jeopardized but viable myocardial tissue, ^{201}Tl can be used to indicate the probable success of revascularization or angioplasty and for prognostic stratification of patients preoperatively. A normal ^{201}Tl scan indicates a benign outcome, even in patients with documented IHD. Transient defects (redistribution) indicate hemodynamically significant coronary lesions with the risk of cardiac death.

Nuclear imaging in conjunction with stress testing provides further information on myocardial perfusion and function. ^{99m}Tc-sestamibi may be used in combination with ^{201}Tl to assess rest and stress myocardial perfusion sequentially in 1 day. The patient's rest study is done first with ^{201}Tl; imaging is started immediately after tracer injection and is completed within about 45 min. Stress testing (pharmacologically or with exercise) is begun after the rest study, and ^{99m}Tc-sestamibi is injected at peak cardiac stress.

Since ^{99m}Tc-sestamibi emits higher energy photons than ^{201}Tl, its images are not subject to cross-interference from the previously administered ^{201}Tl. Both ^{201}Tl and ^{99m}Tc-sestamibi undergo first-pass extraction from blood by myocardial cells; both provide a *stop-frame* image of regional myocardial blood flow at the time of tracer injection. ^{99m}Tc-sestamibi does not leak appreciably from myocardial cells, thus imaging may be delayed to allow blood and lung concentrations to diminish. Consequently, ^{99m}Tc-sestamibi imaging can be completed between 1–4 hr after tracer injection without significantly reducing diagnostic reliability.

The clinically most important application of myocardial perfusion imaging is detection of an AMI. Images are interpreted qualitatively and quantitatively and report the myocardial perfusion to the different areas as normal, defect, reversible defect, fixed defect, or reverse redistribution. Myocardial perfusion imaging may also be used for the assessment of thrombolytic therapy effectiveness and early risk stratification of patients presenting with AMI. ECG-gated myocardial perfusion SPECT studies enhance the interpretive confidence and accuracy and provide information critical for the diagnosis, prognosis, and management decisions, including global left ventricular function and regional wall motion and thickening.

Noninvasive Stress Testing

Exercise Stress Testing

In patients with chronic stable CAD who are capable of physical exercise, myocardial perfusion imaging is used in conjunction with exercise testing. Physical exercise is performed using a graded exercise protocol on a treadmill or upright bicycle. The most widely used protocol is the Bruce protocol. Nonimaging endpoints include reproduction of anginal symptoms, exhaustion, hypertension or 20 mmHg decrease in systolic blood pressure, ventricular arrhythmias, or severe ST-segment depression on ECG. Exercise allows for several useful measurements including the duration of exercise, total workload, maximum heart rate, exercise-induced symptoms, ECG changes, and blood pressure response. Limitations include patients with orthopedic, neurological, or peripheral vascular problems. Patients receiving agents that may blunt heart rate response to exercise (beta-blockers or nondihydropyridine calcium channel blockers) may not be able to achieve optimal test goal.

Pharmacologic Stress Testing

Patients who are unable to exercise may be *stressed* pharmacologically using either (1) vasodilating agents such as adenosine or dipyridamole or (2) positive inotropic agents such as dobutamine. Both modalities produce a hyperemic (vasodilatory response or increased blood flow) response leading to heterogeneity of myocardial blood flow between vascular areas supplied by normal and significantly stenosed coronary arteries. Heterogeneity is visualized with radionuclide myocardial perfusion agents.

Adenosine is an endogenous vasodilator. Coronary vasodilation is mediated through the activation of A_{2a} receptors. Dipyridamole blocks the cellular reabsorption of endogenous adenosine. Vasodilation, by both adenosine and dipyridamole, increases coronary blood flow in normal arteries 3–5 times baseline with little or no increase in blood flow to stenotic arteries. Dobutamine increases myocardial oxygen demand by increasing myocardial contractility, heart rate, and blood pressure. Following dobutamine administration, coronary blood flow in normal arteries is increased 2–3 times baseline, which is similar to that achieved

MINICASE 3

GEORGE S., A 57-YEAR-OLD MALE, previously had been in good health. On the evening of January 21, 2003, after drinking approximately eight cans of beer, he awoke with severe chest pain and diaphoresis. He was driven to the local emergency treatment center by his wife, who noted that he may have "lost consciousness a couple of times" in route.

At the emergency treatment center, George S.' pulse was in the 30s. His ECG showed a 3° AV block in addition to acute ST-segment elevation in the inferior leads (II, III, and aVF). George S. received atropine 2 mg, aspirin 325 mg, and streptokinase 1.5 million units over 1 hr, which increased his heart rate and resolved his ST-segment elevation within approximately 30–60 min.

George S. was then transferred on IV nitroglycerin and heparin to the hospital's cardiovascular ICU. At admission, his ECG showed normal sinus rhythm with developing Q waves in leads II, III, and aVF. The admission laboratory showed normal electrolytes and hematological test results, except for an elevated leukocyte count of 14,800 cells/mm^3 (4800–10,800 cells/mm^3), aPTT of 65 sec (21–45 sec), PT of 17 sec (10–13 sec), and INR of 2.2. In addition, his AST was slightly elevated at 103 IU/L. His blood alcohol level at the local hospital was 168 mg%. Over the next 2 days, his cardiac enzymes rose rapidly as follows:

HOSPITAL		CK	CK-MB	CK-MB INDEX
Day	Time	(40–200 IU/L)	(0–5.9 ng/mL)	(0–1.9%)
1	0148	722	54.8	7.6
	1031	1694	145.7	8.6
	1836	1428	88.5	6.2
2	0710	276	9.7	3.5

Question: How should Goerge S.' findings and laboratory values be interpreted?

Discussion: This patient represents a classic case of inferior wall AMI. His symptoms and ECG changes represent inferior wall location and are consistent with AMI. In addition, his initial ECG showed that he was in 3° AV block with bradycardia (about 30 beats/min), as is commonly seen with inferior AMI.

George S. received a thrombolytic agent, resulting in rapid reperfusion of his occluded artery. As a result, his CK enzymes peaked earlier than usual (within 12 hr of symptom onset) and returned to normal more rapidly (by about 24–30 hr compared to 2–3 days).

In addition to these factors, the leukocytosis was consistent with AMI. George S.' aPTT and PT were elevated because he received the thrombolytic and was on heparin. His AST was probably elevated because of chronic alcohol ingestion. Despite thrombolytic therapy, he experienced significant myocardial injury, as reflected by the enzyme rise and Q waves on his ECG 1 day after his AMI.

---

with exercise. Since myocardial uptake of thallium-201 is directly proportional to coronary blood flow, administration of the above pharmacologic agents causes relatively less thallium-201 uptake in myocardial areas supplied by stenotic arteries. Therefore, a greater difference is seen between tissue supplied by normal arteries and tissue supplied by stenotic arteries.

Computed Tomography

Computed tomography (CT) involves an intense, focused electron beam that is swept along target rings by electromagnets. When the electron beam strikes the target ring, a fan of x-rays is produced and moves around the patient. CT of the heart is limited by cardiac motion, which may be overcome by gating of the CT scan with a simultaneous ECG recording. Alternatively, Ultrafast CT (cine-CT) allows scanning in real time without gating. The main advantage of CT is enhanced resolution and special definition of structures.

CT scanning is useful in the diagnosis and assessment of aortic disease (e.g., dissection or aneurysm) and pericardial effusions. It is not a primary diagnostic procedure for cardiac diseases and has a limited role in the evaluation of patients with ischemic heart disease and ACS.

Magnetic Resonance Imaging

Magnetic resonance imaging (MRI) is a noninvasive imaging technique capable of detailed tissue characterization and blood flow measurements. The procedure involves placing patients in a device generating a powerful magnetic field and aligning the protons of the body's hydrogen atoms relative to the magnetic field. Radio waves pulsed through the field force the protons to shift their orientation. When the radio waves stop, the protons return to their previous orientation, releasing energy in the form of radio waves. The waves are detected by a scanner and converted into images. The images are physiologically gated to an ECG.

During the procedure, the patients are required to remain motionless. Claustrophobic patients may not be able to undergo the procedure. Sedation may be necessary. In addition, patients with metal prostheses (e.g., pacemakers and ferromagnetic intracerebral clips) should not undergo MRI.

Clinical uses of cardiac MRI include assessment of congenital, aortic, and pericardial diseases, tumors, and intravascular thrombus. MRI is only available at some medical centers because of the cost, scan time, and need for specialized equipment and personnel.

Positron Emission Tomography

Positron emission tomography (PET) is a nuclear imaging technique capable of measuring myocardial blood flow and cellular metabolism of substrates such as fatty acids, glucose, and oxygen in vivo. PET uses the properties of short-lived, positron-emitting, isotope-labeled compounds (nitrogen-13, oxygen-15, carbon-11, or fluorine-18) coupled with mathematical models of physiological function. Its most relevant clinical use for cardiovascular evaluation is detection of ischemic, but viable (or *hibernating*) myocardium that appears irreversibly necrotic by other diagnostic tests.

Blood Pool Imaging

Blood pool scintigraphy is used to evaluate ventricular wall motion and function as well as left ventricular volume. Human serum albumin or the patient's red blood cells are tagged with Tc-99m and injected IV into the patient. A scintillation camera records the radioisotope as it passes through the ventricle. Imaging can be gated or linked with a simultaneous ECG recording. Multiple images are taken and are combined to produce a cine film permitting the evaluation of ventricular chamber size, wall motion, filling defects, and ventricular ejection fraction.

SUMMARY

The heart is a muscular pump that circulates blood to the lungs for oxygenation and throughout the vascular system to supply oxygen and nutrients to every cell in the body. Many diseases affect the heart's function including ACS.

The classic laboratory workup for ACS includes the measurement of serum cTnI or cTnT, and/or CK-MB, a more specific isoenzymes of CK. Other biochemical markers such as myoglobin and CK-MB isoforms may be used. Classic ECG changes such as T-wave inversion, ST-segment elevation, and Q-wave appearance may also be present and useful in characterizing AMI. In addition to confirming an equivocal diagnosis, imaging techniques may localize and estimate the size of myocardial infarctions. After an AMI, LVEF may be determined for prognostic information.

The clinician must have knowledge of the methods used to diagnose and assess AMI and its complications. These determinations have a significant impact on decisions regarding medical, percutaneous intervention, or surgical management of the patient with ACS.

REFERENCES

1. Braunwald E. Unstable angina: an etiologic approach to management (editorial). *Circulation*. 1998; 98:2219–22.

2. World Health Organization. Nomenclature and criteria for diagnosis of ischemic heart disease. Report of the Joint International Society and Federation of Cardiology/World Health Organization task force on standardization of clinical nomenclature. *Circulation*. 1979; 59(3):607–9.

3. The Joint European Society of Cardiology/American College of Cardiology Committee: Myocardial infarction redefined: a consensus document of the Joint European Society of Cardiology/American College of Cardiology Committee for the redefinition of myocardial infarction. *J Am Coll Cardiol*. 2000; 36(3):959–69.

4. Adams JE III, Abendschein DR, Jaffe AS. Biochemical markers of myocardial injury: is MB creatine kinase the choice for the 1990s? *Circulation*. 1993; 88(2):750–63.

5. Wu AH, Apple FS, Gibler WB, et al. National Academy of Clinical Biochemistry Standards of Laboratory Practice: recommendations for the use of cardiac markers in coronary artery diseases. *Clin Chem*. 1999; 45:1104–21.

6. Braunwald E, Antman EM, Beasley JW, et al. ACC/AHA guidelines for the management of patients with unstable angina and non–ST-segment elevation myocardial infarction: a report of the American College of Cardiology/American Heart Association Task Force on Practice Guidelines (Committee on the Management of Patients With Unstable Angina). *J Am Coll Cardiol*. 2000; 36:970–1062.

7. Adams JE III, Bodor GS, Davila-Roman VG, et al. Cardiac troponin I: A marker with high specificity for cardiac injury. *Circulation*. 1993; 88:101–6.

8. Apple FS. Tissue specificity of cardiac troponin I, cardiac troponin T and creatine kinase-MB. *Clin Chim Acta*. 1999; 284:151–9.

9. Mair J, Morandell D, Genser N, et al. Equivalent early sensitivities of myoglobin, creatine kinase MB mass, creatine kinase isoform ratios, and cardiac troponins I and T for acute myocardial infarction. *Clin Chem*. 1995; 41:1266–72.

10. Antman EM. Decision making with cardiac troponin tests. *N Engl J Med*. 2002; 346 (26):2079–82.

11. Muller-Bardorff M, Hallermayer K, Schroder A, et al. Improved troponin T ELISA specific for cardiac troponin T isoform: assay development and analytical and clinical validation. *Clin Chem*. 1997; 43(3):458–66.

12. Hallermayer K, Klenner D, Vogel R. Use of recombinant human cardiac troponin T for standardization of third generation troponin T methods. *Scand J Clin Lab Invest Suppl*. 1999; 230:128–31.

13. Christenson RH, Duh SH, Apple FS, et al. Standardization of cardiac troponin I assays: round Robin of ten candidate reference materials. *Clin Chem*. 2001; 47(3):431–7.

14. Wu AH, Feng YJ, Moore R, et al. American Association for Clinical Chemistry Subcommittee on cTnI Standardization. Characterization of cardiac troponin subunit release into serum after acute myocardial infarction and comparison of assays for troponin T and I. *Clin Chem*. 1998; 44(6):1198–208.

15. Apple FS, Maturen AJ, Mullins RE, et al. Multicenter clinical and analytical evaluation of the AxSYM troponin-I immunoassay to assist in the diagnosis of myocardial infarction. *Clin Chem*. 1999; 45:206–12.

16. Laurino JP. Troponin I: an update on clinical utility and method standardization. *Ann Clin Lab Sci*. 2000; 30(4):412–21.

17. Venge P, Lagerqvist B, Diderholm E, et al. Clinical performance of three cardiac troponin assays in patients with unstable coronary artery disease (a FRISC II substudy). *Am J Cardiol*. 2002; 89(9):1035–41.

18. Hamm CW, Goldmann BU, Heeschen C, et al. Emergency room triage of patients with acute chest pain by means of rapid testing of cardiac troponin T or troponin I. *N Engl J Med*. 1997; 337:1648–53.

19. Antman EM, Tanasijevic MJ, Thompson B, et al. Cardiac-specific troponin I levels to predict the risk of mortality in patients with acute coronary syndromes. *N Engl J Med*. 1996; 335:1342–9.

20. Ohman EM, Armstrong PW, Christenson RH, et al. Cardiac troponin T levels for risk stratification in acute myocardial ischemia. GUSTO IIA Investigators. *N Engl J Med*. 1996; 335:1333–41.

21. Hamm CW, Braunwald E. A classification of unstable angina revisited. *Circulation*. 2000; 102:118–22.

22. Watnick S, Perazella MA. Cardiac troponins: utility in renal insufficiency and end-stage renal disease. *Semin Dial*. 2002; 15(1):66–70.

23. Aviles RJ, Askari AT, Lindahl, et al. Troponin T levels in patients with acute coronary syndromes, with or without renal dysfunction. *N Engl J Med*. 2002; 346:2047–52.

24. Fuchs S, Gruberg L, Singh S, et al. Prognostic value of cardiac troponin I re-elevation following percutaneous coronary intervention in high-risk patients with acute coronary syndromes. *Am J Cardiol*. 2001; 88(2):129–33.

25. Gruberg L, Fuchs S, Waksman R, et al. Prognostic value of cardiac troponin I elevation after percutaneous coronary intervention in patients with chronic renal insufficiency: a 12-month outcome analysis. *Catheter Cardiovasc Interv*. 2002; 55(2):174–9.

26. Tsung SH. Several conditions causing elevation of serum CK-MB and CK-BB. *AM J Clin Pathol*. 1981; 75:711–5.

27. Puleo PR, Meyer D, Wathen C, et al. Use of a rapid assay of subforms of creatine kinase-MB to diagnose or rule out acute myocardial infarction. *N Engl J Med*. 1994; 331(9):561–6.

28. Zimmerman J, Fromm R, Meyer D, et al. Diagnostic marker cooperative study for the diagnosis of myocardial infarction. *Circulation*. 1999; 99(13):1671–7.

29. Weissler AM. Diagnostic marker cooperative study for the diagnosis of myocardial infarction (letter). *Circulation*. 2000; 102(6):E40.

30. De Lemos JA, Antman EM, Giugliano RP, et al. Very early risk stratification after thrombolytic therapy with a bedside myoglobin assay and the 12-lead electrocardiogram. *Am Heart J*. 2000; 140(3):373–8.

31. Srinivas VS, Cannon CP, Gibson CM, et al. Myoglobin levels at 12 hr identify patients at low risk for 30-day mortality after thrombolysis in acute myocardial infarction: a Thrombolysis in Myocardial Infarction 10B substudy. *Am Heart J.* 2001; 142(1):29–36.

32. Ardissino D, Merlini PA, Gamba G, et al. Thrombin activity and early outcome in unstable angina pectoris. *Circulation.* 1996; 93(9):1634–9.

33. Becker RC, Cannon CP, Bovill EG, et al. Prognostic value of plasma fibrinogen concentration in patients with unstable angina and non-Q-wave myocardial infarction (TIMI IIIB Trial). *Am J Cardiol.* 1996; 78(2):142–7.

34. Morrow DA, Rifai N, Antman EM, et al. C-reactive protein is a potent predictor of mortality independently of and in combination with troponin T in acute coronary syndromes: a TIMI 11A substudy. Thrombolysis in Myocardial Infarction. *J Am Coll Cardiol.* 1998; 31(7):1460–5.

35. Oltrona L, Ardissino D, Merlini PA, et al. C-reactive protein elevation and early outcome in patients with unstable angina pectoris. *Am J Cardiol.* 1997; 80(8):1002–6.

36. Haverkate F, Thompson SG, Pyke SD, et al. Production of C-reactive protein and risk of coronary events in stable and unstable angina. European Concerted Action on Thrombosis and Disabilities Angina Pectoris Study Group. *Lancet.* 1997; 349(9050):462–6.

37. Morrow DA, Rifai N, Antman EM, et al. Serum amyloid A predicts early mortality in acute coronary syndromes: A TIMI 11A substudy. *J Am Coll Cardiol.* 2000; 35(2):358–62.

38. Biasucci LM, Vitelli A, Liuzzo G, et al. Elevated levels of interleukin-6 in unstable angina. *Circulation.* 1996; 94(5):874–7.

39. Soler NG, Frank S. Value of glycosylated hemoglobin measurements after acute myocardial infarction. *JAMA.* 1981; 246(15):1690–3.

40. Husband DJ, Alberti KG, Julian DG. "Stress" hyperglycaemia during acute myocardial infarction: an indicator of pre-existing diabetes? *Lancet.* 1983; 2(8343):179–81.

41. Morris F, Brady WJ. ABC of clinical electrocardiography: acute myocardial infarction-Part I. *BMJ.* 2002; 324:831–4.

42. Popp RL. Echocardiography (second of two parts). *N Engl J Med.* 1990; 323(3):165–72.

43. ACC/AHA guidelines for percutaneous coronary intervention (revision of the 1993 PTCA guidelines). A report of the American College of Cardiology/American Heart Association Task Force on Practice Guidelines (Committee to Revise the 1993 Guidelines for Percutaneous Transluminal Coronary Angioplasty). *J Am Coll Cardiol.* June 2001; 37(8):2239i-lxvi.

quickview – troponins I and T

PARAMETER	DESCRIPTION	COMMENTS
Common reference ranges	Troponin I: <1.5 ng/mL Troponin T: <0.1 ng/mL	Assay dependent
Critical value	Troponin I: >1.5 ng/mL Troponin T: >0.1 ng/mL	Assay dependent
Natural substance?	Yes	Regulatory proteins found in muscle cells
Inherent activity?	Yes	Regulates calcium-medicated interaction of actin and myosin
Location	Cardiac and skeletal muscle	Cardiac troponins I and T and skeletal muscle troponins I and T have different amino acid sequences
Major causes of... High results	Myocardial infarction Unstable angina	
Associated signs and symptoms	Chest pain, nausea, vomiting, diaphoresis	Decreased or increased heart rate and BP, anxiety, and confusion, depending on AMI size, location, and duration
Low results	Normal finding	No lower limit for normal
Associated signs and symptoms	None	Does not cause signs and symptoms
After AMI, time to... Initial elevation or positive result	4 hr	Time course studies of release needed
Peak values	12 hr–2 days	
Normalization	5–14 days	
Drugs often monitored with test	None	
Causes of spurious results	Table 11-2	

quickview – CK

PARAMETER	DESCRIPTION	COMMENTS
Common reference ranges Adults Pediatrics	Males: 40–200 IU/L Females: 35–150 IU/L >6 weeks = adult value	Females have lower values due to smaller muscle mass
Critical value	150–200 IU/L without signs and symptoms warrants further evaluation	At >70 IU/L, some laboratories automatically test for CK-MB
Natural substance?	Yes	Muscle enzyme
Inherent activity?	Yes	Catalyzes transfer of high-energy phosphate groups
Location Production	Skeletal and cardiac muscle and brain	
Storage	Not stored as such	
Secretion/excretion	Excreted via glomerular filtration	Elimination may decrease in renal failure
Major causes of... High results	Myocardial infarction	Table 11-4

Continued

Continued

PARAMETER	DESCRIPTION	COMMENTS
Associated signs and symptoms	AMI: chest pain, nausea, vomiting diaphoresis	Decreased or increased heart rate and BP, anxiety, and confusion, depending on AMI size, location, and duration
	Signs and symptoms of underlying disorder	High CK does not cause signs and symptoms directly
Low results	Abnormally low muscle mass	Cachexia and neuromuscular disease
Associated signs and symptoms	Causes of abnormally low muscle mass	Does not cause signs and symptoms directly
After AMI, time to... **Initial elevation**	6–8 hr	Sooner with non-Q-wave myocardial infarction or early use of thrombolytic agent
Peak values	24 hr	Sooner with non-Q-wave myocardial infarction or early use of thrombolytic agent
Normalization	3–4 days	Sooner with non-Q-wave myocardial infarction or early use of thrombolytic agent
Drugs often monitored with test	None	
Causes of spurious results	Table 11-4	Assay dependent

PARAMETER	DESCRIPTION	COMMENTS
Common reference ranges **Adults**	<12 IU/L <3–6% of total CK 0–5.9 ng/mL	Assay dependent
Critical value	≥12 IU/L >6% of total CK >5.9 ng/mL	Assay dependent
Natural substance?	Yes	Muscle enzyme
Inherent activity?	Yes	Catalyzes transfer of high-energy phosphate groups
Location **Production**	Primarily cardiac muscle	Release from traumatized skeletal muscle can be incorrectly interpreted as cardiac
Storage	Small amounts in skeletal muscle	
Secretion/excretion	Excreted via glomerular filtration	Eliminated at slightly faster rate than total CK
Major causes of... **High results**	Myocardial infarction	Table 11-5
Associated signs and symptoms	AMI: chest pain, nausea, vomiting diaphoresis	Decreased or increased heart rate and BP, anxiety, and confusion, dpending on AMI size, location, and duration
Low results	Not significant	No lower limit for normal
Associated signs and symptoms	None	Does not cause signs and symptoms

Continued

PARAMETER	DESCRIPTION	COMMENTS
After AMI, time to...		
Initial elevation	3–12 hr	Sooner with non-Q-wave myocardial infarction or early use of thrombolytic agent
Peak values	12–20 hr	Sooner with non-Q-wave myocardial infarction or early use of thrombolytic agent
Normalization	2–3 days	Sooner with non-Q-wave myocardial infarction or early use of thrombolytic agent
Drugs often monitored with test	None	
Causes of spurious results	Table 11-5	Assay dependent

PARAMETER	DESCRIPTION	COMMENTS
Common reference ranges		
Adults	0.5–1 U/L	CK-MB$_2$ and CK-MB$_1$ in equilibrium
Critical value	CK-MB$_2$:≥1 U/L CK-MB$_2$:CK-MB$_1$ ratio:≥1.5	CK-MB$_2$ and ratio increase soon after AMI until new equilibrium reached
Natural substance?	Yes	CK-MB$_2$ found in myocardial cells CK-MB$_1$ formed from CK-MB$_2$ in plasma after in vivo loss of terminal lysine
Inherent activity?	CK-MB$_2$: yes CK-MB$_1$: unknown	Catalyzes final step of glycolysis
Location		
Production	Heart and skeletal muscle	
Storage	Not stored	
Secretion/excretion	Excreted via glomerular filtration	
Major causes of...		
High results	AMI	Table 11-5
Associated signs and symptoms	Chest pain, nausea, vomiting, diaphoresis	Decreased or increased heart rate and BP, anxiety, and confusion, depending on AMI size, location, and duration
Low results	Normal finding	No lower limit for normal
Associated signs and symptoms	None	Does not cause signs and symptoms
After AMI, time to...		
Initial elevation	2–4 hr	Sooner with non-Q-wave myocardial infarction as early use of thrombolytic agent
Peak values	6–8 hr	Sooner with non-Q-wave myocardial infarction or early use of thrombolytic agent
Normalization	10–14 days	Sooner with non-Q-wave myocardial infarction or early use of thrombolytic agent
Drugs often monitored with test	None	
Causes of spurious results	False-positive elevations likely in muscular dystrophy Severe skeletal muscle damage	Table 11-5

Chapter **12**

LIVER AND GASTROENTEROLOGY TESTS

Joshua Farkas, Paul Farkas, and Douglas Hyde

Hepatic and other gastrointestinal (GI) diseases are fascinating areas of human physiology and medicine, and several major medical advances have recently occurred in this field. This chapter covers the common liver function studies and their relationship to various hepatic and nonhepatic problems. The tests are divided into those associated with (1) general liver function, (2) cholestasis, (3) hepatocellular injury, (4) bilirubin metabolism, (5) ammonia, (6) viral hepatitis, and other liver diseases.

This classification is not exact because many interclass relationships exist. In addition, except for serological tests for hepatitis, these tests are often nonspecific; accurate diagnosis of liver disease is possible only with a complete history and physical examination. Furthermore, diagnosis usually requires additional radiographic testing or, ultimately, a biopsy of the liver.

This chapter also describes several nonhepatic tests such as assays for the causative agent of most peptic ulcer disease, tests for pseudomembranous colitis, and tests used to diagnose and assess pancreatitis.

OBJECTIVES

After completing this chapter, the reader should be able to

1. Discuss how the anatomy and physiology of the liver and pancreas affect interpretation of pertinent laboratory test results.
2. Discuss and interpret tests associated with the liver's synthetic ability.
3. Compare and contrast tests that facilitate assessment of cholestatic and hepatocellular diseases.
4. Explain how hepatic and other diseases, as well as drugs and analytical interferences, cause abnormal laboratory test results for bilirubin.
5. List diseases that may alter laboratory test results for ammonia.
6. Given a case study, describe important patterns of results from multiple tests used in diagnosing and monitoring hepatobiliary disorders.
7. Discuss temporal relationships of the appearance and magnitude of hepatitis markers.
8. Discuss the role of *Helicobacter pylori* in peptic ulcer disease and the tests used to diagnose it.
9. Discuss tests and procedures that are used to evaluate pseudomembranous and similar forms of colitis.
10. Given a case study, interpret laboratory test results for assessing the pancreas.

ANATOMY AND PHYSIOLOGY OF LIVER AND PANCREAS

Liver

The liver is the largest solid organ in the human body. Weighing between 1200 and 1500 g, it is located in the right upper quadrant of the abdomen.[1] The liver has two sources of blood supply:

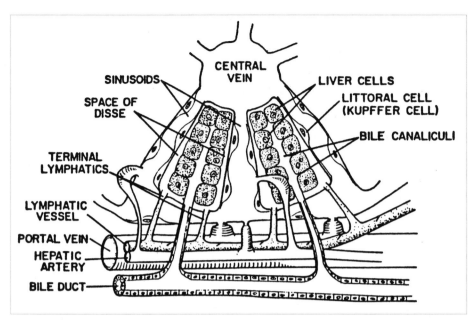

Figure 12-1. Basic structure of a liver lobule including the lymph flow system comprised of the spaces of Disse and interlobular lymphatics. (Reproduced, with permission, from Guyton AC. *Medical Physiology.* 5th ed. Philadelphia, PA: W. B. Saunders; 1976.)

1. The hepatic artery, originating from the aorta, supplies arterial blood rich in oxygen.
2. Portal veins shunt the venous out flow of the intestines and spleen, blood with less oxygen but rich in nutrients, to the liver.

The liver is divided into thousands of lobules (Figure 12-1). Each lobule is comprised of plates of hepatocytes (liver cells) that radiate from the central vein much like spokes in a wheel. Between the plates of liver cells are small bile canaliculi. The hepatocytes continually form and secrete bile into these canaliculi, which empty into terminal bile ducts. Subsequently, like tiny streams forming a river, these bile ducts empty into larger and larger ducts until they ultimately merge into the common duct. Bile then drains into either the gallbladder or the duodenum.

The liver is an extremely complex organ with many functions.[1] It produces bilirubin, a product of hemoglobin (Hgb) breakdown. Bilirubin is excreted via the bile ducts into the intestinal tract, where it plays a crucial role in digestion. Salts of bilirubin aid in making ingested fats more soluble to facilitate their absorption. The liver also plays a major role in amino acid and carbohydrate metabolism. It produces many crucial proteins including coagulation factors and albumin. The liver breaks down some amino acids to yield urea, which is then excreted by the kidneys.

Most lipid and lipoprotein metabolism, including cholesterol synthesis, occurs in the liver. Hepatocytes synthesize cholesterol, which is then excreted into the bile. Therefore, cholesterol may be high in patients with cholestatic disorders and low in patients with cirrhosis or liver failure.

The liver is the primary location for most drug and hormone metabolism including barbiturates, certain tranquilizers, sex hormones, histamine$_2$-blockers, and many narcotics. Thus, in patients with liver failure, standard dosing of some medications can lead to dangerously high serum concentrations and toxicity.

With its double blood supply, large size, and critical role in regulating body metabolic pathways, the liver is affected by many systemic diseases. Although numerous illnesses affect the liver, it has a tremendous reserve capacity and can often maintain its function in spite of significant disease. Furthermore, the liver is one of the few human organs capable of regeneration.

Pancreas

The pancreas is an elongated gland located in the retroperitoneum. Its head lies in close proximity to the duodenum, and the pancreatic ducts empty into the duodenum. The pancreas has both exocrine glands, which secrete into the ducts, and endocrine glands, which secrete into the circulation.

A 50-YEAR-OLD WOMAN, J. M., presented to her physician complaining of increasing fatigue and a 20-lb weight loss over the past 4 months. Initial evaluation showed an albumin of 2 g/dL (3.5–5 g/dL) and a PT of 18 sec (10–13 sec). J. M. was referred for evaluation of possible cirrhosis. On further questioning, she denied any history of hepatitis, exposure to hepatotoxins, alcohol use, family history of liver disease, and liver disease.

The patient's physical examination did not suggest liver disease; there was no evidence of ascites, palmar erythema, asterixis, hepatomegaly, splenomegaly, or spider angiomata. It was noted that she had pedal edema. Liver function studies were otherwise normal: alanine aminotransferase (ALT), 12 IU/L (3–30 IU/L); aspartate aminotransferase (AST), 20 IU/L (8–42 IU/L); total bilirubin, 1 mg/dL (0.3–1.0 mg/dL); and alkaline phosphatase (ALP), 56 IU/L.

An IM dose of vitamin K 10 mg corrected the PT (12 sec) within 48 hr. Workup showed that J. M. had malabsorption due to sprue, a disease of the small bowel. With proper dietary management, her symptoms resolved and she gained weight. At a follow up visit 3 weeks later, her albumin concentration was 3.7 g/dL and her edema had resolved.

Question: Why did this patient develop a low albumin and a prolonged PT? What caused her pedal edema?

Discussion: This case demonstrates that while low albumin and a prolonged PT suggest advanced liver disease, other causes need to be considered. Administration of vitamin K promptly corrected J. M.'s PT, suggesting malabsorption of vitamin K. If she had had cirrhosis, her PT would not have corrected with the vitamin K. Similarly, her hypoalbuminemia was not due to her liver's inability to synthesize albumin but to the malabsorptive disorder that was interfering with protein absorption. Therefore, J. M. had a low albumin and elevated PT in the absence of liver disease. Her pedal edema was due to hypoalbuminemia secondary to malabsorption.

The pancreatic exocrine glands produce primarily enzymes or proenzymes (enzymes requiring further breakdown in the duodenum) that aid in digestion. These enzymes include trypsin, chymotrypsin, lipase, and amylase. Insufficient enzyme production (i.e., pancreatic insufficiency) is associated with malabsorption of nutrients, leading to progressive weight loss and severe diarrhea.

The pancreatic endocrine glands produce many hormones including insulin and glucagon. Insufficient insulin production leads to diabetes mellitus. Thus, the pancreas plays an important role in digestion and absorption of food as well as metabolism of sugar. Like the liver, the pancreas has a tremendous reserve capacity; over 90% glandular destruction is required before diabetes or pancreatic insufficiency develops.

Pancreatitis—inflammation of the pancreas—is the most common disease of this gland. Although the clinical presentation is often the same, pancreatitis can have many causes: gallstones, hypercalcemia, hyperlipidemia, medications, alcoholism, trauma, collagen vascular diseases, and penetrating duodenal ulcers.

TESTS OF LIVER SYNTHETIC CAPABILITIES

The term *liver function test* (LFT) is overused. Most so-called LFTs really measure hepatic or biliary inflammation. Hepatic synthetic reserves are such that, even with massive inflammation, the liver may be able to perform its synthetic functions normally.

To determine the actual functional capabilities of the liver, its synthetic products must be measured. The human liver produces albumin, prealbumin, fibrinogen, prothrombin, haptoglobin, transferrin, and other proteins. The two factors most often used to assess liver function are albumin and prothrombin time (PT). Occasionally, total protein and globulin are measured with albumin. Additionally, an elevated ammonia may indicate liver failure, but the value of this test is controversial.

Albumin

Normal range: 3.5–5 g/dL (35–50 g/L)

Albumin, synthesized by the liver, is involved in maintaining plasma osmotic pressure and the binding and transport of numerous hormones, anions, drugs, and fatty acids.[2] The normal serum half-life of albumin is about 20 days,[3] but this time can be shortened in hypermetabolic (catabolic) states.

Albumin reflects the liver's synthetic ability, and, thus, its concentration may remain normal in many liver diseases when liver function is preserved. However, as the liver is progressively damaged and its synthetic capabilities impaired (e.g., patients with severe hepatitis or cirrhosis), the albumin concentration progressively declines. Because of albumin's long half-life, serum albumin measurements are slow to fall after the onset of hepatic dysfunction. Complete cessation of albumin production results in only a 25% decrease in serum concentrations after 8 days.[1] Largely for this reason, levels are usually normal in acute viral hepatitis, drug-related hepatotoxicity, and obstructive jaundice.[4] However, albumin is commonly reduced in patients with chronic liver disorders such as cirrhosis and usually reflects severe liver damage (given that a healthy liver is capable of producing at least twice the basal synthetic rate).[5,6] Low concentrations (<2.5 g/dL) in liver disease are associated with a poor prognosis.

Some nonhepatic causes of hypoalbuminemia include protein malnutrition, malabsorption, protein loss from the kidney or gut (as in nephrotic syndrome or protein-losing enteropathy, respectively), increased volume of distribution (as in ascites or overhydration), pregnancy, burns, trauma, alcohol use, and inflammatory states.[5,7,8,9] Depending on the assay methods used, albumin concentrations may also be lowered in supine patients (≤1.5 g/dL), icteric patients, or patients on penicillin.[1]

Hypoalbuminemia itself is usually not associated with specific symptoms or findings until concentrations become quite low. At very low concentrations (2–2.5 g/dL), patients can develop peripheral edema, ascites, or pulmonary edema. Albumin normally generates osmotic pressure, which holds fluid in the vasculature. Under conditions of low albumin, fluid leaks from the intravascular into the interstitial spaces of subcutaneous tissues or into the body cavities. Finally, low albumin concentrations affect the interpretation of total serum calcium and concentrations of drugs that are highly protein bound (e.g., phenytoin and salicylates; Chapters 6 and 7).

Hyperalbuminemia is seen in patients with marked dehydration (which concentrates their serum), where it is associated with concurrent elevations in blood urea nitrogen (BUN) and hematocrit. Patients taking anabolic steroids may demonstrate truly increased albumin concentrations, but those on heparin or ampicillin may have falsely elevated results with some assays. Hyperalbuminemia does not cause any symptoms or findings.

Prealbumin (Transthyretin)

Normal range: 16–40 mg/dL

Prealbumin is similar to albumin in several respects. It is synthesized primarily by the liver and is involved in the binding and transport of various solutes (thyroxin and retinol). It is decreased in severe liver disease, pregnancy, burns, and protein malnutrition (as may be caused by malabsorption, nephrotic syndrome, protein-losing enteropathy, or malignancy).

However, differences between prealbumin and albumin make these two tests useful in addressing different questions. Prealbumin has a short half-life (2 days, compared to 20 days for albumin) and a smaller body pool than albumin, making it respond more rapidly than albumin.[10] Additionally, prealbumin is more sensitive to protein nutrition than albumin,

A 16-YEAR-OLD, A. S., was found by her pediatrician to be slightly jaundiced during a routine school physical. She denied any history of liver disease, abdominal pain, alcohol use, and abdominal trauma. Lab evaluation showed a moderately elevated bilirubin of 2.3 mg/dL (0.3–1.0 mg/dL) along with ALP and GGTP concentrations of about 4 times normal. Her AST was 23 IU/L (8–42 IU/L).

A. S. denied being on any medications (except for vitamins), taking illicit drugs, and being exposed to toxins. Nothing suggested the possibility of a neoplastic or infectious process (temperature of 98.9 °F [37.2 °C] and white blood cell [WBC] count of 7.5 x 103 cells/mm^3 [4.8–10.8 x 103 cells/mm^3]). Ultrasound of the liver and biliary system was normal, with no evidence of biliary dilation.

The patient's parents then took her to a pediatric hepatologist. After much discussion (and threat of a liver biopsy), A. S. tearfully revealed that she had gone to a local family planning clinic and was using birth control pills.

Question: How might oral contraceptives cause a cholestatic picture? What was the importance of the ultrasound? What is the usual outcome of patients who develop jaundice while taking oral contraceptives?

Discussion: This case demonstrates that oral contraceptives, primarily because of their estrogen content, can cause alterations in cholestatic test results (manifested by an elevated bilirubin, GGTP, and ALP) with relatively normal aminotransferases. The ultrasound helped to distinguish between intra- and extrahepatic cholestasis. The absence of biliary dilation suggested intrahepatic cholestasis. The normal AST suggested that jaundice was not due to hepatitis.

Cholestasis from oral contraceptives is generally benign and reverses promptly when the medication is withdrawn. Patients often omit mentioning their use of birth control pills.

---

due to its high percentage of tryptophan and essential amino acids, and is less affected by liver disease than albumin.[11] Thus, prealbumin is most frequently used to access nutritional status, although its rapid response time may also be useful in evaluating acute liver failure. Finally, prealbumin is not involved in osmoregulation and is not affected by hydration state.

Prealbumin is routinely used to monitor patients receiving parenteral and enteral nutrition as it may reveal malnutrition before other biochemical assays or clinical examination would.[12] Similarly, when malnourished patients are fed, prealbumin concentrations rise before albumin concentrations. Optimal refeeding leads to increases of greater than 1mg/dL/day. After maintenance rates of parenteral nutrition (or therapeutic enteral feedings) are reached, a goal for prealbumin concentrations in malnourished, hospitalized patients might be an increase of at least 3–5 mg/dL/week until 20 mg/dL is achieved. Concentrations of less than 10.7 mg/dL are associated with severe malnutrition; those between 10.7 and 16 mg/dL are associated with moderate malnutrition.

Prealbumin may be increased by renal insufficiency (reduced catabolism) and acute alcohol intoxication (due to leakage from hepatocytes) or decreased by inflammation, major surgery, or zinc deficiency. Levels of prealbumin may be increased in patients on corticosteroids or with hypothyroidism, sex hormone administration, oral contraceptives, and progestational agents. Caution should be employed in interpretation as some authors believe that the number of confounding factors is large enough to render the test unreliable.[13] However, prealbumin is generally regarded as the best biochemical predictor of nutritional status, and its usefulness in detecting malnutrition has been validated and recommended in clinical settings.[14,15]

Globulin

Normal range: 2–3 g/dL or 20–30 g/L

Globulin refers to the total measurement of immunoglobulins in the serum. Immunoglobulins (also referred to as antibodies) are not actually synthesized by the liver but rather by B cell lymphocytes located throughout the body.

There are many causes of low globulin concentrations including immunodeficiency syndromes, protein malnutrition, malabsorption, and protein-losing enteropathy (similar to albumin; see above). Because most globulins are synthesized outside the liver, hepatocellular dysfunction does not lower globulin concentrations unless associated with malabsorption or malnutrition.

Elevation of globulin concentrations is a sign of inflammation and may be present in hepatitis, especially in chronic viral and autoimmune hepatitis. IgM concentrations are often elevated in primary biliary cirrhosis (as discussed further in the section on primary biliary cirrhosis), and alcoholic hepatitis and cirrhosis may be associated with marked elevations in IgA. Additionally, most types of cirrhosis are associated with increases in IgG and IgM due to decreased first-pass metabolism of antigens absorbed from the gut, allowing these antigens to enter the systemic circulation and provoke an immune response. In this manner cirrhosis (which does not necessarily involve inflammation of the liver itself) may lead to elevation of globulin concentrations.

Nonhepatic causes of elevated globulin concentrations include chronic infections, chronic inflammatory states, and some hematologic diseases (most notably multiple myeloma). In these situations, globulin concentrations may increase disproportionately to albumin concentrations. Thus, the albumin/globulin ratio may be elevated to more than 1 (normally about 0.6). For further information on globulins, see Chapters 15 and 16.

Total Protein

Normal range: 5.5–8.3 g/dL or 55–83 g/L

Since albumin and globulin comprise the majority of serum proteins, total protein primarily reflects the sum of these two factors. In practice, total protein and albumin are often measured, and globulin is calculated by subtracting albumin from total protein. Therefore, if albumin is already known, total protein only provides "new" information regarding globulin, and as such is principally useful in diagnoses such as multiple myeloma based on marked changes in globulin levels.[16,17] The value of obtaining a total protein concentration is limited if albumin and globulin results are already known. The conditions and confounders that affect total protein are a combination of those affecting albumin and globulin as discussed above.

Prothrombin Time

Normal range: 10–13 sec; INR = 1–2

The liver is required for the synthesis of a number of clotting factors, most of which require a Vitamin K cofactor for their activation. Therefore, hepatic impairment or vitamin K deficiency may lead to a deficiency in coagulation factors, causing an increase in the prothrombin time (PT; the time required for a certain set of reactions in the extrinsic coagulation cascade to occur). The activated partial thromboplastin time (aPTT), the time required for a different set of reactions in the intrinsic coagulation cascade to occur, also may become prolonged. The PT is measured either in seconds or in terms of an international normalized ratio (INR), which controls for variability between different laboratories. Further information regarding blood coagulation and the INR may be found in Chapter 15.

The prolongation of PT alone is not specific for liver disease. It can be seen in many situations, most of which interfere with the utilization of vitamin K, a cofactor required for the proper posttranslational modification of clotting factors II, VII, IX, and X. Inadequate vitamin K in the diet or fat malabsorption as caused by cholestasis (vitamin K being a fat-soluble vitamin) may cause hypovitaminosis.[4] Tetracyclines may eliminate vitamin K-producing flora in the gut. The anticoagulant agent warfarin interferes directly with vitamin K.

Clinically, the approach to an elevated PT of uncertain etiology is to provide vitamin K (10 mg) parenterally. If the PT is prolonged due to malabsorption, warfarin, perturbed gut flora, or the absence of vitamin K in the diet, the PT usually corrects by at least 30% within 24 hr.[9] If the PT remains prolonged despite parenteral vitamin K, it is considered a sign of extensive liver damage with a poor prognosis (as with hypoalbuminemia)[2] (Figure 12-2). However, other factors may also be responsible for a pro-

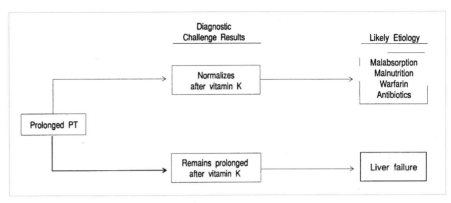

Figure 12-2. Evaluation of a prolonged PT.

longed PT that does not respond to parenteral vitamin K. These include systemic lupus erythematosus (where anticoagulants are in circulation), inherited clotting factor deficiencies, and disseminated intravascular coagulation (DIC, wherein widespread clots deplete clotting factors).

Because clotting factors are produced in excess of need and because the liver has tremendous synthetic reserves, only substantial hepatic impairment (>80% loss of synthetic capability) leads to decreased synthesis of these factors and subsequent clotting abnormalities.[5] Thus, PT lacks sensitivity and may remain normal in the face of substantial liver damage.[2] However, it has considerable prognostic value if liver damage is sufficient to affect it. Unlike albumin (which responds slowly to hepatic insult), PT responds quickly (within 24 hr) to changes in hepatic status due to the short half-life of certain clotting proteins.[18] Thus, the PT may become elevated days before other manifestations of liver failure and, likewise, may normalize prior to other evidence of clinical improvement.[6]

In addition to serving as a liver function test, PT has direct clinical relevance in accessing the patient's tendency to bleed spontaneously, or due to surgical or diagnostic procedures. Bleeding is a dramatic complication of hepatic failure. When the PT is significantly elevated, bleeding may be controlled or at least diminished by fresh frozen plasma, which contains the needed clotting factors and often corrects the PT temporarily.

TESTS TO ASSESS CHOLESTATIC DISEASE AND HEPATOCELLULAR INJURY

Liver diseases tend to fall into two broad categories: cholestatic and hepatocellular. In cholestatic diseases, there is primary interference with the metabolism or secretion of bilirubin anywhere from its initial production in the hepatocytes to its secretion into the duodenum. Therefore, *cholestasis* is defined as the failure of normal amounts of bile to reach the duodenum and implies an obstruction either to bilirubin synthesis or secretion.

In hepatocellular diseases, the hepatocytes are inflamed or damaged. Examples include viral and drug-induced hepatitis. These two categories often overlap, however, and patients with cirrhosis can have elements of both hepatocellular and cholestatic processes.

Cholestatic Liver Disease

Clinically, in cholestatic liver disease, there is an accumulation of substances normally excreted by the liver into the bile. This accumulation can result in jaundice (from bilirubin), pruritus (from bile salts), or xanthomas (from lipid deposits in skin). Weight loss can be caused by anorexia and reduced intestinal absorption (malabsorption) of nutrients (predominantly fat and the fat-soluble vitamins A, D, E, and K), partly due to a lack of bile salts. Other manifestations include (1) osteomalacia secondary to failure to absorb vitamin D and (2) PT elevation due to either intrinsic liver disease or failure to absorb vitamin K.

Cholestatic syndromes may be subclassified as either[19]

- Intrahepatic—the problem is in the liver cells or the bile ducts *within* the liver.
- Extrahepatic—the obstruction is in the major bile ducts *outside* the liver.

Intrahepatic Cholestasis

Intrahepatic cholestasis can be seen in patients with viral hepatitis (especially type A), alcoholic hepatitis, or acquired immunodeficiency syndrome (AIDS). Certain drugs can cause cholestatic jaundice (Table 12-1). Cholestasis also occurs in patients with severe bacterial infections or those receiving parenteral hyperalimentation. Other causes are liver diseases such as primary biliary cirrhosis, sclerosing cholangitis, cholangiocarcinoma, benign recurrent cholestasis, and cholestasis of pregnancy. Cirrhosis also can present with a cholestatic picture.

Extrahepatic Cholestasis

Extrahepatic cholestasis involves obstruction of the large bile ducts outside of the liver, a situation previously only remediable with surgery. Causes include obstruction by strictures (after surgery), stones, or tumors (of pancreas, ampulla of Vater, duodenum, or bile ducts). Another cause is sclerosing cholangitis, a disease causing diffuse inflammation of the bile ducts, often both intrahepatic and extrahepatic. Although previously referred to as "surgical cholestasis," extrahepatic cholestasis can now often be treated (or at least palliated) using endoscopic means (e.g., dilation of strictures).

Tests Associated with Cholestasis

Laboratory tests do not distinguish between intra- and extrahepatic cholestasis. This distinction is usually made clinically (assessment of a history of drug use, hepatitis exposure, etc.) or radiographically. In most instances of extrahepatic cholestasis, a "damming" effect on the bile ducts above the obstruction causes their progressive dilation. This condition can be demonstrated with either computed tomography (CT) scanning or ultrasound. Occasionally, contrast dye is injected into the ducts to demonstrate the dilation and to determine the etiology of the obstruction. This dye can be injected either through the liver, as with a percutaneous cholangiogram, or through the bile ducts, as with an endoscopic retrograde cholangiogram (ERCP).

The laboratory tests most often used to diagnose and monitor cholestatic diseases include alkaline phosphatase (ALP), 5′-nucleotidase, and γ-glutamyl transpeptidase (GGTP or GGT). Other tests that may be abnormally elevated in this situation, but will not be reviewed here, include serum cholesterol (Chapter 14), bile acid levels, leucine aminopeptidase, and hepatic copper levels.

Alkaline Phosphatase (ALP)

Normal range: varies with assay

Alkaline phosphatase (ALP) refers to a group of enzymes whose exact function remains unknown. These enzymes are found in many body tissues including the liver, bone, small intestine, kidneys, placenta, and leukocytes. In adults, most serum ALP comes from the liver and bone (~80%), with the remainder contributed by the small intestine. Different tissues produce slightly different isoenzymes; the liver isoenzyme has a serum half-life of 3 days, while the bone isoenzyme has a half-life of 1–2 days.

Normal ALP concentrations vary primarily with age. In children and adolescents, elevated ALP concentrations result from bone growth, which may result in elevations as high as 3 times normal. Similarly, the increase during late pregnancy is due to placental ALP.[20,21]

TABLE 12-1

SELECTED DRUGS THAT MAY CAUSE INTRAHEPATIC CHOLESTASIS

Amiodarone
Chlorpropamide
Erythromycin
Estrogens
Gold salts
Methyltestosterone
Niacin
Penicillamine
Phenothiazines
Rifampin
Sulfa drugs
Sulindac

Table 12-1. Selected Drugs that May Cause Intrahepatic Cholestasis

In the third trimester, concentrations often double and may remain elevated for 3 weeks postpartum (consistent with placental ALP's half-life of 7 days).[22] In adults younger than 50 years, ALP tends to be higher in males than females, but this difference evens out following menopause (Chapter 1).[6,7]

The mechanism of hepatic ALP release into the serum in patients with cholestatic disease remains unclear. Bile accumulation appears to increase hepatocyte synthesis of ALP, which eventually leaks into the serum.[8,23] ALP concentrations persist until the obstruction is removed and then return to normal within 2–4 weeks.

Clinically, ALP elevation is associated with cholestatic disorders and, as mentioned previously, does not help to distinguish between intra- and extrahepatic disorders. ALP concentrations more than 4 times normal suggest a cholestatic disorder, and 75% of patients with primarily cholestatic disorders have ALP concentrations in this range (Table 12-2). Marked ALP elevations are also typical in any infiltrative process involving the liver including granulomatous diseases, amyloidosis, neoplasia, and abscesses. Concentrations of 3 times normal or less are nonspecific and can occur in all types of liver disease. Even at the highest concentrations seen in the serum, ALP has no toxicological activity, and, thus, reflects tissue damage without *causing* symptoms.

TABLE 12-2

ALP	GGTP	AMINOTRANSFERASES (ALT AND AST)	DIFFERENTIAL DIAGNOSIS
Mildly elevated	Within normal limits	Within normal limits	Pregnancy; nonhepatic causes (Table 12-3)
Moderately elevated[a]	Markedly elevated	Within normal limits or minimally elevated	Cholestatic syndromes
Mildly elevated[b]	Mildly elevated	Markedly elevated	Hepatocellular disease

[a]Usually greater than 4 times normal limits.
[b]Usually less than 4 times normal limits.

Table 12-2. Initial Evaluation of Elevated ALP Concentrations in Context of Other Test Results

When faced with an elevated ALP concentration, a clinician must determine whether it is coming from the liver. One approach is to fractionate the ALP isoenzymes using electrophoresis, but this method is expensive and often unavailable. Thus, the approach usually taken is to measure other indicators of cholestatic disease, 5´-nucleotidase or GGTP. If ALP is elevated, an elevated 5´-nucleotidase or GGTP indicates that at least part of the elevated ALP is of hepatic origin. Alternatively, a normal 5´-nucleotidase or GGTP suggests a nonhepatic cause. However, isolated or disproportionately elevated ALP may occur due to partial bile duct obstruction or infiltrative diseases of the liver.[6]

Nonhepatic causes of elevated ALP include bone disorders (e.g., healing fractures, osteomalacia, Paget's disease, rickets, tumors, hypervitaminosis D, or vitamin D deficiency as caused by celiac sprue), hyperthyroidism, hyperparathyroidism, sepsis, diabetes mellitus, and neoplasias (which may synthesize ALP ectopically, outside tissues that normally contain ALP) (Table 12-3). In children, benign transient hyperphosphatasemia should also be considered.[24] Mild elevations (usually <1.5 times normal) can be seen in normal patients. Some families have inherited elevated concentrations (2–4 times normal), usually as an autosomal dominant trait.[25] Moderate elevations may also result from sec-

TABLE 12-3

BONE DISORDERS	OTHER DISORDERS AND DRUGS
Healing fractures	Acromegaly
Osteomalacia	Anticonvulsant drugs (e.g.,
Paget's disease	phenytoin and phenobarbital)
Rickets	Hyperthyroidism
Tumors	Lithium (bone isoenzymes)
	Neoplasia
	Oral contraceptives
	Sepsis

Table 12-3. Some Nonhepatic Causes of Elevated ALP

ondary liver injury due to congestive heart failure, Hodgkin's disease, myeloid metaplasia, intra-abdominal infections, or osteomyelitis.[6] Markedly elevated concentrations (greater than 4 times normal) are generally seen only in cholestasis, Paget's disease, or infiltrative diseases of the liver. ALP concentrations can be falsely elevated in patients of blood type O or B whose blood is drawn 2–4 hr after a fatty meal due to a rise in intestinal ALP.[26]

ALP concentrations can be lowered by a number of conditions including scurvy, hypothyroidism, milk-alkali syndrome, Wilson's disease with hemolysis, pernicious anemia, zinc or magnesium deficiency, and hypophosphatemia.[8] ALP may also be confounded by a variety of drugs.

5′-Nucleotidase

Normal range: varies

Although 5′-nucleotidase is found in many tissues (including liver, brain, heart, and blood vessels), serum 5′-nucleotidase is elevated only in hepatic diseases. It has a response profile parallel to ALP and similar utility in differentiating between parenchymal and obstructive liver disease. Since it is not elevated in nonhepatic situations where ALP may be elevated—as in bone disorders, bone growth, and pregnancy—it is useful in distinguishing a hepatic origin of elevated ALP. Usually, an elevated ALP with a normal 5′-nucleotidase is not associated with liver disease, although liver disease may occasionally manifest by an elevation of only one of the tests.[27] 5′-nucleotidase may also be increased due to rheumatoid arthritis and certain cancers.[5]

γ-Glutamyl Transpeptidase

Normal range: varies

γ-Glutamyl transpeptidase (GGTP or GGT), a biliary excretory enzyme, can also help determine whether an elevated ALP is of hepatic etiology. Similar to 5′-nucleotidase because GGT has no origin in bone or placenta, it is not elevated in disorders of these tissues. An elevated ALP associated with a normal GGT points to a nonhepatic etiology (Table 12-2). As mentioned previously, ALP concentrations may be normally elevated in pregnant or young patients, especially during growth spurts. An elevated GGT in such patients may reflect underlying hepatobiliary disease.

Generally, GGT parallels ALP and 5′-nucleotidase levels in liver disease. However, GGT concentrations are usually elevated in patients who abuse alcohol or have alcoholic liver disease. Therefore, this test is potentially useful in differential diagnosis with a GGT/ALP ratio greater than 2.5 being highly indicative of alcohol abuse.[28] With abstinence, GGT concentrations often decrease by 50% within 2 weeks.

Although GGT is often regarded as the most sensitive test for cholestatic disorders, unlike 5′-nucleotidase it lacks specificity. In one study of nonselected patients, only 32% of GGT elevations were of hepatic origin.[6] GGT is found in the liver, kidneys, pancreas, spleen, heart, brain, and seminal vesicles. Elevations may occur in pancreatic diseases, myocardial infarction, severe chronic obstructive pulmonary diseases, some renal diseases, SLE, hyperthyroidism, certain cancers, rheumatoid arthritis, and diabetes. GGT may be confounded in patients on a variety of medications, some of which overlap with the medications that confound ALP test results. Thus, elevated GGT (even with concomitant elevated ALP) does not necessarily imply liver injury when 5′-nucleotidase is normal, but rather both elevations in GGT and ALP may be due to a common confounding medication (e.g., phenytoin) or medical conditions (e.g., myocardial infarction).

Hepatocellular Injury

The aminotransferases and lactate dehydrogenase (LDH) are used to assess hepatocellular inflammation or hepatocellular injury (hepatitis). These enzymes are primarily intracellular, where they assist with various metabolic pathways. To the best of our knowledge, they have no true role in the serum, and, thus, are only present at low levels (perhaps related to the normal turnover of cells in the body). These enzymes are released into the serum in greater quantities when there is cell damage. Elevation of aminotransferases suggests damage to hepatocytes. (Similarly, there is no role for ALP or GGTP in the serum; these enzymes are only elevated if there is damage to the biliary tract or to an ongoing cholestatic process.) Although elevations of these enzymes (aminotransferases and LDH) usually lead to a diagnosis of hepatitis, they do not reliably correlate with the degree of inflammation, type of hepatitis, or prognosis. In most forms of hepatic injury, the prognosis is best related to albumin concentrations and PT, which are more direct measurements of hepatic function.

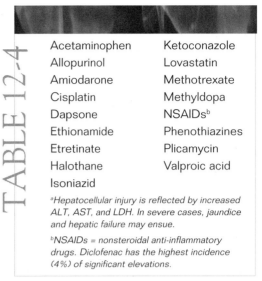

TABLE 12-4	
Acetaminophen	Ketoconazole
Allopurinol	Lovastatin
Amiodarone	Methotrexate
Cisplatin	Methyldopa
Dapsone	NSAIDs[b]
Ethionamide	Phenothiazines
Etretinate	Plicamycin
Halothane	Valproic acid
Isoniazid	

[a]Hepatocellular injury is reflected by increased ALT, AST, and LDH. In severe cases, jaundice and hepatic failure may ensue.

[b]NSAIDs = nonsteroidal anti-inflammatory drugs. Diclofenac has the highest incidence (4%) of significant elevations.

Table 12-4. Selected Drugs Noted for Causing Hepatocellular Injury[a]

There are multiple causes of hepatitis. One common type is viral hepatitis, which is classified A, B, C, D (delta hepatitis), or E based on the causative virus. These viruses, and the tests for them, are discussed in detail in the Viral Hepatitis section. Other forms of viral hepatitis may be caused by the Epstein-Barr virus or cytomegalovirus.

Hepatitis may also be caused by various medications, and such drug-induced hepatitis can be either acute or chronic.[29] Some drugs commonly implicated in cellular hepatotoxicity are listed in Table 12-4. In addition, elevation of aminotransferases has been reported in patients receiving heparin.[30] ALT is elevated in up to 60% of these patients, with a mean maximal value of 3.6 times the baseline. Virtually, every drug can cause hepatic injury. Moreover, drugs extensively metabolized by the liver are particularly likely to cause these problems. Although numerous drugs may result in aminotransferase elevations, such elevations are usually minor, not associated with any symptoms, transient, and of no clinical consequence.[31]

Some other causes of hepatic inflammation are listed in Table 12-5.

It is often difficult to determine the exact etiology of hepatic inflammation (hepatitis). A careful history—especially for exposure to drugs, alcohol, or toxins—and detailed physical examination are crucial. Additional laboratory studies are usually necessary to distinguish one form of hepatitis from another. Radiological testing or liver biopsy may be indicated.

Aminotransferases and LDH, therefore, serve principally as an indication of hepatic inflammation even though they may be somewhat elevated in patients with cholestatic syndromes (Table 12-2). These tests do not indicate the etiology or severity of the inflammation. Since these enzymes do not have any inherent toxicological activity, they do not cause signs or symptoms; their increased serum concentrations only reflect a prior insult to tissues. Figure 12-3 is an algorithm for the differential diagnosis of suspected hepatitis.

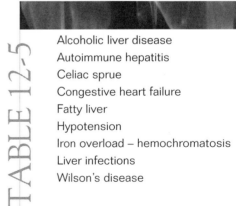

TABLE 12-5
Alcoholic liver disease
Autoimmune hepatitis
Celiac sprue
Congestive heart failure
Fatty liver
Hypotension
Iron overload – hemochromatosis
Liver infections
Wilson's disease

Table 12-5. Some Nondrug Causes of Hepatic Inflammation

Clinical/Laboratory Finding   **Possible Diagnosis**

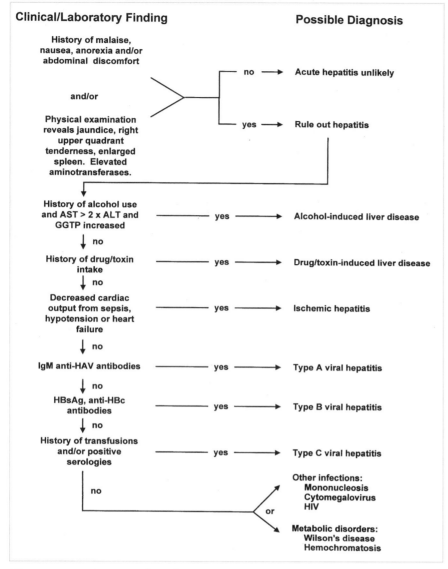

Figure 12-3. Algorithm for differential diagnosis of suspected hepatitis.

Tests Associated with Hepatocellular Injury

Aminotransferases (AST and ALT)

Aspartate aminotransferase (AST), normal range: 8–42 IU/L for adults but varies with assay

Alanine aminotransferase (ALT), normal range: 3–30 IU/L for adults but varies with assay

The aminotransferases, formerly called transaminases, are the most frequently measured indicators of hepatic disease. Both AST and ALT (previously referred to as SGOT and SGPT, respectively) are very sensitive nonspecific indicators of hepatic injury with serum half-lives of 17 and 47 hr, respectively. The enzymes may be released from hepatocytes into the circulation by necrosis or by changes in cell membrane permeability that allow the enzymes to leak out of the cells.[32]

Higher concentrations do not necessarily indicate a greater level of liver damage or a poorer prognosis. For example, in some patients on drugs such as methotrexate, complete hepatic failure can develop despite minimally elevated aminotransferase concentrations, and patients with cirrhosis or chronic HCV may also have normal values.[5] Additionally, a sharp drop in aminotransferase concentrations in fulminant hepatitis may reflect a depletion of viable hepatocytes and poor prognosis.[6] Markedly elevated concentrations (>1000 IU/L) are usually associated with acute viral hepatitis, severe drug or toxic reactions, or ischemic hepatitis. Lower elevations are caused by a greater number of pathologies and are less useful in diagnosis.[33] There are no important causes of depressed ALT or AST, although activities may be suppressed in patients deficient in vitamin B_6 (which is a cofactor for both enzymes).

The ratio of AST to ALT may be of value in diagnosing alcoholic liver disease, where the AST is generally at least twice the ALT and the ALT is rarely above 300 IU/L. In alcoholic liver disease, a mitochondrial isoform of AST with a relatively long half-life (87 hr) is released from hepatocytes, increasing the AST/ALT ratio. Additionally, deficiency of pyridoxine (vitamin B_6), often present in alcoholics, decreases ALT activity more than it decreases AST activity, even though this effect may be masked by certain tests that add pyridoxine in vitro.[7,8]

MINICASE 3

A 36-YEAR-OLD EXECUTIVE, D. D., was referred to a prominent medical center for a second opinion. Her physician had found an elevated AST of 180 IU/L (8–42 IU/L) on a routine screening exam. D. D. had no symptoms; her physical examination had been normal, without any signs of liver disease or hepatomegaly.

Additional studies showed an ALT of 60 IU/L (3–30 IU/L), a markedly elevated GGTP of 380 IU/L (<60 IU/L), and a minimally elevated ALP of 91 IU/L (26–88 IU/L). The patient's WBC count was elevated at 20 x 10³ cells/mm³ (4.8–10.8 x 10³ cells/mm³). After much discussion, she revealed that she was drinking 1 pint of vodka a day.

D. D. then enrolled in Alcoholics Anonymous and stopped drinking. Three months later, all of her tests were normal: ALT, 28 IU/L; GGTP, 54 IU/L; and ALP, 54 IU/L.

Question: What findings suggested alcoholic liver disease? Why did all of D. D.'s numbers return to normal? What else might have happened in this situation?

Discussion: This case demonstrates several aspects of alcoholic liver disease. The diagnosis was suggested by an elevated AST out of proportion to the ALT, as well as by a markedly elevated GGTP with a normal (or virtually so) ALP. An elevated MCV, if present, also would have supported this diagnosis. Patients with alcoholic liver disease may have markedly elevated WBC counts.

Alcoholic liver disease tends to have several different stages. The earliest manifestation may be just a "fatty liver," which is generally reversible with cessation of alcohol intake. Alcoholic hepatitis and cirrhosis can follow with excessive alcohol intake. Unfortunately, alcoholic cirrhosis can develop without any warning signs. If D. D. had alcoholic cirrhosis, stopping alcohol consumption probably would not have significantly altered her abnormal test results.

Clinicians should remember that a patient does not need to be a "skid row" alcoholic to develop alcoholic cirrhosis. Women are more susceptible to the hepatotoxic effects of alcohol than are men, and as few as two or three drinks a day can cause significant liver disease in susceptible persons.

ALT and AST are not solely located in hepatocytes but rather are also found in cardiac muscle, skeletal muscle, kidneys, brain, pancreas, lungs, leukocytes, and erythrocytes. Consequently, they may be elevated due to a variety of conditions including musculoskeletal diseases (e.g., muscular dystrophy, dermatomyostitis, trichinosis, gangrene, and muscle damage secondary to hypothyroidism), intestinal injury, pericarditis, myocardial infarction (although this may act in part via hepatic ischemia), renal infarction or failure, pancreatitis, brain trauma or cerebral infarction, hemolysis, pulmonary embolus, necrotic tumors, burns, and celiac sprue.[5–7] ALT is more localized to the liver than AST, so it is more specific to liver injury. Elevation of AST without concomitant of elevated ALT suggests cardiac or muscle disease.[18] A muscular origin of aminotransferases may also be indicated by increases in aminotransferases below 300 IU/L with concomitant increases in serum creatine kinase (CPK) activity or aldolase activity.[26,34] While elevated aminotransferases are generally associated with hepatocellular disease, they may be significantly elevated (although transiently) in some cholestatic syndromes, and they may rise into the thousands within 24–48 hr following common bile duct obstruction, after which they decline rapidly.

Measurement of AST may be affected by a bewildering variety of medications. Almost any prescription drug (as well as various herbal compounds and illegal drugs) can cause an elevation of aminotransferases.[26] Furthermore, the in vitro assay may be confounded by a variety of factors including in vivo uremia, calcium dust in the air (caused by construction), hyperlipidemia, and hemolysis.[35] False elevations in the in vitro test may be also seen in patients on acetaminophen, levodopa, methyldopa, tolbutamide, p-aminosalycylic acid, erythromycin, or in patients with diabetic ketoacidosis when the automated chemistry profile SMA 12/60 is used.[8,36,37]

Other factors may interfere with the test's accuracy. Serum concentrations of aminotransferases follow a diurnal pattern, varying 10–15% of the daily mean with a maximum around 4 p.m. and a minimum around 8 a.m.[38] Furthermore, levels may be elevated to 2–3 times normal by vigorous exercise in males and decreased to about half following dialysis.[7] Complexing of AST with immunoglobulin (known as *macro-AST*) may occasionally produce a clinically irrelevant elevation of AST. Additionally, unexplained false positives often occur. In healthy individuals, an isolated elevated ALT returns to normal in repeat studies one-half to one-third of the time.[39] For this reason, prior to a workup for mildly elevated aminotransferases, a practitioner should see either elevation of more than one test (i.e., both AST and ALT) or repeated elevations of a single test.

Lactate Dehydrogenase

Normal range: 100–225 IU/L for adults but varies with assay

Lactate dehydrogenase (LDH) is found in most human tissues but primarily in myocardium, liver, skeletal muscle, brain, lung, kidneys, and red blood cells (RBCs). An elevated LDH can be seen in a patient with myocardial infarction (Chapter 10), myocarditis, cardiac failure, hemolysis (including in vitro) or reabsorption of extravasated blood, renal disease or infarction, certain anemias, malignancy, muscle disease, burns, hypothyroidism, trauma, or pulmonary embolus. Therefore, an elevated LDH is not a very specific finding. Fortunately, however, LDH has five isoenzymes, one of which (type 5 or LDH_5) corresponds with liver disease although it may also be increased in muscle disease (Table 12-6).

TABLE 12-6

ISOENZYME	TISSUE WITH INCREASED AMOUNT OF ENZYME[a]	TYPICAL PERCENTAGE OF TOTAL LDH IN ADULT	TYPICAL REFERENCE RANGE (IU/L)
LDH^1	Heart, brain, RBCs	33	22–85
LDH^2	Heart, brain, RBCs	45	30–100
LDH^3	Brain, kidneys, lungs	18	15–65
LDH^4	Liver, muscle, kidneys	3	5–25
LDH^5	Liver, muscle, ileum	1	2–25

[a] These tissues are richest in the indicated enzymes. However, significant amounts of LDH_1 also are found in the renal cortex; LDF_3 is also found in the lymphocytes, spleen, and pancreas.

Table 12-6. Isoenzymes of LDH

Although LDH_5 is less sensitive to liver disease than the aminotransferases, elevated concentrations occur in patients with hepatitis, biliary obstruction, metastatic liver disease, hepatic ischemia, or exacerbation of cirrhosis. In certain situations, LDH_5 may be elevated when total LDH is normal, and, according to some clinicians, an LDH_5 concentration significantly greater than LDH_4 is suggestive of primary or secondary liver disease. LDH may be useful in diagnosing ischemia (characterized by a massive, transient increase) or malignancy (characterized by a sustained elevation).[6] The ratio of ALT to LDH may also be useful in indicating pancreatic necrosis in biliary pancreatitis and differentiating between acute viral hepatitis (>1.5) and shock liver (acute ischemic hepatitis) and acetaminophen toxicity (<1.5).[39,40]

One advantage of LDH compared to aminotransferases is that it is affected by fewer medications. There are no important causes of a truly low LDH. (LDH is discussed from the cardiac perspective in Chapter 11.)

BILIRUBIN METABOLISM

After reaching senescence, RBCs are taken up and destroyed primarily in the spleen. The hemoglobin released from these cells is ultimately broken down to bilirubin. This conversion occurs primarily at the site of RBC destruction and yields unconjugated (water insoluble) bilirubin. Unconjugated bilirubin is also produced by premature destruction of erythroid cells in the bone marrow and turnover of hemoproteins throughout the body.[6] This unconjugated bilirubin is bound to albumin while being transported to the liver. Unconjugated bilirubin is taken up by the liver and covalently conjugated with glucuronic acid by the enzyme glucorynyl transferase, rendering it water soluble.

Conjugated (water soluble) bilirubin is excreted into the bile and, ultimately, the gut. There it is broken down to urobilinogen, some of which is reabsorbed in the terminal ileum and excreted by the kidneys or excreted again by the liver into the gut. The remaining bilirubin, urobilinogen, and various other breakdown products are excreted in the feces (some of these metabolites are responsible for coloring feces brown). With liver damage, urinary urobilinogen may increase; with obstruction, it is usually absent or reduced.[41]

Total Bilirubin

Normal range: 0.3–1 mg/dL or 5–17 μmol/L but varies with assay and age

Total bilirubin refers to the sum of conjugated and unconjugated bilirubin. Conjugated bilirubin reacts quickly in the van den Bergh reaction due to its solubility and, thus, is occasionally called "direct-reacting" or "direct" bilirubin; alternatively, unconjugated bilirubin requires the presence of dissolving agents and is called "indirect-reacting" or "indirect" bilirubin.

Although it is still widely used, the van den Bergh method does not accurately reflect the true values of direct and indirect bilirubin, especially at low total serum bilirubin concentrations. It tends to overestimate the conjugated (a.k.a., soluble or direct) bilirubin. More accurate assessment requires liquid chromatography, which reveals that almost 100% of serum bilirubin is unconjugated in normal individuals. This makes sense because unconjugated bilirubin represents bilirubin in transit to the liver; conjugated bilirubin is normally excreted from hepatocytes into the bile and does not enter the blood.

The hallmark of hyperbilirubinemia is a yellowish skin color (a.k.a., jaundice or icterus). Quinine derivatives (e.g., quinacrine) and carotenes can cause a similar skin discoloration. With excess carotenes the sclerae of the eyes remain their normal color, while in jaundice the sclerae turn yellow. Jaundice usually becomes visible when the total bilirubin concentration is 2–4 mg/dL. Low concentrations are often missed in clinical settings with artificial light because they are best observed in natural light.

In infants, elevated concentrations of unconjugated bilirubin (often >20 mg/dL) can lead to bilirubin encephalopathy or kernicterus. Kernicterus can present as lethargy and low-grade fevers and can progress to spasticity, seizures, and death, if untreated. Survivors may develop mental retardation and spastic paraplegia. In adults, bilirubin has considerably less toxicity, although in certain cases it may cause encephalopathy.[42]

An elevated total serum bilirubin concentration is not a sensitive indicator of hepatic dysfunction or prognosis. Furthermore, an elevated bilirubin can be seen in conditions other than liver disease (e.g., hemolysis and ineffective RBC production). In vitro elevation or depression can also occur due to a variety of drugs. Finally, if specimens are exposed to bright light, bilirubin may degrade by as much as 30%/hr.[37]

Unconjugated (Insoluble) Hyperbilirubinemia

Normal range: 0.2–0.7 mg/dL or 3.4–12 μmol/L

Based on the pathways of biliary metabolism, unconjugated hyperbilirubinemia is expected to result from increased production of bilirubin by extra-hepatic sources or impaired uptake and processing by the liver.[6] Patients with primarily unconjugated hyperbilirubinemia (>70% by the van den Bergh assay) often have no signs or symptoms of liver disease and have normal aminotransferase concentrations. These patients have one of four conditions discussed below or may be experiencing decreased liver uptake due to rifampin or similar drugs.[42]

A 19-YEAR-OLD COLLEGE STUDENT, J. N., anxiously reported to the infirmary when his girlfriend noticed that he was becoming yellow. He felt well and had a normal physical examination. On discussion, he indicated that he had recently embarked on a rigorous crash diet in anticipation of winter break in Florida.

Evaluation showed an elevated total bilirubin of 4.8 mg/dL (0.3–1.0 mg/dL), of which 90% was unconjugated (4.3 mg/dL). The absence of hemolysis was established by microscopic examination of a blood smear, normal reticulocyte count, and LDH, which was 112 IU/L (100–225 IU/L). J. N.'s other LFTs were normal: ALT, 21 IU/L (3–30 IU/L); and ALP, 76 IU/L (21–91 IU/L).

Question: What was the most likely cause of this young man's signs and symptoms? How should his condition be managed? What is his prognosis?

Discussion: Elevated bilirubin concentrations do not necessarily indicate severe liver disease. The normal ALT and ALP ruled out hepatocellular and cholestatic liver diseases. AST, if done, would have been normal. The normal LDH, RBC microscopic exam, and reticulocyte count ruled out hemolysis (Chapter 15) as a cause of the elevated bilirubin. The normal LDH was also consistent with a lack of intrinsic liver disease.

J. N. should be reassured that he has Gilbert's syndrome and might become somewhat jaundiced with fasting or acute or chronic illness. Gilbert's disease is not associated with any symptoms, is totally benign, and requires no treatment. When a patient has an elevated bilirubin, a practitioner should always obtain LFTs before either providing a diagnosis or performing unnecessary tests.

Hemolysis. Increased *hemolysis*, or the destruction of RBCs with release of unconjugated bilirubin, may exceed the liver's ability for conjugation and excretion. Generally, bilirubin is 85% unconjugated in pure hemolysis (by the van den Bergh assay) and rarely exceeds 5 mg/dL.

Increased hemolysis may be due to a variety of conditions including sickle cell disease, spherocytosis, hematomas, or transfusions of old blood.[4] Additionally, a picture similar to hemolysis can be seen in patients with pernicious anemia or other conditions of ineffective erythropoiesis such as myelofibrosis and metastatic replacement of bone marrow (Chapter 14 presents more information on the evaluation of hemolysis.)

Gilbert's syndrome. This syndrome is an inherited, entirely benign trait that may be present in 3–5% of the population. It involves intermittent elevation (increased with fasting, stress, or illness) of unconjugated bilirubin due to mild impairment of conjugation within hepatocytes (rarely >4 mg/dL; Minicase 4).[4]

Crigler-Najjar syndrome. This syndrome is a rare congenital disease, stemming from absent or deficient conjugating enzymes in the liver. Infants with this disease develop a deep jaundice (bilirubin >20 mg/dL) and can suffer brain damage (kernicterus), although some patients with a less severe variant of this syndrome may have few symptoms other than persistent jaundice.

Neonatal jaundice. The onset of jaundice, usually 2–5 days after birth, is common and generally benign and transient. In some instances, neonatal jaundice requires phototherapy to reduce bilirubin concentrations and avoid encephalopathy or kernicterus. The mechanism of neonatal jaundice remains unclear, but it is felt to involve immaturity of the hepatocytes and a relative deficiency of enzymes involved in the uptake and conjugation of bilirubin.

Conjugated (Soluble) Bilirubin

Normal range: 0.1–0.3 mg/dL or 1.7–5 μmol/L by van den Bergh assay; undetectable by liquid chromatography

Conjugated hyperbilirubinemia is defined as greater than 50% of the total bilirubin being conjugated bilirubin, although absolute levels of unconjugated bilirubin may also be elevated.[18] Based on the normal pathways of bilirubin metabolism, increases in serum levels of conjugated bilirubin are expected to occur from obstruction of the biliary tract, with "regurgitation" as the obstructed flow of bile increases pressures at the cellular or canicular levels and results in regurgitation into the serum, or from damaged hepatocytes or bile ducts.[6] Clinically, excretion of excess conjugated bilirubin by the kidneys may cause dark, almost brown urine (as opposed to unconjugated bilirubin, which is bound to albumin, and, thus, not removed by the kidneys). Conjugated bilirubin in the urine can also be detected with a dipstick test, which is more sensitive than measuring conjugated bilirubin via the van den Bergh method (which tends to overestimate conjugated bilirubin).[5] Although rare, congenital disorders can present with primarily conjugated hyperbilirubinemia (Dubin-Johnson and Rotor's syndromes). Conjugated hyperbilirubinemia is generally associated with elevations of other hepatic enzymes and, as such, reflects underlying hepatobiliary disease (Table 12-7).

Conjugated hyperbilirubinemia may result from hepatocellular or cholestatic liver disease. In cholestatic diseases the bilirubin is primarily conjugated, while hepatocellular diseases may cause increases in both conjugated and unconjugated bilirubin. One sign of obstructive jaundice is light colored stools, although this may also occur in hepatocellular diseases.[4,9] Another indication may be the extent of bilirubinemia, which tends to be greater (as high as 25–30 mg/dL) in hepatocellular disease than cholestatic disease since the conjugated bilirubin produced during cholestatic disease is readily excreted in urine.[18] More reliable tests to determine the cause of bilirubinemia include evaluation of the concentrations of ALT, AST, ALP, and GGTP, as described elsewhere in this chapter.

TABLE 12-7

TOTAL BILIRUBIN	DIRECT BILIRUBIN	INDIRECT BILIRUBIN	ALT, AST, GGTP	DIFFERENTIAL DIAGNOSIS
Moderately elevated	Within normal limits or low	Moderately elevated	Within normal limits	Hemolysis,[a] Gilbert's syndrome,[a] Crigler-Najjar syndrome,[b] neonatal jaundice
Moderately elevated	Moderately elevated	Within normal limits	Within normal limits	Cogenital syndromes[c]: Dubin-Johnson[d] Rotor's
Mildly elevated	Mildly elevated	Moderately elevated	Moderately elevated	Liver disease

[a]Usually indirect bilirubin is less than 4 mg/dL but may increase to 18 mg/dL.
[b]Usually indirect bilirubin is greater than 12 mg/dL and may go as high as 45 mg/dL.
[c]These syndromes are distinguished in the laboratory by liver biopsy.
[d]Usually direct bilirubin is 3–10 mg/dL.

Table 12-7. Evaluation of Elevated Bilirubin Concentrations in Context of Other Test Results

AMMONIA

Normal range: 30–70 µg/dL or 17–41 µmol/L but varies with assay

The majority of serum ammonia originates from the large intestine where it is formed by bacterial catabolism of protein (whether from food or blood). Normally, the majority of this ammonia is absorbed by the liver during portal circulation, where it is converted to urea and later excreted by the kidneys. A secondary mode of ammonia excretion involves the production of glutamine by the muscles, brain, and liver, which is deaminated in the kidneys with excretion of ammonia into the urine.

Liver diseases may interfere with the removal of ammonia from the blood. This may be a result of primary hepatocellular disease or portal hypertension (where the blood is shunted around the liver, avoiding first-pass detoxification). Accumulation of ammonia and other toxins due to these disorders may cause a progressive deterioration in mental functioning ranging from subtle personality changes to complete coma. The exact cause of this deterioration, referred to as *hepatic encephalopathy*, remains unclear. It seems to be toxin related because the encephalopathy rapidly clears with improved liver function or following liver transplantation. Ammonia is not the only postulated toxin,[43] and ammonia levels do not correlate well with encephalopathy between patients, indicating that other factors are involved (including poor correlation between serum and CSF ammonia).[5,44]

Nonetheless, ammonia concentrations are commonly used to diagnose hepatic encephalopathy, where they are significantly elevated in 90% of cases.[39] Their greatest value is in the evaluation of the altered mental status of a patient with suspected liver disease. In such patients, a normal concentration may suggest other causes of encephalopathy (e.g., head trauma, drugs, or infection), while an elevated concentration implies hepatic origin. Serial ammonia concentrations may also be used to follow the course of hepatic encephalopathy in a particular patient, although the usefulness of this application is debated. Ammonia concentrations decline with proper therapy for hepatic encephalopathy (e.g., lactulose or neomycin); the concentrations, along with mental status, may be used as a guide to drug therapy.

Serum ammonia concentrations are best measured with arterial blood samples because venous serum concentrations may be falsely elevated by muscular amino acid metabolism, seizures, or prolonged tourniquet placement.[5] Generally, however, venous concentrations are used because they are the easiest to obtain and practitioners hesitate to do arterial sampling in patients who may have an underlying coagulopathy from liver disease. Since blood ammonia increases rapidly at room temperature (due to erythrocyte metabolism), all test specimens must be placed on ice immediately and processed rapidly.

Ammonia concentration may also be elevated in patients with Reye's syndrome, inborn disorders of the urea cycle, rare pediatric metabolic disorders, various medications (most notably valproic acid), impaired renal function, uterosigmoidostomy, or urinary tract infections with bacteria that convert urea to ammonia. In infants receiving large amounts of parenteral nutrition or with erythroblastosis fetalis, ammonia may also be elevated. In cirrhotic patients or patients with mild liver disease, elevated ammonia and hepatic encephalopathy may be precipitated by such factors as increased dietary protein, GI bleeding, constipation, *Helicobacter pylori*, and infections.[7] The test may be falsely elevated following smoking or exercise.

VIRAL HEPATITIS

The onset of acute viral hepatitis may be quite dramatic and present as an overwhelming infection, or it may pass unnoticed by the patient. In the usual prodromal period, the patient has a nonspecific illness that may include nausea, vomiting, fatigue, malaise, or a flu-like syndrome. This period may be followed by clinical hepatitis with jaundice. During this time, the most abnormal laboratory studies are usually the aminotransferases, which can be in the thousands (normally <50 IU/L). Bilirubin may be quite elevated, while ALP only mildly so.

The major types of viral hepatitis are reviewed here, but they are often clinically indistinguishable. Thus, serologic studies of antibodies, molecular assays to detect viral genetic material, and knowledge of the epidemiology and risk factors for different viruses (Table 12-8) are central to diagnosis.

Type A Hepatitis

Hepatitis A virus, spread primarily by fecal-oral route (by contaminated food or water or by person-to-person contact), has an incubation period of 3–5 weeks with a several-day prodrome before the onset of jaundice and malaise. Hepatitis A is responsible for about

TABLE 12-8

HEPATITIS A VIRUS

Contacts with infected persons
Daycare workers and attendees
Institutionalized persons
Unvaccinated international travelers
Military personnel
Male homosexuals
IV drug users

HEPATITIS B VIRUS

Contacts of infected persons
Unvaccinated health care professionals
  and morticians
Hemodialysis patients
Male homosexuals
IV drug users
Multipartner heterosexuals
Tattooed persons
Newborns of HBsAg-carrier mothers

HEPATITIS C VIRUS

Dialysis patients
Health care professionals
IV drug users
Multipartner heterosexuals
Recipients of transfusion or organ
  transplant before July 1992
Tattooed persons
Children born to HCV-positive mothers

HEPATITIS D VIRUS

Health care professionals lacking
  HBV vaccination
Institutionalized persons
IV drug users
Multiply transfused patients

HEPATITIS E VIRUS

Contacts with infected persons
Travelers to Latin America, Egypt, India,
and Pakistan

Table 12-8. Groups at Higher Risk of Infection by Various Hepatitis Viruses

50% of acute hepatitis in the United States (more than all other hepatotrophic viruses combined), generally due to person-to-person contact within community-wide outbreaks.[45,46]

Unlike the B, C, and D hepatitis, the hepatitis A virus (HAV) does not cause chronic disease. Many patients who get type A hepatitis never become clinically ill. Perhaps 10% of all patients become symptomatic, and only 10% of those patients become jaundiced.[47] The majority of patients have a full recovery, but there is a substantial mortality risk in elderly patients, as well as in patients with chronic hepatitis B or C and patients with chronic liver disease of other etiologies.[48,49]

Presently, the only two tests available measure antibodies to the hepatitis A virus, either IgM or all isotypes of antibody. Detection of IgM is the more clinically relevant test as it reveals acute or recent infection. These antibodies are present at the onset of jaundice and decline within 12 (usually 6) months.[49] Total antibody (antibody of all isotypes) against HAV indicates present or previous infection or immunization (Figure 12-4).

Type B Hepatitis

Hepatitis B virus (HBV) is a DNA virus spread by bodily fluids, most commonly via contaminated needles, blood products, sexual intercourse, or vertical transmission (transmission from mother to child, generally at birth). The incubation period of hepatitis B varies from 2–4 months, much longer than that of hepatitis A.

The clinical illness is generally mild and self-limited but can be quite severe. Unfortunately, 10% of infected adults and 90% of infected neonates develop a chronic illness. Chronic HBV is often mild but may progress to cirrhosis, liver failure, or hepatocellular carcinoma, thereby contributing to premature death in 15–25% of cases.[46]

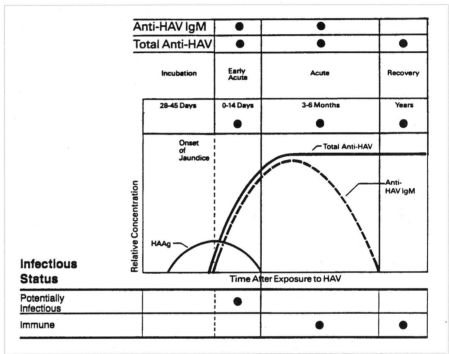

Figure 12-4. Temporal relationships of serologies for hepatitis A with onset of jaundice and infectious status. Anti-HAV IgM is the IgM antibody against the hepatitis A virus. HAAg is the hepatitis A antigen (virus). Total anti-HAV is primarily IgG antibodies (and some IgM in acute phase) against hepatitis A virus. (Adapted, with permission, from educational material of Abbott Laboratories, North Chicago, IL.)

Antigenic Compounds and Their Antibodies

Three HBV antigens are relevant to diagnosis and management. The hepatitis B virus surface antigen (HBsAg) is present on the surface of the virus, and neutralizing antibodies directed against this protein are central to natural and vaccine-induced immunity (Figure 12-5). Neither the core protein (HBcAg) nor the e antigen (HBeAg) are on the surface of the virion, and, thus, antibodies against these antigens are not protective. Nevertheless, antibodies are directed against these proteins and may serve as markers of infection. Of these antigens, only HBsAg and HBeAg can be detected in the serum by conventional techniques.[50] HBsAg is detected for a greater window of time during infection and reveals active infection. Detection of HBeAg indicates large amounts of circulating hepatitis B virus; these patients are 5–10 times more likely to transmit the virus than are HBeAg negative persons.[51]

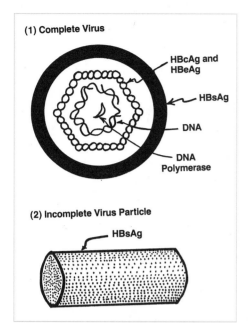

Figure 12-5. Hepatitis B virus and its antigenic components. The complete and infectious virus (1), originally known as the Dane particle, is composed of the outer layer (HBsAg) and inner nucleo-capsid core. The inner core is comprised of HBcAg intermeshed with HBeAg and encapsulates the viral DNA. HBeAg may be an internal component or degradation product of the nucleocapsid core. An incomplete and noninfectious form (2) is composed exclusively of HBsAg and is cylindrical in shape.

In response to infection with HBV, the body produces antibodies to the antigens: antisurface antibody (anti-HBs), anticore antibody (anti-HBc), and anti-e antibody (anti-HBe). All of these antibodies can be detected in clinical laboratories, and in the case of anti-HBcAg separate tests reveal IgM or total antibody (all isotypes). As shown in Figures 12-6 and 12-7, levels of antigens and antibodies show complex patterns in the course of HBV infection, and, thus, can yield considerable information about the infection's course and chronology (Table 12-9).

In addition to serological tests, sensitive molecular assays may be used to detect HBV DNA, revealing active viral replication in either acute or chronic infection.[52] These assays may be useful for early detection, as in screening blood donors, since DNA is detectible an average of 25 days before seroconversion.[46] Additionally, some assays allow the quantification of serum viral load, which may be used in the decision to treat and, subsequently, monitor therapy. For the details of these assays (PCR, RNA:DNA hybrid capture assay, nucleic acid cross-linking assay, and branched DNA assay), the reader is referred to a recent review by Pawlotsky, et al.[53]

Acute Hepatitis B

HBsAg titers usually develop within 4–12 weeks of infection and may be seen even before elevation of aminotransferases or clinical symptoms (see Figure 12-6). Subsequently, HBsAg levels decline as anti-HBs titers develop, which indicates resolution of the acute symptomatic infection and development of immunity. In between the decline of HBsAg and the rise of anti-HBs, there is often a window when neither is present during which time anti-HBcAg may be used to diagnose infection. IgM anti-HBcAg may be used to reveal acute infection as opposed to a flair of chronic HBV.[52]

Chronic Hepatitis B

Chronic hepatitis is defined as persistently elevated LFTs for 6 months. The development of chronic hepatitis B is suggested by the persistence of elevated LFTs (aminotransferases) and is supported by persistence of HBsAg for more than 5 months after acute infection. Persistence of HBeAg also suggests chronic infection, but some chronically infected patients produce anti-HBeAg and, subsequently, clear HBeAg well after the acute phase is over (late seroconversion; see Figure 12-7). Although chronically infected individuals usually lack anti-HBs, in some cases low levels of non-neutralizing antibodies may be present. Additionally, low levels of IgM anti-HBcAg may persist.[48]

Hepatitis B Vaccine

The HBV vaccine consists of recombinant HBsAg, which stimulates the production of protective anti-HBs. Vaccination may be dis-

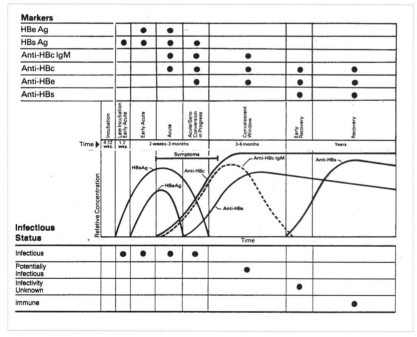

Figure 12-6. Serological profile, including temporal relationships integrated with infectious status and symptoms, in 75–85% of patients with *acute* type B hepatitis. (Adapted, with permission, from educational material of Abbott Laboratories, North Chicago, IL.)

tinguished from previous infection by the absence of antibodies against other antigens (e.g., HBcAg).

Type C Hepatitis

Hepatitis C virus (HCV) is an RNA virus mainly spread parenterally, although it may also be transmitted vertically and sexually. While 70–80% of acute infections are asymptomatic, 70–80% of patients develop chronic disease.[46] Given the mildness of the acute attack and the tendency to develop into chronic hepatitis, it is understandable why many patients with this disease first present with cirrhosis or (more commonly) chronic elevations of aminotransferases.

In chronic hepatitis C, the LFTs are usually minimally elevated with ALT and AST values commonly in the 60–100 IU/L range. These values can fluctuate and occasionally return to normal for a year or more, only to rebound when next checked.[54] The main clinical concern in chronic HCV is that if untreated, within 20 years 20–30% of patients develop cirrhosis and 1–5% develop hepatocellular carcinoma.[46]

The first screening test used is often ELISA (also referred to as anti-HCV), which detects antibodies against a cocktail of HCV antigens. Due to possible cross-reactivity with one of the antigens in the assay, this test has a considerable false-positive rate and, thus, positive results are usually confirmed with a more specific assay. One such assay is the recombinant immunoblot assay (RIBA), which is similar to ELISA in principle but tests antibody reactivity to a panel of antigens individually; binding to two or more antigens is considered a positive test.[48]

Alternatively, qualitative RT-PCR (reverse transcriptase polymerase chain reaction, often referred to as just PCR) to detect viral RNA in the blood is a very sensitive assay that may be used in diagnosis. RT-PCR has several advantages compared to serologic tests. It can detect HCV within 1–2 weeks of exposure and weeks before seroconversion, symptoms, or the elevation of LFTs. This may be useful because seroconversion has only occurred in 70–80% of patients at the onset of symptoms, and it may never occur in immunosuppressed patients.[54] Furthermore, unlike serologic assays, RT-PCR is not confounded by passively acquired antibodies that may be present in uninfected infants, and RT-PCR can distinguish between resolved and chronic infection.

Once a diagnosis of HCV infection is established, various quantitative molecular assays that monitor viral load may be useful in following viral titers during treatment or accessing likelihood of response to therapy. These tests are not preferred for initial diagnosis since they are less sensitive than qualitative RT-PCR. They include a quantitative PCR assay and a branched-chain DNA assay (for more information, see Pawlotsky, et al.).[53]

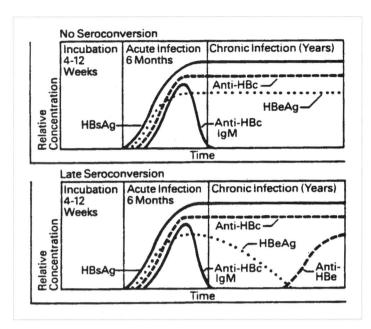

Figure 12-7. Serological profiles of patients who chronically carry hepatitis B virus. (Reproduced, with permission, from Abbott Laboratories, North Chicago, IL.)

TABLE 12-9

HBsAg	ANTI-HBs	ANTI-HBc	INTERPRETATION
Positive	Negative	Positive	Acute infection or chronic hepatitis B
Negative	Positive	Positive	Resolving hepatitis B or previous infection
Negative	Positive	Negative	Resolving or recovered hepatitis B or patient after vaccination

Table 12-9. Interpretation of Common Hepatitis B Serological Test Results

MINICASE 5

A 47-YEAR-OLD ALCOLHOLIC, S. F., was admitted after being found on a park bench surrounded by empty beer bottles. Known to have cirrhosis, S. F. was thought to be showing signs of hepatic encephalopathy as he slowly lapsed into a deep coma over the first 4 days of hospitalization. His physical examination was significant in that he had hepatomegaly and splenomegaly.

Lab evaluation showed a normal urine drug screen for central nervous system (CNS) depressants with glucose normal at 120 mg/dL. All serum electrolytes also were normal: sodium, 140 mEq/L; potassium, 4 mEq/L; chloride, 98 mEq/L; carbon dioxide, 25 mEq/L; and magnesium, 1.5 mEq/L. S. F.'s blood alcohol concentration on admission was 150 (normal: 0). His serum GGTP was 321 IU/L (<60 IU/L), and his AST was 87 IU/L (8–42 IU/L).

Unfortunately, efforts at treating hepatic encephalopathy did not reverse the patient's coma. When it was noted that his ammonia concentration was normal at 48 µg/dL (30–70 µg/dL), further examination and testing were undertaken. A large bruise was then noticed on the side of S. F.'s head, and a CT scan revealed a large subdural hematoma. With surgical treatment of the hematoma, he promptly awoke and began asking for more beer.

Question: How does one establish the diagnosis of hepatic encephalopathy for this patient? What is the role of the serum ammonia concentration in the diagnosis?

Discussion: This case demonstrates that the diagnosis of hepatic encephalopathy is not always straightforward. Hepatic encephalopathy is only one cause of altered mental function in patients with advanced liver disease. Other causes may include drug accumulation, head trauma, hypoglycemia, delirium tremens, and electrolyte imbalance. The diagnosis of hepatic encephalopathy is suggested by

- Elevated ammonia concentrations.
- Presence (in early stages) of asterixis or a flapping tremor of the hands.
- Absence of other causative factors.
- Characteristic electroencephalographic findings (rarely used).

The response to therapy (usually correction of electrolyte imbalances, rehydration, and lactulose or neomycin) further supports this diagnosis.

Serum ammonia concentrations, therefore, are just one piece of this puzzle. An elevated concentration suggests, but does not establish, this diagnosis. Furthermore, although normal ammonia concentrations may cause one to question the diagnosis of hepatic encephalopathy, they can occur in this condition.

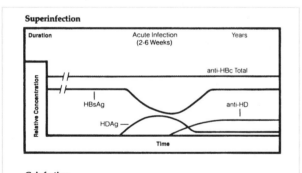

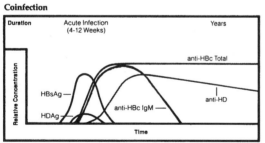

- Infection exists only in presence of HBsAg
- Incubation period 2-6 weeks
- Illness more serious in superinfection
- Most patients present symptoms
- High incidence of fulminant hepatitis
- Route of transmission similar to HBV

Figure 12-8. Two serological profiles of patients infected with the hepatitis D virus. HDAg = hepatitis D antigen (the virus); anti-HD = antibodies against hepatitis D virus. (Reproduced, with permission, from Abbott Laboratories, North Chicago, IL.)

There are six major genotypes of the type C virus. Viral genotype determination may be useful since genotype is known to affect the likelihood of response to certain treatments. Additionally, while the treatment for the most common genotypes found in the US (type 1) is 1 year in duration, current recommendations suggest that some other genotypes (notably 2 or 3) can be successfully treated with only 6 months of therapy. Genotype determination may be done via direct sequencing or hybridization of PCR amplification products.[53]

Type D Hepatitis

Hepatitis D virus (HDV) is caused by a defective virus that requires the presence of hepatitis B surface antigen (HBsAg) to cause infection. Therefore, people can only contract type D hepatitis concomitantly with HBV infection (coinfection) or if chronically infected with HBV (superinfection). Coinfection presents as an acute infection that may be more severe than

A 45-YEAR-OLD EXECUTIVE, M. C., presented to his physician after noticing that he was turning yellow. Other than increased fatigue, he felt well. His physical examination was normal except for his jaundice and tenderness over a slightly swollen liver. Initial laboratory studies showed elevations of the aminotransferases with an ALT of 1235 IU/L (3–30 IU/L) and an AST of 2345 IU/L (8–42 IU/L). His total bilirubin was 18.6 mg/dL (0.3–1.0 mg/dL).

The tentative diagnosis was acute hepatitis. However, M. C. had not had any transfusions, used parenteral drugs, or had recent dental work. No exposure to medications or occupational exposure accounted for the disease, and there was no family history of liver disease. Careful review of the patient's history offered no explanation for his development of hepatitis.

Ultimately, serologies showed a positive HBsAg and anti-HBc antibody. A diagnosis of acute type B hepatitis was established. After much questioning, M. C. revealed that he had a "brief encounter" with a prostitute on a recent business trip. His wife was treated with the vaccine and hepatitis B immunoglobulin, a gamma-globulin with high concentrations of antibodies to HBsAg. Although M. C.'s wife did not develop hepatitis, she did divorce the patient after learning that his secretary developed type B hepatitis about 3 months later.

Question: How was this diagnosis established? How should this patient be followed and what is the likely outcome?

Discussion: This case demonstrates why a determination of the etiology of hepatitis is often difficult. The practitioner must obtain a detailed history of exposures to medicines, drugs, alcohol, infected people, family members with similar illness, and ongoing medical illness. In this case, the exposure to the prostitute put M. C. at risk for hepatitis B, C, and D and for human immunodeficiency virus (HIV). The diagnosis was established by the serologies. Had just the anti-HBc antibody been present, this patient could have

- Been in the "window" phase of the acute disease where this antibody is positive and HBsAg is negative.
- Previously recovered from hepatitis B.
- Been a chronic carrier.

Although the additional presence of HBsAg helped to secure the diagnosis, the clinical picture still had to be considered; both of these tests also can be positive in patients with chronic hepatitis B (Table 12-9). Determination of the type of hepatitis has prognostic value and, in this case, made it possible to administer prophylactic medications to people who might have been exposed.

There is no generally accepted drug therapy for acute viral hepatitis. M. C. should have repeated examinations and LFTs (specifically albumin, PT, AST, ALT, and bilirubin). There is a less than 1% chance that he will develop fulminant hepatitis and die. Most likely, he will recover completely, with his LFTs normalizing over 1–2 months. However, there is a 10–20% chance that he will develop either chronic persistent hepatitis, generally considered benign, or chronic active hepatitis, which could lead to cirrhosis.

The prostitute probably had chronic active hepatitis, but her HIV status was unknown. Unfortunately, even after this case was reported to the public health department, nothing could be done to prevent the prostitute from spreading these diseases to other contacts.

HBV infection alone.[46] Alternatively, the picture of superinfection is that of a patient, with known or unknown chronic HBV, who develops an acute flare with worsening liver function and increases in HBsAg.[48] Acute coinfection is usually self-limited with rare development of chronic hepatitis, while superinfection becomes chronic in more than 75% of cases and increases the risk of negative sequelae such as cirrhosis. Transmission of HDV is generally by parenteral routes, although no obvious cause can be determined in some cases.

HDV testing is usually only indicated in known cases of HBV infection. The single, widely available assay detects anti-HDV antibodies of all isotypes. This test is unable to distinguish between acute, chronic, or resolved infection and lacks sensitivity since only about 38% of infected patients have detectable anti-HDV within the first 2 weeks of illness.[52] Because seroconversion may occur as late as 3 months after infection, testing may be repeated if the clinical picture suggests HDV.[45]

Type E Hepatitis

Like the hepatitis A virus, the hepatitis E virus (HEV) is spread via a fecal-oral route, often by contaminated food or water or person-to-person contact. Clinically, this disease resembles type A and is characterized by a mild course without development of chronic disease. Fulminant hepatitis has occurred in women in their third trimester of pregnancy, occasionally in large outbreaks. The disease is rare in the United States, and most cases are imported by travelers to regions where HEV is endemic.

Although tests are not commercially available, antibodies to hepatitis E can be measured in research facilities and at the CDC.[46]

Primary Biliary Cirrhosis—Antimitochondrial Antibody (AMA)

Primary biliary cirrhosis (PBC) is a chronic disease involving progressive destruction of small intrahepatic bile ducts leading to cholestasis and progressive fibrosis. Over a period of decades, it can progress to cirrhosis and liver failure, necessitating transplantation. Ninety percent of affected individuals are female, with onset occurring between the early twenties and late eighties.[55,56] The etiology of the disease is unknown, although it clearly involves an autoimmune component, and PBC is associated with a variety of autoimmune disorders including Sjorgen's syndrome, rheumatoid arthritis, and scleroderma. In certain situations it appears that the disease may be triggered by environmental agents or medications, particularly drugs that may cause cholestasis.[57]

The initial symptoms of the disease are often those of progressive cholestasis with fatigue, pruritus, jaundice, and deficiencies in fat soluble vitamins, although PBC may also occasionally present with variceal bleeding or osteoporosis (in part to vitamin D deficiency).[56] Due to routine blood chemistries or evaluation of a coexisting autoimmune disorder, 60–70% of patients are diagnosed at an asymptomatic stage.[55,58]

Diagnosis

The most useful laboratory test in diagnosing PBC is the detection of antimitochondrial antibody (AMA) by ELISA or indirect immunofluorescence, with a sensitivity of 95%.[59] This assay is also highly specific, although patients with autoimmune and drug-induced hepatitis occasionally have low antibody titers. The quoted specificity is ~98%, but it could be even higher since patients with antimitochondrial antibodies, who are otherwise normal, tend to subsequently develop biochemical and histological evidence of PBC.[57] However, there is a subset of patients with histologic and biochemical changes of PBC who lack antimitochondrial antibodies and may instead have antinuclear or antismooth muscle antibodies.[60] PBC patients also tend to have elevated levels of IgM (but not IgG or IgA).[55]

PBC usually presents with a cholestatic laboratory picture (i.e., elevated alkaline phosphatase, GGTP, and later an elevated bilirubin). Aminotransferases tend to be minimally elevated or normal. Diagnosis generally requires a liver biopsy but is strongly suggested by elevated levels of IgM and positive antimitochondrial antibody.

Hepatocellular Carcinoma

Hepatocellular carcinoma (HCC, hepatoma, or primary liver cancer) is the most common malignancy in some parts of the world and is less frequent in the developed Western world, although its prevalence is rising. HCC is most often associated with chronic liver disease, especially cirrhosis, with an estimated annual incidence of 3–6% in cirrhotic patients.[61] The rising incidence of this disease in the United States is largely attributable to the increasing prevalence of Hepatitis C, and 30–50% of HCC diagnosed in the United States are related to HCV infection (roughly 2–7% of individuals with HCV are predicted to develop HCC, although this may be averted with successful therapy for HCV).[62] HCC is also associated with Hepatitis B, hemochromatosis, α-1-antitrypsin deficiency, alcoholic cirrhosis, porphyria cutanea tarda, and other liver diseases that cause cirrhosis.

Early diagnosis and treatment of HCC is crucial and provides the main chance for curative treatment, as there are no treatments that improve survival at the advanced stages of disease.[61] Left untreated, the 5-year survival rate is less than 5%.[63] Current recommendations include screening cirrhotic patients with hepatic ultrasound and serum alpha-fetoprotein (AFP) every 6 months.

Alpha-Fetoprotein

Normal range: 10–20 ng/mL

Alpha-fetoprotein (AFP) is so named because it is a fetal protein normally not found in non-pregnant adults. In adults AFP is a tumor marker that is elevated in 70–80% of patients with HCC, limiting the test's sensitivity since many tumors produce no AFP.[64,65] The test's specificity is a function of the cutoff value with moderate elevations (10–500 ng/mL) seen in pregnancy, chronic viral hepatitis, cirrhosis, and other primary tumors of the GI tract.[66] Levels of AFP above 500 ng/mL are 95% specific for HCC (although similar levels may be caused by gonadal tumors) at the cost of lowering the sensitivity to 60%.[62] Although the test has been criticized as lacking sensitivity and specificity (with positive predictive values reported as ranging from 9–32%), it is generally recommended as a useful adjunct to radiographic tumor detection.[67] Serial monitoring to detect trends is more revealing than single measurements and is particularly useful in following the response of an AFP-positive tumor to treatment.[66,64]

TESTS TO ASSESS THE PANCREAS

The tests discussed in this section, amylase and lipase, are primarily used to diagnose pancreatitis. Pancreatitis, or inflammation of the pancreas, can be acute or chronic. It generally presents with severe midepigastric abdominal pain often radiating to the back. The pain tends to be continuous and can last for several days.

This condition is often associated with nausea and vomiting; in severe cases, fever, ileus, and hypotension can occur. Ultimately, there can be progressive anemia, hypocalcemia, hypoglycemia, hypoxia, renal failure, and death. The clinician faces the challenge of establishing this diagnosis, because many conditions (e.g., ulcers, biliary diseases, myocardial infarctions, and intestinal ischemia) can present in a similar manner.

Gallstones and alcohol abuse are causative factors in 60–80% of pancreatitis cases.[68] Medications can also cause acute pancreatitis (Table 12-10) Often, however, it is impossible to determine the definite cause of a patient's attack.

TABLE 12-10

Asparaginase	Nitrofurantoin
Azathioprine	Pentamidine
Cimetidine	Ranitidine
Didanosine	Steroids
Estrogens	Sulfonamides
Furosemide	Sulindac
Mercaptopurine	Tetracycline
Methyldopa	Thiazides
Metronidazole	Valproic acid

Table 12-10. Selected Drugs That May Cause Pancreatitis

Amylase

Normal range: 44–128 IU/L but varies with assay

Amylase helps break starch into its individual glucose molecules. It is secreted by the pancreas and salivary glands to aid in digestion. The enzyme's most frequent clinical use is in the diagnosis of acute pancreatitis.

As with any serum protein, concentrations result from the balance between entry into circulation and rate of clearance. Most circulating amylase originates from the pancreas and salivary glands (responsible for approximately 40% and 60% of serum amylase, respectively).

However, the enzyme is also found in the lungs, liver, fallopian tubes, ovary, testis, small intestine, skeletal muscle, adipose, thyroid, tonsils, and certain cancers, and various pathologies may increase secretion from these sources. The kidneys are responsible for about 25% of the metabolic clearance, with the remaining extrarenal mechanisms being poorly understood. The serum half-life is between 1–2 hr.[69,70] Although there is no amylase activity in neonates and only small amounts at 2–3 months of age, concentrations increase to the normal adult range by 1 year.

Amylase concentrations rise within 2–6 hr after the onset of acute pancreatitis and peak after 12–30 hr if the underlying inflammation has not recurred. In uncomplicated disease, these concentrations frequently return to normal within 3–5 days. More prolonged, mild elevations occur in up to 10% of patients with pancreatitis and may indicate ongoing pancreatic inflammation or associated complications (e.g., pancreatic pseudocyst).

Although serum amylase concentrations do not correlate with disease severity or prognosis, a higher amylase may indicate a greater likelihood that the patient has pancreatitis.[71] For example, serum amylase concentrations may increase up to 25 times the upper limit of normal in acute pancreatitis compared to elevations from opiate-induced spasms of the sphincter of Oddi being 2–10 times normal. Unfortunately, the magnitude of enzyme elevation can overlap in these situations, and ranges are not very specific.

Amylase has a relatively low sensitivity, with about 20% of patients with acute pancreatitis having normal levels. Additionally, amylase has relatively low specificity and may be elevated in a wide variety of conditions. These include a variety of diseases of the pancreas, salivary glands, gastrointestinal system (including hepatobiliary injury, perforated peptic ulcer, and intestinal obstruction or infarction), and gynecologic system (e.g., ovarian or fallopian cysts), as well as pregnancy, trauma, renal failure, various neoplasms, and diabetic ketoacidosis. A variety of medications and alcohol may also cause increased values. In diagnosis, other useful laboratory tests include lipase (since it is confounded by fewer factors) and fractionation into pancreatic and salivary isoenzymes (although its utility has been questioned).[72,73]

Another condition that may cause elevated amylase concentrations is macroamylasemia, a benign condition present in 2–5% of patients with hyperamylasemia.[74] In this condition, amylase molecules are bound by immunoglobulins or complex polysaccharides, forming complexes that are too large to enter the glomerular filtrate and be cleared by the kidneys. This results in serum concentrations up to 10 times the normal limit.[75] Macroamylasemia can be detected by fractionating serum amylase or by measuring urine amylase.

Urine amylase concentrations (normal range: <32 IU for 2-hr collection or <384 IU for 24-hr collection) usually peak later than serum concentrations, and elevations may persist for 7–10 days. This is useful if a patient is hospitalized after acute symptoms have subsided at which point serum amylase may already have returned to normal, leaving only urinary amylase to indicate pancreatitis (as discussed below, lipase may also persist after serum amylase levels decline). Urine amylase levels may also be useful in revealing macroamylasemia (in which case serum amylase is elevated while urinary amylase is normal or decreased).[73] However, this pattern of elevated serum amylase without elevated urinary amylase is also consistent with renal failure.

One cause of amylase's relatively low sensitivity is that marked hypertriglyceridemia may cause amylase measurements to be artificially low, masking elevation in serum amylase. This finding is clinically relevant since hypertriglyceridemia (>800 mg/dL) is a potential cause of acute pancreatitis. Fortunately, however, urinary amylase and serum lipase would typically be abnormal in this situation.

A 48-YEAR-OLD WOMAN, K. M., received a notice 2 weeks after donating blood that it could not be used because her aminotransferases were elevated and a test for hepatitis C was positive. She was referred to a specialist who found that her ALT was 87 IU/L (3–30 IU/L) and her AST was 103 IU/L (8–42 IU/L). Her bilirubin was 0.8 mg/dL (0.3–1.0 mg/dL).

A liver biopsy demonstrated chronic active hepatitis. After considerable discussion, K. M. was placed on interferon and ribavirin. Even after 3 months of therapy, however, her aminotransferases were not responding and she was referred for a second opinion.

Type C hepatitis was excluded when the patient's RIBA and RT-PCR studies were negative. Additional history then was obtained. K. M. had been reluctant to tell her local family physician that, about 6 months previously, she had a positive skin test for tuberculosis (TB) after discovering that her partner was HIV positive. Being embarrassed, she had sought treatment in a nearby city and been placed on isoniazid. Although she had finished the prescriptions, she had never returned to the clinic.

Question: What are the roles of the second- and third-generation tests in the diagnosis of hepatitis C? What other nonviral forms of hepatitis can present as chronic hepatitis?

Discussion: This case demonstrates several points. Many patients with chronic active hepatitis remain totally asymptomatic, their disease first being detected during routine blood work or when symptoms of cirrhosis or liver failure develop. Now that all blood donors are checked for hepatitis C and abnormal aminotransferases, many patients with chronic liver disease are detected before symptoms are present. Unfortunately, however, the blood banks tend to use the less expensive and less accurate ELISA test for hepatitis C, which (as in this case) gives many false-positive results. Before starting interferon therapy or establishing a diagnosis of type C hepatitis, a practitioner should confirm the diagnosis with either a RIBA or RNA polymerase.

There are many nonviral causes of chronic hepatitis including medications such as isoniazid, methyldopa, furantoins, and dantroline. A similar picture also may be seen in autoimmune hepatitis, Wilson's disease, α-1 antitrypsin deficiency, and hemochromatosis. Isoniazid, a common medication for TB, can cause serious liver damage that may be clinically and histologically indistinguishable from viral chronic active hepatitis. Therefore, aminotransferases need to be carefully monitored in patients on this drug. This problem tends to occur in patients over the age of 50, particularly women.

The aminotransferases may be only minimally elevated, as in this patient. Generally, hepatitis develops after about 2–3 months of drug therapy. With withdrawal of the medication, the numbers usually return to normal over an additional 1–2 months. When the diagnosis of chronic active hepatitis is considered, a patient's medications must be very carefully reviewed.

Lipase

Normal range: <1.5 U/mL but varies with assay

Lipase aids in fat digestion by catalyzing the hydrolysis of triglycerides into fatty acids and glycerol. Although mostly secreted by the pancreas, lipase can also be found in the tongue, esophagus, stomach, small intestine, leukocytes, adipose tissue, lung, milk, and liver. In healthy individuals, serum lipase tends to be mostly of pancreatic origin.[76]

Lipase initially parallels amylase levels in acute pancreatitis, increasing rapidly and peaking at 12–30 hr. However, lipase has a half-life of 7–14 hr so that it declines much more slowly, typically returning to normal after 8–14 days. Thus, one utility of lipase (similar to urinary amylase) is the detection of acute pancreatitis roughly 3 or more days after onset at which point amylase levels are no longer elevated. As with amylase, peak lipase concentrations typically range from 3–5 times the upper limit of the reference range.

A comparison of the sensitivity and specificity of amylase vs. lipase, and the utility of these tests alone or in combination remains under debate. This issue is complicated by the fact that the sensitivity and specificity of any laboratory test vary depending on where the cutoff is chosen (e.g., choosing a higher cutoff increases specificity at the cost of lower sensitivity). In general, serum lipase appears to be superior, particularly with respect to specificity.[72–74,77–79] However, simultaneous determination of both lipase and amylase may increase overall specificity because different factors confound the different assays.[80] For example, an elevated amylase with a normal lipase suggests amylase of salivary origin, or may represent macroamylasemia. Similarly, an elevated lipase with normal amylase has been shown to often not be due to pancreatitis, although in the case of pancreatitis it could be caused by delayed laboratory evaluation or artificial lowering of amylase levels by hypertriglyceridemia.[81]

Lipase concentrations may be elevated in patients with nonpancreatic abdominal pain such as a ruptured abdominal aortic aneurysm, a variety of disorders of the alimentary tract and liver (note the enzyme's location in these organs), renal failure, nephrolithiasis, diabetic ketoacidosis, and alcoholism. In these situations, elevations tend to be less than 3 times normal. In the condition of macrolipasemia, similar to macroamylasemia but far less frequent, macromolecular complexes of lipase to immunoglobulin prevent excretion and elevate serum lipase concentrations.[82]

Other Test Results In Pancreatitis

In severe cases of acute pancreatitis, occasionally several days after the insult, fat necrosis may result in the formation of "organic soaps" that bind calcium. Serum calcium concentrations then decrease (low albumin may also contribute), sometimes enough to cause tetany. When pancreatitis is of biliary tract origin, typical elevations in ALP, bilirubin, AST, and ALT are seen. Some researchers believe that in acute pancreatitis an increase of ALT to 3 times baseline or higher is relatively specific for gallstone-induced pancreatitis.[83]

Pancreatitis also may be associated with hemoconcentration and subsequent elevations of the BUN or hematocrit. Depending on the severity of the attack, lactic acidosis, azotemia, anemia, hyperglycemia, hypoalbuminemia, and hypoxemia also may occur.

Despite the perfection of amylase and lipase assays for acute pancreatitis, the sensitivity and specificity of these tests are often regarded as unsatisfactory, and in many patients pancreatitis is only diagnosed on autopsy. For this reason, several new tests have been investigated (e.g., serum trypsin and trypsinogen), although they are not yet widely available.[79,84] CT scanning may be of value in demonstrating pancreatitis when serum markers are not helpful.

ULCER DISEASE

Up to 10% of the US population will develop *ulcers* at some point in life. In 1975, about 4 million Americans had ulcer disease for a total cost of 3.2 billion dollars.[85] Until recently, ulcers were believed to be primarily due to acid. Traditional therapy with antacids, H_2-blockers, and even proton pump inhibitors has been effective in treating ulcers, but it is not as effective in preventing recurrences.

Helicobacter Pylori

Helicobacter pylori was identified as a cause of ulcer disease relatively recently, and studies into its detection and treatment are still in a state of rapid development. *H. Pylori* is a gram-negative bacillus that establishes lifelong colonization of the gastric epithelium in affected individuals. Transmission seems to be via a fecal-oral or oral-oral route. Prevalence increases with age and correlates with poor sanitation.[86] In developed countries about 40–50% of people harbor these bacteria by the age of 50, whereas in developing countries the prevalence is over 90% by this age.[87]

A 24-YEAR-OLD MALE, B. W., was admitted to the hospital with a 5-day history of excruciating midepigastric pain radiating to the back and associated nausea and vomiting. He described a long history of recurring pancreatitis of undetermined etiology with similar symptomatology as his acute complaints. On admission, he had stable vital signs but appeared very uncomfortable. His physical examination was unremarkable except for fairly impressive tenderness in his epigastrium.

All of the patient's admission blood work was normal:

- WBC count of 10,000 cells/mm³ (4800–10,800 cells/mm³) with normal differential.
- AST of 20 IU/L (8–42 IU/L).
- ALT of 25 IU/L (3–30 IU/L).
- ALP of 80 IU/L (26–88 IU/L).
- Bilirubin of 1 mg/dL (0.3–1.0 mg/dL).
- Glucose of 80 mg/dL (70–110 mg/dL fasting).
- Calcium of 9 mg/dL (8.5–10.8 mg/dL).
- Serum amylase of 95 IU/L (44–128 IU/L).
- Lipase of 1.3 U/mL (<1.5 U/mL).

However, urinary amylase concentrations were markedly elevated, with over 1000 IU/2-hr specimen (<32 IU) on two determinations.

Radiographic workup, including abdominal ultrasound and computer-assisted tomography, was normal. Nevertheless, B. W. continued to require large amounts of narcotics to control his pain. One night, a nurse observed him expectorating into his urine specimen. A fractionation of the urinary amylase showed that the elevated amylase concentrations in the urine specimen were of salivary origin. When his narcotics were withdrawn, he signed out against medical advice to begin his search for the next gullible physician.

Question: What symptoms of B. W.'s were consistent with the diagnosis of pancreatitis? Which were not? What was the source of this patient's hyperamylasuria?

Discussion: This patient, clearly seeking narcotics, knew the signs and symptoms of acute pancreatitis. His symptom of epigastric pain radiating to the back was consistent with the diagnosis he suggested (led the doctors to believe) when giving a history of previous pancreatitis attacks. The elevated urinary concentrations of amylase further supported this diagnosis.

The diagnosis of pancreatitis, however, was not supported by the normal serum concentrations of amylase and lipase, lack of a fever, normal WBC count, and normal radiographic tests. After the nurse made her observation, it became clear that the amylase elevation in the urine was salivary amylase due to B. W. deliberately expectorating into the specimen cup. Saliva, as the patient no doubt had learned, has a very large amount of amylase.

H. pylori infection may be found in 90% of patients with duodenal ulcers and 80% of patients with gastric ulcers.[86] Furthermore, the bacteria have been associated with the development of antral gastritis, gastric cancer, and certain types of gastric lymphoma.[47,48,88–90] However, most infected individuals (>70%) are asymptomatic, and eradication therapy is not recommended for asymptomatic infection.[87]

Diagnosis

The diagnostic tests for *H. Pylori* are classified as *noninvasive* (serology, urea breath test, and stool antigen test) or *invasive* (histology, culture, and rapid urea test), depending on whether they require upper endoscopy and biopsy.

The serological test for *H. pylori* detects circulating IgG antibody against bacterial proteins. It has a relatively low sensitivity and specificity (both 80–95%) with the advantage of being widely available and inexpensive.[87,91,92] However, it may not be used to monitor the success of eradication therapy as antibody titers decrease slowly in the absence of bacteria.

The urea breath test is based on the ability of the bacteria to break down urea, releasing ammonia and carbon dioxide. In a breath test, [13]C- or ^{14}C-labeled urea is given by mouth. If the bacteria are present, the radiolabeled urea is metabolized to radiolabeled CO_2, which may be measured in exhaled air. The tests have high sensitivity and specificity (both 90–95% for ^{13}C and 86–95% for ^{14}C).[87,91] However, the ^{13}C isotope has the drawback of being radioactive, and the ^{14}C isotope requires the use of sophisticated detection methods such as isotope ratio mass spectrometry (although samples are stable and may be mailed away for analysis).[93]

The fecal antigen test detects *H. pylori* proteins in stool via ELISA. It has high sensitivity and specificity (both 90–95%) and, like the urea breath test, is a very accurate noninvasive measure that is used primarily to monitor the success of eradication therapy, although it may be used as a test for infection when endoscopy is not indicated.[94]

Upper endoscopy with biopsy of gastric tissue and subsequent histological examination has high sensitivity and specificity (88–95% and 90–95%) with the added advantage of allowing for detection of gastritis, metaplasia, or other histological features. Although not commonly done, biopsy specimens may also be used to culture *H. pylori*. By performing various tests on the cultured bacteria, this test may be rendered highly specific (95–98%), but the bacteria is difficult to culture making this the least sensitive test (80–90%).[86,87,95] The main advantage of culture is that it allows for antibiotic sensitivity testing, which may be useful in addressing treatment failure. Rapid urease tests involve incubating a biopsy specimen in the presence of urea. As mentioned above, *H. pylori* metabolizes urea releasing ammonia, which in this case may be detected by its effect of increasing the pH. This test allows for rapid results (e.g., 1-hr incubation time following endoscopy), high sensitivity and specificity (both 90–95%), and low cost.[87,96] One other invasive test requires a nasogastric catheter; PCR detection of *H. pylori* DNA may be performed on gastric juice extracted from the catheter.[86]

These tests tend to be confounded by a common set of factors that lower bacterial burden. In patients with achlorhydria or patients being treated with antisecretory drugs (e.g., proton pump inhibitors), increased stomach pH decreases bacterial levels and may lead to false-negative results.[93,95,97] Similarly, use of antibiotics (including recent, unsuccessful eradication therapy) may decrease test sensitivity. GI bleeding may also confound the rapid urea test and fecal antigen test.[94]

PSEUDOMEMBRANOUS COLITIS

Colitis—acute inflammation of the colon—often presents quite dramatically with profound diarrhea, urgency, and abdominal cramping. It is generally distinguished from other causes of diarrhea by

- White blood cells in the stools.
- A positive test for occult blood in the stool.
- An elevated WBC count in the blood.

There are many causes of colitis. Infectious colitis is caused by invasive organisms including *Campylobacter jejuni*, *Shigella*, *Salmonella*, and invasive *Escherichia coli*. Amoeba can present in this manner as can certain complications of AIDS (cytomegalovirus infection). Noninfectious colitis includes ischemic colitis (insufficient blood flow to the colon), drug-induced colitis (as with gold salts), NSAID colitis, inflammatory bowel disease (Crohn's or ulcerative colitis), and radiation injury.

CLOSTRIDIUM DIFFICILE

Pseudomembranous colitis is almost always caused by a bacterium, *Clostridium difficile*, an organism that may cause disease ranging from mild diarrhea to life threatening pseudomembranous colitis with toxic megacolon or perforation.[98] Pseudomembranous colitis can occur spontaneously, but it commonly follows the use of antibiotics that distort the gut's normal bacterial flora and only became common following the widespread use of broad-spectrum antibiotics in the 1960s and 1970s.[99] Almost any antimicrobial agent may predispose to infection (including the antibiotics used to treat *C. difficile* infection), in particular, broad spectrum antibiotics and agents active on anaerobic flora.[98,100–102] Surprisingly, even one antibiotic dose (as used prior to surgery) may cause this condition. Antineoplastic agents with antimicrobial activity, laxatives, stool softeners, antacids, immunosuppressive drugs, and enemas also occasionally predispose to disease.[103,104] Although clinical manifestations may start as early as the first or second day of antibiotic treatment, they may not appear until weeks after the regimen is completed.[98,101]

Infection is usually acquired nosocomially as a result of ingestion of *C. difficile* spores. Spores can survive extreme environmental conditions and remain viable for months or years, which is part of the explanation of why *C. difficile* is the most common enteric pathogen and the most common cause of diarrhea in hospitalized patients.[98,99] Neonates are commonly colonized with the bacteria, which may be due to the fact that they have not established a stable gut bacterial flora.[102] However, susceptibility to *C. difficile* associated disease does not develop until ages 1–2 at which point *C. difficile* prevalence has decreased.

Less than 3% of healthy adults are carriers, but about 15–25% of antibiotic-treated hospitalized patients are colonized with this bacterium.[101] Most infected hospital inpatients are asymptomatic. This is in part due to the fact that pathogenic strains of *C. difficile* produce a toxin that causes colitis, but 25% of *C. difficile* isolates neither produce toxins nor cause disease. Other factors that differentiate between symptomatic and asymptomatic infection may include bacterial load (which is lower in healthy carriers than colitis patients) and the presence of protective toxin-neutralizing antibodies (which are higher in carriers).[105]

Diagnosis

Although sigmoidoscopy may demonstrate pathognomonic pseudomembranes, it has low sensitivity since it may be falsely negative if the disease is in the more proximal colon. In one study, up to one-third of the patients only had one lesion in the right colon.[106] Therefore, colonoscopy may be required for endoscopic diagnosis, but it is contraindicated by the risk of perforation in cases involving colonic dilation. Overall, sigmoidoscopy or colonoscopy are not generally indicated as other tests or approaches may be more practical, although endoscopy may be helpful in certain clinical situations requiring rapid diagnosis.[102]

C. difficile may be cultured from stools with selective medium and identified on the basis of colony morphology, fluorescence, odor, gram stain, and/or signature gas liquid chromatography. Culture is the most sensitive test for the organism, but is not usually used for clinical diagnosis because it takes 2–3 days and must be accompanied with testing stool or cultured bacteria for toxin production (to avoid confounding with nontoxic *C. difficile* strains).[104]

Two toxins of *C. difficile* have been identified and are generally present together: endotoxin and cytotoxin (known as Toxins A and B, respectively). The gold-standard test for pathogenic *C. difficile* is the detection of toxin B in stool samples by demonstration of its cytopathic effect in cell cultures and inhibition of cytopathic effect by specific antiserum.[98] This assay has high specificity (99%) and sensitivity (94–100%).[100,107] The cytotoxicity assay remains the single best method for diagnosing *C. difficile* diarrhea, even though it is expensive and results are not obtained for 1–3 days.[108]

J. T. PRESENTED TO HER PHYSICIAN after several days of crampy abdominal pain, diarrhea, fevers up to 102.5 °F (39.2 °C), and chills. On physical examination, she was noted to be well-hydrated. Her abdomen was soft and nontender. Stools were sent for pathogenic bacterium cultures including *Shigella, Salmonella, Campylobacter*, entero-invasive *E. coli*, and *Yersinia*; meanwhile, J. T. was given a prescription for diphenoxylate.

Twenty-four hours later, the patient presented to the emergency room doubled over with severe abdominal pain. Her abdomen was distended and tender with diffuse rigidity and guarding. Clinically, she was dehydrated. Her WBC count was elevated at 23,000 cells/mm^3 (4800–10,800 cells/mm^3), and her BUN was 34 mg/dL (8–20 mg/dL). Abdominal x-rays showed a dilated colon (toxic megacolon) and an ileus. The emergency room physician then learned that, about 6 weeks earlier, J. T. had taken two or three of her sister's amoxicillin pills because she had thought she was developing a urinary tract infection.

Although pseudomembranous colitis was tentatively diagnosed, J. T. could not take oral medication because of her ileus. Therefore, IV metronidazole was started. This patient continued to get sicker, however; early the next day, her colon was removed and an ileostomy was created.

Question: What is the time course of pseudomembranous colitis? Did the use of diphenoxylate influence the outcome?

Discussion: Pseudomembranous colitis can occur even after only one or two doses of a systemic antibiotic or after topical antibiotic use. Moreover, it can occur up to 6 weeks later. A complete history of antibiotic use is critical when dealing with diarrhea patients.

Diphenoxylate or loperamide use in the face of colitis is associated with a risk, although small, of toxic megacolon. In this medical emergency, the colon has no peristalsis; together with the inflammation in the colon wall (colitis), this condition leads to progressive distention. If untreated, perforation and death ensue. The development of a megacolon or ileus in this patient is especially worrisome because the best treatment—oral antibiotics—would be of little benefit. However, IV metronidazole is excreted into the bile in adequate bactericidal levels to eradicate the bacteria.

ELISA tests, which are the most commonly used laboratory tests for detecting pseudomembranous colitis, can detect toxin A or both toxins in stool samples with the advantage of being rapid and inexpensive. They have high specificity (typically >95%), but their sensitivity is considerably lower than the cytotoxicity assay and varies widely (60–95%). Following up a negative test with repeat stool specimens may increase sensitivity to the 90% range.[101,107] Testing for both toxins has a diagnostic advantage over testing for toxin A, because some pathogenic strains are toxin A-negative and toxin-B positive.[103]

Cytotoxicity assays, ELISA tests, and PCR to amplify toxin genes may also be performed on cultured bacteria with greater sensitivity than with stool, although these tests are not as yet routine laboratory procedures.[100,102] Alternatively, in situations that clearly point to a diagnosis of *C. difficile* (e.g., the clinical signs of pseudomembranous colitis combined with a history of antibiotic use) and especially if the patient is at acute risk of complications, the disease may be treated on an empirical basis.

SURVEILLANCE AFTER COLON CANCER RESECTION

Currently, laboratory tests do not play a significant role in the initial detection of colorectal cancer, which is usually achieved by endoscopic or radiographic means. In particular, colonoscopy is generally regarded as the most accurate test for detection of colon cancer detection due to its ability to examine the entire colon and simultaneously remove premalignant polyps. However, the CEA test plays a central role in surveillance for cancer recurrence or metastasis following surgical resection of stage II or III tumors.

CEA (Carcinoembryonic Antigen)

Normal range: <3 ng/mL (<5 ng/mL in smokers)

Carcinoembryonic antigen, or CEA, is an oncofetal antigen that is normally expressed in low levels in the gastrointestinal mucosa but is greatly upregulated in 90% of colorectal carcinomas.[109,110] CEA levels tend to increase as the tumor develops and is not elevated early enough in tumor development to be useful in screening or initial diagnosis of colorectal cancer.[111] Thus, the major use of CEA is after diagnosis, in following response to treatment (e.g., surgery or chemotherapy), and detecting recurrence. Persistence of an elevated CEA after treatment suggests persistence of the cancer and may be useful in redirecting or discontinuing therapy.[110]

CEA is generally regarded as the best test for early detection of liver metastasis after surgery (with sensitivity and specificity in the range of 95%), which is relevant because 40% of colorectal cancer deaths are due to liver metastasis, and early removal of isolated liver metastases may be curative.[112] Because it is less sensitive in revealing anastomotic recurrences and metachronous cancers, it does not preclude colonoscopic follow-up. Unlike alpha-fetoprotein, CEA may be useful in detecting liver metastasis from a CEA-negative colorectal tumor because CEA-negative status is often due to hepatic first-pass metabolism of CEA rather than the CEA status of the tumor.[111]

Increasing CEA levels may be confounded by nonmalignant liver disease due to decreased clearance, as well as a variety of other benign diseases.[112] However, in these cases CEA does not progressively increase and is rarely greater than 10 ng/mL. CEA may also be elevated by other cancers, as well as in treatment with 5-fluouracil and levamisole.[109]

The use of CEA testing remains controversial because the number of patients whose lives are successfully prolonged by CEA-directed treatment is relatively low. However, it is suggested that careful surveillance using the CEA test can be life-saving, and the test is recommended by the American Society of Clinical Oncology.[113]

SUMMARY

Solving the etiology of a given liver or other GI disease is much like putting together a puzzle. A detailed patient history and physical examination are two important pieces. Perhaps even more important is the appropriate use of laboratory studies.

The extent of liver injury or synthetic ability can best be evaluated by measuring the products of the liver including albumin, prealbumin, and PT (an indirect assay of liver production of coagulation factors). Serum bilirubin is also useful as a marker of liver function since it reflects liver uptake, conjugation, and excretion. Although bilirubin can be elevated in some congenital diseases and hemolysis, it may indicate the degree of liver inflammation.

The degree of hepatocellular inflammation is best evaluated with the aminotransferases (ALT and AST), which leak into the blood after damage to liver (and other) cells. Concentrations greater than 8–10 times normal are characteristic of viral hepatitis or drug- or toxin-induced hepatic necrosis. The presence of cholestasis is best detected with ALP, 5'-nucleotidase, and GGTP, although they are not totally specific for liver disease. Elevations in serum ammonia may indicate severe liver disease as well as explain altered mental status in patients with cirrhosis. Various serological tests are available to help distinguish among the many forms of viral hepatitis.

Some other aspects of gastroenterology are also reviewed in this chapter: elevated amylase and lipase tests are used to diagnose acute pancreatitis; ulcer disease is believed to be related to the bacterium *H. pylori*; diagnosis with serological and biopsy tests can aid in curing and preventing relapse of this disease; and antibiotics play a role in causing colitis, and tests for pseudomembranous colitis can confirm this diagnosis.

REFERENCES

1. Sherlock S, Dooley J. *Diseases of the Liver and Biliary System*. 9th ed. London, England: Blackwell Scientific; 1993.

2. Johnson PJ, McFarlane IG. *The Laboratory Investigation of Liver Disease*. London, England: Bailliere Tindall; 1989.

3. Chopra S, Griffin PH. Laboratory tests and diagnostic procedures in evaluation of liver disease. *Am J Med*. 1985; 79:221–30.

4. Beckingham IJ, Ryder SD. Investigation of liver and biliary disease. *Br Med J*. 2001; 322:33–6.

5. Johnston DE. Special considerations in interpreting liver function tests. *Am Fam Phys*. 1999; 59: 2223–30.

6. Pratt DS, Kaplan MM. Evaluation of the liver: laboratory tests. In: Schiff ER, ed. *Schiff's Diseases of the Liver*. 8th ed. Philadelphia, PA: Lippincott; 1999.

7. Dufour DR, Lott JA, Nolte FS, et al. Diagnosis and monitoring of hepatic injury I: performance characteristics of laboratory tests. *Clin Chem*. 2000; 46:2027–49.

8. Aranda-Michael J, Sherman KE. Tests of the liver: use and misuse. *Gastroenterologist*. 998; 6:34–43.

9. Gopal DV, Rosen HR. Abnormal findings on liver function tests. *Postgrad Med*. 2000; 107:100–14.

10. Neyra NR, Hakim RM, Shyr Y, et al. Serum transferrin and serum prealbumin are early predictors of serum albumin in chronic hemodialysis patients. *J Renal Nutr*. 2000; 10:184–90.

11. Spiekerman AM. Nutritional assessment (protein nutriture). *Anal Chem*. 1995; 67:429R–36R.

12. Spiekerman AM. Proteins used in nutritional assessment. *Clin Lab Med*. 1993; 13:353–69.

13. Klein S, Jeejeebhoy KN. The malnourished patient: nutritional assessment and management. In: *Slesinger and Fordtran's Gastrointestinal and Liver Disease*. 6th ed. Philadelphia, PA: W. B. Saunders Company; 1997.

14. Mittman N, Avram MM, Oo KK, et al. Serum prealbumin predicts survival in hemodialysis and peritoneal dialysis: 10 years of prospective observation. *Am J Kidney Dis*. 2001; 38:1358–64.

15. Beck FK, Rosenthal TC. Prealbumin: a marker for nutritional evaluation. *Am Fam Phys*. 2002; 65:1575–8.

16. Hayden K, Heyningen CV. Measurement of total protein is a useful inclusion in liver function test profiles. *Clin Chem*. 2001; 47:793–4.

17. Watts B, Burnett L, Chesher D. Measurement of total protein is not a useful inclusion in liver function test profiles. *Clin Chem*. 2000; 46:1022–3.

18. Kamath PS. Clinical approach to the patient with abnormal liver test results. *Mayo Clin Proc*. 1996; 71:1089–95.

19. Knapp AB, Farkas PS. *Diagnostic Diagrams: Gastroenterology*. Baltimore, MD: Williams & Wilkins; 1985.

20. Reichling JJ, Kaplan MM. Clinical use of serum enzymes in liver disease. *Dig Dis Sci*. 1988; 33:1601–14.

21. Birkett DJ, Done J, Neale FC, et al. Serum alkaline phosphatase in pregnancy: an immunologic study. *Br Med J*. 1966; 1:1210–2.

22. Moss DW, Henderson AR. Clinical enzymology. In: Burtis CA, Ashwood ER, eds. *Tietz Textbook of Clinical Chemistry*. 3rd ed. Philadelphia, PA: W. B. Saunders Company; 1999.

23. Bakerman S, Bakerman P, Strausbauch P. *ABC's of Interpretive Laboratory Data*. 3rd ed. Myrtle Beach, SC: Interpretive Laboratory Data; 1994.

24. Carroll AJ, Coakley JC. Transient hyperphosphatasasemia: an important condition to recognize. *J Paediatr Child Health*. 2001; 37:359–62.

25. Wilson JW. Inherited elevation of alkaline phosphatase activity in the absence of disease. *N Engl J Med*. 1979; 301:983–4.

26. Pratt DS, Kaplan MM. Evaluation of abnormal liver-enzyme results in asymptomatic patients. *N Engl J Med*. 2000; 342:1266–71.

27. Pagani F, Panteghini M. 5'-Nucleotidase in the detection of increased activity of the liver form of Alkaline Phosphatase. *Clin Chem*. 2001; 47:2046–8.

28. Kaplan MM, Matloff DS, Selinger MJ, et al. Biochemical basis for serum enzyme abnormalities in alcoholic liver disease. In: Chang NC, Chan NM, eds. *Early Identification of Alcohol Abuse. NIAAAA Research Monograph 17*. Rockville, MD: U.S. Department of Health and Human Services; 1985:186–98.

29. Ockner RK. Drug induced liver disease. In: Zakim D, Boyer TD, eds. *Hepatology: A Textbook*. Philadelphia, PA: W. B. Saunders Company; 1982: 691–723.

30. Dukes GE, Sanders SW, Russo J, et al. Transaminase elevations in patients receiving bovine or porcine heparin. *Ann Intern Med*. 1984; 100:646–50.

31. Jick H. Drug-associated asymptomatic elevations of transaminase in drug safety assessments. *Pharmacotherapy*. 1995; 15(1):23–5.

32. Fregia A, Jensen D. Evaluation of abnormal liver tests. *Compr Ther*. 1994; 20(1):50–4.

33. Whitehead MW, Hawkes ND, Hainsworth I, et al. A prospective study of the causes of notably raised aspartate aminotransferase of liver origin. *Gut*. 1999; 45:129–33.

34. Ayling RM. Pitfalls in the interpretation of common biochemical tests. *Postgrad Med J*. 2000; 76:129–32.

35. Cohen GA, Goffinet JA, Donabedian RK, et al. Observations on decreased serum glutamic oxaloacetic transaminase (SGOT) activity in azotemic patients. *Ann Intern Med*. 1976; 84:275–80.

36. Glynn KP, Cefaro AF, Fowler CW, et al. False elevations of serum glutamic oxaloacetic transaminase due to para-aminosalicylic acid. *Ann Intern Med*. 1970; 72:525–7.

37. Young DS. *Effects of Drugs on Clinical Laboratory Tests*. 3rd ed. Washington, DC: American Association for Clinical Chemistry Press; 1990.

38. Rivera-Coll A, Fuentes-Arderiu X, Diez-Noguera A. Circadian rhythms of serum concentrations of 12 enzymes of clinical interest. *Chronobiol Int*. 1993; 10:190–200.

39. Friedman LS, Martin P, Munoz SJ. Liver function tests and the objective evaluation of the patient with liver disease. In: Zakim D, Boyer TD, eds. *Hepatology: A Textbook of Liver Disease*. Philadelphia, PA: W. B. Saunders Company; 1996.

40. Isogai M, Yamaguchi A, Hori A, et al. LDH to AST ratio in biliary pancreatitis—a possible indicator of pancreatic necrosis: preliminary results. *Am J Gastro*. 1998; 93:363–7.

41. Rosalki SB, Dooley JS. Liver function profiles and their interpretation. *Br J Hosp Med*. 1994; 51:181–6.

42. Berg CL, Crawford JM, Gollan JL. Bilirubin metabolism and the pathophysiology of jaundice. In: Schiff ER, ed. *Schiff's Diseases of the Liver*. 8th ed. Philadelphia, PA: Lippincott; 1999.

43. Gammal SH, Jones EA. Hepatic encephalopathy. *Med Clin North Am*. 1989; 73:793–813.

44. Zieve L. The mechanism of hepatic coma. *Hepatology*. 1981; 1:360–5.

45. Saab S, Martin P. Tests for acute and chronic viral hepatitis. *Postgrad Med*. 2000; 107:123–30.

46. Wolk DM, Jones MF, Roesnblatt JE. Laboratory diagnosis of viral hepatitis. *Infect Dis Clin N Am*. 2001; 15:1109–26.

47. Lemon SM. Type A viral hepatitis: new developments in an old disease. *N Engl J Med*. 1985; 313:1059–67.

48. Waite J. The laboratory diagnosis of the hepatitis viruses. *Int J STD AIDS*. 1996; 7:400–8.

49. Lemon SM. Type A viral hepatitis: epidemiology, diagnosis, and prevention. *Clin Chem*. 1997; 43:1494–9.

50. Mahoney FJ. Update on diagnosis, management, and prevention of Hepatitis B virus infection. *Clin Microbiol Reviews*. 1999; 12:351–66.

51. Alter HJ. Transmission of hepatitis C virus—route, dose, and titer. *N Engl J Med*. 1994; 330:784–6.

52. Sjogren MH. Serologic diagnosis of viral hepatitis. *Med Clin N Am*. 1996; 80:929–56.

53. Pawlotsky JM. Molecular diagnosis of viral hepatitis. *Gastroenterology*. 2001; 122: 554–68.

54. Moyer LA, Mast EE, Alter MJ. Hepatitis C: routine serologic testing and diagnosis. *Am Fam Phys*. 1999; 59:79–88.

55. Nishio A, Keeffe EB, Gershwin ME. Primary biliary cirrhosis: lessons learned from an organ-specific disease. *Clin Exp Med*. 2001; 1:165–78.

56. Heathcote J. Update on primary biliary cirrhosis. *Can J Gastroenterol*. 2000; 14:43–8.

57. Lazarczyk DA, Duffy MC. Erythromycin-induced primary biliary cirrhosis. *Dig Dis Sci*. 2000; 45:1115–8.

58. Nishio A, Keeffe EB, Ishibashi H, Gershwin EM. Diagnosis and treatment of primary biliary cirrhosis. *Med Sci Monit*. 2000; 6:181–93.

59. Worman JH. Molecular biological methods in diagnosis and treatment of liver diseases. *Clin Chem*. 1997; 43:1476–86.

60. Lacerta MA, Ludwig J, Dickson ER, et al. Antimitochondrial antibody-negative primary biliary cirrhosis. *Am J Gastro*. 1995; 90:247–9.

61. Llovet JM, Bruix J. Early diagnosis and treatment of hepatocellular carcinoma. *Baillere's Best Prac Res Gastroenterol*. 2000; 14:991–1008.

62. Jagannath S, Thuluvath PJ. Hepatocellular carcinoma. *Pract Gastroenterol*. 2002; May:33–54.

63. Ulmer SC. Hepatocellular Carcinoma. *Postgrad Med*. 2000; 107:117–24.

64. Befeler AS, Bisceglie AM. Hepatocellular carcinoma: diagnosis and treatment. *Gastroenterol*. 2002; 122:1609–19.

65. Sherman M. Surveillance for hepatocellular carcinoma. *Sem Oncol*. 2001; 28:450–9.

66. Johnson PJ. The role of serum alpha-fetoprotein estimation in the diagnosis and management of hepatocellular carcinoma. *Clin Liver Dis*. 2001; 5:145–59.

67. Khakoo SI, Grellier LFL, Soni PN, et al. Etiology, screening, and treatment of hepatocellular carcinoma. *Med Clin N Am*. 1996; 80:1121–45.

68. Gregory PB. Diseases of pancreas. *Sci Am Med*. 1994; 4(V):1–15.

69. Soergel K. Acute pancreatitis. In: Sleisenger MH, Fordtran JS, eds. *Gastrointestinal Disease*. 5th ed. Philadelphia, PA: W. B. Saunders Company; 1993:1638–9.

70. Pieper-Bigelow C, Strocchi A, Levitt MD. Where does serum amylase come from and where does it go? *Gastroenterol Clin North Am*. 1990; 19:793–810.

71. Lankisch PG. Underestimation of acute pancreatitis: patients with only a small increase in amylase/lipase levels can also have or develop severe acute pancreatitis. *Gut*. 1999; 44:542–4.

72. Treacy J, Williams A, Bais R, et al. Evaluation of amylase and lipase in the diagnosis of acute pancreatitis. *ANZ J Surg*. 2001; 71: 577–82.

73. Ransom JH. Diagnostic standards for acute pancreatitis. *World J Surg*. 1997; 21:136–42.

74. Vissers RJ, Abu-Laban RB, McHugh DF. Amylase and lipase in the emergency department evaluation of acute pancreatitis. *J Emerg Med*. 1999; 17:1027–37.

75. Gumaste VV. Diagnostic tests for acute pancreatitis. *Gastroenterologist*. 1994; 2:119–30.

76. Gumaste VV, Dave P, Sereny G. Serum lipase: a better test to diagnose acute alcoholic pancreatitis. *Am J Med*. 1992; 92:239–42.

77. Rogers AI. Elevated lipase levels always means pancreatitis? *Postgrad Med*. 2002; 111:104.

78. Gumaste VV, Roditis N, Mehta D, et al. Serum lipase levels in nonpancreatic abdominal pain versus acute pancreatitis. *Am J Gastroenterol*. 1993; 88:2051–5.

79. Munoz A, Katerndahl DA. Diagnosis and management of acute pancreatitis. *Am Fam Phys*. 2000; 62:164–74.

80. Keim V, Teich N, Fiedler F, et. al. A comparison of lipase and amylase in the diagnosis of acute pancreatitis in patients with abnormal pain. *Pancreas*. 998; 16:45–9.

81. Frank B, Gottlieb K. Amylase normal, lipase elevated: Is it pancreatitis? *Am J Gastro*. 1999; 94:463–9.

82. Bode C, Riederer J, Brauner B, et al. Macrolipasemia: a rare cause of persistently elevated serum lipase. *Am J Gastroenterol.* 1990; 85:412–6.

83. Ros E, Navarro S, Bru C, et al. Occult microlithiasis in "idiopathic" acute pancreatitis: prevention of relapses by cholecystectomy or ursodeoxycholic acid therapy. *Gastroenterology.* 1991; 101:1701–9.

84. Kemppainen EA, Hedstrom JI, Puolakkainen PA, et al. Advances in the laboratory diagnostics of acute pancreatitis. *Ann Med.* 1998; 30:169–75.

85. Von Haunalter G, Chandler W. Cost of ulcer disease in the United States. Stanford Research Institute Project 5894. In: Sleisenger MH, Fordtran JS, eds. *Gastrointestinal Disease.* 4th ed. Philadelphia, PA: W. B. Saunders Company; 1989:814–78.

86. Nakamura RM. Laboratory tests for the evaluation of *Helicobacter pylori* infections. *J Clin Lab Anal.* 2001; 15:301–7.

87. Logan RP, Walker MM. Epidemiology and diagnosis of *Helicobacter pylori* infection. *Brit J Med.* 2001; 323:920–2.

88. Vaira D, Gatta L, Rici C, Miglioli M. Review article: diagnosis of *Helicobacter pylori* infection. *Ailment Pharmacol Ther.* 2002a; 16:16–23.

89. Nomura A, Stemmermann GN, Chyou PH, et al. *Helicobacter pylori* infection and gastric carcinoma among Japanese Americans in Hawaii. *N Engl J Med.* 1991; 325:1132–6.

90. Parsonnet J, Friedman GD, Vandersteen DP, et al. Helicobacter pylori infection and the risk of gastric carcinoma. *N Engl J Med.* 1991; 325:1127–31.

91. Vaira D, Vakli N. Blood, urine, stool, breath, money, and *Helicobacter pylori.* *Gut.* 2001; 28:287–9.

92. Vakil N. Review article: the cost of diagnosing Hellicobacter pylori infection. *Ailment Pharmacol Ther.* 2001; 15:10–15.

93. Savarino V, Vigneri S, Celle G. The 13C urea breath test in the diagnosis of *Helicobacter pylori* infection. *Gut.* 1999; 45:I18–22

94. Gisbert JP, Pajares JM. Diagnosis of *Helicobacter pylori* infection by stool antigen determination: a systematic review. *Am J Gastro.* 2001; 96:2829–38.

95. Vaira D, Vakil N, Menegatti M, et al. The stool antigen test for detection of *Helicobacter pylori* after eradication therapy. *Ann Int Med.* 2002b; 136:280–7.

96. Marshall BJ, Warren JR, Francis GJ, et al. Rapid urease test in the management of Campylobacter pyloridis associated gastritis. *Am J Gastroenterol.* 1987; 82:200.

97. Hebrick P, van Doorn LJ. Serological methods for diagnosis of *Helicobacter pylori* infection and monitoring of eradication therapy. *Eur J Clin Microbiol Infect Dis.* 2000; 19:164–73.

98. Tabaqchali S, Jumaa P. Diagnosis and management of Clostridium difficile infection. *Brit J Med.* 1995; 310:1375–80.

99. Kelly CP, LaMont JT. Clostridium difficile infection. *Ann Rev Med.* 1998; 49:375–90.

100. Delmee M. Laboratory diagnosis of Clostridium difficile disease. *Clin Micro Infect.* 2001; 7:411–5.

101. Yassin SY, Young-Fadok TM, Zein NN, et al. Clostridium difficile-associated diarrhea and colitis. *Mayo Clin Proc.* 2001; 76:725–30.

102. Kyne L, Farrell RJ, Kelly CP. Clostridium difficile. *Gastro Clin N Am.* 2001; 30:753–77.

103. Brazier JS. The diagnosis of clostridium difficile-associated disease. *J Antimirco Chemother.* 1998; 41:29–40.

104. Mylonakis E, Ryan ET, Calderwood SB. Clostridium difficile-associated diarrhea. *Arch Intern Med.* 2001; 161:525–533.

105. Fekety R, Shah AB. Diagnosis and treatment of Clostridium difficile colitis. *JAMA.* 1993; 269:71–5.

106. Robesin SE, Levine MS, Glick SN, et al. Pseudomembranous colitis with rectosigmoid sparing on barium studies. *Radiology.* 1989; 170:811.

107. Kelly CP, Pothoulakis C, LaMont JT. Current concepts: clostridium difficile colitis. *N Engl J Med.* 1994; 330:257–62.

108. Barbut F, Kajzer C, Planas N, et al. Comparison of three enzyme immunoassays, a cytotoxicity assay, and toxigenic culture for diagnosis of Clostridium difficile associated diarrhea. *J Clin Microbiol.* 1993; 31:963–7.

109. Mitchell EP. Role of carcinoembryonic antigen in the management of advanced colorectal cancer. *Semin Oncol.* 1998; 25:12–20.

110. MacDonald JS. Carcinoembryonic antigen screening: pros and cons. *Sem Oncol.* 1999; 25:556–60.

111. Adams WJ, Morris DL. Carcinoembronic antigen in the evaluation of therapy of primary and metastatic colorectal cancer. *Aust N Z J Surg.* 1996; 66:515–9.

112. Duffy MJ. Carcinoembryonic antigen as a marker for colorectal cancer: is it clinically useful? *Clin Chem.* 2001; 47:624–30.

113. Desch CE, Benson AB III, Smith TJ, et al. Recommended colorectal cancer surveillance guidelines by the American Society of Clinical Oncology. *J Clin Oncol.* 1999; 17:1312–21.

PARAMETER	DESCRIPTION	COMMENTS
Common reference ranges		
Adults	3.5–5 g/dL	
Pediatrics	2–3.6 g/dL	<1 year old
	2.6–4.2 g/dL	1–3 years old
Critical value	<2.5 g/dL	In adults
Natural substance?	Yes	Blood protein
Inherent activity?	Increases oncotic pressure of plasma; carrier protein	
Location		
Production	Liver	
Storage	Serum	
Secretion/excretion	Broken down in liver	Half-life of about 20 days
Major causes of...		
High or positive results	Dehydration	
	Anabolic steroids	
Associated signs and symptoms	Limited to underlying disorder	No toxicological activity
Low results	Decreased hepatic synthesis	Seen in liver disease
	Malnutrition or malabsorption	Substrate deficiency
	Protein losses	Via kidney in nephrotic syndrome or via gut in protein-losing enteropathy
	Pregnancy or chronic illness	
Associated signs and symptoms	Edema, pulmonary edema, ascites	At levels <2–2.5 g/dL
After insult, time to...		
Initial depression or positive result	Days	
Lowest values	Weeks	Half-life of about 20 days
Normalization	Days	Assumes insult removed and no permanent damage
Drugs often monitored with test	Parenteral nutrition	Goal is increased levels
Causes of spurious results **Falsely elevated**	Ampicillin and heparin	
Falsely lowered	Supine patients, icterus, penicillin	

PARAMETER	DESCRIPTION	COMMENTS
Common reference ranges **Adults and pediatrics**	INR: 1–2 PT: 10–13 sec	
Critical value	>15 sec	Unless on warfarin
Natural substance?	Yes	
Inherent activity?	Indirect measurement of coagulation factors	
Location		
Production	Coagulation factors produced in liver	

Continued

Continued

PARAMETER	DESCRIPTION	COMMENTS
Storage	Carried in bloodstream	
Secretion/excretion	None	
Major causes of...		
Prolonged elevation	Liver failure	Liver unable to produce coagulation factors; does not correct with vitamin K
	Malabsorption or malnutrition	Vitamin K aids in synthesis of coagulation factors and is not absorbed; defect corrects with parenteral vitamin K
	Warfarin	Corrects with vitamin K
	Antibiotics	Interfere with vitamin K production or metabolism
Associated signs and symptoms	Increased risk of bleeding and ecchymoses	Easy bruising
Low results	None	
After insult, time to...		
Initial elevation or positive result	6–12 hr	
Peak values	Days to weeks	Depends on etiology
Normalization	4 hr if vitamin K responsive (due to malabsorption, maldigestion, warfarin, etc.) but 2–4 days if due to liver disease and liver disease reverses	
Drugs often monitored with test	Warfarin	
Causes of spurious results	Improper specimen collection	

PARAMETER	DESCRIPTION	COMMENTS
Common reference ranges		
Adults	Varies with assay	Elevated in pregnancy
Pediatrics	Varies; can be 2- to 3-fold higher than in adults	Elevated with developing bone
Natural substance?	Yes	Metabolic enzyme (intracellular)
Inherent activity?	Elevation alone causes no symptoms	Intracellular activity only
Location		
Production	Intracellular enzyme	
Storage	Liver, placenta, bone, small intestine, leukocytes	These tissues are rich in ALP
Secretion/excretion	None	
Major causes of...		
High or positive results	Cholestasis	Hepatic; associated with elevation of GGTP
	Bone	Paget's disease, bone tumors, rickets, osteomalacia, healing fracture
	Pregnancy	Placental ALP
	Childhood	Related to bone formation

Continued

PARAMETER	DESCRIPTION	COMMENTS
Associated signs and symptoms	Limited to underlying disorder	Reflects tissue or organ damage
Low results	Vitamin D intoxication Scurvy Hypothyroidism	
Associated signs and symptoms	Limited to underlying disorder	
After insult, time to... Initial elevation or positive result	Hours	
Peak values	Days	
Normalization	Days	Assumes insult removed and no ongoing damage
Drugs often monitored with test	None	
Causes of spurious results	Blood drawn after fatty meal and prolonged serum storage	

PARAMETER	DESCRIPTION	COMMENTS
Common reference ranges Adults	8–42 IU/L	Varies with assay
Newborns/infants	20–65 IU/L	Varies with assay
Critical value	>80 IU/L	2 times upper limit of normal
Natural substance?	Yes	Metabolic enzyme
Inherent activity?	None in serum	Intracellular activity only
Location Production	Intracellular enzyme	
Storage	Liver, cardiac muscle, kidneys, brain, pancreas, lungs	These tissues are rich in AST
Secretion/excretion	None	
Major causes of... High or positive results	Hepatitis	Elevated in any disease with hepatocyte inflammation (liver cells)
	Hemolysis Muscular diseases Myocardial infarction Renal infarction Pulmonary infarction Necrotic tumors	Elevated in any disease with damage to tissues rich in enzyme
Associated signs and symptoms	Varies with underlying disease	Reflects tissue or organ damage
Low results	None	

Continued

PARAMETER	DESCRIPTION	COMMENTS
After insult, time to... **Initial elevation or positive result**	2–6 hr	
Peak values	24–48 hr (without further cell damage)	With extensive liver or cellular damage, levels can go up to thousands
Normalization	24–48 hr	Assumes insult removed and no ongoing damage
Drugs often monitored with test	Isoniazid and cholesterol-lowering agents (e.g., lovastatin, allopurinol, ketoconazole, valproic acid, and methotrexate)	Monitoring frequency varies with drug
Causes of spurious results **Falsely elevated**	Heparin, levodopa, methyldopa, tolbutamide, *p*-aminosalicylic acid, erythromycin, diabetic ketoacidosis	
Falsely lowered	Metronidazole, trifluoperazine, vitamin B$_6$ deficiency	

PARAMETER	DESCRIPTION	COMMENTS
Common reference ranges **Adults**	3–30 IU/L	Varies with assay
Newborns	3–60 IU/L	Decreases to adult values within a few months
Critical value	>60 IU/L	Greater than 2 times normal limit
Natural substance?	Yes	Metabolic enzyme
Inherent activity?	None in serum	Intracellular activity only
Location **Production**	Intracellular enzyme	
Storage	Liver, muscle, heart, kidneys	These tissues are rich in ALT
Secretion/excretion		Normally contained intracellularly but, with cell damage, serum concentrations increase
Major causes of... **High or positive results**	Hepatitis	Elevated in any disease with hepatocyte inflammation (liver cells)
	Hemolysis Muscular diseases Myocardial infarction Renal infarction	Elevated in any disease with damage to tissues rich in enzymes
Associated signs and symptoms	Varies with underlying disease	Reflects tissue or organ damage
Low results	Patients deficient in Vitamin B$_6$	
Associated signs and symptoms	None	

Continued

PARAMETER	DESCRIPTION	COMMENTS
After insult, time to... Initial elevation or positive result	2–6 hr	
Peak values	24–48 hr (without further cell damage)	With extensive liver or cellular damage, levels can go up to thousands
Normalization	24–48 hr	Assumes insult removed and no ongoing damage
Drugs often monitored with test	Isoniazid and cholesterol-lowering agents (e.g., lovastatin, allopurinol, ketoconazole, valproic acid, and methotrexate)	Monitoring frequency varies with drug
Causes of spurious results	Heparin (false elevation)	

PARAMETER	DESCRIPTION	COMMENTS
Common reference ranges Adults	0.3–1.0 mg/dL	Varies slightly with assay
Pediatrics	2–6 mg/dL 6–8 mg/dL 0.3–1.3 mg/dL	24-hr infant 48-hr infant >1 month old
Critical value	>4 mg/dL	In adults
Natural substance?	Yes	By-product of Hgb metabolism
Inherent activity?	Yes	CNS irritant or toxin in high levels in newborn (not adult)
Location Production	Liver	
Storage	Gallbladder	Excreted into bile
Secretion/excretion	Stool and urine	Bilirubin and urobilinogen
Major causes of... High or positive results	Liver disease, both hepatocellular and cholestatic Hemolysis Metabolic abnormalities (e.g., Gilbert's syndrome)	
Associated signs and symptoms	Jaundice	
Low results	No important causes	
After insult, time to... Initial elevation or positive result	Hours	
Peak values	3–5 days	Assumes insult not removed
Normalization	Days	Assumes insult removed and no evolving damage
Drugs often monitored with test	None	
Causes of spurious results	Fasting, levodopa, phenelzine, methyldopa, ascorbic acid (false elevation)	

PARAMETER	DESCRIPTION	COMMENTS
Common reference ranges		
Adults and pediatrics	30–70 µg/dL	Varies with assay
Newborns	90–150 µg/dL	Varies with assay
Critical value	Varies, generally 1.5 upper limit of normal	
Natural substance?	Yes	Product of bacterial metabolism of protein (in gut)
Inherent activity?	Probably	Progressive deterioration in neurologic function
Location		
Production	In gut (by bacteria)	
Storage	None	
Secretion/excretion	Liver metabolizes to urea	Urea cycle; diminished in cirrhosis
Major causes of...		
High or positive results	Liver failure Reye's syndrome Metabolic abnormalities (urea cycle)	
Associated signs and symptoms	Hepatic encephalopathy	
Low results	No important causes	
After insult, time to...		
Initial elevation or positive result	Hours	
Peak values	No peak value; rises progressively	
Normalization	Days	After appropriate therapy or resolution of underlying liver disease
Drugs often monitored with test	Valproic acid	
Causes of spurious results	Sensitive test (discussed in text)	

Chapter **13**

ENDOCRINE DISORDERS

Eva M. Vivian

The endocrine system consists of hormones, that serve as regulators, which stimulate or inhibit a biological response to maintain homeostasis within the body. Endocrine disorders often result from a deficiency or excess of a hormone, resulting in an imbalance in the physiological functions of the body. Usually, negative feedback mechanisms regulate hormone concentrations (Figure 13-1). Therefore, laboratory assessment of an endocrine disorder is based on concentrations of a plasma hormone as well as on the integrity of the feedback mechanism regulating that hormone. In this chapter, the evaluation of the function of the thyroid, adrenal, and parathyroid glands serves as an example of these concepts.

This chapter also discusses how the relationship between a hormone (insulin) and a target substrate (glucose) serves as the basis for maintaining glycemic control. The relationship between vasopressin (antidiuretic hormone) and serum and urine osmolality is used to demonstrate the basis for the water deprivation test in diagnosing diabetes insipidus.

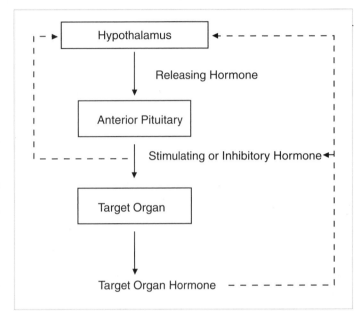

Figure 13-1. The hypothalamus may secrete a releasing hormone in response to low levels of stimulating, inhibitory or target organ hormone. This releasing hormone causes the release of a stimulating or inhibitory hormone that in turn controls the release of target organ hormone.

OBJECTIVES

After completing this chapter, the reader should be able to

1. Determine which patients should be screened for diabetes mellitus and what diagnostic tests should be employed.
2. Identify the subjective and objective data consistent with a diagnosis of type 1 and type 2 diabetes mellitus and relate this data to the pathogenesis of type 1 and type 2 diabetes mellitus.
3. Identify common medications or chemicals that may induce hyperglycemia or hypoglycemia.
4. Describe the use of glycosylated hemoglobin (A1C) and fructosamine tests as therapeutic monitoring tools.
5. Describe the actions of thyroxine (T_4), triiodothyronine (T_3), and thyroid-stimulating hormone (TSH) as well as the feedback mechanisms regulating them.
6. Explain the major differences between laboratory values found in diabetic ketoacidosis and in a hyperosmolar hyperglycemic state.
7. List the signs and symptoms associated with abnormally high and low concentrations of thyroid hormones.
8. Given a case description including thyroid function test results, identify the type of thyroid disorder and describe how tests are used to monitor and adjust related therapy.
9. Describe the relationship between urine osmolality, serum osmolality, and antidiuretic hormone.

DIABETES MELLITUS

This section discusses tests that assess glucose homeostasis as it relates to diabetes mellitus. The factors that can cause glucose concentrations to increase or decrease are also covered. Disorders assessed by these tests, normal glucose metabolism and homeostasis will be discussed.

Glucose Homeostasis

Glucose serves as the fuel for most cellular functions and is necessary to sustain life. Carbohydrates ingested from a meal are metabolized in the body into glucose. Glucose is absorbed from the gastrointestinal tract into the bloodstream where it is utilized in skeletal muscle for energy.

Glucose is also stored in the liver in the form of glycogen (glycogenesis) and is converted in adipose tissue to fats and triglycerides (lipogenesis). Insulin, which is produced, stored, and released from beta cells of the pancreas, facilitates these anabolic processes. The liver, skeletal muscle, and adipose tissue are the main tissues affected by insulin. To induce glucose uptake, insulin must bind to specific cell-surface receptors. Most secreted insulin is taken up by the liver, while the remainder is metabolized by the kidneys. About 80% of glucose uptake is independent of insulin. These insulin-independent cells include nerve tissue, red blood cells (RBCs), mucosal cells of the gastrointestinal (GI) tract, and exercising skeletal muscle.

In the fasting state, insulin levels decrease, resulting in an increase in glycogen breakdown by the liver (glycogenolysis) and an increase in free fatty acids into ketone bodies (lipolysis).

When glucose concentrations fall below 70 mg/dL, an event known as *hypoglycemia* occurs resulting in the release of glucagon by the alpha cells of the pancreas. Glucagon stimulates the formation of glucose in the liver (gluconeogenesis) and glycogenolysis. Glucagon also facilitates the breakdown of stored triglycerides in adipose tissue into fatty acids (lipolysis), which can be used for energy in the liver and skeletal muscle. In addition to glucagon secretion, hypoglycemia leads to secretion of counterregulatory hormones such as epinephrine, cortisol, and growth hormone. Glucagon and, to a lesser degree, epinephrine promote an immediate breakdown of glycogen and the synthesis of glucose by the liver. Cortisol increases glucose levels by stimulating gluconeogenesis. Growth hormone inhibits the uptake of glucose by tissues when glucose levels fall below 70 mg/dL.

In summary, glucose concentrations are affected by any factor that can influence glucose production, insulin production, or secretion. Fasting suppresses the rate of insulin secretion, and feasting generally increases insulin secretion. Increased insulin secretion lowers serum glucose concentrations, while decreased secretion raises glucose concentrations.[1-4]

Hyperglycemia

The classification of diabetes mellitus is standardized. This disorder may be divided into

- Type 1 diabetes mellitus (type 1 DM) (formally known as insulin-dependent diabetes mellitus (IDDM).
- Type 2 diabetes mellitus (type 2 DM) (formerly known as adult onset or noninsulin dependent diabetes mellitus).[5]

Type 1 DM is characterized by a lack of endogenous insulin, predisposition to ketoacidosis, and an abrupt onset. Some patients present with ketoacidosis after experiencing polyuria, polyphagia, and polydipsia for several days. Typically, this type of diabetes mellitus is diagnosed in juveniles but may also occur at a later age. In contrast, patients with type 2 DM are not normally dependent on exogenous insulin to sustain life and are not ketosis prone,

TABLE 13-1

CHARACTERISTICS	TYPE 1	TYPE 2
Age of onset	Childhood or adolescence	>40 years old
Rapidness of onset	Abrupt	Gradual
Family studies	Increased prevalence of type 1	Increased prevalence of type 2
Body weight	Usually thin and undernourished	Obesity is common
Islet cell antibodies and pancreatic cell-mediated immunity	Yes	No
Ketosis	Common	Uncommon; if present associated with severe stress or infection
Insulin	Markedly diminished early in disease or totally absent	Levels may be low, normal or high (indicating insulin resistance)
Symptoms	Polyuria, polydipsia, polyphagia, weight loss	May be asymptomatic; polyuria, polydipsia, polyphagia may be present

Table 13-1. General Characteristics of Type 1 and Type 2 Diabetes

but they are usually obese and are more than 40 years old. There is an alarming increase in the number of juveniles diagnosed with type 2 DM. Although there is a genetic predisposition to the development of type 2 DM, environmental factors such as high-fat diets and sedentary lifestyles contribute to the disorder. Type 2 DM patients are both insulin deficient and insulin resistant (Table 13-1).

Many type 2 DM patients are asymptomatic so diagnosis often depends on laboratory studies. Concentrations of ketone bodies in the blood and urine are typically low or absent, even in the presence of hyperglycemia. This finding is common because the lack of insulin is not severe enough to lead to abnormalities in lipolysis and significant ketosis or acidosis.

Because of the chronicity of asymptomatic type 2 DM, many patients with type 2 DM present with evidence of microvascular complications (neuropathy, nephropathy, and retinopathy) and macrovascular complications (coronary artery, cerebral vascular, and peripheral vascular disease) at the time of diagnosis. Type 2 DM is often identified incidentally during glucose screening sponsored by hospitals and other health care institutions.[1,2]

Patients with gestational diabetes, a third type of glucose intolerance, develop this condition during pregnancy. Patients with gestational diabetes have a 30%–50% chance of developing type 2 DM.[6] A woman with diabetes who becomes pregnant is not included in this category.

Pathophysiology

Type 1 DM usually develops in childhood or early adulthood and accounts for up to 10% of all patients with diabetes. Patients are usually thin, have an absolute lack of insulin and require exogenous insulin to prevent diabetic ketoacidosis (DKA) and sustain life. Genetics as well as environmental and immune factors are the major factors thought to cause type 1 diabetes.

Over 90% of all type 1 DM patients have a combination of human leukocyte antigen (HLA)-DQ coded genes, which increase the risk of developing type 1 DM. Type 1 DM may result from a trigger, which could be environmental or viral. Viral infections may stimulate monocytes and macrophages that activate T cells, which attack beta cells, thereby decreasing insulin production. Bovine serum albumin has also been identified as an environmental

TABLE 13-2

Diuretics	Steroids/hormones
Chlorthalidone	Estrogens
Loop diuretics[a]	Glucocorticoids
Metolazone	Oral contraceptives[d]
Thiazides	Thyroid hormones
Antihypertensives	**Miscellaneous drugs**
Calcium antagonists[b]	Amiodarone[b]
Clonidine[b]	L-Asparaginase
Diazoxide	Epinephrine[e]
	Lithium[b]
Phenothiazines[b]	Nicotinic acid
	Pentamidine[f]
Pyriminil[c]	Phenytoin
	Streptozocin

[a] Loop diuretics are furosemide, bumetanide, and ethacrynic acid. Torsemide has less effect on glucose concentrations.[52]
[b] Clinical significance is less clear.
[c] A rodenticide.
[d] Progestin-only products do not affect glucose tolerance.
[e] Oral sympathomimetics, such as those found in decongestants, are unlikely to be more of a cause of increased glucose than the "stress" from the illness for which they are used.
[f] After initial hypoglycemia, which occurs in about 4–14 (average 11) days.

Table 13-2. Medications and Chemicals that May Cause Hyperglycemia[11–14,46]

trigger. Therefore, it is believed that exposure to cow's milk may increase the risk of developing type 1 DM in patients with a genetic predisposition. An immunologic attack against insulin may also occur. The combination of an autoimmune attack on beta cells and on circulating insulin results in insulin insufficiency.[7–9]

Type 2 DM occurs due to insulin resistance and insulin deficiency. During the early stages of type 2 DM, the ability of insulin to facilitate the diffusion of glucose into the cell is impaired. Defects in insulin receptor function, insulin receptor-signal transduction pathway, glucose transport and phosphorylation, and glucogen synthesis and oxidation contribute to muscle insulin resistance. The pancreas compensates for this deficiency by secreting larger amounts of insulin. Patients remain euglycemic until the pancreatic beta cells are no longer able to compensate for the insulin resistance. Hence, insulin is unable to suppress hepatic glucose production and hyperglycemia results (Figure13-2).[1,10,11]

Insulin resistance of muscle tissue and impaired hepatic glycogen production contribute almost equally to the excessive postprandial increase in the plasma glucose level. Impaired insulin secretion also plays a major role in the pathogenesis of glucose intolerance. In summary, patients with type 2 DM are characterized by defects in both insulin action at target tissues and insulin secretion.[1]

Secondary Causes

Diabetes mellitus may be the result of other pancreatic and hormonal diseases, medications, and abnormalities of the insulin receptor.[11]

Pancreatic cell destruction may be related to diseases, such as cystic fibrosis, or autoimmune conditions. It can be related to drugs (e.g., L-asparaginase, streptozocin, and pentamidine). Similarly, hyperglycemia may result from hormonal disease in which concentrations of circulating catecholamines and glucocorticoids are increased (e.g., catecholamine-secreting pheochromocytoma and Cushing's disease, respectively).[7]

Various medications or chemicals may induce hyperglycemia and glucose intolerance. However, potassium-sparing diuretics have little or no effect on glucose levels. Beta-adrenergic blocking agents may increase or impair insulin secretion in patients with diabetes. Beta-adrenergic blocking agents may decrease glycogenolysis and gluconeogenesis. Diazoxide and phenytoin may decrease insulin secretion resulting in increased glucose levels. Thiazides and loop diuretics may cause hyperglycemia by an unknown mechanism.

Estrogen products influence glucose tolerance to varying degrees, depending on the formulation. In one study, women taking combination oral contraceptives for at least 3 months had plasma glucose concentrations 43–61% higher than controls.[12] Monophasic and triphasic com-

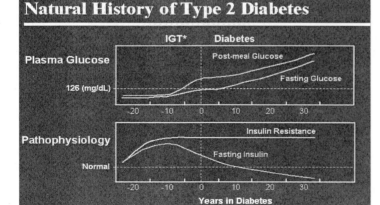

Natural History of Type 2 Diabetes

*IGT = impaired glucose tolerance.
Adapted from International Diabetes Center (IDC), Minneapolis, Minnesota.

Figure 13-2. In the early stages of type 2 DM, the pancreatic beta cells compensate for insulin resistance by secreting more insulin. Over time, these cells burn out resulting in insulin deficiency and hyperglycemia.

bination products diminished glucose tolerance, whereas progestin-only products did not. Insulin resistance was the proposed mechanism, and fasting plasma glucose concentrations were not adversely affected. Table 13-2 lists medications with the potential to cause hyperglycemia.

Laboratory Tests to Assess Glucose Control

The two most common methods used for evaluating glucose homeostasis are the fasting plasma glucose and 2-hr postprandial glucose tests. The oral glucose tolerance test is mainly used to assess equivocal results from these two tests. Glycosylated hemoglobin (A1C) and fructosamine tests are used to monitor long- and medium-term glucose control, respectively. Urine glucose monitoring in patients with diabetes mellitus has been replaced by fingerstick blood glucose tests. Therefore, discussion of this test is relatively brief.

With all of these tests, proper collection and storage of the sample and performance of the procedure are important; improper collection and storage of samples for glucose determinations can lead to false results and interpretations. After collection, RBCs and white blood cells (WBCs) continue to metabolize glucose in the sample tube. This process occurs unless (1) the RBCs can be separated from the serum using serum separator tubes, or (2) metabolism is inhibited using sodium fluoride-containing (gray-top) tubes or refrigeration. Without such precautions, glucose concentration drops by 5–10 mg/dL (0.3–0.6 mmol/L) per hour and does not reflect the patient's fasting plasma glucose at collection time. In vitro, metabolic loss is hastened in samples of patients with leukocytosis or leukemia.[13]

Fasting Plasma Glucose and 2-Hr Postprandial Glucose

The categories of fasting plasma glucose (FPG) values are as follows:

- FPG <110 mg/dL (5.5 mmol/L) represents normal fasting glucose.
- FPG ≥100 (5.5 mmol/L) and <126 mg/dL (7.0 mmol/L) represents *prediabetes* (previously termed *impaired fasting glucose IFG*).
- FPG ≥126 mg/dL (7.0 mmol/L) represents provisional diagnosis of diabetes (the diagnosis must be confirmed as described below).[5]

A fasting plasma glucose concentration is the best indicator of glucose homeostasis. This test measures the ability of endogenous or exogenous insulin to prevent fasting hyperglycemia by regulating glucose anabolism and catabolism. Fasting plasma glucose may be used to monitor therapy in patients being treated for glucose abnormalities. For this test, the patient maintains his or her usual diet, and the assay is performed on awakening (before breakfast). This timing usually allows for an 8-hr fast.

TABLE 13-3

Level of Glucose Tolerance	**VENOUS PLASMA GLUCOSE**[a] **(mg/dL)**			
	Fasting Plasma Glucose	OGTT Value at 30, 60, or 90 min	OGTT Value at 2 hr	OGTT Value at 3 hr
"Normal"	<100	<200	<140	
Prediabetes	100–125	>200	140–199	
Diabetes mellitus	>126	>200	≥200	
Gestational diabetes	<95	>180 (1 hr)	>155	>140

[a] *Multiply number by 0.056 to convert glucose to International System (SI) units (mmol/L).*

Table 13-3. Diagnosis of Glucose Tolerance Based on Fasting Plasma Glucose Concentration and Oral Glucose Tolerance Test (OGTT)[5]

A fasting plasma glucose greater than 126 mg/dL (>7.0 mmol/L), found on at least two occasions, is diagnostic for diabetes mellitus (Table 13-3).

The diagnosis of diabetes mellitus usually can be made if the 2-hr postprandial glucose is equal to or greater than 200 mg/dL (>11.2 mmol/L), especially if previous tests reveal fasting hyperglycemia (Table 13-3).[14]

The ADA recommends that adults ≥45 years of age should be screened for diabetes mellitus every 3 years. Individuals who have a body mass index ≥25 kg/m² with additional risk factors such as polycystic ovary syndrome, vascular disease, hypertension, dyslipidemia, as well as members of high-risk groups (e.g., Native-Americans, Latino/Hispanics, African-Americans, Pacific Islanders, and women with a prior history of gestational diabetes mellitus) should be screened at an earlier age.[5,6] The American College of Endocrinology recommends screening individuals from high-risk groups at 30 years of age.[15]

Oral Glucose Tolerance Test

The categories for the oral glucose tolerance test (OGTT) are as follows:

- 2-hr postload glucose (PG), 140 mg/dL represents normal glucose tolerance.
- 2-hr PG 140–200 mg/dL represents prediabetes (previously termed impaired glucose tolerance (IGT).
- 2-hr PG ≥200 mg/dL represents provisional diagnosis of diabetes (the diagnosis must be confirmed as described above).

The oral glucose tolerance test is used to assess patients who have signs and symptoms of diabetes mellitus but whose FPG is normal or suggests prediabetes (<126 mg/dL or <7.0 mmol/L). The oral glucose tolerance test measures both the ability of the pancreas to secrete insulin following a glucose load and the body's response to insulin action. Interpretation of the test is based on the plasma glucose concentrations drawn before and during the exam. This exam may also be used in diagnosing diabetes with onset during pregnancy if the disease threatens the health of the mother and fetus. The oral glucose tolerance test is not required for patients who have fasting plasma glucose greater than 126 mg/dL on at least two separate occasions as such values confirm the diagnosis of diabetes mellitus.

The oral glucose tolerance test is performed by giving a standard 75-g dose of an oral glucose solution over 5 min following an overnight fast. The pediatric dose is 1.75 g/kg up to a maximum of 75 g. Blood samples commonly are drawn before the test, between 0 and 2 hr, and at 2 hr. The samples should be collected into tubes containing sodium fluoride, unless the assay will be performed immediately.[13]

If the patient vomits the test dose, the exam is invalid and must be repeated. The oral glucose tolerance test is diagnostic for diabetes mellitus if the 2-hr plasma glucose is at least 200 mg/dL (11.2 mmol/L). The patient is considered to have prediabetes if the 2-hr concentration is 140–200 mg/dL (7.8–11.2 mmol/L).

In pregnant women, a screening test is performed that measures plasma glucose 1 hr after a 50g oral glucose load. If the plasma glucose level is >130 mg/dL, then a 100-g oral glucose load is performed after an overnight fast. Plasma glucose concentrations are drawn before the test (fasting) and at 1-, 2-, and 3-hr intervals.[6] The threshold values for the fasting and the 1-, 2-, and 3-hr levels are 95 mg/dL, 180 mg/dL, 155 mg/dL, and 140 mg/dL, respectively. If two or more of the serum plasma glucose levels exceed the threshold, then a diagnosis of gestational diabetes can be made.

The oral glucose tolerance test should not be performed on individuals who are chronically malnourished, consume inadequate carbohydrates (<150 g/day), or are bedridden. Alcohol consumption and medications that cause hyperglycemia (Table 13-2) should be stopped 3 days prior to the examination. Coffee and smoking are not permitted during the test.[11]

Glycosylated Hemoglobin

Normal range: 4–6%

A1C (formally referred to as HbA_{1c}), also known as glycosylated or glycated A1C, is a component of the hemoglobin molecule. During the 120-day lifespan of an RBC, glucose is irreversibly bound to the hemoglobin moieties in proportion to the average serum glucose. The process is called *glycosylation*. Measurement of A1C is, therefore, indicative of glucose control during the preceding 2–3 months. The entire hemoglobin A_1 molecule—composed of A_{1a}, A_{1b}, and A_{1c}—is not used because subfractions A_{1a} and A_{1b} are more susceptible to nonglucose adducts in the blood of patients with opiate addiction, lead poisoning, uremia, and alcoholism.[15] Because the test is for hemoglobin, the specimen analyzed are RBCs and not serum or plasma.

Results are not affected by daily fluctuations in the blood glucose concentration, and a fasting sample is not required. Results can reflect overall patient compliance to various treatment regimens. With most assays, 95% of normal individuals' hemoglobin is 4–6% glycated. An A1C greater than 7% suggests poor glucose control. However, patients with persistent hyperglycemia may have an A1C up to 20% (Table 13-4).[16]

The mean daily plasma glucose concentration can be estimated with the formula $10 \times (A1C + 4)$.[15] Reference ranges and interpretations vary with the assay method.

A few situations confound interpretation of test results. False elevations in A1C may be noted with uremia, chronic alcohol intake, and hypertriglyceridemia.[17] Patients who have diseases with chronic or episodic hemolysis (e.g., sickle cell disease and thalassemia) generally have spuriously low A1C concentrations caused by the predominance of young RBCs (which carry less A1C) in the circulation. In splenectomized patients and those with polycythemia, A1C is increased. If these disorders are stable, the test still can be used, but values must be compared with the patient's previous results rather than published normal values. Both falsely elevated and falsely lowered measurements of A1C may also occur during pregnancy. Therefore, it should not be used to screen for gestational diabetes.

Affinity chromatography and colorimetric assay methods measure total glycosylated hemoglobin including subfractions A_{1a} and A_{1b}. Ion-exchange chromatography and high-performance liquid chromatography only measure the subfraction. The Cholestech GDX® and Metrika's A1CNow® are portable analyzers, which provide A1C results within 5–8 min.[19]

The ADA recommends A1C testing 1–2 times a year for patients with good glycemic control and quarterly in patients with poor control or whose therapy has changed.[5]

TABLE 13-4

A1C (%)	MEAN PLASMA GLUCOSE (mg/dL)	mmoL/L
5	100	5.5
6	135	7.5
7	170	9.5
8	205	11.5
9	240	13.5
10	275	15.5
11	310	17.5
12	345	19.5

ᵃAdapted from Reference 20.

Table 13-4. Correlation between A1C Level and Mean Plasma Glucose Levels

Fructosamine

Normal range: <285 μmol/L but varies

Fructosamine is a general term that is applied to any glycosylated protein. Unlike the A1C test, only glycosylated proteins in the serum or plasma (e.g., albumin)—not erythrocytes—are measured. In nondiabetics, the unstable complex dissociates into glucose and protein. Therefore, only small quantities of fructosamine circulate. In patients with diabetes, higher glucose concentrations favor the generation of more stable glycation, and higher concentrations of fructosamine are found.

Fructosamine has no known inherent toxicological activity but can be used as a marker of medium-term glucose control. Fructosamine correlates with glucose control over 2–3 weeks based on the half-lives of albumin (14–20 days) and other serum proteins (2.5–23 days). As a result, high fructosamine concentrations may alert caregivers to deteriorating glycemic control earlier than increases in Hgb A_{1c}.

Several limitations to this test exist. Falsely elevated results may occur when

- Serum (not whole blood) hemoglobin concentrations are greater than 100 mg/dL (normally <15 mg/dL).

- Serum bilirubin is greater than 4 mg/dL.
- Serum ascorbic acid is greater than 5 mg/dL.[20]

Methyldopa and calcium dobesilate (the latter is used outside the United States) to minimize myocardial damage after an acute infarction may also cause falsely elevated results. Serum fructosamine concentrations are lower in obese patients with diabetes compared to lean patients with diabetes.[21] Some clinicians advocate the use of fructosamine concentrations as a monitoring tool for short-term changes in glycemic control (e.g., gestational DM). More clinical studies are required to determine if this test provides useful clinical information.[22,23]

Urine Glucose

Normal range: negative

Glucose "spills" into the urine when the serum glucose concentration exceeds the renal threshold for glucose reabsorption (normally 180 mg/dL). However, poor correlation exists between urine glucose and concurrent serum glucose concentrations. This poor correlation occurs because urine is "produced" hours before it is tested, unless the inconvenient double-void method (urine is collected 30 min after emptying of the bladder) is used. Furthermore, the renal threshold varies among patients and tends to increase in diabetes over time, especially if renal function is declining.

Urine testing gradually has been replaced by convenient fingerstick blood sugar testing, Urine glucose testing should be recommended only if the patient is unable or unwilling to perform blood glucose monitoring.[24]

The presence and amount of glucose in the urine can be determined by two different techniques. Commercial products that use copper-reducing methods (e.g., Clinitest®) provide the most quantitative estimate of the degree of glycosuria. Therefore, this method is preferred for patients who spill large quantities of glucose into the urine. The two-drop method can detect higher quantities of glucose (3–5%) than the five-drop method, which can quantitate up to only 2%. Generally, copper-reducing products have poor specificity for glucose.

Contrary to popular belief, isoniazid, methyldopa, and ascorbic acid do not interfere with Clinitest®. The literature is unclear on whether chloral hydrate, nitrofurantoin, probenecid, and nalidixic acid interfere with this method.

Patients should be aware that a "pass-through" phenomenon occurs with this test when more than 2% glucose is in the urine. During the test, a fleeting orange color may appear at the climax of the reaction and fade to a greenish-brown when the reaction is complete. The latter color (0.75–1%) may be incorrectly used to assess glucose levels, and the glucose concentration actually may be underestimated.

The second method of urine glucose testing is specific for glucose and provides a more qualitative assessment of it in the urine. Commercial products of this type (e.g., Tes-Tape®, Clinistix®, Diastix®, and Chemstrip®) consist of plastic dipsticks with paper pads that have been impregnated with glucose oxidase. These tests are sensitive to 0.1% glucose (100 mg/dL). Substances that may cause false-negative results with this type of test include ascorbic acid (high dose), salicylates (high dose), and levodopa. Interference also has been reported with phenazopyridine and radiographic contrast media, but the likelihood is less clear.[25]

Self-Monitoring Tests

Glucometers and reagent strips are commercially available so that patients may perform blood glucose monitoring at home. These systems are also used frequently in hospitals, where nurses rely on quick results for determining insulin requirements. The glucometers currently marketed are lightweight, relatively inexpensive, accurate, and user-friendly. These glucometers and reagent strips are based on the ability of glucose oxidase to generate hydrogen peroxide. The reagent strips may be used with or without a colorimeter. Manual or automatic lancet injectors are used to obtain a capillary blood sample from a fingerstick. The blood droplet is placed on a reagent strip, and the color that appears is compared to a color chart corresponding to specific blood glucose values. Use of a colorimeter eliminates the need to estimate the color match and provides the result on a digital display.

Glucometers can be divided into two generations: reflectance photometry and electrochemical. The first generation glucometers use a photometric analysis that is based on a dye-related reaction. This method, also termed reflectance photometry, light reflectance, or enzyme photometric, involves a chemical reaction between the capillary blood and a chemical on the strip that produces a change in color. The amount of color reflected from the strip is measured photometrically. The reflected color is directly related to the amount of glucose in the blood. The darker color the test strip, the higher the glucose concentration. First generation glucometers include Glucometer Encore®, SureStep®, One Touch Basic®, Accucheck-Easy®, One Touch Profile®, and Accucheck Instant® (Table 13-5).

Second generation glucometers utilize an electrochemical or enzyme electrode process, which determine glucose levels by measuring an electric charge produced by the glucose-reagent reaction. These second generation glucometers can further be subdivided according to the electrochemical principle used: colorimetry or amperometry. Amperometry biosensor technology requires a large sample size (4–10 µL). Furthermore, alterations in temperature or hematocrit levels may result in inaccurate results with this method. Glucometers that employ the amperometry method include the following: Glucometer Elite®, Accu-Check Complete®, and Accu-Check Advantage F Exact Tech R.S.G® (Table 13-5).

The colorimetry method involves converting the glucose sample into an electrochemical charge, which is then captured for measurement. An advantage of this system is that a small amount of blood (e.g., 0.3 mL) is enough to determine the blood glucose level. The colorimetry method is not influenced by changes in temperature and hematocrit levels. These monitors can use blood samples extracted from the arm and thigh too. At these alternative sites, there are fewer capillaries and nerve endings, allowing for a less painful stick. Some examples of second generation glucometers that use the colorimetry method include the following: Amira Atlast®, One Touch Ultra®, Freestyle®, and Softtact® (Table 13-5).

The GlucoWatch® is a new blood glucose device that is worn on the wrist like a watch. This device is virtually painless because it measures fluid (interstitial fluid) directly beneath the skin where there are few nerve endings. Blood glucose readings (based on the enzyme electrode method) are provided every 20 min for up to 12 hr. Blood glucose values are displayed on the device. The Glucowatch® will alarm if there is a critically low or high reading. Although this system requires daily calibration with a conventional glucometer and warm-up periods up to 3 hr, it provides continuous measurement for up to 12 hr.[26,27]

While new glucometers report plasma values, older meters may report whole blood values, which are approximately 10–15% lower than plasma values. The ADA recommends whole blood fasting readings of 80–120 mg/dL and bedtime readings between 100–140 mg/dL. Plasma fasting readings should be between 90–130 mg/dL and bedtime readings between 110–140 mg/dL.

Most, if not all, hydrogen peroxide-based blood glucometers are not affected by ascorbic acid, hemoglobin, acetaminophen, serum creatinine, bilirubin, uric acid, heparin, and high-lipid concentrations. The only exception is high-dose ascorbic acid, which may falsely suppress glucose readings with some equipment (e.g., Glucostix). With some machines, swabbing the finger with iodine can falsely elevate the reading. Conversely, dopamine infusions can lead to falsely low readings. The ExacTech Pen®, Companion®, Pen 2®, Companion 2®,

TABLE 13-5

TYPE OF GLUCO-METER	NAME & MANUFACTURER	WEIGHT (oz.)	RANGE (mg/dL)	TEST STRIP USED	TEST TIME (in sec.)	PLASMA vs. WHOLE BLOOD
Reflectance	Accu-Chek Active *RD	1.56	10–600	Accu-Chek Active	5	Plasma
Electrochemical	Accu-Chek Advantage *RD	2.10	10–600	Accu-Chek Advantage or *CC	26	Plasma
Reflectance	Accu-Chek Compact *RD	4.2	10–600	Accu-Chek Compact	15	Plasma
Electrochemical	Accu-Chek Complete *RD	4.4	10–600	Accu-Chek Advantage or *CC	26	Plasma
Electrochemical	Accu-Chek Voicemate *RD	10.94	10–600	Accu-Chek *CC	30	Plasma
Electrochemical	Ascensia DEX 2 Diabetes *CSBC	2.8	20–600	Ascensia Autodisc	30	Plasma
Electrochemical	Ascensia Elite Diabetes *CSBC	1.75	20–600	Ascensia Elite	30	Plasma
Electrochemical	Ascensia Elite XL Diabetes *CSBC	2.1	20–600	Ascensia Elite	30	Plasma
Electrochemical	Assure (Hypoguard)	5.3	30–550	Assure	35	Plasma
Electrochemical	Assure II (Hypoguard)	2.2	30–550	Assure II	30	Plasma
Reflectance	CardioChek (Polymer Technology Systems, Inc.)	4.3	20–600	PTS Panel Glucose	30–60	Plasma
Reflectance	Checkmate Plus Blood Glucose (QuestStar Medical)	3.5	25–500	Focus	15–35	Plasma or Whole Blood
Electrochemical	Freestyle (Therasense)	2.4	20–500	Freestyle	15	Plasma
Electrochemical	Freestyle Tracker (Therasense)	1.3	20–500	Freestyle	15	Plasma
Electrochemical	Hypoguard Advance (Hypoguard)	1.5	20–600	Hypoguard Advance	15	Plasma
Electrochemical	Precision Q.I.D. (Abbott Laboratories)	1.7	20–600	MediSense 2 or Precision Q.I.D.	20	Plasma
Electrochemical	Prec. Q.I.D. Pen Sensor *AL	1.1	20–600	MediSense 2 or Precision Q.I.D.	20	Plasma
	MiniMed CGMS (Cont. Glucose Monitoring Syst.) (Medtronic MiniMed)	4.0	40–400	None	300	Plasma
Reflectance	OneTouch Basic (Lifescan)	4.1	0–600	One Touch	45	Whole Blood
Electrochemical	One Touch FastTake	1.6	20–600	One Touch FastTake	15	Plasma
Electrochemical	One Touch InDuo (Lifescan)	4.4	20–600	One Touch Ultra	5	Plasma
Reflectance	One Touch Profile (Lifescan)	4.5	0–600	One Touch	45	Whole Blood
Reflectance	One Touch Surestep (Lifescan)	3.8	0–500	Surestep	15–30	Plasma
Electrochemical	One Touch Ultra (Lifescan)	1.5	20–600	One Touch Ultra	5	Plasma
Reflectance	Prestige IQ (Home Diag.)	3.6	25–600	Prestige Smart System	10–15	Plasma or Whole Blood
Reflectance	Prestige LX (Home Diag.)	4.9	25–600	Prestige Smart System	10–50	Plasma or *WB
Electrochemical	Precision Xtra (*AL, MediSense Prod.)	2.76	20–500	Precision Xtra	20	Plasma
Reflectance	QuickTek (Hypoguard)	2.1	20–600	QuickTek	10–30	Plasma
Electrochemical	Reli-On (Wal-Mart Pharm.)	1.5	20–600	ReliOn	20	Plasma or *WB
Electrochemical	Sof-Tact Diabetes Mgt. System (Abbott Laboratories, MediSense Products)	11	30–450	Sof-Tact	20	Plasma
Reflectance	Supreme II (Hypoguard)	4.7	30–600	Supreme	50	Plasma or *WB

KEY for Abbreviations

*AL = Abbott Laboratories   ***CC** = Comfort Curve   ***CSBC** = Care System (Bayer Corporation)   ***RD** = Roche Diagnostics
*WB = Whole Blood

Continued on next page

CLEANING REQUIRED	MEMORY (# of READINGS)	FEATURES
Yes	200	Fast test time (5 sec), small sample size, meter turns on automatically with the insertion of the test strip
No	100	Small sample size, memory includes date and time
Yes	100	Storage of drum inside monitor, fast test time (15 sec), memory includes date and time, 7 day test average, downloads into Accu-Chek Compass software
No	1000	Two step test procedure, good memory storage (1000), software available to upload data into personal computer
No	100	For blind or visually impaired, clear step-by-step, voice-activated guide; touchable strips, portable, time/date displayed; identifies Lilly brand of insulin
No	100	Disc-based monitor eliminates test strip handling, performs 10 tests without reloading, automatic calibration for every 10 tests, sensor automatically draws just enough blood needed, downloads memory for PC tracking, provides average daily values
No	20	No buttons, turns on when strip inserted, 3-min automatic shutoff, instructional videotape available on request
No	120	No buttons, turns on when strip inserted, 3-min automatic shutoff, 14-day average, instructional videotape available on request
No	180	Data management system, biosensor technology, large touch screen display, download memory for PC tracking
No	10	Large display, 2 step testing, automatic on/off, large test strip, capillary action, small sample size
Yes	300	Multiple blood chemistry testing including glucose, total cholesterol, ketones, triglycerides, and HDL; internal result storage and review, 3 step procedure, auto or manual shutoff, sold over-the-counter
Yes	225	Hands-off automation calibration, display has word prompts for guidance, automatic hematocrit and temperature corrections for accuracy, automatically accuracy, automatically checks sample volume check, averages glucose test results, stores results with date and time, insulin type and dosage, dataport allows for PC downloading; prompts in 10 different languages
Yes	250	Small sample size, arm or finger testing
Yes	250	Combines a blood glucose meter, diabetes manager, and personal digital assistant (PDA) in one compact device, small sample blood glucose testing for painless monitoring, tracks and stores diabetes information, displays data in various formats to enable easier under standing and management, provides easy access to a 2500 item food list with serving sizes and carbohydrate values
No	100	Large display, 2 step test, automatic on/off, compact meter with carrying case, 14 day average; results can be downloaded for PC use
No	10	Credit card size, very large display window, biosensor technology, automatic start with hands-off testing, individually wrapped test strips
No	10	Biosensor technology, automatic star with hands-off testing, pen size, individually wrapped tested strips
Yes	864	**For physician-supervised use, not long-term self-care;** sensor may be used up to 3 days, test glucose for continuous monitoring with an average glucose every 5 min; device worn like a pager; system not affected by sweat, temperature, or drug use; data is retrospective and cannot be assessed while patient is wearing the device
Yes	75	Optimal display of date and time, 3 step testing; large, easy-to-handle test strips, single button coding
No	150	Date and time displayed, 14 day average, alternate site testing
No	150	Combined glucose and insulin dosing testing system, alternate testing sites (arm or finger), small sample size, 14–30 day testing average, has dataport for PC downloading
Yes	250	Large display in 17 different languages (including English and Spanish); 3 step testing, notifies patient when monitor needs to be cleaned, 14–30 day test average, insulin programming
Yes	150	Single button testing, blue dot confirms sample test, touchable test average, data downloading ability
No	150	Less painful alternate site testing, fast test time (5 sec), tiny blood sample, small meter size, memory includes date and time, 14 and 30 day test averaging, warning to check ketones at 240–600 mg/dL
Yes	365	Large display, 14–30 day test average, sample size confirmation on back of test strip; internet upload ability so patients can graph, track, record, and share their results
Yes	365	Large display, 3 step procedure, sample size confirmation on the back of test strip
No	450	Measures glucose and ketones, fill-trigger ensures proper sample size, not affected by common medications, lighting features for low lit areas; memory includes date and time with 1-, 2-, and 4-week average; can measure ketone levels
Yes	250	Large display, compact meter, memory includes date and time, 2 step procedure; results can be downloaded to PC
No	365	Biosensor testing, wallet size carrying case automatic start; no dataport available
Yes	450	Testing can be done on forearm and upper arm, memory includes date and time with a 1-, 2-, and 4-week average, preload feature allow patients to preload test strips 8 hr in advance; no separate lancing device; results can be downloaded to PC
Yes	100	Large display, universal symbols

[a]Adapted from *Blood glucose monitors and data management. Diabetes Forecast Resource Guide 2003. Pages 43–53.*

Table 13-5. Blood Glucose Monitors[a]

LAURA O., A 5-FT 5-IN, 195-LB., 58-YEAR-OLD FEMALE, visited a community walk-in clinic for the first time with complaints of weakness and polyuria worsening over the past few weeks. Because she had to go to the bathroom often during the past few nights, she did not sleep much and was exhausted. She has no steady health care provider in the area. Her past medical history included hypertension (treated with hydrochlorothiazide 25 mg daily) and a 10-year history of glaucoma (treated with timolol 0.5% eye drops). She also had taken estrogen and calcium carbonate for the past 8 years. She gained 30 pounds over the past year, and a calorie estimate revealed that she took in about 2800 kcal/day.

Laura O. had no known family history of diabetes. Her physical exam was normal, except for slightly dry skin, legs cool to touch with weak pedal pulses, and slightly diminished pedal pinprick sensation. Her vital signs were BP 110/60, temperature 97.5 °F (36.4 °C), HR 60/min, and respiration rate 20/min. A dipstick of her urine was normal, except for 1+ (30 mg/dL) protein and trace (100 mg/dL) glucose. A fingerstick blood glucose was 180 mg/dL 2 hr after breakfast.

Four days later, Laura O. visited the clinic again because her symptoms were not any better even though she followed directions. Her fasting plasma glucose (no food for 8 hr) was 210 mg/dL. Her BUN and SCr from the previous visit were normal at 15 and 1.2 mg/dL, respectively, as were all other chemistries (including uric acid and lipids). Her urine glucose was 250 mg/dL with negative ketones, and she still had 1+ proteinuria. Her specific gravity was normal at 1.010.

Question: Is there enough evidence for a definitive diagnosis of diabetes at this time? Are there any factors contributing to the hyperglycemia that may be corrected in the short-term? In the long-term?

Discussion: Laura O. seems to have symptoms associated with diabetes. Her picture is clear based solely on the first two criteria for diagnosis of diabetes mellitus. She had classic symptoms and a blood glucose concentration of 180 mg/dL on her first visit. She was spilling small amounts of glucose then and slightly more on the second visit. This spilling apparently was enough to cause an osmotic diuresis and polyuria/nocturia.

Laura O. had a fasting plasma glucose greater than 126mg/dL (>7.0 mmol/L) on only one occasion. The polyuria could have been caused by the diuretic. However, the dose had not changed for years and low doses of thiazide diuretics do not significantly increase glucose levels. Her weight gain could contribute to insulin resistance resulting in hyperglycemia. The fact that Laura O. has some signs of type 2 DM complications indicates that she has had a subclinical form of the disease (referred to as prediabetes) for many years. These signs include legs cool to the touch and weak pedal pulses (evidence of macrovascular disease), slightly diminished pedal pinprick sensation (evidence of early neuropathy), and microalbuminuria (evidence of early stages of microvascular nephropathy). The random glucose level of 180 mg/dL, accompanied by classic signs of hyperglycemia followed by a fasting glucose level, confirm the diagnosis of diabetes mellitus.

Laura O.'s management should include diet and exercise control, which will lead to weight loss in addition to oral antidiabetic therapy. A glycosylated hemoglobin should be obtained to determine her glycemic control over the last 3 months. A urinalysis test specific for microalbuminuria should be performed to identify incipient nephropathy. She should be started on an angiotensin converting enzyme inhibitor (e.g., lisinopril) or an angiotensin receptor antagonist (e.g., losartan) to slow the progression of nephropathy.

and Ascensia® use an amperometric measurement and are smaller than the other devices. These devices, except Ascensia®, do not require wiping of the blood from the strip before inserting it in the machine because the end of the strip that contains the blood does not enter the meter. Most products take 0.5–1.5 min to run through the procedure and can read glucose concentrations of 20–600 mg/dL.

Generally, blood glucose concentrations determined by these methods are clinically useful estimates of corresponding plasma glucose concentrations measured by the laboratory. Therefore, home blood glucose monitoring is preferred to urine testing. Home blood testing clarifies the relationship between symptomatology and blood glucose concentrations. The best meter for a patient is an individual decision. The patient should be encouraged to try different brands of meters to find the device with which he or she is most comfortable.[26,27]

Quality control, which consists of control solution testing, calibration, and system maintenance, is a necessary component of accurate glucose testing. Most manufacturers supply control solutions with glucometers that can be used to assess the accuracy of the meter. This method of verifying accuracy operates the same way that the patient analyzes a drop of blood. A few glucometers require manual calibration prior to use, but most have an automatic calibration mode for ease of use. The blood sample intended for the strip may come in contact with the meter and soil the optic window resulting in inaccurate results. Pharmacists should guide patients through the instructions for cleaning the meter that is usually provided by the manufacturer.

Factors affecting glucose readings. Environmental factors such as temperature, humidity, altitude, and light may influence the accuracy of glucose readings. Exposing glucometers to extremes of temperature can alter battery life and performance. Therefore, glucometers should be stored at room temperature to assure accuracy. Humidity may decrease the shelf life of test strips resulting in inaccurate test results. Test strips should not be stored in areas of high humidity such as a bathroom. Individually wrapped strips are now available but are more expensive. Individuals should check the expiration date of the reagents. Because reagents are costly, patients are often tempted to use expired reagents that result in inaccurate readings.[28]

At higher altitudes, changes in oxygen content and temperature alter glucose testing results. Results of studies evaluating the accuracy of glucometers at altitudes greater than 10,000 feet have revealed major alterations in blood glucose levels. These changes were attributed to variations in metabolic rate, hydration, diet, physical exercise, hematocrit, and temperature associated with higher altitudes. Patients should be educated on how to use glucometers at high altitudes. Changes in light exposure can also alter results with photometric glucometers.

User error is the most common reason for inaccurate results. Some of the most common errors include not putting enough blood on the reagent. Patients should be asked periodically to demonstrate how they operate the meter.[26–28]

Glucose monitoring requirements may vary based on the pharmacologic therapy administered. Patients who are well-controlled on oral medications should monitor blood glucose levels at least twice a week and more frequently if there are any changes in drugs or drug doses. Patients who are poorly controlled on oral medications should monitor blood glucose levels 2–4 times daily. Patients taking insulin injections twice a day should check blood glucose levels at least twice a day. Patients on intensive insulin therapy should monitor blood glucose levels 3–4 times a day. In general, premeal glucose measurements are needed to monitor the effectiveness of the basal insulin dose (e.g., glargine or ultralente). Two-hour postprandial glucose readings are needed to monitor rapid acting insulins (e.g., lispro and aspart). Oral antidiabetic agents, such as metformin, thiazolidinediones, and glipizide, are evaluated using the 2-hr postprandial readings. Insulin pump therapy requires monitoring blood glucose levels 4–6 times per day to determine the effectiveness of the basal and bolus doses. Pregnancy requires frequent monitoring of blood glucose levels 4–6 times a day to ensure tight control, and premeal testing is required during acute illness to determine the need for supplemental insulin.[29,30]

Diagnosis of Hyperglycemia

The diagnosis of patients with hyperglycemia commonly falls into one of three categories: (1) diabetes mellitus or prediabetes, (2) diabetic ketoacidosis, and (3) hyperosmolar hyperglycemia syndrome.

Diabetes Mellitus or Glucose Intolerance

Goals of therapy. Once diabetes mellitus is diagnosed, the clinician needs to establish a therapeutic goal with respect to glucose control. The ideal goal would be to maintain concentrations at normal physiological levels. For type 1 patients, this effort requires tight control. Tight control could include preprandial plasma glucose concentrations of 90–130 mg/dL (5.0–7.3 mmol/L) and postprandial concentrations of less than 140 mg/dL (<7.8 mmol/L). Tight control requires intensive therapy and monitoring (three or more insulin injections per day and self-monitoring of glucose concentrations).[5]

Recent data from the Diabetes Control and Complications Trial (DCCT) suggest that this approach leads to significant health benefits.[31] Overall, the study showed that intensive therapy delays the onset and slows progression of diabetic retinopathy, nephropathy, and neuropathy in patients with type 1 DM. Microvascular diseases (e.g., retinopathy, neuropathy, and nephropathy) were diminished as were macrovascular diseases (e.g., large vessel, peripheral vascular diseases, stroke, and ischemic heart disease). The difference in macrovascular complications, however, did not reach statistical significance. No difference existed between the conventional and intensive therapy groups with respect to absolute risk for cardiac events. Statistical significance may not have been reached due to the short follow-up period (6.5 years) and the young average age of patients studied (34 years). In type 1 patients, the peak frequency for development of coronary disease is age 55.

The United Prospective Diabetes Study (UKPDS 33)[34] compared the effects of intensive drug therapy with a sulfonylurea (e.g., chlorpropamide and glipizide) insulin and conventional therapy (diet) in 3867 newly diagnosed type 2 patients with diabetes from 1977 until 1991. The results of the UKPDS show that intensive drug therapy decreased the risk of microvascular complications in type 2 patients with diabetes when compared with conventional therapy. The investigators reported that patients in the intensive group with a 1% median reduction in HbA_{1c} had a 25% reduction in risk of microvascular complications (p=0.0099).

Impact of exogenous insulin on glucose concentrations. Basal secretion of insulin from the pancreas occurs at a rate of 0.5–1 U/h. Bolus secretions of insulin occur when blood sugar levels are above 100 mg/dL after ingestion of food. Therefore, the normal physiologic release pattern of insulin is one of valleys or basal secretion and peaks or bolus secretions (Figure 13-3a). The normal pancreas secretes 25–50 units of insulin daily.

Because the most common and effective means to manage insulin deficiency is with insulin, the importance of the relationship between insulin injection and interpretation of glucose concentrations is briefly discussed. In general, 1 unit of any type of insulin produces the same metabolic response as another. Every 1–2-unit increase in the insulin dose usually leads to a 30–50-mg/dL decrease in the glucose concentration. Although the amount of *total* activity is equal for any given number of units of any insulin, the activity is not elicited evenly over time. A clinician must know the activity-over-time profiles of various insulin types at various injection sites for various species to anticipate correctly a dose's effect on glucose concentrations at a particular time (Table 13-6).

The starting dose of insulin is based on clinical assessment of insulin deficiency and insulin resistance, as well as the patient's lifestyle (i.e., eating patterns, exercise, and waking/sleep patterns).

In general, insulin requirements for type 1 patients with diabetes with a BMI less than 25 are 0.5–1.0

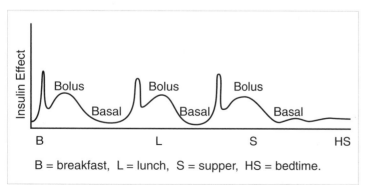

Figure 13-3a.
Adapted, with permission, from Reference 35.

TABLE 13-6

INSULIN	ONSET (MIN)	PEAK ACTION (h)	DURATION (h)
Rapid acting			
Lispro/Aspart	5–15	1–2	4–6
Short acting			
Human Regular	30–60	2–4	6–10
Intermediate Acting			
Human NPH/Lente	60–120	4–8	10–20
Combinations			
70/30; 50/50; 75/25	30–60	2–8	14–18
Long Acting			
Ultralente	120–240	Unpredictable	16–20
Glargine	60–120	Peakless	~24

Table 13-6. Comparisons of Human Insulins and Insulin Analogues

U/kg/day. Insulin requirements may vary during illness or stress. Insulin requirements may decrease during the "honeymoon phase," a remission period that occurs early in the course of the disease.[33] Insulin requirements for type 2 patients with diabetes vary based on the degree of insulin resistance and insulin deficiency. In general, a single or bedtime dose of insulin can be given to type 2 patients with diabetes who have failed oral agents. The oral agents should be continued at the same dose. Patients with a BMI less than 25 kg/m^2 can be started on 5–10 units of intermediate-acting insulin at bedtime. Patients with a BMI greater than 25 kg/m^2 should be started on 10–15 units of intermediate (NPH) at bedtime or combination insulin (70/30) before dinner.[34]

The goal of insulin therapy for the type 1 patients with diabetes is to mimic the body's natural physiologic response to hormonal or glucose loads due to food ingestion. This type of pattern can only be obtained with intensive therapy (greater than 3 injections daily).

Figures 13-3b and 13-3c illustrate the use of short-acting (regular) or rapid-acting (lispro or aspart) insulin before breakfast, lunch, and dinner and a long-acting basal insulin (ultralente or glargine) given at bedtime. This regimen, often referred to as "the poor man's pump," is ideal for patients with unusual schedules. Figures 13-3d and 13-3e illustrate insulin therapy administered by an insulin pump. The pump is programmed to administer insulin (rapid or short acting) throughout the day, and the patient activates the pump to give a bolus of insulin prior to meals. Intensive regimens require more frequent monitoring and are accompanied by an increased risk of hypoglycemia.

In a single, daily injection regimen (Figure 13-3f), one injection (intermediate or long acting) is administered at bedtime. This regimen is ideal for a type 2 DM patient that has failed to obtain glycemic control on oral agents. The oral agents can be continued and long-acting insulin can be administered at bedtime.

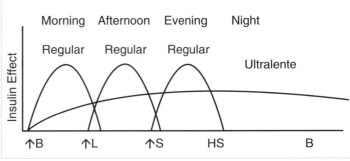

Figure 13-3b.
Adapted, with permission, from Reference 35.

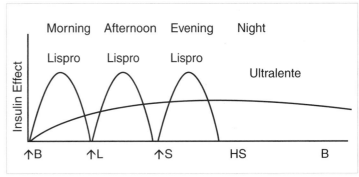

Figure 13-3c.
Adapted, with permission, from Reference 35.

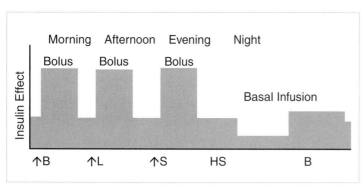

Figure 13-3d.
Adapted, with permission, from Reference 35.

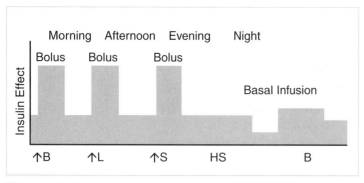

Figure 13-3e.
Adapted, with permission, from Reference 35.

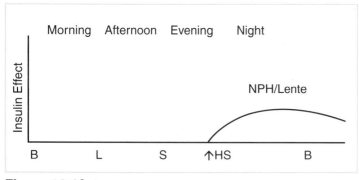

Figure 13-3f.
Adapted, with permission, from Reference 35.

In a twice-a-day injection regimen (Figure 13-3g), an injection of intermediate-acting insulin is administered before breakfast and bedtime. The administration of intermediate-acting insulin before bedtime decreases risk of hypoglycemia in the early morning.

An average regimen (Figure 13-3h) combines a mixed injection of intermediate-acting and regular insulin given before breakfast, an injection of regular insulin at dinner, and another injection of intermediate-acting insulin given before bedtime, which provides safer, more effective overnight glucose control. Without regular insulin administered before dinner, however, glucose concentrations may become unacceptably high after dinner.

Regular insulin should be given 30–45 min before meals unless the preprandial glucose concentration is below 70 mg/dL (<3.9 mmol/L). If the concentration is less than 70 mg/dL, the patient should consume 15 g of carbohydrates (e.g., 4 ounces of orange juice, regular soda, or milk) immediately, and check glucose levels 15 min later. In all regimens, regular insulin doses are adjusted on the basis of self-monitored preprandial glucose concentrations. Lispro and aspart insulin should be given 5–15 min before a meal. Insulin should be used along with diet, exercise, and stress management for best effects.[33-35]

Oral Agents in the Management of Type 2 DM

Currently, there are six classes of oral agents in the United States for the management of diabetes (Table 13-7):

1. Sulfonylureas—first and second-generation agents stimulate the secretion of insulin from pancreatic beta cells.
2. Benzoic acid derivative—repaglinide stimulates the secretion of insulin from pancreatic beta cells.

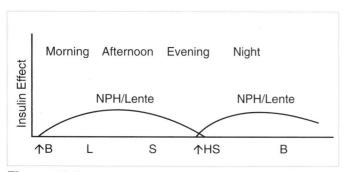

Figure 13-3g.
Adapted, with permission, from Reference 35.

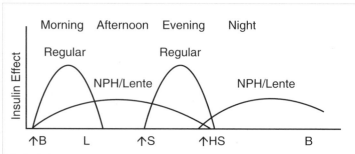

Figure 13-3h.
Adapted, with permission, from Reference 35.

3. D-phenylalanine derivative—nateglinide stimulates the secretion of insulin from pancreatic beta cells.
4. Biguanide—metformin inhibits gluconeogenesis by the liver.
5. Thiazolidinediones—rosiglitazone and pioglitazone increase insulin sensitivity in muscles.
6. Alpha-glucosidase inhibitors—acarbose and miglitol inhibit alpha glucosidase, an enzyme responsible for facilitating the absorption of carbohydrates from the gastrointestinal tract into the circulation.

Agents on the Horizon

Recent technological advances have made it possible to deliver insulin to the alveolar space where it is rapidly absorbed into the alveolar capillaries and distributed into the blood stream. When the inhaler is activated, the blister package, which stores the powdered formulation of insulin, is released into the alveolar space. This form of insulin has produced consistent results, only 30% of the drug reaches the blood stream. However, this may result in more frequent dosing and increased drug cost. Inhaled insulin is expected to be available by the year 2004.[36]

Pramlintide is a synthetic version of the hormone amylin. Amylin is secreted by the pancreatic beta cells in response to a glucose load. Amylin inhibits gastric emptying and suppresses glucagon secretion resulting in a reduction in post prandial glucose concentrations. It is administered subcutaneously 15 min prior to a meal and can be combined with insulin if administered immediately. Pramlintide is scheduled to be approved by the FDA soon.[37] As with the other antidiabetic agents currently marketed, fasting plasma glucose levels and A1C values will be required to assess the effectiveness of these new agents in the patient.

Diabetic Ketoacidosis

Insulin deficiency after ingestion of a meal can result in impaired glucose utilization by peripheral tissues and the liver. Prolonged insulin deficiency results in protein breakdown and increased hepatic glucose production (gluconeogenesis) by the liver and increased release of counterregulatory hormones such as glucagon, catecholamines (e.g., epinephrine and norepinephrine), cortisol, and growth hormones. In the face of lipolysis, free fatty acids are converted by the liver to ketone bodies (beta-hydroxybutyric acid and acetoacetic acid), which results in metabolic acidosis. Diabetic ketoacidosis, which occurs most commonly in patients with type 1 diabetes, is initiated by insulin deficiency. The most common causes of diabetic ketoacidosis are[38]

- Infections, illness, and emotional stress.
- Noncompliance or inadequate insulin dosage.
- Undiagnosed type 1 DM.
- Unknown or no precipitating event.

Clinically, patients with diabetic ketoacidosis typically present with dehydration, lethargy, acetone-smelling breath, abdominal pain, tachycardia, orthostatic hypotension, tachypnea, and, occasionally, mild hypothermia and lethargy or coma. Because of the patient tendency toward low body temperatures, fever strongly suggests infection as a precipitant of diabetic ketoacidosis.

Chemically, diabetic ketoacidosis is characterized by a high glucose concentration. This concentration is typically >300 mg/dL or 16.8 mmol/L. The plasma glucose concentration is not related to the severity of diabetic ketoacidosis. Patients—who have continued to administer insulin, are pregnant, have not eaten adequately, or have vomited excessively—generally present with lower glucose concentrations. As insulin is given, the glucose concentrations decline at a rate of about 75–100 mg/dL/hr.

TABLE 13-7

CLASS	AGENT	MECHANISM	SIDE EFFECTS	DOSAGE RANGE
Sulfo-nylureas		Increases insulin secretion by binding to sulfonylurea receptor on pancreatic β-cell and blocking ATP-K channels	Hypoglycemia, weight gain, water retention, hematologic reactions, skin reactions (particularly rashes), purpura, nausea, vomiting and cholestasis, constipation, headache, photosensitivity	
	1st Generation: Chlorpropamide *Diabinese®*		Disulfiram-like reaction when combined with alcohol; avoid in patients with renal insufficiency	100–500 mg
	Tolazmide *Tolinase®*			100–1000 mg
	Acetohexamide *Dymelor®*		Avoid in patients with renal insufficiency	250–1500 mg
	Tolbutamide *Orinase®*			500–2500 mg
	2nd Generation: Glipizide *Glucotrol®*		Increased risk of rash over other sulfonylureas	5–10 mg daily; titrate to maximum dose of 40 mg daily; usually not above 20 mg/day; give 20 min before meals
	Glyburide *Dia-beta®, Glynase®, Micronase®*		Dizziness, blurred vision, avoid in patients with renal insufficiency	5 mg daily; titrate to maximum dose of 20 mg daily
	Glimepiride *Amaryl®*		Mild incidence of hypogly-cemia, fullness, heartburn, blood dyscrasias	1–2 mg daily; titrate to maintenance
D-phen-lalanine derivative	Nateglinide *Starlix®*	Increases insulin secretion by blocking ATP-K channels on the pancreatic β-cells	Mild hypoglycemia (primarily postprandial), nausea, diarrhea	60–360 mg daily
Meglitinide	Repaglinide *Prandin®*	Increases insulin secretion by blocking ATP-K channels on the pancreatic β-cells	Mild hypoglycemia (primarily postprandial), nausea, diarrhea, upper respiratory infection, headache, rhinitis, bronchitis, back pain, tooth disorder, chest pain, hyperglycemia, heartburn, epigastric fullness	0.5–2 mg (maximum of 4mg) should be taken 15 min prior to meals but may vary from immediately preceding a meal to as long 30 min prior; dosed up to 4 times daily in response to meal pattern; max = 16 mg/day
Biguanide	Metformin *Glucophage®*	Inhibits gluconeo-genesis, increases insulin sensitivity by increasing tyrosine kinase activity, increases glycogen synthesis	Gastrointestinal side effects including abdominal dis-comfort and diarrhea are most common, interference with B^{12} absorption, rare incidence of lactic acidosis (esp. in hypoperfusion disease states such as renal impairment and heart failure/CHF)	500 mg once a day to start (decreases incidence of diarrhea), increase by 500 mg increments per week as tolerated; given in divided dose every 8 to 12 hr; maximum dose = 2550 mg/day
Alpha-glucosidase inhibitors		Inhibits α-glucosi-dase enzyme, which metabolizes complex carbohydrates and sucrose (cane sugar)	Bloating, abdominal discomfort/pain, diarrhea and flatulence in up to 30% of patients; abnormal liver function tests	25 mg daily with first bite of food; titrate *slowly* to 3 times a day; maximum dose 50 mg tid for patients <60 kg and 100 mg tid for patients >60 kg; do not take without a meal
	Acarbose (*Precose®*)			
	Miglitol *Glyset®*)		Skin rash, no reports of hepatic toxicity to date	

Continued on next page

TABLE 13-7

CLASS	AGENT	MECHANISM	SIDE EFFECTS	DOSAGE RANGE
Thiazoli-dinediones		Facilitates muscle cell response to insulin by acting on the peroxisome pro-liferative activated receptor (PPAR), thereby allowing glucose to diffuse into the cell more effectively	Hepatotoxicity, edema (contraindicated in NYHA class III or IV cardiac status), rash, weight gain, decrease in hemoglobin and hematocrit, possible increase in LDL cholesterol	
	Rosiglitazone *Avandia*®			4 mg daily; maximum dose of 8 mg daily; (4 mg bid more effective than 8 mg qd)
	Pioglitazone *Actos*®			15–30 mg daily; maximum dose 45 mg
Combination Agents	Metaglip® (metformin/ glipizide)			1–2 tablets once to twice a day; start 2.5/250 qd if initial treat-ment and 2.5/500 bid or 5/500 bid if 2nd line; max = 20/2000 per day; take with meals
	Glucovance® (metformin/ glyburide)			1–2 tablets twice a day; start 1.25/250 qd if initial treatment and 2.5–5/500 bid if 2nd line; max = 20/2000 per day; take with meals
	Avandamet® (rosiglitazone/ metformin)			1–2 tablets twice a day; start 2/500 twice a day if initial treatment; max = 8/2000 per day

Table 13-7. Oral Antidiabetic Agents

Diabetic ketoacidosis is also characterized by low venous bicarbonate 0–15 mEq/L) and pH (<7.20). Hyperglycemia can lead to osmotic diuresis resulting in hypotonic fluid losses, dehydration, and electrolyte loss. Sodium and potassium concentrations may be low, normal, or high. Sodium concentrations are reflective of the amount of total body water and sodium lost and replaced. In the presence of hyperglycemia, sodium concentrations may be decreased because of the movement of water from the intracellular space to the extracellular space. The potassium level reflects a balance between the amount of potassium lost in the urine and insulin deficiency, which causes higher concentrations of extracellular potassium. Elevated potassium levels are due to extracellular movement of potassium due to insulin deficiency. Hypertonicity and acidosis can cause potassium to move from the intracellular space to the extracellular space resulting in elevated potassium levels. However, total potassium depletion always occurs regardless of the initial potassium level. Patients with low or normal potassium levels should be monitored closely because treatment can result in severe total body potassium that may place the patient at risk for cardiac dysrhythmia.

The phosphate level is usually normal or slightly elevated.[39,40] Creatinine and blood urea nitrogen (BUN) are usually elevated due to dehydration. These levels usually return to normal after rehydration unless there was pre-existing renal insufficiency. Hemoglobin, hematocrit, and total protein levels are mildly elevated due to decreased plasma volume and dehydration. Amylase levels may be increased due to increased secretion by the salivary glands. And liver function tests are usually elevated but return to normal in 3–4 weeks.

MINICASE 2

EUGENE T., A 45-YEAR-OLD MALE with a 30-year history of type 1 DM, was brought into the emergency department after his wife found him to be "out of it" when attempting to wake him. Five days ago, he developed fever, nasal congestion, polyuria, and increasing nausea and abdominal aches. He took no medications except for insulin, captopril 25 mg twice a day for hypertension, multivitamins, and, recently, phenylephrine nasal spray. Over the past 3 days, he did not eat much.

To "adjust" for his decreased caloric intake, Eugene T. stopped injecting his usual insulin dose despite seeing increasing blood sugars with his glucometer (according to his meter's memory, fasting glucoses of 145, 180, 200, and 250 mg/dL). Physical examination revealed a lethargic male with a BP of 115/65 (which dropped to 95/50 when sitting), HR 105, respiratory rate 30 (deep and regular), and oral temperature 101.4 °F (38.6 °C). His skin turgor was poor, and his mucous membranes were dry. Eugene T. had a fruity aromatic odor to his breath and was disoriented and confused. His lab results were as follows:

- Sodium, 143 mEq/L (136–145 mEq/L).
- Potassium, 3.5 mEq/L (3.5–5.0 mEq/L).
- Chloride, 99 mEq/L (96–106 mEq/L).
- BUN, 38 mg/dL (8–20 mg/dL).
- SCr, 2.8 mg/dL (0.7–1.5 mg/dL).
- Phosphorus, 2.7 mg/dL (2.6–4.5 mg/dL).
- Amylase, 350 IU/L (44–128 IU/L).
- pH, 7.15 (7.36–7.44).
- Bicarbonate, 9.0 mEq/L (24–30 mEq/L).
- Hct, 52% (42–52%).
- WBCs, 16×10^3 cells/mm^3 ($4.8–10.8 \times 10^3$ cells/mm^3).
- Calcium, 9 mg/dL (8.5–10.8 mg/dL).
- Glucose, 650 mg/dL (70–110 mg/dL).
- Ketones, 3+ @1:8 serum dilution (normal = 0).
- Osmolality, 335 mOsm/kg (280–295 mOsm/kg).
- Triglycerides, 174 mg/dL (10–160 mg/dL).
- Lipase, 1.4 U/mL (<1.5 U/mL).
- Magnesium, 2 mEq/L (1.5–2.2 mEq/L).

A urine screen with Multistix indicated a "large" (160 mg/dL) amount of ketones, the highest designation on the strip.

Question: Based on clinical and lab findings, what is the most likely diagnosis for Eugene T.? What precipitated this metabolic disorder? Can interpretation of any results be influenced by his acidosis or hyperglycemia? Are there potential drug interferences with any lab tests?

Discussion: Eugene T., a type 1 DM patient, developed diabetic ketoacidosis from an infection and discontinuation of his insulin. Diabetic ketoacidosis rarely occurs in patients with type 2 DM. Clinically, the patient's presentation is classic. His decreased skin turgor, dry mucous membranes, tachycardia (HR of 105), and orthostatic hypotension are consistent with dehydration, a common condition in patients with diabetic ketoacidosis. His breathing is rapid and deep. Although he is not comatose, he is lethargic, confused, and disoriented.

Chemically, Eugene T. probably has a *total body* deficit of sodium and potassium despite *serum* concentration results within normal limits. Orthostatic hypotension is consistent with decreased intravascular volume, causing hemoconcentration of these minerals. Therefore, these values do not reflect total body stores, and the clinician can expect them to decline rapidly if unsupplemented fluids are infused. Although the patient's phosphorus concentration is in the normal range (lower end), it likely will decrease after rehydration and insulin. Serial testing should be done every 3–4 hr during the first 24 hr.

Serial glucose, ketones, and acid-base measurements, typical of diabetic ketoacidosis, should show gradual improvement with proper therapy. With use of the sodium correction factor (addition of 2 mEq/L to the sodium result for every 100 mg/dL of glucose above 200 mg/dL), Eugene T.'s sodium would have been

152 mEq/L had his glucose been normal, a value more consistent with the BUN and Hct concentrations. Another correction factor can be applied to adjust potassium. For reasons described in Chapter 7, Eugene T.'s potassium would have been 5.5–6.0 mEq/L had he not been acidemic. In other words, if his acidosis were corrected without rehydration, his potassium probably would rise above the normal range to 5.5–6.0 mEq/L. This situation does not occur in practice because rehydration is addressed concurrently.

Decreased intravascular volume has led to hemoconcentrated Hct and BUN. BUN is also elevated by decreased renal perfusion (prerenal azotemia), although intrinsic renal causes should be considered if SCr is also elevated. Fortunately, as is probably the case with Eugene T., high SCr may be an artifact caused by the influence of ketone bodies on the assay (Chapter 7). If so, SCr concentrations should decline with ketone concentrations.

Eugene T. also exhibits the typical leukocytosis that often accompanies diabetic ketoacidosis, even in the absence of infection. His osmolarity based on the osmolarity estimation formula would be (2 x 143) + (650/18) + (38/2.8) = 335.7 mOsm/L, approximately equal to the laboratory result. This value is slightly higher than normal for diabetic ketoacidosis (300–320 mOsm/kg).

Finally, Eugene T. had a 3+ serum ketone reading at a dilution of 1:8, not unexpected given the overall severity of his diabetic ketoacidosis. A urine screen also indicated the presence of ketones. Even if the captopril he was taking had falsely "elevated" the urine ketone screen, the results still would have to be interpreted as real and significant, given the serum ketones and all of the other signs and symptoms. For academic purposes, the impact of the drug could be tested (Chapter 4) after the diabetic ketoacidosis resolves.

A serum amylase and lipase were measured to rule out pancreatitis, usually suspected with abdominal pain. However, elevated amylase probably originated from the salivary glands because Eugene T.'s lipase was normal. This finding is seen in 20% of diabetic ketoacidosis patients (Chapter 12).

Initially, potassium concentrations may also be elevated due to metabolic acidosis (Chapter 7). Correction of acidosis elicits the opposite effect. Potassium shifts intracellularly and out of the serum with insulin therapy, leading to a decrease in serum potassium concentrations.

Serum osmolality is typically elevated at 300–320 mOsm/kg (normally, 280–295 mOsm/kg). Serum osmolarity (milliosmoles per liter), which is practically equivalent to osmolality (milliosmoles per kilogram), can be estimated by serum osmolarity (mOsm/L) = (2 x sodium) + glucose/18 + BUN/2.8 where glucose and BUN units are milligrams per deciliter.

Ketones are present in the blood and urine of patients in diabetic ketoacidosis, as the name of this disorder implies. Formation of ketone bodies acetoacetate, acetone, and beta-hydroxybutyrate, is the main cause of acidosis in diabetic ketoacidosis. The usual, nitroprusside-based (nitroferricyanide) assays (Acetest®, Ketostix®, Labstix®, and Multistix®) do not detect beta-hydroxybutyrate and are 15 to 20 times more sensitive to acetoacetate than to acetone. In a few situations (e.g., severe hypovolemia, hypotension, low partial pressure of oxygen [PO$_2$], and alcoholism) where beta-hydroxybutyrate predominates, assessment of ketones may be falsely low. As diabetic ketoacidosis resolves, beta-hydroxybutyric acid is converted to acetoacetate, the assay-reactive ketone body. Therefore, a stronger reaction may be encountered in laboratory results. However, this reaction does not necessarily mean a worsening of the ketoacidotic state.[41]

Clinicians must keep in mind that ketonuria may also result from starvation, high-fat diets, fever, and anesthesia, but these conditions are not associated with hyperglycemia. Levodopa, mesna,[42] acetylcysteine (irrigation),[43] methyldopa, phenazopyridine, pyrazinamide, valproic acid, captopril,[44,45] and high-dose aspirin may cause false-positive results with urine ketone tests.[46] The influence of these drugs on serum ketone tests has not been studied extensively. If the ketone concentration is increased, a typical series of dipstick results is

1. Negative.
2. Trace or 5 mg/dL.
3. Small or 15 mg/dL.
4. Moderate or 40 mg/dL.
5. Large or 80 mg/dL.
6. Very large or 160 mg/dL.

Outside of diabetic ketoacidosis, urine ketone testing is done by type 1 DM patients when their fasting blood glucose concentration exceeds 240 mg/dL (>13.5 mmol/L) or when physiological (or emotional) stress is unusually high (e.g., during an acute infection). If ketonuria is present, serum ketones should be measured to assess the severity of the ketosis. Ketones in the blood are measured or assayed by mixing serum with an equal volume of water or saline sequentially to achieve dilutions of 1:1, 1:2, 1:4, 1:8, etc. The tests are semiquantitative, with readings from 1+ to 4+. A positive nitroprusside ketone test at a dilution of 1:8 or higher should be interpreted as a clinically important degree of ketonemia.

Hyperosmolar Hyperglycemia State

Hyperosmolar hyperglycemia state (HHS) is a condition that occurs most frequently in elderly type 2 patients with diabetes. HHS is usually precipitated by stress or illness when such patients do not drink enough to keep up with osmotic diuresis. Patients usually present with severe hyperglycemia (glucose concentrations >600 mg/dL or >33.3 mmol/L); decreased mentation (e.g., lethargy, confusion, dehydration); neurologic manifestations (e.g., seizures and hemisensory deficits); and an absence of ketosis. Insulin deficiency is not as severe in HHS. Therefore, lipolysis—which is necessary for the formation of ketone bodies—does not occur. The absence of ketosis results in significantly milder gastrointestinal symptoms than patients with diabetic ketoacidosis. Therefore, patients often fail to seek medical attention. Patients with HHS are usually more dehydrated on presentation than patients with DKA due to impairment in the thirst mechanism, which results in prolonged diuresis and dehydration.

In some cases, patients are taking drugs that cause glucose intolerance (e.g., diuretics, steroids, and phenytoin). Stroke and infection are nondrug predisposing factors. Initially, electrolytes are within normal ranges, but BUN routinely is elevated. Serum osmolalities characteristically are higher than those in diabetic ketoacidosis—in the range of 320–400 mOsm/kg. Serum electrolytes (e.g., magnesium, phosphorus, and calcium) are typically abnormal and should be monitored until stable.[39-41]

Hypoglycemia

Hypoglycemia is defined as a blood glucose level of 70 mg/dL (39 mmol/L) or lower. The classification of hypoglycemia is based on the individual's ability to self-treat. Mild hypoglycemia is characterized by symptoms such as sweating, trembling, shaking, rapid heartbeat, heavy breathing, and difficulty concentrating. The symptoms associated with mild hypoglycemia vary in severity and does not imply that the symptoms experienced by the individual are minor or easily tolerated. While a patient may experience profuse sweating, dizziness, and lack of coordination, they still may be able to self-treat. These symptoms resolve after consuming carbohydrates (e.g., fruit juice, milk, or hard candy).

Severe hypoglycemia is characterized by an inability to self-treat due to mental confusion or unconsciousness. Emergency medical treatment is required to raise the blood glucose level out of a dangerously low range.

Increased release of counterregulatory hormones is responsible for most hypoglycemic symptoms. Most of the early signs of hypoglycemia (e.g., trembling, shaking, rapid heart beat, fast pulse, heavy breathing, and changes in body temperature) are mediated by the adrenergic system and sweating, another cardinal sign of hypoglycemia is mediated by the cholinergic system.

Glucagon and epinephrine are the primary counterregulatory hormones responsible for increasing blood glucose concentrations in the presence of hypoglycemia. Glucagon enhances glycogenolysis and epinephrine increases gluconeogenesis and inhibits glucose utilization by tissues. Defects in hormonal counterregulation can diminish autonomic symptoms resulting in hypoglycemia unawareness. Glucagon secretion may become impaired after the first few years of type 1 DM, resulting in epinephrine as the primary mechanism for raising low blood glucose levels. Frequent episodes of hypoglycemia can cause temporary deficits in epinephrine response, resulting in an absence of autonomic symptoms for several days. Epinephrine response returns to normal when patients avoid low blood glucose levels over a period of 3–6 weeks. Patients with diabetes must be taught the importance of maintaining a balanced diet and monitoring their blood glucose levels regularly to decrease the risk of developing hypoglycemia.[47,48]

Neuroglycopenia occurs during hypoglycemic episodes due to decreased glucose supply to the central nervous system. The earliest signs of neuroglycopenia include slow thinking and difficulty concentrating and reading. Patients report that it takes more effort to perform routine tasks (e.g., brushing teeth, combing hair, or taking a bath). As the blood glucose levels decrease further, mental confusion, disorientation, slurred or rambling speech, irrational behavior, and extreme fatigue and lethargy may occur. Neuroglycopenia is usually the cause of physical injuries and accidents that occur during hypoglycemic episodes. Most patients with deficits in epinephrine will only experience signs of neuroglycopenia. Patients should be taught the early warning signs of neuroglycopenic symptoms (e.g., slow thinking, blurred vision, slurred speech, numbness, trouble concentrating, dizziness, fatigue, and sleepiness).

Patients should be encouraged to keep a symptom diary and record their symptoms whenever they measure their blood glucose in order to identify their own most reliable symptoms.

Hypoglycemic episodes are usually caused by excess in blood glucose lowering medications (e.g., insulin and insulin secretagogues), physical activity, or inadequate carbohydrate intake. It is important to carefully examine the individual's insulin regimen. Hypoglycemia frequently occurs when insulin action is peaking. Hypoglycemia can also occur when an individual has not eaten for several hours or after strenuous exercise. Individuals should check their blood glucose levels after exercising. Alcohol consumption in the absence of food intake may also result in hypoglycemia.[49]

Sulfonylureas used concomitantly with sulfa-type antibiotics (e.g., Bactrim, TMP-SMX, and Septa) can cause severe and refractory hypoglycemia. Patients with diabetes must be educated to inform their health care provider if they are taking a sulfonylurea if a sulfa-type antibiotic is prescribed.

Individuals with diabetes should be taught how to treat a hypoglycemic episode. Educate patients that consumption of a high-fat meal may slow gastric emptying and the absorption of carbohydrates. Therefore eating a high fat, low carbohydrate meal after an insulin injection may result in hypoglycemia.

Individuals should be taught that all blood glucose levels below 70 mg/dL (3.9 mmol/L) should be treated, even in the absence of symptoms. Patients should eat or drink 10–15 g of glucose or carbohydrate containing food or beverage, which should increase blood glucose levels by 30–45 mg/dL. Foods and beverages, which contain 15 g of carbohydrate, include 4 ounces of fruit juice, 4 ounces of nondiet soda, 8–10 lifesaver candies, or 3–4 glucose tablets. Avoid drinks and foods that are high in fat (e.g., chocolate or whole milk) that may slow absorption of carbohydrates and take longer to raise blood glucose levels. Adding protein such as meat will not treat hypoglycemia and will not raise blood glucose levels. Test blood glucose levels 15–20 min later. If blood glucose levels are still low, repeat the treatment.

Patients should be informed not to miss meals and to have a bedtime snack if blood glucose levels are less than 120 mg/dL.[47-49]

Other Laboratory Tests Used In the Management of Diabetes

The leading cause of death in patients with diabetes is cardiovascular disease. Control of hypertension and dyslipidemia is necessary to decrease the risk of macrovascular complications.

Patients with diabetes tend to have a unique type of dyslipidemia, which consists of an elevated low-density lipoprotein (LDL) levels, reduced high-density lipoprotein (HDL) levels, elevated triglycerides, and increased platelet adhesiveness, all of which can contribute to the development of arteriolar sclerosis. Aggressive treatment of dyslipidemia will reduce the risk of cardiovascular disease in patients with diabetes. Primary therapy should focus on obtaining LDL goals of less than 100 mg/dL, triglycerides less than 150 mg/dL, and HDL greater than 45 mg/dL for men and greater than 55 mg/dL for women.[50]

Both systolic and diastolic hypertension increases the risk of microvascular and macrovascular complications in patients with diabetes. Aggressive treatment of hypertension can attenuate the progression of complications. The American Diabetes Association (ADA) currently recommends a goal blood pressure of <130/80 mmHg.[51]

Urinalysis for protein should be obtained in patients with diabetes on a yearly basis. This should begin at diagnosis in patients with type 2 diabetes and 5 years after diagnosis in patients with type 1 diabetes.[52] A quantitative test for urine protein should follow a positive result on urinalysis. If urinalysis for protein is negative, a test for microalbuminuria should be obtained. Microalbuminuria indicates glomerular damage and is predictive of clinical nephropathy.

There are three methods available for screening of microalbuminuria. One method is by measuring the urine albumin to creatinine ratio in a spot urine sample. This method is convenient in the clinical setting, as it only requires one urine sample. A morning sample is preferred to take into account the diurnal variation of albumin excretion. A second method is a 24-hr urine collection of albumin. This method may be tedious and accuracy relies on proper collection techniques. An advantage of this method is that renal function can simultaneously be quantified. A third alternative method to the 24-hr collection is a timed urine collection for albumin. Microalbuminuria is defined as a urinary albumin excretion of 30–299 μg/mg on a spot urine sample, 30–299 mg/24 hr on a 24-hr urine collection, or 20–199 μg/min on a timed urine collection. Transient rises in albumin excretion can be associated with exercise, hyperglycemia, hypertension, urinary tract infection, heart failure, and fever. Therefore, if any of these conditions are present, they may result in false positives on screening tests. Variability exists in the excretion of albumin, thus, microalbuminuria must be confirmed in two repeated tests in a 3–6 month period. Two of three positive screening tests for microalbuminuria confirm the diagnosis.[51,52]

THYROID

Anatomy and Physiology

The thyroid gland is a butterfly-shaped organ composed of two connecting lobes that span the trachea. The thyroid produces the hormones thyroxine (T_4) and triiodothyronine (T_3). Approximately 80 and 30 μg of T_4 and T_3, respectively, are produced daily in normal adults. T_4 is produced solely by the thyroid gland, but only about 20–25% of T_3 is directly secreted by this gland. Approximately 80% of T_3 is formed by hepatic and renal deiodination of T_4.

T_4 has a longer half-life than T_3, approximately 7 vs. 1 day, respectively. At the cellular level, however, T_3 is 3–4 times more active physiologically than T_4.[1-3] When the conversion of T_4 to T_3 is impaired, a stereoisomer of T_3, known as reverse T_3, is produced; it has no known biological effect.

Thyroid hormones have many biological effects, both at the molecular level and on specific organ systems. These hormones stimulate the basal metabolic rate and can affect protein, carbohydrate, and lipid metabolism. They are also essential for normal growth and development. Thyroid hormones act to

- Stimulate neural and skeletal development during fetal life.
- Stimulate oxygen consumption at rest.
- Stimulate bone turnover by increasing bone formation and resorption.
- Promote the conversion of carotene to vitamin A.
- Promote chronotropic and inotropic effects on the heart.
- Increase the number of catecholamine receptors in heart muscle cells.
- Increase basal body temperature.
- Increase the production of RBCs.
- Increase the metabolism and clearance of steroid hormones.
- Alter the metabolism of carbohydrates, fats, and protein.
- Control the normal hypoxic and hypercapnic respiratory drives.

The synthesis of thyroid hormones depends on iodine and the amino acid tyrosine. The thyroid gland, using an energy-requiring process, transports dietary iodide (I^-) from the circulation into the thyroid follicular cell. Iodide is oxidized to iodine (I_2) and then combined with tyrosyl residues within the thyroglobulin molecule to form thyroid hormones (iodothyronines). Thus, the thyroid hormones are formed and stored within the thyroglobulin protein for release into the circulation.[53-56]

T_4 and T_3 circulate in human serum bound to three proteins: the majority to thyroxine-binding globulin (TBG), thyroid-binding prealbumin (TBPA), and albumin. Only 0.02% of T_4 and 0.2% of T_3 circulate unbound,[57] free to diffuse into tissues. The "free" fraction is the metabolically active component. Total and free hormones exist in an equilibrium state in which the protein-bound fraction serves as a reservoir for making the free fraction available to tissues.[58]

Thyroid hormone secretion is regulated by a feedback mechanism involving the hypothalamus, anterior pituitary, and thyroid gland itself (Figure 13-4). The release of T_4 and T_3 from the thyroid gland is regulated by thyrotropin, also called TSH, which is secreted by the

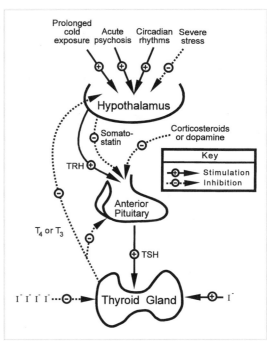

Figure 13-4. The hypothalamic-pituitary-thyroid axis. (Adapted, with permission, from Katzung BG, ed. *Basic and Clinical Pharmacology*. 4th ed. Norwalk, CT: Appleton & Lange; 1989.)

anterior pituitary. The intrathyroidal iodine concentration also influences thyroid gland activity. TSH secretion primarily is regulated by a dual negative feedback mechanism:

1. Thyrotropin-releasing hormone (TRH) or protirelin is released by the hypothalamus, which stimulates the synthesis and release of TSH from the pituitary gland. Basal TSH concentrations in persons with normal thyroid function are about 0.3–5.0 mU/L. The inverse relationship between TSH and free T_4 is logarithmic. A 50% decrease in free T_4 concentrations leads to a 50-fold increase in TSH concentrations and vice versa.[59]

2. Unbound T_4 and T_3 (mainly the concentration of intracellular T_3 in the pituitary) directly inhibit pituitary TSH secretion. Consequently, increased concentrations of free thyroid hormones cause decreased TSH secretion, and decreased concentrations of T_4 and T_3 cause increased TSH secretion.[60]

Prolonged exposure to cold and acute psychosis may activate the hypothalamic-pituitary-thyroid axis, whereas severe stress may inhibit it. While TRH stimulates pituitary TSH release, somatostatin corticosteroids and dopamine inhibit it. Small amounts of iodide are needed for T_4 and T_3 production, but large amounts inhibit their production and release.

Most recent evidence based on the most sensitive assays suggests that no physiologically relevant change in serum TSH concentrations occurs in relation to age.[60]

Thyroid Disorders

Patients with a normally functioning thyroid gland are said to be in a euthyroid state. When this state is disrupted, thyroid disease may result. It occurs 4 times more often in women than in men and may occur at any age, but it peaks between the third and sixth decades of life. A family history of this disease often is present, especially for the autoimmune thyroid diseases.

Diseases of the thyroid usually involve an alteration in the quantity or quality of thyroid hormone secretion and may manifest as hypothyroidism or hyperthyroidism. In addition to the signs and symptoms discussed below, thyroid disease may produce an enlargement of the thyroid gland known as goiter.

Hypothyroidism

Hypothyroidism results from a deficiency of thyroid hormone production, causing body metabolism to slow down. This condition affects about 2% of women and 0.2% of men and the incidence increases with age. Symptoms include lethargy; constipation; dry, coarse skin and hair; paresthesias and slowed deep tendon reflexes; facial puffiness; cold intolerance; decreased sweating; impaired memory, confusion, and dementia; slow speech and motor activity; and anemia and growth retardation in children. Interestingly, these typical signs and symptoms have been observed in as few as 25% of elderly hypothyroid patients.[61]

Hypothyroidism is usually caused by one of three mechanisms. Primary hypothyroidism is failure of the thyroid to produce thyroid hormone, secondary hypothyroidism is failure of the anterior pituitary to secrete TSH, and tertiary hypothyroidism is failure of the hypothalamus to produce TRH. Most patients with symptomatic primary hypothyroidism have TSH concentrations greater than 20 mU/L. Patients with mild signs or symptoms (usually not the reason for the visit to the doctor) have TSH val-

TABLE 13-8

Primary
Iodide deficiency

Excessive iodide intake (e.g., kelp and contrast dyes)

Thyroid ablation: surgery, post ^{131}I treatment of thyrotoxicosis, radiation of neoplasm

Hashimoto's thyroiditis

Subacute thyroiditis

Genetic abnormalities of thyroid hormone synthesis

Drugs: propylthiouracil, methimazole, potassium perchlorate, thiocyanate, lithium, amiodarone

Food: excessive intake of goiterogenic foods (e.g., cabbage and turnips)

Secondary
Hypopituitarism: adenoma, ablative therapy, pituitary destruction, sarcoidosis hypothalamic dysfunction

Other
Abnormalities of T_4 receptor

Table 13-8. Classification of Hypothyroidism by Etiology[53,63,64]

ues of 10–20 mU/L. Patients with secondary and tertiary hypothyroidism may have a low or normal TSH, but other hormones (e.g., prolactin, cortisol, and gonadotropin) can be measured to confirm pituitary insufficiency. Table 13-8 outlines the numerous etiologies of hypothyroidism.

Thyrotoxicosis

Thyrotoxicosis results when excessive amounts of thyroid hormones are circulating and is usually due to hyperactivity of the thyroid gland (hyperthyroidism). Signs and symptoms include nervousness; fatigue; weight loss; heat intolerance; increased sweating; tachycardia or atrial fibrillation; muscle atrophy; warm, moist skin; and, in some patients, exophthalmos. These signs and symptoms occur much less frequently in the elderly, except for atrial fibrillation, which occurs 3 times more often.[61] Table 13-9 summarizes the specific causes of hyperthyroidism.

Nonthyroid Laboratory Tests in Patients with Thyroid Disease

Both hypo- and hyperthyroidism may cause pathophysiology outside the thyroid gland. Table 13-10 lists nonthyroid laboratory tests that may indicate a thyroid disorder. The influence on these tests reflects the widespread effects of thyroid hormones on peripheral tissues. Findings from these tests cannot be used alone to diagnose a thyroid disorder. However, they may support a diagnosis of thyroid dysfunction when used with specific thyroid function tests and the patient's presenting signs and symptoms.

TABLE 13-9

Overproduction of thyroid hormone
Graves' disease[a]
TSH-secreting pituitary adenomas
Hydatidiform moles/choriocarcinomas[b]
Multinodular goiter

"Leaking" thyroid hormone due to thyroid destruction
Lymphocytic thyroiditis
Granulomatous thyroiditis
Subacute thyroiditis
Radiation

Drugs
Thyroid-replacement drugs (excessive), amiodarone, iodinated radiocontrast agents, kelp[c]

Ovarian teratomas with thyroid elements

Metastatic thyroid carcinoma

[a] Most frequent cause. The mechanism is production of thyroid-stimulating antibodies; usually associated with diffuse goiter and ophthalmopathy.
[b] Tumor production of chorionic gonadotropin, stimulating the thyroid.
[c] Patients at risk of hyperthyroidism from these agents usually have some degree of thyroid autonomy.

Table 13-9. Classification of Hyperthyroidism by Etiology[53,61,63,64]

Thyroid Function Tests

Tests more specific for thyroid status or function can be categorized as those that (1) measure the concentration of products secreted by the thyroid gland, (2) evaluate the integrity of the hypothalamic-pituitary-thyroid axis, (3) assess inherent thyroid gland function, and (4) detect antibodies to thyroid tissue.[66] Tests that directly or indirectly measure the concentrations of T_4 and T_3 include

- Free T_4.
- Total serum T_4.
- Serum T_3 resin uptake.
- Free T_4 index.
- Total serum T_3.

The integrity of the hypothalamic-pituitary-thyroid axis is assessed by measuring

- TSH.
- TRH.

Free Thyroxine

Normal range: 0.8–1.5 ng/dL

This test measures the unbound T_4 in the serum and is the most accurate reflection of thyrometabolic status. The low concentration of free T_4 in the serum (<1% of total T_4)

TABLE 13-10

HYPOTHYROIDISM	HYPERTHYROIDISM
Decreased	
Hgb/hematocrit (Hct)[a]	Granulocytes
Serum glucose	Hgb/Hct
Serum sodium	Serum cholesterol
Urinary excretion of 17-hydroxysteroids	Serum triglycerides
Urinary excretion of 17-ketosteroids	
Increased	
Aspartate aminotransferase (SGOT/AST)	Alkaline phosphatase (ALP)
	Lymphocytes
Capillary fragility	Serum ferritin
Cerebrospinal fluid protein	Urinary calcium excretion
Lactate dehydrogenase (LDH)	
Partial pressure of carbon dioxide (pCO_2)	
Serum carotene	
Serum cholesterol	
Serum creatine phosphokinase (CPK)	
Serum prolactin	
Serum triglycerides	

[a]Associated with normocytic and/or macrocytic anemias.

Table 13-10. Nonthyroid Laboratory Tests Consistent with Thyroid Disorders[53,56,63,64]

makes accurate measurement a difficult and laborious process. Therefore, free T_4 is assayed primarily when T_4-binding globulin alterations or nonthyroidal illnesses confound interpretation of conventional tests (Tables 13-11 and 13-12).

Several methods can determine free T_4. Some methods perform well only in otherwise healthy hypo- and hyperthyroid patients and in euthyroid patients with mild abnormalities of TBG. However, in patients with severe alterations of T_4 binding to carrier proteins (e.g., severe nonthyroidal illness), only the direct equilibrium dialysis method maintains accuracy[67] (Table 13-12).

A decreased direct equilibrium dialysis free T_4 with an elevated TSH is diagnostic of primary hypothyroidism, even in patients with severely depressed TBG. Conversely, an increased direct equilibrium dialysis free T_4 with a TSH of less than 0.01 mU/L is consistent with nonpituitary hyperthyroidism.[44] Decreased direct equilibrium dialysis free T_4 with normal or decreased TSH concentrations may be seen in patients on T_3 therapy. Although free T_4 assays are becoming widely available (Table 13-11), most clinicians initially rely on the traditional total serum T_4 measurement by radioimmunoassay (RIA).

Total Serum Thyroxine

Normal range: 4–12.5 µg/dL

Although ultrasensitive TSH and free T_4 assays are gradually supplanting this RIA methodology, total serum T_4 still is the standard initial screening test to assess thyroid function because of its wide availability and quick turnaround time. In most patients, the total serum T_4 level is a sensitive test for the functional status of the thyroid gland. It is high in 90% of hyperthyroid patients and low in 85% of hypothyroid patients. This test measures both bound and free T_4 and is, therefore, influenced by any alteration in the concentration or binding affinity of thyroid-binding protein.

Conditions that increase or decrease thyroid-binding protein result in an increased or decreased total serum T_4, respectively, but do not affect the amount of metabolically active free T_4 in the circulation. Therefore, thyrometabolic status may not always be truly represented by the results. To circumvent this problem, most clinicians concomitantly obtain the T_3 resin uptake test (discussed later) so they can factor out this interference. Table 13-13 lists factors that alter thyroid-binding protein.

Increased total serum thyroxine. An increased total serum T_4 may indicate hyperthyroidism, elevated concentrations of thyroid-binding proteins, or nonthyroid illness. Total serum T_4 elevations have been noted in patients, particularly the elderly, with relatively minor illnesses. These transient elevations may be due to TSH secretion stimulated by a low T_3 concentration. Similarly, up to 20% of all patients admitted to psychiatric hospitals have had transient total serum T_4 elevation on admission.[58,70] Thus, the differential diagnosis for a patient with this elevation must include nonthyroid illness vs. hyperthyroidism if other signs and symptoms of thyroid disease are absent or inconsistent.

TABLE 13-11

DIAGNOSIS	FREE T$_4$ INDEX OR DIRECT EQUILIBRIUM DIALYSIS FREE T$_4$	TSH (mU/L)
Hyperthyroidism		
Primary		
Normal	↓	↑
On dopamine or glucocorticoids	↓	↓
Secondary or tertiary— functional hypopituitarism		
Recent thyroid withdrawal	↓	<0.10
Recently treated hyperthyroidism	↓	<0.10
Hyperthyroidism	↑	<0.10[b]
With severe nonthyroidal illness	↓/WNL/↑[c]	<0.10[b]
Euthyroid states	WNL	WNL
Low total T$_4$ of nonthyroidal illness	↓/WNL↑[d]	WNL/↑
After T$_3$ therapy	↓	WNL/↓
After T$_4$ therapy	WNL	WNL
High total T$_4$ of nonthyroidal illness	↑	WNL/↑
High total T$_4$ from amiodarone or iodinated contrast media	↑	↑
Decreased T$_4$-binding proteins	↓/WNL[e]	WNL

[a]↑ = increased; ↓ = decreased; WNL = within normal limits.
[b]Usually absent TSH response to TRH; also may be normal with hyperthyroidism from TSH-secreting tumors.
[c]Normal or low using free T$_4$ index estimation; increased using the direct equilibrium dialysis free T$_4$ assay.
[d]Decreased using free T$_4$ index estimation; normal to high using the direct equilibrium dialysis free T$_4$ assay.
[e]Decreased using free T$_4$ index estimation; normal using the direct equilibrium dialysis free T$_4$ assay.
(Adapted from Reference 55.)

Table 13-11. Free T$_4$ and TSH in Thyroidal and Nonthyroidal Disorders[a]

TABLE 13-12

ASSAY	% OF EUTHYROID PATIENTS WITH SEVERE TBG DEPRESSION OR SEVERE NONTHYROIDAL ILLNESS IN WHICH ASSAY UNDERESTIMATES FREE T$_4$	COMMENTS
Free T$_4$ index[a] or single-step immunoassays	50–80%[55]	Available in most clinical labs
Immunoextraction or radioimmunoassay[b]	10–30%[55]	Available in some clinical labs
Direct equilibrium dialysis[c]	0–5%[68,d]	Available in reference labs and large medical center labs; gold standard
Ultrafiltration[c]	0–5%[68]	Available only in research labs

[a]Corrects total T$_4$ values using an assessment of T$_4$-binding proteins.
[b]Uses a T$_4$ analog or two-step-back titration with solid-phase T$_4$ antibody but does not use membranes to separate free from bound hormone.
[c]Uses minimally diluted serum that separates free T$_4$ from bound T$_4$ using a semipermeable membrane.
[d]May be underestimated in about 25% of patients on dopamine.[69]

Table 13-12. Performance and Availability of Free T$_4$ Methods

TABLE 13-13

FACTORS THAT INCREASE THYROID-BINDING PROTEIN	FACTORS THAT DECREASE THYROID-BINDING PROTEIN
Acute infectious hepatitis	Acromegaly
Acute intermittent porphyria	Androgen therapy
Chronic active hepatitis	L-Asparaginase
Clofibrate	Cirrhosis
Estrogen-containing oral contraceptives	Danazol
Estrogen-producing tumors	Salsalate
Estrogen therapy	Genetic deficiency of total binding protein
5-Fluorouracil	Glucocorticoid therapy (high dose)
Genetic excess of total binding protein	High-dose furosemide
Heroin	Hypoproteinemia
Methadone maintenance	Malnutrition
Perphenazine	Nephrotic syndrome
Pregnancy	Salicylates
Tamoxifen	Testosterone-producing tumors

[a]Factors have the opposite effect on T_3 resin uptake (Serum Triiodothyronine Resin Uptake section).

Table 13-13. Factors Altering Thyroid-Binding Protein[53,56,58,60,63,a]

TABLE 13-14

MECHANISM	INCREASE TOTAL SERUM T_4 AND FREE T_4	DECREASE TOTAL SERUM T_4 AND FREE T_4
Interference in central regulation of TSH secretion at hypothalamic-pituitary level	Amphetamines	Glucocorticoids (acutely)
Interference with thyroid hormone synthesis and/or release from thyroid	Amiodarone[b] Iodides[b]	Aminoglutethimide Amiodarone[b] Iodides[b] Lithium carbonate 6-Mercaptopurine Sulfonamides
Altered thyroid hormone metabolism	Amiodarone[a] Iopanoic acid Ipodate Propranolol (high dose)	Phenobarbital
Inhibition of gastrointestinal absorption of exogenous thyroid hormone	Nadolol	Antacids Cholestyramine Colestipol Iron Sodium polystyrene sulfonate Soybean flour (infant formulas) Sucralfate

[a]In true alterations, the concentration change is not due to assay interference or alteration in thyroid-binding proteins.
[b]May increase or decrease total serum T_4 and free T_4.
(Compiled, in part, from References 53, 56, 58, 60, and 63.)

Table 13-14. Medications that Cause a True Alteration[a] in Total Serum T_4 and Free T_4 Measurements

Decreased total serum thyroxine. A decreased total serum T_4 may indicate hypothyroidism, decreased concentrations of thyroid-binding proteins, or nonthyroid illness (also called *euthyroid sick syndrome*). Nonthyroid illness may lower the total serum T_4 concentration with no change in thyrometabolic status. Typically in this syndrome, total serum T_4 is decreased (or normal), total serum T_3 is decreased, reverse T_3 is increased, and TSH is normal. Neoplastic disease, diabetes mellitus, burns, trauma, liver disease, renal failure, prolonged infections, and cardiovascular disease are nonthyroid illnesses that can lower total serum T_4 concentrations.

Several mechanisms probably contribute to this low T_4 state. The concentration of serum-binding proteins may diminish hormone-binding capacity. Moreover, the conversion of T_4 to T_3 may be inhibited, causing an increase in the production of reverse T_3. Another theory suggests that a circulating thyroid hormone inhibitor may bind to the thyroid-binding protein.

In general, a correlation exists between the degree of total serum T_4 depression and the prognosis of the illness (i.e., the lower the total serum T_4, the poorer the disease outcome). Since severely ill patients may appear to be hypothyroid, it is important to differentiate between patients with serious nonthyroid illnesses and those who are truly hypothyroid.[47,51] The TSH concentration Laboratory Diagnosis of Hypothalamic-Pituitary-Thyroid Axis Dysfunction section often can be helpful in making this distinction.

Drugs causing true alterations in total serum thyroxine. Medications can cause a true alteration in total serum T_4 and a corresponding change in free T_4 concentrations (Table 13-14). In such cases, the total serum T_4 (and free T_4) result remains a true reflection of thyrometabolic status. High-dose salicylates and phenytoin also may lower total serum T_4 significantly via decreased binding in vivo. Phenytoin may lower free T_4, and salicylates may increase it.[71]

As noted in Table 13-15, iodides can significantly alter thyroid status. They have the potential to inhibit thyroid hormone release and to impair the organification of iodine. In healthy individuals, this effect lasts only 1–2 weeks. However, individuals with subclinical hypothyroid disease may develop clinical hypothyroidism after treatment with iodides. Iodide-induced hypothyroidism has also been noted in patients with cystic fibrosis and emphysema.[58]

Iodides may also *increase* thyroid function. A previously euthyroid patient may develop thyrotoxicosis from exposure to increased quantities of iodine. Supplemental iodine causes autonomously functioning thyroid tissue to produce and secrete thyroid hormones, leading to a significant increase in T_4 and T_3 concentrations. This phenomenon commonly occurs during therapeutic iodine replacement in patients who live in areas of endemic iodine deficiency.

Similarly, patients with underlying goiter who live in iodine-sufficient areas may develop hyperthyroidism when given pharmacological doses of iodide. The heavily (37%) iodinated antiarrhythmic medication amiodarone may induce hyperthyroidism (1–5% of patients) as well as hypothyroidism (6–10% of patients).[6,19] Table 13-15 lists iodine-containing compounds.

TABLE 13-15

Oral radiopaque agents
Diatrizoate
Iocetamic acid
Iopanoic acid
Ipodate
Tyropanoate

Expectorants
Iodinated glycerol[a]
Potassium iodide solution
SSKI (supersaturated potassium iodide)

Parenteral radiopaque agents
Diatrizoate meglumine
Iodamide meglumine
Iopamidol
Iothalamate meglumine
Metrizamide

Miscellaneous compounds
Amiodarone
Kelp-containing nutritional supplements

[a]No longer available; most products reformulated with guaifenesin.
(Compiled, in part, from References 58 and 63.)

Table 13-15. Iodine-Containing Compounds that May Influence Thyroid Status

Although antithyroid drugs such as propylthiouracil and methimazole are not listed in Table 13-15, they are used in hyperthyroid patients to decrease hormone concentrations. Both T_4 and T_3 concentrations decrease more rapidly with methimazole than propylthiouracil.[73]

Serum Triiodothyronine Resin Uptake

Normal range: 25–34%

The T_3 resin uptake test indirectly estimates the number of binding sites on thyroid-binding protein occupied by T_3. This result is also referred to as the *thyroid hormone-binding ratio*. The T_3 resin uptake is usually high when the thyroid-binding protein is low and the reverse.

In this test, radiolabeled T_3 is added to endogenous hormone. An aliquot of this mixture is then added to a resin that competes with endogenous thyroid-binding proteins for the free hormone. Radiolabeled T_3 binds to any free endogenous thyroid-binding protein; at the saturation point, the remainder binds to the resin. The amount of thyroid-binding protein can be estimated from the amount of radiolabeled T_3 taken up by the resin. The T_3 resin uptake result is expressed as a percentage of the total radiolabeled T_3 that binds to the resin. The T_3 resin uptake can verify the clinical significance of measured total serum T_4 and T_3 concentrations because it is an indicator of thyroid-binding protein-induced alterations of these measurements.

Elevated T_3 resin uptake concentrations are consistent with hyperthyroidism, while decreased concentrations are consistent with hypothyroidism. However, this test is never used alone for diagnosis. The T_3 resin uptake is low in hypothyroidism because of the increased availability of binding sites on the thyroid-binding globulin. However, in nonthyroidal illnesses with a low T_4, the T_3 resin uptake is elevated. Therefore, the test may be used to differentiate between true hypothyroidism and a low T_4 state caused by nonthyroid illness.

All of the disease states and medications listed in Table 13-13 can influence thyroid-binding protein and, consequently, alter T_3 resin uptake results. Radioactive substances taken by the patient also will interfere with this test. In practice, the T_3 resin uptake test is used only to calculate the free T_4 index.

Free Thyroxine Index

Normal range: 1.0–4.0 units

The free T_4 index is the product of total serum T_4 multiplied by the percentage of T_3 resin uptake:

$$\text{free } T_4 \text{ index} = \text{total serum } T_4 \text{ (mg/dL)} \times T_3 \text{ resin uptake (\%)}$$

The free T_4 index adjusts for the effects of alterations in thyroid-binding protein on the total serum T_4 assay. The index is high in hyperthyroidism and low in hypothyroidism. Patients taking phenytoin or salicylates have low total serum T_4 and high T_3 resin uptake with a normal free T_4 index. Pregnant patients have high total serum T_4 and low T_3 resin uptake with a normal free T_4 index. Patients taking therapeutic doses of levothyroxine may have a high free T_4 index, because total serum T_4 and T_3 resin uptake are high. In addition to affecting total serum T_4 and free T_4 (Table 13-14), propranolol and nadolol block the conversion of T_4 to T_3, which may cause mild elevations in the free T_4 index.

Total Serum Triiodothyronine

Normal range: 78–195 ng/dL or 1.2–3.0 nmol/L

This RIA measures the highly active thyroid hormone T_3. Like T_4, almost all of T_3 is protein bound. Therefore, any alteration in thyroid-binding protein influences this measurement.

As with the total serum T_4 test, changes in thyroid-binding protein increase or decrease total serum T_3 but do not affect the metabolically active free T_3 in the circulation. Therefore, the patient's thyrometabolic status remains unchanged.

The total serum T_3 is primarily used as an indicator of hyperthyroidism. This measurement is usually made to detect T_3 toxicosis when T_3, but not T_4, is elevated. Generally, the serum T_3 assay is not a reliable indicator of hypothyroidism because of the lack of reliability in the low to normal range.

Drugs that affect T_4 concentrations (Table 13-14) have a corresponding effect on T_3 concentrations. Additionally, propranolol, propylthiouracil, and glucocorticoids inhibit the peripheral conversion of T_4 to T_3 and cause a decreased T_3 concentration (T_4 usually stays normal).[74]

Total serum T_3 concentrations can be low in euthyroid patients with conditions (e.g., malnutrition, cirrhosis, and uremia) in which the conversion of T_4 to T_3 is suppressed. T_3 is low in only half of hypothyroid patients because these patients tend to produce relatively more T_3 than T_4. A patient with a normal total serum T_4, a low T_3, and a high reverse T_3 has euthyroid sick syndrome.

Thyroid-Stimulating Hormone (TSH)

Normal range: 0.25–6.7 μU/mL
text describes interpretation of first- and second-generation assays

TSH is a glycoprotein with two subunits, alpha and beta. The alpha subunit is similar to those of other hormones secreted from the anterior pituitary: follicle-stimulating hormone, human chorionic gonadotropin (HCG), and luteinizing hormone. The beta subunit of TSH is unique and renders its specific physiological properties.

Although the older, "first-generation" TSH assays have been useful in diagnosing primary hypothyroidism, they have not been useful in diagnosing hyperthyroidism. Almost all patients with symptomatic primary hypothyroidism have TSH concentrations greater than 20 mU/L; those with mild signs or symptoms have TSH values of 10–20 mU/L. TSH concentrations often become elevated before T_4 concentrations decline. All assays can accurately measure *high* concentrations of TSH.

The first-generation TSH assays, however, cannot distinguish low-normal from abnormally low values because their lower limit of detection is 0.5 mU/L, while the lower limit of basal TSH is 0.2–0.3 mU/L in most euthyroid persons. This distinction can usually be ascertained with the second-generation assays, which can accurately measure TSH concentrations as low as 0.05 mU/L. Occasionally, some euthyroid patients have concentrations of 0.05–0.5 mU/L. Therefore, supersensitive, third-generation assays have been developed; they can detect TSH concentrations as low as 0.005 mU/L. Concentrations below 0.05 mU/L are almost always diagnostic of primary hyperthyroidism in patients younger than 70 years.

Some clinicians feel that neither a low basal TSH concentration nor a blunted TSH response to TRH discussed later is a reliable predictor of hyperthyroidism in elderly patients.[75] Although third-generation assays are usually not required to make or confirm this diagnosis, they provide a wider margin of tolerance so that discrimination at 0.1 mU/L can be assured even when the assay is not performing optimally.[70]

Use in therapy. In patients with primary hypothyroidism, TSH concentrations are also used to adjust the dosage of levothyroxine replacement therapy. In addition to achieving a clinical euthyroid state, the goal should be to lower TSH into the midnormal range (Minicase 3). TSH concentrations reflect long-term thyroid status, while serum T_4 concentrations reflect acute changes. Patients with long-standing hypothyroidism often notice an improvement in well-being 2–3 weeks after starting therapy. Significant improvements in heart rate

AMY T., AN 18-YEAR-OLD FEMALE, visited her physician with complaints of weakness, fatigue, weight gain, hoarseness, cold intolerance, and unusually heavy periods worsening over the past 2–3 months. Her pulse was 50, and her blood pressure (BP) was 110/70. Her physical exam was normal, except for a mildly enlarged thyroid gland, pallor, and diminished tendon reflexes. She denied taking any medications or changing her diet.

The patient's chemistry results were sodium 130 mEq/L (136–145 mEq/L), potassium 3.8 mEq/L (3.5–5.0 mEq/L), carbon dioxide 28 mEq/L (24–30 mEq/L), calcium 9.5 mg/dL (8.5–10.8 mg/dL), magnesium 2 mEq/L (1.5–2.2 mEq/L), glucose 80 mg/dL (70–110 mg/dL), blood urea nitrogen (BUN) 20 mg/dL (8–20 mg/dL), serum creatinine (SCr) 1.1 mg/dL (0.7–1.5 mg/dL), and cholesterol 235 mg/dL (<200 mg/dL). The cholesterol concentration was elevated since a screening 6 months ago. A test for mononucleosis was negative. Hematocrit (Hct) was low at 35% (37–47%)—close to her usual. Her total serum T_4 was 8 µg/dL (4–12 µg/dL), her T_3 resin uptake was 15% (25–35%), and her free T_4 index was 1.2 (1.2–4.2).

Question: How should these results be interpreted? Are confirmatory tests needed?

Discussion: Clinically, all of the history and physical findings point to hypothyroidism. The pallor and weakness are also consistent with anemia, but an Hct of 35% is unlikely to cause such significant symptoms. Amy T.'s cholesterol recently became elevated, consistent with primary hypothyroidism.[33] Classically, both the total serum T_4 and T_3 resin uptake should be low in hypothyroid patients. In Amy T., only the T_3 resin uptake is low, and the free T_4 index is borderline normal, making laboratory diagnosis unclear. Confirmatory tests should prove useful.

A few days later, Amy T. revisited her physician for additional tests. When questioned, she admitted that she has been taking oral contraceptives and would like to continue. The following day, her TSH was 25 mU/L (0.3–5.0 mU/L), her thyroid microsomal antibody was greater than 1:500, and her thyroglobulin antibody was greater than 1:1000.

Question: Does this information help to elucidate the diagnosis?

Discussion: The high titers of antibodies confirm that Amy T. has Hashimoto's thyroiditis, which has manifested as hypothyroidism. An elevated TSH confirms primary hypothyroidism. The reason for equivocal total serum T_4 and T_3 resin uptake is now apparent—the estrogens in the birth control pills. Estrogens elevate total serum T_4 and thyroid-binding protein and lower T_3 resin uptake. If Amy T. had not been taking estrogens, her total serum T_4 probably would have been below normal and her T_3 resin uptake probably would have been higher (but still below normal). The diagnosis would have been clear earlier. If oral contraceptive use had been identified at the first visit, a TSH concentration should have been performed then.

Amy T. was started on levothyroxine 0.2 mg/day, and her TSH was 6 mU/L 3 weeks later. Clinically, she improved but was not fully back to normal. Six weeks after starting therapy, she complained of jitteriness, palpitations, and increased sweating. Her TSH was less than 0.3 mU/L. Her physician lowered the dose of levothyroxine to 0.1 mg/day, and Amy T. became asymptomatic after about 2 weeks. Eight weeks later, her TSH was 1.5 mU/L and she remained asymptomatic. Her cholesterol was 100 mg/dL, sodium was 138 mEq/L, and Hct was 40%.

Question: Which test(s) should be used to determine proper dosing of levothyroxine? How long after a dosage change should clinicians wait before repeating the test(s)?

Discussion: Although total serum T_4, T_3 resin uptake, and free T_4 index can be used to monitor and adjust doses of thyroid supplements in patients with a hypothyroid disorder, the highly sensitive TSH is most reliable. Chemically, the goal is to achieve a TSH in the normal range, as was ultimately achieved in Amy T. (TSH of 1.5 mU/L). Because of her continued use of birth control pills, TSH is the best test for this patient. The newer TSH assays make it possible to determine whether TSH secretion is being excessively suppressed by thyroid replacement (<0.3 mU/L).

With the increased availability of this sensitive test, TSH is becoming the standard for adjusting thyroid replacement therapy in most patients. The 0.2-mg levothyroxine dose was excessive, given the "hyperthyroid" symptoms and the fully suppressed TSH. Eight weeks later, after T_4 steady state was reached on the 0.1-mg/day dose and after the hypothalamic-pituitary-thyroid axis reached homeostasis, TSH was within the desired range. Amy T.'s cholesterol, sodium, and Hct also normalized as she became euthyroid.

(HR), weight, and puffiness are seen early in therapy, but hoarseness, anemia, and skin/hair changes may take many months to resolve.[76]

Unless undesirable changes in signs or symptoms occur, it is rational to wait at least 6–8 weeks after starting or changing therapy to repeat TSH and/or T_4 concentrations to refine dosing.[55,77] The hypothalamic-pituitary axis requires this time to respond fully to changes in circulating thyroid hormone concentrations.

This slow readjustment can be exploited elsewhere. One study[78] found that greater than 50% of TSH elevations in patients being treated with levothyroxine were attributed to noncompliance; with counseling alone, TSH normalized on subsequent visits. Noncompliant hypothyroid patients who take their levothyroxine pills only before being tested may have elevated TSH concentrations despite a normal T_4 concentration.[70]

Because of slow axis readjustment, patients given antithyroid drugs (e.g., methimazole) may maintain low TSH concentrations for 2–3 months after T_4 and T_3 concentrations have returned to normal. Single, daily doses of 10–20 mg of methimazole usually lead to euthyroidism within several weeks.[79] Treatment should not be adjusted too early using (low) TSH concentrations alone. However, the dose should be reduced within the first 8 weeks if TSH concentrations become elevated.

Patients with thyroid cancer are often treated with TSH suppressive therapy, usually levothyroxine. The therapeutic endpoint is a basal TSH concentration of about 0.1 mU/L.[80] Some clinicians suggest more complete suppression with TSH concentrations less than 0.005 mU/L, while others think that it leads to toxic effects of over-replacement (e.g., accelerated bone loss) (Minicase 3).[70,78]

Potential misinterpretation and drug interference. Some TSH assays may yield falsely high results whenever HCG concentrations are high to the similarity in structure of these two proteins.

Most patients who have secondary or tertiary hypothyroidism have a low or normal TSH concentration. In patients with nonthyroid illness, TSH may be suppressed by factors other than thyroid hyperfunction. As mentioned previously, the TSH concentration typically is normal in patients with the euthyroid sick syndrome.

Thyroid function tests are known to be altered in depressed patients. With the advent of the third-generation TSH assays, investigators hoped that TSH concentrations could help to determine various types of depression and response to therapies. Unfortunately, neither TSH nor its response to TRH has proven useful in this way.[82]

Because endogenous dopamine inhibits the stimulatory effects of TRH, any drug with dopaminergic activity can inhibit TSH secretion. Therefore, levodopa, glucocorticoids, bromocriptine, and dopamine are likely to lower TSH results. The converse is also true—the dopamine antagonists (metoclopramide) may increase TSH concentrations.

Thyrotropin-Releasing Hormone (TRH) Stimulation Test

TRH, a hormone secreted by the hypothalamus, regulates TSH secretion from the pituitary. The TRH test measures the ability of injected TRH to stimulate the pituitary to release TSH (and prolactin). This test has been the most reliable

TABLE 13-16

DYSFUNC-TIONING TISSUE OR GLAND	TSH BEFORE TRH CHALLENGE	TSH AFTER TRH CHALLENGE
Thyroid	High	Exaggerated
Pituitary	Low/absent	No response
Hypothalamus	Low	Sluggish response

[a] *Patients with hyperthyroidism have a suppressed pretest TSH and no response or a blunted response to TRH infusion.*

Table 13-16. Differentiation of Hypothyroid Disorders Based on TSH and TRH Challenge Test Results[a]

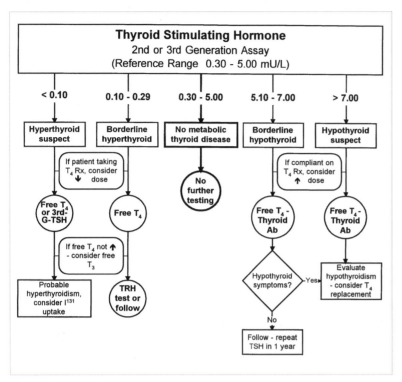

Figure 13-5. Algorithm for investigation of thyroid disease using second-third-generation TSH assay as an initial test in patients without pituitary or neuropsychiatric disease. (Adapted, with permission, from Reference 70.)

indicator of hyperthyroidism in patients whose other thyroid function tests are equivocal, primarily with the older, less sensitive TSH assays. With second- and third-generation TSH assays becoming more widely available, this TRH test is infrequently required. Nevertheless, it still is useful to distinguish primary from secondary hypothyroidism (Table 13-16).

This test is performed by drawing a baseline serum TSH concentration and then administering approximately 200–400 µg of TRH (synthetic protirelin) intravenously (IV) over 30–60 sec. TSH concentrations are drawn at 30–60 min. A normal response, indicative of the euthyroid state, is defined as a TSH rise of 5 µU/mL over baseline. A significant increase virtually rules out hyperthyroidism. A blunted or absent TSH response suggests hyperthyroidism. However, a rise of less than 5 µU/mL can be seen in euthyroid men over age 40, in depressed patients, and in patients with glucocorticoid excess. A blunted response may occur in euthyroid patients receiving adequate thyroid suppression therapy, dopamine, glucocorticoid, somatostatin, or L-dopa therapy.

Endogenous TRH secretion is enhanced by norepinephrine and serotonin. As mentioned previously, the need for this test should decrease with the advent of the sensitive TSH immunometric assays. Patients with basal TSH concentrations less than 0.1 µU/mL typically do not have a TSH increase after a TRH challenge.

Radioactive Iodine Uptake Test

This test is used to detect the ability of the thyroid gland to trap and concentrate iodine and, thereby, produce thyroid hormone. In other words, this test assesses the intrinsic function of the thyroid gland. This test is not specific, and its reference range must be adjusted to the local population. Therefore, its use is declining. In patients with a normal thyroid gland, 12–20% of the radioactive iodine is absorbed by the gland after 6 hr and 5–25% is absorbed after 24 hr. The radioactive iodine uptake test is an indirect measure of thyroid gland activity and should not be used as a basic screening test of thyroid function. This test is most useful in distinguishing hyperthyroidism caused by subacute thyroiditis with absent or reduced uptake of iodine.[64,83,84]

A high radioactive iodine uptake is noted with[52,71,72]

- Thyrotoxicosis.
- Iodine deficiency.
- Post-thyroiditis.
- Withdrawal rebound after thyroid hormone or antithyroid drug therapy.

A low test result occurs in[64,83,84]

- Acute thyroiditis.
- Euthyroid patients who ingest iodine-containing products.
- Patients on exogenous thyroid hormone therapy.
- Patients who are taking antithyroid drugs such as propylthiouracil.
- Hypothyroidism.

TABLE 13-17

DISEASE	TOTAL SERUM T_4	TOTAL SERUM T_3	T_3 RESIN UPTAKE	FREE T_4 INDEX[a]	RAIU	TSH	COMMENT
Hypothyroidism	↓	↓	↓	↓	↓	↑/↓[b]	
Hyperthyroidism	↑	↑	↑	↑	↑	↓	
T_3 thyrotoxicosis	No change	↑	No change	No change	No change/↑	↓	T_3 resin uptake may be slightly increased
Euthyroid sick syndrome	No change/↓	↓	↑	Variable	No change	No change	
Corticosteroids	↓	No change/↓	↑	No change	↓	No change/↓	
Phenytoin/aspirin	↓	↓	↑	No change	↓	No change	Large salicylate dose
Radiopaque media	No change/↑	No change/↓	No change	No change/↑ ↓		No change	

[a]RAIU = radioactive iodine uptake test; ↑ = increased; ↓ = decreased.
[b]Increased TSH diagnostic of primary hypothyroidism. TSH is decreased in secondary and tertiary types.

Table 13-17. Test Results Seen in Common Thyroid Disorders and Drug Effects on Test Results[55,66,70,86,87,a]

The radioactive iodine uptake test is affected by the body's store of iodine. Therefore, the patient should be carefully questioned about the use of iodine-containing products prior to the test. This test is contraindicated during pregnancy.

Antithyroid Antibodies

Normal range: varies with antibody

Antibodies that "attack" various thyroid tissue can be detected in the serum of patients with autoimmune disorders such as Hashimoto's thyroiditis and Graves' disease. Thyroid microsomal antibody is found in 95% of patients with Hashimoto's thyroiditis, 55% of patients with Graves' disease, and 10% of adults without thyroid disease. In patients who have nodular and hard goiters, high antibody titers strongly suggest Hashimoto's thyroiditis as opposed to cancer. In Grave's disease, hyperthyroidism is caused by antibodies, which activate TSH receptors. In chronic autoimmune thyroiditis, hypothyroidism may be caused by antibodies competitively binding to TSH receptors, thereby blocking TSH from eliciting a response.[85]

If a significant amount of antibodies is present in the blood, agglutination (clumping) occurs. The test for this antibody is based dopamine antagonists metoclopramide. Results are reported as the highest titer causing agglutination. Titers in excess of 1:100 are significant and usually can be detected even during remission.

Antibodies (>1:10) to thyroglobulin are present in 60–70% of adults with active Hashimoto's thyroiditis but typically are not detected during remission. Titers above 1:1000 are found only in Hashimoto's thyroiditis or Graves' disease (25 or 10%, respectively). Lower titers may be seen in 4% of the normal population, although the frequency increases with age in females. The thyroid microsomal antibody and thyroglobulin antibody serological tests may be elevated or positive in patients with nonthyroidal autoimmune disease.

Anti-TSH receptor antibodies are present in virtually all patients with Graves' disease, but the test is usually not necessary for diagnosis. These antibodies mostly stimulate TSH receptors but also may compete with TSH and, thus, inhibit TSH stimulation. High titers allow a confirmation of Graves' disease in asymptomatic patients, such as those whose only manifestation is exophthalmos (Minicase 3).

Laboratory Diagnosis of Hypothalamic-Pituitary-Thyroid Axis Dysfunction

The laboratory diagnosis of primary *hypothyroidism* can be made with a low free T_4 index and an elevated TSH concentration. The presence of a low free T_4 index and a normal or low serum TSH concentration indicates secondary or tertiary hypothyroidism or nonthyroid illness. In such patients, the T_3 resin uptake may differentiate between hypothyroidism and a low T_4 state due to nonthyroid illness. An elevated reverse T_3 concentration also suggests nonthyroid illness. The TRH test may be used to pinpoint the thyroid axis defect (Table 13-16). T_3 is of limited usefulness in diagnosing hypothyroidism because it may be normal in up to one-third of hypothyroid patients.[64,66,83,84] With the availability of ultrasensitive TSH assays, many clinicians begin their evaluations with this test. One such approach is illustrated in Figure 13-5 and Minicase 3.

The newer TSH assay can also be used to diagnose *hyperthyroidism* (<0.1 mU/L). The total serum T_4 and free T_4 or free T_4 index still are commonly used here and are increased in almost all hyperthyroid patients. Usually, both T_3 and T_4 are elevated. However, a few (<5%) hyperthyroid patients exhibit normal T_4 with elevated T_3 (T_3 toxicosis). Second-line tests such as antithyroid antibody serologies are necessary to diagnose autoimmune thyroid disorders. Table 13-17 summarizes test results seen with common thyroid disorders.

Adrenal Disorders

The adrenal glands are located extraperitoneally at the upper poles of each kidney. The adrenal medulla, which makes up 10 % of the adrenal gland, secretes catecholamines (e.g., epinephrine and norepinephrine). The adrenal cortex, which comprises 90 % of the adrenal gland, is divided into three areas:

1. The outer layer of the adrenal gland, known as the zona glomerulosa, makes up 15% of the adrenal gland and is responsible for production of aldosterone, a mineralocorticoid that regulates electrolyte and volume homeostasis.
2. The zona fasciculata, located in the center of the adrenal gland, occupies 60% of the gland and is responsible for glucocorticoid production. Cortisol, a principal end product of glucocorticoid production, regulates fat, carbohydrate, and protein metabolism. Glucocorticoids maintain the body's homeostasis by regulating bodily functions involved in stress as well as normal activities.
3. The zona reticularis makes up 25% of the adrenal gland and is responsible for adrenal androgens such as testosterone and estradiol. These hormones influence the development of the reproductive system.[62]

Cushing's Syndrome

Cushing's syndrome, first described 70 years ago, is the result of excessive concentrations of cortisol. In most cases, hypercortisolism is the result of overproduction by the adrenal glands due to an adrenocorticotropic hormone (ACTH) secreting pituitary tumor. Adrenal tumors and long-term use of glucocorticoids can also result in hypercortisolism.

Patients with hypercortisolism generally present with facial plethora as a result of atrophy of the skin and underlying tissue. A common sign of hypercortisolism is fat accumulation in the dorsocervical area often referred to as "buffalo hump." Other cardinal signs and symptoms include hypertension, osteopenia, glucose intolerance, myopathy, bruising, and depression. Hyperpigmentation is present in patients with ACTH-secreting pituitary tumors. Hair loss, acne, and oligomenorrhea are also the result of superfluous cortical secretion.

Diagnostic Tests

Several tests are employed to identify patients with Cushing's syndrome. The most frequently used test to identify patients with hypercortisolism is the 24-hr urine free cortisol (UFC) test. UFC measures free cortisol levels and creatinine in a urine sample, which is collected over a 24-hr period. Cortisol levels greater than 200 µg suggest hypercortisolism. Physiological levels of cortisol usually decline between 8:00 a.m. and 11:00 p.m. Midnight serum cortisol levels greater than 7.5 µg/mL indicates Cushing's syndrome. Of the suppression tests, the overnight dexamethasone-suppression test is the least laborious test to perform. The patient is given 1 mg of dexamethasone at 11:00 p.m. followed by a plasma cortisol assay at 8 a.m. the next morning. Patients with Cushing's disease will have high cortisol concentrations (>5 µg/mL) due to an inability to suppress the negative-feedback mechanism of the HPA axis.

Once hypercortisolism is confirmed, additional tests should be performed to identify the source of hypersecretion. Additional tests should be performed to confirm the diagnosis since other factors (starvation, topical steroid application, and acute stress) influence the results of the abovementioned tests.

Plasma ACTH concentrations can be measured by radioimmunoassay procedures. Interpretation of the results is as follows:

⇒ ACTH concentrations less than 5 µg/mL indicate an ACTH independent adrenal source such as an adrenal tumor or long-term use of steroids.

⇒ ACTH levels between 5–10 µg/mL should be followed by a corticotropin-releasing hormone (CRH) test.

⇒ Levels greater than 10 µg/mL indicate an ACTH-dependent Cushing's syndrome.

The CRH test can be employed to determine if the source of hypercortisolism is pituitary or ectopic (extra-pituitary). Baseline ACTH and CRH levels are obtained. Then, ACTH and cortisol levels are measured 30–45 min after the administration of a 1 µg/mL dose of CRH. A 50% increase from baseline in ACTH levels indicates ACTH-dependent syndrome.

The overnight high dose dexamethasone suppression test is also used to identify the source of hypercortisolism. A baseline plasma cortisol level is obtained the morning prior to the test. Patients are given dexamethasone 8 mg at 11:00 p.m. Plasma cortisol levels are obtained at 8:00 a.m. the following morning. Plasma cortisol levels less than 50% of baseline indicate ACTH-dependent syndrome.[88,89]

Pharmacologic Treatment

Treatment of Cushing's syndrome involves inhibition of steroid synthesis. Mitotane is the most frequently prescribed agent for the treatment of this disorder. Mitotane inhibits steroid biosynthesis as well as inhibits peripheral steroid metabolism and cortisol release. Metyrapone, aminoglutethimide, and ketoconazole are adrenal enzyme inhibitors that inhibit enzymes necessary for the conversion of cholesterol into steroid hormones, which is a necessary step for the production of cortisol. Cyproheptadine is a neuromodulatory agent that has used to decrease ACTH secretion. Due to a low response rate of less than 30%, cyproheptadine is reserved for patients who fail conventional therapy.[88,89]

Adrenal Insufficiency or Addison's Disease

Adrenal insufficiency (Addison's disease or primary adrenal insufficiency) is the result of an autoimmune attack, resulting in destruction of all regions of the adrenal cortex. Tuberculosis, fungal infections, acquired immunodeficiency syndrome, metastatic cancer, and lymphomas can also precipitate adrenal insufficiency. Adrenal insufficiency results in deficiencies in cortisol, aldosterone, and androgens. Patients usually present with weakness, weight loss, increased pigmentation, hypotension, gastrointestinal symptoms, postural dizziness, and vertigo.

Secondary adrenal insufficiency can result from the use of high doses of exogenous steroids, which suppress the hypothalamic-pituitary axis resulting in a decrease in the release of ACTH. Patients with secondary adrenal insufficiency maintain normal aldosterone levels and do not exhibit signs of hyperpigmentation.

Diagnostic Tests

The cosyntropin stimulation test is used to diagnose patients with low cortisol levels. Patients are administered 250 μg of synthetic ACTH or cosyntropin intravenously or intramuscularly. Serum cortisol levels are drawn at the time of injection and 30 min and 1 hr after the injection. Cortisol levels greater than 20 μg/dL indicate an adequate response from the adrenal gland, thus ruling out adrenal insufficiency.

Pharmacologic Treatment

Corticosteroids are used to treat adrenal insufficiency. The agents of choice include prednisone 5 mg/day, hydrocortisone 20 mg/day, and cortisone 25 mg/day given in the morning and evening. Additional mineralocorticoid (e.g., fludrocortisone acetate 0.05–2.0 mg daily) should be given to patients with primary adrenal insufficiency since there is a concomitant depletion of aldosterone levels. The end point of therapy is the reversal of signs and symptoms of adrenal insufficiency, particularly excess pigmentation.[91]

DIABETES INSIPIDUS

Diabetes insipidus is a syndrome in which the body's inability to conserve water manifests as excretion of very large volumes of dilute urine. This section explores related pathophysiology, types of diabetes insipidus, and interpretation of test results to evaluate this disorder.

Physiology

Normally, serum osmolality is maintained around 285 mOsm/kg and is determined by the amounts of sodium, chloride, bicarbonate, glucose, and urea in the serum. The excretion of these solutes along with water is a primary factor in determining urine volume and concentration. In turn, the amount of water excreted by the kidneys is determined by renal function and antidiuretic hormone (ADH), also known as vasopressin.

ADH is synthesized in the hypothalamus and stored in the posterior pituitary gland. This hormone is released into the circulation following physiological stimulation, such as a change in serum osmolality or blood volume detected by the osmoregulatory centers in the hypothalamus.[92] Congestive heart failure lowers the osmotic threshold for ADH release, while nausea—but not vomiting—strongly stimulates ADH. In general, alpha-adrenergic agonists stimulate ADH release while beta-adrenergic agonists inhibit release. ADH acts on the distal renal tubule and the collecting duct to cause water reabsorption. Chlorpropamide potentiates the effect of ADH on renal concentrating ability. When ADH is lacking or the renal tubules do not respond to the hormone, polyuria ensues. If the polyuria is severe enough, a diagnosis of diabetes insipidus is considered.

Clinical Diagnosis

Diabetes insipidus (DI) should be differentiated from other causes of polyuria such as osmotic diuresis (e.g., hyperglycemia, mannitol, and contrast media), renal tubular acidosis, diuretic therapy, and psychogenic polydipsia. Patients usually excrete 16–24 L of dilute urine in 24 hr. The urine specific gravity is less than 1.005 and urine osmolality is less than 200 mOsm/kg.[93,94]

DI is usually caused by a defect in the secretion (neurogenic, also called central) or renal activity (nephrogenic) of ADH. It can also be caused by a defect in thirst (dipsogenic) or psychological function (psychogenic), with resultant excessive intake of water. Although DI typically does not lead to significant morbidity, the underlying cause should be sought to

HELEN T., A 32-YEAR-OLD FEMALE being assessed for infertility, was found to have a TSH concentration of 8.2 µU/mL (0.3–5.0 µU/mL) as measured by a second-generation assay. Her physical exam revealed no abnormalities, and she was clinically euthyroid. Her total serum T_4 was 10 µg/dL (4–12 µg/dL). She was treated with 0.125 mg/day of levothyroxine for 1 month, and a repeat TSH was 6.8 µU/mL. Her dose was increased to 0.2 mg/day.

After 2 months, Helen T.'s TSH was 8.8 µU/mL, while her total serum T_4 was 15 µg/dL, her total serum T_3 was 200 ng/dL (78–195 ng/dL), her TBG was 32 nmol/L (14–41 nmol/L), and her free T_3 was 4.7 pmol/L (3.2–5.1 pmol/L). She was slightly hyperthyroid. Levothyroxine therapy was stopped and, on that day, a TRH challenge (200 µg IV) evoked only minimal increases in TSH concentrations. Magnetic resonance imaging (MRI) of the hypothalamic-pituitary area was normal.

Question: What could have caused Helen T.'s initial elevated TSH?

Discussion: TSH is classically elevated in patients with primary hypothyroidism. However, Helen T. did not have any clinical signs or symptoms of this disorder. Inappropriate elevation of TSH can be caused by a TSH-secreting pituitary tumor, thyroid hormone resistance, or assay interference. Tumor was ruled out by the normal MRI. Hormone resistance is not consistent with the patient's picture. If Helen T. had pituitary-confined resistance, persistent secretion of TSH and thyroid hormones would have led to clinical hyperthyroidism. If resistance had been general, she would have been euthyroid (as she was), but T_4 and T_3 concentrations would have been elevated along with TSH.[35]

Finally, transiently elevated TSH may be found in patients recovering from major physiological stress (e.g., intensive care illnesses and trauma), which was not the case here. Thyroid status should be evaluated after major medical problems have stabilized. The TRH challenge showed essentially no response, a finding that reflects the iatrogenic hyperthyroidism at the time. Therefore, by exclusion, Helen T.'s elevated TSH concentration most likely is an artifact, probably interfering antibodies. This condition is rare but has been described.[36]

---

ensure proper prognosis and therapy. The specific type of DI often can be identified by the clinical setting. If the diagnosis is equivocal, a therapeutic trial with an antidiuretic drug or measurement of plasma ADH is necessary.[62,94]

Clinically, the easiest way to make the diagnosis is to perform a dehydration test, where the patient is deprived of water for 8–12 hr. Urine osmolality, urine volume, and body weight is taken before and after the subcutaneous administration of desmopressin acetate. As compared to patients with nephrogenic diabetes insipidus whose urine osmolality will not rise above 300 mOsm/kg, patients with central diabetes insipidus have an immediate rise in urine osmolality with a decrease in urine volume when challenged with a subcutaneous injection of desmopressin.

Patients can be challenged with a test dose of ADH. Urine osmolality greater than 750 mOsm/kg in response to an ADH test dose confirms the diagnosis of central DI. A hypertonic saline solution can also be administered intravenously in an attempt to raise plasma osmolality to 300 mOsm/kg. A direct measurement of ADH can be done to determine response to hypertonic plasma. Patients with nephrogenic DI will have normal ADH levels compared to patients with central DI who will have a negligible response to hypertonic plasma due to a decrease or lack of endogenous ADH.[95]

Central Diabetes Insipidus

Central diabetes insipidus (ADH deficiency) may be the result of any disruption in the pituitary-hypothalamic regulation of ADH. Patients often present with a sudden onset of polyuria (in the absence of hyperglycemia) and preference for iced drinks. Tumors or metastases in or around the pituitary or hypothalamus, head trauma, neurosurgery, genetic abnormalities, Guillain-Barré syndrome, meningitis, encephalitis, toxoplasmosis, cytomegalovirus, tuber-

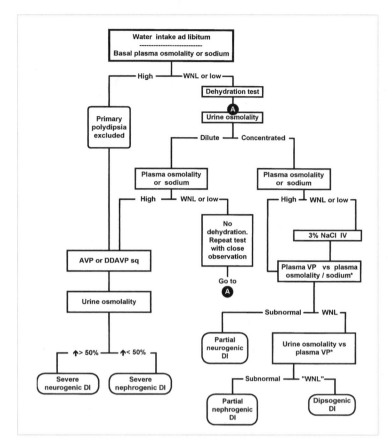

Figure 13-6. Evaluation of diabetes insipidus if diagnosis is ambiguous based on the clinical setting and basal plasma vasopressin concentrations. Plasma osmolality and sodium are considered high if they exceed the upper limit of normal for the laboratory (usually 295 mOsm/kg and 145 mEq/L, respectively). Urine is considered diluted if its osmolality is less than 300 mOsm/kg; it is concentrated if its osmolality is greater than 300 mOsm/kg. If indicated, hypertonic saline is infused at 0.1 mL/kg/min for 2 hr. The vasopressin (aqueous Pitressin, AVP) dose is 1 unit, while the DDAVP dose is 1 µg subcutaneously. WNL = within normal limits; VP = vasopressin = ADH; DI = diabetes insipidus. Interpretation of plasma VP vs. plasma osmolality/sodium and urine osmolality vs. plasma VP requires use of a nomogram. (Adapted, with permission, from Reference 92.)

culosis, and aneurysms are some of the known causes. In addition, phenytoin and alcohol inhibit ADH release from the pituitary. In response to deficient secretion of ADH and subsequent hyperosmolality of the plasma, thirst is stimulated. Thirst induces water intake, which leads to polyuria in the absence of effective ADH.

Nephrogenic Diabetes Insipidus

In nephrogenic diabetes insipidus (ADH resistance), the secretion of ADH is normal, but the renal tubule does not respond to ADH. Causes of nephrogenic diabetes insipidus include chronic renal failure, pyelonephritis, hypokalemia, hypercalciuria, malnutrition, genetic defects, and sickle cell disease. Additionally, lithium toxicity, colchicine, glyburide, demeclocycline, cidofovir, and methoxyflurane occasionally cause this disorder.

Lithium leads to polyuria in about 20% of patients. Typically, polyuria occurs after 2–3 months of therapy. This antimanic drug appears to exert its nephrotoxicity by entering collecting duct cells through sodium channels. Lithium impairs ADH's ability to produce cyclic adenosine monophosphate (AMP), resulting in resistance to the renal effects of ADH on the collecting duct and water loss. Sodium reabsorption in the cortical diluting and distal tubules results in increased urine output. Amiloride, a potassium-sparing diuretic, is useful at doses of 5 mg/day in lithium-induced diabetes insipidus because it closes the sodium channels in the collecting duct cells and decreases lithium accumulation. Chlorpropamide potentiates ADH's effect on the collecting tubules. Chlorpropamide is usually given in doses of 125–500 mg daily; patients should be monitored for hypoglycemia. Thiazides can be used to block sodium reabsorption in the cortical diluting tubule and the distal tubule, thereby, decreasing urine output. Hydrochlorothiazide 50–100 mg daily or an equivalent dose of another thiazide diuretic can be used. Patients who are treated with thiazide diuretics must be monitored because these agents can cause hypokalemia and hypomagnesemia.

Diabetes Insipidus of Pregnancy

A transient diabetes insipidus, originally thought to be a form of nephrogenic diabetes insipidus, may develop during late pregnancy from excessive vasopressinase (ADHase) activity. This kind of diabetes insipidus is associated with preeclampsia with liver involvement. Fortunately, vasopressinase does not metabolize DDAVP (or desmopressin acetate), which is, therefore, the treatment of choice.[95]

Laboratory Diagnosis

Some clinicians avoid dehydration testing and rely on measuring plasma ADH concentrations to distinguish neurogenic from nephrogenic forms. In otherwise healthy adults, the average basal plasma ADH concentration is 1.3–4.0 pg/mL or ng/L.

Based on medical history, symptoms, and signs, an elevated basal plasma ADH level almost always indicates nephrogenic diabetes insipidus. If the basal plasma ADH concentration is low (<1 pg/mL) or immeasurable, the result is inconclusive and a dehydration test should be done. If the diagnosis is ambiguous based on clinical setting and basal plasma ADH concentrations, the plan in Figure 13-5 should elucidate the diagnosis, even in a patient with a less common form of diabetes insipidus.

The theory behind the water deprivation test is that, in normal individuals, dehydration stimulates ADH release and the urine becomes concentrated. An injection of vasopressin at this point does not further concentrate the urine. In contrast, the urine of patients with central diabetes insipidus will not be maximally concentrated after fluid deprivation but will be after vasopressin injection.

To perform the test, patients are deprived of fluid intake (up to 18 hr) until the urine osmolality of three consecutive samples varies by no more than 30 mOsm/kg. Urine osmolality and/or specific gravity are measured hourly. At this time, 5 units of aqueous vasopressin are administered subcutaneously, and urine osmolality is measured 1 hr later. Plasma osmolality is measured before the test, when urine osmolality has stabilized, and after vasopressin has been administered.

In healthy individuals, fluid deprivation for 8–12 hr results in normal serum osmolality and a urine osmolality of about 800 mOsm/kg. The urine osmolality plateaus after 16–18 hr. Patients with central diabetes insipidus have an immediate rise in urine osmolality to approximately 600 mOsm/kg, with a corresponding decrease in urine output. Patients with nephrogenic DI are unable to increase urine osmolality above 300 mOsm/kg. In nephrogenic diabetes insipidus, the vasopressin injection has little effect.

In addition to being inconvenient and expensive, dehydration procedures are reliable only if the diabetes insipidus is severe enough that—even with induced dehydration—the urine still cannot be concentrated. Table 13-18 presents a summary of typical results of a water deprivation test.

Accurate interpretation requires consideration of potential confounding factors. If the laboratory cannot ensure accurate and precise plasma (not serum) osmolality measurements, plasma sodium should be used. Patients should be observed for nonosmotic stimuli, such as vasovagal reactions, that may affect ADH release. Lastly, if the patient has previously received ADH therapy, ADH antibodies may cause false-positive results suggestive of nephrogenic diabetes insipidus.[95]

TABLE 13-18

DIAGNOSIS	URINE SPECIFIC GRAVITY	AVERAGE URINE OSMOLALITY (mOsm/kg)	PLATEAU URINE OSMOLALITY (mOsm/kg)	AVERAGE SERUM OSMOLALITY (mOsm/kg)	CHANGE IN URINE OSMOLALITY AFTER VASOPRESSIN
Normal individuals	>1.015	300–800	<1600	280–295	Little change
Central diabetes insipidus	<1.010 <1.005	<300	<300	Normal or increased	Increases
Nephrogenic diabetes insipidus	<1.010 <1.005	<300	<300	Normal or decreased	Little change

Table 13-18. Differential Diagnosis of Diabetes Insipidus Based on Water Deprivation Test[90,91,95]

SUMMARY

Endocrine disorders often result from a deficiency or excess of a hormone. Laboratory tests that measure the actual hormone, precursors, or metabolites can help to elucidate whether and why a hormonal or metabolic imbalance exists. Tests used to assess thyroid, adrenal, parathyroid, glucose, sex hormone, and water homeostasis or receptors have been discussed.

The fasting plasma glucose and the 2-hr postprandial glucose concentrations are the most commonly performed tests for evaluation of glucose homeostasis. If elevated (>126 mg/dL) blood glucose persists, diabetes mellitus is likely. However, other causes of hyperglycemia (e.g., drugs) should be considered. Glycated hemoglobin (A1C) assesses average glucose control over the previous 2–3 months, while fructosamine assesses average control over the previous 2–3 weeks.

Diabetic ketoacidosis and hyperosmolar nonketotic hyperglycemia are the most severe disorders along the continuum of glucose intolerance. Extreme hyperglycemia (600–2000 mg/dL) with insignificant ketonemia/acidosis is consistent with hyperosmolar nonketotic hyperglycemia, while less severe (350–650 mg/dL) hyperglycemia with ketonemia and acidosis is characteristic of diabetic ketoacidosis. Conversely, hypoglycemia (glucose <50 mg/dL) most often is seen in patients with type 1 DM who have injected excessive insulin relative to their caloric intake.

Thyroid tests can be divided into those that (1) measure the concentration of products secreted by the thyroid gland (T_3 and T_4), (2) evaluate the integrity of the hypothalamic-pituitary-thyroid axis (TSH and TRH), (3) assess inherent thyroid gland function (radioactive iodine uptake test), and (4) detect antibodies to thyroid tissue (thyroid microsomal antibody). TSH concentrations are usually undetectable or less than 0.3 mU/L (newer assays), and T_4 concentrations are usually high in patients with overt hyperthyroidism. TSH concentrations are low or undetectable in patients with hypothyroidism from hypothalamic or pituitary insufficiency and in patients with nonthyroidal illness. In contrast, TSH concentrations are high and T_4 concentrations are low in patients with primary hypothyroidism.

Glucocorticoids maintain the body's homeostasis by regulating bodily functions involved in stress and normal activities. Cortisol, androgens, aldosterone, and estrogens are all produced in the adrenal glands. Cushing's syndrome is the result of excessive cortisol in the body. Addison's disease occurs when there is a deficiency in cortisol production.

Diabetes insipidus is a syndrome in which the body's inability to conserve water manifests as excretion of very large volumes of dilute urine. It most often is caused by a defect in the secretion (neurogenic, also called central) or renal activity (nephrogenic) of antidiuretic hormone. Urine and plasma osmolality are key tests. With the advent of high-performance assays, the use of plasma vasopressin concentrations to distinguish neurogenic from nephrogenic may obviate the need for iatrogenic dehydration procedures.

REFERENCES

1. Buse, JB. Progressive use of medical therapies in type 2 diabetes. *Diabetes Spectr.* 2000; 13(4):211–20.
2. DeFronzo R. Pharmacological therapy for type 2 diabetes. *Ann Inter Med.* 1999; 17:281–303.
3. Gerich JE. Matching treatment to pathophysiology in type 2 diabetes. *Clin Ther.* 2000; 23:646–59.
4. Dinneen S, Gerich J, Rizza R. Carbohydrate metabolism in non-insulin-dependent diabetes mellitus. *N Engl J Med.* 1992; 327:707–13.
5. American Diabetes Association. Standards of Medical Care for Patients with Diabetes Mellitus. *Diabetes Care.* 2003; 26 (suppl 1) S33–49.
6. American Diabetes Association. Gestational Diabetes Mellitus. *Diabetes Care.* 2003; 26 (suppl 1):S103–5.
7. Redondo MJ, Fain PR, Eisenbarth GS. Genetics of type 1A diabetes. *Recent Pro Horm Res.* 2001; 56:69–89.
8. Ong KK, Dunger DB. Thrifty genotypes and phenotypes in the pathogenesis of type 2 diabetes. *J Pediatr Endocrinol Metab.* 2000; 13(suppl 6):1419–24.
9. Tripathy D, Carlsson AL, Lehto M, et al. Insulin secretion and insulin sensitivity in diabetic subgroups: studies in the prediabetic and diabetic state. *Diabetologia.* 2000; 43:1476–83.

10. Froguel P, Velho G. Genetic determinants of type 2 diabetes. *Recent Prog Horm Res*. 2001; 56:91–105.

11. Bennett PH. Definition, diagnosis, and classification of diabetes mellitus and impaired glucose tolerance. In: Kahn CR, Weir GC, eds. *Joslin's Diabetes Mellitus*. 13th ed. Philadelphia, PA: Lea & Febiger; 1994: 193–200.

12. Godsland IF, Crook D, Simpson R, et al. The effects of different formulations of oral contraceptive agents on lip and carbohydrate metabolism. *N Engl J Med*. 1990; 323:1375–81.

13. Howanitz PJ, Howanitz JH. Carbohydrates. In: Henry JB, ed. *Clinical Diagnosis and Management by Laboratory Methods*. 17th ed. Philadelphia, PA: W. B. Saunders; 1984: 165–203.

14. American Diabetes Association. Screening for Diabetes. *Diabetes Care*. 2004; 27(suppl 1):S11–4.

15. American Association of Clinical Endocrinologists Conference on the Insulin Resistance Syndrome: August 25–26, 2002; Washington, DC. http://www.aace.com/pub/BMI/findings.php.

16. Goldstein DE, Little RR, Wiedmeyer HM, et al. Glycated hemoglobin: methodologies and clinical applications. *Clin Chem*. 1986; 32(suppl 10):B64–70.

17. Yarrison G, Allen L, King N, et al. Lipemic interference in Beckman Diatrac hemoglobin A_{1c} procedure removed. *Clin Chem*. 1993; 39:2351–2.

18. Goldstein DE, Parker M, England JD, et al. Clinical application of glycosylated hemoglobin measurements. *Diabetes*. 1982; 31(suppl 3):70–8.

19. American Diabetes Association. *Resource Guide 2003: Glycohemoglobin Tests Diabetes Forecast*. Alexandria, VA: American Diabetes Association; 2003: (suppl 1)67.

20. American Diabetes Association. Tests of glycemia in diabetes. *Diabetes Care*. 2003; 26(suppl 1):S106–8

21. Ardawi MS, Nasrat HA, Bahnassy AA. Fructosamine in obese normal subjects and type 2 diabetes. *Diabet Med*. 1994; 11:50–6.

22. Cefalu WT, Ettinger WH, Bell-Farrow AD, et al. Serum fructosamine as a screening test for diabetes in the elderly: a pilot study. *J Am Geriatr Soc*. 1993; 41:1090–4.

23. Tahara Y., Shima K. Kinetics of HbA_{1c}, glycated albumin, and fructosamine and analysis of their weight functions against preceding plasma glucose level. *Diabetes Care*. 1995; 18(4)440–7

24. Smolowitz JL, Zaldivar A. Evaluation of diabetic patients' home urine glucose testing technique and ability to interpret results. *Diabetes Educ*. 1992; 18:207–10.

25. Rotblatt MD, Koda-Kimble MA. Review of drug interference with urine glucose tests. *Diabetes Care*. 1987; 10:103–10.

26. Mehta M, Vincze G, Lopez D. Emerging technologies in diabetes care. *US Pharmacist [serial online]*. 2002; 27:11. Available at: http://www.uspharmacist.com/index.asp?show=article&page=8_995.htm. Accessed January 12, 2003.

27. Gadsden, RH Sr. Sources of variation in blood glucose testing. In: *Challenges in Diabetes Management/Milestone in Monitoring, Health Education Technologies*. New York, NY: 1988; 63–6.

28. Sylvester AC, Price CP, Burrin JM. Investigation of the potential for interference with whole blood glucose strips. *Ann Clin Biochem*. 1994; 31:94–6.

29. Avignon A, Radauceanu A, Monnier L. Nonfasting plasma glucose is a better marker of diabetic control than fasting plasma glucose. *Diabetes Care*. 1997; 20:1822–6.

30. Bell D, Ovalle F, Shadmany S. Postprandial rather than preprandial glucose levels should be used for adjustment of rapid-acting insulins. *Endocrine Practice*. 2000; 6:477–8

31. The Diabetes Control and Complications Trial Research Group. The effect of intensive treatment of diabetes on the development and progression of long-term complications in insulin-dependent diabetes mellitus. *N Engl J Med*. 1993; 329:977–86.

32. UK Prospective Diabetes Study Group. Intensive blood glucose control with sulphonylureas or insulin compared with conventional treatment and risk of complications in patients wit type 2 diabetes (UKPDS 33). *Lancet*. 1998; 352:837–53.

33. Skyler JS, ed. *Medical Management of Type 1 Diabetes*. 3rd ed. Alexandria, VA: American Diabetes Association; 1998.

34. Zimmerman BR, ed. *Medical Management of Type 2 Diabetes*. 4th ed. Alexandria, VA: American Diabetes Association; 1998.

35. Skyler JS. Insulin treatment. In: Lebovitz HE, ed. *Therapy for Diabetes Mellitus and Related Disorders*. 3rd ed. Alexandria, VA: American Diabetes Association; 1998: 186–203.

36. White JR Jr, Campbell RK. Inhaled insulin: an overview. *Clinical Diabetes*. 2001; 19:13–6.

37. Thompson RG, Peterson J, Gottlieb A, et al. Effects of pramlintide, an analogue of human amylin, on the plasma glucose profiles in patients with IDDM: results of a multicenter trial. *Diabetes*. 1997; 46 632–6.

38. DeFronzo RA, Matsuda M, Barrett E. Diabetic ketoacidosis: a combined metabolic-nephrologic approach to therapy. *Diabetes Rev*. 1994; 2:209–38.

39. Matz R. Hyperosmolar nonacidotic diabetes (HNAD). In: Porte D Jr, Sherwin RS, eds. *Diabetes Mellitus: Theory and Practice*. 5th ed. Amsterdam: Elsevier; 1997: 845–60.

40. Burge MD, Hardy KJ, Schade DS. Short-term fasting is a mechanism for the development of euglycemic ketoacidosis during periods of insulin deficiency. *J Clin Endocrinol Metab*. 1993; 76:1192–8.

41. American Diabetes Association. Hyperglycemic crises in patients with diabetes mellitus. *Diabetes Care*. 2002; 25(suppl 1): S100–8.

42. Goren MP, Pratt CB. False-positive ketone tests: a bedside measure of urinary mesna. *Cancer Chemother Pharmacol*. 1990; 25:371–2.

43. Holcombe BJ, Hopkins AM, Heizer WD. False-positive tests for urinary ketones (letter). *N Engl J Med*. 1994; 330:578.

44. Graham P, Naidoo D. False-positive Ketostix in a diabetic on antihypertensive therapy. *Clin Chem*. 1987; 33:1490.

45. Warren SE. False-positive urine ketone test with captopril. *N Engl J Med*. 1980; 303:1003–4.

46. Young DS. *Effects of Drugs on Clinical Laboratory Tests*. 3rd ed. Washington, DC: American Association for Clinical Chemistry Press; 1990.

47. Cryer PE. Hypoglycemia: the limiting factor in the management of IDDM. *Diabetes*. 1994; 43:1378–89.

48. Cox DJ, Gonder-Frederick L, Antoun B, et al. Perceived symptoms in the recognition of hypoglycemia. *Diabetes Care*. 1993; 6:519–27.

49. Cryer, PE. *Hypoglycemia: Pathophysiology, Diagnosis and Treatment*. New York, NY: Oxford University Press; 1997.

50. American Diabetes Association. Management of dyslipidemia in adults with diabetes. *Diabetes Care*. 2003; (suppl 1);S83–6.

51. Consensus Development Conference on the Treatment of Hypertension in Diabetes. Detection and management of lipid disorders in diabetes. *Diabetes Care*. 1996; 19:S96–113.

52. Moorhead JF. Lipids and progressive kidney disease. *Kidney International*. 1991; 39 (suppl 31):35–40.

53. Petrone LR. Thyroid disorders. In: Arcangelo VP, Peterson AM, eds. *Pharmacotherapeutics for Advanced Practice, A Practical Approach*. 1st ed. Philadelphia, PA: Lippincott Williams & Wilkins; 2001: 666–81.

54. Surks, MI, Sievert, R. Drugs and thyroid function. *N Engl J Med*. 1995; 333: 1688–94.

55. Kaptein EM. Clinical application of free thyroxine determinations. *Clin Lab Med*. 1993; 13:653–72.

56. Thomas JA, Keenan EJ. Thyroid and antithyroidal drugs. In: Thomas JA, Keenan EJ, eds. *Principles of Endocrine Pharmacology*. New York, NY: Plenum; 1986: 69–91.

57. Nelson JC, Wilcox RB, Pandin MR. Dependence of free thyroxine estimates obtained with equilibrium tracer dialysis on the concentration of thyroxine-binding globulin. *Clin Chem*. 1992; 38:1294–1300.

58. Singer PA. Thyroid function tests and effects of drugs on thyroid function. In: Lavin N, ed. *Manual of Endocrinology and Metabolism*. Boston, MA: Little, Brown; 1986: 341–54.

59. Klee GG, Hay ID. Assessment of sensitive thyrotropin assays for an expanded role in thyroid function testing: proposed criteria for analytic performance and clinical utility. *J Clin Endocrinol Metab*. 1987; 64:461–71.

60. Ingbar SH, Woeber KA. The thyroid gland. In: Williams RH, ed. *Textbook of Endocrinology*. 6th ed. Philadelphia, PA: W. B. Saunders; 1981: 117–248.

61. Mokshagundam S, Barzel US. Thyroid disease in the elderly. *J Am Geriatr Soc*. 1993; 41:1361–9.

62. Reasner CA, Talbert RL. Thyroid disorders. In: DiPiro JT, Talbert RL, Yee GC, eds. *Pharmacotherapy: A Pathophysiologic Approach*. 5th ed. New York, NY: McGraw-Hill; 2002: 1359–78.

63. Safrit H. Thyroid disorders. In: Fitzgerald PA, ed. *Handbook of Clinical Endocrinology*. Greenbrae, CA: Jones Medical Publications; 1986: 122–69.

64. Hershman JM. Hypothyroidism and hyperthyroidism. In: Lavin N, ed. *Manual of Endocrinology and Metabolism*. Boston, MA: Little, Brown; 1986: 365–78.

65. Tunbridge WM, Evered DC, Hall R, et al. The spectrum of thyroid disease in a community: the Whickham survey. *Clin Endocrinol (Oxf)*. 1977; 7:481–93.

66. Becker DV, Bigos ST, Gaitan E, et al. Optimal use of blood tests for assessment of thyroid function. *JAMA*. 1993; 269:2736–7.

67. Spencer CA. Thyroid profiling for the 1990s: free T_4 estimate or sensitive TSH measurement. *J Clin Immunoassay*. 1989; 12:82–5.

68. Surks MI, Hupart KH, Pan C, et al. Normal free thyroxine in critical nonthyroidal illnesses measured by ultrafiltration of undiluted serum and equilibrium dialysis. *J Clin Endocrinol Metab*. 1988; 67:1031–9.

69. Wong TK, Pekary AE, Hoo GS, et al. Comparison of methods for measuring free thyroxine in nonthyroidal illness. *Clin Chem*. 1992; 38:720–4.

70. Klee GG, Hay ID. Role of thyrotropin measurements in the diagnosis and management of thyroid disease (review). *Clin Lab Med*. 1993; 13(3):673–82.

71. Young DS. *Effects of Drugs on Clinical Laboratory Tests*. 3rd ed. Washington, DC: American Association for Clinical Chemistry Press; 1990.

72. Khanderia U, Jaffe CA, Theisen V. Amiodarone-induced thyroid dysfunction. *Clin Pharm*. 1993; 12:774–9.

73. Okamura K, Ikenoue H, Shiroozu A, et al. Reevaluation of the effects of methylmercaptomidazole and propylthiouracil in patients with Graves' hyperthyroidism. *J Clin Endocrinol Metab*. 1987; 65:719–23.

74. Franklyn JA. The management of hyperthyroidism. *N Engl J Med*. 1994; 330:1731–8.

75. Finucane P, Rudra T, Hsu R, et al. Thyrotropin response to thyrotropin-releasing hormone in elderly patients with and without acute illness. *Age Ageing*. 1991; 20:85–9.

76. Toft AD. Thyroxine therapy. *N Engl J Med*. 1994; 331:174–80.

77. Nicoloff JT, Spencer CA. The use and misuse of the sensitive thyrotropin assays. *J Clin Endocrinol Metab*. 1990; 71:553–8.

78. McClelland P, Stott A, Howel-Evans W. Hyperthyrotropinaemia during thyroxine replacement therapy. *Postgrad Med J*. 1989; 65:205–7.

79. Reinwein D, Benker G, Lazarus JH, et al. A prospective randomized trial of antithyroid drug dose in Graves' disease therapy. *J Clin Endocrinol Metab*. 1993; 76:1516–21.

80. Liewendahl K, Helenius T, Lamberg BA, et al. Free thyroxine, free triiodothyronine, and thyrotropin concentrations in hypothyroid and thyroid carcinoma patients receiving thyroxine therapy. *Acta Endocrinol*. 1987; 116:418–24.

81. Stall GM, Harris S, Sokoll LJ, et al. Accelerated bone loss in hypothyroid patients overtreated with L-thyroxine. *Ann Intern Med*. 1990; 113:265–9.

82. Vanelle JM, Poirier MF, Benkelfat C, et al. Diagnostic and therapeutic value of testing stimulation of thyroid-

stimulating hormone by thyrotropin-releasing hormone in 100 depressed patients. *Acta Psychiatr Scand.* 1990; 81:156–61.

83. Ingbar SH. Diseases of the thyroid. In: Braunwald E, Isselbacher KJ, Petersdorf RG, et al, eds. *Harrison's Principles of Internal Medicine.* 11th ed. New York, NY: McGraw-Hill; 1987: 1732–52.

84. Hershman JM, Chopra IJ, Van Herle AJ, et al. Thyroid disease. In: Hershman JM, ed. *Endocrine Pathophysiology: A Patient-Oriented Approach.* 2nd ed. Philadelphia, PA: Lea & Febiger; 1982: 34–68.

85. Utiger RD. Thyrotropin-receptor mutations and thyroid dysfunction. *N Engl J Med.* 1995; 332:183–5.

86. Sacher RA, McPherson RA. *Widman's Clinical Interpretation of Laboratory Tests.* 10th ed. Philadelphia, PA: F. A. Davis; 1991.

87. Wallach J. *Interpretation of Diagnostic Tests: A Synopsis of Laboratory Medicine.* 5th ed. Boston, MA: Little, Brown; 1992.

88. Findling JW, Raff H. Newer diagnostic techniques and problems in Cushing's disease. *Endocrinol Metab Clin North Am.* 1999; 28:191–210.

89. White PC. Mechanisms of disease: disorders of aldosterone biosynthesis and action. *N Engl J Med.* 1994; 331:250–8.

90. Fitzgerald PA. Pituitary disorders. In: Fitzgerald PA, ed. *Handbook of Clinical Endocrinology.* Greenbrae, CA: Jones Medical Publications; 1986: 22–9.

91. Ramsay DJ. Posterior pituitary gland. In: Greenspan FS, Forsham PH, eds. *Basic and Clinical Endocrinology.* 2nd ed. Los Altos, CA: Lange Medical Publications; 1986:132–42.

92. Robertson GL. Differential diagnosis of polyuria. *Ann Rev Med.* 1988; 39:425–42.

93. Lightman SL. Molecular insights into diabetes insipidus. *N Engl J Med.* 1993; 328:1562–3.

94. Krege J, Katz VL, Bowes WA Jr. Transient diabetes insipidus of pregnancy. *Obstet Gynecol Surv.* 1989; 44:789–95.

95. Sowers JR, Zieve FJ. Clinical disorders of vasopressin. In: Lavin N, ed. *Manual of Endocrinology and Metabolism.* Boston, MA: Little, Brown; 1986: 65–74

quickview—total serum T_4

PARAMETER	DESCRIPTION	COMMENTS
Common reference ranges		
Adults and children	4–12 mg/dL (51–154 nmol/L)	Affected by TBG changes with nonthyroidal illness SI conversion factor = 12.87 (nmol/L)
Newborn/3–5 days	16–26/9–20 µg/dL	Affected by TBG changes with nonthyroidal illness SI conversion factor = 12.87 (nmol/L)
Critical value	Not established	Extremely high or low values should be reported quickly, especially in newborns
Natural substance?	Yes	Only 0.02% of T_4 is unbound
Inherent activity?	Only free portion	*Total* assumed to correlate with *free* T_4 activity
Location		
Production and storage	Thyroid gland	Bound mostly to thyroglobulin
Secretion/excretion	From thyroid to blood	About 33% converted to T_3 outside thyroid
Major causes of...		
High results	Hyperthyroidism	Not truly a cause but a reflection of high result
	T_4 supplements Other causes	
Associated signs and symptoms	Signs and symptoms of hyperthyroidism	Nervousness, weight loss, heat intolerance, HR increase, diaphoresis
Low results	Hypothyroidism	Not truly a cause but a reflection of low result
	Other causes (Table 13-9)	
Associated signs and symptoms	Signs and symptoms of hypothyroidism	Lethargy, constipation, dry skin, cold intolerance, slow speech, confusion
After insult, time to...		
Initial elevation or depression	Weeks to months	Increases within hours in *acute* T_4 overdose
Peak values	Weeks to months	Increases within hours in *acute* T_4 overdose
Normalization	Usually same time as onset	Assumes insult removed or effectively treated
Drugs often monitored with test	Levothyroxine (T_4)	Other drugs (Tables 13-8 and 13-9)
Causes of spurious results	Increased or decreased TBG leads to falsely increased or decreased total serum T_4 Nonthyroidal illness leads to falsely increased or decreased total serum T_4	Factors affecting TBG (Table 13-13)

quickview—total serum T_3

PARAMETER	DESCRIPTION	COMMENTS
Common reference ranges		
Adults and children	78–195 ng/dL (1.2–3.0 nmol/L)	Affected by TGB changes SI conversion factor = 0.0154 (nmol/L)
Critical value	Not established	Extremely high or low values should be reported quickly
Natural substance?	Yes	Only 0.2% of T_3 is unbound
Inherent activity?	Only free portion	*Total* assumed to correlate with *free* T_3 activity

Continued

Continued

quickview—total serum T$_3$

PARAMETER	DESCRIPTION	COMMENTS
Location		
Production and storage	Liver and kidneys; thyroid gland	Bound mostly to thyroglobulin
Secretion/excretion	From thyroid, liver, and kidneys to blood	
Major causes of...		
High results	Hyperthyroidism	Not truly a cause but a reflection of high result
	T$_4$/T$_3$ supplements Other causes (Table 13-9)	
Associated signs and symptoms	Signs and symptoms of hyperthyroidism	Nervousness, weight loss, heat intolerance, tachycardia, diaphoresis
Low results	Hypothyroidism	Not truly a cause but a reflection of low result
	Other causes (Table 13-9) Propranolol Propylthiouracil Glucocorticoids	
Associated signs and symptoms	Signs and symptoms of hypothyroidism	Lethargy, constipation, dry skin, cold intolerance, slow speech, confusion
After insult, time to...		
Initial elevation or depression	Weeks to months	Increases within hours in *acute* T$_4$ or T$_3$ overdose
Peak values	Weeks to months	Increases within hours in *acute* T$_4$ or T$_3$ overdose
Normalization	Usually same time as onset	Assumes insult removed or effectively treated
Drugs often monitored with test	Levothyroxine (T$_4$) and triiodothyronine (T$_3$)	Other drugs (Tables 13-8 and 13-9)
Causes of spurious results	Increased or decreased TBG leads to falsely increased or decreased total serum T$_3$ Nonthyroidal illness leads to falsely increased or decreased total serum T$_3$	Factors affecting TBG (Table 13-13)

quickview—free T$_4$

PARAMETER	DESCRIPTION	COMMENTS
Common reference ranges		
Adults and children	0.8–2.7 ng/dL (10–35 pmol/L)	Higher in infants <1 month; direct equilibrium dialysis assay not affected by TBG changes or severe nonthyroidal illness SI conversion factor = 12.87 (pmol/L)
Critical value	Not established	Extremely high or low values should be reported quickly
Natural substance?	Yes	Only 0.02% of T$_4$ is unbound
Inherent activity?	Probably	Some influence on basal metabolic rate; T$_3$ most active

Continued

Continued

PARAMETER	DESCRIPTION	COMMENTS
Location **Production and storage**	Thyroid gland	Bound mostly to thyroglobulin
Secretion/excretion	From thyroid to blood	33% converted to T$_3$ outside thyroid
Major causes of... **High results**	Hyperthyroidism	Not truly a cause but a reflection of high result
	T$_4$ supplements Other causes	
Associated signs and symptoms	Signs and symptoms of hyperthyroidism	Nervousness, weight loss, heat intolerance, tachycardia, diaphoresis
Low results	Hypothyroidism	Not truly a cause but a reflection of low result
	Other causes	
Associated signs and symptoms	Signs and symptoms of hypothyroidism	Lethargy, constipation, dry skin, cold intolerance, slow speech, confusion
After insult, time to... **Initial elevation or depression**	Weeks to months	Increases within hours in *acute* T$_4$ overdose
Peak values	Weeks to months	Increases within hours in *acute* T$_4$ overdose
Normalization	Usually same time as onset	Assumes insult removed or effectively treated
Drugs often monitored with test	Levothyroxine (T$_4$)	Other drugs (Tables 13-8 and 13-9)
Causes of spurious results	Rare with direct equilibrium dialysis assay (Table 13-12)	Decreased direct equilibrium dialysis assay for free T$_4$ with decreased or normal TSH may occur in patients taking T$_3$

PARAMETER	DESCRIPTION	COMMENTS
Common reference ranges **Adults and children**	0.3–5.0 µU/mL	Sometimes reported in mU/L
Critical value	Not established	Extremely high or low values should be reported quickly
Natural substance?	Yes	
Inherent activity?	Yes	Stimulates thyroid to secrete hormone
Location **Production and storage**	Anterior pituitary	
Secretion/excretion	Unknown	
Major causes of... **High results**	Primary hypothyroidism	Causes of primary hypothyroidism
	Antithyroid drugs	
Associated signs and symptoms	Signs and symptoms of hypothyroidism	Lethargy, constipation, dry skin, cold intolerance, slow speech, confusion

Continued

PARAMETER	DESCRIPTION	COMMENTS
Low results	Primary hyperthyroidism	Must be ≤0.05 for definitive diagnosis of (primary hyperthyroidism); may be decreased or normal in secondary or tertiary hypothyroidism
	Other causes (Table 13-9)	
Associated signs and symptoms	Signs and symptoms of hyperthyroidism	Nervousness, weight loss, heat intolerance, HR increase, diaphoresis
After insult, time to...		
Initial elevation or depression	Weeks to months	Decreases within hours in *acute* T_4 over dose
Peak values	Weeks to months	Decreases within hours in *acute* T_4 over dose
Normalization	Usually same time as onset	Assumes insult removed or effectively treated
Drugs often monitored with test	Levothyroxine (T_4) and triiodothyronine (T_3)	Also antithyroid drugs (methimazole and propylthiouracil)
Causes of spurious results	Increased TSH: dopamine antagonists	Metoclopramide and domperidone
	Decreased TSH: dopamine agonists	Dopamine, bromocriptine, levodopa, glucocorticoids
	Above TSH measurements are accurate here	But may confound diagnosis
		These drugs affect TSH, but the change is not reflective of primary hypo- or hyperthyroidism; therefore, the results are not truly spurious

PARAMETER	DESCRIPTION	COMMENTS
Common reference ranges		
Adults and children	Fasting: 70–110 mg/dL (3.9–6.1 mmol/L)	Multiply by 0.056 for SI units (mmol/L)
	2-hr postprandial: <140 mg/dL (8.4 mmol/L)	
	Full-term infant normal: 20–90 mg/dL	
Critical value	No previous history: >200 mg/dL Anytime: <50 mg/dL	In known diabetic, increased glucose is not immediate concern unless symptomatic; increased glucose is not critical if decreasing in series
Natural substance?	Yes	Always present in blood
Inherent activity?	Yes	Major source of energy for cellular metabolism
Location		
Production/intake	Liver and muscle	Dietary intake
Storage	Liver and muscle	As glycogen
Secretion/excretion	Mostly metabolized for energy	Levels >180 mg/dL spill into urine

Continued

Continued

PARAMETER	DESCRIPTION	COMMENTS
Major causes of...		
High results	Diabetes mellitus Drugs Excess intake	Type 1 and type 2 Steroids, thiazides, adrenalin
Associated signs and symptoms	Polyuria, polydipsia, polyphagia, weakness	Long-term: damage to kidneys, retina, neurons, and vessels
Low results	Insulin secretion/dose excessive relative to diet Sulfonylureas Insulinomas	Most common in diabetics
Associated signs and symptoms	Hunger, sweating, weakness, trembling, headache, confusion, seizures, coma	From neuroglycopenia and adrenergic discharge
After insult, time to...		
Initial elevation or depression	Type 1 DM: months to elevation Type 2 DM: years to elevation After insulin: minutes to decrease After meal: 15–30 min to elevation After epinephrine or glucagon: minutes After steroids and growth hormone: hours	
Normalization	After insulin: minutes After exercise: minutes to hours	Depends on insulin type Depends on intensity and duration
Drugs often monitored with test	Insulin, sulfonylureas, biguanides (e.g., metformin), thiazolididiones (e.g., rosiglitazone)	Also, diazoxide, L-asparaginase, total parenteral nutrition
Causes of spurious results	High dose vitamin C Metronidazole	With some glucometers With some automated assays

PARAMETER	DESCRIPTION	COMMENTS
Common reference ranges		
Adults and teenagers	4–6%	Fasting not required; represents average glucose levels past 8 weeks
Critical value	Not applicable	Reflects long-term glycemic control; >13% suggests poor control
Natural substance?	Yes	Subunit of Hgb
Inherent activity?	Yes	Oxygen carrier; also carries glucose
Location		
Production	Bone marrow	In newborns in liver and spleen
Storage	Not stored	Circulates in blood
Secretion/excretion	Older cell removed by spleen	Transformed to bilirubin
Major causes of...		
High results	Diabetes mellitus Chronic hyperglycemia	Any cause of prolonged hyperglycemia
Associated signs and symptoms	Signs and symptoms of diabetes	
Low results	Not clinically useful	

Continued

Continued

PARAMETER	DESCRIPTION	COMMENTS
After insult, time to...		
Initial elevation	2–4 months	Initial insult is chronic hyperglycemia
Normalization	2–4 months	Assumes sudden and persistent euglycemia
Drugs often monitored with test	Insulin, sulfonylureas, biguanides	Also diet and exercise
Causes of spurious results	Alcoholism, uremia, increased triglycerides, hemolysis, polycythemia	Also seen in pregnant and splenectomized patients

Chapter **14**

LIPID DISORDERS

Jill S. Burkiewicz

Hyperlipidemia, or an abnormal serum lipid profile, is a major risk factor in the development of coronary artery disease. With over 12 million people in the United States affected by coronary heart disease—accounting for nearly 1 million deaths annually— preventative efforts are key to decrease associated morbidity and mortality.[1] Practitioners are being asked to assess the lipid panel in an effort to decrease overall cardiovascular risk.

Over 100 million Americans have cholesterol levels above the desirable range.[1] As a 10% decrease in total cholesterol levels may result in an estimated 30% reduction in the incidence of coronary heart disease, lipid monitoring is warranted and effective treatments are indicated in selected patients.[1] While there are millions of people with hyperlipidemia, many go untreated due to lack of physician recognition.[2] While 95% of physicians are aware of guidelines that classify lipid levels, it is estimated that less than 40% of patients achieve low-density cholesterol (LDL) goals.[3] Some experts note that often patients who have not achieved goal are not treated with high doses, and a more aggressive approach to LDL reduction is required.[3]

This chapter primarily covers the physiology of cholesterol and triglyceride metabolism, their actions as part of lipoproteins, disorders of lipids and lipoproteins, and consequences of elevated lipid levels. The effects of diet, exercise, and drugs on these lipid values are also discussed. A detailed interpretation of test results and drug therapy with regard to cardiovascular risk is beyond the scope of this chapter, but references provide additional information.[4–7]

OBJECTIVES

After completing this chapter, the reader should be able to

1. List primary and secondary causes of hyperlipidemia.
2. Outline the pathophysiology of lipid metabolism and correlate lipid levels to the risk of atherosclerotic cardiovascular disease.
3. Calculate low-density lipoprotein (LDL) when provided with total cholesterol (TC), high-density lipoprotein (HDL), and triglyceride (TG) values.
4. Given a case study, interpret laboratory results from a lipid profile and discuss how they should guide treatment choices.

PHYSIOLOGY OF LIPID METABOLISM

The major plasma lipids are cholesterol, triglycerides, and phospholipids. The regulation of serum lipids is determined by the synthesis and metabolism of lipoproteins. An understanding of this regulation is necessary for proper diagnosis and treatment of hyperlipidemia in efforts to reduce overall cardiovascular risk.

Cholesterol serves as a structural component of cell wall membranes and is a precursor for the synthesis of steroid hormones and bile acids. It may be dietary in origin or synthesized in the liver and intestine. Cholesterol is continuously undergoing synthesis, degradation, and recycling. Approximately 40% of cholesterol consumed in the diet is absorbed.[8] Dietary cholesterol directly contributes relatively little to serum cholesterol levels. However, diets high in calories and saturated fat promote endogenous cholesterol biosynthesis. Approxi-

The contribution of material written by Diana Laubenstein and Scott L. Traub in previous editions of this book is acknowledged.

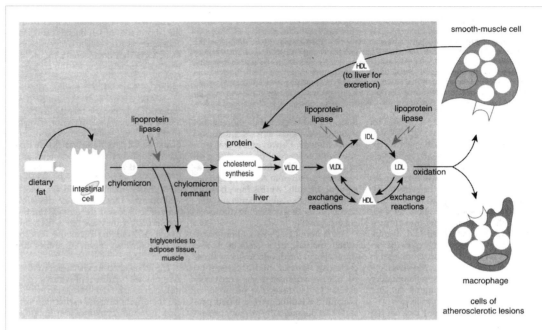

Figure 14-1. Lipid Metabolism. (Reprinted, with permission, by American Scientist, magazine of Sigma Xi, The Scientific Research Society.)

mately 90% of serum cholesterol is derived from cholesterol synthesis. Most cholesterol synthesis occurs during the night.[9] The rate-limiting step in the cholesterol synthesis is the conversion of hepatic hydroxymethylglutaryl-coenzyme A (HMG-CoA) to mevalonic acid. This conversion is catalyzed by the enzyme HMG-CoA reductase and is inhibited by drugs designed to reduce cellular synthesis of cholesterol (Figure 14-1).[10]

Intestinal cholesterol absorption, hepatic cholesterol synthesis, and excretion of cholesterol and bile acids regulate serum cholesterol concentrations.[8] An inhibitory feedback mechanism modulates cholesterol synthesis. Presence of cholesterol in hepatic cells leads to decreased biosynthesis of cholesterol. Conversely, when hepatic cholesterol concentrations decrease, there is a resulting increase in hepatic cholesterol biosynthesis.

Triglycerides, the esterified form of glycerol and fatty acids, constitute the main form of lipid storage in humans. Triglycerides serve as a reservoir of fatty acids to be used as fuel for gluconeogenesis or for direct combustion as an energy source. Triglycerides, like cholesterol, can either be synthesized by the liver or absorbed. Endogenous triglycerides are mainly synthesized in the liver from accumulated fatty acids. Dietary fat is incorporated into chylomicrons in the small intestine and is known as exogenous triglyceride.

Phospholipids are lipid molecules that contain a phosphate group. Like cholesterol, phospholipids become constituents of cell wall membranes. In contrast to cholesterol and triglycerides, dietary phospholipids are not absorbed. Most phospholipids originate in the liver and intestinal mucosa, but they may be synthesized by most body tissues. Phospholipids act as donors of phosphate groups for intracellular metabolism and blood coagulation.

Triglycerides, cholesterol, and phospholipid molecules are complexed with specialized proteins (apoproteins) to form lipoproteins, the transport form in which lipids are measured in the blood. As lipids are insoluble in aqueous plasma, they are formed into complexes with an outer hydrophilic coat of phospholipids and proteins and an inner core of fatty cholesterol and triglycerides. There are many ways to classify these lipoproteins, but, most frequently, lipoproteins are classified by their density and chemical composition. Table 14-1 summarizes the characteristics of triglycerides and cholesterol in terms of lipoprotein density.[7,11–13]

TABLE 14-1

LIPOPROTEIN	TRIGLYCERIDES (%)	CHOLESTEROL (%)	PHOSPHOLIPID (%)	ORIGIN	COMMENTS
Chylomicrons	80–95	3–7	3–9	Intestines	Primarily triglycerides
Very low-density lipoproteins (VLDL)	45–65	16–24	10–20	Liver and intestines	Primarily triglycerides
Intermediate-density lipoproteins (IDL) or remnants	15–32	30–50	15–25	Chylomicrons and VLDL	Transitional forms
Low-density lipoproteins (LDL)	4–10	46–58	20–25	End-product VLDL	Major carrier of cholesterol
High-density lipoproteins (HDL)	2–7	18–25	20–30	Intestines and liver	Removes cholesterol from atherosclerotic plaques in arteries

Table 14-1. Characteristics of Lipoproteins[7,11–13]

There is a strong correlation between hyperlipidemia and the development of atherosclerotic vascular disease. Atherosclerotic vascular disease may be manifested by coronary heart disease, stroke, and peripheral vascular disease. There is a positive relationship between serum cholesterol levels and risk for coronary heart disease.[14,15] For all age groups, the higher the total cholesterol level, the greater the risk. Proper diagnosis and treatment of hyperlipidemia can be an important preventative strategy. Numerous trials of effective treatment of hyperlipidemia have demonstrated reductions in cardiovascular events, stroke, and total mortality in patients with a prior history of atherosclerotic vascular disease (secondary prevention)[16–19] and in patients with asymptomatic hyperlipidemia (primary prevention).[20,21]

Primary Lipid Disorders

Hyperlipidemias, or elevated concentrations of any lipoprotein type, are classified by etiology into primary or secondary disorders. Primary disorders are caused by genetic defects in the synthesis or metabolism of the lipoproteins. Table 14-2 shows the characteristics of the major familial hyperlipoproteinemias. Familial, or genetic, disease should be strongly suspected in a patient with an elevated total serum cholesterol concentration greater than 300 mg/dL (>7.8 mmol/L) or in a patient with LDL cholesterol greater than or equal to 190 mg/dL (≥4.9 mmol/L). In such cases, family members should be screened.

Secondary Lipid Disorders

Secondary hyperlipidemias are disorders precipitated by other disease states, medications, or lifestyle (Table 14-3). When a secondary cause is likely responsible for hyperlipidemia, it may be necessary to treat the underlying cause prior to initiating drug therapy for hyperlipidemia.

The most common disease-related causes of hyperlipidemia are diabetes and thyroid disorders, with links to endocrine abnormalities. Patients with diabetes may have elevated LDL cholesterol and TG levels as well as decreased HDL cholesterol levels. Optimization of glycemic control is an important step in management of elevated triglycerides in patients with diabetes. Total cholesterol and LDL cholesterol concentrations increase in hypothyroidism, as a result of decreased catabolism of LDL particles. In addition to these endocrine disorders, nephrotic syndrome and chronic liver disease should be excluded by patient history, physical examination, and laboratory data. Laboratory tests such as fasting blood glu-

TABLE 14-2

GENETIC DISORDER	ELEVATED LIPOPROTEIN	PLASMA CHOLESTEROL (mg/dL)	PLASMA TRIGLYCERIDE (mg/dL)	CLINICAL MANIFESTATIONS AND GENETICS
Familial lipoprotein lipase deficiency (type 1)	Chylomicrons	Normal[a]	>1000[a]	Abdominal pain and/or pancreatitis; hepatosplenomegaly; eruptive xanthomas; lipemia retinalis Monogenic, recessive
Familial hypercholester-olemia (type 2a)	LDL	>300	Normal	Premature atherosclerosis and tendinous xanthomas Monogenic, dominant
Familial dysbetalipopro-teinemia (type 3)	LDL	>300	>300	Coronary and peripheral atherosclerosis; tuberous xanthomas; tendinous xanthomas; palmar and plantar xanthomatous streaks; glucose intolerance (25%); hypothyroid (25%) Monogenic, recessive
Familial hypertriglycer-idemia (type 4)	VLDL	Normal	200–500	Commonly associated with obesity, hyperglycemia, and insulin resistance Adult onset; monogenic, dominant
Familial hyperlipopro-teinemia (type 5)	Chylomicrons and VLDL	>300	>500	Pancreatitis and eruptive xanthomas; rare Monogenic, dominant
Familial combin-ed hyperlipidemia (types 2a, 2b, 4, and 5)	LDL and VLDL	250–600	200–600	Premature atherosclerosis Monogenic, dominant
Polygenic hypercholes terolemia (type 2b)	LDL and VLDL (inconsistent)	>300	Normal or >300	Premature atherosclerosis Monogenic, dominant

[a]Conversion factor for cholesterol in International System (SI) units (millimoles per liter) is 0.026. Conversion factor for triglyceride in SI units (millimoles per liter) is 0.011.

Table 14-2. Characteristics of Familial Hyperlipoproteinemias[7,8]

cose, thyroid stimulating hormone (TSH), alkaline phosphatase, and urinalysis for proteinuria are useful on diagnosis of hyperlipidemia to exclude common secondary causes of hyperlipidemia.

In drug-induced hyperlipidemia, withdrawal of the precipitating medication usually leads to reversal of secondary hyperlipidemia. Antihypertensive agents are frequently administered to patients with cardiovascular risk. Beta-blocking agents, except agents with intrinsic sympathomimetic activity such as pindolol, may increase triglyceride concentrations and reduce HDL cholesterol concentrations.[22] Thiazide diuretics increase total cholesterol, LDL cholesterol, and triglyceride concentrations.[23] Thiazide effects on the lipid panel are most pronounced with higher dosages (50 mg or more daily).[23] The effects of beta-blockers and diuretics may be short-term, with a return to baseline levels at 1 year.[24] In contrast, calcium channel blockers and angiotensin-converting enzyme (ACE) inhibitors have no clinically significant effect on the lipid profile, while alpha-agonists and alpha-antagonists may actually improve the lipid profile.[23]

While it is important to realize the effect of antihypertensive agents on the lipid profile, agents that adversely affect the lipid profile are not contraindicated in patients with hyperlipidemia. Careful consideration of the patient-specific factors is warranted. For example,

TABLE 14-3

DISORDER OR CONDITION[a]	DRUG OR DIET[a]
Acute hepatitis (↑TG)	Alcohol (↑TG)
Cholestasis (↑LDL)	Amiodarone (↑TG)
Diabetes mellitus (↑LDL, ↓HDL, ↑TG)	Antipsychotics (↑TG)
Glycogen storage disease (↑TG)	Beta-blockers (↑TG, ↓HDL)
Hypothyroidism (↑LDL, ↓HDL, ↑TG)	Contraceptives (estrogen and progestin)[b] (↑TG)
Nephrotic syndrome (↑LDL, ↓HDL, ↑TG)	Corticosteroids (↑LDL)
Obesity (↑LDL, ↓HDL, ↑TG)	Cyclosporine (↑LDL, ↑TG)
Pregnancy (↑TG)	Danazol (↑LDL, ↓HDL)
Sedentary lifestyle (↑LDL, ↓HDL, ↑TG)	Diet high in saturated fats and cholesterol (↑LDL, ↑TG)
Systemic lupus erythematosus (↑TG)	Estrogens (↑HDL, ↓LDL, ↑TG)
Uremia (↑TG)	Isotretinoin (↑LDL, ↓HDL, ↑TG)
	Parenteral lipid emulsions (↑TG)
	Progestins (↑LDL, ↓HDL, ↑TG)
	Tamoxifen (↓LDL, ↓HDL, ↑TG)
	Thiazide diuretics (↑LDL, ↑TG)
	Sirolimus (↑LDL, ↑TG)

[a]↑=increase; ↓=decrease, LDL=low-density lipoprotein, HDL=high-density lipoprotein, TG=triglycerides.

[b]Effect on HDL, LDL depends on specific components.

Table 14-3. Secondary Causes of Hyperlipidemia and Major Associated Changes in Lipoprotein Component[7,25,27]

hypertension in a patient with a history of myocardial infarction and hyperlipidemia is appropriately treated with a beta-blocker. While beta-blockers may adversely affect the lipid profile, beta-blockers are preferred due to documented decreases in mortality postmyocardial infarction.

Various oral contraceptives affect lipoproteins differently. Combination oral contraceptives do not routinely cause an increase in total serum cholesterol, but they do increase triglyceride concentrations. Effects on LDL and HDL are variable, depending on oral contraceptive components.[25–27] Oral contraceptives with "second generation" progestins may increase LDL cholesterol levels and decrease HDL cholesterol levels. However, combined oral contraceptives with "third generation" progestins may favorably decrease LDL levels and increase HDL.[25]

Unopposed estrogen replacement therapy generally has a beneficial affect on the lipid profile with increases in HDL cholesterol, decreases in LDL cholesterol and in total cholesterol, but increases in triglycerides. Oral estrogen replacement therapy results in increases in HDL, but the same effect is not observed with transdermal therapy. With combined hormone replacement therapy, estrogen/progestin therapy maintains beneficial effects on LDL and HDL cholesterol. However, the effects of unopposed estrogen on HDL cholesterol are diminished and effects on triglycerides are variable.[25] The selective estrogen receptor modulators, such as tamoxifen and raloxifene, have similar effects on the lipid panel as unopposed estrogen but with no changes in HDL cholesterol observed.

Protease inhibitors are known to cause lipodystrophy, characterized by central adiposity, hyperlipidemia, insulin resistance, and a peripheral fat wasting.[28] The hyperlipidemia is characterized by elevations in triglycerides and reductions in HDL cholesterol concentrations.[29] It is estimated that three out of four patients on long-term therapy with protease inhibitors develop hyperlipidemia.[30]

A summary of drugs with effects on the lipid profile is listed in Table 14-3. Immunosuppressive drugs such as cyclosporine, sirolimus, and corticosteroids adversely affect the lipid profile, but tacrolimus does not impact the lipid profile with the same magnitude.[25] Another immunosuppressive drug, mycophenolate mofetil, does not affect the lipid profile.[25] Some of the agents listed, such as antipsychotics and parenteral lipids, mainly elevate triglyceride levels. Though drug-associated adverse effects on the lipid profile have not been correlated with increased risk for CHD, it is important to assess these effects in considering laboratory data and the appropriate treatment plan for the patient.

Lifestyle modification (diet and exercise) also may affect lipoprotein concentrations. Besides being an independent risk factor for coronary heart disease, obesity causes an increase in serum triglycerides, primarily VLDL. Likewise, a sedentary lifestyle may increase serum triglyceride concentrations by decreasing peripheral utilization of fat and glucose and by increasing VLDL production by the liver.[12] In contrast, exercise increases HDL, a beneficial type of cholesterol; exercise independently increases longevity.[31]

A diet that is high in saturated fats and cholesterol increases total serum cholesterol concentrations and LDL. In fact, age-adjusted coronary heart disease mortality rates have declined by 50% over the past four decades, probably because of decreases in animal fats in the diet along with better control of hypertension and smoking cessation.[12] Cigarette smoking is associated with increases in triglycerides and decreases in HDL cholesterol.[32] Light to moderate alcohol intake (one to two glasses of beer or wine or 1–2 ounces of liquor per day) increases HDL and is associated with lower mortality from coronary heart disease as compared with abstention from alcohol.[33,34] However, light to moderate alcohol consumption is associated with increases in triglycerides, especially in patients predisposed to hypertriglyceridemia. Since evidence to date is epidemiologic in nature, alcohol is not recommended until data from controlled clinical trials is available.[35]

LABORATORY TESTS FOR LIPIDS AND LIPOPROTEINS

Hypercholesterolemia and hypertriglyceridemia are major contributors to coronary artery disease and peripheral vascular disease. Fortunately, several laboratory tests can be used to assess the concentrations of various lipids in the blood, making early detection and monitoring possible. Identification of patients at risk for coronary artery disease and peripheral vascular disease is a two-part process. First, a laboratory assessment of the lipid profile must occur. Second, an assessment of the risk determinants of coronary artery disease must occur.

The third report of the Expert Panel on Detection, Evaluation and Treatment of High Blood Cholesterol in Adults (Adult Treatment Panel III, or ATP III) by the National Cholesterol Education Program (NCEP) outlines screening recommendations for the detection of hyperlipidemia.[36] A fasting lipoprotein profile is recommended once every 5 years in all adults older than 20 years of age. If the screening was nonfasting, then only the total cholesterol and HDL cholesterol data will be useable. In this case, if the TC >200 mg/dL or HDL <40 mg/dL, the patient should return for a fasting lipoprotein profile to determine the appropriate plan for treatment.

The fasting lipoprotein profile includes: TC, TG, HDL, and calculated LDL. A typical sample is collected following a 9–12 hr fast. Patients must avoid food, as well as beverages with caloric content such as juices, sodas, or alcohol drinks, during the fasting period. Ideally, the patient should remain seated 5 min prior to phlebotomy to avoid hemoconcentration, which may cause falsely elevated lipid levels. Serum samples are collected in collection tubes without anticoagulant; plasma samples are collected in tubes with ethylenediaminetetraacetic acid (EDTA).[37]

A number of factors may cause variation in obtained lipid values including sample type and tourniquet application. Plasma concentration lipid values are approximately 3% lower than those values associated with serum measurements. Prolonged tourniquet application may cause venous stasis and increases in total serum cholesterol concentrations by 5–10%. Methods used to assay total serum cholesterol vary. It is important to become familiar with the method of lipid profile measurement used by the laboratory that the clinician uses regularly.

In addition to factors specific for laboratory methods, patient-specific factors may interfere with the proper lipid panel results. The preferred lipid panel is obtained in the absence of any acute illness. This provides levels that are not affected by deviation from a baseline stable condition. Vigorous physical activity (within the last 24 hr), pregnancy, recent weight loss, and acute illness result in levels that are not representative of the patient's usual value. Measurement of plasma lipids in the setting of acute coronary syndrome usually provides LDL values that are lower than baseline by 24 hr after an event.[38] The LDL values may continue to be decreased for weeks following the event. While these values are not representative of baseline values, recommendations are to use these values to guide initiation of LDL-lowering therapy to reduce cardiovascular risk and continue to follow lipids postdischarge.[39,40]

Total Serum Cholesterol

For nonfasting adults >20 years[36]:

desirable, <200 mg/dL or <5.17 mmol/L;

borderline high, 200–239 mg/dL or 5.17–6.18 mmol/L;

or high, ≥240 mg/dL or >6.20 mmol/L

In all patient populations, including the elderly,[36,41] lowering elevated serum cholesterol concentrations decreases death from coronary artery disease[42] and results in regression of atherosclerotic lesions.[43,44] In young healthy adults, total serum cholesterol is a strong predictor of clinically evident cardiovascular events occurring 25 or more years later.[45]

Despite popular belief, a fasting sample is not necessary because total serum cholesterol is not affected by a single meal. Factors that may interfere with accurate assessment include pregnancy, recent weight loss, vigorous exercise, and acute myocardial infarction. Although low total serum cholesterol is usually considered a sign of good health, it can be a sign of hyperthyroidism, malnutrition, chronic anemia, cancer, or severe liver disease.

Methods used to assay total serum cholesterol vary greatly among laboratories. Therefore, clinicians should become familiar with the method used by their laboratory as well as with potential causes of misleading or erroneous results. Serum or heparinized plasma is the typical specimen collected.

Triglycerides

For adults >20 years[36]:

normal, <150 mg/dL or <1.69 mmol/L;

borderline high, 150–199 mg/dL or 1.69–2.25 mmol/L;

high, 200–499 mg/dL or 2.26–5.63 mmol/L;

or very high, ≥500 mg/dL or ≥5.64 mmol/L

Disorders leading to hypertriglyceridemia involve dysregulation of chylomicrons and/or VLDL. Chylomicrons and intermediate-density lipoproteins are present only in postprandial or pathological states, while VLDL, LDL, and HDL are present in the fasting state. Triglycerides in the form of chylomicrons appear in the plasma as soon as 2 hr after a meal, reach a maximum at 4–6 hr, and persist for up to 14 hr.[13] To avoid falsely elevated concentrations, measurement of triglycerides and lipoproteins is recommended after an overnight fast. Triglyceride concentrations occasionally become transiently or persistently elevated in patients receiving intermittent or constantly infused intravenous lipids, respectively. However, lipid emulsion regimens are not usually changed unless there is risk of pancreatitis. Heparin, a common additive to parenteral nutrition solutions, may facilitate faster metabolism of chylomicrons and reduce triglyceride concentrations by a stimulatory effect on lipoprotein lipase.

As a secondary disorder, hypertriglyceridemia is associated with obesity, uncontrolled diabetes mellitus, liver disease, alcohol ingestion, and uremia. Combination oral contraceptives, corticosteroids, antihypertensive agents, and isotretinoin may also elevate triglyceride concentrations (Table 14-3).

Extremely high concentrations of triglycerides—concentrations in excess of 2000 mg/dL—may also lead to eruptive cutaneous xanthomas on the elbows, knees, and buttocks. The xanthomas may disappear once triglyceride concentrations fall below 2000 mg/dL (<22.6 mmol/L). Hypertriglyceridemia may also manifest as lipemia retinalis (a whitish cast in the vascular bed of the retina). This sign is due to triglyceride particles scattering light in the blood and is seen in the retinal vessels during an eye exam. In patients with lipemia retinalis, triglyceride concentrations may be 3000 mg/dL (34 mmol/L) or greater.[46,47] A concentration this high requires immediate action because it causes hyperviscosity of the blood with the risk of thrombus formation.

Hypertriglyceridemia, without other lipid abnormalities, is established as an independent risk factor for coronary heart disease.[36] In addition to increased risk of cardiovascular disease, hypertriglyceridemia (concentrations >500 mg/dL or >5.64 mmol/L) may precipitate pancreatitis (Chapter 12). In fact, many patients with hypertriglyceridemia have intermittent episodes of epigastric pain due to recurrent pancreatic inflammation. In patients with very high triglycerides (concentrations >500 mg/dL or 5.64 mmol/L), the initial goal of therapy is to prevent pancreatitis through a very low-fat diet (≤15% of calories from fat), weight reduction, increased physical activity, and drug therapy. In patients with a triglyceride concentration of 250–750 mg/dL (2.8–8.5 mmol/L), a 10–20-lb weight loss usually leads to a marked reduction in triglyceride concentrations and an increase in HDL (if low). The drugs of choice for lowering triglycerides are fibrates or nicotinic acid. An alternative approach to drug therapy in patients with borderline high or high triglycerides is to intensify therapy with an LDL-lowering drug, such as a statin, which will provide some reduction in triglycerides.

Most patients with a high triglyceride concentration are inactive and obese. The majority of patients encountered in clinical practice with elevated triglycerides have similar lipid and nonlipid risk factors of metabolic origin termed *metabolic syndrome*.[48] The metabolic syndrome is characterized by abdominal obesity, insulin resistance, hypertension, low HDL, and elevations in triglycerides. The metabolic syndrome is managed by correcting underlying causes, such as obesity, with lifestyle changes and by treating associated lipid risk factors.

Since hypertriglyceridemia is an independent risk factor for CHD, this suggests that triglyceride-rich lipoproteins may be atherogenic.[36] VLDL is a triglyceride-rich lipoprotein. There is recent evidence that VLDL, like LDL particles, is atherogenic. In patients with high triglycerides, the sum of atherogenic particles (both VLDL and LDL) may be estimated by calculating non-HDL cholesterol. The lowering of non-HDL cholesterol (total cholesterol [LDL + VLDL] – HDL) is a secondary target of therapy in all persons with high triglycerides (≥200 mg/dL). VLDL is estimated to be the plasma triglyceride level divided by five. The non-HDL cholesterol target of therapy is set at 30 mg/dL greater than the LDL goal. For example, if a patient with CHD has an LDL goal of less than 100 mg/dL, the non-HDL goal will be set at <130 mg/dL. If triglycerides are less than 200 mg/dL, then lifestyle modifications are appropriate. If triglycerides are 200–499 mg/dL, then the non-HDL goal should be the target of therapy. This underscores the need to assess non-HDL as a marker of atherosclerotic risk in all patients with serum triglycerides greater than 200 mg/dL. VLDL levels are not routinely measured in practice or targeted in therapy. The triglyceride rich lipoprotein is assessed by use of TG or non-HDL levels instead.

There are several triglyceride assay interferences regarding triglyceride measurement. The triglyceride assay itself is susceptible to interference by glycerol, which may be a component of medications or used as a lubricant in laboratory equipment.[49] An excess of triglycerides in the blood can lead to errors in other laboratory measurements. Lipemic samples can cause falsely low serum amylase results, underestimation of electrolytes, and erratic interferences with many other tests.[50] The potential interference with amylase is especially clinically relevant since high triglyceride concentrations can cause pancreatitis, and accurate amylase concentrations are crucial to diagnosis.

Fortunately, most technologists can identify lipemic samples as the serum specimen will appear milky. The appearance of a patient's serum sample before and after 12–16 hr of refrigeration can indicate triglyceride-rich serum. If the sample shows a uniform turbidity or opalescence, VLDL has increased without a concurrent increase in chylomicrons. A "cream" supernatant layer atop a clear solution indicates chylomicronemia, without an excess of both chylomicrons and VLDL.

Low-Density Lipoprotein Cholesterol

For fasting adults >20 years[36]:

optimal, <100 mg/dL or <2.58 mmol/L;

near or above optimal, 100–129 mg/dL or 2.58–3.33 mmol/L;

borderline high, 130–159 mg/dL or 3.36–4.11 mmol/L;

high, 160–189 mg/dL or 4.13–4.88 mmol/L;

or very high, ≥190 mg/dL or 4.91 mmol/L

Since total cholesterol concentrations include both the "good" (HDL) and "bad" (LDL) cholesterol, the primary goals of therapy are stated in terms of only the "bad" cholesterol, or low-density lipoprotein cholesterol (LDL). The LDL must be measured while the patient is in a fasting state. Low-risk patients whose LDL cholesterol is less than individualized goal (without drug therapy) should have their fasting lipoprotein profile measured every 5 years. More frequent measurement may be desired in patients with multiple risk factors or patients with low-risk (0–1 risk factor) (but with previous LDL values only slightly below individualized goal). The total fasting lipid profile includes total cholesterol, HDL, LDL, and triglycerides. Direct measurement of LDL is not commonly performed due to labor-intensive centrifugation. Instead, LDL cholesterol concentrations can be estimated indirectly by a method determined by Friedewald.[51] The formula subtracts the HDL and VLDL cholesterol from the total plasma cholesterol. The VLDL is estimated to be the plasma triglyceride level divided by five. Using the following formula (all in milligrams per deciliter), LDL may be estimated in patients with a triglyceride concentration less than 400 mg/dL (<4.52 mmol/L) and without type 3 hyperlipoproteinemia (see Table 14-2):

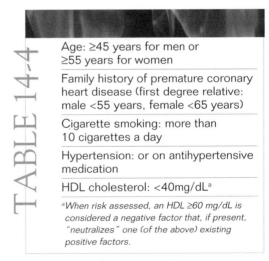

TABLE 14-4

Age: ≥45 years for men or ≥55 years for women
Family history of premature coronary heart disease (first degree relative: male <55 years, female <65 years)
Cigarette smoking: more than 10 cigarettes a day
Hypertension: or on antihypertensive medication
HDL cholesterol: <40mg/dL[a]

[a]When risk assessed, an HDL ≥60 mg/dL is considered a negative factor that, if present, "neutralizes" one (of the above) existing positive factors.

Table 14-4. Risk Factors for Atherosclerotic Vascular Disease from High Cholesterol (Primarily LDL)[36]

$$LDL = \text{total serum cholesterol} - HDL - (\text{triglycerides}/5)$$

If a patient's serum triglyceride concentration exceeds 400 mg/dL (4.5 mmol/L), LDL cholesterol cannot be calculated with this formula. A direct LDL measurement by laboratory would provide an LDL value. However, since treatment of hypertriglyceridemia would take priority in such a patient, most clinicians would treat hypertriglyceridemia through lifestyle modifications and medications first. Once triglyceride values have decreased to <400 mg/dL (<4.52 mmol/L), a fasting lipid panel would provide LDL cholesterol data.

TABLE 14-5

CHD or CHD Risk Equivalents[a]	Risk Factors[b]	Initiate Lifestyle Changes LDL (mg/dL)[c]	Consider Drug Therapy LDL (mg/dL)[c]	LDL Goal
No	None or one	≥160 (≥4.14)	≥190 (≥4.92)	<160 (<4.14)
No	Two or more	≥130 (≥3.36)	10-year risk <10% ≥160 (≥4.14)	<130 (<3.36)
			10-year risk 10–20% ≥130 (≥3.36)	
Yes	None or any	≥100 (≥2.60)	≥130 (≥3.36)	<100 (<2.60)

[a]Coronary heart disease (CHD) includes angina, myocardial infarction, and coronary angioplasty. CHD risk equivalents include diabetes, peripheral arterial disease, TIA/stroke and a 10-year risk >20%.
[b]Risk factors in Table 14-4. An increased (≥60 mg/dL) HDL concentration is a negative risk factor discussed previously) and negates one of the positive risk factors.
[c]Amount in parentheses is in SI units of millimoles per liter.

Table 14-5. LDL-Based Treatment Recommendations of the Expert Panel of the National Cholesterol Education Program[36]

Table 14-5 lists the treatment recommendations from the 2001 report of the expert panel of the National Cholesterol Education Program.[36] LDL cholesterol lowering is the primary goal of therapy in patients with hyperlipidemia. Based on epidemiologic data, when LDL cholesterol levels are maintained below 100 mg/dL, the risk for atherogenesis is nearly absent. Therefore, LDL cholesterol levels are considered *optimal* when maintained below 100 mg/dL. The actual goal LDL for an individual patient is defined by a risk evaluation. If a patient has CHD or a CHD risk equivalent, the goal LDL is less than 100 mg/dL. Examples of patients with CHD include a patient with a history of myocardial infarction, unstable angina, stable angina, or coronary angioplasty. Diabetes, peripheral arterial disease, history of transient ischemic attack, and stroke are examples of CHD risk equivalents.

In patients without CHD or a CHD risk equivalent, an assessment of the patient's number of risk factors must be done (Table 14-4). For patients with two or more risk factors, a Framingham risk score is calculated to determine the patient's CHD risk (Figure 14-2).[36] The Framingham score takes into account data from the Framingham study used to weight individual risk factors. If a patient is determined to have a 10-year risk of CHD of greater than 20%, this patient is said to have a CHD risk equivalent and treated to a goal LDL of less than 100 mg/dL. In patients with two or more risk factors and a 10-year risk of CHD of 20% or less, an LDL goal of less than 130 mg/dL is desired. However, drug therapy may be initiated earlier in those patients with a risk of greater than 10%. In those patients with lower risk (0–1 risk factors), the goal LDL is set at less than 160 mg/dL.

Lifestyle modifications are appropriate for all patients with hyperlipidemias. Detailed education should be provided to patients regarding the adoption of a low saturated fat and low cholesterol diet, maintenance of a healthy weight, and regular physical activity. Reducing saturated fat in the diet to <7% of calories gives an approximate LDL cholesterol reduction of 8–10%, while an intake of <200 mg/day of dietary cholesterol would provide an additional 3–5% reduction in LDL.[52] A weight reduction by 10 pounds due to moderate physical activity and dietary changes may provide an approximate LDL reduction of 5–8%. Dietary supplementation with soluble fiber and the use of plant stanols and sterols are therapeutic dietary options to lower LDL cholesterol. Drug therapy is generally initiated when lifestyle modifications have been inadequate in addressing elevations in LDL, particularly if the LDL remains greater than 30 mg/dL over the patient's individual goal.

Estimate of 10-Year Risk for **Men**
(Framingham Point Scores)

Age, y	Points
20-34	-9
35-39	-4
40-44	0
45-49	3
50-54	6
55-59	8
60-64	10
65-69	11
70-74	12
75-79	13

Total Cholesterol, mg/dL	Points				
	Age 20-39 y	Age 40-49 y	Age 50-59 y	Age 60-69 y	Age 70-79 y
<160	0	0	0	0	0
160-199	4	3	2	1	0
200-239	7	5	3	1	0
240-279	9	6	4	2	1
≥280	11	8	5	3	1

	Points				
	Age 20-39 y	Age 40-49 y	Age 50-59 y	Age 60-69 y	Age 70-79 y
Nonsmoker	0	0	0	0	0
Smoker	8	5	3	1	1

HDL, mg/dL	Points
≥60	-1
50-59	0
40-49	1
<40	2

Systolic BP, mm Hg	If Untreated	If Treated
<120	0	0
120-129	0	1
130-139	1	2
140-159	1	2
≥160	2	3

Point Total	10-Year Risk, %
<0	<1
0	1
1	1
2	1
3	1
4	1
5	2
6	2
7	3
8	4
9	5
10	6
11	8
12	10
13	12
14	16
15	20
16	25
≥17	≥30

Estimate of 10-Year Risk for **Women**
(Framingham Point Scores)

Age, y	Points
20-34	-7
35-39	-3
40-44	0
45-49	3
50-54	6
55-59	8
60-64	10
65-69	12
70-74	14
75-79	16

Total Cholesterol, mg/dL	Points				
	Age 20-39 y	Age 40-49 y	Age 50-59 y	Age 60-69 y	Age 70-79 y
<160	0	0	0	0	0
160-199	4	3	2	1	1
200-239	8	6	4	2	1
240-279	11	8	5	3	2
≥280	13	10	7	4	2

	Points				
	Age 20-39 y	Age 40-49 y	Age 50-59 y	Age 60-69 y	Age 70-79 y
Nonsmoker	0	0	0	0	0
Smoker	9	7	4	2	1

HDL, mg/dL	Points
≥60	-1
50-59	0
40-49	1
<40	2

Systolic BP, mm Hg	If Untreated	If Treated
<120	0	0
120-129	1	3
130-139	2	4
140-159	3	5
≥160	4	6

Point Total	10-Year Risk, %
<9	<1
9	1
10	1
11	1
12	1
13	2
14	2
15	3
16	4
17	5
18	6
19	8
20	11
21	14
22	17
23	22
24	27
≥25	≥30

Figure 14-2. Framingham Point Scores.[36]

High-Density Lipoprotein Cholesterol

For fasting adults >20 years[36]:

low, >40 mg/dL or >1.03 mmol/L;

high, ≥60 mg/dL or 1.55 mmol/L

Based on epidemiological evidence, HDL acts as an antiatherogenic factor and is often termed the "good cholesterol."[53,54] While a high HDL concentration is associated with cardioprotection, low levels are associated with increased risk of coronary artery disease. Every 1% increase in HDL cholesterol is associated with a decrease in coronary heart disease by 2% in men and 3% in women.[55] The Framingham Study demonstrated that HDL levels were predictive of cardiovascular risk independent of elevations in LDL. Examples of this atherogenic potential are best illustrated with the coronary arteries. Concentrations less than 40 mg/dL (<1.03 mmol/L) are associated with an increased risk of myocardial infarction. Similarly, low HDL is also associated with an increased risk of coronary angioplasty restenosis.[54,56] Generally, the ideal LDL:HDL ratio is less than 3. An LDL:HDL ratio greater than 4 is considered atherogenic, but lowering this ratio has not been a primary target of therapy.[36,46] While it is reasonable to desire lower LDL:HDL ratios, NCEP panel guidelines emphasize reduction of LDL with non-HDL as a secondary target of therapy instead. The blood need not be drawn after a 12-hr fast. However, a fast is usually required because HDL is often ordered in combination with LDL.

MINICASE 1

HENRIETTA F., A 42-YEAR-OLD FEMALE, had her lipid profile results forwarded to the clinic after attending a local health fair. Her nonfasting total and HDL cholesterol levels were 232 mg/dL and 52 mg/dL, respectively. She follows a reasonable, low-fat diet, and hikes for exercise often. She has a 20 pack/year history of smoking but rarely drinks alcohol. She takes vitamins, calcium, and an antihistamine for seasonal allergies. She does not have a family history of diabetes, hyperlipidemias, pancreatitis, or coronary heart disease. At her office visit, she has a normal physical exam. Her fasting glucose was 90 mg/dL; electrolyte, hematology, liver, renal, and thyroid tests are all normal. She is 5-ft 8-in, 135 pounds, and premenopausal.

Question: How should the lipid results be interpreted? What should be done next?

Discussion: Henrietta F. is young, asymptomatic, and premenopausal; watches her cholesterol intake; is active; is not hypertensive; and has no familial risk factors. Her habit of cigarette smoking is a major risk factor for coronary heart disease. Henrietta F. has no evident secondary causes of hyperlipidemia. She has no occult thyroid, renal, or liver disease. She is not using drugs that can cause an elevation in lipids. Though a fasting lipoprotein profile is recommended to screen for hyperlipidemia, the total cholesterol and HDL cholesterol values of the nonfasting screening may be used in this initial evaluation. Her total cholesterol is in the *borderline high* category, but her HDL is not in the *low* or *high* category. Since her total cholesterol was elevated, the measurement should be repeated in the fasting state. This would allow for determination of LDL and TG to assess her cardiovascular risk.

Henrietta F. returns for a fasting lipoprotein profile. After a 12-hr fast, the following laboratory results are obtained: total cholesterol 224 mg/dL, HDL cholesterol 54 mg/dL, triglycerides 105 mg/dL, LDL cholesterol 149 mg/dL.

Question: How should the follow-up lipid results be interpreted? What should be done next?

Discussion: The total cholesterol measurement has varied from the previous measurement, which is expected. Total cholesterol concentrations vary from day to day, usually by 2–3%. Henrietta F's total cholesterol remains in the *borderline high* category. However, her triglycerides and HDL are within the normal range. Since Henrietta F. has only one CHD risk factor (cigarette smoking, Table 14-4), her desired LDL goal is less than 160 mg/dL (Table 14-5). As direct LDL measurements are not often obtained from the laboratory, the LDL was calculated using the Friedewald formula: LDL = total serum cholesterol – HDL – (triglycerides/5).

$$LDL = 224 \text{ mg/dL} - 54 \text{ mg/dL} - (105 \text{ mg/dL} /5) = 149 \text{ mg/dL}$$

Reinforce Henrietta F's low-fat, low-cholesterol diet and physical activity. To reduce cardiovascular risk, she should also be advised to stop smoking and provided with guidance to assist her reach this goal. Since her LDL is below the desired goal of 160 mg/dL, no drug therapy is required. A repeat fasting lipid profile is desired in 5 years. However, some clinicians may chose to follow-up sooner since her LDL of 149 mg/dL was only slightly below the goal of less than 160 mg/dL.

MINICASE 2

GEORGE L., A 58-YEAR-OLD, 5-FT 9-IN, 250-LB. MALE, just transferred physicians due to changes in his health plan. He presents to the clinic for a routine physical examination. His past medical history is significant for a myocardial infarction (MI) at age 56 and hypertension. He does not have a history of diabetes or thyroid disorder. Current medications include a beta-blocker (metoprolol), ACE inhibitor, and low-dose aspirin daily. He has never taken cholesterol-lowering medication. Since his MI, he has quit smoking. George L. states he tries to follow a low-fat, low-cholesterol diet, but he often eats out at restaurants. He did very little exercise prior to his MI, but he has tried to walk once weekly since the event. His father died of a heart attack at age 58. He has no family history of diabetes or lipid disorders.

His blood pressure at the office was 150/86, heart rate 88. Fasting lipid profile was as follows: total cholesterol 225 mg/dL; triglycerides 140 mg/dL, LDL 159 mg/Dl, and HDL 38 mg/dL. Fasting glucose is 100 mg/dL; electrolyte, hematology, liver, renal, and thyroid tests are all normal.

Question: Was it appropriate to order a lipid profile? How should the lipid profile be interpreted?

Discussion: All patients with coronary artery disease (myocardial infarction or angina) should have a lipid profile performed. It is unknown whether George L.'s previous physician had performed lipid panels and if the results were within desired range.

Even before his myocardial infarction at age 56, George L. was at high risk for atherosclerotic disease. At that time he was an overweight, male smoker—older than 45 years—who lived a sedentary lifestyle. His father died prematurely of atherosclerotic vessel disease, although his age at death (58) does not meet the official criteria for a risk factor (<55 years old).

George L. has no evidence of disease-related secondary causes of hyperlipidemia (diabetes, hypothyroidism, obstructive liver disease, chronic renal failure). However, there are potential medication-related secondary causes of hyperlipidemia in George L.'s case. Beta-blockers may impact the lipid profile by causing decreases in HDL and increases in triglycerides. George L.'s HDL cholesterol value is indeed low. However, discontinuation of the beta-blocker is not warranted as the benefits of beta-blockers in reducing mortality postmyocardial infarction outweigh the impact on the lipid profile. Further, George L.'s LDL cholesterol is elevated and will be the primary target of therapy.

Currently, George L. has three risk factors for cardiovascular disease: hypertension, age ≥45, and low HDL <40 mg/dL. It is not necessary to calculate George L.'s Framingham risk score, as with a history of myocardial infarction George L. has CHD. All patients with CHD have an LDL goal set at less than 100 mg/dL. Therapeutic lifestyle changes (TLC) are appropriate for George L., including a greater emphasis on reducing saturated fat and cholesterol intake in the diet and increasing physical activity. While lifestyle therapy should definitely be initiated, even if George L. adheres strictly to a therapeutic lifestyle change (TLC) diet, only a 10–15% decrease in LDL cholesterol is expected. George L. needs to obtain a 37% reduction in his LDL cholesterol to bring his current LDL cholesterol of 159 mg/dL to a goal of less than 100 mg/dL. Therefore, drug therapy should also be initiated. Statins, bile acid sequestrants, and nicotinic acid are all considered LDL lowering drug therapy appropriate for George L. Depending on the selection of an agent, appropriate baseline laboratory values should be obtained. A fasting lipid profile should be checked in 6 weeks to determine if goals have been met or changes in drug therapy are warranted.

Most patients with low HDL levels have concomitant elevated triglyceride levels. In these patients, lifestyle therapy or drug therapy to decrease triglycerides usually results in a desirable increase in HDL. However, there are also patients with isolated low HDL cholesterol. Since LDL is the primary goal of therapy in the National Cholesterol Education Panel guidelines, there is no specific goal for raising HDL, which is negatively correlated with triglycerides, smoking, and obesity. In contrast, HDL is positively correlated with physical activity and smoking cessation (Minicases 1–3).

Emerging Risk Factors

A number of emerging lipid risk factors for coronary artery disease are being investigated to varying degrees: lipoprotein remnants and lipoprotein (a), small LDL particles, HDL subspecies, and apolipoproteins, such as apolipoprotein B and apolipoprotein AI.[13,57,58] Stan-

MINICASE 3

LISA M. IS A 56-YEAR-OLD, 5-FT 6-IN, 180-LB. FEMALE who had a recent lipid panel drawn for routine screening. The results of a lab, drawn yesterday, are now available, and her health-care provider calls her to follow-up on the results. Her past medical history is significant for hypertension and allergic rhinitis. She has no family history of cardiovascular disease, but her mother has a history of pancreatitis. Medications include hydrochlorothiazide 12.5 mg, a multivitamin, and calcium daily. Her diet consists of hamburgers, steak, and pasta, with 2–3 glasses of wine each night. Physical activity is minimal. Lisa M. denies abdominal pain, epigastric tenderness, and fever. She also denies nausea and vomiting. Fasting lab results are as follows: total cholesterol 190 mg/dL, triglycerides 600 mg/dL, HDL 58 mg/dL, and glucose 88 mg/dL.

Question: How should the lipid results be interpreted? What should be done next?

Discussion: The first action the clinician should take is to confirm that the lab result is indeed a fasting lipid profile. Often high triglyceride values create unnecessary panic because the patient misunderstood directions and failed to fast. In this case, as the glucose value of 88 mg/dL suggests, the lipids were drawn in the fasting state. An LDL value is unavailable since LDL can only be calculated with the Friedewald formula when triglycerides are less than 400 mg/dL.

Lisa M. has *very high* triglycerides with a triglyceride level greater than 500 mg/dL. Lisa M. has no physical signs of symptoms of pancreatitis, but she does have a positive family history. To prevent acute pancreatitis, triglycerides should be lowered though a very low-fat diet with ≤15% of caloric intake from fat, weight reduction, and increased physical activity. Lisa M.'s current diet is high in saturated fat in cholesterol. Abstention from all alcohol intake is an important step to minimize the risk of pancreatitis. Though low to moderate intake of alcohol intake may be associated with a decreased risk of cardiovascular disease, Lisa M.'s current alcohol intake is too high. A triglyceride-lowering drug, such as a fibrate or nicotinic acid, may also be considered. If Lisa M. experiences epigastric pain, it may be prudent to check amylase and lipase levels (Chapter 12) and proceed with further evaluation. Once triglyceride levels have been lowered to less than 500 mg/dL, then attention can be turned to repeating a fasting lipid panel to assess LDL. Keep in mind that unless an institution has direct LDL measurement available, an indirect value cannot be calculated if triglycerides remain above 400 mg/dL.

dardized laboratory techniques have not been developed for the measurement of these lipoproteins. Moreover, measurements are not readily available in clinical practice. At this time, measurement of these risk factors is primary employed by specialists until more evidence linking them to cardiovascular risk and more refined laboratory methods are available.

Nonlipid emerging risk factors are also under investigation.[58–61] Plasma homocysteine levels, thrombogenic factors, and inflammatory markers, such as C-reactive protein, all have been linked to coronary heart disease. Like the emerging lipid risk factors, there are no recommendations at this time to routinely monitor this laboratory data in patients.[36]

Point-of-Care Testing Options

In addition to laboratory monitoring, there is a home testing kit available to the patient for determination of total cholesterol.[62] The clinical applicability of this testing method, which utilizes a fingerstick for obtaining a sample, is limited since total cholesterol alone is no longer recommended as a screening tool by NCEP.[36] In addition to home testing methods, there are relatively inexpensive compact devices for point-of-care testing outside the laboratory that are waived from the Clinical Laboratory Improvement Amendments (CLIA). These devices enable testing for total cholesterol, HDL cholesterol, and triglycerides. The LDL is calculated either by the user or the device using the Friedewald formula. Separate cartridges are available for testing of ALT. Generally, the devices meet accuracy standards of ±3% set by NCEP devices, which vary, but do not necessarily meet the precision standard of ±3%.[63–65]

One important consideration when evaluating studies of point-of-care testing devices is to be aware that some variability may be explained by the fact that different samples types are often compared. For example, a fingerstick provides a sample with capillary blood and a venous draw provides venous whole blood. Nevertheless, the point-of-care testing devices are accepted methods for screening for hyperlipidemia and are frequently used in clinical practice for patient care.[63,64] In one study, despite variability, patients were classified into appropriate risk groups with few misclassifications based on NCEP recommendations.[63] In this study, values near NCEP cut points were repeated. In any point-of-care testing setting, quality control, quality assessment, and proper training of personnel can work to improve the accuracy of testing.[66] One of the overwhelming benefits of point-of-care testing is that it involves the patient in the laboratory process, which has been identified by NCEP as an intervention to improve patient adherence.[36] The laboratory visits become opportunities for the clinician to provide the patient with feedback on progress and reinforce the steps needed to achieve goals.

EFFECTS OF HYPOLIPEMIC MEDICATIONS

Clinicians must be aware of how antihyperlipidemic drugs can influence laboratory test results. The two principal approaches to management of hyperlipidemia are lifestyle intervention and drug therapy. In high-risk patients, drug therapy is immediately initiated along with lifestyle interventions and is always concurrently used with drug therapy. In most patients, when lifestyle interventions do not result in appropriate reductions, drug therapy is considered. The ultimate goal of therapy is to reduce cardiovascular risk, or, in the case of elevated triglycerides alone, reduce the risk of pancreatitis. In general, statins, bile acid sequestrants, and niacin are considered LDL-lowering drug therapy. Fibrates and niacin are considered drugs for lowering triglycerides or raising HDL. Specific actions of the drugs are reviewed below.

Bile Acid Sequestrants

Agents that bind bile acids (e.g., cholestyramine, colesevelam, and colestipol) lower LDL concentrations by 15–30% but may raise triglycerides, especially if hypertriglyceridemia exists.[4] Because these products stay within the enterohepatic circulation, they do not directly cause other systemic effects that may be reflected in laboratory data. They do, however, interfere with the absorption of fat-soluble vitamins and drugs (e.g., digoxin, thyroid supplements, and warfarin) and may affect serum concentrations of these drugs or prothrombin times. Bile acid sequestrants may increase triglyceride levels and are not recommended in individuals with triglycerides greater than 200 mg/dL and are contraindicated in patients with triglycerides greater than 400 mg/dL. In clinical trials, bile acid sequestrants are associated with reduced major coronary events and CHD deaths.[36]

Niacin

Although niacin, or nicotinic acid, is associated with more bothersome side effects (e.g., flushing, pruritus, and gastrointestinal distress) than other agents, it has desirable effects on the lipid profile. In therapeutic doses, this B vitamin lowers total serum cholesterol, LDL (by 5–25%), and triglycerides (by 20–50%) and tends to raise HDL (by 15–35%).[4] Niacin may increase serum glucose, uric acid, and liver function tests (LFTs) and decrease serum thyroxine (T_4) and thyroxine-binding globulin without causing clinical hypothyroidism.[5,67] Flushing can be minimized by taking aspirin before each dose or by taking niacin with a meal. Sustained-release formulations may also minimize flushing. However, hepatotoxicity, detected by increase in LFTs greater than 3 times the upper limit of normal, is more often associated with sustained-release preparations of niacin.[5] Niacin is associated with reductions in major coronary events and possibly reductions in total mortality.[36]

Statins

By inhibiting the enzyme that catalyzes the rate-limiting step in cholesterol synthesis, statins, or 3-hydroxy-3-methylglutaryl coenzyme A reductase inhibitors (HMG-CoA reductase inhibitors) lower total cholesterol and LDL (18–55%, depending on the drug and dose) and may raise HDL as much as 15%.[4,36] Statins may also decrease triglyceride concentrations (by 7–30%). The degree of TG lowering with the statins depends on the degree on initial elevation in triglycerides.[5] With all statins, maximum effects usually are seen after 4–6 weeks.

Patients on these agents may develop increases in transaminases and creatine phosphokinase (CPK) (Chapter 11) with muscle pain. Laboratory monitoring of LFTs for potential hepatotoxicity of the statins and CPK for myopathy is required. General recommendations for monitoring are that LFTs be performed before the initiation of therapy, at 6 and 12 weeks after initiation, and then semiannually. If transaminases (aspartate aminotransferase and alanine aminotransferase) rise to 3 times the upper limit of normal or higher, withdrawal of the drug is recommended. Myalgia, muscle pain, tenderness and/or weakness, occurs in 2–7% of patients on statins.[68] Myopathy occurs in 0.1–0.2% of patients on statins. Increased risk of myopathy is associated with the use of high-dose statins, renal insufficiency, concurrent use of fibrates, and concurrent use of cytochrome P450 inhibitors.[68] All patients should have baseline CPK drawn prior to initiation of statin therapy. In patients with complaints of muscle pain, tenderness or weakness, serum CPK should be drawn. Elevations in CPK and myalgia together are termed *myopathy*. In some cases, rhabdomyolysis has been reported. Most clinicians will discontinue the drug when CPK levels are greater than 10 times the upper limit of normal. Routine monitoring of CPK is not warranted.

Numerous trials document the clinical benefits of statins. The agents are associated with reductions in major coronary events, CHD deaths, need for coronary procedures, stroke, and total mortality.[36]

Fibric Acid Derivatives

Fibrates, gemfibrozil, fenofibrate, and clofibrate reduce triglycerides by 20–50% and increase HDL by 10–20%.[4] In patients with moderately elevated triglycerides, LDL may be decreased 5–20% by fibrates. However, in patients with very high triglycerides, treatment with a fibrate may increase LDL concentrations. Gemfibrozil or fenofibrate is preferred to clofibrate, which is avoided by clinicians due to evidence of increased total mortality with this agent in one trial.[69] Like the statins, the agents are associated with transaminase and CPK elevations (with myositis and flu-like symptoms). Baseline, week 6, week 12, and then periodic (every 6–12 months) LFTs should be done in patients receiving these drugs. CPK should be monitored in patients with complaints of muscle ache. A higher risk of myopathy is observed in patients on combination therapy with fibrates and statins.[70] Prothrombin time monitoring is required in patients on warfarin as fibrates displace warfarin from protein-binding sites.[4] Fibric acid derivatives in clinical trials have demonstrated reductions in major coronary events.[36]

Ezetimibe

By selectively inhibiting the intestinal absorption of cholesterol, ezetimibe monotherapy reduces LDL cholesterol by approximately 17%.[71] Adding ezetimibe to therapy with a statin provides LDL reductions greater than the statin alone.[72] In patients with primary hypercholesterolemia, ezetimibe reduces triglycerides by approximately 8%.[73] Ezetimibe is generally well-tolerated. When ezetimibe is coadministered with a statin, routine liver function tests should be performed as with statin therapy alone. The incidence of increased transaminases from coadministration of ezetimibe and a statin (1.3%) is higher than the incidence for patients treated with statins alone (0.4%).[73]

SUMMARY

All adults, age 20 years or older, should have a fasting lipoprotein profile checked once every 5 years. The fasting profile consists of total cholesterol, LDL cholesterol, HDL cholesterol, and triglycerides. If total serum cholesterol and triglycerides are lowered and HDL is raised, death from coronary artery disease decreases. Additionally, hypertriglyceridemia increases the risk of pancreatitis. Hyperlipidemia may be primary (genetic or familial) or secondary to other diseases or drugs. Measurement of the specific lipoproteins (LDL, HDL, and VLDL), which carry cholesterol and triglycerides, assists with diagnostic, prognostic, and therapeutic decisions. While lowering LDL is the primary goal of therapy, decreasing non-HDL is a secondary target of therapy, particularly in patients with elevated triglycerides. When diet and exercise fail to correct the lipid disorder, hypolipemic agents are used to impact the lipid profile.

REFERENCES

1. American Heart Association. *2002 Heart and Stroke Statistical Update*. Dallas, TX: American Heart Association; 2001.

2. McBride P, Schrott HG, Plane MB, et al. Primary care practice adherence to National Cholesterol Education Program guidelines for patients with coronary heart disease. *Arch Intern Med*. 1998; 158:1238–44.

3. Pearson TA, Laurora I, Chu H, et al. The lipid treatment assessment project (L-TAP): a multicenter survey to evaluate the percentages of dyslipidemic patients receiving lipid-lowering therapy and achieving low-density lipoprotein cholesterol goals. *Arch Intern Med*. 2000; 160:459–67.

4. Gotto AM. Management of dyslipidemia. *Am J Med*. 2002; 112(suppl 8A):10S–18S.

5. Knopp RH. Drug treatment of lipid disorders. *N Engl J Med*. 1999; 341:498–511.

6. Lousberg TR, Denham AM, Rasmussen JR. A comparison of clinical outcome studies among cholesterol-lowering agents. *Ann Pharmacother*. 2001; 35:1599–607.

7. Ginsberg HN, Goldberg IJ. Disorders of lipid metabolism. In: Braunwald E, Fauci AS, Kasper DL, et al, eds. *Harrison's Principles of Internal Medicine*. 15th ed. New York, NY: McGraw-Hill; 2001: 2245–57.

8. Duell PB, Illingworth DR, Connor WE, et al. Disorders of lipid metabolism. In: Felig P, Frohman LA, eds. *Endocrinology & Metabolism*. 4th ed. New York, NY: McGraw-Hill Health Professions Division; 2001: 993–1075.

9. Jones PJ, Schoeller DA. Evidence for diurnal periodicity in human cholesterol synthesis. *J Lipid Res*. 1990; 31:667–73.

10. Hajjar DP, Nicholson AC. Atherosclerosis. *American Scientist*. 1995; 83:460.

11. Ginsberg HN. Lipoprotein physiology. *Endocrinol Metab Clin North Am*. 1998; 27:503–19.

12. Schaefer EJ, Lichtenstein AH, Lamon-Fava S, et al. Lipoproteins, nutrition, aging, and atherosclerosis. *Am J Clin Nutr*. 1995; 61:726S–40S.

13. Koay ES. Plasma lipid profiles: the expanding repertoire of tests, their clinical significance and pitfalls. *Ann Acad Med Singapore*. 1989; 18:436–43.

14. Stamler J, Wentworth D, Neaton JD. Is relationship between serum cholesterol and risk of premature death from coronary heart disease continuous and graded? Findings in 356,222 primary screenees of the Multiple Risk Factor Intervention Trial (MRFIT). *JAMA*. 1986; 256:2823–8.

15. Neaton JD, Blackburn H, Jacobs D, et al. Serum cholesterol level and mortality findings for men screened in the Multiple Risk Factor Intervention Trial. Multiple Risk Factor Intervention Trial Research Group. *Arch Intern Med*. 1992; 152:1490–500.

16. Scandinavian Simvastatin Survival Study Group. Randomised trial of cholesterol lowering in 4444 patients with coronary heart disease: the Scandinavian simvastatin survival study (4S). *Lancet*. 1994; 344:1383.

17. The Long-Term Intervention with Pravastatin in Ischaemic Disease (LIPID) Study Group. Prevention of cardiovascular events and death with pravastatin in patients with coronary heart disease and a broad range of initial cholesterol levels. *N Engl J Med*. 1998; 339:1349.

18. Sacks FM, Pfeffer MA, Moye LA, et al. The effect of pravastatin on coronary events after myocardial infarction in patients with average cholesterol levels. Cholesterol and Recurrent Events Trial investigators. *N Engl J Med*. 1996; 335:1001–9.

19. Miettinen T, Pyorala K, Olsson AG, et al. Cholesterol-lowering therapy in women and elderly patients with myocardial infarction or angina pectoris. Findings from the Scandinavian Simvastatin Survival Study (4S). *Circulation*. 1997; 96: 4211–8.

20. Shepherd J, Cobbe SM, Ford I, et al. Prevention of coronary heart disease with pravastatin in men with hypercholesterolemia. West of Scotland Coronary Prevention Study Group. *N Engl J Med*. 1995; 333: 1301–7.

21. Downs JR, Clearfield M, Weis S, et al. Primary prevention of acute coronary events with lovastatin in men and women with average cholesterol levels: results of AFCAPS/TexCAPS. Air Force/Texas Coronary Atherosclerosis Prevention Study. *JAMA*. 1998; 279:1615–22.

22. Krone W, Nagele H. Effects of antihypertensives on plasma lipids and lipoprotein metabolism. *Am Heart J*. 1988; 116:1729–34.

23. Kasiske BL, Ma JZ, Kalil RS, et al. Effects of antihypertensive therapy on serum lipids. *Ann Intern Med.*1995; 122:133–41.

24. Lakshman MR, Reda DJ, Materson BJ, et al. Diuretics and beta-blockers do not have adverse effects at 1 year on plasma lipid and lipoprotein profiles in men with hypertension. Department of Veterans Affairs Cooperative Study Group on Antihypertensive Agents. *Arch Intern Med.* 1999; 159:551–8.

25. Mantel-Teeuwisse AK, Kloosterman JM, Maitland-van der Zee AH, et al. Drug-Induced lipid changes: a review of the unintended effects of some commonly used drugs on serum lipid levels. *Drug Saf.* 2001; 24:443–56.

26. Teichmann A. Metabolic profile of six oral contraceptives containing norgestimate, gestodene, and desogestrel. *Int J Fertil Menopausal Stud.* 1995; 40 (suppl 2):98–104.

27. Henkin Y, Como JA, Oberman A. Secondary dyslipidemia. Inadvertent effects of drugs in clinical practice. *JAMA.* 1992; 267:961–8.

28. Carr A, Samaras K, Burton S, et al. A syndrome of peripheral lipodystrophy, hyperlipidaemia, and insulin resistance in patients receiving HIV protease inhibitors. *Aids.* 1998; 12:F51–8.

29. Echevarria KL, Hardin TC, Smith JA. Hyperlipidemia associated with protease inhibitor therapy. *Ann Pharmacother.* 1999; 33:859–63.

30. Carr A, Samaras K, Thorisdottir A, et al. Diagnosis, prediction, and natural course of HIV-1 protease-inhibitor-associated lipodystrophy, hyperlipidaemia, and diabetes mellitus: a cohort study. *Lancet.* 1999; 353:2093–9.

31. Lee IM, Hsieh CC, Paffenbarger Jr RS. Exercise intensity and longevity in men. The Harvard Alumni Health Study. *JAMA.* 1995; 273:1179–84.

32. Dallongeville J, Marecaux N, Richard F, et al. Cigarette smoking is associated with differences in nutritional habits and related to lipoprotein alterations independently of food and alcohol intake. *Eur J Clin Nutr.* 1996; 50:647–54.

33. Gaziano JM, Buring JE, Breslow JL, et al. Moderate alcohol intake, increased levels of high-density lipoprotein and its subfractions, and decreased risk of myocardial infarction. *N Engl J Med.* 1993; 329:1829–34.

34. Suh I, Shaten BJ, Cutler JA, et al. Alcohol use and mortality from coronary heart disease: the role of high-density lipoprotein cholesterol. The Multiple Risk Factor Intervention Trial Research Group. *Ann Intern Med.* 1992; 116:881–7.

35. Goldberg IJ, Mosca L, Piano MR, et al. AHA Science Advisory: Wine and your heart: a science advisory for healthcare professionals from the Nutrition Committee, Council on Epidemiology and Prevention, and Council on Cardiovascular Nursing of the American Heart Association. *Circulation.* 2001; 103:472–5.

36. Executive Summary of The Third Report of The National Cholesterol Education Program (NCEP) Expert Panel on Detection, Evaluation, And Treatment of High Blood Cholesterol In Adults (Adult Treatment Panel III). *JAMA.* 2001; 285:2486–97.

37. Myers GL, Cooper GR, Sampson EJ. Traditional lipoprotein profile: clinical utility, performance requirement, and standardization. *Atherosclerosis.* 1994; 108 (suppl):S157–69.

38. Faulkner MA, Hilleman DE, Destache CJ, et al. Potential influence of timing of low-density lipoprotein cholesterol evaluation in patients with acute coronary syndrome. *Pharmacotherapy.* 2001; 21:1055–60.

39. Spin JM, Vagelos AR. Early use of statins in acute coronary syndromes. *Curr Cardiol Rep.* 2002; 4:289–97.

40. Henkin Y, Crystal E, Goldberg Y, et al. Usefulness of lipoprotein changes during acute coronary syndromes for predicting postdischarge lipoprotein levels. *Am J Cardiol.* 2002; 89:7–11.

41. Grundy SM, Cleeman JI, Rifkind BM, et al. Cholesterol lowering in the elderly population. Coordinating Committee of the National Cholesterol Education Program. *Arch Intern Med.* 1999; 159:1670–8.

42. Kane JP, Malloy MJ, Ports TA, et al. Regression of coronary atherosclerosis during treatment of familial hypercholesterolemia with combined drug regimens. *JAMA.* 1990; 264:3007–12.

43. Jukema JW, Bruschke AV, van Boven AJ, et al. Effects of lipid lowering by pravastatin on progression and regression of coronary artery disease in symptomatic men with normal to moderately elevated serum cholesterol levels. The Regression Growth Evaluation Statin Study (REGRESS). *Circulation.* 1995; 91:2528–40.

44. Haskell WL, Alderman EL, Fair JM, et al. Effects of intensive multiple risk factor reduction on coronary atherosclerosis and clinical cardiac events in men and women with coronary artery disease. The Stanford Coronary Risk Intervention Project (SCRIP). *Circulation.* 1994; 89:975–90.

45. Klag MJ, Ford DE, Mead LA, et al. Serum cholesterol in young men and subsequent cardiovascular disease. *N Engl J Med.* 1993; 328:313–8.

46. Brewer HB Jr. Clinical significance of plasma lipid levels. *Am J Cardiol.* 1989; 64:3G–9G.

47. Consensus conference: Treatment of hypertriglyceridemia. *JAMA.* 1984; 251:1196–200.

48. Grundy SM. Hypertriglyceridemia, insulin resistance, and the metabolic syndrome. *Am J Cardiol.* 1999; 83:25F–29F.

49. Klotzsch SG, McNamara JR. Triglyceride measurements: a review of methods and interferences. *Clin Chem.* 1990; 36:1605–13.

50. Hulley SB, Newman TB. Cholesterol in the elderly. Is it important? *JAMA.* 1994; 272:1372–4.

51. Friedewald WT, Levy RI, Fredrickson DS. Estimation of the concentration of low-density lipoprotein cholesterol in plasma, without use of the preparative ultracentrifuge. *Clin Chem.* 1972; 18:499–502.

52. Jenkins DJ, Kendall CW, Axelsen M, et al. Viscous and nonviscous fibres, nonabsorbable and low glycaemic index carbohydrates, blood lipids and coronary heart disease. *Curr Opin Lipidol.* 2000; 11:49–56.

53. Kwiterovich PO Jr. The antiatherogenic role of high-density lipoprotein cholesterol. *Am J Cardiol.* 1998; 82:13Q–21Q.

54. Rader DJ. Pathophysiology and management of low high-density lipoprotein cholesterol. *Am J Cardiol.* 1999; 83:22F–24F.

55. Gordon DJ, Probstfield JL, Garrison RJ, et al. High-density lipoprotein cholesterol and cardiovascular disease. Four prospective American studies. *Circulation.* 1989; 79:8–15.

56. Johansen O, Abdelnoor M, Brekke M, et al. Predictors of restenosis after coronary angioplasty. A study on demographic and metabolic variables. *Scand Cardiovasc J.* 2001; 35:86–91.

57. Seman LJ, McNamara JR, Schaefer EJ. Lipoprotein(a), homocysteine, and remnantlike particles: emerging risk factors. *Curr Opin Cardiol.* 1999; 14:186–91.

58. Wood D. Established and emerging cardiovascular risk factors. *Am Heart J.* 2001; 141:S49–57.

59. Lagrand WK, Visser CA, Hermens WT, et al. C-reactive protein as a cardiovascular risk factor: more than an epiphenomenon? *Circulation.* 1999; 100:96–102.

60. Nygard O, Nordrehaug JE, Refsum H, et al. Plasma homocysteine levels and mortality in patients with coronary artery disease. *N Engl J Med.* 1997; 337:230–6.

61. Farmer JA, Torre-Amione G. Atherosclerosis and inflammation. *Curr Atheroscler Rep.* 2002; 4:92–8.

62. Home testing of cholesterol. *Med Lett Drugs Ther.* 1994; 36:85–6.

63. Volles DF, McKenney JM, Miller WG, et al. Analytic and clinical performance of two compact cholesterol-testing devices. *Pharmacotherapy.* 1998; 18:184–92.

64. Stein JH, Carlsson CM, Papcke-Benson K, et al. Inaccuracy of lipid measurements with the portable Cholestech L.D.X analyzer in patients with hypercholesterolemia. *Clin Chem.* 2002; 48:284–90.

65. Cobbaert C, Boerma GJ, Lindemans J. Evaluation of the Cholestech L.D.X. desktop analyser for cholesterol, HDL-cholesterol, and triacylglycerols in heparinized venous blood. *Eur J Clin Chem Clin Biochem.* 1994; 32:391–4.

66. du Plessis M, Ubbink JB, Vermaak WJ. Analytical quality of near-patient blood cholesterol and glucose determinations. *Clin Chem.* 2000; 46:1085–90.

67. Shakir KM, Kroll S, Aprill BS, et al. Nicotinic acid decreases serum thyroid hormone levels while maintaining a euthyroid state. *Mayo Clin Proc.* 1995; 70:556–8.

68. Hamilton-Craig I. Statin-associated myopathy. *Med J Aust.* 2001; 175:486–9.

69. W.H.O. cooperative trial on primary prevention of ischaemic heart disease using clofibrate to lower serum cholesterol: mortality follow-up. Report of the Committee of Principal Investigators. *Lancet.* 1980; 2:379–85.

70. Rader DJ, Haffner SM. Role of fibrates in the management of hypertriglyceridemia. *Am J Cardiol.* 1999; 83:30F–35F.

71. Dujovne CA, Ettinger MP, McNeer JF, et al. Efficacy and safety of a potent new selective cholesterol absorption inhibitor, ezetimibe, in patients with primary hypercholesterolemia. *Am J Cardiol.* 2002; 90:1092–7.

72. Gagne C, Bays HE, Weiss SR, et al. Efficacy and safety of ezetimibe added to ongoing statin therapy for treatment of patients with primary hypercholesterolemia. *Am J Cardiol.* 2002; 90:1084–91.

73. Zetia® (ezetimibe) package insert. North Wales, PA: Merck/Schering-Plough Pharmaceuticals; 2002.

quickview—serum triglycerides

PARAMETER	DESCRIPTION	COMMENTS
Common reference ranges Adults	Desirable: <150 mg/dL Borderline high: 150–199 mg/dL High: 200–499 mg/dL Very high: ≥500 mg/dL	SI conversion factor: 0.0113 (mmol/L)
Pediatrics	1–9 years: 25–125 mg/dL 10–19 years: 25–140 mg/dL	
Critical value	≥500	High risk of pancreatitis
Natural substance?	Yes	Required
Inherent activity?	No, but intermediary for other active substances	Needed for formation of other lipids and fatty acids
Location Production	Liver and intestines	From ingested food
Storage	Fat	
Secretion/excretion	Excreted in bile	Also recycled to liver
Major causes of... High results	Excess fat intake Genetic defects Drugs Alcohol	Associated with obesity, diabetes, steroids, estrogens, and renal disease
Associated signs and symptoms	Pancreatitis, xanthomas, lipemia retinalis	Atherosclerotic vascular disease
Low results	Not clinically important	Usually considered sign of good health
Associated signs and symptoms	None	
After insult, time to... Initial elevation	Days to weeks	Single meal has major effect on triglyceride concentration within 2 hr
Peak values	Days to weeks	Increases with aging
Normalization	Days to weeks	After diet changes or drugs
Drugs often monitored with test	Hypolipidemics	Statins, niacin, fibric acids
Causes of spurious results	Glycerol, recent meal, alcohol, lipid emulsion	

quickview—total serum cholesterol

PARAMETER	DESCRIPTION	COMMENTS
Common reference ranges Adults	Desirable: <200 mg/dL Borderline high: 200–239 mg/dL High: ≥240 mg/dL	SI conversion factor: 0.0259 (mmol/L)
Pediatrics	0–1 month: 45–100 mg/dL 1–9 years: 45–240 mg/dL 10–19 years: 115–215 mg/dL	
Critical value	Not acutely critical	Depends on risk factors, LDL, and HDL
Natural substance?	Yes	Required

Continued

Continued

PARAMETER	DESCRIPTION	COMMENTS
Inherent activity?	No, but intermediary for other active substances	Needed for cell wall, steroid, and bile acid production
Location		
Production	Liver and intestines	Ingested in diet
Storage	Fat	
Secretion/excretion	Excreted in bile	Also recycled to liver
Major causes of...		
High results	Excess fat intake (especially saturated fats) Genetic defects Drugs	Tables 14-2 and 14-3
Associated signs and symptoms	Atherosclerotic vascular disease	Angina, myocardial infarction, stroke
Low results	Hyperthyroidism Malnutrition Anemia Liver disease	Usually considered sign of good health
Associated signs and symptoms	None	
After insult, time to...		
Initial elevation	Days to weeks	Single meal has little effect on total cholesterol concentration
Peak values	Days to weeks	Can increase with aging; does not change acutely
Normalization	Weeks to months	After diet changes or drugs
Drugs often monitored with test	Hypolipidemics	Statins, niacin, fibric acids, binding resins
Causes of spurious results	Prolonged tourniquet application	Causes venous stasis (increase 5–10%)

Chapter **15**

HEMATOLOGY: RED AND WHITE BLOOD CELL TESTS

Paul R. Hutson

This chapter reviews the basic functions and expected laboratory values of erythrocytes and leukocytes. It also discusses, in an introductory manner, selected disorders of these two cellular components of blood. It must be remembered that the ability of laboratory medicine to discriminate between leukocytes is increasing, and many methods—considered investigational in this edition—may become a routine component of blood examination in the future.

OBJECTIVES

After completing this chapter, the reader should be able to

1. Describe the physiology of blood cell development and bone marrow function.
2. Discuss the interpretation and alterations of hemoglobin (Hgb), hematocrit (Hct), and various RBC indices in the evaluation of macrocytic; microcytic; and normochromic, normocytic anemias.
3. Describe the significance of abnormal erythrocyte morphology, including sickling, anisocytosis, and nucleated erythrocytes.
4. Interpret results of the erythrocyte sedimentation rate (ESR) test.
5. Name the different types of leukocytes and their primary functions.
6. Calculate the absolute number of various types of leukocytes from the WBC count and differential.
7. Interpret alterations in the WBC count, differential, and CD_4 lymphocyte count in acute bacterial infections, parasitic infections, and human immunodeficiency virus (HIV) infection.
8. Identify potential causes of neutrophilia.

PHYSIOLOGY OF BLOOD CELLS AND BONE MARROW

The cellular components of blood are derived from pluripotential stem cells located in the bone marrow (Figure 15-1). Bone marrow is a highly structured and metabolically active organ of both hematopoietic and reticuloendothelial systems. It normally produces 2.5 billion RBCs, 1 billion granulocytes, and 2.5 billion platelets/kg of body weight daily.[1] Production can vary greatly, from nearly zero to 5–10 times normal. Usually, however, levels of circulating cells remain in a relatively narrow range.[2]

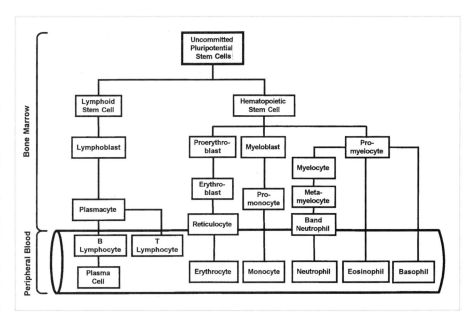

Figure 15-1. Schematic diagram of hematopoiesis.

In the fetus and children, blood cell formation or hematopoiesis occurs in the marrow of virtually all bones. With maturation, the task of hematopoiesis shifts to flat bones of the axial skeleton such as the cranium, ribs, pelvis, and vertebrae. The long bones, such as the femur and humerus, do not produce a large amount of blood cells in adulthood as the marrow is gradually replaced by fatty tissue. Radiation directed to large portions of hematopoietic bones can lead to deficient hematopoiesis in patients treated for cancerous lesions. Similarly, preparation for a bone marrow transplant will often include total body irradiation (TBI) to destroy the hematopoietic cells of the recipient in the bone, spleen, and other sites so that the grafted cells will not be destroyed by residual host defenses.

Although the majority of hematopoiesis occurs in the marrow, modern methods of identifying cellular characteristics have demonstrated that pluripotential cells—identified by a positive test for the surface marker CD34—also normally circulate in the blood. The number of circulating pluripotential stem cells can be greatly increased by treatment with small doses of alkylating chemotherapy agents (e.g., cyclophosphamide) or with stem cell stimulating drugs (e.g., recombinant granulocyte- or granulocyte-macrophage colony-stimulating factor [G-CSF or GM-CSF]).[3,4]

Although the majority of this chapter discusses laboratory analysis of blood obtained from the vein (peripheral venipuncture), an analysis of the bone marrow itself may be needed to diagnose or monitor various disease states, most commonly the leukemias discussed later in the chapter. Bone marrow sampling is usually made in the ileal crest of the pelvis or, less commonly because of increased risk, at the sternum. Bone marrow sampling can involve an aspirate, a core biopsy, or both. After penetrating the bone, a small aspiration is made to provide a cell count. A separate penetration is used for a biopsy using a special coring needle to cut a sample of the bone marrow matrix for removal and examination. The biopsy provides the advantage of examining the structure of the marrow stroma, as well as the spatial relationship of the various hematopoietic cells.[5]

In the bone marrow, stem cells become increasingly differentiated or specialized until they are committed to develop further into erythrocytes, platelets, or various leukocytes (Figure 15-1). Many regulatory proteins are involved in the maintenance of hematopoiesis, but their functions and interrelationships are not yet fully understood. In addition to the colony-stimulating factors mentioned above, proteins that stimulate hematopoiesis include erythropoietin, thrombopoietin, and various interleukins. Inhibitors of hematopoiesis are not as well-defined but include interferons and lymphotoxins. In considering differences in the peripherally measured response to exogenously administered hematopoietic stimulants, it is important to recall that their activity in vivo involves local production of a combination of signaling proteins in the hematopoietic clusters in the marrow, and that they are directed toward adjacent or closely approximated differentiating cells.[4]

Unipotential or committed stem cells undergo further differentiation in the bone marrow until they develop into mature cells. Many developmental stages along the way can be identified by differing morphological characteristics. Generally, only mature cellular forms are found in the circulating blood, and it is from this blood that clinical specimens are usually taken.

COMPLETE BLOOD COUNT

The complete blood count (CBC) is, perhaps, the most commonly ordered laboratory test. It supplies useful information regarding the concentration of the different cellular and noncellular elements of blood and applies to multiple disorders. CBC is a misnomer since concentrations, not counts, are measured and provided. Functionally, the CBC can be thought of as a complete blood analysis because a series of tests are performed. Moreover, information besides concentrations is reported.

Most clinical laboratories utilize an automated method to determine the CBC. Results are usually accurate, reproducible, and rapidly obtained. Numerous measured and calculated values are included in a CBC (Table 15-1). These results traditionally include

- Erythrocyte (RBC) count.
- Leukocyte (WBC) count.
- Hemoglobin (Hgb).
- Hematocrit (Hct).
- RBC indices [mean cell volume (MCV), mean cell Hgb (MCH), mean cell Hgb concentration (MCHC)], and RBC distribution width (RDW).
- Reticulocyte count.
- Platelet count and mean platelet volume (MPV).

When a "CBC with differential" is ordered, the various types of WBCs are also analyzed (White Blood Cell Count and Differential section). The reliability of the results can be doubtful if (1) the integrity of the specimen is questionable (inappropriate handling or stor-

TABLE 15-1

TEST NAME	REFERENCE RANGE[a]	SI UNITS	COMMENTS
RBC	Males 4.5–5.9 x 10^6 cells/µl Females 4.1–5.1 x 10^6 cells/µl	4.5–5.9 x 10^{12} cells/L 4.1–5.1 x 10^{12} cells/L	
Hemoglobin (Hgb)	Males 14–17.5 g/dL Females 12.3–15.3 g/dL	140–175 g/L 123–153 g/L	Amount of Hgb in given volume of whole blood; indication of oxygen-transport capacity of blood; elevated in hyperlipidemia
Hematocrit (Hct)	Males 42–50% for males Females 36–45% for females	0.42–0.51 0.36–0.45	Percentage volume of blood comprised of erythrocytes; usually approximately 3 times Hgb
RBC indices Mean cell volume (MCV)	80–96 fL/cell		Hct/RBC: increased in vitamin B_{12} and folate deficiency, cold agglutinins, reticulocytosis, hyperglycemia, and leukemic cells; decreased in iron deficiency
Mean cell Hgb (MCH)	27.5–33.2 pg/cell		Hgb/RBC: increased in vitamin B_{12} and folate deficiency, cold agglutinins, and hyperlipidemia; decreased in iron deficiency
Mean cell Hgb concentrations (MCHC)	33.4–35.5 g/dL	334–355 g/L	Hgb/Hct: amount of Hgb in terms of percentage volume of cell; increased in hyperlipidemia and cold agglutinins; decreased in iron deficiency
Reticulocyte count	0.5–2.5% of RBCs	0.005–0.025	Increased in acute blood loss and hemolysis; decreased in untreated iron, vitamin B_{12}, and folate deficiency
RBC distribution width (RDW)	11.5–14.5 %	0.115–0.145 %	Measure of variation in red cell volumes: the larger the percent, the greater the variation in size of red cells; increased in early iron deficiency anemia and mixed anemias
White blood cell (WBC) count	4.4–11.3 x 10^3 cells/µL	4.4–11.3 x 10^9 cells/L	Elevated by large numbers of giant platelets and platelet clumps; decreased with cold agglutinins
Platelet count	150,000–450,000/µL	150–450 x 10^9/L	Elevated in presence of red cell fragments and microcytic erythrocytes; decreased in presence of large numbers of giant platelets and platelet clumps
Mean platelet volume (MPV)	6.8–10.0 fL		

[a]Modified from References 8 and 9.

Table 15-1. Reference Ranges and Interpretive Comments on Common Hematological Tests (Typical CBC)

age), or (2) the specimen contains substances that interfere with the automated analysis. Grossly erroneous results are usually flagged for verification by another method. Manual microscopic review of the blood smear is used to resolve unusual automated results.[1]

Red Blood Cell Count

Normal adult range, males: $4.5–5.9 \times 10^6$ cells/μL or $4.5–5.9 \times 10^{12}$ cells/L;
females: $4.1–5.1 \times 10^6$ cells/μL or $4.1–5.1 \times 10^{12}$ cells/L

The red blood cell count (RBC) is the number of red corpuscles in a given amount of blood. The International Unit for reporting blood cells is for a one liter volume, but it is still common to see values reported in cells/microliter (μL), or less commonly in cells/cubic millimeter (mm^3). The count is now done by automated methods so that results are accurate, reproducible, and quickly derived. After puberty, females have slightly lower counts (and Hgb) than men, partly because of their menstrual blood loss and because of higher concentrations of androgen (an erythropoietic stimulant) in men. The RBC count in all anemias is by definition below the normal range. This decrease causes a proportionate decrease in Hct and Hgb.

Mature erythrocytes have a median lifespan of 120 days under normal conditions. They are removed from the circulation by macrophages in the spleen and other reticuloendothelial organs. The erythrocytes are tested for flexibility, size, and integrity in these organs as the cells pass through areas of osmotic, pH, or hypoxic stress.[6]

Variability in the size of red cells is termed *anisocytosis*, and any variation in the normal biconcave disc shape is termed *poikilocytosis*. Such abnormalities are seen with iron deficiency or periods of increased erythrocyte production and/or damage.[7]

White Blood Cell Count

Normal range: $4.4–11.3– \times 10^3$ cells/mm^3 or $4.4–11.3– \times 10^9$ cells/L

The white blood cell count (WBC) is an actual count of the number of leukocytes in a given amount of blood. Unlike RBCs, leukocytes have a nucleus and mature into several different forms. The various percentages of immature and mature WBCs, also called the WBC differential, are discussed later in this chapter.

Hemoglobin

Normal range, males: 14–17.5 g/dL or 140–175 g/L;

females: 12.3–15.3 g/dL or 123–153/L

The hemoglobin (Hgb) value is the amount of this metalloporphyrin-protein contained in a given volume (100 mL or 1 L) of whole blood. The Hgb concentration provides a direct indication of the oxygen-transport capacity of the blood. As a substance contained in RBCs, Hgb is proportionately low in patients with anemia.

Hematocrit

Normal range, males: 42–50% or 0.42–0.50;

females: 36–45% or 0.36–0.45

Hematocrit (Hct) is the percentage volume of blood that is composed of erythrocytes. It is also known as the packed cell volume. To manually perform the Hct test, a blood-filled capillary tube is centrifuged to settle the erythrocytes. Then, the percentage volume of the tube that is composed of erythrocytes is calculated.[5] The Hct is usually about 3 times the value of the Hgb, but disproportion can occur when cells are substantially abnormal in size or shape. Like Hgb, Hct is low in patients with anemia.

Red Blood Cell Indices

Because the following laboratory tests specifically assess red blood cell counts, they are called *RBC indices*. These indices are useful in the evaluation of anemias, polycythemia, and nutritional disorders. Essentially, they assess the size and Hgb content of the RBC. They are not measured but are calculated from Hgb, RBC count, and Hct using predetermined formulas.

Mean Cell Volume

Normal range: 80–96 fL/cell

The mean cell volume (MCV) is an estimate of the average volume of RBCs and is the most clinically useful of the RBC indices. It is calculated by dividing the hematocrit by the RBC count. Abnormally large cells have an increased MCV and are called *macrocytic*. Vitamin B_{12} and/or folate deficiency cause the formation of macrocytic erythrocytes and correspond to a true increase in MCV. In contrast, reticulocytosis—an increase in the number of reticulocytes in the peripheral blood—causes a false increase in MCV. Reticulocytes are larger than mature erythrocytes so an increase in circulating reticulocytes can lead to an increased MCV.[5]

Likewise, cold agglutinins that cause clumping (agglutination) of erythrocytes also cause false elevations when automated methods interpret these clumps to be individual cells. The MCV may also be falsely increased in hyperglycemia. When erythrocytes are mixed with diluting fluids to perform the test, the cells swell because the fluids are relatively hypotonic compared to the patient's blood.

Abnormally small cells (with a decreased MCV) are called *microcytic*. A decrease in the MCV implies some abnormality in Hgb synthesis. The most common cause of microcytosis is iron deficiency.[8]

Mean Cell Hemoglobin

Normal range: 27–33 pg/cell

Mean cell hemoglobin (MCH) is the amount of hemoglobin per RBC. It is calculated by dividing the Hgb by the RBC count. MCH can be falsely increased in patients with hyperlipidemia, but it can be truly increased in the presence of folate deficiency. As expected, MCH is decreased in iron deficiency when the iron is insufficient to manufacture the usual amount of Hgb in RBCs. A low MCH corresponds with hypochromic (pale) RBCs, as seen in iron deficiency anemia.

Mean Cell Hemoglobin Concentration

Normal range: 33.4–35.5 g/dL or 334–355 g/L

The mean cell hemoglobin concentration (MCHC) is the hemoglobin divided by the hematocrit. As mentioned previously, this calculation is usually around 33 g/dL (330 g/L) because the Hct is usually 3 times the Hgb. Iron deficiency is the only anemia in which the MCHC is *routinely* low, although it can also be decreased in other disorders of Hgb synthesis.[8,9] Like MCH, it can be falsely elevated in hyperlipidemia due to specimen turbidity. It must be considered that the Wintrobe indices are averages for the patient's blood, and that normal values may be reported by automated methods even in the presence of a mixed (normal + abnormal) erythrocyte population.

Red Blood Cell Distribution Width

Normal range: 11.5–14.5% or 0.115–0.145

The red blood cell distribution width (RDW) is an indication of the variation in red cell size, termed *anisocytosis*.[8] The RDW is reported as the coefficient of variation of the MCV (standard deviation/mean value). This value is used primarily with other tests to diagnose iron deficiency anemia from thalassemias. The RDW increases in early iron deficiency, often before other tests show signs of this kind of anemia. However, it is not specific for iron deficiency anemia.

Reticulocyte Count

Normal range: 0.5–2.5% of RBCs or 0.005–0.025

The reticulocyte is the cell form that precedes the mature RBC or erythrocyte. During the entire maturation process, hemoglobin (Hgb) is produced and incorporated into the cell. The reticulocyte does not contain a nucleus but possesses nucleic acids that can be considered remnants of the nucleus or endoplasmic reticulum. The mature erythrocyte contains neither an organized nucleus nor nucleic acids. Reticulocytes persist in the circulation for 1–2 days before maturing into erythrocytes.[2]

In anemia, the reticulocyte count or reticulocyte index (RI) reflects not only the level of bone marrow production but also a decline in the total number of mature erythrocytes that normally dilute the reticulocytes. Therefore, the reticulocyte count would double in a person whose bone marrow production is unchanged but whose Hct has fallen from 46 to 23%. A corrected reticulocyte count is one that has been adjusted to a normal Hct to eliminate the increase in count seen on the basis of changes in the dilution effect alone, as illustrated in the following equation[11]:

$$RI = \% \text{ Reticulocytes} \times \frac{\text{Actual Hct}}{\text{Normal Hct}}$$

In persons with anemia secondary to *acute* blood loss or hemolysis, even the corrected reticulocyte count is increased.[6] This increase reflects an attempt by the bone marrow to compensate for the lack of circulating erythrocytes. Because RBC production is increased to far above basal activity, more reticulocytes escape into the circulation earlier than normal. In contrast, persons with *untreated* anemia secondary to iron, folate, or vitamin B_{12} deficiency are unable to increase their reticulocyte count appropriate to the degree of their anemia.

The reticulocyte count can be useful in identifying drug-induced bone marrow suppression where the percentage of circulating reticulocytes should be close to zero. It can also be used to monitor an anemic patient's response to vitamin or iron therapy. In such patients, supplementation of the lacking factor causes rapid (5–7 days) elevation of the reticulocyte count.

ERYTHROCYTE SEDIMENTATION RATE

Normal range, males: 1–15 mm/hr; females: 1–20 mm/hr
(increases with age)

Numerous physiological and disease states are associated with the rate at which erythrocytes settle from blood, termed the *erythrocyte sedimentation rate* (ESR). Erythrocytes normally settle slowly in plasma but settle rapidly when they aggregate because of electrostatic forces. Each cell normally has a net negative charge and repels other erythrocytes because like charges repel each other. Many plasma proteins are positively charged and are attracted to the surface charge of one or more erythrocytes, thereby promoting erythrocyte aggregation.[12] Anemia, pregnancy, multiple myeloma, and various inflammatory diseases (including infections) can elevate the ESR (Table 15-2). Sickle cell disease, high doses of cor-

INCREASED ESR	DECREASED ESR
Advanced age	Congestive heart failure
Female sex	Corticosteroids
Infection	Microcytic anemia
Macrocytic anemia	Sickle cell anemia
Normocytic anemia	
Pregnancy	
Rheumatoid arthritis	

TABLE 15-2

Table 15-2. Conditions that may alter ESR

ticosteroids, liver disease, microcytosis, carcinomas, and congestive heart failure can also decrease the ESR.[8]

Although the ESR may be used to confirm a diagnosis supported by other tests, it is rarely used alone for a specific diagnosis. Rather, the ESR is useful for monitoring the activity of inflammatory conditions (e.g., temporal arteritis, polymyalgia rheumatica, rheumatoid arthritis, and osteomyelitis).[12] The ESR is often higher when the disease is active and falls when the intensity of the disease decreases.

The ESR is usually measured using either the Wintrobe or the Westergren method. Anticoagulated blood is diluted and placed in a glass tube of standard size. After 1 hr, the distance from the meniscus to the top of the erythrocyte column is recorded as the ESR in millimeters per hour.[12] A corrected sedimentation rate, called the *zeta-sedimentation rate* or *ratio*, has been developed to eliminate the effect of anemia on the ESR.[13] The patient's blood is spun in a special centrifuge, and the level of erythrocytes in the centrifuged tube is recorded as if it were the Hct. This value is called the *zetacrit*, and its normal range is 40–52%. It is linearly related to increases in the fibrinogen concentration.[8] Elevations above the normal range are interpreted in the same manner as an elevated ESR by traditional methods.

Platelet Count and Mean Platelet Volume

Normal ranges: 150,000–450,000/μL

The platelet count, often included routinely in the CBC with differential, is discussed with other coagulation tests in Chapter 16.

LABORATORY ASSESSMENT OF ANEMIA

The functions of the erythrocyte are to transport and protect Hgb, the molecule used for oxygen and carbon dioxide transport. Anemia can be defined as a decrease in either the RBC count or the Hgb concentration below the normal range for age and sex. Anemia is not a disease in itself but one manifestation of an underlying disease process. Appropriate treatment of the anemic patient depends on the exact cause of the condition. Signs and symptoms of anemia depend on its severity and the rapidity with which it has developed. Severe, acute blood loss results in more dramatic symptoms than an anemia that took months to develop because there may not have been time for adequate compensatory adjustments. Patients with mild anemia are often asymptomatic (i.e., absence of pallor, weakness, and fatigue), but severely symptomatic patients manifest shortness of breath, tachycardia, and palpitations even at rest. This contrast should be kept in mind when interpreting test results.

Anemia can be caused by decreased production and/or increased destruction of erythrocytes as well as acute blood loss. Use of erythrocyte morphology is one common method to "narrow down" the possible etiology of anemia. This method is useful because different causes of anemia lead to different erythrocyte morphology. Figure 15-2 outlines this approach. Only a few common causes of anemia are included, but others can be fit into this outline. Other laboratory tests that are useful in differentiating the anemias are listed in their appropriate locations. Usual laboratory findings are also included in each section (Table 15-3).

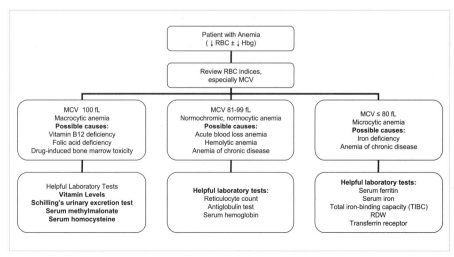

Figure 15-2. Use of erythrocyte morphology in differential diagnosis of anemia.

TABLE 15-3

	VITAMIN B₁₂ DEFICIENCY	FOLATE DEFICIENCY	IRON DEFICIENCY	ACUTE BLOOD LOSS	HEMOLYTIC ANEMIA	ANEMIA OF CHRONIC DISEASE
RBC	⇓	⇓	⇓	⇓	⇓	⇓
Hgb	⇓	⇓	⇓	⇓	⇓	⇓
Hct	⇓	⇓	⇓	⇓	⇓	⇓
MCV	⇑	⇑	⇓			⇓⇓
MCH	⇑	⇑	⇓			⇓⇓
MCHC	⇔	⇔	⇔		⇓⇓	
RDW			⇑		⇑	⇔
Reticulocyte count	⇓	⇓		⇑	⇑	⇓ ⇔
Serum vitamin B₁₂	⇓	⇔				
Serum folate	⇔	⇓				
Serum methylmalonate	⇑	⇔				
Serum homocysteine	⇑	⇑				
Ferritin			⇓			⇔
Serum iron			⇓			⇓
TIBC			⇑			⇓
Serum haptoglobin					⇓	
Plasma hemoglobin					⇑	
Autoantibodies					+	

* Some tests with no change (⇔) are left empty for clarity.
+ Autoantibodies positive for antibody-mediated immune hemolysis.

Table 15-3. Qualitative Laboratory Findings for Various Types of Anemia

Macrocytic Anemia

Macrocytic anemia is a lowered hemoglobin value associated with abnormally enlarged erythrocytes. The two most common causes are vitamin B₁₂ and/or folic acid deficiencies. Drugs that cause macrocytic anemia mainly interfere with proper utilization, absorption, and metabolism of these vitamins (Table 15-4).

Vitamin B₁₂ Deficiency

Vitamin B_{12} is also known as cobalamin. The normal daily requirement of vitamin B_{12} is 2–5 μg.[14] It is stored primarily in the liver, which contains approximately 1 μg of vitamin/g of liver tissue. Overall, the body has B_{12} stores of approximately 2–5 mg. Therefore, if vitamin B_{12} absorption suddenly ceased in a patient with normal liver stores, several years would pass before any abnormalities occurred due to vitamin deficiency.

The absorption of vitamin B_{12} is complex, and the mechanisms responsible are still being defined. Cobalamin (vitamin B_{12}) is ingested in meats, eggs, and dairy products. Strict vegans, who avoid all such foods in their diet, may over time develop vitamin B_{12} deficiency if supplements are not ingested. Some forms of B_{12}, such as those made by the blue-green algae *Spirulina*, are active vitamins in bacterial assays but are not active vitamins for humans. Other cobamides structurally related to cobalamin are found in plasma after ingesting other animal and plant-based foods. Only the cobamide with an attached 5,6-dimethylbenzimidazole group is correctly termed *cobalamin* and is active in humans.[14]

Dietary B_{12} or cobalamin is usually bound nonspecifically to proteins, and gastric acid and pepsin are required to hydrolyze the vitamin from the protein. Aging patients with decreasing stomach acid production may be less able to free vitamin B_{12} from meat protein. Freed B_{12} is bound with very high affinity to protein R, which is a large protein secreted in saliva. The cobalamin-protein R complex moves to the duodenum where proteases denature protein R and allow the freed vitamin to bind to intrinsic factor, which is secreted in the stomach and is resistant to the intestinal proteases. Patients may develop autoantibodies to intrinsic factor, and, thereby, develop vitamin B_{12} deficiency. The cobalamin-intrinsic factor complex is transported into the ileal epithelium, dissociates, and the cobalamin enters the circulation on the basolateral side of the cell bound to transcobalamin, which is largely homologous with intrinsic factor. Clearly, there are several steps in the absorption of Vitamin B_{12} that may be responsible for a deficiency.

Clinical and laboratory diagnosis. Vitamin B_{12} is necessary for deoxyribonucleic acid (DNA) synthesis in all cells, for the synthesis of neurotransmitters, and for metabolism of homocysteine. B_{12} deficiency, therefore, leads to symptoms involving many organ systems.[14,15] The most notable symptoms involve

- Gastrointestinal (GI) tract (e.g., loss of appetite, smooth and/or sore tongue, and diarrhea or constipation).
- Central nervous system (CNS) (e.g., paresthesias in fingers and toes, loss of coordination of legs and feet, tremors, irritability, somnolence, and abnormalities of taste and smell).
- Hematopoietic system (anemia).

A maturation arrest occurs in the immature cells in the bone marrow. The morphological result is that larger cells are produced, and they have characteristics specific to this maturation arrest. The anemia that results is called a *macrocytic, megaloblastic* (both morphological characteristics of maturation arrest) *anemia*.[15] Visual inspection of smears of both peripheral blood and bone marrow reveals characteristic megaloblastic changes in the appearance of erythrocytes and WBCs. The development of neutrophils is also affected, resulting in macrocytic cells with hypersegmentation (>3 nuclear lobes). A mild pancytopenia—decreased numbers of all blood elements—also occurs. The usual laboratory test results found with vitamin B_{12} deficiency are listed in Table 15-3.

Serum cobalamin concentrations were in the past measured using a microbiologic assay and a cobalamin-dependent organism. The assay has largely been replaced by a competitive displacement assay using radioactive cobalamin and intrinsic factor. Unfortunately, because of cross-reactivity with other cobamides, approximately 5% of patients will have cobalamin concentrations that appear to be within the normal range yet can be shown to have hematologic and/or neurologic signs of deficiency. There is increasing acceptance of the use of serum homocysteine and methylmalonate as more sensitive indicators of cobalamin deficiency. In the presence of inadequate cobalamin, these two compounds accumulate because of the cobalamin-dependence of their metabolizing enzymes, methionine synthase, and

TABLE 15-4

Marrow toxicity and interference with folate metabolism
Alcohol

Marrow Toxicity
Antineoplastic Agents
Zidovudine

Altered Folate Absorption
Phenytoin

Altered Folate Metabolism
Primidone, Phenobarbital
Methotrexate
Oral contraceptives
Pentamidine
Sulfasalazine
Sulfamethoxazole
Triamterene
Trimethoprim

Vitamin B_{12} Malabsorption
Colchicine
Neomycin
Para-aminosalicylic acid

Vitamin B_{12} Inactivation
Nitrous oxide

Table 15-4. Examples of Causes of Drug-Induced Macrocytic Anemia[20]

methylmalonyl-CoA-mutase, respectively. An elevated serum methylmalonate concentration in the presence of normal RBC folate and plasma homocysteine is strongly indicative of a pure deficiency of cobalamin.

A deficiency of cobalamin (vitamin B_{12}) raises the question of whether the patient has inadequate intake of the vitamin, or a deficiency of the intrinsic factor required for the effective ileal absorption of the vitamin. The Schilling test is used to determine if impaired absorption is the reason for the deficiency. Cyano-(^{57}Co)-cobalamin is administered orally and is allowed to be absorbed, if possible. An unlabelled, intravenous injection of cobalamin follows and will displace some radioactive ^{57}Co-cobalamin from transcobalamin and into the urine. If oral absorption is normal (e.g., the deficiency was caused by inadequate dietary intake), >8% of the radioactive cobalamin will be excreted in the urine. If abnormal, the test can be repeated at a later date (stage II test), adding exogenous intrinsic factor to the dose of oral labeled CN-(^{57}Co)-cobalamin to determine if inadequate urinary excretion secondary to poor absorption was due to a relative lack of the protein.[15]

If a deficiency of intrinsic factor is found to explain the poor absorption of cobalamin, oral doses of animal intrinsic factor can be administered with the vitamin. This is not favored, in part, because of erratic absorption but also because of the potential for sensitization to the animal protein. Intramuscular injections of vitamin B_{12} obviate the need for intrinsic factor and are favored in patients with impaired cobalamin absorption, regardless of the cause. For this reason, there is little rationale to perform the second stage of the Schilling test with intrinsic factor.[15]

Inadequate dietary intake is a rare cause of vitamin B_{12} deficiency, usually occurring only in vegans[14] who abstain from all animal food including milk and eggs. On the other hand, defective production of intrinsic factor is a common cause of the deficiency.[16] The gastric mucosa can fail to secrete intrinsic factor because of atrophy, especially in the elderly.

Pernicious anemia is a separate disease characterized by atrophic gastritis associated with antibodies against intrinsic factor and gastric parietal cells. It is not clear whether the gastritis results from or is caused by antibody formation. Gastrectomy, removal of all or part of the stomach, can also lead to vitamin B_{12} deficiency because the procedure removes the production site of intrinsic factor. Achlorhydria from gastrectomy or drugs can decrease the release of cobalamin from meat. Defective or deficient absorption of the intrinsic factor–vitamin B_{12} complex can be caused by inflammatory disease of the small bowel, ileal resection, and bacterial overgrowth in the small bowel.[17,18] Administration of colchicine, neomycin, and para-aminosalicylic acid can lead to impaired absorption of vitamin B_{12} (Table 15-4).

Folic Acid Deficiency

Normal range, serum folate: 5–25 µg/L; RBC folate: 166–640 µg/L

Folic acid is also called pteroylglutamic acid. Folates refer to folic acid or reduced forms of folic acid that may have variable numbers of glutamic acid residues attached to the folic acid molecule. The folates present in food are mainly in a polyglutamic acid form and must be hydrolyzed in the intestine to the monoglutamate form to be absorbed efficiently. The liver is the chief storage site. Adult daily requirements are approximately 50 µg of folic acid, equivalent to about 400 µg of food folates. Folate stores are limited, and anemia arising from a folate-deficient diet occurs in 4 to 5 months.[14]

Inadequate dietary intake is the major cause of deficiency. Folates are found in green, leafy vegetables such as spinach, lettuce, and broccoli. Inadequate intake can have numerous causes: alcoholics classically have poor nutritional intake of folic acid; certain physiological states such as pregnancy require an increase in folic acid; malabsorption syndromes (mentioned in the section on vitamin B_{12}) can also lead to defective absorption of folic acid; and celiac sprue can lead to folate malabsorption.[17]

Certain medications (e.g., methotrexate, trimethoprim-sulfamethoxazole, and triamterene) can act as folic acid antagonists by interfering with the conversion of folic acid into its metabolically active form, tetrahydrofolic acid. Phenytoin and phenobarbital administration can interfere with the intestinal absorption or utilization of folic acid (see Table 15-4).[19]

Folic acid is required as the intermediate for one-carbon transfers in several biochemical pathways. After absorption, folate is reduced to tetrahydrofolate, and a carbon in one of several oxidation states is attached for transfer. Most transfer processes allow facile regeneration. However, the formation of methyltetrahydrofolate requires vitamin B_{12} as a cofactor for the methyl group transfer. Methyltetrahydrofolate is required for the conversion of homocysteine to methionine, which is subsequently used as a methyl donor in many synthetic pathways that include the production of critical neurotransmitters and amino acids.

MINICASE 1

FREDERICK M., A 41-YEAR-OLD MALE ALCOHOLIC, was admitted to the hospital because of pneumonia. His physical exam revealed an emaciated patient with ascites, dyspnea, fever, cough, and weakness. No cyanosis, jaundice, or peripheral edema was evident. His peripheral neurologic exam was within normal limits as were his serum electrolytes, urea nitrogen, creatinine, and glucose. The following CBC was obtained:

TEST NAME	RESULT	REFERENCE RANGE
RBC	3.1×10^6 cells/µL	$4.1–5.1 \times 10^6$ cells/µL for females
WBC	4.6×10^3 cells/µL	$4.4–11.3 \times 10^3$ cells/µL
Hgb	12.3 g/dL	12.3–15.3 g/dL for females
Hct	33.9 %	36–45% for females
MCV	110.8 fL/cell	80–96 fL/cell
MCH	40.2 pg/cell	27–33 pg/cell
RDW	15.4%	11.5–14.5%
Platelet count	174,000/µL	150,000–450,000/µL
Neutrophils	68%	45–73%
Bands	6%	3–5%
Monocytes	11%	2–8%
Eosinophils	2%	0–4%
Basophils	2%	0–1%

Question: What abnormalities are present? What is the likely cause?

Discussion: The most remarkable finding is the macrocytic anemia, evidenced by the low RBC, Hbg, and Hct, and the markedly increased MCV and MCH. These findings are typical of folic acid deficiency, a common finding in alcoholics.

Clinical and laboratory diagnosis. Since folic acid is necessary for DNA synthesis, a deficiency causes a maturation arrest in the bone marrow similar to that caused by vitamin B_{12} deficiency. Folic acid deficiency is also characterized by a macrocytic, megaloblastic anemia.[20] However, with folic acid deficiency, pancytopenia does not develop as consistently as it does with vitamin B_{12} deficiency.

Folate concentrations in both serum and in erythrocytes (RBCs) are used to assess folate homeostasis. A low serum folate indicates negative folate balance and can be expected to lead to folate deficiency when hepatic folate stores are depleted. Folate deficiency is indicated if both the serum and RBC folate concentrations are low.

Folate supplementation in patients with a folate deficiency will provide folate for the nonmethyl transfer steps that do not require vitamin B_{12}. These processes include RNA and DNA synthesis and can often, at least partially, reverse megaloblastic anemia. However, without adequate vitamin B_{12}, the lack of methionine synthesis will lead to potentially serious and irreversible neurological damage. It is not yet clear whether this damage is due to a deficiency in the methionine-dependent neurotransmitters and amino acids or to accumulation of homocysteine. Regardless, although folate deficiency is more common and easily treated, it is critical to correctly identify the cause of a megaloblastic anemia so that any vitamin B_{12} deficiency is appropriately treated.

Microcytic Anemia

Causes

Microcytic anemia is associated with abnormally small erythrocytes. Iron deficiency is the primary cause of microcytic anemia, but a decreased MCV is a late indicator of the deficiency (Figure 15-2). Daily requirements are approximately 1 mg of elemental iron for each 1 mL of RBCs produced, so daily requirements are approximately 20–25 mg for erythropoeisis.[21] Most iron needed within the body is obtained by recycling of metabolized hemoglobin. RBCs have a lifespan of approximately 120 days. When old or damaged erythrocytes are taken up by macrophages in the liver, spleen, and bone marrow, the hemoglobin molecule is broken down and iron is extracted and stored with proteins. Only about 5% of the daily requirement (1 mg) is newly absorbed to compensate for losses due to fecal and urinary excretion, sweat, and desquamated skin.

Menstruating women require more iron because of increased losses. Iron requirements vary among women, but 2 mg/day is probably an average. Orally ingested iron is absorbed in the GI tract, which should permit just enough to prevent excess or deficiency. Typically, 5–10% of oral intake is absorbed (normal daily dietary intake: 10–20 mg).[21]

Iron deficiency is usually due to inadequate dietary intake and/or increased iron requirements. Poor dietary intake, especially in situations that require increased iron (e.g., pregnancy), is a common cause. Other causes of iron deficiency include

- Blood loss due to excessive menstrual discharge.
- Peptic ulcer disease.
- Hiatal hernia.
- Gastrectomy.
- Gastritis due to the ingestion of alcohol, aspirin, and non-steroidal anti-inflammatory drugs (NSAIDs).
- Bacterial overgrowth of the small bowel.
- Inflammatory bowel disease.
- Occult bleeding from GI carcinoma.

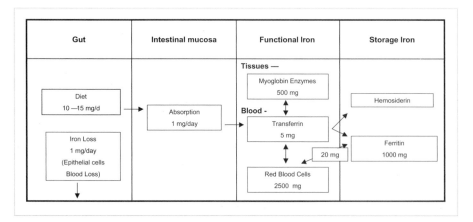

Figure 15-3. Intake, loss, and recycling of iron and iron storage forms.

Ionized, soluble iron is toxic because of its ability to mediate the formation

MINICASE 2

DONNA T. IS A 25-YEAR-OLD WOMAN seen in a community health clinic for a routine checkup. Her family history includes a sister with sickle cell disease. She has not been affected personally but has not been tested to determine her sickling genotype. She describes painful menstrual periods and takes aspirin for them. She also admits to a pica of ingesting cornstarch throughout the day. The following laboratory tests were done:

TEST NAME	RESULT	REFERENCE RANGE
RBC	3.3×10^6 cells/μL	$4.1–5.1 \times 10^6$ cells/μL for females
WBC	5.1×10^3 cells/μL	$4.4–11.3 \times 10^3$ cells/μL
Hgb	10.1 g/dL	12.3–15.3 g/dL for females
Hct	30%	36–45% for females
MCV	78 fL/cell	80–96 fL/cell
MCH	25 pg/cell	27–33 pg/cell
RDW	16.1%	11.5–14.5%
Platelet count	195,000/μL	150,000–450,000/μL
Neutrophils	52%	45–73%
Bands	3%	3–5%
Monocytes	2%	2–8%
Eosinophils	1%	0–4%
Basophils	0%	0–1%
Serum iron	54 μg/dL	50–150 μg/dL
TIBC	451 μg/dL	250–410 μg/dL
Transferrin saturation	14%	30–50%
Serum ferritin	5.2 μg/L	10–20 μg/L

Question: What hematologic abnormalities are apparent from these results?

Discussion: This patient demonstrates an anemia as manifested by the decreased hematocrit, hemoglobin, and RBC. Her WBC and platelet counts are normal. The MCV and MCH are both low, indicating a microcytic, hypochromic form of anemia most likely due to iron deficiency. This is corroborated by the iron studies, which indicate a low serum iron and transferrin saturation. Serum ferritin is also decreased, indicating that her iron stores are markedly reduced. The TIBC is increased both because of increased transferrin production and decreased iron available to bind to the protein.

Three may be multiple causes of Donna T.'s iron deficiency. Most commonly, the combination of low dietary iron and blood loss from menstruation increases the frequency of iron deficiency anemia in women. An additional possibility is occult blood loss from gastrointestinal ulcerations caused by the aspirin. An exacerbating factor for this woman is her starch pica, or craving for abnormal food. In addition to the high caloric intake associated with this particular pica, the starch decreases the bioavailability of ingested iron, decreasing the ability of the patient to absorb dietary or supplemental iron. Given the pica, she would likely best be treated with a parenteral iron product.

of oxidative species. Iron is, therefore, bound to proteins both in and outside of cells. The iron-protein complex within the macrophage is known as *ferritin* (Figure 15-3). In the normal adult, approximately 500–1500 mg is stored as ferritin and 2500 mg of iron is contained in Hgb.[21] When the total quantity of extracted iron exceeds the amount that can be stored as ferritin, the excess iron is stored in an insoluble form called *hemosiderin*.

While ferritin is primarily stored in macrophages, small amounts can be found in plasma and can be measured. Therefore, serum ferritin concentration reflects total body iron stores and is the most clinically useful method to evaluate patients for iron deficiency. Since the protein is an acute phase reactant, serum ferritin concentrations can be increased by chronic infections, fever, and inflammatory reactions.

The transport of iron in plasma and extracellular fluid occurs with two ferric ions bound to the protein transferrin, which when not binding iron is termed *apotransferrin*. Transferrin binds to specific membrane transferrin receptors where the complex enters the cell and releases the iron. Apotransferrin is released when the apotransferrin-receptor complex returns to the surface of the cell.

The tendency of ferritin to be falsely elevated with inflammatory processes has led to recent interest in using soluble transferrin receptor concentrations as an alternative marker of iron deficiency. The circulating receptor fragment is considered to reflect total body receptor expression and is elevated in times of increased erythropoiesis such as sickle cell anemia, thalassemias, and chronic hemolysis. If such causes of increased erythropoiesis can be excluded, elevated concentrations of circulating transferrin receptor are thought to reflect iron deficiency. The use of transferrin receptor concentrations may help determine if decreased ferritin concentrations are due to iron deficiency or to anemia of chronic (inflammatory) disease.

Clinical and laboratory diagnosis. The first change observed in the development of iron deficiency anemia is a loss of storage iron (hemosiderin). If the deficiency continues, a loss of plasma iron occurs. The decrease in plasma iron stimulates an increase in transferrin synthesis. When enough iron has been depleted that supplies for erythropoiesis are inadequate, anemia develops. The RBCs are smaller than usual (microcytic—low MCV) and not as heavily pigmented as normal RBCs (hypochromic—low MCH) because they contain less Hgb than normal erythrocytes. Clinically, patients present with progressively worsening weakness, fatigue, pallor, shortness of breath, tachycardia, and palpitations. Numbness, tingling, and glossitis may exist.[10] Laboratory results for iron deficiency anemia are listed in Table 15-3. With adequate iron therapy, the maximal daily rate of Hgb regeneration is 0.3 g/dL.

Serum ferritin (normal range: >10–20 ng/mL or >10–20 μg/L). Loss of storage iron (hemosiderin) was traditionally evaluated by a liver or bone marrow biopsy. Serum ferritin has largely replaced these invasive tests as an indirect measure of iron stores. Serum ferritin concentrations are markedly reduced in iron deficiency anemia (3–6 μg/L).

Serum iron (normal range: 50–150 μg/dL or 9–26.9 μmol/L) and total iron-binding capacity (TIBC) (normal range: 250–410 μg/dL or 45–73 μmol/L). The serum iron concentration measures iron bound to transferrin. This value represents about one-third of the TIBC of transferrin.[21] The TIBC measures the iron-binding capacity of transferrin protein. In iron deficiency anemia, TIBC is increased due to a compensatory increase in transferrin synthesis.[22] This increase leads to a corresponding decrease in the percent saturation that can be calculated. For example, a person with a serum iron concentration of 100 μg/dL and a TIBC of 300 μg/dL has a transferrin saturation of 33%. Iron deficient erythropoiesis exists whenever the percent saturation is 15% or less.

Other disease states besides iron deficiency that can alter serum iron and TIBC are infections, malignant tumors, and uremia.[9,10] Serum iron and TIBC both decrease in these disorders, unlike in iron deficiency anemia where serum iron decreases but TIBC increases. Anemia from these diseases is sometimes called *anemia of chronic disease*.

Normochromic, Normocytic Anemia

This classification encompasses numerous etiologies. Three causes are discussed: acute blood loss anemia, hemolytic anemia, and anemia of chronic disease.

Acute Blood Loss Anemia

Patients who suffer from acute hemorrhage can have a dramatic drop in their RBC count. In this situation, the Hct is not a reliable indicator of the extent of anemia. It is a measure of the concentration of Hgb, not the total body amount of Hgb. The RBC count can be mark-

MINICASE 3

BRIAN O., A 39-YEAR-OLD MALE with a long history of alcohol abuse, cirrhosis, and esophageal varices, was brought to the emergency department by concerned family members. The family said that he suddenly began coughing up bright red blood. As Brian O. was moved to a bed in the emergency department, he began coughing and vomiting large amounts of bright red blood. A stat CBC revealed the following:

TEST NAME	RESULT	REFERENCE RANGE
RBC	2.91×10^6 cells/µL	4.5–5.9×10^6 cells/µL for males
WBC	6.6×10^3 cells/µL	4.4–11.3×10^3 cells/µL
Hgb	8.9 g/dL	14–17.5 g/dL for males
Hct	29.6%	42–50% for males
MCV	92.4 fL/cell	80–96 fL/cell
MCH	30.6 pg/cell	27–33 pg/cell
RDW	14.1%	11.5–14.5%
Platelet count	80,000/µL	150,000–450,000/µL

Question: What does this CBC indicate?

Discussion: The presence of bright blood (as opposed to dark, "coffee ground" material) in the emesis indicates an acute bleed, either from a gastric ulcer or from esophageal varices. The CBC is consistent with acute blood loss. At the onset of bleeding, the RBC, Hgb, and Hct may show minimal changes. Here, the RBC, Hbg, and Hct are all markedly decreased, and the red cell indices are within normal limits, supporting a recent history of blood loss. The platelet count is also decreased, which may have led to the increasing blood loss. As could be anticipated from his history of alcohol abuse, the bleeding was found to arise from a ruptured esophageal varix.

---

edly reduced, while the Hct may be normal or even slightly increased. Usually, however, it is decreased. Hemorrhage evokes vasoconstriction, and it initially prevents extravascular fluid from replacing intravascular fluid loss.

In patients with normal bone marrow, the production of RBCs increases in response to hemorrhage, resulting in reticulocytosis. If the patient is transfused, each unit of packed RBCs administered should increase the Hgb by 1 g/dL if the bleeding has stopped. Table 15-3 shows the usual laboratory findings in acute blood loss anemia.

Hemolytic Anemia

Hemolysis is the lysis of erythrocytes. If hemolysis is rapid and extensive, severe anemias can develop, yet RBC indices remain unchanged. Patients with normal bone marrow respond with an increase in erythrocyte production to replace the lysed cells, and reticulocytosis is present. Specialized tests, called *antiglobulin tests*, can be useful in determining immune causes of hemolytic anemia.[22]

Plasma (free) Hgb measures the concentration of Hgb circulating in the plasma unattached to RBCs. It is almost always elevated in the presence of intravascular hemolysis. Haptoglobin, an acute-phase reactant, binds free Hgb and carries it to the reticuloendothelial system. In the presence of intravascular hemolysis, haptoglobin is decreased. Concomitant corticosteroid therapy may confound interpretation since many diseases associated with in vivo hemolysis are treated with steroids. Serum haptoglobin may be normal or elevated in hemolysis if the patient is receiving steroids. If the increase in serum haptoglobin is from steroids, other acute-phase reactants such as prealbumin will often be elevated. Serum haptoglobin is also elevated in patients with biliary obstruction and nephrotic syndrome. It is variably decreased in folate deficiency, sickle cell anemia, thalassemia, hypersplenism, liver disease, and estrogen therapy or pregnancy.[8]

Immune hemolytic anemias are caused by the binding of antibodies and/or complement components to the erythrocyte cell membrane with subsequent lysis. The method used to detect autoantibodies already bound to erythrocytes is a direct antiglobulin test (DAT), sometimes referred to as the direct Coombs' test. The method used to detect antibodies present in serum is an indirect antiglobulin test (IAT, indirect Coombs'). The DAT is performed by combining a patient's RBCs with rabbit or goat antihuman globulin serum, which contains antibodies against human immunoglobulins and complement.[22] If the patient's RBCs are coated with antibody or complement, the antibodies in the antiglobulin serum bind to the immunoglobulins coating the RBCs, leading to the agglutination of the RBCs. The DAT is the only test that provides definitive evidence of immune hemolysis.[23] The DAT can also be used to investigate possible blood transfusion reactions.[22]

The IAT detects antibodies in the patient's serum. Patient serum is combined with several types of normal erythrocytes of known antigenic expression. Any antibodies able to bind to the antigens expressed on these sample RBCs will adhere after the serum is washed away. Antihuman immune globulin is then added and will bind to any of the patient's immune globulin that is present on the erythrocytes, followed by agglutination.[22,23]

The antiglobulin tests are very sensitive, but a negative result does not eliminate the possibility of antibodies bound to erythrocytes. An estimated 100–150 molecules of antibody must be bound to each erythrocyte for detection by the antiglobulin test.[22] Smaller numbers of antibodies give a false-negative reaction.

Numerous conditions and medications can be associated with immune hemolytic anemia (Table 15-5). Medications can induce antibody formation by three mechanisms that result in a hemolytic anemia.

Autoimmune type. Methyldopa, an infrequently used antihypertensive drug, can induce the formation of antibodies directed specifically against normal RBC proteins. This autoimmune state can persist for up to 1 month after drug administration has been discontinued. This mechanism is known as a true autoimmune type of antibody formation and is detected using the direct antiglobulin test.[24]

Innocent bystander type. Antibodies to the drugs quinine and quinidine are examples of the immune complex (innocent bystander) mechanism.[19] Each drug forms a drug-protein complex with plasma proteins to which antibodies are formed. This drug–plasma protein–antibody complex attaches to erythrocytes and fixes complement, which leads to lysis of the RBCs.[22] In this situation, the RBC is an innocent bystander. Examples of drugs implicated in causing this type of hemolytic anemia are listed in Table 15-5.

Hapten type 1. The hapten (penicillin) type 1 mechanism is involved when a patient has produced antibodies to penicillin. If the patient receives high-dose penicillin at a future date, some penicillin can bind to the RBC membrane. The antipenicillin antibodies, in turn, bind to the penicillin bound to the RBC, and hemolysis can result.

G6PD Deficiency Anemia

Glucose-6-phosphate dehydrogenase (G6PD) is an intracellular enzyme that forms the NADPH needed by the erythrocyte to synthesize the antioxidant glutathione. Variants of this enzyme are more commonly found in African Black (Gd^{A-}) and Mediterranean/Asian

TABLE 15-5

Neoplasm
Chronic lymphocytic leukemia
Lymphoma
Multiple myeloma

Collagen Vascular Disease
Systemic lupus erythematosus
Rheumatoid arthritis

Medication
Auto-immune type
Levodopa, mefenamic acid, methyldopa, procainamide
Innocent bystander type
Cefotaxime, ceftazidime, ceftriaxone, chlorpromazine, doxepin, fluorouracil, isoniazid, quinidine, quinine, rifampin, sulfonamides, thiazides
Hapten type 1
Cephalosporins, penicillins

Infections
Mycoplasma
Viruses

Table 15-5. Causes of Immune Hemolytic Anemia

populations (Gd^Med) than in Caucasians. These variants have an impaired ability to resist the oxidizing effect of drugs and of collateral oxidative exposure to the granulocytic response to infections. Thus, exposure of patients with G6PD deficiency to oxidizing drugs or to an infection can lead to a dramatic, nonimmunologic hemolysis. Drug-induced hemolysis is less likely in the Gd ^A- variant, but both variants are susceptible to infection-induced hemolysis.[26] Assessment of at-risk patients for signs of hemolysis (anemia, hemoglobinemia, dark urine, and back pain) is appropriate. Future, routine genotyping of patients will aid in drug selection and monitoring of at-risk population.

Anemia of Chronic Disease

Mild to moderate anemia often accompanies numerous infections, inflammatory traumatic illnesses, or neoplastic diseases that last over 1–2 months.[27] Chronic infections include pulmonary abscesses, tuberculosis (TB), endocarditis, pelvic inflammatory disease, and osteomyelitis. Chronic inflammatory illnesses (e.g., rheumatoid arthritis and systemic lupus erythematosus) and hematological malignancies (e.g., Hodgkin's disease, leukemia, and multiple myeloma) are also associated with anemia. Because these disorders as a group are common, anemia due to chronic disease is also quite common. While anemia of chronic disease is more commonly associated with normocytic, normochromic anemia, it can also cause microcytic anemia. Table 15-3 shows the usual laboratory results found in anemia of chronic disease.

The pathogenesis of this anemia is not totally understood. Various investigations have found that the erythrocyte lifespan is shortened and that the bone marrow does not increase erythrocyte production to compensate for the decreased longevity. Iron utilization is also impaired. Although erythrocytes are frequently normal size, microcytosis can develop. One distinguishing feature between early iron deficiency anemia and a microcytic anemia of chronic disease is the normal serum ferritin that is present in the latter.[27]

Hemoglobinopathies

Several diseases arise from abnormal synthesis of the α or β subunits of hemoglobin. The most common types of anemias related to these hemoglobinopathies include *sickle cell trait/ disease* and *thalassemias*. Sickle cell trait is caused by the substitution of a valine amino acid for glutamate on the beta chain of hemoglobin. The heterozygous carrier state is thought to provide a resistance to clinical manifestations and sequelae of malaria. Homozygous persons with both beta-chains carrying the valine substitution are at increased risk of developing a sickling of erythrocytes. This occurs most commonly under circumstances of hypoxia, infection, dehydration, or acidosis. The hemoglobin molecules polymerize into a rod-like structure within the RBC, deforming the cell into a rigid, arched, sickled cell. These erythrocytes are not able to deform and pass through the capillaries or reticuloendothelial system. Hypoxia, ischemia, and even infarction occur in tissues downstream of these sites of impaired erythrocyte flow. Severe pain is usually present during these "sickle crises," and opiate analgesics are often needed in addition to hydration and other treatments. Diagnosis is made by inspection of the peripheral blood smear and by electrophoresis of the patient's hemoglobin.[28,29]

Thalassemias are a more diverse group of hemoglobinopathies most commonly associated with persons of ancestry arising in the Mediterranean region. Unlike the chemical change caused by the valine substitution in sickle cell patients, thalassemias are characterized by a deficiency or absence of one of the subunits of the hemoglobin. Since there are two alpha and two beta hemoglobin subunits in the normal hemoglobin tetramer, an inability to produce adequate amounts of one of the subunits would clearly lead to difficulty in synthesizing intact, complete hemoglobin molecules.[30]

Thalassemias are often diagnosed by a peripheral blood smear, which shows small, pale erythrocytes. Some of the RBCs are nucleated, reflecting the intense pressure on erythropoiesis in the bone marrow to provide oxygen carrying capacity to the body even if it requires releasing immature, nucleated erythrocyte precursors. The type of thalassemia present is determined using electrophoresis.

WHITE BLOOD CELL COUNT AND DIFFERENTIAL

White blood cells are divided into two general classifications:

1. Granulocytes or phagocytes (leukocytes that engulf and digest other cells).
2. Lymphocytes (leucocytes involved in the recognition of nonself cells or substances).

The functions of these general leukocyte classes are interrelated. For example, immunoglobulins produced by B lymphocytes are needed to coat or opsonize encapsulated bacteria so that neutrophils can more effectively identify, adhere, and engulf them for destruction.

When a WBC count and differential is ordered for a patient, the resulting laboratory report is a tally of the total WBCs in a given volume of blood plus the relative percentages each cell type contributes to the total. Therefore, the percentages of the WBC subtypes must add up to 100%. If one cell type increases, percentages of all other types must decrease proportionately. This decrease is not necessarily associated with any pathology. Table 15-6 is a general breakdown of the different types of WBCs and their usual percentages in peripheral blood.

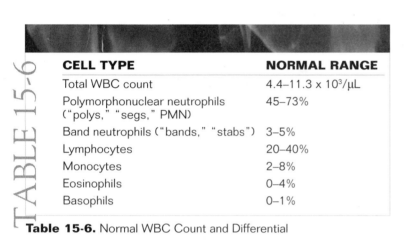

TABLE 15-6

CELL TYPE	NORMAL RANGE
Total WBC count	4.4–11.3 x 10³/µL
Polymorphonuclear neutrophils ("polys," "segs," PMN)	45–73%
Band neutrophils ("bands," "stabs")	3–5%
Lymphocytes	20–40%
Monocytes	2–8%
Eosinophils	0–4%
Basophils	0–1%

Table 15-6. Normal WBC Count and Differential

Absolute counts are sometimes calculated and compared with reference ranges. For example, the absolute segmented neutrophil count is the percentage of neutrophils and bands multiplied by the WBC count. The reference range for absolute counts can be estimated by multiplying the normal range of percentages for the particular type of WBC by the upper and lower limits of the total WBC count.

The WBC count and differential is one of the most widely performed clinical laboratory tests. In the past, differentials were determined by a manual count of a standard number of cells. In addition to being labor-intensive and slow, this method is imprecise and inaccurate when compared to automated methods.[31] Currently, clinical laboratories commonly use automated methods for determining the WBC differential. These instruments count thousands of cells and can report not only the relative percentages of the various WBC types but also the absolute numbers, RBC, platelets, and red cell indices. When reviewing a WBC differential, one must be aware of not only the relative percentages of cell types but also the absolute numbers. The percentages viewed in isolation can lead to incorrect conclusions. Minicase 4 demonstrates this principle.

False-negative results can occur. Lymphoma cells, atypical lymphocytes, and various types of immature granulocytes may not be detected in small numbers. Likewise, false-positive results can occur. However, positive results generally provoke a warning, requiring subsequent manual review of the blood smear.

Granulocytes

Granulocytes are phagocytes (eating cells) and derive their name from the presence of granules within the cytoplasm. The granules store lysozymes and other chemicals needed to oxidize and enzymatically destroy foreign cells. Granulocytic leukocytes include neutrophils,

MINICASE 4

DAVID D., A 46-YEAR-OLD MALE, presented to the emergency department with a temperature of 104 °F (40 °C), diarrhea, and abdominal pain. Urine and blood cultures were obtained, and he was given broad spectrum antibiotics. The following CBC was obtained:

TEST NAME	RESULT	REFERENCE RANGE
RBC	3.18×10^6 cells/µL	$4.5-5.9 \times 10^6$ cells/µL for males
WBC	118.9×10^3 cells/µL	$4.4-11.3 \times 10^3$ cells/µL
Hgb	9.9 g/dL	14–17.5 g/dL for males
Hct	29.5%	42–50% for males
MCV	92.8 fL/cell	80–96 fL/cell
MCH	30 pg/cell	27–33 pg/cell
RDW	14.1%	11.5–14.5%
Platelet count	69,000/µL	150,000–450,000/µL
Neutrophils	21%	45–73%
Bands	12%	3–5%
Metamyelocytes	5%	0%
Myelocytes	5%	0%
Promyelocytes	8%	0%
Lymphocytes	6%	20–40
Atypical lymphocytes	0%	0%
Monocytes	2%	2–8%
Eosinophils	1%	0–4%
Basophils	10%	0–1%
Blasts	30%	0%

Question: What does his CBC reveal?

Discussion: This CBC is grossly abnormal, showing marked leukocytosis with elevations in the absolute neutrophil and lymphocyte counts. Note that the percentages of these cells are markedly decreased, but a neutrophilia is revealed when the absolute numbers are calculated (e.g., $118.9 \times 10^3 \times 21\%$ = 25,000 cells/µL; normal range 2200–8000/µL). Bands are also neutrophilic leukocytes and may be included in the absolute neutrophil count at some sites. He has a normochromic, normocytic anemia and thrombocytopenia.

At first, one might expect that David D.'s condition could be consistent with an overwhelming infection. However, he has a marked number of immature WBC forms in the peripheral blood—metamyelocytes, myelocytes, promyelocytes, and blasts. These forms are normally found only in the bone marrow and not in circulation.

A bone marrow biopsy reveals that he has chronic myelogenous leukemia with a blast (myeloblast) crisis. The anemia is likely myelophthistic, which occurs in part by the "crowding out" of red cell precursors by the neoplastic and immature WBC cells in the bone marrow. This is also likely the cause of his normochromic, normocytic anemia.

eosinophils, basophils, and monocytes. Monocytes mature into macrophages, which are predominantly found in tissue rather than in the circulation. When a peripheral smear of blood is prepared, three types of granulocytes are named by the staining characteristics of their cytoplasmic granules[8]:

1. Neutrophils retain neutral stains and appear light tan.
2. Eosinophils retain acidic dyes and appear red-orange.
3. Basophils retain basic dyes and appear dark blue to purple.

Granulocytes are formed in large numbers from the pluripotential stem cells in the bone marrow. They undergo numerous differentiation and proliferation steps in the marrow and are usually released into the peripheral blood in their mature form. A common exception is the appearance of band cells during an infection, as discussed below. Neutrophils, eosinophils, and basophils die in the course of destroying ingested organisms or particles, yielding pus. On the other hand, monocytes and macrophages do not usually need to sacrifice themselves when destroying target cells.

Neutrophils

Normal range, PMN leukocytes: 45–73%; bands: 3–5%

Neutrophils are also termed segmented neutrophils (or "segs") or polymorphonuclear cells (PMNs or "polys"). The less-mature form of the neutrophil with a crescent-shaped nucleus is a band or stab cell. Bands derive their name from the morphology of their nucleus, which has not yet segmented into multiple lobes. Less mature forms of the neutrophil, such as the metamyelocyte and myelocyte, are normally not in the peripheral blood. The neutrophil is a phagocytic cell that exists to ingest and digest foreign proteins (e.g., bacteria and fungi).

Under normal conditions, about 90% of the neutrophils are stored in the bone marrow. When released, neutrophils will still predominantly marginate or adhere and roll along the endothelium. Infections, glucocorticosteroids, epinephrine, or intense exercise can all cause a demargination of neutrophils and other marginating granulocytes. This dynamic process of margination and demargination causes large shifts in the measured neutrophil count, since only the granulocytes that are circulating at the time are measured by a venipuncture. Neutrophils spend only about 6–8 hr in circulation after which they move through the endothelium into the tissue. Unless used to engage a foreign body or sustained by the cytokine milieu, neutrophils then undergo programmed cell-death, a noninflammatory process termed *apoptosis*.[32]

During an acute infection there is an increase in the percentage of neutrophils as they are released from the bone marrow and demarginate from the endothelium.[33,34] Less mature band forms may also be released, but these immature neutrophils are still considered to be active. The appearance of band cells in infections is termed a *left shift*. This may be due to the traditional order in which the differential was reported. It may also arise from the use of a left-to-right sequence in figures describing the process of neutrophil differentiation from the stem cell (see Figure 15-1).

When the neutrophils and/or bands are elevated, the percentage of lymphocytes usually decreases proportionately. Only 10–15% lymphocytes may appear in these patients, but the *lymphopenia* is not necessarily real because of a concomitant increase in total WBCs. An exception is a neutrophilia caused by glucocorticoid treatment, which will cause a drop in the absolute lymphocyte count because of its lymphotoxic effect while increasing the absolute neutrophil count due to demargination.

Eosinophils and Basophils

Normal range, eosinophils: 0–4%; basophils: 0–1%

The functions of eosinophils and basophils are not completely known. Eosinophils are present in large numbers in the intestinal mucosa and lungs, two locations where foreign proteins enter the body.[11] Eosinophils can phagocytize, kill, and digest bacteria and yeast. Elevations of eosinophils counts are highly suggestive of parasitic infections.

Basophils are present in small numbers in the peripheral blood and are the most long-lasting granulocyte in blood with a circulating lifespan of approximately 2 weeks.[2] They contain heparin, histamine, and leukotriene B_4.[35,36] Many signs and symptoms of allergic responses can be attributed to specific mast cell and basophil products.[35] Basophils are probably involved in immediate hypersensitivity reactions (e.g., extrinsic, or allergic, and asthma) in addition to delayed hypersensitivity reactions. Basophils may be increased in chronic inflammation and leukemia.

Monocytes/Macrophages

Normal range, monocytes: 2–8%

Monocytes leave the circulation in 16–36 hr and enter the tissues where they mature into macrophages. Macrophages are present in lymph nodes, alveoli of the lungs, spleen, liver, and bone marrow.[37] These tissue macrophages participate in the removal of foreign substances from the body. In addition to attacking foreign cells, they are involved in the destruction of old erythrocytes, denatured plasma proteins, and plasma lipids. Tissue macrophages also salvage iron from the hemoglobin of old erythrocytes and return the iron to transferrin for delivery to the bone marrow. Under appropriate stimuli, monocytes/macrophages are transformed into antigen-presenting cells (APC, also termed *dendritic cells*). These transformed macrophages are an important component of both cell-mediated (T lymphocytes) and soluble (B lymphocyte) immune activity against antigens.[37]

Lymphocytes and Plasma Cells

Normal range, lymphocytes: 20–40%

Lymphocytes make up the second major group of leukocytes. They are characterized by a far less granular cytoplasm and relatively large, smooth nuclei. These cells give specificity and memory to the body's defense against foreign invaders.[38] The three subgroups of lymphocytes are

1. T lymphocytes (T cells).
2. B lymphocytes (B cells).
3. Natural killer cells (NK cells)

Lymphocytes are not phagocytic, but the NK and T cell subtypes are cytotoxic by virtue of complement activation and antibody-dependent cellular cytotoxicity (ADCC). Morphologic differentiation of lymphocytes is difficult; visual inspection of a blood smear cannot uniformly distinguish between T, B, and NK cells. Fortunately, lymphocytes can be distinguished by the presence of lineage-specific membrane markers, historically termed *clusters of differentiation* (CD). Thus, mature T cells are CD4 or CD8, B cells have CD20, and NK cells have CD56 membrane markers.[36,39] In fact, the individual CD moieties may be surface proteins, enzymes, or adhesion molecules, to name a few. Labeled antibodies to specific CD molecules will identify the lineage of the lymphocyte, either in blood or in tissue.

Identification of the subtype of lymphocytes is not a routine clinical hematology test at present; they are reported simply as lymphocytes by automated counting instruments. However, in research applications and for the diagnosis of leukemias and lymphomas, subtypes can both be counted and sorted by an automated process termed *fluorescence-activated cell sorting* (FACS). The white cell layer is separated by centrifugation and exposed to one or more CD-antibodies that contain fluorescent dyes. The labeled cells are given an electrostatic charge and flow individually by a laser that induces the labeled cells to glow. These fluorescing cells are counted and can be sorted as they fall past the detector into collection vessels by using electrostatic charges to push or pull the charged cell in the desired direction. This method is very general and can be used to count and sort virtually any cell that can be labeled with a fluorescent tag.[40]

With the help of T cells, B cells recognize foreign substances and are transformed into plasma cells, capable of producing antibodies (discussed later). Table 15-6 lists the types of disorders in which lymphocytes are increased or decreased.

T Lymphocytes

T lymphocytes are responsible for cell-mediated immunity and are the predominant lymphocytes in circulation and in tissue. They require partial maturation in the embryonic thymus, hence the name T cell. In addition to identifying infections, they oversee delayed hypersensitivity (seen with skin tests for TB, mumps, and *Candida*) and rejection of transplanted organs.[36] In order for a foreign antigen to be recognized by T cells, it must be "presented" by macrophages or dendritic cells on one of two complex, individualized molecules termed *major histocompatibility complexes* (MHC1 and MHC2).

T cells can be further divided into helper and cytotoxic (or suppressor) cells, which, respectively, express the CD4 and CD8 markers. CD4 helper cells are not cytotoxic, but on recognizing an antigen will activate and produce cytokines such as IL-2 that stimulate nearby immune cells such as macrophages and CD8 T cells, B cells, and NK cells.

CD4 T-helper cells can again be divided into T_{H1} and T_{H2} subtypes. The T_{H1} subtype mediates the activation of macrophages and the delayed hypersensitivity response, while the T_{H2} subtype appears primarily responsible for B cell activation. The cellular specificity of these subtypes appears to arise primarily from their distinct pattern of cytokine production.

The HIV virus binds specifically to the CD4 receptor but does not elicit the desired antiviral response in most patients. This infection leads to destruction of this subset of T cells and an imbalance of the remaining T cells. The CD4 lymphocyte count and viral burden measured by viral RNA are inversely related and seem to correlate with overall prognosis. Although the CD4 count remains a useful surrogate marker in monitoring the course and treatment of HIV-infected patients, viral loads are also increasingly measured. The lack of adequate numbers of active T-helper cells that activate other immune cells leads to an increased susceptibility to numerous opportunistic infections and cancer, yielding a syndrome that is well-known as AIDS.[41,42] T cells are the primary mediator for host rejection of transplanted solid organs such as heart, lung, kidney, liver, and/or pancreas grafts. The peri- and postoperative treatment of solid organ graft recipients is directed toward minimizing the antigraft T cell response while not ablating the T cell population to the point of causing life-threatening infections. In practice, this is a narrow path plagued by viral and fungal infections that cause substantial morbidity and mortality in graft recipients.

Typically, T cell populations in graft recipients are not measured, and drug titration is based on biopsies of the transplanted organ, drug concentrations of the immunosuppressants, and blood counts. Anti-T-cell treatments employed in transplant recipients include corticosteroids; OKT3 antibody directed against the CD3 marker found on T cells; anti-human lymphocyte immunoglobulin; and inhibitors of T cell activation such as tacrolimus or mycophenolate. Since the immunoglobulins are typically obtained from nonhuman species, they can cause severe allergic reactions and are usually effective for only a short period.

B Lymphocytes and Plasma Cells

B cells are named after similar avian lymphocytes that required maturation in an organ termed the *Bursa of Fabricus*. There is no equivalent organ in humans, and maturation of B lymphocytes occurs in the bone marrow. Quiescent, circulating B cells express one form of antibody, immunoglobulin M. When stimulated by activated T cells or antigen-presenting cells (APC, or dendritic cells), B cells are transformed into plasma cells that will produce one of five immunoglobulin types: IgA, IgD, IgE, IgG, or IgM.[36]

The two antibodies most commonly associated with the development of immunity to foreign proteins, viruses, and bacteria are IgM and IgG. IgE is associated with the development of allergic phenomena. IgA is secreted into the lumen of the GI tract and helps avoid sensitization to foodstuffs, and IgD is bound to the lymphocyte cell membrane.[36]

Natural killer cells (NK) are derived from T cell lineage but are not as restricted in requiring MHC identification of the target cell. NK cells are thought to be particularly important for cytotoxic effects on virally-infected cells and cancer cells.

Lymphopenia and hypogammaglobulinemia (a decrease in the total quantity of immunoglobulin) are seen as a consequence of steroid treatment, transplant rejection prophylaxis, and anticancer treatment but can also be a consequence of the tumor itself. In general, lymphopenia is more common in chemotherapy regimens that include high doses of glucocorticosteroids. Glucocorticosteroids bind to the receptor of lymphocytes and are lymphotoxic, even to the point of initiating cellular apoptosis.[39] Interestingly, although HIV-1 virus infections lead to lymphopenia, other viral infections (e.g., infectious mononucleosis, hepatitis, mumps, varicella, rubella, herpes simplex, herpes zoster, and influenza) often increase the number of circulating lymphocytes (lymphocytosis).[43,44]

Leukocyte Disorders

Patients can suffer from three major classes of leukocyte disorders: functional, quantitative, and myeloproliferative. *Functional* disorders involve defects in recognition, metabolism, cytotoxic effects, signaling, and other related activities. Routine laboratory values are not intended to evaluate these abnormalities and will not be discussed further here.

Quantitative disorders involve too few or too many leucocytes. Possible causes are listed in Table 15-7. Neutropenia is usually considered to exist when the neutrophil count is less than 1500 or 1800 cells/μL.[45] When the neutrophil count is less than 500 cells/μL, normal defense mechanisms are greatly impaired and the patient is at increased risk of bacterial and fungal infections. A neutrophil count less than 100/μL is termed *agranulocytosis* or *absolute neutropenia*. This is usually encountered after chemotherapy is administered, especially following regimens intended to ablate the bone marrow in preparation for a stem cell transplant. An infection is probable if agranulocytosis is prolonged, so patients at risk are often given prophylactic antibiotics. When infections do occur in such patients, they can be very difficult to successfully treat—even with normally effective antibiotics—because the number and phagocytic activity of the neutrophils are impaired.

Agranulocytosis may be caused by aplastic anemias that reflect inadequate myelopoiesis. Aplastic anemias have multiple causes including drug, toxin, or radiation exposure, congenital defect, or age-related fatty or fibrotic displacement. The *anemia* in this term is misleading since production of one or all other blood cell types can also be affected. These myelodysplastic anemias are typically classified by the FAB RAEB system based on the marrow morphology identified from a marrow biopsy. The usual treatment course is a stem cell transplant in patients for whom this is feasible.[46]

Neutrophilia (increased neutrophils) is usually caused by a shift of marginated cells into the circulation. As mentioned earlier this shift, which can be caused by acute infections, trauma, or administration of epinephrine or corticosteroids, is reversible. Chronic neutrophilia may be due to sustained overproduction caused by chronic bacterial infections.[34] Iatrogenic neutrophilia will arise from excessive use of granulocyte (G-CSF) or granulocyte-macrophage (GM-CSF) colony-stimulating factor.

Myeloproliferative disorders involve an abnormal proliferation of bone marrow cells. Tumors of erythrocyte progenitors can be seen, leading to polycythemia vera. More commonly,

TABLE 15-7

WBC ABNORMALITY	TYPICAL THRESHOLD (CELLS/L)	POSSIBLE CAUSES
Neutrophilia	>12,000	Acute bacterial infection Trauma Myocardial infarction Chronic bacterial infection Epinephrine, lithium, G-CSF, GM-CSF, glucocorticosteroids

Neutropenia	<1500	Radiation exposure
		Medications:
		   Antineoplastic cytotoxic agents
		   Captopril
		   Cephalosporins
		   Chloramphenicol
		   Ganciclovir
		   Methimazole
		   Penicillins
		   Phenothiazines
		   Procainamide
		   Ticlopidine
		   Tricyclic antidepressants
		   Vancomycin
		   Zidovudine
		Overwhelming acute bacterial infection
		Vitamin B_{12} or folate deficiency
		Salmonellosis
		Pertussis

Eosinophilia	>350	Allergic disorders/asthma
		Parasitic infections
		Leukemia
		Medications
		   Angiotensin-converting enzyme inhibitors
		   Antibiotics (or any allergic reaction to a drug)

Eosinopenia	<50	Acute infection
Basophilia	>300	Chronic inflammation Leukemia
Monocytosis	>800	Recovery state of acute bacterial infection Tuberculosis (disseminated) Endocarditis Protozoal or rickettsial infection Leukemia
Lymphocytosis	>4000	Infectious mononucleosis Viral infections (e.g., rubella, varicella, mumps, cytomegalovirus) Pertussis Tuberculosis Syphilis Lymphoma
Lymphopenia	<1000	HIV Type 1 Radiation exposure Glucocorticosteroids Lymphoma (Hodgkin's disease) Aplastic anemia

Table 15-7. Quantitative Disorders of White Blood Cells[18–9,21–22]

neoplasms of the myeloproliferative stem cells occur that involve a leukocyte progenitor line. Leukemias are usually classified as myeloblastic (granulocytic lineage) or lymphoblastic (lymphocytic lineage).[47] The clinical courses and biology of various leukemias varies but can be characterized by the following categorization:

- Acute myelogenous (AML).
- Acute lymphocytic (ALL).
- Chronic myelogenous (CML).
- Chronic lymphocytic (CLL).
- Multiple myeloma (plasma cell).

Although the clinical course will vary among these neoplasms, a common denominator is the proliferation of the neoplastic line and displacement of normal myelopoiesis. The neoplastic cells may arise from stem cells of varying levels of differentiation, so morphologies and CD membrane markers will vary among individuals but be uniform for a given patient. The morphology and CD markers of cells obtained from the diagnostic bone marrow biopsy are used to assign an FAB classification of M1 through M7 to characterize the subtype of AML. Somewhat similar morphologic and surface marker methods are used to characterize the other leukemias.

Multiple myeloma is notable in that it is a plasma cell neoplasm. The monoclonal neoplastic plasma cells produce a single immunoglobulin. Other laboratory findings associated with multiple myeloma include Bence Jones proteins in urine, hypercalcemia, increased ESR, and findings consistent with normochromic, normocytic anemia, and coagulopathies.[48]

CML is characterized by a chromosomal translocation (t9:22, "Philadelphia chromosome") that creates a fusion product (BCR-ABL) resulting in an autonomous tyrosine kinase growth signaling enzyme. Some patients with no Philadelphia chromosome have been thought to have CML. However, new techniques suggest that the translocation is fundamental to the diagnosis of CML, and that in its absence these individuals are more likely to have some other myeloproliferative disorder.[49]

Patients with chronic leukemias may live for several years with minimal treatment because of the indolent nature of the disease. However, most will at some point develop a transformation of their disease into a life-threatening accelerated phase or blast crisis. Although the chronic leukemias are less aggressive than the acute leukemias, they are less curable with chemotherapy, and stem cell transplantation is sought when possible.

Lymphomas. A lymphoma is a neoplasm of a lymphocytic line predominating in the lymph nodes rather than the bone marrow. The cytology of the neoplasia maybe similar to that seen in CLL, and a malignant lymphoma with circulating lymphoblasts is often difficult to differentiate from CLL without the use of immunohistologic markers. Lymphomas are categorized somewhat simplistically as Hodgkin's lymphoma and non-Hodgkin's lymphoma (NHL). NHL has been further defined by the "Working Group Criteria" into several other categories that are based on the cellular size, morphology, and distribution/association within the cancerous lymph node.[50] Non-Hodgkin's lymphomas can also be practically divided into aggressive and indolent forms. The aggressive lymphomas grow and spread quickly but are generally more likely to be eradicated with current, intensive chemotherapy. In contrast, the slower-growing, indolent lymphomas are not as responsive and are more difficult to cure.

Lymphomas predictably involve T or B lymphocyte precursors, and many express CD markers characteristic of mature lymphocytes. Identification of the CD20 marker on B cell lymphomas provides an opportunity to treat these patients with recombinant antibodies specific to this surface marker.

The favorable response of patients with CD20+ lymphomas to target monoclonal antibody drugs such as rituximab can be considered a portent of the future of treating myeloproliferative diseases.[51] An increasing number of characteristic surface markers or genetic abnormalities such as the BCR-ABL fusion gene in CML are being identified and are the targets for innovative treatments. Although at present most leukemias and lymphomas are defined by morphology, it is not unrealistic to anticipate that they will be increasingly identified and treated based on their immunohistochemical and genetic pattern.

SUMMARY

This chapter has presented a brief characterization of the lineage and utility of red and white blood cells. Normal values have been presented, but it is important to realize that normal ranges will vary depending on the laboratory conducting the analysis and the population being studied.

In hematology, as in most medical sciences, it is important to consider the background and context of the tests used. For example, the RBC indices were characterized at a time when the iron-transporting proteins and vitamin needs of erythrogenesis were unknown. In most cases, abnormalities of the indices reflect a long-term inadequacy of iron, folate, or vitamin B_{12}. Biochemical markers such as circulating ferritin, transferrin receptors, folate, homocysteine, and methylmalonate are likely to take on an increasing importance in the early detection of such deficiencies.

Similarly, the definition of lineage specific markers (CD phenotypes) on leukocytes has revolutionized our ability to diagnose and treat leukemias. General diagnoses such as acute myelogenous leukemia (AML) will likely continue to be used, but increasingly specific characterization of the surface markers, biochemistry, and genetics of such cells will provide new opportunities to more effectively treat such diseases.

Novelties notwithstanding, the importance of understanding the fundamentals of clinical hematology cannot be discounted. Infections and chronic leukemias will continue to be diagnosed and monitored from an elevated WBC, and anemias will be caught and treated through routine blood examinations. Old and new technologies will continue to complement one another in clinical hematology.

REFERENCES

1. Gulati GL, Ashton JK, Hyun BH. Structure and function of the bone marrow and hematopoiesis. *Hematol Oncol Clin North Am.* 1988; 2:495–511.
2. Finch CA, Harker LA, Cook JD. Kinetics of the formed elements of the human blood. *Blood.* 1977; 50:699–707.
3. Kipps TJ. The cluster of differentiation antigens. In: Beutler E, Coller BS, Lichtman MA, et al, eds. *William's Hematology.* 6th ed. New York, NY: McGraw-Hill; 1999: 141–52.
4. Quesenberry PJ, Colvin GA. Hematopoietic stem cells, progenitor cells, and cytokines. In: Beutler E, Coller BS, Lichtman MA, et al, eds. *William's Hematology.* 6th ed. New York, NY: McGraw-Hill; 1999: 153–74.
5. Ryan DH. Examination of the marrow. In: Beutler E, Coller BS, Lichtman MA, et al, eds. *William's Hematology.* 6th ed. New York, NY: McGraw-Hill; 1999: 17–25.
6. Beutler E. Production and destruction of erythrocytes. In: Beutler E, Coller BS, Lichtman MA, et al, eds. *William's Hematology.* 6th ed. New York, NY: McGraw-Hill; 1999: 355–68.
7. Bull BS. Morphology of the erythron. In: Beutler E, Coller BS, Lichtman MA, et al, eds. *William's Hematology.* 6th ed. New York, NY: McGraw-Hill; 1999: 271–88.
8. Perkins SL. Examination of the blood and bone marrow. In: Lee GR, Foerster J, Lukens J, et al, eds. *Wintrobe's Clinical Hematology.* 10th ed. Baltimore, MD: Williams & Wilkins: 1999: 9–35.
9. Morris MW, Davey FR. Basic examination of the blood. In: Henry JB, ed. *Clinical Diagnosis and Management by Laboratory Methods.* 19th ed. Philadelphia, PA: W. B. Saunders; 1996: 549–94.
10. Massey AC. Microcytic anemia: differential diagnosis and management of iron deficiency anemia. *Med Clin North Am.* 1992; 76:549–66.
11. Gulati GL, Hyun BH. The automated CBC. A current perspective. *Hematol Oncol Clin North Am.* 1994; 8:593–603.
12. Sox HC, Liang MH. The erythrocyte sedimentation rate: guidelines for rational use. *Ann Intern Med.* 1986; 104:515–23.
13. Bull BS, Brailsford JD. The zeta sedimentation ratio. *Am J Clin Pathol.* 1972; 40:550–9.
14. Lee GR, Herbert V. Nutritional factors in the production and function of erythrocytes. In: Lee GR, Foerster J, Lukens J, et al, eds. *Wintrobe's Clinical Hematology.* 10th ed. Baltimore, MD: Williams & Wilkins: 1999: 840–51.

15. Babior BM. The megaloblastic anemias. In: Beutler E, Coller BS, Lichtman MA, et al, eds. *William's Hematology*. 6th ed. New York, NY: McGraw-Hill; 1999: 425–47.

16. Bunting RW, Bitzer AM, Kennedy RM, et al. Prevalence of intrinsic factor antibodies and vitamin B_{12} malabsorption in older patients admitted to a rehabilitation hospital. *J Am Geriatr Soc*. 1990; 38:743–7.

17. Phillips DL, Keeffe EB. Hematologic manifestations of gastrointestinal disease. *Hematol Oncol Clin North Am*. 1987; 1:207–28.

18. Ravel R. Clinical laboratory medicine: Factor deficiency anemia. In: Ravel R, ed. *Clinical Laboratory Medicine: Clinical Application of Laboratory Data*. 6th ed. St Louis, MO: Mosby; 1995: 22–34.

19. Troutman WG. Drug-induced diseases. In: Anderson PO, Knoben JE, Troutman WG, eds. *Handbook of Clinical Drug Data*. 10th ed. New York, NY: McGraw-Hill; 2002: 817–29.

20. Colon-Otero G, Menke D, Hook CC. A practical approach to the differential diagnosis and evaluation of the adult patient with macrocytic anemia. *Med Clin North Am*. 1992; 76:581–97.

21. Erslev AJ, Gabuzda TG. *Pathophysiology of Blood*. Philadelphia, PA: W. B. Saunders; 1985.

22. Henry JB, Beadling WV. Immunohematology. In: Henry JB, ed. *Clinical Diagnosis and Management by Laboratory Methods*. 19th ed. Philadelphia, PA: W. B. Saunders; 1996: 748–92.

23. Tabara IA. Hemolytic anemias. Diagnosis and treatment. *Med Clin North Am*. 1992; 76:649–68.

24. Thomas AT. Autoimmune hemolytic anemias. In: Lee GR, Foerster J, Lukens J, et al, eds. *Wintrobe's Clinical Hematology*. 10th ed. Baltimore, MD: Williams & Wilkins: 1999: 1233–63.

25. Blum MD, Graham DJ, McCloskey CA. Temafloxacin syndrome: review of 95 cases. *Clin Infect Dis*. 1994; 18:946–50.

26. Lux SE. Hereditary defects in the membrane or metabolism of the red cell. In: Bennett JC, Plum JF, eds. *Cecil Textbook of Medicine*. 20th ed. Philadelphia, PA: W. B. Saunders; 1996: 851–9.

27. Lee GR. The anemia of chronic disorders. In: Lee GR, Foerster J, Lukens J, et al, eds. *Wintrobe's Clinical Hematology*. 10th ed. Baltimore, MD: Williams & Wilkins; 1999: 1193–210.

28. Fixler J, Styles L. Sickle cell disease. *Pediatr Clin North Am*. 2002; 49:1193–210.

29. Wang WC, Lukens JN. Sickle cell anemia and other sickling syndromes. In: Lee GR, Foerster J, Lukens J, et al, eds. *Wintrobe's Clinical Hematology*. 10th ed. Baltimore, MD: Williams & Wilkins: 1999; 1346–97.

30. Lo L, Singer ST. Thalassemia: current approach to an old disease. *Pediatr Clin North Am*. 2002 Dec; 49:1165–91.

31. Krause JR. The automated white blood cell differential. A current perspective. *Hematol Oncol Clin North Am*. 1994; 8:605–16.

32. Gottlieb. Apoptosis. In: Beutler E, Coller BS, Lichtman MA, et al, eds. *William's Hematology*. 6th ed. New York, NY: McGraw-Hill; 1999: 125–9.

33. Strausbaugh LJ. Hematologic manifestations of bacterial and fungal infections. *Hematol Oncol Clin North Am*. 1987; 1:185–206.

34. McKenzie SB, Laudicina RJ. Hematologic changes associated with infection. *Clin Lab Sci*. 1998; 11:239–51.

35. Serafin WE, Austen KF. Mediators of immediate hypersensitivity reactions. *N Engl J Med*. 1987; 317:30–4.

36. Roitt IM, Brostoff J, Male D. *Immunology*. 6th ed. New York, NY: Mosby; 2001: 21–100.

37. Ganz T, Lehrer RI. Production, distribution, and fate of monocytes and macrophages. In: Beutler E, Coller BS, Lichtman MA, et al, eds. *William's Hematology*. 6th ed. New York, NY: McGraw-Hill; 1999: 873–6.

38. Baird SM. Morphology of lymphocytes and plasma cells. In: Beutler E, Coller BS, Lichtman MA, et al, eds. *William's Hematology*. 6th ed. New York, NY: McGraw-Hill; 1999: 911–9.

39. Kipps TJ, Carson DA. Composition and biochemistry of lymphocytes and plasma cells. In: Beutler E, Coller BS, Lichtman MA, et al, eds. *William's Hematology*. 6th ed. New York, NY: McGraw-Hill; 1999: 819–25.

40. Young NS. Acquired aplastic anemia. *Ann Int Med*. 2002; 136:534–46.

41. Ho DD, Pomerantz RJ, Kaplan JC. Pathogenesis of infection with human immunodeficiency virus. *N Engl J Med*. 1987; 317:278–86.

42. Mindel A, Tenant-Flowers M. ABC of AIDS: natural history and management of early HIV infections. *BMJ*. 2001; 322:1290–3.

43. Baranski B, Young N. Hematologic consequences of viral infections. *Hematol Oncol Clin North Am*. 1987; 1:167–83.

44. Friedman AD. Hematologic manifestations of viral infections. *Pediatric Ann*. 1996; 25:555–60.

45. Dale DC. Neutropenia and neutrophilia. In: Beutler E, Coller BS, Lichtman MA, et al, eds. *William's Hematology*. 6th ed. New York, NY: McGraw-Hill; 1999: 823–34.

46. Paraskevas F. Clinical flow cytometry. In: Lee GR, Foerster J, Lukens J, et al, eds. *Wintrobe's Clinical Hematology*. 10th ed. Baltimore, MD: Williams & Wilkins: 1999: 56–71.

47. Wetzler M, Byrd JC, Bloomfield CD. Acute and chronic myeloid leukemia. In: Braunwald E, Fauci AS, Kasper DL, et al, eds. *Harrison's Principles of Internal Medicine*. 15th ed. New York, NY: McGraw-Hill; 2001: 706–14.

48. Barlogie B, Shaughnessy J, Munshi N, et al. Plasma cell myeloma. In: Beutler E, Coller BS, Lichtman MA, et al, eds. *William's Hematology*. 6th ed. New York, NY: McGraw-Hill; 1999: 1279–304.

49. Lichtman MA, Liesveld JL. Chronic myelogenous leukemia and related disorders. In: Beutler E, Coller BS, Lichtman MA, et al, eds. *William's Hematology*. 6th ed. New York, NY: McGraw-Hill; 1999: 1085–124.

50. Banks PM. Pathology of malignant lymphoma. In: Beutler E, Coller BS, Lichtman MA, et al, eds. *William's Hematology*. 6th ed. New York, NY: McGraw-Hill; 1999: 1207–14.

51. Maloney DG, Smith B, Rose A. Rituximab: mechanism of action and resistance. *Semin Oncol*. 2002; 29(suppl):2–9.

Chapter **16**

HEMATOLOGY: BLOOD COAGULATION TESTS

James B. Groce III and Julie B. Leumas

Normal hemostasis results from a complex interaction among the vascular subendothelium, platelets, coagulation factors, and proteins that promote clot formation and subsequent degradation as well as inhibitors of these substances. Bleeding can result from acquired or inherited deficiencies of coagulation factors or physiological disorders of platelets. Excessive clotting can result from abnormalities of the vascular endothelium, alterations in blood flow, or deficiencies in clotting inhibitors—characterized as hypercoagulable states that may give rise to thromboembolism.[1,2]

Practitioners routinely monitor coagulation tests for patients receiving anticoagulants, though thrombolytics are not routinely monitored by single endpoint tests since most of the tests used to assess fibrinolytic activity are used as part of a panel and not as a single endpoint. Antiplatelet agents (i.e., the drugs themselves) are not routinely monitored, although there have been studies to suggest that monitoring may have clinical utility. Certain bleeding abnormalities are associated with primary coagulopathies and numerous drugs. Therefore, coagulation tests should be monitored periodically for patients in these situations.

This chapter reviews normal coagulation physiology, common tests used to assess coagulation and hypercoagulable states, and, finally, factors (including drugs) that alter coagulation tests.

OBJECTIVES

After completing this chapter, the reader should be able to

1. Discuss normal platelet physiology and the role of platelets in hemostasis.
2. Describe the coagulation cascade system, including the intrinsic, extrinsic, and common pathways.
3. Discuss normal physiology of coagulation inhibition.
4. Discuss the fibrinolytic system and how it promotes clot degradation.
5. List the laboratory tests used to assess platelets and discuss factors, such as drugs, that may influence their results.
6. List the laboratory tests used to assess coagulation and explain their use in evaluating anticoagulant therapy.
7. List the laboratory tests used to assess hypercoagulable states.
8. Define International Normalized Ratio (INR) and recognize both the advantages and disadvantages of INR determinations.
9. List the laboratory tests used to assess clot degradation and disseminated intravascular coagulation (DIC) and discuss their limitations.
10. Given results of laboratory tests used for evaluating coagulation and anticoagulant therapy in a case description, properly interpret the results and suggest follow-up action.
11. Briefly discuss the availability and use of bedside testing devices for anticoagulant therapy.

PHYSIOLOGICAL PROCESS OF HEMOSTASIS

Coagulation is the process that halts bleeding following vascular injury. Normal hemostasis involves the complex relationship among substances that promote clot formation (platelets and the coagulation cascade), inhibit coagulation, and dissolve the formed clot. Each substance is briefly reviewed.

Clot Formation

Platelets

Platelets are 2–4 microns, disk-shaped structures that are nonnucleated and do not reproduce themselves. Platelets contain mitochondria and glycogen granules that provide energy. Lysosomal granules, nonribosomal endoplasmic reticulum, and contractile actinomycin are found within platelets.

Most platelets are formed in the extravascular spaces of bone marrow from megakaryocytes. The lungs and other tissues can retain megakaryocytes and produce platelets.[3] The megakaryocytes produce 35,000 platelets/µL of blood per day and up to 8 times this amount during stress. Megakaryocyte production and maturation are promoted by the hormone thrombopoietin, which recently was purified and cloned.[4] Two-thirds of the platelets are found in the circulation and one-third in the spleen (in splenectomized patients, however, nearly 100% are in the circulation).

The average platelet lifespan is 8–12 days, and about 10% turn over each day.[3] Transfused platelets have a shorter lifespan (4–5 days). The size of platelets does not change as they age. On aging, platelets are destroyed by the spleen, liver, and bone marrow. Additionally, platelet function is affected by numerous factors[5]:

- Drugs.
- Common foods.
- Vitamins.
- Spices.
- Systemic conditions such as chronic renal disease and hematological disorders (e.g., myeloproliferative and lymphoproliferative diseases, dysproteinemias, and the presence of antiplatelet antibodies).

The surface of normal blood vessels does not stimulate platelet adhesion. However, vascular injury is often caused by rheological damage, trauma, or the rupture of plaque from the vessel wall, resulting in endothelial damage. Subendothelial structures, such as collagen, basement membrane, and fibronectin, then become exposed (Figure 16-1). Collagen is a potent stimulator of platelet adhesion.[6–10] Circulating von Willebrand factor acts as a binding ligand between the subendothelium and glycoprotein Ib receptors on the platelet surface and contributes to platelet adhesion.

Once adhesion occurs, platelets change shape and activation occurs.[6,8] Collagen, adenosine diphosphate (ADP), thrombin, thromboxane A_2, and prostaglandin H_2 stimulate the change in platelet shape from ovoid disks to spheres with pseudopods.[8] These stimulators cause the platelets to aggregate, change shape, and release their contents, which include ADP, serotonin (5HT), platelet factor 3 (PF3), and platelet factor 4 (PF4). Following platelet adhesion to the subendothelium, platelet aggregation completes the formation of the hemostatic plug. Platelets bind to one another at glycoprotein IIa/IIIb receptor sites with fibrinogen acting as the primary binding ligand.

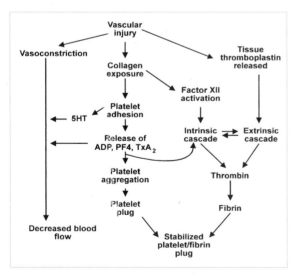

Figure 16-1. Relationship between platelets and the clotting cascade in the generation of a stabilized fibrin clot. 5HT = serotonin; ADP = adenosine diphosphate; PF4 = platelet factor 4; TxA_2 = thromboxane A_2.

ADP and thromboxane A_2 recruit additional platelets, which aggregate to the platelets that are already bound to the subendothelial tissues. In addition to promoting aggregation, thromboxane A_2, 5HT, and other substances are potent vasoconstrictors that limit blood flow to the damaged site. When vascular damage is minimal, the vasoconstriction and platelet aggregation (formation of a platelet plug) may be sufficient to limit bleeding.

However, the platelet plug is not stable and can be dislodged. To form a more permanent hemostatic plug, the clotting system must be stimulated. By releasing PF3, platelets initiate the clotting cascade and concentrate clotting factors at the site of the vascular (endothelial) injury.

Prostaglandins play an important role in platelet function. Figure 16-2 displays a simplified version of the complex arachidonic acid pathways that occur in platelets and on the vascular endothelium. Thromboxane A_2, a potent stimulator of platelet aggregation and vasoconstriction, is formed in platelets. In contrast, prostacyclin (PG2) (located on the vessel surface) is a potent inhibitor of platelet aggregation and a potent vasodilator that limits excessive platelet aggregation.

Cyclooxygenase and PG2 are clinically important. An aspirin dose of 80 mg/day acetylates and inhibits cyclooxygenase in the platelet irreversibly because the platelet cannot regenerate this enzyme.[9,10] Platelets are rendered incapable of forming arachidonic acid and prostaglandins. This effect of low-dose aspirin lasts for the lifespan of the exposed platelets (up to 12 days).

Vascular endothelial cells also contain cyclooxygenase, which converts arachidonic acid to PG2. Aspirin in high doses inhibits the production of PG2. However, because the vascular endothelium can regenerate PG2, aspirin's effect there is much shorter than its effect on platelets. Thus, aspirin's effect at high doses may both inhibit platelet aggregation (antiplatelet effect) and block the aggregation inhibitor PG2. This phenomenon is the rationale for using low doses of aspirin 80–325 mg/day to help prevent myocardial infarction.

In summary, a complex interaction between the platelet and blood vessel wall maintains hemostasis. Once platelet adhesion occurs, the clotting cascade may become activated. After thrombin and fibrin are generated, the platelet plug becomes stabilized with insoluble fibrin at the site of vascular injury.

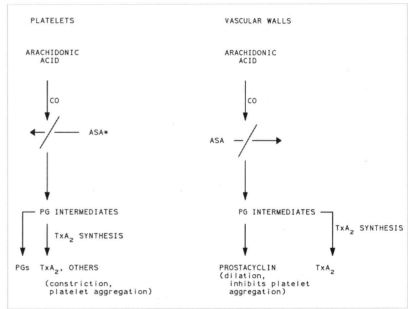

Figure 16-2. Formation of thromboxane A_2 (TxA$_2$), prostaglandins (PGs), and prostacyclin in platelets and vascular endothelial cells. CO = cyclooxygenase; ASA* = low-dose, irreversible, inactivation of platelet cyclooxygenase; ASA/ = high-dose inactivation of platelet cyclooxygenase.

Coagulation Cascade

The coagulation cascade (Figure 16-3) generates fibrin, which forms an insoluble mesh surrounding the platelet plug. Platelets concentrate clotting factors at the site of vascular injury. The platelet surface has receptors that bind and activate factors XII, XI, IX, and X; prekallikrein; and prothrombin.[11]

The coagulation system is called a *cascade* because each activated factor serves as a catalyst to the next reaction. Therefore, small amounts of activated clotting factors early in the cascade result in very large concentrations of thrombin and fibrin. The nomenclature for

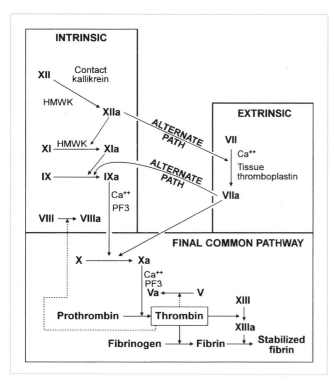

Figure 16-3. Coagulation cascade. Dotted lines indicate thrombin's feedback action, which modifies factors V and VIII. HMWK = high molecular weight kininogen. (Reproduced, with permission, from Reference 11.)

the coagulation proteins is shown in Table 16-1. The coagulation cascade is typically divided into the intrinsic, extrinsic, and common pathways.

Intrinsic pathway. All components for initiation of the intrinsic pathway are present in the blood in their inactive forms. In this pathway, factor XII becomes activated when exposed to collagen in damaged vascular subendothelium. In the presence of prekallikrein and a kininogen, activated factor XII activates factor XI; in the presence of calcium, factor XI activates factor IX. Activated factor IX, in turn, activates factor X in the presence of platelet membrane lipoprotein, factor VIII, and calcium.

Extrinsic pathway. The extrinsic pathway is initiated when tissue thromboplastin is released from damaged cells and then activates factor VII in the presence of calcium. Tissue thromboplastin is a complex mixture of substances located in the vascular intima.[11] It activates factor VII and, in the presence of calcium, factor X.

Common pathway. Both the intrinsic and extrinsic pathways activate factor X in the final common pathway. Prothrombinase, with a phospholipid (e.g., PF3), is a complex that forms when factors Xa and V, platelet phospholipid, and calcium combine to become an enzyme-like substance.[11] This complex converts prothrombin to thrombin. In addition to the direct effects and feedback mechanisms of thrombin shown in Figure 16-3, thrombin also stimulates platelet aggregation and activates protein C and the fibrinolytic system. Thrombin cleaves other prothrombin molecules to form additional thrombin. It also cleaves fibrinogen in several steps that eventually result in a stable, insoluble fibrin plug. This fibrin plug is strengthened by cross-linking between factor XIII and fibrin.

Inhibition of Coagulation

Numerous mechanisms limit coagulation.[12–15] Factors V and VIII are destroyed by protein C, which is activated by negative feedback from high concentrations of thrombin. Thrombin activates protein C by cleaving a heavy chain from the molecule.[15] Normal blood flow also dilutes activated clotting factors and results in their degradation in various tissues (e.g., liver) and by proteases. However, in areas of low flow or venous stasis, clotting factors may not be readily cleared. Other mechanisms that limit coagulation include natural inhibitors and the fibrinolytic system.

Antithrombin (previously antithrombin III) and proteins C and S are naturally occurring inhibitors of coagulation. These substances are, in part, responsible for preventing uncontrolled coagulation of blood. Most patients who are deficient in these proteins have recurrent thromboem-

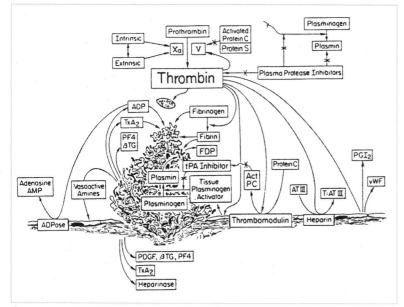

Figure 16-4. Mechanisms for limiting coagulation. Adenosine AMP = cyclic adenosine monophosphate; vWF = plasma cofactor VIII/von Willebrand factor; PDGF = platelet-derived growth factor; bTG = b-thromboglobulin; PF4 = platelet factor 4; TxA_2 = thromboxane A_2. (Reproduced, with permission, from Reference 9.)

bolic events, often at a young age.[1,2,12–17]

The complex mechanisms that limit thrombus formation are shown in Figure 16-4. Coagulation (thrombus extension) is limited due to resistance of intact endothelium to thrombus formation. Platelet aggregation is prevented by active clearance of vasoactive amines, complexation of thrombin with antithrombin, and the explosive thrombin-mediated synthesis and release of the platelet aggregation inhibitor PG2. The effects of thrombin are also limited to the injury site by protease inhibitors, enhancement of the thrombin-antithrombin complex, and binding of thrombin to thrombomodulin. This, in turn, activates protein C to inactivate factors Va and VIIIa and also induces the release of tissue plasminogen activator (tPA) from the endothelium. Therefore, thrombin initiates negative feedback mechanisms controlling its own generation.

TABLE 16-1

COAGULATION FACTOR	NAMES	HALF-LIFE (HR)
I	Fibrinogen	90
II	Prothrombin and prethrombin	60
III	Tissue factor and tissue thromboplastin	
IV	Calcium	
V	Proaccelerin and accelerator globulin	12–36
VI	Not assigned	
VII	Proconvertin and serum prothrombin conversion accelerator	4–6
VIII	Antihemophilic factor and platelet cofactor I	12
IX	Plasma thromboplastin component, Christmas factor, antihemophilic factor B, platelet cofactor II	24
X	Stuart-Prower factor, Stuart factor, autoprothrombin III	45–72
XI	Plasmin thromboplastin anticedent and antihemophilic factor C	48–84
XII	Hageman factor, glass factor, contact factor	48–52
XIII	Fibrin stabilizing factor and fibrinase	72–124
	Prekallikrein and Fletcher factor	35
	High molecular weight kininogen and Fitzgerald factor	156

[a] Adapted, with permission, from Reference 11.

Table 16-1. International Nomenclature and Corresponding Half-Lives for Hemostatic

Antithrombin, a naturally occurring glycoprotein, inactivates thrombin. Heparin (either natural or exogenous) serves as a cofactor for the reaction between antithrombin and serine proteases in the clotting cascade that includes thrombin and activated factors IX–XII (discussed previously).[1,12] Heparin and antithrombin combine one-to-one, and the complex almost instantaneously neutralizes the activated clotting factors and inhibits the coagulation cascade.

Protein C, a vitamin K-dependent protein, inactivates factors Va and VIIIa in the presence of phospholipid and calcium ions.[11,12,15] Circulating protein S increases the rate at which activated protein C inactivates factor Va. Before this reaction can occur, protein C must be activated. Thrombin binds to thrombomodulin and forms a complex that markedly accelerates the activation of protein C. Since thrombomodulin is located on the endothelial cell surface, it is not present at the site of vascular injury.[12] However, thrombomodulin at adjacent, noninjured tissue activates protein C and prevents the propagation of the clot onto normal tissues. Activated protein C also increases fibrinolysis. It neutralizes an inhibitor of the naturally occurring fibrinolytic protein, tPA, which results in enhanced conversion of plasminogen to plasmin (Clot Degradation section).[15]

Studies have found that the uncommon complication of skin necrosis may occur when warfarin is started in patients with depressed concentrations of protein C.[2,15] Protein C has a very short half-life (6 hr). Clotting factors IX and X are associated with the antithrombotic effects of warfarin, but their half-lives are 20–30 hr.[1,2] Therefore, initiation of warfarin de-

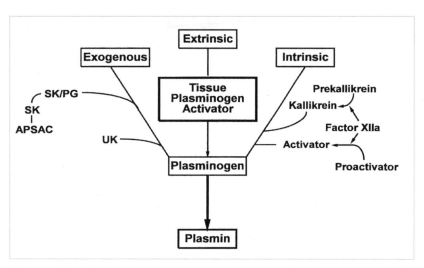

Figure 16-5. Exogenous, extrinsic, and intrinsic pathways for activation of plasminogen. APSAC = anistreplase; SK = streptokinase; SK/PG = streptokinase-plasminogen complex; UK = urokinase. (Reproduced, with permission, from Reference 18.)

presses protein C more rapidly than factors IX and X. This inequity results in a relative hypercoagulable state that may manifest as skin necrosis.

Other thrombin inhibitors include a_1-proteinase inhibitor and heparin cofactor II as well as a_2-macroglobulin, which inhibits both thrombin and plasmin.[12]

Clot Degradation

Fibrinolysis is the mechanism by which formed thrombi are lysed to prevent excessive clot formation and vascular occlusion. As discussed previously, fibrin is formed in the final common pathway of the clotting cascade. During fibrinolysis, fibrin in a formed clot is broken down. A natural or extrinsic activator of the fibrinolytic system, tPA, is produced by the vascular endothelial cells. Drugs or exogenous activators (e.g., streptokinase, anistreplase, urokinase, and recombinant tPA) also activate fibrinolysis. Various other activators of plasminogen are referred to as *intrinsic* (e.g., kallikrein). They include activated factor XII, activated protein C, and a plasma protein termed *activator* (Figure 16-5).

Plasmin is the enzyme that eventually breaks down fibrin into fibrin degradation products (FDPs). However, plasmin must first be formed from plasminogen (Figure 16-5).[10,18] The fibrin located in the clot binds circulating plasminogen. The release of tPA from the adjacent vascular endothelium is stimulated by thrombin, causing the conversion of plasminogen to plasmin (Figure 16-4). Plasmin that is released from the clot enters the circulation and is rapidly inactivated by a_2-antiplasmin and a_2-macroglobulin.[11] Pharmacological inhibitors of fibrinolysis include tranexamic acid, aminocaproic acid, and aprotinin.

TESTS TO EVALUATE HEMOSTASIS

For the purpose of discussion, bleeding and clotting disorders are divided into tests to assess

- Platelets.
- Coagulation.
- Clot degradation.
- Hypercoagulable state.

Tests to assess platelets include platelet count, volume (mean platelet volume [MPV]), function (e.g., bleeding time [BT] and platelet aggregation), and others. Thrombin time (TT), reptilase time, prothrombin time (PT)/INR, activated partial thromboplastin time (aPTT), activated clotting time (ACT), fibrinogen assay, and others are laboratory tests that assess coagulation. Clot degradation is assessed with tests for FDPs and the D-dimer. Fibrinolysis also is monitored with the euglobulin lysis test.

A hypercoagulable state workup may include activated protein C resistance and the factor V Leiden mutation, anticardiolipin antibody, antiphospholipid antibody, antiplasmin, antithrombin, C-reactive protein, heparin neutralization, homocystine, lipoprotein, plasminogen, plasminogen activator inhibitor 1 (PAI1), platelet hyperaggregation, Proteins C&S, Prothrombin G20210A Mutation, Reptilase Time and Thrombin Time. These tests are often performed in panels since the presence of more than one predisposition to thrombosis further increases the risk for thrombosis.[19,20]

TABLE 16-2

DISORDER OR DRUG	PLATELET COUNT	BT	PT	aPTT	COMMENTS
Thrombocytopenic purpura	*Low*	*Prolonged*	WNL	WNL	
Glanzmann's thrombasthenia	*WNL*	WNL or prolonged	WNL	*WNL*	*Platelets appear normal*
von Willebrand's disease	WNL	*Prolonged or WNL*	WNL	*WNL or prolonged*	
Fibrinogen deficiency	WNL	WNL	*Prolonged*	Prolonged	BT prolonged if severe, *fibrinogen levels decreased*, TT prolonged
Wafarin therapy	WNL	WNL	*Prolonged*	WNL or prolonged	BT prolonged if overdosed
Heparin therapy	WNL	WNL or prolonged	WNL or prolonged	*Prolonged*	Platelet count may decrease[b]
Vascular purpura	WNL	WNL	WNL	WNL	

[a] Italic type indicates most useful diagnostic or therapeutic tests; WNL = within normal limits.
[b] Significant thrombocytopenia may occur as a heparin side effect in 1–5% of patients.

Table 16-2. Summary of Coagulation Tests Done in Hemorrhagic Disorders and Anticoagulant Drug Monitoring[a]

In addition, general hematological values such as hemoglobin (Hgb), hematocrit (Hct), red blood cell count, and white blood cell count should be obtained when evaluating blood and coagulation disorders (Chapter 15). Even the results of urinalysis and stool guaiac tests may be important. Table 16-2 is a summary of common tests used to evaluate bleeding disorders and monitor anticoagulant therapy.

Platelet Tests

Platelet Count

Normal range: 140,000–440,000/µL

The only test to determine the number (actually, the concentration) of platelets in a blood sample is the platelet count, although various methods are used. Platelet counts can be performed by manual or automated methods. When the platelet count is 50,000–500,000/µL, the automated methods are more accurate. Values outside this range exceed the accuracy of the instrumentation. In such cases, manual counts using phase-contrast microscopy are the most reliable.[21] Hematocrit values below 20 or above 50 also cause a loss of reliability and necessitate manual platelet counts. The coefficient of variation (CV) is 16% for phase-contrast microscopy and may be up to 25% for ordinary light microscopy.

Automated platelet counts can be performed on anticoagulated whole blood or platelet-rich plasma. Most instrumentation that performs hematological profiles provides platelet counts. Platelets are passed through a tube, generating an electric pulse each time one passes, and each pulse is counted. When the platelet count is 50,000–500,000/µL, the CV may be as low as 4%.[21]

Thrombocythemia. An abnormal platelet count can have many causes. Stress or infection is associated with thrombocytosis, an elevation in the platelet count. Additionally, thrombocytosis may be caused by

- Splenectomy.
- Trauma.
- Asphyxiation.
- Rheumatoid arthritis.
- Iron-deficiency anemia.
- Posthemorrhagic anemia.
- Cirrhosis.
- Chronic pancreatitis.
- Tuberculosis.
- Recovery from bone marrow suppression.

Values of 500,000–800,000/μL are not uncommon.

Thrombocythemia refers to an excess of platelets, often greater than 800,000/μL of whole blood. Thrombocythemia may be seen with essential thrombocythemia, polycythemia vera, chronic myelogenous leukemia, or myelosclerosis. In addition to arterial and venous thrombosis, patients with thrombocythemia may have abnormalities in platelet function studies as well as spontaneous bleeding.

Thrombocytopenia. The definition of thrombocytopenia is a platelet count below 150,000/μL. Several diseases, such as thrombotic thrombocytopenic purpura (TTP), idiopathic thrombocytopenic purpura (ITP), disseminated intravascular coagulation (DIC), and hemolytic-uremic syndrome, result in rapid destruction of platelets.[21] TTP and hemolytic-uremic syndrome[22] have been associated with several drugs including antineoplastic agents.[23] Diseases such as aplastic anemia, leukemia, and metastatic carcinoma may decrease the production of platelets.

Numerous drugs have been associated with thrombocytopenia (Table 16-3). However, heparin and antineoplastics are common causes. Thrombocytopenia is also common with radiation therapy. Autoimmune diseases such as ITP result from antibodies to platelets that lead to their destruction. Many drugs associated with thrombocytopenia alter platelets by the formation of antibodies to platelets (e.g., heparin, penicillin, and gold).

Immunoassay techniques can now measure drug-directed platelet antibodies, but these methods are not commonly used to assess drug-induced thrombocytopenia. Other causes of thrombocytopenia include viral infections; pernicious, aplastic, and folate/B$_{12}$-deficiency anemias; complications of pregnancy; massive blood transfusions; exposure to dichlorodiphenyltrichloroethane (DDT); and human immunodeficiency virus (HIV) infections.

When the platelet count falls below 20,000/μL, the patient is at risk of spontaneous bleeding. Therefore, therapy with platelet concentrations is often initiated. Bleeding may occur at higher platelet counts (e.g., 50,000/μL) if trauma occurs.

In the past, heparin had been associated with thrombocytopenia (heparin-induced thrombocytopenia or HIT) in up to 30% of patients who receive the drug.[1,2] Reliable estimates of the inci-

TABLE 16-3

Aldesleukin	Nalidixic acid
Allopurinol	Penicillamine
Amphotericin B	Penicillins
Amrinone	Pentamidine
Antineoplastics	Phenylbutazone
Antiviral agents	Phenytoin
Azathioprine	Propylthiouracil
Carbamazepine	Quinacrine
Cephalosporins	Quinidine
Chloramphenicol	Quinine
Chlorpropamide	Radiation
Etretinate	Sulfonamides
Gold compounds	Tamoxifen
Griseofulvin	Thiazide diuretics
H$_2$ antagonists	Tolbutamide
Heparin	Trimethoprim
Interferons·	Trimetrexate
Methimazole	Valproic acid

a Most drugs listed cause an idiosyncratic, drug-induced thrombocytopenia. Exceptions include amrinone, antineoplastics, and possibly amphotericin B, which cause a direct toxic effect that may be dose related.

Table 16-3. Partial List of Agents Associated with Thrombocytopenia[a]

dence are 1–5%, although the frequencies of HIT antibody formation and clinical HIT vary in different clinical settings (e.g., patients undergoing surgery are more likely to develop HIT than are medically ill patients).[24] Recent studies indicate that the frequency of HIT is <1% when either unfractionated heparin or LMWH is given for no more than 5–7 days. Because of this finding, a platelet count should be checked between day 3 and day 5 of therapy. If heparin is administered for a longer period, another platelet count should be checked between day 7 and day 10 and another at day 14.[25] Heparin induced thrombocytopenia (HIT) is an antibody-mediated, adverse reaction to heparin, which can cause venous and arterial thrombosis. HIT is manifested both by clinical and serological features. HIT antibody formation accompanied by otherwise unexplained fall in platelet count >50% (even if the nadir remains $>150 \times 10^9$/L) or skin lesions at injection sites are manifestations of the HIT syndrome.[24]

Although much less common, cases of thrombocytopenia associated with low-dose heparin prophylaxis (5000 U every 8–12 hr subcutaneously) have been reported. There may be no difference in the risk of drug-induced thrombocytopenia with heparin derived from either bovine lung or porcine intestine.[26] Recent evidence also suggests that the incidence of heparin-induced thrombocytopenia is lower with a low molecular weight heparin (LMWH) since it binds less to platelets.[24] LMWHs should be used cautiously when patients have HIT.[27] Direct thrombin inhibitors such as Refludan®, Argatroban, and Angiomax®, may be used as alternative anticoagulants for patients with HIT.[25]

In all patients receiving heparin, platelet counts should be monitored at least every 2–3 days. Some experts recommend daily platelet counts for the first 3 weeks. Shorter treatment courses of heparin and warfarin dosed concomitantly on day 1 may eliminate this requirement. If the platelet count falls below 100,000/μL, heparin may be discontinued by some practitioners.

Mean Platelet Volume

Normal range: 7–11 fL but varies with laboratory

Mean platelet volume (MPV), the relationship between platelet size and count, is most likely to be used by clinicians in assessing disturbances of platelet production. MPV is useful in distinguishing between hypoproductive and hyperdestructive causes of thrombocytopenia (Figure 16-6). Despite the widespread availability of platelet indices, many clinicians do not use them in clinical decision making. In the past, this disuse was attributed to difficulties with the laboratory measurement of indices. Laboratory measurement has now overcome methodological problems that once stymied the role of MPV determinations in the diagnosis of pathological thrombopoiesis.[28]

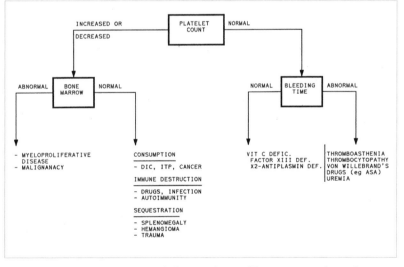

Figure 16-6. Assessment of abnormalities of homeostasis based on platelet count, bone marrow exam, and BT.

Many laboratories routinely report the MPV as part of the complete blood count (CBC) (Chapter 15), especially if a differential is requested. In general, lower platelet counts are common with higher platelet volumes (i.e., an inverse relationship exists between the platelet count and the MPV). Although MPV is most valuable in distinguishing hypoproductive from hyperdestructive causes of thrombocytopenia, a definitive diagnosis cannot be made based on MPV alone. In thrombocytopenia, an elevated MPV suggests no problem with platelet production (in fact, production is reflexively increased). Conversely, a normal or low MPV suggests impaired thrombopoiesis.

Determination of MPV requires a blood collection tube containing an anticoagulant. Usually, such tubes contain the anticoagulant ethylenediamine tetraacetic acid (EDTA).[29] Heparin should not be used because it may interfere with the method of measuring platelet volume by causing platelets to clump. Citrated anticoagulants also should not be used because platelets tend to maintain their normal discoid shape within citrated anticoagulant tubes.[30]

<table>
<tr><td colspan="2"></td></tr>
<tr><td>**INCREASE IN MPV**</td><td>**DECREASE IN MPV**</td></tr>
<tr><td>Diabetes</td><td>Host chemotherapy</td></tr>
<tr><td>Hereditary</td><td>Hyperplasia</td></tr>
<tr><td>Hyperthyroidism</td><td>Hypersplenism</td></tr>
<tr><td>Immune thrombocytopenic purpura</td><td>Hypothyroidism</td></tr>
<tr><td>Myocardial infarction</td><td>Marrow aplasia</td></tr>
<tr><td>Pregnancy-induced hypertension</td><td>Reactive thrombocytosis</td></tr>
<tr><td>Renal failure</td><td></td></tr>
<tr><td>Respiratory disease</td><td></td></tr>
<tr><td>Sepsis</td><td></td></tr>
</table>

a Reference ranges for MPV vary among laboratories and are inversely proportional to the platelet count; however, a common reference range is 7–11 fL in patients with a normal platelet count.[21]

Table 16-4. Conditions that Alter MPV[a]

Currently, MPV is not widely used but may evolve into a valuable screening test for the disorders listed in Table 16-4. Interesting data relating MPV to these disorders are now surfacing. For example, the MPV is often elevated at the time of myocardial infarction, although it is not specific enough to be of diagnostic value. Two recent studies[31,32] suggested that a high MPV at 6 months postinfarction is a predictor of re-infarction. Moreover, the magnitude of the changes was similar to established coronary risk factors such as fibrinogen.

MPV is also altered in the presence of other disease states. For example, a fall in MPV is common in patients with enlarged spleens (hypersplenism) due to preferential sequestering of larger platelets within the spleen. Hypersplenism is associated with slightly low MPVs, whereas elevated MPVs are seen with immune thrombocytopenic purpura.[33] In myeloproliferative disorders, MPVs usually stay within the reference range.[33] Concomitant increases in large and small platelets account for an overall net zero increase in size. During the third trimester of pregnancy, an increase in platelet size in preeclamptic patients results from increased platelet consumption.[34] Finally, MPV is elevated in hyperthyroid patients and declines to normal as they become euthyroid. Hypothyroid patients often have a high platelet count and a low MPV.[35,36]

The inverse relationship of a high MPV and a low platelet count is demonstrated in other conditions including respiratory disease,[37] renal failure,[38] and sepsis.[39] Unlike most other conditions that demonstrate the inverse relationship of MPV and platelet count, both are low in HIV infection. These decreases suggest an impairment of synthesis and maturation of megakaryocytes as well as enhanced platelet destruction in the bloodstream.[40] Administration of erythropoietin stimulates megakaryocyte cell line production that leads to an increase in MPV. Thrombopoietin probably causes the same effect.[41-44] The role of thrombopoietin has lead to advances in the treatment of thrombocytopenia caused by deficient production of platelets (e.g., in patients undergoing bone marrow transplantation or cancer chemotherapy).[44]

Platelet Function

Abnormalities of platelet function may be either *inherited* or *acquired*. Bleeding as a result of an inherited vs. acquired abnormality may be difficult to prove. Common bleeding sites in patients with inherited disorders of platelet function include ecchymosis of the skin, epistaxis, gingival bleeding, and menorrhagia.[5] Less common bleeding disorders are gastrointestinal hemorrhage and hematuria. Hematomas and hemarthroses (the predominant sites of bleeding in patients with inherited familial clotting disorders) are rare, except after trauma.[45]

Although the *sites* of bleeding are predictable, the *severity* is not predictable in patients with inherited disorders of platelet function.[45] Unfortunately, the risk of bleeding and bleeding patterns in patients with acquired platelet dysfunction are less predictable and more

TABLE 16-4

difficult to distinguish. Because both inherited and acquired etiologies increase the risk of bleeding, patients overtly bleeding without a clear cause or without an invasive procedure should be suspect for one of these platelet function disorders.[45]

Bleeding time (normal range: 2–9 min). Tissue and vascular injury causes platelets to aggregate at the site of injury. Various aspects of platelet function can be determined with BT and more specific aggregation studies. Although BT is an indirect test of primarily platelet aggregation, low platelet counts and other factors can prolong test results. The ability of platelets to perform this function can be assessed with the BT test.

Technical difficulty in performing this test may significantly affect results. Though in the past considered as the single best screening test for disorders of platelet function[46] the BT is neither a sensitive or a specific test. This would account for its declining use and elimination from within some institutions clinical laboratory.

Some patients with acquired disorders of platelet function may have deficient platelet aggregation but a normal BT.[4] Conversely, certain systemic disorders, such as chronic renal failure and DIC,[50,51] have been shown to prolong BT. Lastly, patients with coronary artery disease (CAD) undergoing cardiopulmonary bypass have longer than expected BTs relative to their degree of thrombocytopenia.[52]

Most acquired disorders affecting BT are related to drugs that decrease platelet numbers or reduce platelet function. The most notable drug that affects platelet function is aspirin. After the administration of aspirin, some patients appear to have excessive increases in BT.[53] After the ingestion of 650 mg of aspirin, the average BT in normal patients increases and stays increased for as long as 4–7 days. However, this rise occurs in only 50% of persons taking this dose.[54,55]

Aspirin irreversibly acetylates cyclooxygenase (Figure 16-2). Platelets cannot synthesize new cyclooxygenase, and the effect of aspirin persists for the lifespan of the exposed platelets. The prolongation of BT caused by aspirin is somewhat shorter than the platelet lifespan (8–12 days), because platelets formed after aspirin exposure are not affected. In other words, platelets formed after aspirin is no longer present can confer some agreeability before all aspirin-exposed platelets are eliminated. Aspirin's ability to prolong BT is enhanced immediately after alcohol consumption.[56] Heparin may also prolong BT but not by affecting platelet aggregation.[57] Although BT is influenced by some drugs, it is not used to monitor drug therapy.

The increase in BT caused by aspirin may have beneficial effects. Numerous studies examined the use of aspirin to prevent either myocardial infarction (e.g., high-risk patients with unstable angina) or reinfarction in patients who have suffered a myocardial infarction.[58] In one arm of the Physicians' Health Study, otherwise healthy male physicians were given either placebo or 325 mg of aspirin every other day.[59] The risk of myocardial infarctions in the aspirin-treated group was so significantly reduced that investigators terminated this arm of the study early. The role of aspirin in the prevention of *recurrent* myocardial infarction is now universally accepted.

The combined use of warfarin and aspirin may be synergistic and superior to either agent alone in prevention of myocardial infarction. Elevations in activated clotting factor VII are associated with a risk of ischemic heart disease.[60] This clotting factor's activity is most rapidly and extensively reduced by warfarin. Because of this consideration, investigators have speculated that warfarin would be of benefit in myocardial infarction prevention.

Other drugs that may prolong BT are listed in Table 16-5. While nonacetylated salicylates do not impair platelet aggregation or affect BT, all other nonsteroidal anti-inflammatory drugs (NSAIDs) reversibly inhibit platelet cyclooxygenase and inhibit aggregation as long as the drug remains in the plasma. Therefore, the clinician can estimate the time it

TABLE 16-5

Table 16-5. Medications and Drug Classes that May Cause Abnormalities of Platelet Function[a]

	ABNORMALITY	
MEDICATION	ABNORMAL BT	ABNORMAL PLATELET AGGREGATION
Aspirin	√	√
Anticoagulants	√	√
Beta-blocking agents		√
Calcium channel blockers	√	√
Cephalosporins	√	√
Chemotherapeutic agents	√	√
Clofibrate		√
Dextran	√	√
Dipyridamole[b]		
Ethanol	√	√
Nitrofurantoin	√	√
Nitroglycerin	√	√
Nonsteroidal anti-inflammatory agents	√	√
Phenothiazines		√
Quinidine	√	
Thrombolytic agents	√	
Ticlopidine	√	√

[a]Adapted from Reference 5.
[b]This medication has not been demonstrated to cause abnormal platelet function, but it has been used extensively as an antithrombotic agent.

takes for BT to normalize after withdrawing these drugs (by knowing their respective half-lives).

Platelet aggregation. The ability of platelets to aggregate is most commonly measured by preparing a specimen of platelet-rich plasma and warming it to 98.6 °F (37 °C) with constant stirring. This test is performed with an aggregometer that measures light transmission through a sample of platelets in suspension.[19] After a baseline reading is obtained, a platelet-aggregating agonist (e.g., epinephrine, collagen, ADP, or arachidonic acid) is added. As platelets aggregate, more light passes through the sample. The change in optical density can be measured photometrically and recorded as an aggregation curve, which is then printed on a plotter.

Interpretation of platelet aggregation tests involves a comparison of the patient's curves with the corresponding curves of a normal control. Minor differences in the slope (rate) and extent (plateau) of aggregation of as much as 25% are not significant.[61] To eliminate the optical problems of turbidity with lipemia plasma, the patient and the normal control should be fasting. Patients should not take aspirin or NSAIDs because they may interfere with test results.

Lumiaggregometry measures both platelet aggregation and the platelet secretion reaction. This measurement simplifies the diagnosis of platelet dysfunction.[19] The lumiaggregometer measures light transmission through platelets and the emission luminescence generated by adenosine triphosphate during the platelet release reaction. The test is performed with citrated whole blood. The detection method is based on impedance or increased electrical resistance caused by the accumulation of platelet aggregates on the circuit.

The shape of the aggregation curve depends on the agonist(s) used and the type of platelet abnormality. By examining the pattern of aggregation, the shape of the curve, and the platelet release reaction, the laboratory can detect several functional platelet disorders—either inherited or acquired.

More recent technologies, including the Platelet Function Analyzer (PFA-100, Dade Behring), simulate the in vivo hemodynamic conditions of platelet adhesion and aggregation following vascular injury, allowing for rapid and meaningful evaluation of platelet function. The tests can be used to detect platelet dysfunction due to drugs, decreased von Willebrand factor, and other thrombocytopathies (Table 16-2).

Other Platelet Tests

The measurement of platelet-specific substances, such as PF4 and ß-thromboglobulin, can now be performed by radioimmunoassay or enzyme immunoassay.[19] High concentrations of these substances may be observed with CAD, acute myocardial infarction (AMI), and thrombosis, where platelet lifespan is reduced. Since numerous drugs can potentially cause thrombocytopenia, detection of antibodies directed by specific drugs against platelets may help to determine the culprit.

Platelet survival can be measured by injecting radioisotopes that label the platelets. Serial samples can then determine platelet survival, which is normally 8–12 days.

Coagulation Tests

Coagulation tests are useful in the identification of deficiencies of coagulation proteins responsible for bleeding as well as thrombotic disorders. The most commonly performed tests, including the prothrombin time (PT), activated partial thromboplastin time (aPTT), and activated clotting time (ACT), also are used to monitor anticoagulant therapy. There are numerous, highly precise automated laboratory methods available to perform these tests. However, there is an overall lack of standardization across coagulation testing that can lead to considerable variation in test results and their interpretation. Normal and therapeutic ranges established for one test method are not necessarily interchangeable with other methods, especially when differences in endpoint detection or reagents exist. Therefore, it is important to interpret test results based on the specific performance characteristics of the method used to analyze samples.

Careful attention to blood collection technique and sample processing—as well as laboratory quality control—is critical for reliable coagulation test results. Blood is collected in syringes or vacuum tubes that contain heparin, EDTA, or sodium citrate. Because heparin and EDTA interfere with several clotting factors (with few exceptions), only sodium citrate is used for coagulation and platelet tests. Factors that promote clotting and interfere with coagulation studies include[62]

- Tissue trauma (searching for a vein).
- Prolonged use of tourniquet.
- Small-bore needles.
- Vacuum tubes.
- Heparin contamination from indwelling catheters.
- Slow blood filling into collection tube.

Ideally, blood should be collected into vacuum tubes containing 3.2% (109 mM) sodium citrate in a proportion of 9 parts blood to 1 part citrate using appropriate venipuncture technique.[63] The sample should be mixed, by gentle inversion, immediately after collection. When samples must be collected from indwelling catheters, lines that have been previously flushed with heparin should be avoided if possible. The line should be flushed with 5 mL of saline and the first 5 mL of blood or 6 dead space volumes of the catheter discarded.[64]

The maximum time before a sample must be centrifuged and the appropriate storage temperature are critical and dependent on the type of test being performed. Errors in coagulation can be large unless quality assurance is strict with collection, reagents, controls, and equipment.[63,64]

Coagulation tests can assess bleeding or clotting disorders. This discussion focuses on commonly used tests but does not cover outdated ones such as whole blood clotting time. In Minicase 1 the common screening tests are discussed. Other sophisticated tests that might be used to assess a bleeding disorder include assays for specific clotting factors, which are discussed in another chapter.

Coagulation studies may be used to assess certain bleeding disorders; the hemophilias are common. Hemophilia A (factor VIII deficiency) or hemophilia B (factor IX deficiency) occurs in one out of every 5000 males.[65] These deficiencies, inherited sex-linked recessive traits, primarily affect males and cause over 90% of hemophilia cases. Other bleeding disorders include von Willebrand's disease, the most common hereditary bleeding disorder, and deficiencies in fibrinogen or factors II, V, VII, X, XI, XIII, and/or a combination of these factors.

Patients with thrombotic disorders may have their hypercoagulability evaluated with specific assays for[1,2,12]

- Antithrombin.[13]
- Protein C.[15,17]
- Protein S.[14,16]
- Prothrombin G20210A mutation.[66]
- Activated protein C resistance mutation.[67]

Normal reference ranges for antithrombin and proteins C&S tests are often reported as a percent of normal activity. For antithrombin, the normal activity level is 70%–145%. For proteins C and S, normal activity levels are 58%–201% and 83%–167%, respectively. Protein C activity level is performed utilizing a chromogenic assay. Protein S activity level may be performed via an ELISA antigentic assay or via a functional clot-based assay. As alluded to previously, deficiencies result in frequent, recurrent thromboembolic events in most patients with these disorders. Because these deficiencies are rare, their respective assays are not discussed here. Acquired, transient deficiencies of any of these inhibitors may be observed during thrombotic states. Typically, these parameters are assessed after the thrombosis has been resolved when the patient is off of heparin or warfarin.

Prothrombin G20210A mutation is a common hereditary predisposition to venous thrombosis. DNA-based methods, such as the polymerase chain reaction (PCR)-based assay, are used to determine the presence or absence of a specific mutation at nucleoside position 20210 in the prothrombin gene. A normal test would show absence of the G20210A mutation. The test identifies individuals who have the G20210A mutation and reveals whether the affected individual is heterozygous or homozygous for the mutation. The heterozygous form of the mutation is present in 2.3% of the general population and 6.2% of patients with venous thrombosis. It is present in 18% of cases of familial venous thrombosis.[66]

Activated protein C (APC) resistance mutation and the factor V Leiden mutation are conditions leading to hypercoagulable states with increased risks for venous thrombosis. The effect of exogenous APC on the patient's clotting time (usually activated partial thromboplastin time [aPTT] is used to detect presence of resistance to APC as occurs in individuals with the factor V Leiden mutation). Activated protein C is the most prevalent hereditary predisposition to venous thrombosis. It is present in 5% of the general Caucasian population and is less common or rare in other ethnic groups.[67–70]

Activated Protein C resistance accounts for 20% of unselected patients with a first deep vein thrombosis and 50% of familial cases of thrombosis.[71]

APC usually prolongs the aPTT more than 2-fold in controls (normal persons) and less than 2-fold in affected individuals. Presence of lupus anticoagulants, Refludan®, or Argatroban and Angiomax® may cause inaccurate results in the commonly used aPTT clotting-time based assay but do not affect DNA-based tests.[72,73]

Prothrombin Time/International Normalized Ratio

Normal range for PT: 10–13 sec but varies based on reagent-instrument combinations

Therapeutic range for INR: dependent on indication for anticoagulation

The prothrombin time (PT), also called protime, test is used to assess deficiencies of the extrinsic and common pathways (II, V, VII, X). It is the most commonly used test to monitor the effects of oral anticoagulant therapy with vitamin K antagonists including warfarin. The PT, based on Quick's method first described in 1935, is determined by adding calcium chloride and thromboplastin containing both the tissue factor and the phospholipid necessary to promote the activator of factor X by factor VIIa in patient's plasma.[74] The time it takes for clot formation to occur after the addition of the thromboplastin and calcium chloride to the patient's plasma is the prothrombin time, reported in seconds. The endpoint, clot formation, originally performed using a manual tilt tube method, is typically determined using automated optical or mechanical instrumentation.

Assay performance characteristics, standardization and reporting. The prothrombin time is dependent on the tissue thromboplastin source and test method used to detect clotting. Thromboplastin reagents are derived from animal or human sources and include recombinant products. Factor sensitivity is highly dependent on the source of the thromboplastin, even between different lots of the same reagent. Generally, rabbit-based thromboplastins are less sensitive to changes in factor activity than human tissue thromboplastin. This means that it takes a more significant decrease in factor activity to produce a prolongation of the PT when rabbit-based thromboplastin reagents are used compared to human-based reagents. Differences in reagent sensitivity, combined with the influence of end point detection, affect clotting time results both in the normal and therapeutic ranges. Large differences in factor sensitivity between comparative methods can result in conflicting interpretation of results, both in the assessment of factor deficiencies and adequacy of anticoagulation therapy.

In a study conducted by the New York State Department of Health, blood samples were mailed to 340 laboratories. The CVs ranged from 5–6% with mechanical methods and from 7–11% with manual methods.[75]

In recent years, attempts have been made to standardize PT results using an alternative reporting method. Two international committees proposed the use of the International Normalized Ratio (INR). The INR is the PT ratio that would result if the World Health Organization (WHO) international reference thromboplastin were used to test the sample.[76] To convert a PT ratio to an INR, the sensitivity of the thromboplastin must be known. The reagent's sensitivity is expressed as an International Sensitivity Index (ISI). The ISI expresses the sensitivity of the thromboplastin reagent compared to the WHO reference thromboplastin (ISI= 1.0). The ISI also is a factor of the clot detection method used to measure the endpoint. The ISI for a reagent/instrument combination is determined by testing normal donor plasmas and patients who are on stable, oral anticoagulant regimens and comparing PT results to those obtained with the WHO reference thromboplastin using a manual tilt tube method. Reagents that are less sensitive than the WHO reference have corresponding ISI values >1.0. When used as an exponent to the observed PT ratio (a patient's PT in seconds divided by the mean normal PT obtained with a specific reagent/instrument combination; Table 16-6), the ISI theoretically produces the same result that would have been obtained if the primary International Reference Preparation of WHO had been used as the reagent.[77]

The accuracy of manufacturers' ISI calibrations over the last few years has been questioned.[78] The calibration of the ISI value may impact the accuracy of normalizing PTs. In addition, consideration must be given to the variability in PTs caused by differing lab instrumentation when paired with specific reagents. Because of this problem, thromboplastin manufacturers should describe in their product literature the variability introduced by use of their reagent with different instruments for PT determinations.[79] The citrate concentration also may effect the ISI determination of certain reagents. Historically, coagulation samples have been collected into either 3.2% (109 mM) or 3.8% (129 mM) sodium citrate. However, ISI values, unless specifically stated, are determined from samples collected into 3.2% sodium citrate. More recently, the National Committee for Clinical Laboratory Standards (NCCLS) and the International Society of Hemostasis have recommended that all samples for coagulation be anticoagulated using 3.2% citrate. ISI values for North American rabbit brain thromboplastin have been variously reported as 2.2–2.6 and 1.8–2.8.[80,81] For bovine brain, 1.0–1.1 has been reported.[81] Human tissue and recombinant thromboplastins have ISI values similar to bovine thromboplastins.

Additional inaccuracy in normalizing PTs occurs with thromboplastins that have especially high ISI values (>2.0). An Australian study urged caution when interpreting INRs obtained with ISI values greater than 2.0, citing these high values to be the likely cause of bleeding because the overanticoagulation may not be detected.[82] Reagents with ISI values of <1.4 are recommended for use when monitoring patients on oral anticoagulant therapy.

There are other factors that may influence the PT. Lupus anticoagulants sometimes prolong the PT, although both the heterogeneity of these inhibitors combined with widely varying differences in reagent sensitivity makes this prolongation difficult to predict.

Finally, if heparin-sensitive thromboplastin reagents are used, falsely elevated PT/INR values may result. These inaccurate values might suggest sufficient anticoagulation with oral anticoagulation therapy and result in the premature discontinuation of heparin. This additional variability in the response of some thromboplastins introduced by concomitant heparin therapy was just elucidated.[83]

Although the INR system has greatly improved the standardization of the PT, one can still expect differences in INRs reported with two different methods, particularly in the upper therapeutic and supratherapeutic ranges. The greater the differences in the ISI values for two comparative methods, the more likely differences will be noted in the INR. Laboratories and anticoagulation clinics should review the performance characteristics of the prothrombin time method used to evaluate their specific patient populations and report changes in methods to healthcare professionals, particularly those monitoring anticoagulant therapy.

Monitoring warfarin therapy. The PT/INR is used to monitor warfarin therapy. Laboratory monitoring of warfarin therapy is performed by measuring the PT. Because commercially available PT reagents vary markedly in their responsiveness, a standardized reporting system became necessary. Standardization is achieved by converting the PT ratio with any local thromboplastin into the INR (Table 16-6). When warfarin therapy is monitored, INR is used more often to correct for PT ratios obtained with thromboplastin reagents with varying degrees of responsiveness.

Current American College of Chest Physicians' and National Heart, Lung, and Blood Institute guidelines recommend an INR of 2.0–3.0 for all indications (including recurrent systemic embolism) except mechanical prosthetic heart valves (an INR of 2.5–3.5 is recommended).[2,76] Commencing with The Fourth American College of Chest Physicians' Conference consensus report, there was a recommendation that all laboratories convert to the INR system of reporting. Two other documents have cited the reporting of a PT ratio and its corresponding INR as potentially dangerous.[76,84]

Despite this recommendation, some laboratories still report PT ratio values with their reported INR or, worse still, PT percentages or PT in seconds.[81] Therefore, clinicians may continue to use PT ratio values. This situation is unfortunate since variability among reagents and labs still exists.[75]

Heparin may also prolong PT, especially in higher doses.[85–87] Patients who have significant prolongation of their aPTT values (>150 sec) are likely to have their PTs prolonged an average of 2.5 sec. When heparin dosage is therapeutic, minimal prolongation of the PT should be expected (1.2–1.8 sec).[86] These "crossover" effects may have to be considered frequently because oral and parenteral anticoagulants are usually given concomitantly for several days. However, this influence of heparin on PT is infrequently of clinical significance when heparin is dosed to maintain an aPTT in the therapeutic range (0.3–0.7 anti-Xa IU/mL). Numerous drugs, disease states, and other factors prolong PTs in patients receiving warfarin by various mechanisms of action (Table 16-7).

TABLE 16-6

THROMBO-PLASTIN	PATIENT'S PT (SEC)	MEAN NORMAL (SEC)	PT RATIO[a]	ISI	INR[b]
A	16	12	1.3	3.2	2.6
B	18	12	1.5	2.4	2.6
C	21	13	1.6	2.0	2.6
D	24	11	2.2	1.2	2.6
E	38	14.5	2.6	1.0	2.6

[a] $PT\ ratio = \left[\dfrac{patient's\ PT\ (sec)}{mean\ normal\ PT\ (sec)}\right]$

[b] $INR = (PT\ ratio)^{ISI}$

Example: $\left[\dfrac{24\ sec}{11\ sec}\right]^{1.2} = 2.58 \approx 2.6$

Table 16-6. Variability in International Sensitivity Index (ISI) Thromboplastin Reagents Using Blood from Single Patient

Minicase 1 presents each test of blood coagulation that is already described and other tests that follow.

Activated Partial Thromboplastin Time

Normal range: varies by manufacturer

The activated partial thromboplastin time (aPTT) is used to screen for deficiencies and inhibitors in the intrinsic pathway (factors VIII, IX, XI, and XII) as well as factors in the final common pathway (factors II, V, and X). The aPTT is also commonly used as a surrogate assay to monitor unfractionated heparin. The aPTT, reported as a clotting time in seconds, is determined by adding partial thromboplastin (animal, human, or recombinant source phospholipid that mimics platelet phospholipid), calcium chloride, and an activator to the patient's plasma.[88] This activator substance simulates a surface on which contact activation can occur. The activators can be particulate or chemical and commonly include kaolin, diatomaceous earth, silica, or elegiac acid. Normal ranges vary depending on the reagent/instrument combination used to perform the test, but they generally are between 22–38 sec.

Factor and heparin sensitivity as well as the precision of the aPTT test depend both on the reagents and instrumentation.[75,89–91] In addition, some aPTT reagents are formulated for increased sensitivity to lupus anticoagulants. Today more than 30 different reagent instrument combinations are used in the United States. Despite numerous attempts to standardize the aPTT, very little progress has been made. The difficulty in part may reflect differences in opinion as to the appropriate heparin sensitivity, the need to have lupus anticoagulant sensitivity for targeted patient populations, and suitable factor sensitivity to identify deficiencies associated with increased bleeding risk. Normal and therapeutic ranges must be established for each reagent instrument combination, and ranges should be verified with changes in lots of the same reagent. Various multicenter surveys of laboratories have found CVs (coefficient of variation) from 5–17%.[75,91] Generally speaking, precision (as assessed by %CV) has improved significantly, especially with the automated instruments used today. As a consequence, many laboratories do not conduct PT and aPTT tests in duplicate. The use of the ratio of the patient's aPTT to the normal value may reduce the CV.[75]

MINICASE 1

HARRY C., A 36-YEAR-OLD MALE, was hospitalized with a longstanding history of alcohol abuse. Physical examination revealed a cachectic-appearing male with spider-hemangiomas, petechial hemorrhages, and asterixis. The patient was taking cimetidine and phenytoin. He denied taking over-the-counter medications.

The following laboratory parameters were determined for Harry C:

LABORATORY STUDY	NORMAL RESULTS	PATIENT RESULTS
PT	10–13 sec	14.8 sec
INR	–	1.49
aPTT	21–45 sec	54 sec
CBC		
Hgb	14–18 g/dL	11 g/dL
Hct	42–52%	33%
Platelet count	140,000–440,000/μL	87,000/μL
MPV	7–11 fL	19 fL
Aspartate aminotransferase	8–42 IU/L	85 IU/L
(AST)	3–30 IU/L	25 IU/L
Alanine aminotransferase	3.5–5 g/dL	1.4 g/dL
(ALT)		
Albumin		

Question: What specific test(s) may be performed to assess the pertinent patient findings from the physical examination? How might these tests relate to normal hemostasis?

Discussion: Specific studies for bleeding disorders include the PT/INR and aPTT; they should be used as a preliminary screening for Harry C. His elevations above baseline are consistent with coagulopathies common in patients who abuse ethanol. This increase occurs because clotting factors that affect these tests are manufactured in the liver.

Platelet count determination and general hematologic values (Hgb and Hct) are consistent with physical examination findings (petechial hemorrhages), revealing the patient to be thrombocytopenic and anemic. As expected, the lowered platelet count and higher platelet volume demonstrate the inverse relationship that typically exists when thrombocytopenia occurs (MPV section). Liver function tests (LFTs) would further substantiate the suspected etiology of the patient's petechial hemorrhages. The typical AST/ALT "split" (i.e., a doubling of the AST relative to ALT) is consistent with the patient's history of alcohol abuse.

These findings suggest liver impairment and, when paired with Harry C.'s albumin, indicate the possibility of clotting abnormalities (demonstrated objectively by his prolonged PT and aPTT). Table 16-2 summarizes common tests to evaluate bleeding disorders and monitor anticoagulant therapy.

With this patient, history is important. Cimetidine and phenytoin have been associated with thrombocytopenia, which could also account for petechial hemorrhages. Harry C. denies using aspirin, but many patients unknowingly ingest it in over-the-counter products such as brand-name aspirin and cold preparations.

Though used to detect clotting factor deficiencies, today, the aPTT is used primarily for monitoring heparin therapy. The current recommendation for the therapeutic range of heparin is an aPTT ratio of 1.5–2.5 times control. Given the inter- and intrapatient variability that can result from aPTT reagents, alternative means of monitoring heparin therapy are being scrutinized. This 1.5–2.5 aPTT ratio corresponds to [92–93]

- A plasma heparin concentration of 0.2–0.4 U/mL by assay using the protamine titration method.
- A plasma heparin concentration of 0.35–0.7 U/mL by assay using the inhibition of factor Xa.

Causes of aPTT prolongation. In addition to reagent specific issues impacting on aPTT responsiveness, there may be hereditary or acquired causes of aPTT prolongation that may make the aPTT test result prolonged.

Causes of aPTT Prolongation

Hereditary

- Deficiency of factor VIII, IX, XI, XII, prekallikrein, or HMWK (PT is normal).
- Deficiency of fibrinogen or factor II, V, or X (PT is also prolonged).

Acquired

- Lupus anticoagulants (PT usually normal).
- Heparin (PT less affected than aPTT, PT may be normal).
- Refludan®, Angiomax®, or Argatroban (PT usually also prolonged).
- Liver dysfunction (PT affected earlier and more than aPTT).
- Vitamin K deficiency (PT affected earlier and more than aPTT).
- Warfarin (PT affected earlier and more than aPTT).
- Disseminated intravascular coagulation (DIC) (PT affected earlier and more than aPTT).
- Specific factor inhibitors (PT normal except in the rare case of an inhibitor against fibrinogen, factor II, V or X)

Heparin should be given by continuous intravenous (IV) infusion using an individualized, weight-based dosing approach. Various methods may be used.[92–99] Most methods rely on a weight-based approach, typically 15–25 U/kg of body weight per hour. To achieve an immediate anticoagulant effect, an initial heparin bolus (70–100 U/kg) is administered. Coagulation tests (e.g., aPTT) should be drawn 6 hr after continuous IV heparin is begun and after each subsequent dosage adjustment, since this interval approximates four half-lives of heparin (the time to achieve steady-state pharmacokinetics).[97]

Some authors advocate serial aPTT determinations during the initial 24 hr of heparinization.[98] Gusto-III used serial aPTT determinations. GUSTO-III compared the safety and efficacy of reteplase (a plasminogen activator thrombolytic) with alteplase in patients with AMI. An aPTT was drawn before heparin; at 6, 12, and 24 hr after heparin was started; and then daily. Heparin was given in both study groups and was adjusted with a nomogram (Figure 16-7). A similar nomogram was used in earlier trials (GUSTO-I, GUSTO-IIa, and TIMI-9A), but the target aPTT range has been lowered from approximately 60–85 sec to 50–75 sec based on data of the earlier studies.[99–102]

Because use of a nomogram allows quick fine-tuning of anticoagulation by nurses without continuous physician input, many hospitals have adopted one of the GUSTO nomograms as their standard protocol for dosing heparin in patients with AMI. Some hospitals use the nomogram in patients with noncoronary thrombosis (e.g., deep venous thrombosis and pulmonary embolism), although its efficacy and safety have not been well-studied in these disorders. The initial heparin infusion rate has traditionally been 20 mL/hr (1000 U/hr) using a heparin concentration of 50 U/mL. However, the GUSTO-III trial used a starting dose of 800 U/hr (1000 U/hr in patients 80 kg).[3]

GUSTO III Heparin Infusion Adjustment Nomogram				
aPPT (sec)	Heparin Bolis (units)	Stop Drip (min)	Rate Change (cc/hour)	Repeat aPPT
<40	3000	0	+2 (↑100 U/hr)	6 hr
40—49	0	0	+1 (↑50 U/hr)	6 hr
50—75	0	0	0 (no change)	Next a.m.
76—85	0	0	-1 (↓50 U/hr)	Next a.m.
86—100	0	30	-2 (↓100 U/hr)	6 hr
101—150	0	60	-3 (↓150 U/hr)	6 hr
>150	0	60	-6 (↓300 U/hr)	6 hr

Figure 16-7. GUSTO-III trial heparin adjustment nomogram for heparin dilution of 50 U/mL and standard laboratory reagents with a mean control aPTT of 26–36 sec. The infusion rate may be adjusted *only* upward in response to the 6-hr post-thrombolytic aPTT unless overt bleeding is seen or the aPTT is greater than 150.

Subcutaneous doses of heparin, usually 5000 U every 8 hr or 7500 U every 12 hr, have been used for prophylaxis against thromboembolic disease after total hip replacement surgery and in acute spinal cord injury patients.[99] The dosage of subcutaneous heparin in this regimen is sometimes adjusted to keep the aPTT in the upper normal range (31–36 sec) at the midpoint of the dosing interval. However, some clinicians do not adjust subcutaneous heparin requirements with an aPTT value.

aPTT determinations obtained earlier than 6 hr, while not at steady state, may be combined with heparin concentrations for dosage individualization using non-steady-state concentrations. This approach has been demonstrated to reduce the incidence of subtherapeutic aPTT ratios significantly during the first 24 hr of therapy.[92,103] This finding is important because the recurrence rate of thromboembolic disease increased when aPTT values were not maintained above 1.5 times the patient's baseline aPTT during the first 24 hr of treatment.[104,105]

Warfarin effect on aPTT. Although warfarin also elevates the aPTT, aPTT is not used to monitor warfarin therapy. Hauser and Rozek[106] found a strong correlation between the increase in PT and a corresponding increase in aPTT with warfarin therapy. With an average PT ratio of 1.8, aPTT was 1.9 times the aPTT baseline (55 vs. 31 sec). Therefore, if warfarin is started in a patient receiving heparin, the clinician should expect some elevation in aPTT.

Heparin concentration measurements may provide a target plasma therapeutic range, especially in unusual coagulation situations such as pregnancy (where the reliability of clotting studies is questionable). In this setting, shorter than expected aPTT results in relation to heparin concentration measurements may be indicative of increased circulating levels of factor VIII and increased fibrinogen levels.[107] Patients may have therapeutic heparin concentrations measured by whole blood protamine sulfate titration or by the plasma anti-Xa heparin assay. However, they may have aPTTs not significantly prolonged above baseline. This difference has been referred to as a dissociation between the aPTT and the heparin concentration.[108] Many of these patients have very short pretreatment aPTT determinations.

Current recommendations suggest that such patients be managed by monitoring their heparin concentrations using a heparin assay to avoid unnecessary dosage escalation without compromising efficacy.[108,109] These patients, referred to as *pseudo-heparin resistant,* may be identified as having a poor aPTT response (but an adequate heparin concentration >0.3 U/mL via plasma anti-Xa assay) despite high doses of heparin (>50,000 U/24 hr; usual dose is 20,000–30,000 U/24 hr) (Minicase 2).[109] When higher doses of heparin (>1500 U/hr) are required to maintain therapeutic aPTT values, high concentrations of heparin-binding protein or phase reactant proteins bind and neutralize heparin. Additionally, thrombocytosis, or antithrombin deficiency may exist.[108]

Heparin alone has minimal anticoagulant effects; when it is combined with antithrombin (normal range: 70–145%), the inhibitory action of antithrombin on coagulation enzymes results in the inhibition of thrombus propagation. Patients who are antithrombin deficient (<50%) may be difficult to anticoagulate, as seen with DIC (Minicase 3). The DIC syndrome is associated not only with obvious hemorrhage but also with occult diffuse thrombosis.

BRIAN M., A 36-YEAR-OLD MALE with a history of deep vein thrombosis, presented to the emergency department with signs and symptoms of the same condition. A routine heparin regimen was started. The patient had the following laboratory determinations performed 6 hr after initiation of heparin:

LABORATORY STUDY	NORMAL RESULTS	PRETREATMENT PATIENT RESULTS	POSTHEPARIN RESULTS
PT	10–13 sec	11.1 sec	12.3 sec
INR	varies	0.98	1.18
aPTT	21–45 sec	19 sec	23 sec
ATIII	70–145%	57%	50%

Question: What might account for this patient's postheparin elevation in PT? Why was the aPTT not prolonged? What is the role of ATIII here?

Discussion: Brian M. was started on a continuous IV heparin infusion with plans to convert to long-term warfarin, per the institution's protocol. Subsequent postheparin laboratory determinations revealed a hypercoagulable state consistent with thromboembolic disease. Circulating procoagulants account for the patient's low pretreatment aPTT. ATIII—the cofactor with which heparin binds to exert its anticoagulant effect—is depressed, making the patient hypercoagulable. Subsequent to the initiation of heparin, the ATIII concentration declined further. This drop reflected the binding of ATIII to heparin.

Despite a normal dosing protocol for heparin, Brian M.'s initial aPTT value (obtained 6 hr after the loading dose and continuous maintenance infusion of heparin) remained low. One might be suspicious of pseudo-heparin resistance or dissociation of the aPTT responsiveness after adequate treatment with heparin. To assess the likelihood of this situation, a heparin concentration measurement could be obtained (discussed later) to demonstrate adequate heparinization despite a subtherapeutic aPTT determination.

Prior to initiation of concomitant warfarin therapy, Brian M.'s PT increased slightly to 12.3 sec. Minimal prolongation of the PT may be expected from heparin's influence. This degree of elevation is consistent with this observation. The patient's PT/INR should be followed, with the desired endpoint of warfarin therapy being an INR of 2–3.

Another use for heparin concentration is to demonstrate both efficacy and safety with LMWH. For prophylaxis against deep vein thrombosis following hip or knee replacement surgery a LMWH may be used. Low molecular weight heparin has a pharmacokinetic and pharmacodynamic profile making routine monitoring in the setting of prophylaxis unnecessary.[107] PT nor aPTT times are significantly prolonged at recommended doses of LMWHs.[107,110] However, both efficacy and safety can be demonstrated by performing a heparin level (if necessary). A therapeutically effective plasma concentration range is approximately 0.2–0.4 plasma anti-Xa U/mL at prophylaxis doses.[107,117] When using heparin levels for assessment of therapeutic or treatment doses of LMWH, a therapeutically effective concentration range is approximately 0.5–1.1 plasma anti-Xa U/mL when drawn 4 hr after a subcutaneous injection. This therapeutic range is for twice daily subcutaneous dosing of LMWH. For once daily subcutaneous dosing of LMWH, the therapeutic range is less certain but has been recommended to be maintained at approximately 1.0–2.0 U/mL.[112]

Recently, a modified version of the aPTT, the Heptest, was studied. This test measures several clotting factors, but it is specific for anti-Xa activity.[113] The role of this test has not yet been determined for monitoring heparin therapy.

Bleeding risk and test results. The major determinants of bleeding are the

* Intensity of the anticoagulant effect.
* Underlying patient characteristics.
* Use of drugs that interfere with hemostasis (see Tables 16-3 and 16-6).
* Length of therapy.

MINICASE 3

TERESA G., A 36-YEAR-OLD FEMALE in her third trimester of pregnancy, was hospitalized with clinical suspicion of DIC because of acute onset of respiratory failure, circulatory collapse, and shock. The following laboratory values for

Teresa G. were obtained:

LABORATORY STUDY	NORMAL RESULTS	PATIENT RESULTS
PT	10–13 sec	16 sec
aPTT	21–45 sec	59 sec
TT	25–35 sec	36 sec
CBC		
Hgb	12–16 g/dL	9.8 g/dL
Hct	37–47%	27.7%
Platelet count	140,000–440,000/μL	64,000/μL
MPV	7–11 fL	17 fL
FDP (latex)	2–7 μg/mL	120 μg/mL
ATIII	70–145%	57%
D-dimer	<200 ng/mL	2040 ng/mL

Question: What laboratory tests are used to determine if a patient is experiencing DIC? What are the expected laboratory results for these tests?

Discussion: Teresa G.'s PT and aPTT are prolonged. Laboratory findings of DIC may be highly variable, complex, and difficult to interpret. Both PT and aPTT should be prolonged but this may not occur.[107] Because of this consideration, the usefulness of both PT and aPTT determinations may be unreliable. TT is prolonged as expected. The platelet count is typically and dramatically decreased. The patient's MPV is inversely related to her decreased platelet count as expected, suggesting a hyperdestructive phenomenon versus a hypoproliferative state. FDPs are elevated, but this rise is not solely pathognomonic for DIC. ATIII determination reveals a considerable decrease consistent with DIC. Decreased ATIII is useful and reliable for diagnosis of DIC in the absence of D-dimer testing ability. The role of ATIII concentrate (human ATIII, Thrombate III) replacement therapy in congenital ATIII deficiency is well established. The role of the concentrate in acquired ATIII deficiencies by DIC is currently being investigated.

In terms of treatment decision making for anticoagulant therapy, bleeding risk cannot be considered alone. The potential decrease in thrombosis must be balanced against the potential increased bleeding risk.[114] The risk of bleeding associated with continuous IV heparin in patients with acute thromboembolic disease is approximately 5%. Some evidence suggests that this bleeding increases with an increase in heparin concentration. However, evidence also suggests that serious bleeding can occur in patients prone to bleeding even when the anticoagulant response is in the therapeutic range.[114] The risk of bleeding is usually higher earlier in therapy, when both heparin and warfarin are given together, which may be related to excessive anticoagulation. Patients who have a coexisting disease that elevates the PT, the aPTT, or both (e.g., liver disease) are often at much higher risk of bleeding. In these patients, the use and intensity of anticoagulation that should be employed are controversial.

Activated Clotting Time

Normal range: 80–130 sec but varies

Activated clotting time (ACT)[88] (also known as activated coagulation time) is frequently used to monitor heparin therapy[1,115] during procedures that require moderate to high-dose heparin (e.g., cardiopulmonary bypass surgery and angioplasty in which anti-Xa heparin levels are >1.0 IU/mL). Because the ACT device is considered a point-of-care testing apparatus, it may be run directly in the operating room as well as in the angioplasty suite by nonlaboratory-trained personnel. ACTs are performed on whole blood or citrated whole blood rather than plasma. This advantage has placed ACT devices in other locations where rapid bedside testing is desirable (e.g., hemodialysis unit, operating room, and cardiac catheterization laboratories).

ACT responsiveness remains linear in proportion to an increasing dose of heparin. Corresponding ACT values up to 400 sec demonstrate this dose-response relationship, but ACT lacks reproducibility for values in excess of 600 sec. The variability in ACT test results is significantly increased by variations in

- Test method.
- Blood volume to be tested.
- Technique.
- Sample temperature.
- Hemodilution.

In view of the lack of advantages over the aPTT for monitoring of venous thromboembolism, the ACT is not highly recommended for use in this setting. It has been more readily adopted by invasive cardiologists due to the test being readily available at the bedside in the cardiac catheterization suite. A measure of adequate heparinization must be determined based on the indication for which heparin is being administered.[116]

Fibrinogen Assay

Normal range: 200–400 mg/dL

While the PT and aPTT are used to screen for deficiencies in the intrinsic, extrinsic and common pathways, the fibrinogen assay is most commonly used to assess fibrinogen concentration. Fibrinogen assays are performed by adding a known amount of thrombin to a dilution of patient plasma. The fibrinogen concentration is determined by extrapolating the patient's clotting time to a standard curve. Fibrinogen is an acute phase reactant and may be elevated during pregnancy and with coronary disease. Decreased fibrinogen is associated with DIC. Additionally, heparin concentrations greater than 1 U/mL of the patient's blood volume may result in falsely low fibrinogen concentration measurements.

Thrombin time (TT) is the most sensitive test for fibrinogen deficiency, and it is prolonged when fibrinogen concentrations are below 100 mg/dL.[88] However, the actual fibrinogen concentration occasionally must be determined. A common method is the Dade fibrinogen assay. Erroneous results can be caused by (1) improper specimen collection with the wrong blood:anticoagulant ratio, or (2) lack of correction of citrate volume for a low or high Hct. Additionally, heparin concentrations greater than 1 U/mL of the patient's blood volume may result in falsely low fibrinogen concentration measurements.

Thrombin Time

Normal range: 25–35 sec but varies

Also known as thrombin clotting time, the thrombin test (TT) uses human or bovine thrombin mixed with the patient's plasma. TT measures the time required for a plasma sample to clot after the addition of thrombin and is compared to that of a normal plasma control. Deficiencies in both the intrinsic and extrinsic systems do not affect TT, which assesses only the final phase of the common pathway or essentially the ability to convert fibrinogen to a fibrin clot.

TABLE 16-7

GUT	PLASMA	LIVER	HEMOSTATIC PLUG
Anticoagulant effect potentiated	**Anticoagulant effect unchanged**	**Anticoagulant effect potentiated**	**Impaired hemostatic plug formation**
Low vitamin K intake	Displacement of warfarin	Drugs	
Reduced vitamin K absorption in fat malabsorption	from albumin binding does not influence anticoagulant effect of warfarin	Amiodarone	**Impaired coagulation**
		Anabolic steroids	Reduced vitamin K dependent
		Cimetidine	
Anticoagulant effect counteracted		Clofibrate	**Coagulation factors**
Increased vitamin K intake		Disulfiram	
Reduced absorption of warfarin by cholestyramine		Erythromycin	**Reduction in concentration of other coagulation factors**
		Fluconazole	
		Isoniazid	
		Ketoconazole	**Other anticoagulants:**
		Metronidazole	Heparin and ancrod
		Omeprazole	
		Oral fluoroquinolones	**Impaired platelet function**
		Phenylbutazone	Thrombocytopenia
		Phenytoin	Aspirin
		Piroxicam	Other NSAIDs
		Quinidine	
		Sulfinpyrazone	**Ticlopidine**
		Tamoxifen	
		Thyroxine	**Moxalactam**
		Trimethoprim-sulfamethoxazole	
		Vitamin E (mega dose)	**Carbenicillin and high doses of other penicillins**
		Liver disease	
		Hypermetabolic states	
		Pyrexia	
		Thyrotoxicosis	
		Anticoagulant effect counteracted	
		Drugs	
		Barbiturates	
		Carbamazepine	
		Griseofulvin	
		Penicillin	
		Rifampin	
		Alcohol	

[a]Adapted from Reference 78.

Table 16-7. Factors Altering Pharmacokinetics and Pharmacodynamics of Warfarin[a]

Prolongation of TT (e.g., 3 sec beyond the control value) may be caused by afibrinogenemia, dysfibrinogenemia, heparin, or the presence of FDPs that are produced with thrombolytic therapy (e.g., streptokinase).[3] In thrombolytic therapy, laboratory monitoring may not prevent bleeding or ensure thrombolysis. However, some clinicians recommend measuring TT, fibrinogen, plasminogen activation, or FDPs to document that a *lytic state* has been achieved. Typically, TT is greater than 120 sec 4–6 hr after "adequate" thrombolytic therapy.

Reptilase Time

Normal range: 18–22 sec

Additional tests can be performed to rule out the presence of circulating coagulation inhibitors such as heparin.[88] The reptilase time is a variation of the TT test in which venom from the pit viper is used instead of thrombin. Both thrombin and the venom convert fibrinogen to fibrin. FDPs inhibit conversion by reptilase, but heparin does not. Therefore, reptilase time is used to evaluate fibrinogen status in heparinized patients. If heparin is the only cause of a prolonged TT, reptilase time will be normal.

Diagnostic follow-up. If TT, PT, or aPTT is prolonged and if circulating inhibitors or bleeding disorders are suspected, further tests are usually performed. For example, hemophilia or autoimmune diseases may be associated with inhibitors such as antifactor VIII and the lupus anticoagulant. When dysfibrinogenemia or afibrinogenemia causes prolonged TT, PT, and aPTT values (see Table 16-2), it may be necessary to measure fibrinogen.[88] Fibrinogen levels are recommended by some clinicians to measure the lytic state with nonspecific thrombolytic agents (e.g., streptokinase). However, due to nonavailability of the fibrinogen test in many hospitals and delays in turnaround time, this measurement is not routinely done.

Other Coagulation Studies

Assays for specific clotting factors can be performed to determine whether a deficiency exists.[88] Factor assays using the aPTT test include factors VIII, IX, XI, and XII as well as prekallikrein. Factors II, V, VII, and X can be determined with assays that use the PT.

Clot Degradation Tests

Fibrin Degradation Products

Normal range: 2–7 µg/mL but varies

Excessive activation of thrombin leads to overactivation of the fibrinolytic system and increased production of FDPs. Excessive degradation of fibrin and fibrinogen also increases FDPs. This increase can be observed with DIC or thrombolytic drugs—FDP values may be in excess of 40 µg/mL. FDPs can be monitored during thrombolytic therapy, but they may not be predictive of clot lysis.[117,118]

FDPs can be measured by immunological techniques in which immunoglobulins to FDPs are produced in sheep, harvested, and coated onto latex particles.[60] In the semiquantitative Thrombo-Wellco test, the concentration of FDPs is determined by the agglutination of the latex particles. Under normal conditions, FDPs should be below 2 µg/mL of plasma when using this test. However, this test is labor intensive and subject to observer variability.[119] A quantitative, automated assay for FDPs was recently described[118] in which the 95% confidence interval for normal subjects consisted of values between 2 and 7 µg/mL. False-positive reactions may occur in healthy women immediately before and during menstruation and in patients with advanced cirrhosis or metastatic cancer.

D-Dimer

Normal range: <0.5 µg/mL or <200 ng/mL but varies with specific assay

A newer test for DIC is the D-dimer assay. D-dimer is a neoantigen formed when thrombin initiates the transition of fibrinogen to fibrin and activates factor XIII to cross link the fibrin formed. This neoantigen is formed as a result of plasmin digestion of cross-linked fibrin. The D-dimer test is specific for FDPs, whereas the formation of FDPs (discussed previously) may be either fibrinogen or fibrin derived following plasmin digestion (Figure 16-8). Of the common tests used in assessing DIC patients, the D-dimer assay appears to be the most sensitive.[120] Because of this high predictive ability, the D-dimer is commonly used to confirm or rule out DIC. Table 16-9 provides a list of the laboratory parameters, including the D-dimer, used to diagnose DIC (Minicases 3 and 4).

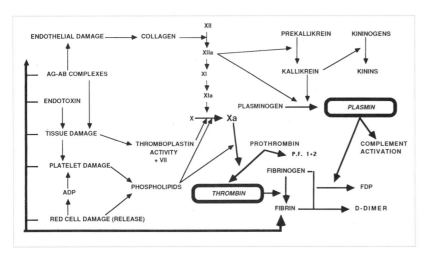

Figure 16-8. Triggering mechanisms for disseminated intravascular coagulation. (Reproduced, with permission, from Reference 117.)

Near-Patient or Point-of-Care Testing Devices

Several bedside/near-patient testing coagulation devices have been introduced over the past several years. Although the point-of-care ACT has been used for nearly 30 years, PT and aPTT tests to monitor oral anticoagulation and unfractionated heparin are now commonly utilized in both inpatient and outpatient care environments. Platelet function tests, fibrinogen, heparin and heparin neutralization assays, and protamine titration methods also are available from some manufacturers. Point-of-care coagulation testing offers specific clinical advantages, especially when used to monitor anti-thrombotic therapy because test results can be combined with clinical presentation to make more timely decisions regarding therapeutic intervention. This is especially significant in cardiac intervention laboratories, surgical settings, and critical care units where immediate turnaround time is essential to patient care decisions. In outpatient settings, point-of-care testing may not only be clinically beneficial, but also more cost effective and convenient than central laboratory testing, particularly in oral anticoagulation clinics and home health care settings.[121] These technologies will become increasingly relevant as new antithrombotic strategies with LMWH, direct thrombin inhibitors, Xa inhibitors and platelet inhibitors as well as thrombolytic agents become standard of care in critical care environments.

By design, point-of-care coagulation testing methods are easy to use by multiple healthcare professionals, adaptable to a number of patient care environments, require minimal to no sample processing, and are an extension of central laboratory testing when rapid turnaround is required. Today, a number of manufacturers provide point-of-care tests and instrumentation. Although some instruments perform only one assay, a number of devices are capable of performing multiple tests including the PT, aPTT, and ACT as well as various specialty tests for heparin titration, LMWH, and direct thrombin inhibitors. These devices typically are used in hospital settings and may be more cost effective than single assay platforms because hospitals can standardize all point-of-care coagulation testing using one system. Like central laboratory testing, none of the PT, aPTT, and ACT methods are standardized and users are required to verify performance characteristics for normal and therapeutic ranges and should have an understanding of the potential limitations due to sample type, sample stability, and volume. Because of a lack of standardization, the use of point-of-care devices for PT and aPTT testing in addition to central laboratory testing can be challenging to the clinician interpreting test results. In these cases, it may be beneficial to use only one method to monitor patients in a particular patient care environment. In most cases this suggestion is not problematic since the point-of-care method is most advantageous and cost effective when targeted to critical care environments where rapid turnaround time is most beneficial to patient care. As patients are transferred out of a critical care unit, rapid turnaround time and clinical monitoring may not be as significant to patient care decisions. In these cases, routine testing, performed by the clinical laboratory may be preferred.

Generally, point-of-care testing is not as precise as a fully automated central laboratory system that requires minimal user intervention, although in most cases the imprecision is an acceptable compromise for rapid turnaround. Point-of-care testing uses whole blood, a sample that may, in fact, be more physiologically relevant and result in a more accurate assessment

MINICASE 4

ALFRED F., A 44-YEAR-OLD MALE had clinical signs and symptoms and electrocardiogram findings consistent with acute anterior-wall myocardial infarction requiring emergent angioplasty. He received intracoronary streptokinase without successful opening of the coronary artery. Subsequently, Alfred F. was heparinized. The following pre- and post-therapy coagulation lab studies were obtained:

LABORATORY STUDY	NORMAL RESULTS	PRETHERAPY	POST-THERAPY
PT	10–13 sec	12.2 sec	17 sec
aPTT	21–45 sec	39 sec	69 sec
Fibrinogen	200–400 mg/dL	300 ng/mL	22 ng/mL
FDP (latex)	2–7 µg/mL	<10 µg/mL	>160 µg/mL
D-dimer	<200 ng/mL	<200 ng/mL	300 ng/mL
Plasminogen	68–150%	70%	22%

Question: What might explain the elevated FDP? What accounts for the fall in the plasminogen level on completion of the lytic therapy? Finally, why is the D-dimer concentration not elevated in proportion to the greatly elevated FDP concentration?

Discussion: The elevated post-therapy PT and aPTT are consistent with heparinization after intracoronary thrombolytic therapy. The FDP concentration is elevated because the streptokinase resulted in fibrinolysis. Many FDPs are generated in this setting. By the nature of thrombolytic therapy, plasminogen is converted to plasmin, accounting for the decline in the plasminogen percentage. Because thrombolytic therapy was unsuccessful in full clot lysis (resulting only in fibrinogen lysis), the D-dimer concentration is not greatly elevated. For this assay to have been more elevated, degradation products arising from cross-linked fibrin would have had to be present.

Fibrinogen concentrations should be followed periodically in patients receiving thrombolytic agents. Low levels may predict clot lysis with streptokinase and urokinase but not tPA (alteplase) or APSAC (anistreplase).[1,108]

of true coagulation potential. Many of these devices have some type of data management system that can interface with the hospital's information system. The more advanced systems can restrict operator access, store lot specific information, manage quality control functions, and flag out of range results. These systems are usually very reliable, but system performance and accuracy of results are reliant on routine maintenance and adherence to manufacturers' guidelines on test procedures and operational environment. A quality assurance program that utilizes recommended quality control materials and troubleshooting measures are essential to all clinical programs using point-of-care devices.

In recent years, choices for antithrombotic therapies have increased tremendously. While many of the newer drugs don't require routine monitoring, the availability of rapid interventional testing may be critical to the selection of certain therapies for target patient populations, particularly when these drugs have a long half-life or cannot be completely reversed. Concomitant therapy is being used increasingly in cardiac patients, especially during cardiac intervention and so the potential for thrombotic or hemorrhagic problems may be increased without the ability to rapidly confirm coagulation potential, both at the initiation of therapy and at the conclusion of a procedure.

In summary, point-of-care coagulation tests are innovative tools that can be used to effectively manage patients requiring antithrombotic therapy. They have contributed to the successful use of unfractionated heparin and oral anticoagulants for more than 30 years. The availability of rapid diagnostic tests to manage LMWH, direct thrombin inhibitors, and platelet inhibitor drugs may influence the adoption of newer therapies for specific patients in certain patient care environments and could improve their effectiveness in a larger population of patients.

SUMMARY

Many factors contribute to normal hemostasis, including interactions among vascular subendothelium, platelets, coagulation factors, natural anticoagulant proteins C and S, and substances that promote clot degradation such as tPA. In the clinical setting, the impact of these and other considerations must be evaluated. Disorders of platelets or clotting factors can result in bleeding, which may necessitate the monitoring of specific clotting tests. The MPV test is useful in distinguishing between hypoproductive vs. hyperdestructive causes of thrombocytopenia.

Coagulation tests such as aPTT, ACT, and PT/INR are used to monitor heparin and warfarin therapies. In general, coagulation tests are used for patients receiving anticoagulants, thrombolytics, and antiplatelet agents. The availability of rapid diagnostic tests to manage LMWH, direct thrombin inhibitors, and platelet inhibitor drugs may influence the adoption of these newer therapies. When fibrinolysis occurs, monitoring of FDPs is necessary. Other indications for routine use of these tests include primary coagulopathies and monitoring of drugs that may cause bleeding abnormalities. Finally, other available tests (e.g., D-dimer and antithrombin level determinations) might improve diagnostic accuracy and resultant therapies.

TABLE 16-8

DIC MONITORING PARAMETER	DIC	PRIMARY FIBRINOLYSIS	TTP	CHRONIC LIVER DISEASE
FDP	↑	↑	WNL to ↑	WNL to ↑
D-dimer	↑	↑	WNL	WNL
PT	↑	↑	WNL	↑
aPTT	↑	↑	WNL	WNL to ↑
Fibrinogen	↓	↓	WNL	Variable
Platelet count	↓	WNL	WNL to ↓	↓
LFTs	WNL	WNL	WNL	↑
Blood urea nitrogen	↑	WNL	↑	WNL

a↓ = decreased; ↑ = increased; WNL = within normal limits.

Table 16-8. Laboratory Differential Diagnosis of DIC[a]

REFERENCES

1. Carter BL, Jones ME, Waickman LA. Pathophysiology and treatment of deep-vein thrombosis and pulmonary embolism. *Clin Pharm.* 1985; 4:279–96.
2. Carter BL. Therapy of acute thromboembolism with heparin and warfarin. *Clin Pharm.* 1991; 10:503–18.
3. Fritsma GA. Platelet production and structure. In: Corriveau DM, Fritsma GA, eds. *Hemostasis and Thrombosis in the Clinical Laboratory.* Philadelphia, PA: J. B. Lippincott; 1988: 206–28.
4. Schick BP. Clinical implications of basic research: hope for treatment of thrombocytopenia. *N Engl J Med.* 1994; 331:875–6.
5. George JN, Shattil SJ. The clinical importance of acquired abnormalities of platelet function. *N Engl J Med.* 1991; 324:27–39.
6. Vermylen J, Verstraete M, Fuster V. Role of platelet activation and fibrin formation in thrombogenesis. *J Am Coll Cardiol.* 1986; 8:2–9B.
7. Heptinstall S, Hanley SP. Blood platelets and vessel walls. In: Bowie EJW, Sharp AA, eds. *Hemostasis and Thrombosis.* London, England: Butterworth & Co.; 1985: 36–74.
8. Brace LD. Platelet physiology. In: Corriveau DM, Fritsma GA, eds. *Hemostasis and Thrombosis in the Clinical Laboratory.* Philadelphia, PA: J. B. Lippincott; 1988: 229–78.
9. Harker LA, Fuster V. Pharmacology of platelet inhibitors. *J Am Coll Cardiol.* 1986; 8:21–32B.
10. Moake JL, Levine JD. Thrombotic disorders. In: Trench AH, ed. *Clinical Symposia.* Vol. 3. Summit, NJ: Ciba-Geigy Corp.; 1985: 3–32.
11. Corriveau DM. Plasma proteins: factors of the hemostatic mechanism. In: Corriveau DM, Fritsma GA, eds. *Hemostasis and Thrombosis in the Clinical Laboratory.* Philadelphia, PA: J. B. Lippincott; 1988: 34–66.
12. High KA. Antithrombin, protein C, and protein S: naturally occurring anticoagulant proteins. *Arch Pathol Lab Med.* 1988; 112:28–36.
13. Maung R, Kelly JK, Schneider MP, et al. Mesenteric venous thrombosis due to antithrombin deficiency. *Arch Pathol Lab Med.* 1988; 112:3–9.
14. Comp PC, Esmon CT. Recurrent venous thromboembolism in patients with a partial deficiency of protein S. *N Engl J Med.* 1984; 311:1525–8.

15. Clouse LH, Comp PC. The regulation of hemostasis: the protein C system. *N Engl J Med*. 1986; 314:1298–1304.

16. Engesser L, Broekmans AW, Briet E, et al. Hereditary protein S deficiency: clinical manifestations. *Ann Intern Med*. 1987; 106:6–82.

17. Hubbard AR. Standardization of protein C in plasma: establishment of an international standard. *Thromb Haemost*. 1988; 59:464–7.

18. Crabbe SJ, Cloninger CC. Tissue plasminogen activator: a new thrombolytic agent. *Clin Pharm*. 1987; 6:33–86.

19. Ridker PM, Hennekens CH, Shelhub J, et al. Interrelation of hyperhomocyst(e)inemia, factor V Leiden, and risk of future venous thromboembolism. *Circulation*. 1997; 95:1777–82.

20. Koelman BPC, van Rumpt D, Hamulyak K, et al. Factor V Leiden: an additional risk factor for thrombosis in Protein S deficient families? *Thromb Haemost*. 1995; 74:580–83.

21. Fritsma GA. Tests of platelet number and function. In: Corriveau DM, Fritsma GA, eds. *Hemostasis and Thrombosis in the Clinical Laboratory*. Philadelphia, PA: J. B. Lippincott; 1988: 278–303.

22. Levin M, Walters MD, Barratt TM. Hemolytic uremic syndrome. *Adv Pediatr Infect Dis*. 1989; 4:51–81.

23. Fields SM, Lindley CM. Thrombotic microangiopathy associated with chemotherapy: case report and review of the literature. *Drug Intell Clin Pharm*. 1989; 23:582–8.

24. Hirsh J, Warkentin TE, Shaughnessy SG, et al. *Chest*. 2001; 119:64S–93S.

25. Hyers TM, Agnelli G, Hull RD, et al. Antithrombotic therapy for venous thromboembolic disease. *Chest*. 2001; 119:176S–193S.

26. Bailey RT, Ursick JA, Helm KL, et al. Heparin-associated thrombocytopenia: a prospective comparison of bovine lung heparin manufactured by a new process and porcine intestinal heparin. *Drug Intell Clin Pharm*. 1986; 20:374–8.

27. Green D, Hirsh J, Heit J, et al. Low molecular weight heparin: a critical analysis of clinical trials. *Pharmacol Rev*. 1994; 46:89–109.

28. Jackson SR, Carter JM. Platelet volume: laboratory measurement and clinical application. *Blood Rev*. 1993; 7(2):104–13.

29. Trowbridge EA, Reardon DM, Hutchinson D, et al. The routine measurement of platelet volume: a comparison of light-scattering and aperture impedance technologies. *Clin Phys Physiol Meas*. 1985; 6:221–38.

30. Thompson CB, Diaz D, Quinn PG, et al. The role of anticoagulation in the measurement of platelet volumes. *Am J Clin Pathol*. 1983; 80:327–32.

31. Martin JF, Bath DM, Burr ML. Influence of platelet size on outcome after myocardial infarction. *Lancet*. 1991; 338:1409–11.

32. Burr ML, Holliday RM, Fehily AM, et al. Hematological prognostic indices after myocardial infarction: evidence from the diet and reinfarction trial (PART). *Eur Heart J*. 1992; 13:166–70.

33. Baynes RD, Lamparelli RD, Bezwoda WR, et al. Platelet parameters, part II. Platelet volume-number relationships in various normal and disease states. *South Afr Med J*. 1988; 73:39–43.

34. Singer CRJ, Walker JJ, Cameron A, et al. Platelet studies in normal pregnancy and pregnancy induced hypertension. *Clin Lab Haematol*. 1986; 8:27–32.

35. Haubenstock A, Panzer S, Vierhapper H. Reversal of hyperthyroidism to euthyroidism leads to increased numbers of small size platelets. *Thromb Haemost*. 1988; 60:346–7.

36. Panzer S, Haubenstock A, Minar E. Platelets in hyperthyroidism: studies on platelet counts, mean platelet volume, 111-indium labeled platelet kinetics and platelet associated immunoglobulins G and M. *J Clin Endocrinol Metab*. 1990; 70:491–6.

37. Wedzicha JA, Cotter FE, Empey DW. Platelet size in patients with chronic airflow obstruction with and without hypoxemia. *Thorax*. 1988; 43:61–4.

38. Michalak E, Walkowiak B, Paradowski M, et al. The decreased circulating platelet mass and its relation to bleeding time in chronic renal failure. *Thromb Haemost*. 1991; 65:11–4.

39. Bessman JD, Gardner FH. Platelet size in thrombocytopenia due to sepsis. *Surg Gynecol Obstet*. 1983; 156:177–80.

40. Koenig C, Sidhu G, Schoentag RA. The platelet volume-number relationship in patients infected with the human immunodeficiency virus. *Am J Clin Pathol*. 1991; 96:500–3.

41. de Sauvage FJ, Hass PE, Spencer SD, et al. Stimulation of megakaryocytopoiesis and thrombopoiesis by the c-Mpl ligand. *Nature*. 1994; 369:533–8.

42. Lok S, Kaushansky K, Holly RD, et al. Cloning and expression of murine thrombopoietin cDNA and stimulation of platelet production in vivo. *Nature*. 1994; 369:565–8.

43. Kaushansky K, Lok S, Holly RD, et al. Promotion of megakaryocyte progenitor expansion and differentiation by the c-Mpl ligand thrombopoietin. *Nature*. 1994; 369:568–71.

44. Wendling F, Maraskovsky E, Debili N, et al. c-Mpl ligand is a humoral regulator of megakaryocytopoiesis. *Nature*. 1994; 369:571–4.

45. George JN, Caen JP, Nurden AT. Glanzmann's thrombasthenia: the spectrum of clinical disease. *Blood*. 1990; 75:1383–95.

46. Rodgers RPC, Levin J. A critical reappraisal of the bleeding time. *Semin Thromb Hemost*. 1990; 16:1–20.

47. Burns ER, Lawrence C. Bleeding time: a guide to its diagnostic and clinical utility. *Arch Pathol Lab Med*. 1989; 113:1219–24.

48. Hassouna HL. Specificity and sensitivity in coagulation testing. *Hematol Oncol Clin North Am*. 1993; 7:1194–1216.

49. Davis GL, Fritsma GA. Platelet disorders. In: Corriveau DM, Fritsma GA, eds. *Hemostasis and Thrombosis in the Clinical Laboratory*. Philadelphia, PA: J. B. Lippincott; 1988: 304–42.

50. Steiner RW, Coggins C, Carvalho ACA. Bleeding time in uremia: a useful test to assess clinical bleeding. *Am J Hematol.* 1979; 7:107–17.

51. Pareti FI, Capitanio A, Mannucci L, et al. Acquired dysfunction due to circulation of "exhausted" platelets. *Am J Med.* 1980; 69:235–40.

52. Holloway DS, Summaria L, Sandesara J, et al. Decreased platelet number and function and increased fibrinolysis contribute to postoperative bleeding in cardiopulmonary bypass patients. *Thromb Haemost.* 1988; 59:62–7.

53. Fiore LD, Brophy MT, Lopez A, et al. The bleeding time responses to aspirin: identifying the hyperresponders. *Am J Clin Pathol.* 1990; 94:292–6.

54. Mielke CH Jr, Kaneshiro MM, Maher IA, et al. The standardized normal ivey bleeding time and its prolongation by aspirin. *Blood.* 1969; 34:204–15.

55. Mielke CH Jr. Influence of aspirin on platelets and bleeding time. *Am J Med.* 1983; 74:suppl(6A)72–8.

56. Deykin D, Janson P, McMahon L. Ethanol potentiation of aspirin-induced prolongation of the bleeding time. *N Engl J Med.* 1982; 306:852–4.

57. Heiden D, Mielke CH Jr, Rodvien R. Impairment by heparin of primary haemostasis and platelet [14C] 5-hydroxy-tryptamine release. *Br J Haematol.* 1977; 36:427–36.

58. Fuster V, Cohen M, Halperin J. Aspirin in the prevention of coronary disease. *N Engl J Med.* 1989; 321:183–5.

59. Steering committee of the Physician's Health Study research group. Final report on the aspirin component of the ongoing Physician's Health Study. *N Engl J Med.* 1989; 321:129–35.

60. Meade TW, Mellows S, Brozovic M, et al. Haemostatic function and ischaemic heart disease: principal results of the northwick park heart study. *Lancet.* 1986; 2:533–7.

61. Manner CE. Laboratory evaluation of platelets. In: Lotspeich-Steininger CA, Stein-Martin EA, Koepke JA, eds. *Clinical Hematology.* Philadelphia, PA: J. B. Lippincott; 1992: 671–9.

62. National Committee for Clinical Laboratory Standards: collection, transport, and processing of blood specimens for coagulation testing and performance of coagulation assays. Document H21–A3. 1998; 18:Document H21–A3.

63. Laxon CJ, Titler MG. Drawing coagulation studies from arterial lines: an integrative literature review. *Am Journ Crit Care.* 1994; 1:16–24.

64. Palkuti HS. Specimen collection and quality control. In: Corriveau DM, Fritsma GA, eds. *Homeostasis and Thrombosis in the Clinical Laboratory.* Philadelphia, PA: J. B. Lippincott; 1988: 6–91.

65. Weiss AE. The hemophilias. In: Corriveau DM, Fritsma GA, eds. *Hemostasis and Thrombosis in the Clinical Laboratory.* Philadelphia, PA: J. B. Lippincott; 1988: 128–68.

66. Van Cott EM, Laposta M. Laboratory evaluation of hypercoagulable state. *Hematol Oncol Clin North Am.* 1998; 12:1141–66.

67. Van der Meer FJ, Koster T, Vandenbroucke JP, et al. The Leiden Thrombophilia Study (LETS). *Thromb Haemost.* 1997; 78:631–5.

68. Poort SR, Rosendal FR, Reitsma PH, et al. A common genetic variation in the 3'-untranslated region of the prothrombin gene is associated with elevated plasma prothrombin levels and an increase in venous thrombosis. *Blood.* 1996; 88:698–703.

69. Rees DC, Cox M, Clegg JB. World distribution of factor V Leiden. *Lancet.* 1995; 346:1133–4.

70. Ridker PM, Miletich JP, Hennekens CH, et al. Ethnic distribution of factor V Leiden in 4047 men and women. *J Am Med Assoc.* 1997; 277:1305–7.

71. Svensson PJ, Dahlback B. Resistance to activated protein C as a basis for venous thrombosis. *N Engl J Med.* 1994; 330:517–22.

72. Akthar MS, Blair AJ, King TC, et al. Whole blood screening test for factor V Leiden using a Russell Viper Venom time-based assay. *Am J Clin Pathol.* 1998; 109:387–91.

73. Martorell JR, Munoz-Castillo R, Gil JL. False-positive activated Protein C resistance due to antiphospholipid antibodies is corrected by platelet extract. *Thromb Haemost.* 1995; 74:796–7.

74. Hirsh J, Dalen JE, Anderson DR, et al. Oral anticoagulants: mechanisms of action, clinical effectiveness, and optimal therapeutic range. *Chest.* 1998; 114(suppl 5):445S–469S.

75. Naghibi F, Han Y, Dodds WJ, et al. Effects of reagent and instrument on prothrombin times, activated partial thromboplastin times and patient/control ratios. *Thromb Haemost.* 1988; 59:455–63.

76. Hirsh J, Dalen JE, Anderson DR, et al. Oral anticoagulants: mechanism of action, clinical effectiveness, and optimal therapeutic range. *Chest.* 2001; 119(suppl 1):8S–21S.

77. Loeliger EA. ICSH/ICTH recommendations for reporting prothrombin time in oral anticoagulant controls. *J Clin Pathol.* 1985; 38:133–4.

78. McKernan A. The reliability of international normalized ratios during short-term oral anticoagulant treatment. *Clin Lab Haematol.* 1988; 10:63–71.

79. Poggio M. The effect of some instruments for prothrombin time testing on the international sensitivity index (ISI) of two rabbit tissue thromboplastin reagents. *Thromb Haemost.* 1989; 62:866–74.

80. Poller L, Thomson JM, Taberner DA. Effect of automation on prothrombin time test in NEQAS surveys. *J Clin Pathol.* 1989; 42:97–100.

81. Bussey HI. Reliance on prothrombin time ratios causes significant errors in anticoagulation therapy. *Arch Intern Med.* 1992; 152:278–82.

82. Moriarty HT, Lamp-Po-Tang PRL, Anastas N, et al. Comparison of thromboplastins using the ISI and INR system. *Pathology.* 1990; 22:71–6.

83. Schuff-Werner P, Schutz E, Gonska BD. Variation in the prothrombin-time ratio during oral anticoagulation. *N Engl J Med.* 1994; 330:570.

84. Poller L. Oral anticoagulants reassessed. *Br Med J.* 1982; 284:1425–6.

85. Sawyer WT, Raasch RH. Effect of heparin on prothrombin time. *Clin Pharm.* 1984; 3:192–4.

86. Lutomski DM, Djuric PE, Draeger RW. Warfarin therapy: the effect of heparin on prothrombin times. *Arch Intern Med.* 1987; 147:432–3.

87. Schultz NJ, Slaker RA, Rosborough TK. The influence of heparin on the prothrombin time. *Pharmacotherapy.* 1991; 11(4):312–6.

88. Fritsma GA. Clot-based assays of coagulation. In: Corriveau DM, Fritsma GA, eds. *Hemostasis and Thrombosis in the Clinical Laboratory.* Philadelphia, PA: J. B. Lippincott; 1988: 92–197.

89. Poller L, Thomson JM, Palmer MK. Measuring partial thromboplastin-time: an international collaborative study. *Lancet.* 1976; 2:842–6.

90. Brandt JT, Triplett DA. Laboratory monitoring of heparin: effects of reagents and instruments on the activated partial thromboplastin time. *Am J Clin Pathol.* 1981; 76:530–7.

91. Gawoski JM, Arkin CF, Bovill T, et al. The effects of heparin on the activated partial thromboplastin time of the College of American Pathologists Survey specimens. *Arch Pathol Lab Med.* 1987; 111:785–90.

92. Groce JB, Gal P, Douglas JB, et al. Heparin dosage adjustment in patients with deep-vein thrombosis using heparin concentrations rather than activated partial thromboplastin time. *Clin Pharm.* 1987; 6:216–22.

93. Hyers TM, Agnelli G, Hull RB et al. Antithrombotic therapy for venous thromboembolic disease. *Chest.* 2001; 119(suppl 1):176S–93S.

94. Brill-Edwards P, Ginsberg JS, Johnston M, et al. Establishing a therapeutic range for heparin therapy. *Ann Intern Med.* 1993; 119:104–9.

95. Hattersley PG, Mitsuoka JC, Ignoffo RJ, et al. Adjusting heparin infusion rates from the initial response to activated coagulation time. *Drug Intell Clin Pharm.* 1983; 17:632–4.

96. Hull RD, Raskob GE, Rosenbloom D, et al. Optimal therapeutic level of heparin therapy in patients with venous thromboembolism. *Arch Intern Med.* 1992; 152:1589–95.

97. Raschke RA, Reilly BM, Guidry JR, et al. The weight-based heparin dosing nomogram compared with a "standard care" nomogram: a randomized controlled trial. *Arch Intern Med.* 1993; 119:874–81.

98. Cipolle RJ, Rodvold KA. Heparin. In: Evans WE, Schentag JJ, Jusko WJ, eds. *Applied Pharmacokinetics.* Vancouver, British Columbia: Applied Therapeutics; 1992: 1–39.

99. Claggett GP, Anderson FA, Heit J. Prevention of venous thromboembolism. *Chest.* 1995; 108(suppl 4):312S–34S.

100. The GUSTO investigators. An international randomized trial comparing four thrombolytic strategies for acute myocardial infarction. *N Engl J Med.* 1993; 329:673–82.

101. The global use of strategies to open occluded coronary arteries (GUSTO) IIa investigators. Randomized trial of intravenous heparin vs. recombinant hirudin for acute coronary syndromes. *Circulation.* 1994; 90:1631–7.

102. Antman EM, for the TIMI 9A investigators. Hirudin in acute myocardial infarction: safety report from the thrombolysis and thrombin inhibition in myocardial infarction (TIMI) 9A trial. *Circulation.* 1994; 90:1624–30.

103. Kandrotas RJ, Gal P, Douglas JB, et al. Rapid determination of maintenance heparin infusion rates with the use of non-steady-state heparin concentrations. *Ann Pharmacother.* 1993; 27:1429–33.

104. Basu D, Gallus A, Hirsh J, et al. A prospective study of the value of monitoring heparin treatment with the activated partial thromboplastin time. *N Engl J Med.* 1972; 287:324–7.

105. Hull RD, Raskob GE, Hirsh J, et al. Continuous intravenous heparin compared with intermittent subcutaneous heparin in the initial treatment of proximal-vein thrombosis. *N Engl J Med.* 1986; 315:1109–14.

106. Hauser VM, Rozek SL. Effect of warfarin on the activated partial thromboplastin time. *Drug Intell Clin Pharm.* 1986; 20:964–7.

107. Groce JB. Heparin and low molecular weight heparin. In: Murphy JE, ed. *Clinical Pharmacokinetics.* 2nd ed. Bethesda, MD: American Society of Health-System Pharmacists; 2001: 165–98.

108. Levine MN, Hirsh J, Gent M, et al. A randomized trial comparing activated partial thromboplastin time with heparin assay in patients with acute venous thromboembolism requiring large doses of heparin. *Arch Intern Med.* 1994; 154:49–56.

109. Hirsh J, Hull RD. Treatment of venous thromboembolism. *Chest.* 1986; 89(suppl 5):426S–33S.

110. Colwell CW, Spiro TE, Trowbridge AA, et al. Use of enoxaparin, a low-molecular-weight heparin, and unfractionated heparin for the prevention of deep venous thrombosis after elective hip replacement. *J Bone Joint Surg.* 1994; 76-A:3–14.

111. Frydman AM, Bara L, LeRoux Y, et al. The antithrombotic activity and pharmacokinetics of enoxaparin, a low molecular weight heparin, in humans given single subcutaneous doses of 20 to 80 mg. *J Clin Pharmacol.* 1988; 28:609–18.

112. Laposta M, Green D, Van Cott EM, et al. College of American Pathologists Conference XXXI on Laboratory Monitoring of Anticoagulant Therapy. The clinical use and laboratory monitoring of low-molecular-weight heparin, danaproid, hirudin and related compounds, and Agatroban. *Arch Pathol Lab Med.* 1998; 122:799–807.

113. Bara L, Combe-Tamzali S, Conard J, et al. Laboratory monitoring of a low molecular weight heparin (enoxaparin) with a new clotting test (Heptest). *Haemostasis.* 1987; 1:12–33.

114. Levine MN, Raskob G, Landefeld S, et al. Hemorrhagic complications of anticoagulant treatment. *Chest.* 2001; 119(suppl 1):108S–121S.

115. Hattersley PG, Mitsuoka JC, Ignoffo RJ, et al. Adjusting heparin infusion rates from the initial response to activated coagulation time. *Drug Intell Clin Pharm.* 1983; 17:632–4.

116. Olson JD, Arkin CF, Brandt JT, et al. College of American Pathologists Conference XXXI on Laboratory Monitoring of Anticoagulant Therapy. Laboratory monitoring of unfractionated heparin therapy. *Arch Pathol Lab Med.* 1998; 122:765–816.

117. Bick RL. Disseminated intravascular coagulation: objective criteria for clinical and laboratory diagnosis and assessment of therapeutic response. *Clin Appl Thrombosis/Hemostasis*. 1995; 1(1):3–25.

118. Conrad J, Samama MM. Theoretic and practical considerations on laboratory monitoring of thrombolytic therapy. *Semin Thromb Hemost*. 1987; 13:212–22.

119. Sigal SH, Cembrowski GS, Shattil SJ, et al. Prototype quantitative assay for fibrinogen/fibrin degradation products: clinical evaluation. *Arch Intern Med*. 1987; 147:1790–3.

120. Bick RL. Disseminated intravascular coagulation: objective criteria for diagnosis and management. *Med Clin North Am*. 1994; 78:511–43.

121. Ansell J, Hirsh J, Dalen J, et al. Managing Oral Anticoagulant Therapy. *Chest*. 2001; 119:(suppl 1):22S–35S.

Chapter **17**

INFECTIOUS DISEASES

Sharon M. Erdman and Keith A. Rodvold

The assessment, diagnosis, and treatment of a patient with an infectious disease may appear to be an overwhelming task to most clinicians. This is likely due to the nonspecific presentation of many infectious processes, the continuous introduction of new antimicrobials to the existing large armamentarium, and the continuously changing taxonomy and diagnostic procedures of infecting organisms. This chapter focuses on one of the aspects in the management of infection, namely, the laboratory tests used for the diagnosis of infectious diseases. It is important to note that the diagnostic tests for many infectious diseases, such as acquired immunodeficiency syndrome (AIDS), are continuously being updated to reflect technological advances in laboratory procedures.

This chapter describes some of the laboratory tests that are utilized in the diagnosis of the most common infectious diseases due to bacteria, viruses, fungi, mycobacteria, and other organisms. Information regarding white blood cells and their role in infection is discussed in Chapter 15 (Hematology: Red and White Blood Cells). Laboratory tests utilized in the diagnosis of viral hepatitis, *Helicobacter pylori* gastrointestinal infection, and *Clostridium difficile* pseudomembranous colitis are addressed in Chapter 12 (Liver and Gastroenterology Tests).

OBJECTIVES

After completing this chapter, the reader should be able to

1. List the laboratory tests that may be utilized in the identification of bacteria.
2. Describe the types of clinical specimens that may be analyzed for the presence of bacteria by the use of a Gram's stain.
3. Discuss the processes involved in staining and culturing a specimen for bacterial growth, including the time required to obtain a result from either method. Analyze the clinical utility of the information obtained from a Gram's stain or a culture.
4. Identify bacteria according to gram-stain results (positive vs. negative), morphology (cocci vs. bacilli), and culture growth characteristics (aerobic vs. anaerobic).
5. Define normal flora and identify those anatomic sites where normal flora are commonly present and those sites that are typically considered "sterile." Identify which bacteria are considered normal flora in each of those sites.
6. Given various anatomic sites of infection, distinguish the most likely pathogens responsible for the infection.
7. Describe the common methods used for determining antimicrobial susceptibility with regard to technique, type of result derived, clinical implications, and limitations of each of the methods. Demonstrate the ability to use this information to make clinical decisions with regard to choosing an appropriate antimicrobial regimen for a patient.
8. Discuss how the culture and susceptibility results from clinical isolates from patients in a hospital can be used to construct a hospital-wide antibiogram. Discuss the utility of the antibiogram when choosing empiric antibiotic therapy for a patient's infection.
9. Define MIC, MIC_{50}, MIC_{90}, MIC susceptibility breakpoints, and MBC.
10. Understand the basic methods used to diagnose systemic fungal infections.

11. Discuss the laboratory tests that are commonly utilized in the diagnosis of *Mycobacterium tuberculosis* and nontuberculous mycobacteria.

12. Discuss the laboratory tests that are commonly utilized in the diagnosis of influenza, herpes simplex virus, cytomegalovirus, and respiratory syncytial virus.

13. Discuss the laboratory tests that are commonly utilized in the diagnosis of human immunodeficiency virus (HIV) and determine which laboratory tests may be utilized in the assessment and monitoring of patients infected with HIV.

14. Understand the laboratory tests that may be performed for the diagnosis of infections due to miscellaneous or uncommon organisms such as *Borrelia burgdorferi*, *Treponema pallidum*, *Legionella pneumophila*, and *Pneumocystis carinii*.

15. Distinguish between the different types of laboratory tests that are routinely performed for the diagnosis of infection in
    a. Cerebrospinal fluid (CSF) when meningitis is suspected.
    b. Respiratory secretions when upper or lower respiratory tract infections are suspected.
    c. Urine, prostatic secretions, or genital secretions when a genitourinary tract infection is suspected.
    d. Otherwise sterile fluid when infection is suspected (e.g., synovial and peritoneal).

BACTERIA

Bacteria are small, unicellular, prokaryotic organisms that contain a cell wall but lack a well-defined nucleus. They are a large and diverse group of microorganisms that exist in different shapes and organizations with varying rates of pathogenicity. Bacteria are a very common cause of infection in both the community and hospital setting, and can cause infection in patients with normal or suppressed immune systems. Bacteria must be considered as a causative pathogen in any patient presenting with signs and symptoms of infection.

The Identification of Bacteria

Several factors must be considered when choosing an appropriate antimicrobial regimen for the treatment of a particular infectious disease. These factors include patient characteristics (e.g., immune status, age, and end-organ function), drug characteristics (e.g., spectrum of activity, pharmacokinetics, and penetration to the site of infection), the type of infection that is suspected or known, and information regarding the infecting organism. Therefore, appropriate diagnosis is a key factor in selecting effective antibiotic therapy for the treatment of an infection. In the case of a suspected infection, appropriate culture specimens should be obtained for laboratory testing (if possible) from the suspected site of infection *before* antibiotics are initiated in an attempt to isolate and identify the causative pathogen. Special attention should be placed on specimen collection and timely submission to the laboratory since the accuracy of the results will be limited by

TABLE 17-1

Aqueous/Vitreous Fluid

Abscess or Wound Exudate, Pus or Fluid—swab or aspirate

Blood

Bone Marrow

Body Fluids—amniotic, abdominal, bile, pericardial, peritoneal, pleural, or synovial by needle aspiration

Bone—biopsy of infected area

Cerebrospinal Fluid—by lumbar puncture or directly from shunt

Cutaneous—skin scrapings, aspiration of leading edge of infection; nail scrapings

Ear—middle ear specimen by myringotomy; outer ear specimen by swab

Eye—swab of conjunctiva, corneal scrapings

Foreign Bodies—IV catheter tips by roll plate method; prosthetic heart valves, prosthetic joint material, IUDs, etc.

Gastrointestinal—gastric aspirate for AFB; gastric biopsy for *H. pylori*, rectal swab for VRE, stool cultures

Genital Tract—cervical, endometrial, urethral, vaginal, or prostatic secretions

Respiratory Tract—sputum, tracheal aspirate, bronchoalveolar lavage, swab of nasopharynx or pharynx

Tissue—biopsy specimen

Urine—clean catch midstream specimen, catheterized specimen, suprapubic aspirate

Table 17-1. Common Biologic Specimens Submitted for Culture[1,5]

the quality and condition of the submitted specimen.[1] Table 17-1 lists common biologic specimens that are submitted to a microbiology laboratory for bacteriologic analysis.

When a specimen from the suspected site of infection is submitted to the microbiology laboratory, a number of different microbiologic tests are performed, which will aid in identification of the infecting bacteria. The most common laboratory tests utilized for the identification of bacteria include direct microscopic examination using specialized stains (Gram stain) and growth of the microorganism using culture techniques. Once a bacterium has been identified, antimicrobial susceptibility testing methods are subsequently performed to determine the sensitivity of the infecting organism to antibiotics.

The Gram Stain

The Gram stain is the most common method of staining biological specimens for the microscopic examination of bacteria, with results typically obtained in a matter of minutes. The Gram stain basically classifies bacteria into two large groups, namely gram-positive and gram-negative, based on their reaction to an established series of dyes and decolorizers. The differences in stain uptake between gram-positive and gram-negative bacteria are primarily due to differences in their bacterial cell wall composition and permeability.[2-5] While this stain does not provide an exact identification of the infecting organism (e.g., *Klebsiella pneumoniae* vs. *Serratia marcescens*), it does provide rapid, preliminary information about the organism, which can be used to guide empiric antibiotic therapy while waiting for the results from the bacterial culture. The Gram stain is useful for characterizing most clinically important bacteria but is unable to detect bacteria that exist intracellularly (e.g., *Chlamydia*), those without cell walls (e.g., *Mycoplasma*), or those that are too small to be visualized with light microscopy (spirochetes).[3,4]

The current methodology utilized in the Gram stain of a biological specimen is a slight modification of the original Gram stain process developed by Hans Christian Gram in the late 19th century.[2-5] The Gram stain procedure involves a number of staining and rinsing steps, which can all be performed in a few minutes. First, a thin smear of a biological specimen is applied, dried, and heat-fixed on a clean glass slide. Once the slide has cooled, it is then rinsed with crystal or gentian violet (a purple dye), Gram's iodine, decolorized with an ethanol or acetone rinse, and then counterstained with safranin (a pink or red dye). A gentle, tap water rinse is performed between each of the steps listed above. Lastly, the slide is blotted dry and examined under a microscope using the oil immersion lens. If bacteria are present, they are observed for their uptake of stain, their shape (round = coccus, rod = bacillus), and their organization (e.g., pairs, clusters, etc.). Gram-positive bacteria stain purple due to retention of the crystal violet-iodine complex in their cell walls, while Gram-negative bacteria stain pink or red since they do not retain the crystal violet and are counterstained by safranin.[2,3,5,6] The results of the Gram stain (e.g., gram-positive cocci in pairs or gram-negative rods) are then utilized to help predict the identification of the infecting organism before the culture results become available. Table 17-2 lists the most likely bacteria present based on Gram stain results.[5,7-9] Therefore, the clinician can use the information from the Gram stain to quickly select an empiric antibiotic regimen for the patient directed against the most likely pathogen before the final culture and susceptibility results are known (which may take days). Once the culture and susceptibility results become available, the initial empiric antibiotic regimen can be changed, if necessary, to target the infecting bacteria.

There are also other pieces of valuable information that can be derived from a Gram stain.[1,4-6,8] First, it is an extremely helpful diagnostic test to determine the presence of bacteria in biological specimens obtained from normally sterile body fluids (e.g., CSF, pleural fluid, synovial fluid, and urine directly from the bladder), as well as from specimens where infection is suspected (e.g., abscess fluid, wound swabs, sputum, and tissue).[5,6] The Gram

TABLE 17-2

GRAM STAIN RESULT	LIKELY BACTERIAL PATHOGEN
GRAM-POSITIVE (Stain PURPLE)	
Gram-positive cocci in clusters	***Staphylococcus* sp**. (*S. aureus, S. epidermidis, S. hominis, S. saprophyticus, S. haemolyticus,* etc.)
Gram-positive cocci in pairs	***Streptococcus pneumoniae***
Gram-positive cocci in chains	**Viridans (α-hemolytic) Streptococci** (*S. milleri, S. mutans, S. salivarius, S. mitis*) β-**Hemolytic Streptococci** (*S. pyogenes, S. agalactiae,* Groups C, F, and G streptococcus) ***Peptostreptococcus* sp.**
Gram-positive cocci in pairs & chains	***Enterococcus* sp.** (*E. faecalis, E. faecium, E. durans, E. gallinarum, E. avium, E casseliflavus, E. raffinosus*)
Gram-positive bacilli ***Non-spore-forming***	***Corynebacterium* sp.** (*C. diphtheriae, C. jeikeium, C. striatum,* etc.) ***Lactobacillus* sp.** ***Listeria monocytogenes*** ***Proprionibacterium* sp.** (*P. acnes*)
Spore-forming	***Bacillus* sp.** (*B. anthracis, B. cereus,* etc.) ***Clostridium* sp.** (*C. perfringens, C. difficile, C. tetani*) ***Streptomyces* sp.**
Branching, filamentous	***Actinomyces* sp.** (*A. israelii*) ***Erysipelothrix rhusiopathiae*** ***Nocardia* sp.** (*N. asteroides,* etc.)
GRAM-NEGATIVE (Stain RED)	
Gram-negative cocci	***Neisseria* sp.** (*N. gonorrhoeae, N. meningitidis,* etc.) ***Veillonella* sp.**
Gram-negative coccobacilli	***Haemophilus* sp.** (*H. influenzae, H. parainfluenzae, H. ducreyi,* etc.) ***Moraxella catarrhalis***
Gram-negative bacilli ***Lactose-fermenting***	***Escherichia coli*** ***Klebsiella pneumoniae*** ***Enterobacter* sp.** (*E. cloacae, E. aerogenes*) ***Citrobacter* sp.** (*C. freundii, C. koseri*) ***Aeromonas hydrophila*** ***Pasteurella multocida*** ***Vibrio cholerae***
Non-lactose-fermenting	***Pseudomonas* sp.** (*P. aeruginosa, P. putida, P. fluorescens*) ***Proteus* sp.** (*P. mirabilis, P. vulgaris*) ***Serratia marcescens*** ***Morganella morganii*** ***Salmonella* sp.** (*S. typhi, S. paratyphi, S. enteritidis, S. typhimurium*) ***Shigella* sp.** (*S. dysenteriae, S. sonnei*) ***Stenotrophomonas maltophilia*** ***Acinetobacter* sp.** ***Alcaligenes* sp.** ***Burkholderia cepacia***
Other gram-negative bacilli	***Helicobacter pylori*** ***Campylobacter jejuni*** ***Bacteroides* sp.** (*B. fragilis, B. thetaiotamicron, B. ovatus, B. disastonis*) ***Brucella* sp.** ***Bordetella* sp.** ***Francisella***
GRAM-VARIABLE (Stain both gram-positive and gram-negative in the same smear)	
Gram-variable bacilli	***Gardnerella vaginalis***

Table 17-2. Preliminary Identification of Medically Important Bacteria Using Gram Stain Results[5,7–9]

stain can also demonstrate the presence of white blood cells; the number or relative quantity of infecting bacteria; and the adequacy of the submitted specimen (e.g., large numbers of epithelial cells in a sputum or urine sample may signify contamination).[1,3–6]

Culture and Identification

The results derived from the Gram stain provide only preliminary information regarding the potential infecting bacteria. In order for the bacteria to be definitively identified, the clinical specimen must also be processed to facilitate bacterial growth in culture and then observed for growth characteristics (e.g., type of media, aerobic vs. anaerobic, and shape and color of colonies) and reactions to biochemical testing. Under normal circumstances, the results of a bacterial culture are typically available within 24–48 hr of specimen set-up and processing.

In order for a bacteria to be grown successfully in culture, the specific nutritional and environmental growth requirements of the bacteria must be taken into consideration.[5,9,10] There are several clinical microbiology textbooks and reference manuals available that can assist the laboratory in selecting the appropriate culture media and environmental conditions (to facilitate the optimal growth of bacteria based on specimen type and suspected bacteria).[5,10–12]

Different types of primary culture media are available and can be used to enhance or optimize bacterial growth, namely, nutritive media (blood or chocolate agar), differential media, selective media, and supplemental broth.[1,5,9,10] The most commonly utilized bacterial growth media are listed in Table 17-3. Blood and chocolate agar plates are *nutritive* media in that they support the growth of many different types of bacteria, both aerobic and anaerobic.

GROWTH MEDIUM	COMPOSITION	USES
Agars		
Blood Agar (SBA)	5% Sheep Blood	The most commonly used all-purpose medium with ability to grow most bacteria, fungi, and some mycobacteria. It is also used for determination of hemolytic reactions.
Chocolate Agar	2% hemoglobin or Iso VitaleX in peptone base	All-purpose medium that supports growth of most bacteria. Especially useful for growth of *Haemophilus sp.* and pathogenic *Neisseria sp.*
Eosin Methylene Blue (EMB) Agar or MacConkey Agar (Mac)	Peptone base with sugars and dyes that yield differentiating biochemical characteristics	Typically included in primary set-up of nonsterile specimens. Selective isolation of gram-negative bacteria, and differentiation between those that are lactose-fermenting and non-lactose fermenting.
Phenylethyl Alcohol Agar (PEA) or Colistin-Nalidixic Acid Agar (CNA)	Nutrient agar bases with supplemental agents to inhibit growth of gram-negative bacteria.	Typically included in primary set-up of nonsterile specimens. Selective solation of gram-positive cocci.
Broths		
Trypticase Soy Broth (TSB)	All purpose enrichment broth.	Used for subculturing bacteria grown on agar plates. Supports the growth of many fastidious and nonfastidious bacteria.
Thioglycollate Broth	Pancreatic digest of casein, soy broth, and glucose.	Supports the growth of aerobic, anaerobic, microaerophilic, and fastidious bacteria.

TABLE 17-3

Table 17-3. Some Commonly Used Bacterial Growth Media[1,5,9,10]

Blood agar is also a *differential* media in that it is also able to distinguish between the different types of hemolysis for streptococci. MacConkey, EMB, CNA, and PEA agar plates are all *selective* media because they preferentially support the growth of one group of organisms (e.g., gram-negative or gram-positive bacteria). Trypticase soy broth (TSB) and thioglycollate broth are considered *supplemental* broths since they are used for subculturing bacteria detected on agar plates or as back-up cultures to agar plates for the detection of small numbers of bacteria in some biological specimens.

Once specimens are processed in appropriate media, the plates must be then incubated in the appropriate environment to support bacterial growth. The environmental factors that should be controlled include oxygen or carbon dioxide content, temperature, pH, and moisture content of the medium and atmosphere.[1,10] Different bacteria have different oxygen requirements for growth. Strict *aerobic* bacteria grow best in ambient air which contains 21% oxygen and a small amount of carbon dioxide (e.g., *Pseudomonas aeruginosa* and *Staphylococcus aureus*.).[1] Strict *anaerobes* are unable to grow in an oxygen-containing environment and require a controlled environment containing 5–10% carbon dioxide for optimal growth (e.g., *Bacteroides sp.*). Facultative anaerobes can grow in the presence or absence of oxygen (e.g., *Escherichia coli* and some streptococci). In addition, most clinically relevant bacteria grow best at a temperature of 35–37 °C (the temperature of the human body), at a pH of 6.5–7.5, and in an atmosphere rich in moisture (agar plates are sealed to trap moisture).[10]

When bacteria are successfully grown in culture, they appear as colonies on agar plates. Tests that are performed to identify the bacteria include the initial evaluation of colony characteristics (size, pigmentation, shape, and surface appearance); the assessment of culture media and environmental conditions which supported the growth of the bacteria; the changes that occurred to the culture media as a result of bacterial growth; the aroma of the bacteria; a Gram stain of individual colonies; and biochemical tests directed at the most likely bacteria.[9,10,13] Biochemical tests can be enzyme-based, where the presence of a specific enzyme is measured (e.g., catalase, oxidase, indole, or urease tests), or based on the presence and measurement of metabolic pathways or byproducts (e.g., oxidative and fermentation tests or amino acid degradation).[9,13] Results that may be derived from biochemical tests include the presence of catalase as an enzyme in the organism or the ability of a bacteria to ferment glucose. Most biochemical tests are now performed using manual or automated commercial identification systems.[13-15] Some of the commercial identification systems consist of multicompartment biochemical tests in a single microtiter tray and allow several biochemical tests to be performed at once.[13-15] The information derived from the macroscopic examination of the bacteria and the results of biochemical tests are then combined to determine the specific identity of the bacteria.

Contamination, Colonization, or Infection

The growth of an organism from a submitted biologic specimen does not always indicate the presence of infection but may represent the presence of bacterial contamination or colonization.[6,8] Some areas of the human body are sterile and should not contain bacteria under any circumstances. These sites are listed in Table 17-4 and include the bloodstream, the cerebrospinal fluid, bone, synovial fluid, etc. There are other body sites, however, that contain a number of microorganisms called *normal flora* that naturally *colonize* their surfaces. Normal bacterial flora can be found on the skin and in the respiratory, gastrointestinal, and genitourinary tracts. The bacteria that typically colonize these body sites are listed in Table 17-5. Normal flora can be located in the same areas of the body as pathogenic bacteria and may provide some benefit by competing with pathogenic bacteria for nutrients, suppressing the growth of potentially patho-

TABLE 17-4

**Bloodstream
Cerebrospinal Fluid
Pericardial Fluid
Pleural Fluid
Peritoneal Fluid
Synovial Fluid
Bone
Urine (directly from the bladder)**

Table 17-4. Normally Sterile Body Sites

genic bacteria and fungi, and stimulating the production of cross-protective antibodies.[8,16] Typically, normal flora are harmless bacteria that rarely cause infection. However, these bacteria may potentially become pathogenic and cause infection in some circumstances, such as in patients with impaired host defenses, or after the translocation of normal flora bacteria to other body sites and tissues during trauma, intravascular line insertion, or surgical procedures (when skin is not adequately cleansed). In addition, *colonization* may also occur with pathogenic bacteria when they inhabit body sites but do not invade tissue, and, hence, they do not cause the signs and symptoms of infection that are listed in Table 17-6.

Skin	Respiratory Tract
Corynebacterium sp.	Viridans streptococci
Proprionibacterium sp.	Anaeroobic streptococci
Staphylococcus sp.	*Haemophilus* sp.
(especially coagulase-negative	*Neisseria* sp.
staphylococci)	
Streptococcus sp.	
Gastrointestinal Tract	**Genital Tract**
Bacteroides sp.	*Lactobacillus* sp.
Clostridium sp.	*Streptococcus* sp.
Escherichia coli	*Staphylococcus* sp.
Klebsiella pneumoniae	*Mycoplasma*
Enterococcus sp.	*Corynebacterium* sp.
Anaerobic streptococci	

Table 17-5. Body Sites with Normal Colonizing Bacterial Flora[8,16]

Contamination occurs when a bacteria is accidentally introduced into a biologic specimen of a patient during specimen collection or processing.[8] Bacteria that cause contamination typically originate from the skin of the patient (especially if not cleansed adequately), the clinician, or the microbiology laboratory technician, but may also come from the environment. A common biologic specimen contaminant is *Staphylococcus epidermidis*, which is an organism that can normally colonize the skin. In addition, the presence of normal vaginal or perirectal flora in the urine culture of a patient without evidence of a urinary tract infection (absence of symptoms or white blood cells) may also be indicative of contamination. In select circumstances, however, these organisms can also cause infection.

Infection occurs when a pathogen invades and damages host tissues, eliciting a host response and symptoms consistent with an infectious process. There are several factors that should be considered when diagnosing the presence of infection, such as the clinical condition of the patient (e.g., fever and purulent discharge), the presence of laboratory signs of infection (e.g., high white blood cell count), and the results of microbiologic cultures.[6] Table 17-6 describes the clinical signs and symptoms and laboratory findings that may be present in a patient with infection.

The diagnosis of infection is usually suspected in a patient with a positive culture from a normally sterile site or a positive culture from a normally nonsterile site—the definitive diagnosis is typically made when the positive culture is accompanied by clinical and laboratory findings suggestive of infection. In clinical practice, there are several situations that may occur that will warrant a thorough investigation to determine if the patient with a positive culture from a biologic specimen is truly infected. Since false-positive cultures can be associated with the use of additional laboratory tests and unnecessary antibiotics, as well as increased length of hospitalization and patient costs, every positive culture result should warrant an evaluation for clinical significance.[17] Since it is known that certain bacteria have a propensity to commonly cause infection in particular body sites and fluids (see Table 17-7), the clinician can determine

CLINICAL
Localized
Pain and Inflammation at site of infection—erythema, swelling, warmth
Purulent discharge (wound, vaginal, urethral discharge)
Sputum production and cough
Diarrhea
Skin lesions
Systemic
Fever
Malaise
Chills, rigors
Tachycardia
Tachypnea
Hypotension
Mental status changes

LABORATORY
Increased white blood cell (WBC) count—occasionally with increase in immature neutrophils (bands or stabs) called a "shift to the left"
Positive gram stain and/or culture from site of infection
Elevated erythrocyte sedimentation rate (ESR) or C-reactive protein
Positive antigen or antibody titers

Table 17-6. Clinical and Laboratory Signs of Infection[8]

TABLE 17-7

Mouth	**Skin & Soft Tissue**	**Bone & Joint**
Peptococcus sp.	*Staphylococcus aureus*	*Staphylococcus aureus*
Peptostreptococcus sp.	*Streptococcus pyogenes*	*Streptococcus pyogenes*
Actinomyces israelii	*Staphylococcus epidermidis*	*Streptococcus* sp.
Treponema pallidum	*Pasteurella multocida*	*Staphylococcus epidermidis*
	Clostridium sp.	*Neisseria gonorrhoeae*
		Gram-negative bacilli
Abdominal	**Urinary Tract**	**Upper Respiratory Tract**
Escherichia coli	*Escherichia coli*	*Streptococcus pneumoniae*
Proteus mirabilis	*Proteus mirabilis*	*Haemophilus influenzae*
Klebsiella sp.	*Klebsiella* sp.	*Moraxella catarrhalis*
Enterococcus sp.	*Enterococcus* sp.	*Streptococcus pyogenes*
Bacteroides sp	*Staphylococcus saprophyticus*	
Clostridium sp.		
Lower Respiratory Tract Community Acquired	**Lower Respiratory Tract Hospital Acquired**	**Meningitis**
Streptococcus pneumoniae	*Klebsiella pneumoniae*	*Streptococcus pneumoniae*
Haemophilus influenzae	*Pseudomonas aeruginosa*	*Neisseria meningitidis*
Moraxella catarrhalis	*Enterobacter* sp.	*Haemophilus influenzae*
Klebsiella pneumoniae	*Citrobacter* sp.	Group B streptococcus
Legionella pneumophila	*Serratia marcescens*	*Escherichia coli*
Mycoplasma pneumoniae	*Acinetobacter* sp.	*Listeria monocytogenes*
Chlamydia pneumoniae	*Staphylococcus aureus*	

Table 17-7. Common Pathogens by Site of Infection[16,18]

if the bacteria isolated in culture is a common pathogen at the particular site of infection.[16,18] For instance, the growth of *Streptococcus pneumoniae* in a patient with signs and symptoms of pneumonia is a significant finding. However, the growth of *Staphylococcus epidermidis* in the cultures (e.g., from the bloodstream or wound) of any hospitalized patient should be evaluated for clinical significance as a true pathogen since it may be a contaminant of the submitted specimens.[8] The information in Table 17-7 can also be used to help guide empiric antibiotic therapy before culture results are available if the clinician chooses an antibiotic with activity against the most common causative bacteria at that site of infection, as illustrated in Minicase 1.

Occasionally, patients with infection may have negative cultures as can be seen in the setting of previous antibiotic use, improper culture methods, or the submission of inadequate specimens. Again, the clinical condition of the patient may establish the presence of infection despite negative cultures.[6]

Antimicrobial Susceptibility Testing

Once an organism has been cultured from a biologic specimen, further testing is performed in the microbiology laboratory to determine the antibiotic susceptibility of the patient-specific infecting organism to help direct and streamline antibiotic therapy. Due to the emergence of bacterial resistance in many organisms, bacterial susceptibility testing is extremely useful in determining which antimicrobial agents could potentially be used for the treatment of the infection. There are a number of different methods that can be utilized to determine the susceptibility of a particular organism to various antibiotics. These methods can either (1) directly measure the activity of an antibiotic against the organism or (2) detect the presence of a specific resistance mechanism in the organism, as outlined in Table 17-8.[19] Microbiology labs often utilize several different methods for susceptibility testing in order to accurately determine the activity of an antibiotic against many different types of bacteria (e.g., aerobic, anaerobic, and fastidious). The National Committee for Clinical Laboratory Standards continuously updates and publishes standards and guidelines for the susceptibility

V. A., A 79-YEAR-OLD MALE, was admitted to the University Hospital from home with a temperature of 102.5 °F, chills, a productive cough, and tachypnea. His physical exam is significant for an increase respiratory rate of 24 breaths/min and decreased breath sounds in the left lower lobe. His laboratory results reveal a total white blood cell count of 16,000 cells/mm³ (4800–10,800 cells/mm³) with 80% polymorphonuclear (PMN) leukocytes (45–73%), 15% bands (3–5%), and 5% lymphs (20–40%). His chest x-ray displays left lower lobe consolidation consistent with pneumonia. The differential diagnosis includes bacterial pneumonia, and a sputum sample is obtained for a Gram stain and culture to hopefully isolate the causative organism. The Gram stain results reveal many white blood cells, few epithelial cells, and many gram-positive cocci in pairs. The physician taking care of the patient asks you to recommend empiric antibiotic therapy to treat this patient's pneumonia before the final culture results are available.

Question: What is the most likely causative organism of this patient's pneumonia, and which empiric antibiotic therapy would you choose based on the gram stain results?

Discussion: This patient most likely has community-acquired pneumonia. The most common causative organisms (Table 17-7) of community-acquired lower respiratory tract infections include *Streptococcus pneumoniae, Haemophilus influenzae, Moraxella catarrhalis*, and atypical bacteria such as *Legionella pneumophila*. Based on the gram stain results (Table 17-2), this patient most likely has community-acquired pneumonia due to *Streptococcus pneumoniae* (which is the most common cause of community-acquired pneumonia overall). Empiric antibiotic therapy should have excellent activity against *Streptococcus pneumoniae* and could include regimens such as ceftriaxone or levofloxacin (since they have activity against >96% of organisms). The antibiotic regimen can be changed to more directed therapy, if possible, once the results of the culture and susceptibility are available.

---

testing of aerobic and anaerobic bacteria, which can assist the microbiology laboratory in determining which specific test and antibiotics should be utilized in a particular situation or against a particular organism.[9,19–23]

Methods that Directly Measure Antibiotic Activity

There are several different tests utilizing various methods that can be used to measure the activity of an antibiotic against a particular bacterium. There are quantitative tests that measure the exact concentration of an antibiotic necessary for inhibiting the growth of the bacteria, as well as qualitative methods that provide an assessment of the comparative activity of several antibiotics against the organism. It is important to note that the test results from each of these methods will be reported based on the methodology that was utilized by the susceptibility test. The advantages and disadvantages of each method are listed in Table 17-9.

Dilution Methods (Macrodilution and Microdilution)

Several dilution methods are available to measure the antibiotic susceptibility of an organism. Broth dilution and agar dilution are both quantitative in vitro measures of the activity of an antibiotic against a particular organism. The main differences between broth

TABLE 17-8

METHODS THAT DIRECTLY MEASURE ANTIBIOTIC ACTIVITY

Dilution Susceptibility Tests—broth macrodilution (tube dilution), broth microdilution, agar dilution
Disk Diffusion—Kirby Bauer
Antibiotic Concentration Gradient Methods—epsilometer test (E-test), spiral gradient endpoint test
Other Specialized Tests:
• *Measure Bactericidal Activity*—minimum bactericidal concentration (MBC) testing, time-kill studies, serum bactericidal test (SBT)
• *Susceptibility Testing of Antibiotic Concentrations (Synergy Testing)*—checkerboard technique, time-kill curve technique, disk diffusion, E-test

METHODS THAT DETECT PRESENCE OF ANTIBIOTIC RESISTANCE MECHANISM

Beta-Lactamase Detection
Detection of High Level Aminoglycoside Resistance (HLAR)
Agar Screens to Detect Methicillin-Resistant Staphylococcus aureus (MRSA) or Vancomycin Resistant Enterococcus (VRE)
Chloramphenicol Acetyltransferase Detection
Molecular Methods Involving Nucleic Acid Hybridization and Amplification

Table 17-8. Antimicrobial Susceptibility Testing Methods[6,8,19,21,27–29]

TABLE 17-9

METHOD	ADVANTAGES	DISADVANTAGES
Broth Macrodilution (Tube Dilution)	An exact MIC is generated The MBC can also be determined, if desired	Each antibiotic is tested individually Method is labor and resource intensive
Broth Microdilution (Automated)	Simultaneously tests several antibiotics at the same time Utilizes less labor and resources Commercially-prepared trays or cards can be used	MIC range (rather than exact MIC) is typically reported Antibiotics and concentrations within the cassettes, trays or cards are predetermined
Agar Dilution	An exact MIC is generated Can test a number of isolates simultaneously on the same plate at a relatively low cost Able to test fastidious bacteria since agar supports their growth	Very time consuming Antibiotic plates need to be prepared manually when needed, and can only be stored for short periods of time Plates are not commercially-available, must be made by the lab
Disk Diffusion (Kirby-Bauer)	Simultaneously tests several antibiotics	Exact MICs cannot be determined Cannot use for fastidious or slow-growing bacteria
E-test	An exact MIC is derived Easy to perform Several antibiotics can be tested on the same plate	Relatively expensive Only certain antibiotics are available as E-test strips
Spiral Gradient Endpoint Test	An exact MIC is derived Easy to perform	Relatively expensive Can only test one antibiotic at a time Plates are not commercially available; must be made by the lab

Table 17-9. Advantages and Disadvantages of the Different Antimicrobial Susceptibility Testing Methods[6,8,19,24–26]

macrodilution and broth microdilution are the volume of broth in which the test is performed, the number of antibiotics that can be tested at the same time, and the manner in which the test results are generated and reported. Agar dilution differs in that it is performed in solid growth media.

Broth macrodilution. Broth macrodilution, or the tube-dilution method, is one of the oldest methods of susceptibility testing and is often considered the gold standard. This method is performed in test tubes in which twofold serial dilutions of the antibiotic being tested (based on achievable serum concentrations in µg/mL) are placed in a liquid growth medium ($\geq$1 mL of broth) to which a standard inoculum (5×10^5 cfu/mL) of the infecting bacteria is added.[19,20,22,24,25] The tests tubes are incubated for 24 hr at 35 °C and then examined macroscopically for the presence of turbidity or cloudiness, which is an indication of bacterial growth.[8,19,22,24,25] The first test tube that appears clear to the unaided eye signifies the lowest antibiotic concentration (in µg/mL), which completely inhibited visible bacterial growth—the concentration in that test tube is then recorded as the Minimum Inhibitory Concentration or MIC (Figure 17-1).[19,22,24,25]

The NCCLS has established interpretive criteria for the MIC results of each bacteria and each antibiotic as *Susceptible*, *Intermediate*, and *Resistant* based on the achievable serum concentrations of the antibiotic after normal dosing, the inherent susceptibility of the organism to the antibiotic, the site of infection, and the results of efficacy trials of the antibiotic against infections due to that organism.[9,19–22,26] The exact MIC concentrations that separate these susceptibility categories are known as *MIC breakpoints*.[19,21,26] The categorization of the MICs as susceptible, intermediate, and resistant is primarily done to help predict the probable response of a patient's infection to a particular antibiotic.[6,21,24,25] Bacteria that are categorized as

"*Susceptible*" to a given antibiotic will, most likely, be eradicated during treatment of the infection, since concentrations of the antibiotic represented by the MIC are easily achieved using standard doses of the antibiotic. "*Intermediately*" susceptible bacteria display higher MICs, and successful treatment may be achieved if higher than normal doses of an antibiotic are utilized. There are rare circumstances in clinical practice where an antibiotic displaying intermediate susceptibility against an organism would be used for treatment of the infection since clinical response is unpredictable. Lastly, organisms that are "*Resistant*" to an antibiotic display extremely high MICs that exceed the achievable serum concentrations of the antibiotic (even if maximal doses are utilized) so that a poor clinical response would be expected.

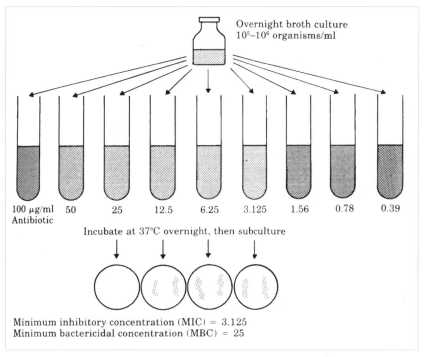

Figure 17-1. Broth macrodilution susceptibility testing for MIC and MBC. (Reprinted, with permission, from Reference 6.)

An additional step can be performed to the MIC determination of broth macrodilution to determine the actual antibiotic concentration that kills 99.9% of the bacterial inoculum (the Minimum Bactericidal Concentration or MBC).[19,27,29] All of the test tubes that did not exhibit visible growth from the MIC determination are subcultured on agar plates and incubated at 35 °C for 24 hr (Figure 17-1).[6,8,27] The plate containing the lowest antibiotic concentration that does not display any bacterial colonies is defined as the MBC. Because a higher concentration of an antibiotic may be necessary to kill the organism rather than just inhibit its growth, the MIC is always equal to or lower than the MBC. The determination of the MBC is not a routine microbiologic test, and there are only rare clinical circumstances in which it may be performed to provide additional information, such as in the treatment of severe or life-threatening infections including endocarditis, meningitis, osteomyelitis, or sepsis in immunocompromised patients.[6,8,19,27–29]

Broth macrodilution is very useful because an exact MIC (and, if needed, an MBC) of the infecting organism can be derived. The test results of broth macrodilution are often reported as the MIC of the antibiotic against the infecting organism with its corresponding interpretive category (susceptible, intermediate, or resistant). Today, broth macrodilution is rarely utilized in microbiology laboratories since the methodology is very resource and labor intensive which makes it impractical for every day use.

Broth microdilution. Broth microdilution susceptibility testing was developed in response to the limitations of the broth macrodilution method and has become the most commonly used method for susceptibility testing of bacteria in microbiology labs.[8,19,22,24,25] Instead of utilizing standard test tubes with twofold serial dilutions of antibiotics, this method utilizes manually or commercially-prepared disposable microtiter cassettes or trays that contain as many as 96 wells, which can test the susceptibility of up to 12 antibiotics at the same time (depending on the product used).[8,19,22,24,25] The wells in the broth microdilution trays contain a small volume of broth (0.05–0.1 mL) to support bacterial growth, as opposed to 1.0 mL or more utilized in the macrodilution method. The microtiter tray is inoculated with a standardized bacterial suspension of the infecting organism and incubated for 16–20 hr. The tray is then examined for bacterial growth by direct visualization (utilizing light boxes

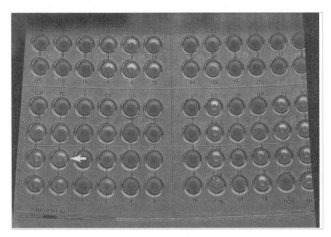

Figure 17-2 (a). Examples of microdilution trays. (Reprinted, with permission, from Reference 19.)

or reflecting mirrors) or computer-assisted readers (automated). The MIC is reported as the lowest antibiotic concentration that did not produce turbidity (e.g., lowest concentration that inhibited visible growth). Several examples of microtiter trays are displayed in Figure 17-2a and 17-2b. There are a number of companies that currently supply preprepared broth microdilution panels including BD Microbiology Systems, AccuMed, and Pasco Laboratories.[19] The most commonly used automated microdilution susceptibility systems are Vitek, Vitek-2, and the Microscan Walkaway System. These systems have also been engineered to help identify bacteria, and often provide rapid susceptibility results within 3–5 hr due to shortened incubation times.[26]

Because of the size constraints of microtiter cassettes, only certain antibiotics and certain concentrations of the antibiotics are incorporated into the trays. Typically, drugs that have inherent activity against the class of bacteria being tested (e.g., gram-positive vs. gram-negative) are included in the trays, and the concentrations incorporated into the wells for each antibiotic concentrations reflect their NCCLS susceptibility breakpoints for the particular organism. For example, when determining the susceptibility of gram-negative bacteria, it is impractical to include antibiotics in the microtiter trays that do not have activity against gram-negative organisms, such as penicillin, nafcillin, or vancomycin. The same holds true for susceptibility testing of gram-positive organisms (e.g., it would be impractical to test the susceptibility of piperacillin or ceftazidime against *Staphylococcus aureus* because these agents have limited antistaphylococcal activity). Microbiology laboratories should consult NCCLS guidelines and standards for guidance in the appropriate testing and reporting of antimicrobial susceptibilities.

The test results of broth microdilution are often expressed as an MIC range ($\leq$ or $\geq$ to a particular MIC) because of the limited antibiotic concentrations that can be tested for each antibiotic. If bacterial growth, for example, is not detected in the lowest concentration tested of a particular agent, the MIC would be reported as less than or equal to that concentration tested. The MIC could be much lower, but an exact MIC sometimes cannot be determined by this method because it does not incorporate all antibiotic concentrations in the wells of the microtiter cassettes. As in broth macrodilution, the test results for broth microdilution will be expressed as the MIC (or MIC range) of the antibiotic against the infecting bacteria with its corresponding interpretive category (susceptible, intermediate, or resistant).

The advantages of broth microdilution include the ability to test the susceptibility of multiple antibiotics at the same time; ease of use when commercially-prepared microtiter trays are utilized; generation of an exact MIC susceptibility result in some circumstances; rapid result reporting with some of the automated methods; and decreased cost and la-

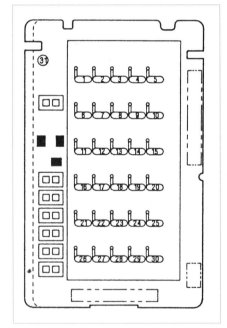

Figure 17-2 (b). Example of microtiter cassette used in automated systems that test for bacterial susceptibilities to various antimicrobials. (Reprinted with permission, from Vitek Systems. Insert No.012416. Hazelwood, MO: Vitek Systems, McDonnell Douglas; 1988.)

bor.[19,22,26] The disadvantages of broth microdilution include the lack of flexibility of antibiotics that are available in the commercially-prepared microtiter cassettes; the limitation on the number of antibiotic concentrations that can be tested due to size constraints of the trays; and the occasional reporting of an MIC range rather than the true MIC against an infecting organism.[8,19,24,26]

Agar dilution. Agar dilution is another quantitative susceptibility testing method that utilizes 2-fold serial dilutions of an antibiotic. Instead of being placed into test tubes or microtiter trays, the different antibiotic concentrations are incorporated into an agar growth medium and placed into individual petri dishes.[19,24–26] The surface of each plate is then inoculated with a droplet of standardized bacterial suspension (1×10^4 cfu/mL) and incubated for 18–20 hr at 35 °C. The susceptibility of several different bacteria can be evaluated simultaneously on these plates. The MIC is represented by the plate with the lowest concentration of antibiotic that does not support visible growth of the bacteria. The advantages of agar dilution include the ability to simultaneously test a number of different bacteria; the ability to perform susceptibility testing of fastidious organisms since the agar is able to adequately support bacterial growth; and the results of the test yield an exact MIC of the infecting bacteria. However, agar dilution is not commonly utilized in most microbiology labs because it is resource and labor intensive. In addition, the antibiotic plates are not commercially available and need to be prepared before each test since they can only be stored for short periods of time.[19,24–26]

Disk Diffusion Method (Kirby-Bauer)

The disk diffusion method is a well-standardized and highly reproducible qualitative method for antimicrobial susceptibility testing. The method was developed by Kirby and Bauer in 1966 (before broth microdilution) in response to the need for a more practical susceptibility test capable of measuring the susceptibility of multiple antibiotics at the same time.[19,23–26] Commercially prepared, filter paper disks impregnated with a fixed concentration of an antibiotic are placed on solid media agar plates that have been inoculated with a standardized inoculum of the infecting organism ($1–2 \times 10^8$ cfu/mL). The plates are large enough to accommodate up to 12 disks (representing 12 different antibiotics) at the same time (see Figure 17-3). The plate is then incubated for 16–18 hr in ambient air at 35 °C. During this incubation time, the antibiotic diffuses out of the disk into the surrounding media (with the highest concentration closest to the disk) as the bacteria multiply on the surface of the plates.[19,25] The bacteria will only grow in areas on the plate where the concentrations of the antibiotic are too low to inhibit bacterial growth. At the end of incubation period, the plates are examined for the inhibition of bacterial growth by measuring the diameter (in millimeters) of the clear zone of inhibition surrounding each filter paper disk. In general, the larger zones of inhibition generally indicate a more active antibiotic against the organism.

The diameter of the zone of inhibition is inversely correlated to the approximate MIC of the antibiotic against the infecting organism.[19,23,26] The NCCLS has developed interpretive criteria based on this relationship to categorize certain zone diameters as susceptible, intermediate, and resistant for each drug and each organism.[5,23] Subsequently, the results of the disk diffusion test are considered qualitative because the report will reveal the category of susceptibility of the antibiotic against the infecting organism rather than an MIC.[24]

The disk diffusion susceptibility test allows the simultaneous testing of a number of antibiotics in a relatively easy and inexpensive manner and also provides flexibility in determining exactly which antibiotics will be included in the susceptibility testing (if a filter paper disk is available). However, the major disadvantages include the inability to generate an exact MIC and the difficulty in determining the susceptibility of fastidious or slow-growing organisms.

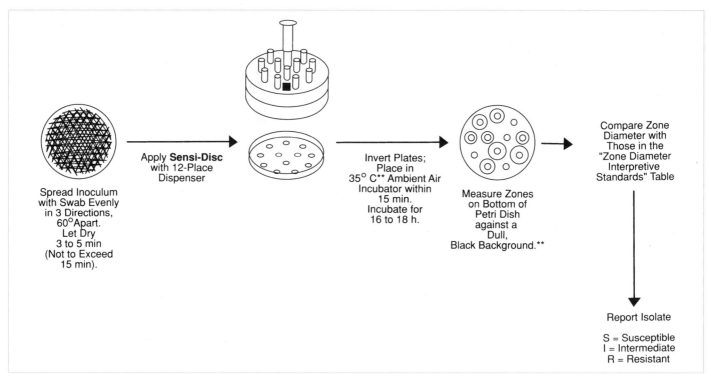

Figure 17-3. Example of a disk diffusion susceptibility test. Typical susceptibility testing using the disk diffusion method. The diameter of zones of growth inhibition around each disk is measured and compared with standards to determine the degree of susceptibility. Additional steps may be performed for methicillin-resistant S. aureus isolates. (Adapted, with permission, from Power DA, McCuen PJ, eds. *Manual of BBL Products and Laboratory Procedures*. Cockeysville, MD: Becton Dickinson Microbiology Systems; 1988: 69.)

Antibiotic Concentration Gradient Methods

Epsilometer test. The Epsilometer test or E-test (AB Biodisk, Solna, Sweden) is a relatively new susceptibility test that combines the benefits of broth microdilution with the ease of disk diffusion.[8,25] The E-test method allows the simultaneous testing of several different concentrations of a single antibiotic on one plastic strip so that an exact MIC can be determined. The plastic strips, called E-test strips, are manufactured by AB Biodisk and are impregnated on one side with a known, prefixed concentration gradient of an antibiotic. The other side of the E-test strip is marked with a numeric scale which depicts the concentration of antibiotic at that location on the reverse side of the test strip.[5,6,19,24,25] Like disk diffusion, the E-test strip is applied onto a solid media agar plate that has been inoculated with a standardized concentration of the infecting bacteria. Several E-test strips can actually be placed on the same agar plate providing simultaneous susceptibility testing of a number of antibiotics.[6,19,24,25] During overnight incubation, bacteria multiply on the agar plates as the antibiotic diffuses out of the E-test strip according to the concentration gradient. Bacterial growth will only occur in areas on the agar plate where drug concentrations are below those required to inhibit growth. An elliptical zone of growth inhibition will form around the E-test strip, and the MIC is read as the drug concentration where the ellipse intersects the plastic strip (see Figures 17-4 and 17-5).[5,19]

The results derived from the E-test are reported as the MIC of the infecting bacteria and the susceptibility interpretation and appear to correlate well with those obtained from other susceptibility testing methods.[6,19,24,26] The E-test method is useful in that the susceptibility of several antibiotics can be tested at the same time; an exact MIC of the infecting bacteria can be determined; the laboratory can choose the antibiotics to be tested; and it is easy to perform. However, the E-test is considerably more expensive than disk diffusion and is limited to testing only those antibiotics in which an E-test strip is commercially available.

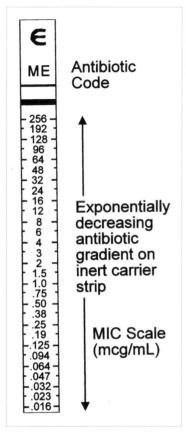

Figure 17-4. Diagram of E test strip and gradient.

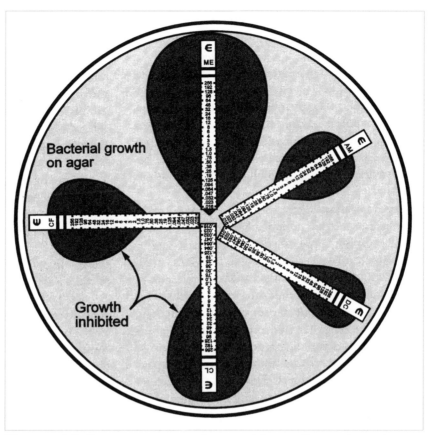

Figure 17-5. E-test strips on agar showing inhibition of bacterial growth.

The E-test is currently used in many labs for the susceptibility testing of fastidious bacteria (e.g., *Streptococcus pneumoniae, Haemophilus influenzae*, and anaerobes) or for those bacteria in which a routine susceptibility test is not available and an MIC result is preferred.[6,24,26]

Spiral gradient endpoint test. The Spiral Gradient Endpoint test (SGE, Spiral Biotech, Norwood, MA) is another antibiotic gradient diffusion test that utilizes agar plates containing a continuous radial concentration gradient of antibiotic in the agar from the center of the plate (where the concentration is the highest) to the edge of the plate (where the concentration is the lowest).[6,26] The plates are not commercially available but can be made by individual labs with specialized equipment. The infecting bacteria is then deposited onto the agar as a radial streak (up to 15 streaks of the bacterial suspension are applied per plate) and incubated. The MIC is determined by measuring the radial distance of the growth transition endpoint from the center of the plate. This measurement is used to compute the concentration of antibiotic at that particular location (which is the MIC).[6,26] Relatively easy to perform, this method generates an exact MIC of the infecting bacteria. However, it is relatively expensive, can only test the susceptibility of one organism and antibiotic at a time, and requires the use of specialized equipment. Therefore, it is not routinely used by most microbiology labs.

Other Specialized Susceptibility Tests

There are a number of other tests that may be performed in the microbiology lab to provide further information on the activity of an antibiotic against an infecting organism. These specialty susceptibility tests may measure the bactericidal activity of the antibiotic (e.g., MBC testing, serum bactericidal tests, and time-kill curves) or may measure the activity of two or more antibiotics in combination against an infecting organism (e.g., checkerboard technique and time-kill). None of these tests, however, are routinely performed in most labs due to potential technical difficulties, complexity in the interpretation of the results, and uncertain clinical applicability.[19, 27–29,30]

Tests measuring bactericidal activity. Several different methods can be used to measure the direct killing activity of an antibiotic against an organism. As noted earlier, there are only a limited number of clinical circumstances where this information may be useful. The information regarding the ability of an antibiotic to kill an organism is probably most useful in the treatment of infections where host defenses are poor or absent, such as in the treatment of endocarditis, meningitis, and life-threatening infections in immunocompromised patients.[6,19,27–29,30]

The MBC (minimum bactericidal concentration) is one test that can be performed to determine the minimum concentration of an antibiotic needed to kill 99.9% of a bacterial inoculum. This methodology and the results derived from this test have been previously described in detail in the section on Broth Macrodilution or Tube Dilution. In the MBC test, a lower number represents better activity against the infecting organism.

The *time-kill study/curve* is another test that may be used to determine the bactericidal activity of an antibiotic. This test allows the measurement of the rate of bacterial killing over time, as opposed to the MBC, which measures the bacterial killing of an agent after a specified amount of time.[19,29,30] A standardized bacterial inoculum is grown in broth and exposed to several concentrations of an antibiotic (usually the MIC and multiples of the MIC). Samples of the antibiotic-broth solutions are obtained at predetermined time intervals to evaluate the number of viable bacterial colonies present over the 24-hr incubation.[8,19,29,30] The number of viable bacteria present at each time point are plotted over time to determine the rate of bacterial killing of the antibiotic against the organism. A 2 to 3 log decrease in bacterial counts within 2–8 hr is indicative of bactericidal activity.[8,29,30] While this test is also not routinely performed in the clinical microbiology lab, it is often used in the research setting.

The *Serum Bactericidal Titer* (SBT, or Schlichter's test) is another measure of bacterial killing that may be performed in the lab. This test evaluates the killing activity of a *patient's serum* against their own infecting organism after they have received a dose of an antibiotic.[6,19,28–31] The methodology is very similar to determining the MIC using broth macrodilution, but instead of using known concentrations of an antibiotic, this test utilizes dilutions of the patient's serum.[6,8,19,29–31] The patient's serum is obtained at predefined intervals after a dose of an antibiotic, namely at the time of expected peak and at the time of expected trough. The patient's serum is then serially diluted and inoculated with a standardized concentration of the infecting organism. The SBT is the highest 2-fold dilution of the patient's serum that kills 99.9% of the standardized bacterial inoculum on agar plates (like the MBC). The results of the SBT are reported as a titer, which represents the number of 2-fold serial dilutions of the patient's serum that led to bacterial killing (e.g., SBT = 1:16), with a higher titer indicating better activity against the organism.[28,30,31] The optimal SBT that should be obtained at peak or trough remains undefined and controversial for many infections.

Methodology standards have been developed by the NCCLS for the SBT. However, this test is also not routinely performed in most microbiology labs due to technical difficulties; limited data available regarding the clinical usefulness of SBTs in guiding therapy (only in endocarditis, osteomyelitis, and febrile neutropenia); the inability of results to directly predict the response to therapy; and limited clinical applicability.[8,27–31] The measurement of the SBT is performed in rare clinical circumstances and may be occasionally utilized to monitor the effectiveness of antimicrobial treatment in serious or life-threatening infections (such as endocarditis, osteomyelitis, or serious infections in neutropenic patients).[6,8,27,29,31]

Tests measuring antibiotic combinations (synergy testing). In the treatment of bacterial infections, there are clinical situations that may arise where combination antimicrobial therapy will be considered and utilized. The decision to use combination therapy may be made based on the severity of infection, the organism being treated, or a particular type of infection.[8] The potential benefits of combination antibiotic therapy include (1) expanding the antimicrobial spectrum of activity, especially for polymicrobial infections or when using empiric therapy for a life-threatening infection; (2) producing synergistic bactericidal activity from the combination that is not achieved with each agent alone (e.g., ampicillin and gentamicin for the treatment of *Enterococcal* endocarditis); and (3) decreasing the emergence of resistant organisms (e.g., in the treatment of tuberculosis).[19,29] Routine antimicrobial susceptibility tests only measure the activity of one antibiotic against a particular organism. There are several tests, however, that may be performed to evaluate the effects of a combination of antibiotics against an infecting organism—the results of which are expressed as one of three types of activity[8,19]:

- *Synergy:* the activity of the antibiotic agents in combination is significantly greater than the additive effects of each agent alone.
- *Indifference:* the activity of the antibiotic agents in combination is similar to the additive effects of each agent alone.
- *Antagonism:* the activity of the antimicrobial agents in combination is less than the additive effects of each agent alone.

Therefore, before an antibiotic combination is utilized, it may be useful to determine the effects of the antimicrobial combination against the infecting organism, especially since some antibacterial combinations may produce suboptimal effects.

Synergy testing of an antimicrobial combination can be performed using the checkerboard technique, the time-kill curve technique, the disk diffusion assay, or the E-test method.[8,19,29] The checkerboard and kill-curve techniques are the tests used most often. Briefly, the checkerboard technique is performed in macrodilution tubes or microtiter plates containing serial dilutions of the antibiotics in combination. The tubes or plates are then inoculated with a standardized inoculum of the infecting bacteria and incubated for 24 hr. The effect of the antibiotic combination is determined by comparing the MICs of the agents when used together with the MICs of each agent when used alone—a synergistic combination displays lower MICs. The time-kill curve method for combination therapy is similar to the time-kill curve method used to determine the rate of bacterial killing of a single agent, except that two antibiotics are added to the tubes in fixed concentrations. The effect of the antibiotic combination is determined by comparing the time-kill rates of combination therapy vs. the time-kill rates of each agent used alone, with a synergistic combination displaying a 100-fold decrease in viable colony counts as compared to the most potent agent tested alone.[8,19]

In the clinical setting, synergy testing methods are not routinely performed due to their tedious, time-consuming methodologies; their expense; and their inability to apply the information to the management of an infection to predict clinical outcome.[8,19,29]

Methods Detecting the Presence of Antibiotic Resistance Mechanisms

Detection of β-Lactamase Activity

There are many different types of β-lactamase enzymes that may be elaborated by infecting bacteria, including inducible and extended spectrum β-lactamases. Typically, these enzymes cause hydrolysis of the amide bond in the β-lactam ring and, depending on the type of enzyme, may result in inactivation of one or numerous β-lactam-containing antibiotics. It is important to understand the consequences of detecting a particular β-lactamase enzyme in an organism because certain enzymes produce resistance only to certain antimicrobials.[19,28]

There are a number of different test methods that can be utilized to detect the presence of a β-lactamase enzyme depending on the organism and the type of β-lactamase enzyme that is suspected. Some tests directly detect the presence of β-lactamase activity, while other β-lactamase enzymes (such as the inducible or extended spectrum β-lactamases) can be suspected based on resistance patterns and MICs derived from routine susceptibility tests.

The assays that directly detect β-lactamase activity in an organism include the acidimetric, iodometric, and chromogenic tests. All of these tests directly measure the presence of β-lactamase enzyme by observing a color change based on reactions to different substrates, and all can be performed in a short period of time with results available within minutes to hours.[5,28] The chromogenic test is the most common direct test utilized by microbiology laboratories due to its reliability in detecting β-lactamase enzymes produced by many different bacteria.[28] These tests utilize chromogenic cephalosporins (nitrocefin or cefesone) incorporated into filter paper disks which produce a colorimetric change if they are hydrolyzed by β-lactamase enzymes present when a sample of the clinical specimen is inoculated onto the disk. A positive reaction using one of these direct β-lactamase tests for *Haemophilus influenzae*, *Moraxella catarrhalis*, and *Neisseria gonorrhoeae* predicts resistance to only penicillin, ampicillin, and amoxicillin (but potentially not to other β-lactam antibiotics that are more stable to the hydrolysis by β-lactamase enzymes).[5] A positive β-lactamase test for *Staphylococcus sp.* predicts resistance to penicillin, ampicillin, amoxicillin, carbenicillin, ticarcillin, and piperacillin.

For some organisms, such as the *Enterobacteriaceae* and *Pseudomonas sp.*, the production of β-lactamase enzyme may be inducible, and the detection of β-lactamase enzyme cannot fully predict the antibiotic susceptibility (or resistance) of the organism.[5,28,32] Therefore, direct β-lactamase testing for these organisms is not recommended. The presence of β-lactamase enzyme in these organisms can be determined using recently developed guidelines by the NCCLS that involve MIC and disk diffusion screening breakpoints for particular antibiotics as well as confirmatory tests using β-lactamase inhibitors.[20–23,28,32]

High-Level Aminoglycoside Resistance

The aminoglycoside antibiotics have relatively poor activity against *Enterococcus* sp. due to poor intracellular uptake. Thus, they cannot be utilized as monotherapy in the treatment of infections due to Enterococci. They may be, however, combined with a β-lactam or vancomycin in order to achieve synergistic bactericidal activity, as in the treatment of Enterococcal endocarditis or Enterococcal osteomyelitis. Gentamicin and streptomycin are the two aminoglycosides most commonly used in this situation, and they are, therefore, the agents most commonly tested for activity. The microbiology laboratory can perform an easy supplemental test to detect the presence of *high-level aminoglycoside resistance* (HLAR), which can be utilized to predict the lack of synergism between gentamicin or streptomycin and cell-wall active agents against *Enterococcus* sp.[5,26,28,32]

The test is most commonly performed with agar screen plates containing high concentrations of gentamicin (500 µg/mL) and streptomycin (2000 µg/mL).[5,28] The plates are inoculated with a standardized concentration of the infecting bacteria and incubated for 24 hr in ambient air.[28] The growth of one or more *Enterococcus* colonies on the agar plate is indicative of HLAR, and the corresponding aminoglycoside cannot be used with a cell-wall active agent to achieve synergistic bactericidal activity. Other methods that are available to detect HLAR include broth microdilution and disk diffusion.[5,28] HLAR to gentamicin also confers resistance to tobramycin, netilmicin, and amikacin, but not necessarily streptomycin, which should be tested independently.[5,28] A modified test using kanamycin may be used to predict HLAR to amikacin and kanamycin for strains of *Enterococcus faecalis*; however, this test is not generally available in most labs.[5,28] Testing for HLAR is usually performed only on Enterococcal isolates that have been derived from an infection that requires combination bactericidal activity, such as bacteremia, endocarditis, osteomyelitis, or meningitis.[26,28]

Agar Screens to Detect MRSA and VRE

There are a number of agar screening tests that can be utilized to detect or confirm the presence of a resistant bacteria. For the detection or confirmation of the presence of methicillin-resistant *Staphylococcus aureus* (MRSA), a commercially-available oxacillin agar screening plate can be utilized. A standard inoculum of the infecting *S. aureus* is inoculated onto an agar plate containing 6 μg/mL of oxacillin and incubated in ambient air for 24 hr.[5,28,32] The presence of growth indicates MRSA, which also confers resistance to nafcillin, oxacillin, cloxacillin, dicloxacillin, and cephalosporins. This test is not recommended for the detection of methicillin-resistance in other *Staphylococcus* sp.[28,32]

A similar test is available for the detection and screening of vancomycin resistance in *Enterococcus* sp. (VRE), namely, the vancomycin agar screening method. In this test, a standard inoculum of the infecting *Enterococcus sp.* is inoculated onto an agar plate containing 6 μg/mL of vancomycin and incubated in ambient air for 24 hr.[5,28,32] The presence of any growth demonstrates the detection of VRE. This test is most useful for detecting acquired vancomycin resistance in *E. faecalis* and *E. faecium*, but is not useful for strains with intrinsic resistance to vancomycin, such as *E. gallinarum* and *E. casseliflavus*. The vancomycin agar screening method test is also useful to detect the presence of a newly emerging resistant pathogen, namely vancomycin-intermediate *Staphylococcus aureus* (VISA).[8,26,28,32]

Special Considerations for Fastidious or Anaerobic Bacteria

It is important to note that the susceptibility of some bacteria (e.g., fastidious organisms such as *Haemophilus influenzae*, *N. gonorrhoeae*, and *Streptococcus pneumoniae*) cannot be performed utilizing standard broth microdilution, disk diffusion, or automated testing methods since these organisms require more complex growth media and environmental conditions to support bacterial growth.[32] The NCCLS has developed and published modified methodologies (broth dilution, disk diffusion, and automated methods) as well as quality control and interpretive breakpoint criteria that should be utilized for the susceptibility testing of these bacteria.[20–25,32]

The clinical significance of anaerobes is more widely appreciated, and the susceptibility patterns of anaerobes to various anti-infective agents is not predictable.[6] The appropriate handling and processing of biologic specimens for anaerobic culture and susceptibility testing are extremely important to the validity of the results since most anaerobic bacteria of clinical importance are intolerant to oxygen.[5,6,33] Specimens should be collected in appropriate anaerobic transport systems (commercially-available vials or tubes) that contain specialized media and atmospheric conditions to support the growth of the anaerobic bacteria until the specimen is processed in the lab.[5,33] Once collected, the specimens should be immediately (within minutes to hours of collection depending on the specimen) transported to the lab and setup for culture in anaerobic jars or chambers in the appropriate growth media and incubated. Acceptable specimens that provide the best yield for anaerobic culture include aspirated material and tissue or biopsy specimens.[5,33]

The identification of anaerobic bacteria by an individual hospital laboratory may be performed in one of three methods: (1) preliminary or presumptive identification of the organism based on Gram stain information, plate and cell morphology, and various rapid spot and disk tests; (2) presumptive or definitive identification based on the results of individual biochemical tests that detect the presence of preformed enzymes in certain anaerobes; and (3) rapid identification of anaerobes using commercially available systems, which also detect the presence of preformed enzymes (within hours) such as the An-Ident (bioMerieux, Inc.), the BBL Crystal Anaerobe ID (Becton Dickinson and Company), the RapID-ANA II (REMEL, Inc.), the Rapid Anaerobe Identification Panel (MicroScan), or the Anaerobe ANI Card (Vitek).[5,34] Many hospital laboratories do not have the commercially-available, anaerobic identification systems, and rely on the first two methods for presumptive identification of the anaerobic bacteria before a decision is made as to whether or not the isolate should be sent to a reference lab for further testing.

Most clinical microbiology labs do not currently offer routine susceptibility testing of anaerobic bacteria for a number of reasons including the uncommon occurrence of pure anaerobic infections; the uncertain role of anaerobes in mixed infections; the previous predictable susceptibility of anaerobic bacteria to antibiotics; the previous lack of standardization of antimicrobial susceptibility testing of anaerobes; and the technical difficulties in performing the tests.[26,34–36] However, it is becoming apparent that routine antimicrobial susceptibility testing of anaerobic bacteria is necessary, especially in light of the increasing incidence of serious infections due to anaerobic bacteria and the emerging resistance in anaerobic bacteria to multiple antibiotic agents.[26,34–37]

The susceptibility testing of anaerobic bacteria has undergone numerous methodologic modifications and standardization over the past several years.[6,35–37] The current recommended methods have been recently outlined in an Approved Standard published by the NCCLS.[37] These guidelines address which clinical isolates should be tested for antibiotic susceptibility, which methods of susceptibility testing should be utilized, when and how surveillance susceptibility reporting should be performed, and which antibiotic agents should be tested for susceptibility.

The current NCCLS guidelines recommend susceptibility testing for anaerobes isolated from patients with serious or life-threatening infections such as endocarditis, brain abscesses, empyema, bone or joint infections, bacteremia, and prosthetic device or vascular graft infections.[6,35,37] Susceptibility testing should also be performed in patients with persistent or recurring anaerobic infection despite what appears to be appropriate antibiotic therapy.[6,35,37] Lastly, periodic susceptibility testing of anaerobes isolated in an individual hospital is recommended to monitor local and regional resistance patterns (surveillance).[35,37]

The two recommended anaerobic susceptibility testing methods include agar dilution (the gold standard reference method) and broth microdilution using supplemented *Brucella* blood agar or broth, either of which can be reliably performed by most clinical microbiology labs.[6,34–37] The agar dilution method can be utilized to test the susceptibility of a number of different anaerobic bacteria, while the broth microdilution method has only been established for antimicrobial susceptibility testing of the *Bacteroides fragilis* group organisms.[37] The broth microdilution method has been modified to allow the preparation and inoculation of the biologic specimen aerobically before being incubated anaerobically, and can actually test the susceptibility of multiple antibiotics simultaneously. Otherwise, the general methodology for each of these tests is similar to those described above for aerobic bacteria. Other methods that can be used for susceptibility testing of anaerobes include agar disk diffusion, broth disk elution, E-test, Spiral Gradient Endpoint (SGE) test, and broth macrodilution, although none of these tests has been adequately validated against the reference agar dilution method.[34–37]

Since routine antimicrobial susceptibility is not performed by all hospital microbiology laboratories or for all anaerobic isolates, antibiotic therapy is usually empirically chosen based on the typical antibiotic susceptibilities of the infecting organism (based on studies published by reference labs).[35] However, if susceptibility testing is performed on an individual anaerobic isolate, the results should be used to guide the anti-infective therapy for the patient.

Methods for Reporting Susceptibility Results

Individual Isolate Report

When a bacterial isolate from a suspected site of infection is sent to the microbiology lab for identification and susceptibility testing, the results are compiled in a report that is typically inserted into the patient's chart. The bacterial identification and antibiotic susceptibility report often contains information including the patient's name, medical record number, the date and time of specimen collection, the site of specimen collection, the bacteria that were identified (if any), and the list of antibiotics tested for susceptibility with their MIC or disk diffusion results and interpretive category, as shown in Figure 17-6.[38,39] In some hospitals, the susceptibility report may also contain information regarding the usual daily doses and costs of the antibiotics that were tested.

| Patient Name: Jane Doe |
| Medical Record Number: 1111111 |
| Specimen Collection Date and Time: October 20, 2002, 0730 |
| Specimen Type: Blood |
| Organism Identification: Staphylococcus aureus |

ANTIMICROBIAL SUSCEPTIBILITY

Antibiotic	MIC (µg/mL)	Interpretive Category
Penicillin	≥16	Resistant
Ampicillin/Sulbactam	≤4	Susceptible
Cefazolin	≤8	Susceptible
Oxacillin	0.5	Susceptible
Trimethoprim/Sulfa	≤10	Susceptible
Vancomycin	≤0.5	Susceptible
Clindamycin	≤0.5	Susceptible
Erythromycin	≤0.5	Susceptible

Figure 17-6. Example of microbiology laboratory report with bacterial identification and antibiotic susceptibility. (Adapted from Reference 38.)

The susceptibility report is often used to guide the choice of *directed* antibiotic therapy since the culture and susceptibility results are known, and an antibiotic can be chosen based on the results to streamline the antimicrobial coverage against the organism isolated. The exact choice of which antibiotic to use is usually based on a number of clinical and economic parameters such as the severity of infection; the site of infection; the end-organ function of the patient; the presence of drug allergies; the activity of the antibiotic against the infecting organism; the proven efficacy from clinical trials of the antibiotic in treating the particular infection; the overall spectrum of activity of the antibiotic (a narrow spectrum agent is preferred); and the daily cost of the antibiotic, etc. The susceptibility report provides some of the information that is required for the antibiotic decision-making process, namely, the site of infection, the identification of the infecting organism, and the susceptibility of the infecting organism to a number of antibiotics.

As seen in the sample susceptibility report in Figure 17-6, there may be a number of antibiotics to which the infecting organism is susceptible, often with differing MICs. It is not always advantageous to choose the antibiotic with the lowest MIC against a particular organism on a susceptibility report because (as previously explained) each antibiotic has different MIC breakpoints for S, I, and R based on achievable serum concentrations of the antibiotic after normal dosing; the inherent susceptibility of the organism to the antibiotic; the site of infection; and the results of efficacy trials of the antibiotic against infections due to that organism. Therefore, different antibiotics typically have different MIC breakpoints for susceptibility. The choice of which antibiotic to use is typically based on the knowledge of those MICs that are good for a particular drug-bug combination as well as the clinical and economic parameters listed above. In the sample report in Figure 17-6, oxacillin (nafcillin) or cefazolin would be suitable choices for the treatment of *Staphylococcus aureus* bacteremia in a patient without drug allergies since these agents are active against the infecting organism; are effective in the treatment of systemic Staphylococcal infections; are relatively narrow-spectrum antibiotics; and are inexpensive. Minicase 2 is another example illustrating the use of a culture and susceptibility report in the antibiotic decision-making process.

The decision regarding which antibiotics will be tested and reported on an individual susceptibility report for a bacterial isolate is typically based on input from the infectious diseases physicians, the infectious disease pharmacists, the Infection Control Committee,

S. D., A 34-YEAR-OLD FEMALE, visits her Internal Medicine physician with complaints of urinary frequency and pain on urination for the past 2 days. She has a history of recurrent urinary tract infections, with three episodes over the past 6 months that have required antibiotic therapy. The patient reports an allergy to penicillin (angioedema). Her current physical exam does not reveal any costovertebral angle tenderness. Because she has a history of recurrent UTIs, a midstream, clean-catch urine sample is obtained for urinalysis and culture/susceptibility. The results of her urinalysis and culture are as follows:

Urinalysis:

Yellow, cloudy; pH 7.0, specific gravity 1.015, protein negative, RBC trace, WBC packed.

Urine Culture and Susceptibility:

>100,000 cfu/mL of *Escherichia coli*

Sensitive to: ampicillin/sulbactam (MIC ≤8 µg/mL), cefazolin (MIC ≤8 µg/mL), ceftriaxone (MIC ≤8 µg/mL), aztreonam (MIC ≤8 µg/mL), imipenem (MIC ≤4 µg/mL), gentamicin (MIC 1 µg/mL), ciprofloxacin (MIC ≤0.5 µg/mL).

Resistant to: ampicillin (MIC >32 µg/mL), ticarcillin (MIC >64 µg/mL), trimethoprim-sulfamethoxazole (MIC >80 µg/mL).

Question: What is an appropriate recommendation for antibiotic therapy for this patient?

Discussion: This patient has a history of recurrent UTIs, which required the acquisition of a urinalysis and culture in order to guide current antimicrobial treatment (her past UTIs and subsequent antibiotic treatment put her at risk for acquiring an infection with a resistant bacteria). Based on her presenting symptoms and the findings on her physical examination, the patient most likely has acute, uncomplicated cystitis. Therefore, she can probably be treated with an oral antibiotic if her organism is susceptible. Based on her serious β-lactam allergy and the results of her urine culture and susceptibility results, the most appropriate treatment for this patient's urinary tract infection is oral ciprofloxacin, which is the only oral agent to which her organism is susceptible.

the Pharmacy and Therapeutics Committee, and the microbiology laboratory of a given hospital.[5] These decisions are often based on which antibiotics are available on the hospital formulary, the level of control of antibiotic use that is desired, and the tests that are utilized by the microbiology laboratory for susceptibility testing. Tables that outline which antibiotics should be routinely tested and reported for certain organisms can be found in the NCCLS Performance Standards and Guidelines for susceptibility testing of bacteria.[20–23]

There are several methods for reporting the antibiotic susceptibility of a given bacteria. Some labs choose to report the susceptibility of all antibiotics that were tested for susceptibility, while other labs choose to report the susceptibility of only those antibiotics that are available for routine use on the hospital formulary or those that are useful for the treatment of a particular organism (*selective reporting*). An example of selective reporting would be the exclusion of cefazolin from the susceptibility report of a CSF sample growing *E. coli* since cefazolin is not a suitable treatment option for meningitis. Other hospital labs choose to report the susceptibility of those agents that they consider to be first-line choices for the treatment of a particular organism or infection, and will only report the susceptibility of what they consider to be second-line agents if the first-line agents are inappropriate for the treatment of the particular infection or if the first-line agents are inactive against the infecting organism. This process is called *cascade reporting* and is occasionally utilized as a method to control the inappropriate use of broad-spectrum or expensive antibiotics.[5,39] An example of cascade reporting would include the reporting of the susceptibility of *Pseudomonas aeruginosa* to amikacin only if the organism is resistant to gentamicin or tobramycin, which are less expensive aminoglycoside agents.

MINICASE 3

R. J. IS A 45-YEAR-OLD-MALE who sustained multiple medical injuries after a motorcycle accident. He has been in the Surgical ICU on a ventilator for the past 10 days. In the last 12 hr, his oxygen requirements have increased on the ventilator, he has spiked a temperature to 39 °C, and the nurse has been suctioning increasing amounts of green respiratory secretions from his endotracheal tube. A portable chest x-ray was performed and demonstrated RLL consolidation consistent with pneumonia. A sputum sample is obtained for Gram stain and culture, with the Gram stain showing many gram-negative rods. You are asked by the Surgical ICU attending to choose an *empiric* antibiotic regimen to treat this patient's ventilator-associated pneumonia while you are waiting for the results of the culture and susceptibility tests. The patient has no known drug allergies, and your hospital antibiogram is pictured in Figure 17-7.

Question: What empiric antibiotic regimen should be used in this patient?

Discussion: Gram-negative, ventilator-associated pneumonia is a potentially life-threatening infection, which will require aggressive antibiotic therapy for treatment. Many clinicians would choose combination therapy, especially while waiting for the results of culture and susceptibility data. Combination antibiotic therapy might provide some antibacterial synergy, as well as provide coverage against a wide range of potential infecting bacteria. Based in the hospital antibiogram, it would probably be prudent to choose antibiotics that have good activity (>85%) against gram-negative bacteria that commonly cause ventilator-associated pneumonia, namely, *Pseudomonas aeruginosa*, *E. coli*, *Klebsiella pneumoniae*, *Serratia marcescens*, and *Enterobacter cloacae*. Some useful combinations would be imipenem plus tobramycin, ceftazidime plus tobramycin, or ceftazidime plus ciprofloxacin.

Hospital Susceptibility Reports (Hospital Antibiograms)

Many hospitals prepare and publish a cumulative report, called an *antibiogram*, of the antimicrobial susceptibility profiles of the organisms that have been isolated from the patients within their hospital. The hospital antibiogram often reflects the antibiotic susceptibility patterns of isolates obtained in the surrounding community as well as in the hospital (nosocomially-acquired). The hospital antibiogram is a useful tool when selecting the most appropriate *empiric* antibiotic therapy based on the organism that is most likely suspected to be causing the patient's infection, as listed in Table 17-7 and discussed in Minicase 3.[39] If the susceptibility results of the infecting organism are not yet known, an antibiotic is then chosen based on the local susceptibility patterns of the most likely infecting organism. In most cases, therapy must be initiated at the suspicion of infection since many infectious diseases are often acute where a delay in treatment may result in significant morbidity or

Antibiotic Formulary Status (Bold = FORMULARY, Upper/Lower = RESERVED)	Acinetobacter calcoacet (11)	Enterobacter aerogenes (12)	Enterobacter cloacae (30)	Escherichia coli (271)	Haemophilus influenzae (63)	Klebsiella pneumoniae (63)	Proteus mirabilis (37)	Pseudomonas aeruginosa (101)	Staphylococcus aureus (153)	Enterococci (gp D strep) (97)	Enterococcus faecium (12)	Usual dose	Cost/day (includes administration costs)	Pharmacy (x2549) / Microbiology (x5529)
AMPICILLIN				73	73		100			97		1-2 gm IV Q6hr	$4 - 5	
AMOXICILLIN - CLAVULANATE				95								250-500 mg PO TID	$4 - 6	
CEFAZOLIN				97		97	100		87			500 mg IV Q8 hr	$6	
CEFOTETAN			63	100		100	100					1-2 gm IV Q12 hr	$18 - 35	
Ceftazidime	100	92						98				1-2 gm IV Q8 hr	$31 - 61	
Ceftriaxone		92	86	100	100	100	100					1-2 gm IV Q24 hr	$25- 50	
Cefuroxime		92	72	99	97	98	100					750 mg IV Q8 hr	$14	
Ciprofloxacin	100	100	100	100		100	100	95	90	78		250-750 mg PO BID	$4 - 9 (only oral form available)	
CLINDAMYCIN									91			600 mg Q8 hr	IV - $9 PO - $8	
ERYTHROMYCIN									72			500 mg Q6 hr	IV - $7 PO - $0.20	
GENTAMICIN	91	100	100	100		100	100	92				80 mg IV Q8 hr	$5	
Imipenem	100	100	100					91				500 mg IV Q8-6 hr	$60 - 79	
METRONIDAZOLE												500 mg Q6 hr	IV - $7 PO - $.50	
OXACILLIN									87			2 gm IV Q6 hr	$10	
NITROFURANTOIN			100	99						99	95	50 - 100 mg PO Q6 hr for urine isolates only	$2 - 3	
PENICILLIN G												1 million units IV Q4 hr	$9	
TETRACYCLINE			85	85			92		92			250-500 mg PO Q6 hr	$0.20	
TICARCILLIN	100	83	63	74			100	89				3 gm IV Q4	$48	
Ticarcillin-clavulanate	Activity superior to ticarcillin vs. staph, most gram neg. rods and anaerobes (including B. fragilis). Activity same as ticarcillin vs. Pseudomonas, Acinetobacter, Enterobacter.											3.1 gm IV Q6 hr	$43	
Tobramycin	100	100						100				80 mg IV Q8 hr	$18	
TRIMETHOPRIM - SULFAMETHOXAZOLE	91	100	97	92	92	90	97		94			20 ml IV Q12 hr / 1 DS Tab PO BID	IV - $3 PO - $0.15	
Vancomycin									99	100	92	1 gm IV Q12 hr	$15	

ANTIBIOTIC SUSCEPTIBILITIES Jan. - Dec. 1993. Numbers are percent susceptible (# isolates).

Figure 17-7. Example of a hospital antibiogram.

TABLE 17-10

1. In order to serve as a continuously useful tool, the cumulative antimicrobial susceptibility report should be compiled and reported at least yearly.

2. Only the first clinical isolate of a given species of bacteria per patient per analysis period (yearly if that is the time frame of the antibiogram) should be included in the cumulative susceptibility report, regardless of site of isolation, susceptibility pattern of the bacteria, or other phenotypic characteristics. The inclusion of duplicate clinical isolates from the same patient will lead to incorrect reporting of actual bacterial resistance patterns.

3. Include in the antibiogram only those species of bacteria where at least 10 isolates have been collected, tested, and reported.

4. Data from isolates recovered during surveillance cultures (e.g., MRSA and VRE), environmental cultures, or other nonpatient sources should not be included in the antibiogram.

5. The cumulative susceptibility report should include all antibiotics that were tested for susceptibility, regardless if they were reported in the final susceptibility report.

6. Only include bacterial isolates where all routine antibiotics were tested for susceptibility. Results of agents selectively tested or supplementally tested should not be included in the cumulative susceptibility report. For example, if only isolates resistant to primary agents were then analyzed for susceptibility to secondary agents, this will bias the resistance results towards higher levels of resistance to the secondary agents.

7. Data may be stratified and reported by age, unit in which the isolate was collected (e.g., MICU and SICU), or by site of collection (e.g., blood isolates, CSF isolates, and urine isolates) as long as duplicate patient isolates are removed and there are a sufficient number of isolates collected (>10) during the time frame of the antibiogram.

Table 17-10. NCCLS Recommendations for Antibiogram Development[39]

mortality (e.g., meningitis and pneumonia). However, once the culture and susceptibility results of the infecting bacteria are known, antibiotic therapy can be streamlined to an agent with more targeted activity against the organism. In order for the hospital antibiogram to be clinically useful, the susceptibility data from patient isolates should be appropriately collected, analyzed, and reported according to the recently published guidelines by the NCCLS, which are outlined in Table 17-10.[39]

The antibiogram usually reports the percent of isolated organisms that were susceptible to the different antibiotics over the time frame of the antibiogram, as illustrated in Figure 17-7.

The information is derived by dividing the number of organisms susceptible to a particular antibiotic by the total number of organisms collected and reported. The denominator is usually based on the highest number of bacteria/antibiotic combinations tested. The calculations can be performed either manually or by using automated systems as long as appropriate definitions are programmed within the computer systems to remove duplicate patient isolates. The antibiogram typically contains separate tables for reporting the susceptibility of gram-positive, gram-negative, and anaerobic bacteria. In addition, for some organisms, the antibiogram will contain information regarding the presence of bacterial resistant mechanisms, particularly when routine susceptibility testing cannot be performed. An example is the reporting of the percentage of isolated *Haemophilus influenzae* that produced β-lactamase during the time period of the antibiogram.

Reporting Surveillance Susceptibility Testing of Large Numbers of Isolates

Surveillance susceptibility testing is a useful method to monitor the susceptibility of bacteria to antimicrobial agents over time, and can be performed in an individual hospital or within a geographic location (e.g., regionally, nationally, and internationally).[38] These surveillance studies typically report the overall susceptibility of the bacteria to particular antimicrobial agents, along with other susceptibility parameters such as the MIC_{50} and the MIC_{90}. The MIC_{50} is the MIC that represents 50% of the isolates tested in the surveillance study. The MIC_{90} is the MIC that represents 90% of the isolates tested in the study. The MIC_{90} value may be higher than the MIC_{50} value. This information may be useful for detecting the emergence of subclinical antibiotic resistance where the MIC_{50} and MIC_{90} of a particular agent may be increasing over time but are still below the MIC susceptibility breakpoint.

Additional Considerations
When Interpreting Susceptibility Results

The successful treatment of a patient's infection involves an understanding of the interactions among the patient, the infecting organism, and the antibiotic. It is important to note that antimicrobial susceptibility testing only measures one of these factors, namely, the activity of the antibiotic against the infecting organism (in a laboratory setting). The current methodologies for antibiotic susceptibility testing are unable to reproduce the interaction between the antibiotic and the bacteria at the site of infection where a multitude of host factors (e.g., immune system function, and concomitant disease states and drugs) and drug factors (e.g., pharmacokinetic parameters including concentration of free drug at the site of infection and protein binding) also interplay.

FUNGI

Fungi are eucaryotic, aerobic organisms that have a well-defined nucleus and rigid cell wall containing chitin, cellulose, or both.[41,42] There are more than 50,000 species of fungi that have been identified, however, only 100 to 150 species are causes of disease in humans and animals.[41] Pathogenic fungi can cause infection in both normal and immunocompromised hosts, while opportunistic fungi usually require some alteration in the host's immune system in order to cause infection. The overall incidence of fungal infections has been steadily increasing over the past two decades due to a number of causes including recent advances in medical technology and medical care (e.g., solid organ and bone marrow transplantation, use of immunosuppressive drugs such as steroids or cytotoxic chemotherapy, use of indwelling catheters and mechanical ventilation, and use of broad spectrum antibiotics) and the emergence of immunosuppressive disease states (e.g., HIV infection).[41,42] Therefore, fungal infections have emerged as a major cause of infection in both immunocompromised and hospitalized patients, and as a leading cause of death due to infection in patients with hematologic malignancy or those undergoing solid organ or bone marrow transplant.

The Identification of Fungi

As mentioned earlier, there are approximately 100 to 150 fungal species that are known to cause infection in humans and animals, with the most common infecting fungi listed in Table 17-11. These pathogenic fungi can be grouped morphologically as yeasts or filamentous molds based on the appearance of growing colonies in culture. Yeasts are monomorphic (always exist as one form), unicellular, oval or round organisms that grow as moist, creamy colonies on agar media. Conversely, filamentous molds grow as multicellular, tube-like (hyphae), branching organisms that grow outward to produce fluffy, matted growth on agar media. In addition, several pathogenic species of fungi exist in either a yeast or mold form depending on the environmental conditions and are considered *dimorphic* fungi.[40–42]

The ability to accurately diagnose the presence of a fungal infection is highly dependent on appropriate selection and collection of biologic specimens for staining and

TABLE 17-11

MONOMORPHIC YEASTS	DIMORPHIC FUNGI	FILAMENTOUS MOLDS
Candida albicans	Blastomyces dermatitidis	Aspergillus fumigatus
Candida parapsilosis	Histoplasma capsulatum	Aspergillus flavus
Candida tropicalis	Coccidioides immitis	Aspergillus niger
Candida krusei	Paracoccidioides brasiliensis	Fusarium sp.
Candida lusitaniae	Sporothrix schenckii	Mucor sp.
Candida guillermondii	Penicillium marneffei	Rhizopus sp.
Torulopsis glabrata		Absidia sp.
Cryptococcus neoformans		Alternaria sp.
Malasezzia furfur		Acremonium sp.
Saccharomyces sp.		Scedosporium prolificans
Trichosporon beigelii		Pseudallescheria boydii
		Tricophyton sp.

Table 17-11. Common Pathogenic Fungi[40,41]

culture. Since different fungi are capable of causing a number of infections, the following biologic specimens may be submitted for fungal culture: respiratory tract secretions (e.g., sputum and bronchial washings), cerebrospinal fluid, blood, urine, tissue, exudate or wound drainage, bone marrow, sterile body fluids, hair, and skin or nail scrapings.[40,41] Biologic specimens for fungal culture should be processed according to specified guidelines shortly after reaching the microbiology lab to prevent the overgrowth of bacteria that may also be present in the specimen.[40,41]

Similar to the processing of a specimen for bacterial culture, biologic specimens submitted for fungal culture are stained and microscopically examined for fungal elements and then plated for fungal culture. However, the stains and culture media are somewhat different. The microscopic examination of a processed specimen for fungal culture is a rapid diagnostic test, which typically involves the use of stains taken up by elements of the fungal cell wall. The most commonly utilized stains for the microscopic examination of fungi include the potassium hydroxide (KOH) stain with or without calcofluor white (rapid detection of fungal elements); the India ink stain (especially useful for the detection of *Cryptococcus neoformans*); the Gomori methenamine silver stain (used primarily for histologic sections of tissue); the Periodic acid-Schiff (PAS) stain (stains fungal elements and hyphae); the acid-fast stain (for detection of *Blastomyces dermatitidis*); and the Wright stain or Giemsa stain (for detection of *Histoplasma capsulatum* and *Cryptococcus neoformans* only).[40,41] In addition, the Gram stain that is typically used for bacterial processing may also allow the detection of most fungi, especially *Candida* sp.

There are a number of culture media that may be utilized for the growth of yeasts and molds, with the decision of which media to utilize being based on the characteristics of the patient, the infection type, the organism suspected, the endemic fungi, and the cost and availability of different media.[40,41] The most common growth media for fungal culture include (1) agar plates with and without antibiotics such as chloramphenicol or gentamicin to inhibit bacterial contamination; (2) agar plates with and without cycloheximide which inhibits the growth of rapidly growing saprophytic fungi; and (3) enriched media with and without blood to ensure the growth of fastidious organisms.[40,41] Most biologic specimens are processed on a number of different growth media in order to ensure adequate recovery of potential pathogenic fungi. Agar plates are preferred over screw-cap tubes containing agar because they provide better aeration and a larger surface area for optimal fungal growth.

Fungal cultures should be incubated at 30 °C (optimal) for 7 days to >8 weeks depending on the fungal organism suspected of causing the infection. Cultures for yeasts only require a 7-day incubation period since they grow rather quickly, while cultures for dimorphic fungi and molds require a 6–8 week incubation before they can be considered negative since they grow at a much slower rate. Culture plates or tubes are typically examined every 2–3 days for the first week and then weekly thereafter during the incubation period. Once fungal growth appears on the culture plates, the organisms are subjected to microscopic examination (looking for characteristic colonial morphologic features), biochemical tests (with commercial identification systems for yeasts), germ-tube tests (for *Candida albicans*), latex agglutination for antigen detection (*Cryptococcus neoformans*), rapid enzyme tests, and molecular detection methods for definitive identification.[40,41] Histologic sections of some biologic specimens (e.g., tissue and bone marrow) submitted for fungal culture are also sent to the pathology lab for microscopic examination for evidence of infection and tissue invasion by fungi.

Due to cost considerations, time constraints, and difficult methodologies for the identification of fungi, diagnostic clinical mycology is performed by only a limited number of clinical microbiology labs and reference labs. Therefore, the decision to fully identify yeasts and molds recovered from biologic specimens is dependent on the clinical condition of the patient, the site of infection, the specific organism recovered, the amount of organism recovered, and the practicality of the diagnostic work-up.[41]

Antifungal Susceptibility Testing

Considerable variation exists in the susceptibility of certain fungi to antifungal agents, even within the same species.[41,43] Antifungal resistance and treatment failures have steadily emerged in the face of the increasing number of fungal infections.[41–43] Therefore, standardized methods for susceptibility testing of fungi were developed to assist in the therapeutic management of fungal infections.

The methods for the susceptibility testing of fungi, however, are not as well-established as those for bacteria. Therefore, most clinical microbiology labs do not routinely perform susceptibility testing for fungi partly because new standardized guidelines have only recently been developed; there is limited correlation between in vitro testing and clinical outcomes; and the current tests only address a limited number of antifungal agents against a limited number of infecting fungi.[41–44]

The NCCLS has recently published standardized guidelines for the susceptibility testing of yeasts using broth macrodilution or microdilution methods.[43,44] These guidelines outline the methodology that should be utilized when performing susceptibility testing of yeasts, as well as the organisms and antifungal agents that should be tested. Susceptibility interpretive breakpoint guidelines have only been established for flucytosine, fluconazole, and itraconazole against *Candida* sp., while testing methods have been standardized for *Cryptococcus neoformans*.[41–44] Susceptibility breakpoints have not yet been established for amphotericin b, caspofungin, or voriconazole. Methods for the susceptibility testing of *Aspergillus* sp., *Fusarium* sp., *P. boydii*, and the Zygomycetes (*Rhizopus* sp.) have also been recently developed.[43,45]

Currently, susceptibility testing of fungi is not routinely recommended and should only be performed in a limited number of circumstances. Susceptibility testing should be considered for patients with refractory oropharyngeal candidiasis; for isolates of non-*albicans* Candida; and to assist in the management of patients with persistent, prolonged fungemia or invasive *Candidal* infections despite apparent appropriate therapy.[41,45] In the future, routine susceptibility testing of fungi may become more useful to aid in the decision regarding appropriate antifungal therapy, especially in light of the increasing number and types of fungal infections, the emergence of resistance to antifungal agents, and the generation of new data that is substantiating the in vitro results with clinical outcome.[41–43]

Skin Testing or Serologic Studies

Several skin tests containing different fungal antigens are available to detect the presence of fungal antibodies after exposure or infection. However, skin tests for the diagnosis of fungal infections, namely the Histoplasmin skin test and Coccidioidomycosis skin test, are not considered to be definitive diagnostic tools because they cannot distinguish between past or present infection.[42] They are typically only employed in epidemiologic studies to determine the presence of infection in an endemic areas (e.g., *Coccidioides* infection in the southwestern US). Skin tests are also available to detect the presence of antibody to *Candida* and *Tricophyton*, but they are only clinically used to detect the presence of an intact immune system in patients suspected of having an immune deficiency (since most patients should have an antibody response to these commonly encountered fungi). Again, a positive skin test in this setting does not distinguish between past or active infection and may just represent asymptomatic exposure to the organism.

Serologic testing for the presence of fungal infection is primarily useful for the detection of *Cryptococcus neoformans*, *Histoplasma capsulatum*, and *Coccidioides immitis*. These serologic tests measure the actual fungal antigen titer or antibody titer and are utilized to aid in the diagnosis of fungal infection, predict the outcome of infection, follow the course of infection, and monitor the response to antifungal therapy.[42]

VIRUSES

There are approximately 73 families and groups of viruses that are known to cause infection in humans and other vertebrate animals.[46] The three major properties that classify viruses into families include (1) the nucleic acid core (either deoxyribonucleic acid [DNA] or ribonucleic acid [RNA], but not both); (2) whether the viral nucleic acid is single- or double-stranded; and (3) the presence or absence of a lipoprotein envelope (Tables 17-12 and 17-13). In addition, the virus families can be further categorized on the basis of morphology (e.g., size, shape, and substructure), mode of replication, and genomic characteristics. The most recent information on the rapidly changing classification and taxonomy of viruses can be obtained from the website database (http://life.bio2.columbia.edu/ICTVdB/) that has been established by The International Committee on Taxonomy of Viruses (ICTV).[47]

The Identification of Viruses

The ability to detect and accurately identify viruses in the clinical laboratory has increased during the last 20 years as a result of wider applicability of diagnostic laboratory techniques, the addition of new antiviral drugs for specific viral infections, and the availability of newer reagents and rapid commercial diagnostic kits.[48,49] It is important to note that all diagnostic tests for the identification of viruses are not available at each institution, and the clinician will need to establish a relationship with the laboratory that will be performing viral testing. In certain clinical situations, samples may need to be sent out for diagnostic testing at either large reference or public health laboratories since they are able to provide the necessary methods that are difficult or impossible to perform in the routine clinical virology laboratory.

TABLE 17-12

FAMILY	NATURE[a]	ENVELOPE	SHAPE	NUCLEOCAPSID, SYMMETRY	EXAMPLES OF SPECIES COMMONLY INFECTING HUMANS	METHOD OF IDENTIFICATION[b]
Adenoviridae	dsDNA, linear	No	Isometric	Icosahedral	Human adenovirus A to F	Cell culture, FA (respiratory samples) EIA, EM (fecal specimens)
Herpesvirdae	dsDNA, linear	Yes	Spherical	Icosahedral	Herpes simplex virus (HSV-1, HSV-2) Varicella-Zoster (VZV) Cytomegalovirus (CMV) Epstein-Barr virus (EBV)	Cell culture, FA, NA Cell culture, FA Cell culture, serology, FA, NA Serology, NA (CNS infection, tumors)
Hepadnaviridae	dsDNA, circular	Yes	Spherical	Icosahedral	Hepatitis B virus	EIA, serology, NA
Papillomaviridae	dsDNA, circular	No	Isometric	Icosahedral	Papillomavirus (warts)	Hybrid capture, histology
Parvoviridae	ssDNA, (-), linear	No	Isometric	Icosahedral	B19 virus (exanthema in children)	NA, serology
Polyomaviridae	dsDNA, circular	No	Isometric	Icosahedral	JC polyomavirus (JCV) BK polyomavirus (BKV)	Serology, NA (compromised host) Serology, NA (compromised host)
Poxviridae	dsDNA, linear	+/-	Brick-shaped or oval	Complex	Smallpox virus Molluscum contagiosum virus	EM, serology, cell culture EM, serology, cell culture

[a] dsDNA, double-stranded DNA; ssDNA, single-stranded DNA; (-), negative stranded.
[b] FA, fluorescence-labeled antibodies; EIA, enzyme immunoassay; EM, electron microscopy; NA, nucleic acid detection assays; CNS, central nervous system.

Table 17-12. Characteristics and Laboratory Diagnosis of Selected DNA Viruses of Medical Importance to Humans

TABLE 17-13

FAMILY	NATURE[a]	ENVELOPE	SHAPE	NUCLEO-CAPSID, SYMMETRY	EXAMPLES OF SPECIES INFECTING HUMANS	COMMON METHODS FOR IDENTIFICATION[b]
Arenaviridae	ssRNA, (-), circular	Yes	Spherical	Helical	Lassa virus	Serology, NA
					Lymphocytic choriomeningitis virus	Serology, NA
					Guanarito virus	Serology
					Junin virus	Serology
					Machupo virus	Serology
					Sabia virus	Serology
Astroviridae	ssRNA, (+), linear	No	Isometric	Icosahedral	Human astrovirus	EM, EIA
Bunyaviridae	ssRNA, (-), linear	Yes	Spherical, pleomorphic	Helical	California encephalitis virus	Serology, antibody detection in CSF
					La Crosse virus	Serology, antibody detection in CSF
					Hantaviruses	Serology, antibody detection in CSF
Caliciviridae	ssRNA, (+), linear	No	Isometric	Icosahedral	Norwalk virus	EM, EIA, NA
					Sapporo virus	EM, EIA, NA
					Hepatitis E virus	EIA, serology
Coronaviridae	ssRNA, (+), linear	Yes	Spherical, pleomorphic	Helical	Human coronavirus	EM
Filoviridae	ssRNA, (-), linear	Yes	Filamentous, pleomorphic	Helical	Ebola virus	EM, cell culture; biosafety level 4
					Marburg virus	EM, cell culture; biosafety level 4
Flaviviridae	ssRNA, (+), linear	Yes	Spherical	Icosahedral	Tick-borne encephalitis virus	Serology, antibody detection (CSF)
					Dengue virus	Serology, antibody detection (CSF)
					Japanese encephalitis virus	Serology, antibody detection (CSF)
					Murray Valley virus	Serology, antibody detection (CSF)
					St. Louis encephalitis virus	Serology, antibody detection (CSF)
					West Nile virus	Serology, antibody detection (CSF)
					Hepatitis C virus	Serology, NA
					Hepatitis G virus	Serology, NA
Orthomyxo-viridae	ssRNA, (-), linear	Yes	Pleomorphic	Helical	Influenzae virus types A-C	Cell culture, EIA, FA stain
Paramyxo-viridae	ssRNA, (-), linear	Yes	Pleomorphic	Helical	Mumps virus	Cell culture, serology
					Measles virus	Cell culture, serology
					Parainfluenza virus	Cell culture, EIA, FA stain
					Human respiratory syncytial virus	Cell culture, EIA, FA stain
Picornaviridae	ssRNA, (-), linear	No	Isometric	Icosahedral	Human enterovirus types A–D	Cell culture, NA, serology
					Rhinovirus types A and B	Cell culture (usually not necessary)
					Hepatitis A virus	Serology
Reoviridae	dsRNA, linear	No	Isometric	Icosahedral	Rotavirus A and B	EIA, latex agglutination
Retroviridae	ssDNA, (+), linear	Yes	Spherical	Icosahedral	Human immuno-deficiency viruses, Types 1 and 2 (HIV-1, HIV-2)	Serology, EIA, NA
					Human T-lympho-tropic viruses, HTLV-1 and HTLV-2	Serology
Rhabdoviridae	ssRNA, (-), linear	Yes	Bullet shaped	Helical	Rabies virus	FA staining, NA
Togaviridae	ssRNA, (+), linear	Yes	Spherical	Icosahedral	Rubella virus	Serology, culture
					Arboviruses including alphaviruses	Serology, antibody detection in CSF

[a] dsRNA, double-stranded RNA; ssRNA single-stranded RNA; (+), positive stranded; (-), negative stranded.
[b] FA, fluorescence-labeled antibodies; EIA, enzyme immunoassay; EM, electron microscopy; NA, nucleic acid detection assays; CSF, cerebrospinal fluid.

Table 17-13. Characteristics and Laboratory Diagnosis of Selected RNA Viruses of Medical Importance to Humans

The ability to accurately diagnose a viral infection is highly dependent on appropriate selection, collection, and handling of biological specimens.[48] In general, the highest titers of viruses are present early in the course of illness and decrease as the duration of illness increases. Therefore, it is very important to collect specimens for the detection of viruses early in the course of an infection. In most cases, identification of viruses is a specimen-driven process. The different types of clinical specimens that can be collected for viral culture and antigen detection include respiratory specimens (e.g., nasopharyngeal swabs, aspirates, and washes; throat swabs; and bronchoalveolar lavage and bronchial washes), blood, cerebrospinal fluid, stool, biopsy tissue, urine, ocular specimens, vesicles and other skin lesions, and amniotic fluid. In addition, specimens for molecular diagnostic testing (e.g., PCR and other nucleic amplification techniques) must be obtained following specific guidelines so that the stability and amplifiability of the nucleic acids are ensured.

Once the sample is collected, it should be promptly transported to the laboratory using the appropriate viral transport media to maximize viral recovery in a sterile, leak-proof container. Every effort should be made to prevent delay between the time of specimen collection and its arrival to the laboratory. When delays are expected, viral samples should be refrigerated at 4° C or frozen at -70 °C. Subsequently, the laboratory will need to follow specific procedures in regards to specimen preparation before diagnostic viral testing is performed.

The laboratory techniques used in the diagnosis of viral infections include cell culture, cytology and histology, electron microscopy, antigen detection, nucleic acid detection, and serologic testing. The following section, as well as Tables 17-12 and 17-13, provide a brief summary of the common methods currently used in diagnostic testing of common viruses.[47,50] For more detailed information, the reader is referred to current published literature and standard reference books.

Cell Culture

The gold standard method for the diagnosis of viral infections in most clinical laboratories has been the use of cell culture to isolate a virus.[48,51] The advantages of cell culture include good specificity and sensitivity, the capability of detecting multiple viruses if present, and the cultivation of the virus for further laboratory testing, if needed. The disadvantages of cell culture include the long time needed for the detection of viruses using conventional cell culture (e.g., days to weeks), the need for cell culture facilities, the expense of performing cell culture, and the methodology is not applicable to all viruses.

There are several different types of cell culture that are available to grow clinically important viruses. Most specimens are inoculated onto two or more types of cell culture based on the most likely viruses associated with the type of clinical specimen that was submitted. The different types of cell cultures can be divided into three categories: primary, diploid (also called semicontinuous), and continuous. Primary cell cultures (e.g., monkey kidney cells or human amnion cells) are prepared from animal or embryo tissue and can withstand only a few generations of passages until the cells die. Diploid cell cultures (e.g., human embryonic lung fibroblast lines such as WI-30 or MRC-5) can undergo 50–100 passages before cells are unable to survive. Continuous cell cultures can undergo an indefinite number of passages and include Hep-2, HeLa, and RK-13 cells.

The growth of a virus from a clinical specimen provides direct evidence that the patient was infected with a virus. The main method for detecting growth from the cell culture method is by microscopic examination of the cultured cells for morphological changes or cytopathic effect (CPE). The characteristics of the CPE (e.g., which cell culture types were affected; what is the resultant shape of the cells; whether the effect is focal or diffuse; the time of its appearance and progression) can be used for primary and/or definitive identification of the virus. Subsequently, fluorescent antibody (FA) staining of cells harvested from the culture is often used to confirm the identification of the virus.

Some viruses will grow in cell cultures without producing CPE so that other methods are utilized to identify and detect these viruses, including hemadsorption and interference. Hemadsorption is used to detect viruses such as influenza and parainfluenza, which can grow rapidly and reach high titers in cell cultures without producing CPE. Hemadsorption involves the removal of the culture medium from the inoculated cell culture, adding a suspension of erythrocytes and examining for hemadsorption with a low-power microscope. Interference, used to detect viruses such as rubella, involves growing a virus that yields a cell culture resistant to other viruses (to which it is normally susceptible). The viruses that produce hemadsorption or interference can, subsequently, be identified by FA staining with specific monoclonal antibodies or antiserum.

Shell vial cultures are used to decrease the amount of time required to grow a virus by conventional cell cultures. This technique makes use of cells grown on microscope coverslips that are placed within shell vials and covered with culture media. After cultures are incubated for 1 to 2 days, FA staining is performed on the cells on the coverslips using specific antibodies to recognize an antigen in the nucleus of infected cells. Shell vial cultures have been applied to the detection of cytomegalovirus (CMV), herpes simplex virus (HSV), varicella-zoster virus (VZV), and the human respiratory viruses.

Cytology and Histology

Cytologic examination can be performed on smears prepared from samples that are applied to a microscope slide, or "touch preps" of tissues.[48,51] Cytologic findings are suggestive of a viral infection. However, the specific virus cannot be identified. Applications of cytology to viral diagnosis include the Tzanck smear for demonstrating the presence of HSV or VZV infection, Papanicolaou staining of cells obtained from the uterine cervix (Pap smear) for providing evidence of human papillomavus (HPV) infection, and cytologic staining of urinary sediments for detecting the presence of either CMV or polyomaviruses JC and BK.

Similar to cytology, histologic examination of tissue provides evidence to suggest a group of viruses that may be causing infection, but it does not identify a specific virus.[48,51] Despite this shortcoming, histopathology has been useful in differentiating between asymptomatic viral shedding and clinically important infections of CMV, and it is now often considered the preferred method for the diagnosis of CMV infections in tissue samples obtained from biopsy or at autopsy. In addition, detection of specific viral antigens by immunohistochemistry (IHC) and detection of specific viral nucleic acids by in situ hybridization (ISH) has allowed specific viruses to be identified by histopathology.

Electron Microscopy

Viruses are the smallest infectious pathogens that range in diameter from 18–300 nm.[47] Direct visualization of a virus with a light microscope can only be performed on pathogens with a diameter greater than 200 nm. The electron microscopy (EC) allows visualization of viruses, and unlike direct detection or molecular methodologies, is capable of detecting the distinctive appearances of multiple viruses, if present.[48,51]

Several techniques have been incorporated to allow the visualization of viruses with EC from various types of clinical specimens. Negative staining is a technique for identification of viruses in fluid samples, stool samples, and blister fluid. Thin sectioning can be performed on tissue samples that have been fixed with specific fixatives for electron microscopy study, and it can be used to visualize the herpesviruses, respiratory viruses, and rabies virus.

Direct Antigen Detection

Antigen detection methods involve the use of virus-specific antibodies directed towards viral antigens in a clinical specimen.[48,51] Examples of viruses that can be identified by direct antigen detection include respiratory syncytial virus, influenza virus, parainfluenza virus, adenovirus, herpes simplex virus, varicella-zoster virus, cytomegalovirus, rotavirus, hepatitis B virus, and measles. The advantages of direct antigen detection include the rapidity of diagnosis (e.g., hours to days), the usefulness for the identification of viruses that are difficult to culture, and the detection of viral specific antigens even if viable virus is not present in the clinical specimen. The disadvantages include the potential for false-positive and false-negative results, the difficulty to perform batch testing, and the lack of sensitivity necessary for diagnostic applications for all viruses (e.g., not applicable for rhinoviruses since there are more than 90 serotypes and cross-reacting antibodies).

The techniques commonly used for antigen detection include fluorescent antibody staining (direct and indirect), immunoperoxidase staining, and enzyme immunoassay (including enzyme-linked immunosorbent assay [ELISA]). More recently, membrane immunoassays have been used for several commercial tests (e.g., Directigen Flu A Test and TestPack A for detecting influenza A).[50] These viral antigen tests have become simple to use and allow for single specimens to be conveniently tested for the presence of influenza in outpatient facilities and physician offices.

Molecular Diagnosis

The detection of specific viral nucleic acids (NA) by molecular diagnostic techniques is revolutionizing the field of diagnostic virology.[48,51,52] The techniques used in viral nucleic acid detection include direct hybridization assays, target (template) amplification (e.g., polymerase chain reaction [PCR], self-sustained sequence replication [3SR] method, strand displacement assay [SDA]), and signal amplification (e.g., branched-chain DNA [bDNA] assay and hybrid capture assay). Among these, PCR has been the most important technique in diagnostic virology because of its versatility in detecting DNA or RNA, as well as being able to provide qualitative and quantitative information on specific viral nucleic acids.

Commercial nucleic acid detection assays have become available for several viruses including hepatitis B and C viruses (HBV and HCV), human immunodeficiency virus (HIV), herpes viruses, and cytomegalovirus (CMV). For certain viral infections, the use of PCR and bDNA has become the standard of care (e.g., HCV and HIV) or the preferred method for the diagnosis of viral infection in certain clinical situations (e.g., enterovirus meningitis, herpes simplex virus encephalitis, Epstein-Barr virus in spinal fluid, or CMV in bronchoalveolar fluid or the blood of immunocompromised hosts).

The advantages of viral nucleic acid detection methods include the rapidity of results, high sensitivity for virus-specific detection and identification, the ability to detect viruses that are difficult to culture, and the ability to detect nucleic acids without viable virus present in the clinical specimen. The disadvantages of these techniques include labor-intense methodology, the commercial assays are not always available, and a potential for PCR contamination that may lead to false-positive results.

Serology

Serologic tests are designed to detect an antibody response in serum samples after an exposure to viral antigens has occurred.[48,51] The major uses of serology for the detection of viral infections include the demonstration of immunity or exposure to a virus, the diagnosis of postinfectious sequelae, and the screening of blood products. In several clinical situations, serologic testing remains the primary means for the laboratory diagnosis of viruses that are difficult to culture or detect by direct methods (e.g., rubella virus, Epstein-Barr virus, hepatitis viruses, human immunodeficiency virus, arboviruses). Serologic testing may also serve as a supportive or adjunctive role in clinical situations where viral cultures or direct detection methods are available.

For viral infections, serologic testing can (1) identify the virus; (2) distinguish the strain or serotype; (3) differentiate between primary infection and reinfection; and (4) determine if the infection is in an acute or convalescent phase. Virus-specific immunoglobulin antibodies (e.g., IgM or IgG) are produced during the time course of a viral infection. In general, virus-specific IgM is detected in serum sooner than virus-specific IgG. The results measure the relative concentration of antibody in the body as a titer, with the titer representing the lowest antibody concentration (or inverse of the greatest dilution; dilution of 1:128 equals a titer of 128) that demonstrates activity in a patient's serum. The exact value for a titer varies with each testing method, the virus involved, and the presence of active disease.

For most viral infections, virus-specific IgM can be detected as soon as 3–7 days after the onset of infection. The presence of virus-specific IgM in a single serum sample shortly after the onset of symptoms (acute phase) is usually indicative of a very recent or current primary infection. Titers of virus-specific IgM usually decline to near undetectable amounts within 1–4 months after the onset of infection. Virus-specific IgG can be detected during the acute phase of infection and will continue to increase for several months before reaching a maximal titer. Thereafter, the IgG titer will decline, but it usually remains detectable in serum for the remainder of a person's life. Seroconversion has occurred when at least a 4-fold increase in IgG titer has occurred between serum samples collected in the acute and convalescent (2–3 weeks afterwards) phases. The presence of virus-specific IgG is also indicative of a past infection.

Serologic tests are also used to assess the immunity or exposure to a virus. The presence of antibody can detect which patients have been previously infected by or vaccinated for a specific virus. For example, a positive result (presence of antibody) for rubella in a woman of childbearing age implies that congenital infection will not occur during subsequent pregnancies. A negative result (absence of antibody) implies susceptibility to infection, and the woman should receive rubella vaccination if she is not pregnant. Some other examples of viruses for which serologic determination of immune status is useful include hepatitis A and B, measles, mumps, parvovirus B19, and varicella-zoster virus.

The techniques commonly used for serologic assays include enzyme immunoassay (EIA), immunofluorescent assay (IFA), and Western blot. In the diagnosis of certain viral syndromes (e.g., central nervous system infections), a serology panel may be helpful so that a battery of antigens is tested for antibody to several viruses. The advantages of viral serology include the assessment of immunity or response of a virus isolated from a nonsterile site, serum specimens are easy to obtain and store, and it can be used to identify viruses that are difficult to culture or detect by immunoassay. The disadvantages include the time to results (e.g., few days to weeks), the potential for cross-reactions between different viruses, and the need for acute and convalescent specimens.

HUMAN IMMUNODEFICIENCY VIRUS

Human immunodeficiency virus (HIV) is the causative agent of acquired immunodeficiency syndrome (AIDS). HIV is an enveloped, positive-strand ribonucleic acid (RNA) virus that belongs to the Retroviridae (retrovirus) family and Lentvirinae subfamily. The virus is about 100 nm in diameter and has a characteristic dense cylindrical nucleoid containing core proteins and genomic RNA. The RNA of HIV is transcribed into proviral DNA by the reverse transcriptase enzyme, and it is then incorporated into the host's DNA resulting in a lifelong latent infection. The virus is transmitted to humans by the exchange of blood or other body fluids through sexual contact; by the exposure to contaminated blood; by the transfusion of contaminated blood and/or blood products; or through contaminated needles (e.g., intravenous drug abusers or accidental needle sticks). In addition, infants can acquire HIV from an infected mother during pregnancy or delivery, as well as through breast-feeding.

There are two distinct serotypes of HIV, namely, HIV-1 and HIV-2. HIV-1 is the most prevalent causative serotype of HIV infections worldwide, while HIV-2 is the most common serotype found in Africa (especially in persons with a direct link to West Africa). Routine diagnostic testing of HIV-2 is not recommended in the United States since its prevalence is extremely low. Thus, the following discussion will focus mainly on laboratory tests for HIV-1. However, HIV-2 testing may be indicated in persons at risk for HIV-2 infection or who have symptoms suggestive of HIV infection, but test results for HIV-1 are negative or indeterminate. In addition, all blood donations in the United States are tested for both HIV-1 and HIV-2

Laboratory Tests for HIV-1 Infection

There are several laboratory tests that are available for the diagnosis and monitoring of patients with HIV-1 infection. The most common virologic testing methods include HIV-1 antibody assays, HIV-1 p24 antigen assays, DNA polymerase chain reaction (DNA-PCR), plasma HIV-1 RNA (viral load) assays, and phenotypic and genotypic assays. In addition, the absolute number of CD4$^+$ lymphocytes and the ratio of helper (CD4$^+$) to inducer (CD8$^+$) lymphocytes (CD4$^+$:CD8$^+$ ratios) are routinely measured to evaluate the patient's immune status and response to antiretroviral therapy. HIV cultures are limited to research studies or when routine HIV testing procedures provide conflicting or confusing results, and they are typically performed only at research, academic, or large reference laboratories due to the expense and the need for highly specialized facilities and laboratory personnel.

The clinical use of laboratory tests for HIV-1 infection fall into three main categories: (1) diagnosing HIV-1 infection, (2) monitoring progression of HIV infection and antiretroviral therapy, and (3) screening blood donors. The selection of these tests is highly dependent on the clinical situation, the patient population, and the specified purpose for the testing, as described in Table 17-14 and Minicase 4. The following section briefly reviews each of the specific tests. Detailed descriptions of the various commercial assays and their clinical applications have been recently reviewed elsewhere.[53,54]

MINICASE 4

D. R. IS A FOURTH YEAR MEDICAL STUDENT who is currently doing a rotation on the General Surgery service. He is holding a clamp during an abdominal surgery case, and the surgical nurse accidentally sticks him with a used scalpel as she is placing it back onto the surgical tray. Because of this exposure, D. R. is instructed to immediately seek attention at Student Health to obtain testing for HIV and hepatitis C. The HIV and hepatitis C status of the patient is unknown. D. R. is advised by the physician at Student Health to submit a blood sample for immediate testing, as well as to return at regular intervals during the next 6 months for additional testing.

Question: How long will D. R. have to wait before he can be certain that he did not acquire HIV from the exposure?

Discussion: The hallmark tests for diagnosing HIV infection include the ELISA and Western Blot. The ELISA test detects the presence of anti-HIV antibodies, which may take several weeks to months before they appear in the blood of a newly infected patient. The HIV status of the source patient is unknown. Therefore, the source patient should be questioned regarding risk factors that may predispose to HIV infection, as well as undergo HIV testing (rapid screen and ELISA). Even if the source patient is currently HIV negative by ELISA, D. R. will need to undergo at least 6 months of testing before HIV infection can be ruled out.

TABLE 17-14

CLINICAL SITUATION	RECOMMENDED TEST(S)	COMMENTS
Diagnosis of HIV infection (excluding infants and acute infection)	Antibody EIA and WB	The combination of EIA and WB testing has a positive predictive value of ~100%
Diagnosis of acute HIV infection	Plasma RNA detection, DNA PCR, or p24 antigen	Plasma HIV RNA the preferred method; when antibody test is negative or indeterminate, plasma HIV RNA establishes the diagnosis
Diagnosis of infant (<18 months of age) born to HIV-infected mother	DNA PCR, plasma RNA detection, or p24 antigen	HIV DNA PCR is the preferred method; for infants with acute HIV infection, plasma RNA detection may be more useful since these assays have been reported more sensitive than HIV DNA PCR
Indeterminate HIV-1 WB result	Repeat HIV-1 antibody EIA and WB; perform HIV-2 antibody EIA and WB; DNA PCR	Careful patient history to assess the risks for HIV-1 or HIV-2 infection; consider testing for HIV-2; perform more sensitive diagnostic tests; repeat HIV-1 antibody testing in 3–6 months
Prognosis	Plasma RNA quantification and CD4+ T cell count	Substantial risk of progression with a HIV RNA level >55,000 copies/mL; increased mortality with CD4+ T cell count <200/μL
Response to therapy	Plasma RNA quantification and CD4+ T cell count	Decisions of drug therapy should be based on laboratory results as well as clinical findings, patient interests, adherence issues, and risks of toxicity and drug interactions
Antiretroviral drug resistance testing	Phenotypic and/or genotypic resistance assays	Recommended for determining virologic failure during therapy and when suboptimal suppression of viral load after therapy is initiated
Blood donor screening	Antibody EIA and WB; p24 antigen; plasma RNA detection	In the United States, the blood from all donors is tested for HIV-1 and HIV-2 antibodies as well as p24 antigen

Table 17-14. Recommended Laboratory Tests for Diagnosis, Monitoring, and Blood Donor Screening for HIV

HIV Antibody Tests

Infection with HIV results in a humoral antibody response to HIV-specific proteins and glycoproteins. For most patients, antibodies to HIV-1 can be detected in the blood by 4–12 weeks after exposure to the virus. However, it may take 6–12 months in some patients. There are a number of tests currently available for the detection of HIV-antibody in infected patients.

The methodology of enzyme immunoassay (EIA; also referred to as an enzyme-linked immunosorbent assay [ELISA]) is widely used as the *initial* screening test to detect HIV-specific antibodies.[53,54] The commercial EIA kits utilized by most diagnostic laboratories can detect both HIV-1 and HIV-2, with a sensitivity and specificity of >99%. However, false-positive and false-negative results can occur. False-positive results from a variety of reasons can occur at a fairly high rate in populations with a low prevalence of HIV infection (e.g., volunteer blood donors). Some causes for false-positive HIV EIA results have included the reactivity of antibodies to human leukocyte antigen, autoimmune diseases, recent influenza vaccination, acute viral infection, alcoholic liver disease, chronic renal failure, lymphoma, hematologic malignancies, rapid plasma reagin positive serum, and improper specimen handling (e.g., heating). Thus, EIA should not be used alone in making a diagnosis of HIV infection, and positive results *must be confirmed* with a more specific test (e.g., Western blot). Several causes have been identified for false-negative results and include immunosuppressive therapy, severe hypogammaglobulinemia, replacement transfusion, and testing when HIV antibody production is low (too early [first 1–2 weeks after infection] or too late in the course of HIV infection).

The results of EIA are reported as reactive (positive) or nonreactive (negative). If the initial result is nonreactive, no further testing for HIV antibodies is performed and the person is considered uninfected unless they are suspected of having acute HIV infection. When the initial result is reported as reactive, the same test should be repeated in duplicate. If the repeated result is nonreactive, then it can be assumed that an assay or laboratory error had occurred with the first test and the patient is considered uninfected. If the duplicate test is also reactive, the results should be reported as "repeatedly reactive" and a more specific supplemental test for confirming the presence of antibodies specific to HIV-1 must be performed in order to confirm the diagnosis of HIV infection.

Western blot (and less commonly, an indirect immunofluorescence assay [IFA]) is the confirmatory test of choice for detecting HIV-specific antibodies by an alternative method.[53,54] The Western blot is a protein electrophoretic immunoblot technique that detects specific antibodies to HIV proteins and glycoproteins. The blots are classified as positive (HIV antibodies present), indeterminate (presence of HIV antibodies cannot be excluded or definite), or negative (no HIV antibodies present). A Western blot result with no bands present for HIV antibodies is considered negative, and it can be assumed that the EIA results were a false positive. A Western blot is considered positive if bands are present for two of three HIV-specific proteins including p24, gp41, and gp120/160. For adults and children older than 18 months of age, the diagnosis of HIV-1 infection can be made if the results of the repeated positive EIA are confirmed by a positive Western blot. The Western blot test is not considered a suitable initial screening test for detecting the presence of HIV antibodies because 4–20% of the test results are reported as indeterminate. Some of the causes for indeterminate Western blot results include testing too early or too late in the course of HIV infection, cross-reaction with HIV-2 infection, or the production of nonspecific antibody reactions. If the Western blot result is indeterminate, then repeat testing of the EIA and Western blot are necessary. In addition, specific antibody testing for HIV-2 or other diagnostic test methods may need to be considered (see Table 17-14). The Western blot test is used only to confirm a positive EIA test because it is technically difficult to perform, is expensive, has a relatively high rate of indeterminate results, and the results are available in 1–2 weeks.

Rapid HIV tests. Recent technological advances have allowed for the development of rapid (e.g., ≤30 min) screening tests for the detection of HIV antibodies.[53–55] Two rapid HIV-1 tests have been approved by the FDA for use in the United States: OraQuick Rapid HIV-1 Antibody Test (OraSure Technologies, Inc., Bethlehem, Pennsylvania) and Single Use Diagnostic System for HIV-1 (SUDS, Murex-Abbott Inc., Norcross, Georgia). Both tests have specificity and sensitivity similar to EIA, require moderate complexity to perform, can be stored at room temperature, and require no specialized laboratory equipment.

The OraQuick test is a lateral flow immunochromatographic strip (e.g., similar to dipsticks for pregnancy testing) designed to be used as a point-of-care test that requires a whole blood sample that can be obtained from a finger stick. In brief, a small drop of blood is added to a vial containing developer solution. The test device is then placed in the vial until the results are directly read from the device at no less than 20 min (however not greater than 60 min). The appearance of two reddish bands is indicative of a reactive (or positive) test for HIV-1 antibodies. A single reddish band at the control location of the device signifies a negative test.

The SUDS test uses a microfiltration enzyme immunoassay involving the addition of serum or plasma to a test cartridge, and it traditionally has been performed in a clinical laboratory from a blood sample obtained by venipuncture. The test reagents and buffer are added to the cartridge at timed intervals with the results being read directly from a membrane on the cartridge. A bluish color is indicative of a reactive (or positive) test of HIV-1 antibodies whereas no color is considered a negative test. A reactive test should be immediately repeated, and if the second result is also reactive, then a preliminary positive test can be reported. Although the test procedure requires about 15 min to perform, the entire procedure takes about 0.75–1.5 hr to complete since blood collection and specimen handling is required.

Rapid HIV testing has proven useful for the detection of HIV infection in a number of clinical settings including during the labor and delivery of a pregnant women at high risk of HIV infection who was never previously tested, at facilities where return rates for HIV test results are low, and when a health care worker has been potentially exposed to HIV infection (e.g., through a needle stick) and immediate decisions regarding postexposure prophylaxis are needed.[54-56] As with other screening tests for HIV-1 antibodies (including EIA), a positive result from a rapid HIV test must be confirmed with an alternative method of testing (e.g., Western blot or IFA) before the final diagnosis of HIV infection can be made. If the results of a rapid HIV test are negative, a person is considered uninfected. However, retesting should be considered in persons with possible exposure to HIV within the previous 3 months since the testing may have been performed too early in the infection to detect antibodies to the virus.

Noninvasive HIV-1 tests. Several tests have been developed for testing antibodies to HIV from oral fluid or urine.[53-55] The Orasure Western blot kit (Epitope Inc., Beaverton, Oregon) uses a cotton fiber pad that is place between the cheek and lower gum for 2 min to collect oral mucosal transudate containing IgG. Orasure HIV-1 oral device is FDA-approved and has a specificity of 99.4% (similar to EIA). Two urine-based HIV-1 tests (EIA and Western blot) have also been FDA-approved for use. The urine tests are associated with a lower sensitivity and specificity than the oral fluid testing. As with EIA testing of blood samples, subsequent testing is required for both types of tests in order to confirm the diagnosis of HIV infection. Noninvasive HIV-1 testing should be considered in persons who are unable to go to health care facilities, have poor venous access, or are reluctant to have their blood drawn. The advantages of these tests include avoidance of blood drawing for sample collection, ease of use, low cost, and stability of samples for up to 3 weeks at room temperature.

Home sample collection tests. Several home sample collection tests for the detection of HIV infection are available over-the-counter.[53-55] A few drops of whole blood are obtained using a finger stick and placed on a blood specimen card. The dried blood spot is mailed to a designated laboratory that then uses EIA to detect HIV-1 antibodies. The person calls for the results (positive or negative for HIV antibodies) over the next 3–7 business days. A telephone counselor provides the test results, telephone support, information, guidance about repeat testing, and referral as needed. The advantages of home sample collection tests include ready access to HIV-1 testing, convenience, lower costs, anonymity, and privacy.

p24 Antigen Tests

The main core protein of HIV is p24, with levels of p24 antigen being elevated during the early and late stages of HIV infection. The direct detection of HIV-1 p24 antigen can be performed using one of several commercial EIA assay kits (two of which are FDA-approved for use).[53,54] Similar to antibody testing, positive results of the initial testing for HIV-1 p24 antigen must be retested in duplicate using the same EIA method. In addition, these results need to be confirmed with a neutralization assay specific for antibodies to HIV-1 p24 antigen. Many of the commercial assay kits have increased their sensitivity by providing the appropriate reagents to allow dissociation of antigen-antibody immune complexes before testing is completed.

The current uses of p24 antigen testing include screening blood donors, detecting growth in viral cultures, and as an alternative diagnostic test for HIV-1 in acute HIV infection or infants less than 18 months of age born to HIV-infected mothers (Table 17-14).[53,54] The advantages of the p24 antigen test include the earlier detection of HIV infection compared to antibody testing (16 days vs. 22 days), easier to perform, low cost, and specificity that approaches 100%. However, the DNA PCR assays and plasma HIV-RNA concentrations demonstrate greater sensitivity and have replaced the p24 antigen tests in many clinical situations.

DNA PCR

DNA polymerase chain reaction (PCR) is an effective technique for early detection of proviral HIV-1 DNA in almost all patients with HIV infection.[53,54,57] This method can detect small amounts of nucleic acid obtained from whole blood, peripheral blood mononuclear cells (PBMCs), or HIV-1 RNA in plasma or serum (after being converted to cDNA with reverse transcription). The advantages of HIV DNA PCR include a high level (>98%) of sensitivity and specificity, the requirement for only a small volume of blood (e.g., 200 µl), and the rapid turnaround time. The disadvantages include the expense, the high level of variability between laboratories performing the assays, and the limited availability of commercial assays (none are FDA-approved).

The current recommended uses for DNA PCR include diagnosis of HIV infection in infants (<18 months of age) born to HIV-infected mothers and any clinical situations where antibody tests are inconclusive or undetectable (Table 17-14).[53,54,57] Antibody tests are not useful for diagnosing HIV infection in infants since maternal HIV antibodies can persist in the infant for up to 18 months after birth. Therefore, infants should be tested with the DNA PCR test at the ages of 48 hr, 1–2 months, and 3–6 months. A negative test at birth can be repeated at 14 days of life since the assay sensitivity is increased by 2 weeks of life. In order to confirm the diagnosis of HIV infection, a positive result at any sampling time needs to be confirmed by a second specimen collected shortly after the first positive result. If two or more negative results (two being at age ≥1 month and one being at age ≥4 months) are obtained, then the diagnosis of HIV infection can be reasonably excluded.

HIV-RNA Concentration

The accurate measurement of plasma HIV-RNA concentrations (also known as the HIV viral load) in conjunction with CD4+ T lymphocyte count has become an essential component in the management of patients with HIV-1 infection.[53,54,56–59] The results of these two laboratory tests provide the clinician with information regarding a patient's virologic and immunologic status, which is needed to make decisions regarding the initiation or changing of antiretroviral therapy as well as to predict the progression of infection towards AIDS. In addition, plasma HIV-RNA concentrations can assist in the diagnosis of HIV infection in selected clinical situations (see Table 17-14).[53,54]

Current methods that are used to measure the amount of HIV-RNA in plasma include coupling reverse transcription to a DNA polymerase chain reaction (RT-PCR), identification of HIV-RNA with signal amplification by DNA branched-chain technique (bDNA), and nucleic acid sequence-based amplification (NASBA). Currently, the RT-PCR assay (Amplicor HIV-1 Monitor, Roche Molecular Diagnostics) is the only method that has been approved by the FDA for the diagnosis of HIV infection. The results of any of the test methods are reported as the number of HIV copies/mL. A plasma HIV-RNA level of 10,000 copies/mL or lower is suggestive of a good prognosis, whereas a level above 100,000 copies/mL suggests a substantial risk of disease progression. In addition, changes in the amount of plasma HIV-RNA (used to monitor the response to antiretroviral therapy) are often reported in log base 10 values. For example, a change from 10,000 to 1000 copies/mL would be considered a 1-log decrease in viral load. Also, these assays have a lower limit of detection of approximately 50 copies/mL. Therefore, if a viral load is reported as "undetectable," it signifies that the plasma HIV-RNA concentrations are below the lower limits of detection of the assay. Viral load testing should not be performed during or within 4 weeks of acute infection, during illnesses, or immediately after immunization since plasma HIV-RNA levels can be increased.

Once the diagnosis of HIV-1 infection has been confirmed, a plasma HIV-RNA level should be measured to assist in the decision to start or defer therapy. Ideally, the plasma HIV-RNA level (and CD4+ T lymphocyte count) is performed on two separate occasions before antiretroviral therapy should be initiated. The decision to start antiretroviral therapy will depend on the clinical findings and symptoms of the patient, the laboratory values for plasma HIV-RNA levels and CD4+ T lymphocyte count, the willingness of the patient to comply with therapy, and the potential risks associated with therapy. Although expert guidelines differ in their recommendations, initiation of therapy is often suggested in asymptomatic infected patients with plasma HIV-RNA levels above 50,000 to 100,000 copies/mL (and any level of CD4+ T lymphocyte count).[58,59] For patients started on drug therapy, current guidelines recommend monitoring plasma HIV-RNA levels at the following time intervals: (1) 2–8 weeks and 3–4 months after starting antiretroviral drug therapy; (2) every 3–4 months while on therapy; and (3) anytime that a clinical event occurs including a significant decline in CD4+ T lymphocyte count. With optimal therapy, plasma HIV-RNA levels should decrease by 3-fold or >0.5 $\log_{10}$ during the first 2–8 weeks after starting therapy and should continue to decline over subsequent weeks. The goal of therapy should be to obtain an undetectable viral load (e.g., <50 copies/mL) by 6 months of therapy. However, every patient responds differently. For patients who are not on therapy, plasma HIV-RNA levels should be monitored every 3–4 months. All testing of plasma HIV-RNA levels should be conducted by the same laboratory and laboratory method so that consistent results are obtained. The reader is encouraged to review the most recent guidelines on HIV-infection since recommendations for different patient populations are continuously being modified as newer data becomes available.[57–60]

CD4+ T Lymphocyte Count

Flow cytometry can be used to identify the various subsets of lymphocytes by their cluster of differentiation (CD) of specific monoclonal antibodies to surface antigens. The CD4+ T lymphocytes are the helper-inducer T cells, whereas the CD8+ T lymphocytes are the cytotoxic-suppresser T cells. HIV infection causes a decrease in the total number of lymphocytes (particularly the CD4+ T lymphocytes) as well as changes in the ratios of the different types of lymphocytes. A person with a CD4+ T lymphocyte count of less than 200 cells/mm^3 (normal count 800–1100 cells/mm^3) or a CD4+ T lymphocyte count of less than 14% of the total lymphocyte count (normal 40% of total lymphocytes) is indicative of severe immunosuppression and at risk for the development of opportunistic infections.

As stated earlier, the CD4+ T lymphocyte count is utilized in conjunction with the plasma HIV-RNA level to provide clinicians with essential information regarding a patient's virologic and immunologic status, progression of infection towards AIDS, and decisions to initiate or change antiretroviral therapy.[58,59] Because of this, most guidelines recommend monitoring CD4+ T lymphocyte counts at a frequency similar to or guided by plasma HIV-RNA levels (see above). Expert guidelines recommend initiation of antiretroviral therapy in asymptomatic, HIV-infected patients with a CD4+ T lymphocyte count <200 cells/mm^3 (and at any value of plasma HIV RNA). When the CD4+ T lymphocyte count is in the range of 200–350 cells/mm^3 or greater, the decision to start therapy in asymptomatic patients is less clear and should be individualized. Therapy may need to be considered in patients with a high rate of decline in CD4+ T lymphocyte (defined as >100 cell/mm^3 per annum) even when current count is 350 cells/mm^3 or greater.

Phenotypic and Genotypic Assays for Drug Resistance

Resistance of HIV-1 to antiretroviral drugs is an important cause for treatment failure. Genotypic assays detect point mutations known to confer drug resistance in the reverse transcriptase (RT) or protease amino acid sequences of HIV-1. Phenotypic assays, particularly those incorporating the insertion of enzymatic activities of RT and protease, measure the concentration of antiretroviral agent needed to inhibit 50% or 90% (IC_{50} or IC_{90}) of viral replication. The ratio of IC values for the test and reference viruses is calculated and used to report the fold-increase in resistance of each antiretroviral agent. The interpretation of results from both assays is complex and requires expert knowledge and consultation.[53,58,59]

The current recommended uses for drug resistance assays include virologic failure during highly active antiretroviral therapy (HAART) and suboptimal suppression of plasma HIV-RNA level after the initiation of antiretroviral therapy.[53,58,59] Resistance testing should also be considered in acute HIV infections. Phenotypic and/or genotypic assays are generally not recommended in patients with chronic HIV-infection who have not started antiretroviral therapy, in patients who have discontinued drug therapy, and or in patients with plasma HIV-RNA levels <1000 copies/mL.

The advantages and disadvantages of genotypic and phenotypic assays for the detection of HIV-1 resistance have been previously described.[53] In brief, the genotypic assay may be preferred over the phenotypic assay because they are more readily available, are clinically relevant, and have a faster turnaround time (1–2 weeks) compared to phenotypic assays (2–6 weeks). Both assays are complex, technically demanding, and expensive, and are not routinely performed in most clinical laboratories.

MYCOBACTERIA

Mycobacteria are nonmotile, nonspore-forming aerobic bacilli that are still considered to be a significant cause of morbidity and mortality, especially in developing countries.[61] Currently, more than 70 species of mycobacteria have been identified, with infections in humans most often caused by only a handful of species including M. *tuberculosis*, M. *leprae*, M. *avium* complex, M. *kansasii*, M. *fortuitum*, M. *chelonae*, M. *marinum*, and M. *abscessus*. Depending on the species, mycobacteria can be nonpathogenic, pathogenic, or opportunistic and, therefore, may cause infection in both normal and immunocom-promised hosts. The common pathogenic mycobacteria species, the infections that they cause, and their environmental sources are listed in Table 17-15.[61–67]

TABLE 17-15

MYCOBACTERIUM SPECIES	ASSOCIATED INFECTIONS	ENVIRONMENTAL SOURCES
Mycobacterium tuberculosis (Tuberculosis, TB, "Consumption")	Pulmonary infection, lymphadenitis, musculoskeletal infection, gastrointestinal infection, peritonitis, hepatitis, pericarditis	Humans
Mycobacterium bovis	Soft tissue infection, gastrointestinal infection	Humans, cattle
Mycobacterium leprae (Leprosy, Hansen's disease)	Skin and soft tissue infections	Humans, armadillos
Mycobacterium avium complex (MAC)	Pulmonary infection, cutaneous ulcers, lymphadenitis, disseminated infection	Soil, water, swine, cattle, birds
Mycobacterium kansasii	Pulmonary infection, musculoskeletal infection, disseminated infection	Water, cattle
Mycobacterium fortuitum	Skin and soft tissue infections, disseminated infection	Soil, water, animals, marine life
Mycobacterium chelonae	Skin and soft tissue infections, osteomyelitis, disseminated infection	Soil, water, animals, marine life
Mycobacterium abscessus	Skin and soft tissue infections, osteomyelitis, disseminated infection	Soil, water, animals, marine life
Mycobacterium marinum	Skin and soft tissue infections	Fish, water

Table 17-15. Pathogenic Mycobacteria and Associated Infections[61–67]

The genus of *Mycobacterium* is typically divided into two groups based on epidemiology and spectrum of disease: (1) the M. *tuberculosis* complex that includes the species M. *tuberculosis*, M. *bovis*, M. *bovis* bacille Calmette-Guerin (BCG), M. *africanum*, and M. *microti*, and (2) nontuberculous mycobacteria (NTM, or also referred to as mycobacteria other than tuberculosis, MOTT), which include all other species of mycobacteria.

The most clinically significant mycobacterial species is *Mycobacterium tuberculosis*, which is the causative organism of tuberculosis or TB. The incidence of tuberculosis in the United States was on a steady decline between 1953 (when it became a notifiable disease) and 1985 as a result of improved diagnostic methods, public health efforts to isolate TB patients, and the introduction of effective antimycobacterial agents.[62] This decline in TB led experts to predict the elimination of the disease by 2010. However, between 1986 and 1992, there was an increase in the incidence of TB in the United States due to deterioration of TB public health programs, the emergence of the HIV epidemic, the increase in immigration, and the emergence of multidrug resistant tuberculosis. Since 1992, the number of cases of TB in the United States has declined steadily in the face of improved public health control strategies. Despite the advances in medical care and treatment, tuberculosis continues to be one of the most common infectious diseases worldwide, causing 8 million new cases and 2 million deaths annually.[61,67] Since TB can be transmitted from person-to-person, rapid diagnosis is necessary to decrease the spread of infection.

The Identification of Mycobacteria

Mycobacteria possess a number of unique characteristics that contribute to some of the difficulty in the growth, identification, and treatment of these organisms. The cell wall of mycobacteria is complex and composed of peptidoglycan, polypeptides, and a lipid-rich hydrophobic layer. This cell wall structure bestows a number of distinguishing properties in the mycobacteria including (1) resistance to disinfectants and detergents; (2) the inability to be stained by many common laboratory identification stains; (3) the inability of mycobacteria to be decolorized by acid solutions (a characteristic which has given them the name of *acidfast* bacilli or AFB); (4) the ability of mycobacteria to grow slowly, and (5) resistance to common anti-infective agents.[61,64] These characteristics have led to the continuous modification and improvement of laboratory practices used in the diagnosis of mycobacterial infections. Many of these laboratory practices involve specialized growth media, identification techniques, specialized environmental conditions (Biosafety Level 3 facilities for M. *tuberculosis*), and susceptibility testing techniques that may be unavailable in some clinical laboratories.[64,66]

The ability to accurately diagnose the presence of a mycobacterial infection is highly dependent on appropriate selection and collection of biologic specimens for staining and culture. Since different mycobacteria are capable of causing a number of infections (as listed in Table 17-15), the following biologic specimens may be submitted for mycobacterial culture depending on the site of infection: respiratory tract secretions (e.g., sputum and bronchial washings, especially for the diagnosis of tuberculosis), gastric lavage specimens (tuberculosis), cerebrospinal fluid, blood (especially for M. *avium* complex), stool (especially for M. *avium* complex), urine, tissue, exudate or wound drainage, bone marrow, sterile body fluids, and skin specimens.[62,64] For the diagnosis of pulmonary tuberculosis, several early morning, concentrated sputum specimens are recommended to improve diagnostic accuracy.[62,66] Biologic specimens for mycobacterial culture should be processed according to specified guidelines shortly after reaching the microbiology lab to prevent the overgrowth of bacteria that may also be present in the specimen. Specimens should also be concentrated to enhance diagnostic capability.[62,64,66]

Similar to the processing of a specimen for bacterial culture, biologic specimens submitted for mycobacterial culture are stained for microscopic examination for mycobacterial elements and also plated for mycobacterial culture. The stains and culture media, however, are somewhat different since mycobacteria are poorly visualized with a Gram stain and take longer to grow than conventional bacteria.

The microscopic examination of a processed specimen for mycobacterial culture is a rapid diagnostic test that typically involves the use of stains that are taken up by elements of the mycobacterial cell wall. Two different acid-fast stains are commonly utilized for the microscopic examination of mycobacteria and include the carbolfuschin stains viewed under light microscopy (Ziehl-Neelsen or Kinyoun method) and fluorochrome stains (auramine-rhodamine) examined under fluorescence microscopy (a more sensitive test). The sensitivity of the staining method is highly dependent on the type of clinical specimen, the species of mycobacteria present, the technique utilized in specimen processing, the staining method, the thickness of the smear, and the experience of the laboratory technologist.[62,64] These methods are able to detect the presence of mycobacteria in the clinical specimen but cannot differentiate which species is present or if the organism is viable. However, several molecular techniques involving nucleic acid amplification (polymerase chain reaction or PCR) are now commercially available to detect M. tuberculosis in acid-fast smear positive specimens (Amplicor Mycobacterium tuberculosis Test by Roche Diagnostic Systems and the Amplified Mycobacterium tuberculosis Direct Test by Gen-Probe).[61,62,64,66–68]

A combination of culture media, including at least one solid medium and one broth medium, is often used for the cultivation of mycobacteria in order to optimize the growth and pigment production of the organism which is needed for identification.[64,67] The preferred commercially-available solid media for the culture of mycobacteria include a serum-based agar medium such as Middlebrook 7H10 and an egg-based medium such as Lowenstein-Jensen. Many labs utilize both media for the culture of mycobacteria in clinical specimens.

There are several liquid medium systems that are available for the culture of mycobacteria, some of which employ continuous monitoring systems for the detection of mycobacterial growth.[64,67,68] These systems typically provide more rapid isolation of acid-fast bacilli when compared to conventional solid media techniques, with results often observed within 10 days as compared to 2–3 weeks using solid medium.[62,64–66] The most commonly used semiautomated systems include the BACTEC 460 TB system (Becton Dickinson Diagnostic Systems), the Septi-Check AFB System (Becton Dickinson Diagnostic Systems), and the Mycobacterial Growth Indicator Tube (MGIT, Becton Dickinson). The fully automated, continuous monitoring systems that are available include the ESP Culture System II (Accumed International), the BACTEC 9000 MB (Becton Dickinson), and the BACTEC MGIT 960 (Becton Dickinson). Once growth is detected using any of these liquid medium systems, an acid-fast stain is performed on the specimen (to confirm the presence of mycobacteria) and then subsequently subcultured on solid media.

Mycobacterial cultures should be incubated at 35 °C (optimal) in the dark in an atmosphere of 5–10% carbon dioxide and high humidity for up to 8 weeks. Cultures for mycobacteria typically require prolonged incubation periods (8 weeks) because most of the more common pathogens grow rather slowly. The rapid growing mycobacteria (M. fortuitum, M. chelonae, M. abscessus) can usually grow on solid media within 7 days, while the slow growing mycobacteria (M. tuberculosis, M. avium complex, M. kansasii, M. marinum) often require longer than 7 days for colonies to appear (up to 7 weeks for some species). Therefore, culture tubes are typically examined weekly during the incubation period.

Once growth appears on the culture plates, the organisms are subjected to microscopic examination (observed for characteristic colonial morphologic features, pigmentation, and growth rate); biochemical tests; and molecular detection methods (PCR methods mentioned above, DNA hybridization using DNA probes, and chromatographic methods such as HPLC or GLC to detect mycobacterial lipids) for definitive identification.[62,64–68] DNA probes are highly sensitive and specific and are now available for the identification of M. tuberculosis, M. gordonae, M. kansasii, and M. avium complex.[65,67] All of the recently developed molecular methods have significantly decreased the identification time of mycobacterial species to within 21 days of specimen receipt (as compared to several weeks or months using traditional identification methods) and have replaced the use of biochemical tests in many laboratories.[62,68]

Susceptibility Testing of Mycobacteria

The choice of which antibiotic or antimycobacterial agents to utilize in the treatment of a mycobacterial infection truly depends on the species of mycobacteria involved. It is important for the clinician to have an understanding of the typical susceptibility pattern of the specific mycobacterial species, the current treatment guidelines regarding which and how many drugs to use, and the methodology available for drug susceptibility testing for the particular mycobacterial species being treated.

Currently, there are standardized guidelines available only for the susceptibility testing of M. tuberculosis. The testing can be performed directly on a smear-positive specimen (direct method) or on isolated colonies (indirect method), with the direct method producing faster but less standardized results.[64,66] There are four conventional methods that can be used for determining the susceptibility of M. tuberculosis isolates to antituberculous agents including the absolute concentration method, the resistance ratio method, the agar proportion method, and the liquid radiometric method (using the BACTEC 460 instrument). Susceptibility testing is initially performed using primary antituberculous agents such as isoniazid, rifampin, ethambutol, streptomycin, and pyrazinamide. However, if resistance to any of these drugs is demonstrated, susceptibility testing is then performed using second-line drugs such as ethionamide, capreomycin, ciprofloxacin, ofloxacin, kanamycin, cycloserine, or rifabutin.[64,66] The proportion method and the BACTEC radiometric method are most often used in the United States.

The proportion method is a modified agar dilution test that evaluates the extent of growth of a standardized inoculum of M. tuberculosis in control and drug-containing agar medium. The organism is considered resistant if its growth is greater than 1% on the agar plate containing critical concentrations of the drug. The results of the proportion method are typically available 21 days after the plates have been inoculated.

The BACTEC radiometric method utilizes liquid growth medium and measures the growth of the organism in the presence and absence of the antituberculous drug. This method generates rapid susceptibility results for the primary antituberculous agents but cannot be used for susceptibility testing of second-line agents. However, this method is recommended as the initial susceptibility test by most experts since the results are often available within 5–7 days after inoculation, and can help guide appropriate therapy without the unnecessary delay of the proportion method.[62,66,67]

There are a number of other susceptibility testing methods that are currently being evaluated for drug susceptibility testing of M. tuberculosis. Many antimycobacterial drugs are now available in E-test strips, including streptomycin, ethambutol, isoniazid, and ethionamide.[68] Several studies have evaluated their performance as compared to the BACTEC radiometric method; however, further studies are needed to validate their use as a suitable, alternative susceptibility testing method. In addition, newer molecular methods for drug susceptibility testing of M. tuberculosis are currently being evaluated that are easier to perform and produce more reliable results in a shorter period of time.[64,66–68] These methods include PCR amplification, DNA sequencing line probe assays, or single-strand conformation polymorphism to detect known drug resistance mutations. Further study, however, is warranted before these newer susceptibility testing methods can replace conventional methods.

Susceptibility testing methods for nontuberculous mycobacteria (NTM) have not been standardized for many species and are only routinely recommended for rapidly growing mycobacteria such as M. *fortuitum*, M. *chelonae*, and M. *abscessus*.[64,65,67,68] Susceptibility testing of M. *avium* complex is recommended on initial blood isolates in patients with disseminated infection and on clinically significant isolates from patients on previous or current macrolide therapy.[65] Depending on the species isolated, the methods that can be utilized for susceptibility testing of NTM include the radiometric BACTEC method (M. *avium* complex and M. *kansasii*), microtiter dilution (M. *avium* complex and M. *kansasii*), the agar proportion method (M. *kansasii*), broth microdilution (M. *fortuitum*, M. *chelonae*, and M. *abscessus*), the E-test method (M. *fortuitum*, M. *chelonae*, and M. *abscessus*), and agar disk elution (M. *fortuitum*, M. *chelonae*, and M. *abscessus*).[62,64,65,68]

Skin Testing

The Mantoux test or tuberculin skin test is the only widely utilized test available for the detection of latent tuberculosis. It involves the intradermal injection of a purified protein derivative (PPD) of the tubercle bacilli, which is obtained from a culture filtrate derived by protein precipitation.[66] Injection of the PPD into previously exposed individuals will elicit a delayed hypersensitivity reaction involving T cells that migrate to the area of intradermal injection (usually the dorsal aspect of the forearm), induce the release of lymphokines, and produce induration and edema within 48–72 hr after injection. Therefore, the diameter of induration should be evaluated by a health care professional between 48–72 hr after injection. There are published guidelines for determining a positive tuberculin skin test reaction based on the size of the induration and a number of clinical and demographic characteristics of the patient.[61,66] An induration of ≥5 mm is considered positive for persons at high risk of developing tuberculous disease if they are exposed to tuberculosis including HIV infected patients; patients on immunosuppressive agents; and patients who have been recently exposed to tuberculosis. An induration of 10 mm is considered positive for patients who are not immunocompromised and possess no other identified risk factors for developing tuberculous disease, such as recent immigrants from high prevalence countries; injection drug users; residents and employees of high-risk settings (e.g., prisons, health-care facilities, and mycobacteria lab personnel); persons with chronic medical conditions of high risk (e.g., diabetes, silicosis, and CRF), and children younger than 4 years of age. An induration of ≥15mm is considered positive for persons at low risk for developing active infection with tuberculosis.

LABORATORY TESTS UTILIZED FOR THE IDENTIFICATION OF UNCOMMON OR MISCELLANEOUS ORGANISMS

There are a number of pathogenic organisms which are difficult to detect or cultivate using the standard microbiologic procedures outlined above. These organisms often pose a diagnostic dilemma since they often require some type of specialized testing for identification. It is beyond the scope of this chapter to describe in detail all of the specialized testing methods that are available to detect these organisms. However, an abbreviated list can be found in Table 17-16.[69–85]

LABORATORY TESTS UTILIZED FOR THE DIAGNOSIS OF SPECIFIC INFECTIONS

Meningitis

Meningitis is one of the few infectious diseases medical emergencies and requires prompt and accurate diagnosis and treatment. Many different pathogens can cause meningitis (e.g., bacteria, viruses, fungi, and mycobacteria) with a resulting clinical presentation of acute or

TABLE 17-16

ORGANISM	TYPE OF ORGANISM	CLINICAL FINDINGS AND INFECTIONS	DIAGNOSTIC METHOD	POSITIVE RESULT	REFER-ENCES
***Bordetella pertussis* (Whooping cough)**	Bacteria	Upper respiratory tract symptoms, characteristic whooping cough, pneumonia	Culture	Growth within 3 to 4 days	69
			PCR	Direct detection in 1 to 2 days	
***Borrelia burgdorferi* (Lyme disease)**	Spirochete	Erythema migrans, pericarditis, arthritis, neurologic disease	Culture	Hold cultures for 6 to 8 weeks	71
			ELISA	Measures antibody responses against *B. burgdorferi* antigens	
			Western Blot	Measures antibody response to specific borrelial antigens	
			PCR	Can detect low numbers of spirochetes	
***Brucella* sp.**	Bacteria	Systemic infection (can involve any organ); spondylitis, arthritis, endocarditis	Culture	Growth within 7 days; but hold cultures for 30 days	72
			Serum agglutination test (SAT)	Detects antibodies to most *Brucella* sp.; titer of ≥ 1:160 is positive	
Chlamydia pneumoniae	Atypical bacteria	Upper respiratory tract infections, pharyngitis, pneumonia	Complement Fixation	Fourfold rise in titer between acute and convalescent sera	69
			Microimmuno-fluorescence (MIF)	Fourfold rise in titer, IgM titer of ≥1:16, or an IgG titer ≥1:512	
***Clostridium difficile* (Pseudo-membranous colitis)**	Anaerobic bacteria	Pseudomembranous colitis, diarrhea	Culture using CCFA growth media	Growth within 48 hr	73
			Cell culture cytotoxin test or Enzyme immunoassay (EIA) toxin test	Detection of toxin A activity	
***Coxiella burnetti* (Q Fever)**	Bacteria	Acute or chronic systemic illness, pneumonia, hepatitis, endocarditis	Indirect immuno-fluorescence	IgM titer of ≥1:50, or an IgG titer ≥1:200	69
Crypto-sporidium parvum	Protozoa	Acute diarrhea (self-limiting to severe), abdominal pain, dehydration	Modified acid faxt staining	Detection of oocysts in stool or intestinal scrapings	74,75
			Immunofluorescent assay using a monoclonal anti-body against oocyst	Detection of oocysts in stool or intestinal scrapings	
			Enzyme immuno-assay (EIA)	Detection of oocysts in stool or intestinal scrapings	

Continued on next page

TABLE 17-16

ORGANISM	TYPE OF ORGANISM	CLINICAL FINDINGS AND INFECTIONS	DIAGNOSTIC METHOD	POSITIVE RESULT	REFER-ENCES
Entamoeba histolytica	Protozoa	Amebiasis: intestinal (colitis, diarrhea) and extraintestinal (liver abscesses)	Stool exam for ova and parasites (O & P) with culture	Detection of trophozoites and/or cysts	74,75
			Enzyme immuno-assay (EIA)	Detection of trophozoites and/or cysts	
			Serology (indirect immunohemag-glutination assay for amebic liver abscesses)	Positive titer (can remain positive for years after initial infection)	
***Erlichia* sp.**	Bacteria	Human monocytotropic ehrlichiosis or HME (fever, severe headache, malaise, chills, myalgias, and arthralgias) which can be moderate to life-threatening	Indirect immuno-fluorescence serology	Single sample IgG titer of >1:128 or a 4-fold rise in titer between acute and convalescent sera	76
Giardia lamblia	Protozoa	Acute diarrhea (self-limiting to severe), malabsorption syndromes	Stool exam for ova and parasites (O & P)	Detection of trophozoites and/or cysts	74,75
			Wet preps or stains of duodenal material	Detection of trophozoites and/or cysts	
			ELISA or immuno-fluorescence assay	Detection of trophozoites and/or cysts	
Helicobacter pylori	Bacteria	Peptic ulcer disease	Urea breath test	Positive test indicative of the presence of organism	77,78
			Serologic tests	Detect IgG and IgA antibodies to *H. pylori*	
			Stool antigen assays (EIA)	Detection of *H. pylori* specific antigens	
			Urease test on antral biopsy specimen	Positive test indicative of the presence of organism	
Legionella pneumophila	Atypical bacteria	Pneumonia	Culture (using specialized media)	Growth in 3–5 days	69,70,85
			Direct fluorescent antibody (DFA) staining	Binds to *L. pneumophila* antigen to produce fluorescence	
			Serology—IFA	Acute and convalescent sera required, 4-fold or greater rise in antibody titer to ≥1:128	
			Urinary antigen detection (EIA, RIA, ICT)	Only detects Legionella serotype 1 antigen	

Continued on next page

TABLE 17-16

ORGANISM	TYPE OF ORGANISM	CLINICAL FINDINGS AND INFECTIONS	DIAGNOSTIC METHOD	POSITIVE RESULT	REFER-ENCES
Leishmania *sp.*	Protozoa	Cutaneous or visceral (Kala-Azar) infection; can infect organs of the reticulo-endothelial system	Giemsa staining and light microscopy	Amastigotes within the tissue specimen	75
			Culture	Growth of promastigotes	
Leptospira *sp.*	Spirochetes	Anicteric leptospirosis (self-limiting with high fevers, headache, aseptic meningitis); icteric leptospirosis (severe with liver, kidney, and/or vascular dysfunction)	Dark-field microscopy or immuno-fluorescence	Detection of motile leptospires	79
			Culture	Growth within 6 weeks	
			Serology using microscopic agglutination	Fourfold or greater rise in agglutinating antibodies	
Mycoplasma *hominis*	Atypical bacteria	Urogenital tract infections including prostatitis, pelvic inflammatory disease, bacterial vaginosis, urethritis; systemic infection in neonates and immunocompromised	Culture using selective media	Growth within 5 days	80
Mycoplasma *pneumoniae*	Atypical bacteria	Pneumonia, tracheobronchitis	Cold agglutinins	Titers >1:128	69
			Complement fixation serology	Fourfold rise in titer between acute and convalescent sera	
Plasmodium *falciparum*, *P. vivax*, *P. ovale*, *P. malariae* **(Malaria)**	Protozoa	Symptoms include high fever (cyclic with *P. vivax*, *P. ovale*, *P. malariae*), chills, nausea, vomiting, severe headache, anemia, abdominal pain; life-threatening with *P. falciparum*	Thick and thin blood films stained with Giemsa or Wright's stain	Presence of malarial parasites	75,81
			Fluorescence microscopy	Detection of fluorescence when dyes are taken up by the nucleus of the parasite	
			PCR (not routine)	Detection of malaria-specific DNA sequences	
Pneumocystis *carinii*	Protozoa or Fungus?	Pneumonia, extrapulmonary infection	Modified Wright-Giemsa stain of induced sputum	Detection of trophozoites or intracystic sporozoites	82
			Direct fluorescent antibody (DFA) stains	Detection of cysts or trophozoites	
			PCR	Detection of *P. carinii*-specific nucleic acid	
Rickettsia *ricksettii* **(Rocky Mountain spotted fever or RMSF)**	Rickettsia	Fever, headache and rash in patient with recent tick bite; myalgias, malaise, nausea, vomiting, abdominal pain, focal neurologic findings	Serology by latex agglutination, indirect fluore-scent antibody test (IFA), or direct fluore-scent antibody testing	Detection of IgM or IgG antibodies to *Rickettsia sp.*	83

Continued on next page

TABLE 17-16

ORGANISM	TYPE OF ORGANISM	CLINICAL FINDINGS AND INFECTIONS	DIAGNOSTIC METHOD	POSITIVE RESULT	REFER-ENCES
Taenia solium	Tapeworm	Neurocysticercosis (infection within brain tissue) causing seizures, headache, focal neurologic deficits; muscular and subcutaneous abscesses	Serology by the enzyme-linked immunoelectro-transfer blot assay (EITB)	Detection of antibodies to *T. solium* glycoprotein antigens	75
			ELISA on CSF	Detection of anticysticercal antibodies or cysticercal antigens	
***Toxoplasmosis gondii* (Toxo-plasmosis)**	Protozoa	Encephalitis, myocarditis, lymphadenitis, polymyositis, chorioretinitis, toxo-plasmosis during pregnancy	Serology	Positive IgG antibody	75,84
			Analysis of CSF or body tissues	Demonstration of tachyzoites	
			PCR	Detection of *T. gondii*-specific DNA	
Ureaplasma urealyticum	Atypical Bacteria	Urogenital tract infections including prostatitis, pelvic inflammatory disease, bacterial vaginosis, urethritis; systemic infection in neonates and immunocompromised	Culture using selective media	Growth within 5 days	80

PCR = Polymerase chain reaction.
ELISA = Enzyme-linked immunosorbent assay.
ICT = Immunochromatographic membrane assay.

Table 17-16. Specialized Laboratory Tests for the Detection of Specific Organisms

chronic meningitis depending on the causative organism. Therefore, in a patient with a suspected CNS infection, a lumbar puncture is performed to obtain a sample of cerebrospinal fluid (CSF) for laboratory analysis to aid in the diagnosis of the infection and the causative organism.[86–91] A lumbar puncture involves the aseptic insertion of a spinal needle into the subarachnoid space (at the lumbar spine level), with the aspiration of CSF (5–20 mL) which is placed into three or four separate sterile screw-cap tubes.[86,87] Once obtained, the CSF specimens should be immediately transported to the laboratory for rapid processing. The first two tubes of CSF are processed for microbiologic (e.g., Gram stain, fungal stains, antigen detection, and culture) and chemical studies (e.g., glucose and protein), while the last two tubes are processed for determination of the cell count and differential as described below. The typical chemistry, hematology, and microbiologic findings in the CSF of patients with several different types of meningitis are listed in Table 17-17. The opening pressure is also measured when initiating the lumbar puncture and may be elevated in patients with meningitis due to the presence of cerebral edema or intracranial foci of infection.[89]

Chemistry and Hematology

The chemistry and hematology results from the CSF analysis correlate directly with the probability of infection, so that negative findings exclude the likelihood of meningitis in almost all cases.[87,90] In patients with meningitis, the CSF protein concentration is elevated (possibly due to disruption of the blood brain barrier), and the CSF glucose concentration is decreased. Patients with acute bacterial meningitis often demonstrate marked abnormalities in the chemistry analysis of the CSF, with protein concentrations of >100 mg/dL and glucose concentrations <45 mg/dL (or a CSF:blood glucose ratio of <0.5).[88,89]

TABLE 17-17

	NORMAL	BACTERIAL MENINGITIS	VIRAL INFECTION	FUNGAL MENINGITIS	TUBERCULOUS MENINGITIS
Opening pressure (mm H$_2$0)	<180	>180			
White blood cells (count/mm^3)	0–5	400–20,000 (mean 800)	5–500 (mean 80)	20–2000 (mean 100)	5–2000 (mean 200)
WBC differential	No predominance	>80% PMNs	>50% Lymphs, < 20% PMNs	>50% Lymphs	>80% Lymphs
Protein (mg/dL)	15–50	>100	30–150	40–150	>50
Glucose (mg/dL)	45–100 (2/3 of serum)	<45 (<1/2 of serum)	30–70	30–70	<40
Gram stain (% positive)	—	60–90	Negative	Negative	37–87 (AFB Smear)

PMNs = polymorphonuclear cells (neutrophils).
Lymphs = lymphocytes.
Monos = monocytes.

Table 17-17. Typical CSF Findings in Patients with Meningitis[87–91]

Hematologic analysis of the CSF involves a determination of the white blood cell count (WBC) and corresponding differential—the results of which can suggest the potential causative organism of the meningitis. Patients with acute bacterial meningitis often demonstrate a high WBC count in the CSF (>400 cells/mm^3) with a predominance of neutrophils (>90%). In contrast, patients with viral, fungal or mycobacterial meningitis often display lower CSF-WBC counts (5–2000 cells/mm^3), with a predominance of lymphocytes.

CSF Stain and Culture

For patients with suspected bacterial meningitis, a Gram stain and culture should be performed on the submitted CSF specimen. The Gram stain is positive (an organism is visualized) in 60–90% of patients with bacterial meningitis and is helpful in choosing empiric antibiotic therapy.[88–91] However, the CSF Gram stain can be negative in those patients who have received antibiotics prior to the lumber puncture (partially treated meningitis). In patients with meningitis due to viruses, fungi, or mycobacteria, the Gram stain is usually negative. In these circumstances, specialized stains should be used for the detection of these organisms, such as the India ink stain for the detection of *Cryptococcus neoformans* or the acid-fast stain for the detection of *Mycobacterium*.

All CSF specimens should be processed for the appropriate cultures based on the type of meningitis (acute vs. chronic) and the organism suspected of causing the infection. In patients with bacterial meningitis, the cultures are often positive within 24–48 hr. In patients with nonbacterial meningitis, culture specimens should be observed for longer periods of time (up to 2–6 weeks) since these organisms often take longer to grow.

Other Specialized Tests

There are a number of specialized tests that may be performed on CSF specimens to aid in the detection of the causative organism. These tests include bacterial antigen detection using latex agglutination, latex fixation or enzyme immunoassay (EIA); fungal antigen detection; antibody detection; and polymerase chain reaction (PCR) assay.[87–91]

Bacterial antigen testing has been employed for many years as a rapid diagnostic test for CSF analysis since the results are available quickly (well before the results of the CSF culture). Some of the tests are commercially available and involve the process of an antibody-coated particles that bind to specific antigens of the most common bacterial pathogens that cause acute meningitis, if present. The tests are performed by mixing the CSF specimen (although it can also be done with urine or serum) with the antibody-coated particles and observing for agglutination, which signifies the presence of the bacterial antigen in the specimen. If visible agglutination does not occur, either the antigen is not present or it is present in amounts too small to cause agglutination. Bacterial antigen tests are available for the detection of *S. pneumoniae*, *Neisseria meningitidis*, *H. influenzae* type B, and group B streptococci. It is important to note that bacterial antigen detection of CSF specimens is no longer routinely recommended since the results rarely impact patient treatment. However, bacterial antigen testing may be useful in patients with negative Gram stains or in patients that have received previous antimicrobial therapy.[87,88,90]

Fungal antigen testing is available for both *Histoplasma capsulatum* and *Cryptococcus neoformans*.[87,91] The antigen testing for *Cryptococcus neoformans* has become an important diagnostic tool, and it is also useful in predicting the course of the disease and for monitoring the response to antifungal therapy.

There are some diagnostic tests available that detect the presence of antibody in the CSF to a specific organism. Antibody tests are available for the detection of antibodies to syphilis (*Treponema pallidum*), Lyme disease (*Borrelia burgdorferi*), and *Coccidioides immitis*.[91]

Polymerase chain reaction assays are the most useful test for the diagnosis of viral infections of the central nervous system. PCR can be used to detect the presence of herpes simplex virus (HSV), cytomegalovirus (CMV), varicella-zoster virus (VZV), Epstein-Barr virus (EBV), and enteroviruses in the CSF.[48,51,52] The PCR assay involves the amplification of small amounts of specific DNA of the target organism, followed by subsequent identification and verification. PCR is also available for the detection of *S. pneumoniae*, *N. meningitidis*, *Listeria monocytogenes*, and *Mycobacterium tuberculosis*; however, the time and expense of performing the PCR assays for these organisms has limited its routine clinical use.[88]

Streptococcal Pharyngitis

Acute pharyngitis is one of the most common infections encountered in medicine and can occur in both children and adults. Acute pharyngitis can be caused by a number of organisms (e.g., bacteria and viruses), with antibiotic therapy only recommended for those patients who develop pharyngitis due to group A streptococci.[92] Because the presenting signs and symptoms of bacterial and viral pharyngitis are similar, and the fact that group A strep pharyngitis comprises only a small percentage of patients with acute pharyngitis, it is important to have a rapid, reliable diagnostic test so that antibiotics will not be used unnecessarily in patients with acute viral pharyngitis.

The major diagnostic test for acute pharyngitis is the throat culture, which typically requires overnight incubation for the final results. Therefore, rapid antigen detection tests (RADT) have been developed to expedite and confirm the diagnosis of group A streptococcal pharyngitis, as well as expedite the initiation of treatment, if positive. There are several RADT tests that are commercially available, with the newer tests employing enzyme immunoassay (EIA), optical immunoassay, or chemiluminescent DNA probes to produce the greatest specificity and sensitivity.[92] However, there is limited data currently available comparing the performance of the different tests to throat culture (the gold standard). Therefore, it is recommended that a negative RADT test in children and adolescents be confirmed with a throat culture.[92]

Pneumonia

There are a number of obstacles that make the bacterial diagnosis of pneumonia quite difficult. First, the respiratory tract is colonized with bacteria that may or may not be contributing to the infectious process. When obtaining a sample for culture, lower respiratory tract secretions can become contaminated with secretions or bacteria colonizing the upper respiratory tract. Therefore, expectorated sputum samples should be evaluated to determine if contamination with saliva or upper respiratory tract flora has occurred (assess the adequacy of the sample).[86,93,94] In addition, if bacteria are isolated in culture, the clinician must determine the relative importance and significance of the organism as a potential cause of pneumonia. Second, adequate sputum specimens that are representative of an infectious process are very difficult to obtain without invasive procedures such as bronchoalveolar lavage (BAL) or protected specimen brush. Invasive procedures are sometimes utilized to aid in the diagnosis of pneumonia in those patients who are not able to expectorate an adequate sample. Lastly, despite the best efforts at obtaining a sputum specimen for culture, as many as 50% of patients with pneumonia have negative cultures.[93,94]

In order to produce a good expectorated sputum sample, the patient should be instructed to provide sputum generated from a deep cough. All expectorated sputum samples should then be screened to assure that the specimen is adequate and has not been contaminated by saliva or upper respiratory tract flora prior to processing for culture.[86,93,94] Information utilized to screen expectorated sputum samples is derived from visualization of the Gram stain of the specimen. Expectorated sputum specimens that contain >25 WBCs/hpf and <10 squamous epithelial cells/hpf are adequate for further processing and culture.[93,94] Samples with >10 epithelial cells/hpf are representative of upper respiratory tract contamination (saliva) and should not be processed for culture.

The sputum Gram stain from an adequate expectorated sputum or sputum derived from an invasive method may be used to guide empiric antibiotic therapy when the specimen is purulent and contains a predominant organism. The antibiotic therapy can then be modified if the culture results reveal an infecting organism. In the case of pneumonia caused by atypical bacteria such as *Legionella pneumophila*, *Mycoplasma pneumoniae*, or *Chlamydia pneumoniae*, antigen detection tests or serologic tests may be performed to aid in the diagnosis since these organisms are difficult to culture in the lab (see Table 17-16).

Genitourinary Tract Infections

Urinary Tract Infections

Urinary tract infections are one of the most common community-acquired and nosocomially-acquired bacterial infections, prompting more than 6 million office visits and 300,000 hospitalizations per year.[95-97] Urinary tract infections are especially common in females due to the close proximity of the urethra (which is shorter than males) to the perirectal and vaginal regions, which are both colonized with bacteria. Because of this anatomic difference, bacteria are able to easily ascend the urethra in females and potentially cause infection in the bladder (cystitis) and upper urinary tract (pyelonephritis). In addition, hospitalized patients (male and female) with indwelling urinary catheters are at increased risk for developing urinary tract infections, with approximately 20% of catheterized patients developing a UTI even with only short-term catheterization.[96]

Under normal circumstances, urine within the bladder is sterile since all anatomic areas above the urethra in the urinary tract are not colonized with bacteria. However, the urethra is colonized with bacteria and introduces some difficulty in obtaining an adequate urine sample, because it must pass through a nonsterile environment for collection if noninvasive specimen collection methods are utilized.[95-97] Therefore, diagnostic criteria have been developed to discriminate between infection, bacterial colonization, or bacterial contamination based on quantitative urine cultures and the presence of inflammatory cells and epithelial cells in the urinalysis.

Urine samples for urinalysis and culture can be collected a number of ways. The most common method involves the collection of a clean-catch, midstream urine sample. Before obtaining a sample, the patient should be instructed to clean and rinse the periurethral area with a mild detergent, and then retract the labial folds or penile foreskin when beginning to urinate. The patient should attempt to collect a midstream urine sample into a sterile cup.

Other methods for urine collection involve more invasive procedures such as straight catheterized urine and suprapubic bladder aspiration. Both of these methods avoid the potential contamination of the urine specimen by the urethra since the urine is collected directly from the bladder. In hospitalized patients with indwelling urinary catheters, urine specimens should be aspirated from the catheter port or tubing (representing freshly voided urine) rather than obtained from the collection bag (urine collected over a period of time).[95-97]

In all cases, urine samples should be immediately transported to the laboratory for processing. The exact processing of the urine sample will typically depend on the infection type. Urine samples from patients with uncomplicated cystitis may only be analyzed using screening tests such as reagent strip testing (dipsticks), while samples from patients with more serious urinary tract infections (e.g., recurrent UTIs and pyelonephritis) are analyzed using microscopic examination and culture.

The urine from a patient with uncomplicated cystitis is usually only evaluated using screening tests. The results of the screening tests are rapidly available and are most useful at excluding the presence of a urinary tract infection.[95] The most common rapid screening tests include commercially available test reagent strips that contain the leukocyte esterase test and the nitrate reductase test, which provide a negative predictive value of 98%.[95-97] The leukocyte esterase test detects the presence and activity of leukocyte esterase, an enzyme produced by neutrophils (pyuria) mobilized in the host's response to infection. The nitrate reductase test detects the presence of urinary nitrite, which is produced by the reduction of nitrate by nitrate-reducing enzymes produced by common urinary tract pathogens.[95-97] Positive results from the leukocyte esterase test and nitrate reductase test warrant treatment for a urinary tract infection without the need for urine culture.

The urine from patients with recurrent or complicated urinary tract infections is typically evaluated using a urinalysis (microscopic examination) and urine culture. The urinalysis is a rapid test which involves the macroscopic and microscopic examination of the urine sample for color, clarity, specific gravity, and the presence of protein, glucose, red blood cells, white blood cells, bacteria, and epithelial cells. The urinalysis is performed either manually or through the use of automated instruments. Urinalysis findings that suggest a urinary tract infection include cloudiness of the specimen and the presence of pyuria (>10 WBC/hpf).[95-97] The detection of hematuria, proteinuria, or bacteriuria in the urinalysis may be an indication of infection but is not specific. The presence of tubular epithelial cells (>2–5 epithelial cells/hpf) in the urine sample suggests poor specimen collection and possible contamination.

The urine culture remains the hallmark for the diagnosis of urinary tract infections, with quantitative cultures providing the most useful data for determining the clinical significance of isolated bacteria. To establish the diagnosis of a urinary tract infection, urine cultures from midstream urine samples or catheterized specimens should display $>10^5$ cfu/mL of a single potential uropathogen along with pyuria. However, colony counts of $>10^3$ cfu/mL with pyuria are considered clinically relevant in urine specimens from men or children.[95] For urine specimens obtained by suprapubic aspiration, the diagnosis of infection is established if the culture displays $>10^2$ cfu/mL with pyuria.[95-97]

Prostatitis

Bacterial prostatitis can present as either an acute or chronic infection and typically occurs in males over the age of 30 years.[97] The diagnosis of acute bacterial prostatitis is often based on the clinical presentation of the patient as well as the presence of bacteria in a urine specimen. Digital palpation of the prostate and prostatic massage to express purulent secretions are not recommended for the diagnosis of acute bacterial prostatitis since it may induce bacteremia. However, the diagnosis of chronic bacterial prostatitis can often not be determined on clinical grounds alone (since the symptoms are nonspecific and the prostate is often not acutely inflamed) but may be established through the analysis of sequential urine and prostatic fluid cultures.[97,98] Initially, two samples of urine are obtained for culture—one sample on initiation of urination (VB-1) and one sample obtained at midstream (VB-2). Next, prostate fluid is obtained for culture by massaging the prostate to produce expressed prostatic secretions (EPS). Lastly, a urine sample (VB-3) is obtained after prostatic secretions have been obtained and sent for culture. The diagnosis of chronic bacterial prostatitis is made when the EPS sample contains greater than 10 times the quantity of bacteria cultured from VB-1 or VB-2, or if the VB-3 contains 10 times the quantity of bacteria cultured from VB-1 or VB-2.[97,98]

Sexually Transmitted Diseases (STDs)

Gonorrhea

Infection due to *Neisseria gonorrhoeae* is the second most common STD reported in the United States.[99] Uncomplicated infections due to *N. gonorrhoeae* typically involve the mucosa of the cervix, the urethra, the rectum, and the pharynx. These infections include localized, uncomplicated genital infections (e.g., cervicitis, endometritis, pelvic inflammatory disease in women, and urethritis or epididymitis in men), pharyngitis, anorectal infections, and disseminated infection (e.g., septic arthritis and meningitis) in both men and women.[99] Women with genital tract infection and patients with pharyngeal infection are often asymptomatic, while men with urethritis often display symptoms of dysuria and urethral discharge. In addition, patients with *N. gonorrhoeae* are often coinfected with other STDs, such as *Chlamydia trachomatis*, syphilis, or *Trichomonas vaginalis*. Therefore, the diagnosis and treatment of all possible STDs in the patient and their sexual partners are important considerations in the control of STDs.

The diagnosis of gonorrheal infections can be made by culture, stained clinical smears, or nonculture techniques (nucleic acid amplification tests) of urethral or cervical/vaginal discharge.[99–101] Urethral and cervical/vaginal specimens for the detection of gonorrhea should be obtained using a urogenital swab and transported to the laboratory in modified Stuart's or Amie's charcoal transport media.[99,100]

Culture on selective media remains the diagnostic standard for the identification of *N. gonorrhoeae*.[99,101] Culture is the recommended method for the diagnosis of gonorrhea from urethral, cervical/vaginal, pharyngeal, or rectal swabs specimens and should be performed on specimens from all patients (and sexual partners) with suspected gonococcal infections.[99] Culture is also used as a confirmatory test in patients who have suspected gonorrhea based on positive-stained smears or nonculture tests (as a confirmatory test) if the specimen has been adequately maintained. Occasionally, positive cultures are processed for antimicrobial susceptibility testing (especially in patients failing apparent appropriate therapy) to guide the choice of antibiotic therapy, as well as for epidemiologic purposes. In either case, patients are typically treated empirically with an antibiotic that demonstrates excellent activity against gonorrhea, keeping in mind that the incidence of ß-lactamase-producing, penicillin-resistant gonococci is increasing.

A presumptive diagnosis of gonorrhea can be made with the use of a Gram stain and oxidase test of a clinical specimen, where gram-negative, oxidase-positive diplococci are demonstrated.[99–101] This test has been found to be sensitive and specific for the presumptive diagnosis of N. gonorrhoeae as a point-of-care test for men with urethral discharge but is not as useful when evaluating endocervical or pharyngeal specimens. Additional tests, such as culture, should be performed to confirm the identification of the organism.

The newest nonculture test used for the detection of N. gonorrhoeae is the Nucleic Acid Amplification tests (NAATs), which are able to amplify organism-specific nucleic acid sequences, even in nonviable organisms.[99] There are a number of commercially-available NAAT tests for the detection of N. gonorrhoeae that have been designed to detect RNA or DNA sequences using amplification techniques, and have been FDA-approved for the detection of N. gonorrhoeae in endocervical swabs from women, urethral swabs from men, and urine samples from men and women.[99,101] These tests are also useful for the detection of N. gonorrhoeae from clinical specimens that have not been adequately maintained during transport or collection for culture methods to be utilized.

Chlamydia trachomatis

Infections due to Chlamydia trachomatis are probably the most common STDs in the United States, with 3–4 million infections occurring annually in sexually active adolescents and adults.[99,100] Infection with Chlamydia trachomatis is now a reportable communicable disease in all 50 of the United States, with a significant increase in reported cases observed from 1987 to 2001. Chlamydia trachomatis can cause a number of infections including cervicitis, endometritis, and pelvic inflammatory disease (PID) in women; and urethritis, epididymo-orchitis, prostatitis, and proctitis (via receptive anal intercourse) in men.[99,102] Infection with C. trachomatis is also thought to contribute to female infertility and ectopic pregnancies. It is estimated that over $2.4 billion is spent annually on the direct and indirect costs of C. trachomatis infections.

Unfortunately, the majority of patients who acquire chlamydial infections are asymptomatic so that screening is necessary to detect the presence of this organism and treat the infection. Because of the asymptomatic nature of Chlamydia, it is thought that the current rates of reporting underestimate the true incidence of infection. Screening for the presence of C. trachomatis is typically performed on specimens obtained from patients presenting with other STDs since Chlamydia often coexists with other STD pathogens.

There are a number of laboratory diagnostic tests that can be utilized for the detection of chlamydial infections, including both culture and nonculture methods. Cell culture of Chlamydia trachomatis involves the inoculation of the biologic specimen onto a confluent monolayer of susceptible cells. These cells become infected with C. trachomatis and develop characteristic intracellular inclusions within 48–72 hr that can be detected using a fluorescent monoclonal antibody stain.[99] This method is not routinely utilized because it is not standardized between labs, is costly, technically demanding, and requires at least 48 hr to yield results. Therefore, other nonculture approaches to the laboratory diagnosis of Chlamydia have been developed, including the direct fluorescent antibody test (DFA) and nucleic acid amplification tests (NAATs).

The direct fluorescent antibody test (DFA) involves the staining of a biologic specimen with a fluorescein-labeled monoclonal antibody that binds to C. trachomatis-specific antigens (elementary bodies). If the patient is infected with C. trachomatis, the antibodies will react with the elementary bodies of the Chlamydia in the secretions to produce fluorescence.

The other nonculture test used for the detection of Chlamydia trachomatis is the nucleic acid amplification test (NAAT), which has largely replaced tissue culture and DFA tests because of greater sensitivity.[99,101] There are a number of commercially-available NAAT tests for the detection of *C. trachomatis* that have been designed to detect RNA or DNA sequences using polymerase chain reaction (PCR), ligase chain reaction ((LCR), and various amplification techniques. These tests have been FDA-approved for the detection of *C. trachomatis* in endocervical swabs from women, urethral swabs from men, and urine samples from men and women.

Syphilis (Treponema pallidum)

The spirochete *Treponema pallidum* is the causative pathogen of another sexually transmitted disease known as syphilis. There are a number of clinical manifestations and stages of syphilis which are based primarily on presenting symptoms and natural history of the infection[103]:

- *Primary syphilis*—characterized by painless genital ulcers called *chancres*, which are typically located at the site of inoculation or initial infection.
- *Secondary syphilis*—characterized by systemic symptoms including fever, weight loss, malaise, and a generalized skin rash often involving the palms or the soles of the feet.
- *Latent syphilis*—occurs after secondary syphilis where the organism is still present, but the patient is without symptoms; this subclinical infection can only be detected by serologic tests.
- *Late/tertiary syphilis*—occurs in approximately 35% of untreated patients up to 10–25 years after initial infection; manifested as progressive disease involving the ascending aorta and/or CNS (neurosyphilis).

Spirochetes cannot be grown in culture in the microbiology lab. Therefore, the diagnosis of syphilis involves the direct detection of the spirochete in biologic specimens by microscopy or the detection of specific antibodies by serologic testing. Direct detection methods involve the acquisition of an appropriate clinical specimen from suspicious genital or skin lesions.

The direct detection of *Treponema pallidum* using dark-field microscopy involves the immediate examination of the biologic specimens under a microscope with a dark-field condenser, looking for the presence of motile spirochetes. *T. pallidum* can be visualized as 8–10 μm, spiral-shaped organisms.[101,103]

Another test for the direct detection of *Treponema pallidum* is the direct fluorescent antibody (DFA-TP) test. The biologic specimen is combined with fluorescein-labeled monoclonal or polyclonal antibodies specific for *T. pallidum* and examined by fluorescence microscopy. The interaction between the antibodies and Treponema-specific antigens will produce fluorescence that can be visualized using microscopy.

There are two types of serologic tests that are utilized for the diagnosis of syphilis, namely, tests that measure the presence of *nontreponemal* or reaginic antibodies such as the Venereal Disease Research Laboratory (VDRL) test and the rapid plasma reagin (RPR) test, and tests that measure the presence of *treponemal* antibodies such as the fluorescent treponemal antibody absorption (FTA-ABS) test and the microhemagglutination (MHA-TP) test.[101,103]

The nontreponemal antibody tests (VDRL, RPR) measure the presence of reaginic antibodies and are both flocculation tests in which visible clumps are produced in the presence of the reagin antibody (*T. pallidum*) in the submitted specimen. Reagin is an antibody-like protein that is produced in patients infected with syphilis. However, reagin is also produced in patients with a number of other illnesses, some of which include leprosy, tuberculosis, malaria, and drug addiction.

To perform the VDRL test, the biologic specimen (serum, CSF) of the patient is combined with the antigen cardiolipin-lecithin coated cholesterol particles on a glass slide and examined microscopically.[103] If the reagin antibody is present in the biologic specimen, visual clumping will occur and be reported as reactive (medium and large clumps). This test can also be quantified by evaluating several dilutions of the biologic specimen for reactivity, with the dilution that produces a fully reactive result being reported as the VDRL titer (e.g., 1:8 or 1:32). Therefore, the VDRL titer is also utilized to monitor a patient's response to therapy. The high titers present in untreated disease (e.g., 1:32) traditionally decrease 4-fold by 6–12 months and become undetectable in 1–2 years.

The RPR test is a modification of the VDRL test and is commercially available as a reaction card. Sera from the patient is placed on the reaction card and observed for clumping. The RPR is easier to perform than the VDRL and is used by many laboratories and blood banks for routine syphilis screening. However, the RPR should not be used for CSF specimens.

Because the nontre-ponemal antibody detection tests are nonspecific, false-positive (up to 1–2%) results can occur in numerous situations (in patient types mentioned above). Because they are relatively nonspecific, they are most useful for *screening* for the presence of syphilis. In addition, since it takes several weeks for the development of reagin antibodies, false-negative results (up to 25% of patients with primary syphilis) can occur in the early stages of the disease.[101]

Nontreponemal tests are useful for screening and monitoring therapeutic response, and a positive result should be confirmed with the FTA-ABS or the MHA-TP test, which both measure the presence of treponemal antibody.

In the FTA-ABS test, the patient's serum is initially absorbed with non *T. pallidum* antigens to reduce cross-reactivity and then combined with a fluorescein-conjugated antihuman antibody for specific antitreponemal antibodies. The amount of fluorescence is subjectively measured by the laboratory technician and reported as reactive, minimally reactive, or nonreactive. Therefore, this test is difficult to standardize among different laboratories. Because this test is also fairly expensive, it is primarily used to verify the results of a positive VDRL or RPR, rather than as a routine screening tool.[103] The FTA-ABS test can detect antibodies earlier in the course of syphilis than nontreponemal tests and, once positive, will remain positive for the life of the patient.

The MHA-TP test is performed utilizing erythrocytes from a turkey, sheep, or other mammal that have been coated with treponemal antigens. These erythrocytes are then mixed with the patient's serum and observed for agglutination, which signifies the presence of antibodies directed against *T. pallidum*. The results are reported as reactive (positive) or nonreactive (negative).

Trichomonas vaginalis

Infection caused by the protozoan, *Trichomonas vaginalis*, is one of the most common and treatable sexually-transmitted diseases in the world.[102,104] The method that is commonly employed for the diagnosis of infection due to *Trichomonas* is microscopic examination of a wet preparation or wet mount of the biologic specimen, looking for motile *Trichomonas* organisms.[101,102,104] Due to low diagnostic sensitivity of the wet prep, other diagnostic tests have been developed to enhance sensitivity and specificity. These methods include enzyme immunoassay, immunofluorescence tests, and polymerase chain reaction (PCR).

Herpes Simplex Virus

Herpes simplex virus is the most common cause of genital ulceration in the United States, with over 45 million patients infected.[101] There are two serotypes of herpes simplex virus that cause infection: HSV type 1 (HSV-1), which is most often associated with oropharyngeal infection (cold sores), and HSV type 2 (HSV-2), which is most commonly associated with genital tract infection. Some patients with genital herpes are asymptomatic, while others experience recurrent vesicular and ulcerative genital lesions typically at the site of initial infection. In either case, HSV can be transmitted to others during reactivation of the infection.

In many patients, the diagnosis of HSV can be made based on the characteristic findings on physical examination (vesicular or ulcerative genital lesions). If lesions are present, the diagnosis can be confirmed by performing a Tzank smear of a specimen obtained by scraping the base of an active lesion, and visualizing the specimen for characteristic viral intranuclear inclusions using microscopy (cytology and histology).[101,105] Viral culture is the gold standard for the diagnosis of HSV and can also be performed on the specimen from the active lesion. However, it may take up to 5–7 days for the virus to grow and be identified.

Other tests that can be used for the diagnosis of HSV infection include HSV antigen detection (e.g., direct immunofluorescence, immunoperoxidase staining, and enzyme immunoassay or EIA); HSV DNA detection; and HSV-PCR. The results from these tests are often available sooner than traditional cell culture and are most useful when rapid detection of HSV is necessary, such as for the diagnosis of encephalitis or before an impending birth.[101] In addition, there are also commercially-available, FDA-approved serology kits for the diagnosis of HSV-1 and HSV-2 that detect antibody produced against specific HSV antigens. HSV serologic tests are primarily used in research; for the diagnosis of genital herpes in patients with suspected genital lesions; for patients with known or suspected exposure to HSV; and for determining the serostatus of pregnant women or patients undergoing organ or bone marrow transplantation.[106]

Assessing Sterile Body Fluids for the Presence of Infection

There are a number of sterile fluids that may be analyzed for the presence of infection including pericardial fluid (pericarditis), pleural fluid (empyema), synovial fluid (septic arthritis), and peritoneal fluid (peritonitis). The specimens should be aseptically obtained by needle aspiration, placed in sterile collection tubes, and immediately transported to the lab. Approximately 1–5 mL of fluid should be obtained when analyzing pericardial, pleural or synovial fluid, while up to 10 mL of peritoneal fluid is required for the diagnosis of peritonitis.[107] All sterile fluids should be processed for cell count (presence of white blood cells with differential), chemistry (protein and glucose), direct microscopic examination including Gram stain (presence of bacteria), and culture. For pleural and synovial fluids, there are specific criteria that are utilized to diagnose the presence of infection (see Tables 17-18 and 17-19).[108-111] In addition, the diagnosis of infection in one of these sterile sites is also made based on the characteristic signs and symptoms of infection (depending on the infection site), the presence of white blood cells in the sterile fluid specimen, and the growth of a pathogenic organism in the cultured material.

TABLE 17-18

	TRANSUDATIVE (suggestive of CHF, cirrhosis)	EXUDATIVE (suggestive of infection such as empyema; malignancy; pancreatitis with esophageal perforation; SLE)
pH	>7.2	<7.2
LDH (IU/Liter)	<200	>200–1000
Pleural fluid LDH to serum LDH ratio	<0.6	>0.6
Protein (g/dL)	<3.0	>3.0
Pleural fluid protein to serum protein ratio	<0.5	>0.5
Glucose (mg/dL)	>60 (same as serum)	<40–60
White blood cells (count/mm³)	<1000	<1000
WBC differential	<50% PMNs	If infectious, depends on pathogen.

PMNs = polymorphonuclear cells (neutrophils).

Table 17-18. Pleural Fluid Findings and Interpretation[108,109]

TABLE 17-19

	NORMAL	NONINFLAMMATORY (osteoarthritis, trauma, avascular necrosis, SLE, early rheumatoid arthritis)	INFLAMMATORY (rheumatoid arthritis, spondylo-arthropathies, viral arthritis, crystal-induced arthritis)	PURULENT (bacterial joint infection, tuberculous joint infection, fungal joint infection)
White blood cells (count/mm³)	<150	<3000	3000–50,000	>50,000
WBC differential	No pre-dominance	<25% PMNs	>70% PMNs, variable	>75 to 90% PMNs
Protein (g/dL)	1.3–1.8	3–3.5	>3.5	>3.5
Glucose (mg/dL)	Normal	Normal	70–90	<40 to 50

PMNs = polymorphonuclear cells (neutrophils).

Table 17-19. Synovial Fluid Findings and Interpretation[109–111]

SUMMARY

Although infectious disease is a rapidly changing field because of new challenges and technological advances, the diagnosis of many infectious illnesses depends on proper performance and interpretation of numerous basic laboratory tests. For example, the Gram's stain is a readily available, invaluable tool for examining clinical specimens for the presence of bacteria. Culture of clinical specimens using appropriate growth media allows the cultivation of many of the usual infecting bacteria in the clinical laboratory. Because empiric antimicrobial therapy is based on the patient's history and clinical condition, information from a Gram's stain and culture are useful in targeting antibiotic therapy towards the infecting organism.

Susceptibility tests for rapidly growing aerobic bacteria are commonly performed using an automated microdilution or a manual disk diffusion method. Bacterial susceptibilities to various antimicrobial agents are reported as susceptible, intermediate, or resistant. National standards for susceptibility testing are available and help guide the performance of the tests, the choice of antimicrobial agents, and the reporting procedures of susceptibility tests by the clinical microbiology laboratory. Moreover, susceptibility information should be considered in conjunction with patient-specific data (e.g., clinical condition, site of infection, drug allergies, and renal function) to design an appropriate antimicrobial drug regimen for a patient.

New testing methods and guidelines have recently become available for the recovery, identification, and susceptibility testing of fungi, mycobacteria, and viruses. These processes may challenge the clinical microbiology laboratory due to their requirements for specialized staining, culturing, and susceptibility testing procedures.

Lastly, several infection types (e.g., meningitis, urinary tract infections, etc.) and certain pathogens (e.g., *Borrelia burgdorferi* and *Legionella pneumophila*) often require specialized laboratory testing to aid in the identification of the infecting organism. The clinician should be aware of the diagnostic tests currently available for these infections.

REFERENCES

1. General issues and role of laboratories. In: Forbes BA, Sahm DF, Weissfeld AS, eds. *Diagnostic Microbiology*. 11th ed. St Louis, MO: Mosby, Inc.; 2002: 2–18.
2. Popescu A, Doyle RJ. The Gram stain after more than a century. *Biotech Histochem.* 1996; 71(3):145–51.
3. Role of microscopy in the diagnosis of infectious diseases. In: Forbes BA, Sahm DF, Weissfeld AS, eds. *Diagnostic Microbiology*. 11th ed. St Louis, MO: Mosby, Inc.; 2002: 119–32.
4. Woods GL, Walker DH. Detection of infection and infectious agents by use of cytologic and histologic stains. *Clin Microbiol Rev.* 1996; 9(3):382–404.

5. Isenberg HD, ed. *Essential Procedures for Clinical Microbiology*. Washington DC: American Society for Microbiology; 1998.

6. Graman PS, Menegus MA. Microbiology laboratory tests. In: Reese RE, Betts RF, eds. *A Practical Approach to Infectious Diseases*. 4th ed. New York, NY: Little, Brown and Company; 1996: 935–66.

7. Bacteria. In: Wilborn JW. *Microbiology*. Springhouse, PA: Springhouse Corporation; 1993: 36–50.

8. Rybak MJ, Aeschlimann JR. Laboratory tests to direct antimicrobial pharmacotherapy. In: DiPiro JT, Talbert RL, Yee GC, et al., eds. *Pharmacotherapy: A Pathophysiologic Approach*. 5th ed. Stamford, CT: McGraw-Hill/Appleton & Lange; 2002: 1797–815.

9. Gill VJ, Fedorko DP, Witebsky FG. The clinician and the microbiology laboratory. In: Mandell GL, Bennett JE, Dolin R, eds. *Principles and Practice of Infectious Diseases*. 5th ed. Philadelphia, PA: Churchill Livingstone; 2000: 184–221.

10. Laboratory cultivation and isolation of bacteria. In: Forbes BA, Sahm DF, Weissfeld AS, eds. *Diagnostic Microbiology*. 11th ed. St Louis, MO: Mosby, Inc.; 2002: 133–47.

11. Busse HJ, Denner EBM, Lubitz W. Classification and identification of bacteria: current approaches to an old problem. Overview of methods used in bacteria systematics. *J Biotechnol*. 1996; 47:3–38.

12. Murray PR, Baron EJ, Pfaller MA, et al., eds. *Manual of Clinical Microbiology*. 6th ed. Washington DC: American Society for Microbiology; 1995.

13. Overview of conventional methods for bacterial identification. In: Forbes BA, Sahm DF, Weissfeld AS, eds. *Diagnostic Microbiology*. 11th ed. St Louis, MO: Mosby, Inc.; 2002: 148–68.

14. Overview of bacterial identification methods and strategies. In: Forbes BA, Sahm DF, Weissfeld AS, eds. *Diagnostic Microbiology*. 11th ed. St Louis, MO: Mosby, Inc.; 2002: 260–83.

15. Stager CE, Davis JR. Automated systems for identification of microorganisms. *Clin Microbiol Rev*. 1992; 5:302–27.

16. Sharp SE. Commensal and pathogenic microorganisms of humans. In: Murray PR, Baron EJ, Pfaller MA, et al., eds. *Manual of Clinical Microbiology*. 7th ed. Washington DC: ASM Press; 1999: 23–32.

17. Bates DW, Goldman L, Lee TH. Contaminant blood cultures and resource utilization: the true consequences of false-positive results. *JAMA*. 1991; 265:365–9.

18. Reese RE, Betts RF. Principles of antibiotic use. In: Reese RE, Betts RF, eds. *A Practical Approach to Infectious Diseases*. 4th ed. New York, NY: Little, Brown and Company; 1996: 1059–97.

19. Laboratory methods for detection of antimicrobial resistance. In: Forbes BA, Sahm DF, Weissfeld AS, eds. *Diagnostic Microbiology*. 11th ed. St Louis, MO: Mosby, Inc.; 2002: 229–50.

20. National Committee for Clinical Laboratory Standards. *Performance Standards for Antimicrobial Susceptibility Testing: Approved Standard M100-S14*. Ferraro MJ, et al. Wayne, PA: NCCLS; 2004.

21. National Committee for Clinical Laboratory Standards. *Development of In Vitro Susceptibility Testing Criteria and Quality Control Parameters: Approved Guideline M23-A2*. Wayne, PA: NCCLS; 2001.

22. National Committee for Clinical Laboratory Standards. *Methods for Dilution Antimicrobial Susceptibility Tests for Bacteria That Grow Aerobically: Approved Standard M7-A5*. Wayne, PA:NCCLS; 2000.

23. National Committee for Clinical Laboratory Standards. *Performance Standards for Antimicrobial Disk Susceptibility Tests: Approved Standard M2-A7*. Wayne, PA: NCCLS; 2000.

24. Jorgensen JH, Ferraro MJ. Antimicrobial susceptibility testing: general principles and contemporary practices. *Clin Infect Dis*. 1998; 26:973–80.

25. Jorgensen JH, Turnridge JD, Washington JA. Antibacterial susceptibility tests: dilution and disk diffusion methods. In: Murray PR, Baron EJ, Pfaller MA, et al., eds. *Manual of Clinical Microbiology*. 7th ed. Washington DC: ASM Press; 1999: 1526–43.

26. Louie M, Cockerill FR. Susceptibility testing: phenotypic and genotypic tests for bacteria and mycobacteria. *Infect Dis Clin North Am*. 2001; 15(4):1205–26.

27. Peterson LR, Shanholtzer CJ. Tests for bactericidal effects of antimicrobial agents: technical performance and clinical relevance. *Clin Microbiol Rev*. 1992; 5:420–32.

28. Swenson JM, Hindler JA, Peterson LR. Special phenotypic methods for detecting antibacterial resistance. In: Murray PR, Baron EJ, Pfaller MA, et al., eds. *Manual of Clinical Microbiology*. 7th ed. Washington DC: ASM Press; 1999:1563–77.

29. DeGirolami PC, Eliopoulos G. Antimicrobial susceptibility tests and their role in therapeutic drug monitoring. *Clin Lab Medicine*. 1987; 7:499–512.

30. National Committee for Clinical Laboratory Standards. *Methods for Determining Bactericidal Activity of Antimicrobial Agents: Approved Standard M26-A*. Wayne, PA: NCCLS; 1998.

31. Reller LB. The serum bactericidal test. *Rev Infect Dis*. 1986; 8:803–8.

32. Jorgensen JH, Ferraro MJ. Antimicrobial susceptibility testing: special needs for fastidious organisms and difficult-to-detect resistance mechanisms. *Clin Infect Dis*. 2000; 30:799–808.

33. Anaerobic bacteriology: overview and general considerations. In: Forbes BA, Sahm DF, Weissfeld AS, eds. *Diagnostic Microbiology*. 11th ed. St Louis, MO: Mosby, Inc.; 2002: 511–9.

34. Anaerobic bacteriology: laboratory considerations. In: Forbes BA, Sahm DF, Weissfeld AS, eds. *Diagnostic Microbiology*. 11th ed. St Louis, MO: Mosby, Inc.; 2002: 520–36.

35. Hecht DW. Susceptibility testing of anaerobic bacteria. In: Murray PR, Baron EJ, Pfaller MA, et al., eds. *Manual of Clinical Microbiology*. 7th ed. Washington DC: ASM Press; 1999: 1555–62.

36. Hecht DW. Evolution of anaerobe susceptibility testing in the United States. *Clin Infect Dis*. 2002;35(suppl 1):S28–S35.

37. National Committee for Clinical Laboratory Standards. *Methods for Antimicrobial Susceptibility Testing of Anaerobic Bacteria: Approved Standard M11-A5*. Wayne, PA: NCCLS; 2001.

38. Laboratory strategies for antimicrobial susceptibility testing. In: Forbes BA, Sahm DF, Weissfeld AS, eds. *Diagnostic Microbiology*. 11th ed. St Louis, MO: Mosby, Inc.; 2002: 251–9.

39. National Committee for Clinical Laboratory Standards. *Analysis and Presentation of Cumulative Antimicrobial Susceptibility Test Data: Approved Guideline M39-A*. Wayne, PA: NCCLS; 2002.

40. Larone DH. *Medically Important Fungi: A Guide to Identification*. 4th ed. Washington DC: ASM Press; 2002.

41. Laboratory methods in basic mycology. In: Forbes BA, Sahm DF, Weissfeld AS, eds. *Diagnostic Microbiology*. 11th ed. St Louis, MO: Mosby, Inc.; 2002: 711–97.

42. Carver, PL. Invasive fungal infections. In: DiPiro JT, Talbert RL, Yee GC, et al., eds. *Pharmacotherapy: A Pathophysiologic Approach*. 5th ed. Stamford, CT: McGraw-Hill/Appleton & Lange; 2002: 2059–88.

43. Pfaller MA, Yu WL. Antifungal susceptibility testing: new technology and clinical applications. *Infect Dis Clin North Am*. 2001; 15:1227–61.

44. National Committee for Clinical Laboratory Standards. *Reference Method for Broth Dilution Susceptibility Testing of Yeasts: Approved Standard M27-A2*. Wayne, PA: NCCLS; 2002.

45. National Committee for Clinical Laboratory Standards. *Reference Method for Broth Dilution Susceptibility Testing of Conidium-Forming Filamentous Fungi: Proposed Standard M38-P*. Wayne, PA: NCCLS; 1998.

46. Melnick JL. Taxonomy and classification of viruses. In: Murray PR, Baron EJ, Pfaller MA, et al., eds. *Manual of Clinical Microbiology*. 7th ed. Washington, DC: ASM Press; 1999: 835–42.

47. Buchen-Osmond C. Taxonomy and classification of viruses. In: Murray PR, Baron EJ, Jorgensen JH, et al., eds. *Manual of Clinical Microbiology*. 8th ed. Washington, DC: ASM Press; 2003: 1217–26.

48. Forman MS, Valsamakis A. Specimen collection, transport, and processing: virology. In: Murray PR, Baron EJ, Jorgensen JH, et al., eds. *Manual of Clinical Microbiology*. 8th ed. Washington, DC: ASM Press; 2003: 1227–41.

49. Menegus MA. Rapid systems and instruments for the identification of viruses. In: Truant AL, ed. *Manual of Commercial Methods in Clinical Microbiology*. Washington, DC: ASM Press; 2002: 84–99.

50. Yolken RH, Smith TF, Waner JL, et al. Algorithms for detection and identification of viruses. In: Murray PR, Baron EJ, Jorgensen JH, et al., eds. *Manual of Clinical Microbiology*. 8th ed. Washington, DC: ASM Press; 2003: 1242–5.

51. Storch GA. Methodologic overview. In: Storch GA, ed. *Essentials of Diagnostic Virology*. New York, NY: Churchill Livingstone; 2000: 1–23.

52. Jungkind D, Kessler HH. Molecular methods for diagnosis of infectious diseases. In: Truant AL, ed. *Manual of Commercial Methods in Clinical Microbiology*. Washington, DC: ASM Press; 2002: 306–23.

53. Hodinka RL. Human immunodeficiency virus. In: Truant AL, ed. *Manual of Commercial Methods in Clinical Microbiology*. Washington, DC: ASM Press; 2002:100–27.

54. Mylonakis E, Paliou M, Lally M, et al. Laboratory testing for infection with the human immunodeficiency virus: established and novel approaches. *Am J Med*. 2000; 109:568–76.

55. Revised guidelines for HIV counseling, testing, and referral. *MMWR*. 2001; 50(RR-19):1–57. Also at http:hivatis.org (see this website for most updated guidelines).

56. Revised recommendations for HIV screening of pregnant women. *MMWR*. 2001; 50(RR-19):63–85. Also at http:hivatis.org (see this website for most updated guidelines).

57. The Working Group on Antiretroviral Therapy and Medical Management of HIV-Infected Children. Guidelines for the use of antiretroviral agents in pediatric HIV infection. At http:hivatis.org (see this website for most updated guidelines).

58. Dybul M, Fauci AS, Bartlett JG, et al. Panel on Clinical Practices for the Treatment of HIV. Guidelines for using antiretroviral agents among HIV-infected adults and adolescents: recommendations of the Panel on Clinical Practices for the Treatment of HIV. *MMWR*. 2002; 51(RR-7):1–55. Also at http:hivatis.org (see this website for most updated guidelines).

59. Yeni PG, Hammer SM, Carpenter CCJ, et al. Antiretroviral treatment for adult HIV infection in 2002: update recommendations of the International AIDS Society-USA Panel. *JAMA*. 2002; 288:222–35.

60. Mofenson LM. US Public Health Service Task Force recommendations for use of antiretroviral drugs in pregnant HIV-1-infected women for maternal health and interventions to reduce perinatal HIV-1 transmission in the United States. *MMWR*. 2002; 51(RR-18):1–38. Also at http:hivatis.org (see this website for most updated guidelines).

61. Mycobacterium. In: Murray PR, Rosenthal KS, Kobayashi GS, et al., eds. *Medical Microbiology*. 4th ed. St Louis, MO: Mosby, Inc; 2002: 366–77.

62. Woods GL. Mycobacteria. In: Henry JB, ed. *Clinical Diagnosis and Management by Laboratory Methods*. 20th ed. Philadelphia, PA: W. B. Saunders Company; 2001:1144–57.

63. Brahmer J, Hwang Y, Sande MA. Other mycobacteria. In: Wilson WR, Sande MA, eds. *Diagnosis and Treatment in Infectious Diseases*. New York, NY: Lange Medical Books/McGraw-Hill; 2001: 653–61.

64. Mycobacteria. In: Forbes BA, Sahm DF, Weissfeld AS, eds. *Diagnostic Microbiology*. 11th ed. St Louis, MO: Mosby, Inc.; 2002: 538–71.

65. American Thoracic Society Committee on Microbiology, Tuberculosis and Pulmonary Infections. Diagnosis and treatment of disease caused by nontuberculous mycobacteria. *Am J Respir Crit Care Med*. 1997; 156:S1–S25.

66. American Thoracic Society Committee on Microbiology, Tuberculosis and Pulmonary Infections. Diagnostic standards and classification of tuberculosis in adults and children. *Am J Respir Crit Care Med*. 2000; 161:1376–95.

67. Hale YM, Pfyffer GE, Salfinger M. Laboratory diagnosis of mycobacterial infections: new tools and lessons to be learned. *Clin Infect Dis*. 2001; 33:834–46.

68. Roberts GD, Hall L, Wolk DM. Mycobacteria. In: Truant AL, ed. *Manual of Commercial Methods in Clinical Microbiology*. Washington DC: ASM Press; 2002:256–73.

69. Hindiyeh M, Carroll KC. Laboratory diagnosis of atypical pneumonia. *Semin Resp Infect*. 2000; 15:101–3.

70. Fields BS, Benson RF, Besser RE. *Legionella* and Legionnaire's disease: 25 years of investigation. *Clin Micro Rev*. 2002; 15:502–26.

71. Dam AP. Recent advances in the diagnosis of Lyme disease. *Expert Rev Mol Diagn*. 2001; 1:413–27.

72. Brucella. In: Forbes BA, Sahm DF, Weissfeld AS, eds. *Diagnostic Microbiology*. 11th ed. St Louis, MO: Mosby, Inc.; 2002: 487–90.

73. Gerding DN, Johnson S, Peterson LR, et al. *Clostridium difficile*-associated diarrhea and colitis. *Infect Control Hosp Epidemiol*. 1995; 16:459–77.

74. Katz DE, Taylor DN. Parasitic infections of the gastrointestinal tract. *Gastroenterol Clin North Am*. 2001; 30:797–815.

75. Laboratory methods for the diagnosis of parasitic infections. In: Forbes BA, Sahm DF, Weissfeld AS, eds. *Diagnostic Microbiology*. 11th ed. St. Louis; Mosby, Inc., 2002: 604–709.

76. Olano JP, Walker DH. Human erlichioses. *Med Clin North Am*. 2002; 86:375–92.

77. Suerbaum S, Michetti P. *Helicobacter pylori* infection. *N Engl J Med*. 2002; 347:1175–86.

78. Passaro DJ, Chosy EJ, Parsonnet J. *Helicobacter pylori*: consensus and controversy. *Clin Infect Dis*. 2002; 35:298–304.

79. Levett PN. Leptospirosis. *Clin Micro Rev*. 2001; 14:296–326.

80. Cell-wall deficient bacteria: *Mycoplasma* and *Ureaplasma*. In: Forbes BA, Sahm DF, Weissfeld AS, eds. *Diagnostic Microbiology*. 11th ed. St Louis, MO: Mosby, Inc.; 2002: 587–94.

81. Moody A. Rapid diagnostic tests for Malaria parasites. *Clin Micro Rev*. 2002;15:66–78.

82. Thomas CF, Limper AH. *Pneumocystis* pneumonia: clinical presentation and diagnosis in patients with and without acquired immune deficiency syndrome. *Semin Resp Infect*. 1998; 13:289–95.

83. Sexton DJ, Kaye KS. Rocky mountain spotted fever. *Med Clin North Am*. 2002; 86:351–60.

84. Montoya JG. Laboratory diagnosis of *Toxoplasma gondii* infections and Toxoplasmosis. *J Infect Dis*. 2002; 185(suppl 1):S73–S82.

85. Murdoch DR. Diagnosis of *Legionella* infection. *Clin Infect Dis*. 2003; 36:64–9.

86. Wilson ML. Clinically relevant cost-effective clinical microbiology. *Am J Clin Pathol*. 1997; 107:154–67.

87. Meningitis and other infections of the central nervous system. In: Forbes BA, Sahm DF, Weissfeld AS, eds. *Diagnostic Microbiology*. 11th ed. St Louis, MO: Mosby, Inc.; 2002: 907–16.

88. Ross GH, Gunderson BW, Ibrahim KH, et al. Central nervous system infections. In: DiPiro JT, Talbert RL, Yee GC, et al., eds. *Pharmacotherapy: A Pathophysiologic Approach*. 5th ed. Stamford, CT: McGraw-Hill/Appleton & Lange; 2002: 1831–47.

89. Tunkel AR, Scheld WM. Acute meningitis. In: Mandell GL, Bennett JE, Dolin R, eds. *Principles and Practice of Infectious Diseases*. 5th ed. Philadelphia, PA: Churchill Livingstone; 2000: 959–97.

90. Thomson RB, Bertram H. Laboratory diagnosis of central nervous system infections. *Infect Dis Clin North Am*. 2001;15: 1047–71.

91. Zunt JR, Marra CM. Cerebrospinal fluid testing for the diagnosis of central nervous system infections. *Neurol Clin North Am*. 1999; 17:675–89.

92. Bisno AL, Gerber MA, Gwaltney JM, et al. Practice guidelines for the diagnosis and management of Group A streptococcal pharyngitis. *Clin Infect Dis*. 2002; 35:113–25.

93. Infections of the lower respiratory tract. In: Forbes BA, Sahm DF, Weissfeld AS, eds. *Diagnostic Microbiology*. 11th ed. St Louis, MO: Mosby, Inc.; 2002: 884–98.

94. Ruiz M, Arosio C, Salman P, et al. Diagnosis of pneumonia and monitoring of infection eradication. *Drugs*. 2000; 60:1289–302.

95. Graham JC, Galloway A. The laboratory diagnosis of urinary tract infections. *J Clin Pathol*. 2001; 54:911–9.

96. Infections of the urinary tract. In: Forbes BA, Sahm DF, Weissfeld AS, eds. *Diagnostic Microbiology*. 11th ed. St Louis, MO: Mosby, Inc.; 2002: 925–38.

97. Coyle EA, Prince RA. Urinary tract infections and prostatitis. In: DiPiro JT, Talbert RL, Yee GC, et al., eds. *Pharmacotherapy: A Pathophysiologic Approach*. 5th ed. Stamford, CT: McGraw-Hill/Appleton & Lange; 2002: 1981–96.

98. Meares EM, Stamey TA. Bacteriologic localization patterns in bacterial prostatitis and urethritis. *Invest Urol*. 1968; 5:492–518.

99. CDC. Screening tests to detect *Chlamydia trachomatis* and *Neisseria gonorrhoeae* infections–2002. *MMWR*. 2002; 51:1–27.

100. Genital tract infections. In: Forbes BA, Sahm DF, Weissfeld AS, eds. *Diagnostic —Microbiology*. 11th ed. St Louis, MO: Mosby, Inc.; 2002:939–53.

101. Knodel LC. Sexually transmitted diseases. In: DiPiro JT, Talbert RL, Yee GC, et al., eds. *Pharmacotherapy: A Pathophysiologic Approach*. 5th ed. Stamford, CT: McGraw-Hill/Appleton & Lange; 2002: 1997–2016.

102. Bowden FJ, Tabrizi SN, Garland SM, et al. Sexually transmitted diseases: new diagnostic approaches and treatments. *Medical Journal of Australia*. 2002; 176:551–7.

103. The spirochetes. In: Forbes BA, Sahm DF, Weissfeld AS, eds. *Diagnostic Microbiology*. 11th ed. St Louis, MO: Mosby, Inc.; 2002: 595–602.

104. Wendel KA, Erbolding EJ, Gaydos CA, et al. *Trichomonas vaginalis* polymerase chain reaction compared with standard diagnostic and therapeutic protocols for the detection and treatment of vaginal trichomoniasis. *Clin Infect Dis*. 2002; 35:576–80.

105. Laboratory methods in basic virology. In: Forbes BA, Sahm DF, Weissfeld AS, eds. *Diagnostic Microbiology*. 11th ed. St Louis, MO: Mosby, Inc.; 2002: 799–863.

106. Ashley RL. Performance and use of HSV type-specific serology test kits. *Herpes*. 2002; 9:38–45.

107. Normally sterile body fluids, bone and bone marrow, and solid tissues. In: Forbes BA, Sahm DF, Weissfeld AS, eds. *Diagnostic Microbiology*. 11th ed. St Louis, MO: Mosby, Inc.; 2002: 985–94.

108. Pierson DJ. Disorders of the pleura, mediastinum, and diaphragm. In: Wilson JD, Braunwald E, Isselbacher KJ, et al., eds. *Harrison's Principles of Internal Medicine*. 12th ed. New York, NY: McGraw Hill, Inc.; 1991: 1111–6.

109. Penn RL, Betts RF. Lower respiratory tract infections (including tuberculosis). In: Reese RE, Betts RF, eds. *A Practical Approach to Infectious Diseases*. 4th ed. New York, NY: Little, Brown and Company; 1996: 258–349.

110. Shmerling RH. Synovial fluid analysis: A critical reappraisal. *Rheum Infect Dis Clin North Am*. 1994; 20:503–12.

111. Smith JW, Hasan MS. Infectious arthritis. In: Mandell GL, Bennett JE, Dolin R, eds. *Principles and Practice of Infectious Diseases*. 5th ed. Philadelphia, PA: Churchill Livingstone; 2000: 1175–82.

Chapter **18**

RHEUMATIC DISEASES

Terry L. Schwinghammer

The diagnosis and management of most rheumatic diseases depend primarily on patient medical history, symptoms, and physical examination findings. A variety of laboratory tests are used to assist in the diagnosis of rheumatologic disorders, but many are nonspecific tests that are not pathognomonic for any single disease. However, the results of some specific laboratory tests may be essential for establishing the diagnosis of some diseases. Consequently, laboratory tests are important diagnostic tools when used in concert with the medical history and other subjective and objective findings. Some laboratory test results are also used to assess disease severity and to monitor the beneficial and adverse effects of pharmacotherapy.

The diagnostic utility of a laboratory test depends on its sensitivity, specificity, and predictive value (Chapter 1). Tests that are highly sensitive and specific for certain rheumatic diseases often have low predictive values because the prevalence of the suspected rheumatic disease is low. The pretest probability of disease, or a clinician's estimated likelihood that a certain disease is present based on history and clinical findings, is the most important determinant of a laboratory test's diagnostic usefulness. As the number of disease-specific signs and symptoms increases and approaches diagnostic confirmation, the pretest probability also increases.

After briefly reviewing pertinent physiology of immunoglobulins, this chapter discusses various tests used to diagnose and assess rheumatic diseases, followed by interpretation of these test results in common rheumatic disorders. Tests used to monitor antirheumatic pharmacotherapy are also described.

OBJECTIVES

After completing this chapter, the reader should be able to

1. Describe the physiologic basis for rheumatologic laboratory tests and the pathophysiologic processes that result in abnormal test results.
2. Understand the appropriate clinical applications for laboratory tests used to diagnose or assess the activity of individual rheumatic diseases.
3. Interpret the results of laboratory tests used to diagnose or manage common rheumatic diseases.
4. Use the results of rheumatologic laboratory tests to make decisions about the effectiveness of pharmacotherapy.
5. Employ laboratory tests to identify and prevent adverse reactions to drugs used to treat rheumatic diseases.

STRUCTURE AND PHYSIOLOGY OF IMMUNOGLOBULINS

Many rheumatologic laboratory tests involve detection of immunoglobulins (antibodies) that are directed against normal cellular components. In order to facilitate understanding of these tests, the structure and functions of immunoglobulins is reviewed briefly.

When the immune system is challenged by a foreign substance (antigen), activated B lymphocytes differentiate into immunoglobulin-producing plasma cells. Immunoglobulins are Y-shaped proteins with an identical antigen-binding site (called *Fab* or *fraction antigenbinding*) on each arm of the Y (Figure 18-1). Each arm is composed of a light amino acid

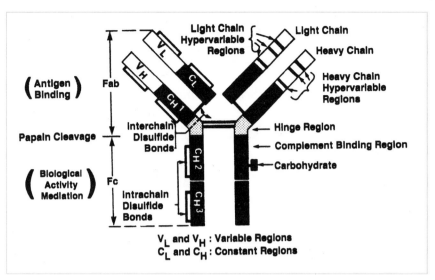

Figure 18-1. Prototypic IgG immunoglobulin. (Adapted from Wasserman RL, Capra JD. Immunoglobulins. In: Horowitz MI, Pigman W, eds. *The Glycoconjugates.* New York, NY: Academic Press; 1977. Reproduced, with permission, from Koopman WJ, Griffin JA. B-lymphocytes. In: Kelley WN, Harris ED Jr, Ruddy S, et al., eds. *Textbook of Rheumatology.* 3rd ed. Philadelphia, PA: W. B. Saunders; 1989.)

chain and a heavy amino acid chain. The terms *light* and *heavy* refer to the number of amino acids in each chain. Because the heavy chain has more amino acids than the light chain, it is longer and has a higher molecular weight.

Both types of chains have a variable region (V_L and V_H) and a constant region (C_L and C_H). The *variable* regions contain the antigen-binding sites and vary in amino acid sequence. The sequences differ to allow immunoglobulins to recognize and bind specifically to thousands of different antigens. The *constant* region of the light chain (C_L) is a single section. Immunoglobulins that have identical constant regions in their heavy chains (e.g., C_H1, C_H2, and C_H3) are of the same class.

The five classes of immunoglobulins are IgA, IgD, IgE, IgG, and IgM. Depending on the immunoglobulin, the constant region of the heavy chain has either three domains and a hinge region (IgA, IgD, and IgG) or four domains without a hinge region (IgE and IgM). Thus, the immunoglobulin's heavy chain determines its class (α heavy chains, IgA; δ heavy chains, IgD; ε heavy chains, IgE; γ heavy chains, IgG; and μ heavy chains, IgM).

In Figure 18-1, the second and third domains (C_H2 and C_H3) of the heavy chain are part of the Fc (fraction crystallizable) portion of the immunoglobulin. This portion has two important functions: (1) activation of the complement cascade (discussed later); and (2) binding of immunoglobulins (which react with and bind antigen) to cell surface receptors of effector cells such as monocytes, macrophages, neutrophils, and natural killer (NK) cells.[1]

TESTS TO DIAGNOSE AND ASSESS RHEUMATIC DISEASES

Blood tests that are relatively specific for certain rheumatic diseases include rheumatoid factors (RFs), antinuclear antibodies (ANAs), antineutrophil cytoplasmic antibodies (ANCAs), and complement. Nonspecific blood and other types of tests include erythrocyte sedimentation rate (ESR), C-reactive protein (CRP), analysis of synovial fluid, and others.

RF and ANAs are the most frequently ordered specific rheumatologic tests. ANCAs are incompletely understood and presently have limited but important clinical significance. Where applicable, the sections that follow discuss *quantitative* assay results (where normal values are reported as a range of concentrations), *qualitative* assay results (where assay results are reported as only positive or negative), and their use in common rheumatic and nonrheumatic diseases.

Rheumatoid Factor

Rheumatoid factors (RFs) are immunoglobulins that are abnormally directed against the Fc portion of IgG. These immunoglobulins do not recognize the IgG as being "self." Therefore, the presence of RFs in the blood indicates an autoimmune process. The RF measured in most laboratories is *IgM-anti-IgG* (an IgM antibody that specifically binds IgG). Like all IgM antibodies, IgM RF is composed of five subunits whose Fc portions are attached to the same base. The variable regions of each IgM antibody can bind up to five IgG molecules at its multiple binding sites, making IgM RF the most stable and easiest to quantify.

RFs are most commonly associated with rheumatoid arthritis (RA) but are not specific for that disease. Other rheumatic diseases in which circulating RFs have been identified include systemic lupus erythematosus (SLE), progressive systemic sclerosis (scleroderma), mixed connective-tissue disease (MCTD), and Sjögren's syndrome.[2] The significance of RFs in these diseases remains unknown.

The presence of RF is not conclusive evidence that a rheumatic disease exists. Patients with various acute and chronic inflammatory diseases as well as normal individuals may be RF positive. Nonrheumatic diseases associated with RFs include mononucleosis, hepatitis, malaria, tuberculosis, syphilis, subacute bacterial endocarditis, cancers after chemotherapy or irradiation, chronic liver disease, hyperglobulinemia, and cryoglobulinemia.

The percentage of individuals with positive RF concentrations and the mean RF concentration of the population increase with advancing age. Although RFs are associated with several rheumatic and many nonrheumatic diseases, the concentrations of RFs in these diseases are lower than those observed in patients with RA.

Quantitative Assay Results

Normal values: <1:20 and ≤20 IU/mL

When a quantitative RF test is performed, results are reported as either a dilutional titer or a concentration in international units per milliliter. RF titers are reported positive as a specific serum dilution. That is, serum is diluted serially (e.g., 1:20, 1:40, 1:80, 1:160, 1:320); the ability to detect RF is tested at each dilution. The greatest dilution that results in a positive test is reported as the endpoint. A titer of ≤1:20 or a concentration >20 IU/mL is generally considered to be positive.

Qualitative Assay Results

The dilutional titer chose to indicate a positive RF excludes 95% of the normal population. Stated another way, at a serum dilution at which 95% of the normal population is RF negative, 70–90% of RA patients will have a positive RF test. The remaining RA patients who have RF titers within the normal range may be described as *seronegative*.

Antinuclear Antibodies

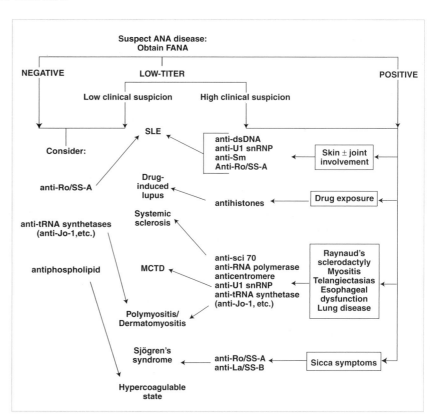

Figure 18-2. Algorithm for the use of ANAs in the diagnosis of connective tissue disorders. (Reproduced, with permission, from Reference 3.)

Antinuclear antibodies (ANAs) are a heterogeneous group of autoantibodies directed against nucleic acids and nucleoproteins within the nucleus and cytoplasm. Intracellular targets of these autoantibodies include deoxyribonucleic acid (DNA), ribonucleic acid (RNA), individual nuclear histones, acidic nuclear proteins, and complexes of these molecular elements.

The ANA test is included in the diagnostic criteria for idiopathic SLE, drug-induced lupus, and MCTD because of its high rate of positivity in these disorders. However, its low specificity makes it unsuitable for use as a screening test for rheumatic or nonrheumatic diseases in asymptomatic individuals.

Figure 18-2 provides guidelines for the use of the ANA test in diagnosing rheumatic disorders. The titer or quantitative value should be considered when evaluating the clinical significance of ANA test results.

Three specific ANAs have high disease specificities. However, these tests have little clinical utility because of their low sensitivity (Table 18-1):

TABLE 18-1

ANA	IMMUNOFLUORESCENT STAINING PATTERN	TARGETED CELLULAR MATERIAL	SENSITIVITY	SPECIFICITY
Anti-dsDNA[b]	Rim	dsDNA	SLE[b] 60–70%	High: SLE >90% if present in high titer
Anti-Sm[b,c] (rarely occurs by itself)	Fine speckled	Nuclear ribonucleoproteins	SLE 25% (Asian/ African 30–40%; Caucasian 10–20%)	High: SLE 98%
Anti-ssDNA[b]	Rim	ssDNA	SLE 90%; RA[b] 60%; Drug-induced lupus 55%	
Antihistone	Homogeneous	Chromatin and DNA-packing protein	Drug-induced lupus 100%; SLE 30%; RA 15–20%	Low
Anti-U$_1$RNP[b]	Fine speckled	Nuclear ribonucleoproteins	MCTD[b] 100%; SLE 30%; Scleroderma 20–30%; Discoid lupus 20–30%; RA 10%; Polymyositis 10%	Low
Anti-Ro[c]/ anti-SSA[d]	Fine speckled	Nuclear ribonucleoproteins	Sjögren's syndrome 90%; SLE 25–50%; Polymyositis 18%; RA 5%; Scleroderma 5%	Low
Anti-La[c]/anti-SSB[d]/Ha[c] (rarely occurs by itself)	Fine speckled	Nuclear ribonucleo-proteins	Sjögren's syndrome 85%; SLE 10–15%	Low
Anticentromere	Discrete large speckled	Chromatin and centromere	Scleroderma 10–15%; CREST[b] 50–90%; Raynaud's disease 15–30%	High: Scleroderma, CREST, or Raynaud's disease >95%
Antitopoiso-merase I (anti-Scl$_{70}$)	Grainy speckled	Chromatin and DNA-catalyzing protein	Scleroderma 15–20%	High: Scleroderma >95%
Anti-Jo-1	Cytoplasmic	Cytoplasm and histidyl tRNA synthetase	Polymyositis 20–30%; Jo-1 syndrome 50%	High: Polymyositis with interstitial lung disease or Jo-1 syndrome

[a] Adapted from References 3–6.

[b] Anti-dsDNA = anti-double-stranded DNA; anti-Sm = an immunoglobulin specific against Sm, a ribonucleoprotein found in the cell nucleus; anti-ssDNA = anti-single-stranded DNA; anti-U$_1$RNP = anti-uridine-rich ribonuclear protein; SLE = systemic lupus erythematosus; RA = rheumatoid arthritis; MCTD = mixed connective-tissue disease; CREST = syndrome characterized by calcinosis, Raynaud's phenomenon, esophageal motility disorder, sclerodactyly, and telangiectasias.

[c] Represents the first two letters of the surname of the patient whose serum was used to identify the reaction in agar diffusion.

[d] Sjögren's syndrome A and B.

Table 18-1. Laboratory and Clinical Characteristics of Antibodies to Nuclear/Cytoplasmic Antigens[a]

1. *Anticentromere* and
2. *Antitopoisomerase I (ScI$_{70}$)*—These two antibodies are highly specific for scleroderma and related diseases such as CREST syndrome (associated with **c**alcinosis, **R**aynaud's phenomenon, **e**sophageal dysmotility, **s**clerodactyly and **t**elangiectasias) and Raynaud's disease.
3. *Anti-Jo-1*—This antibody is highly specific for polymyositis with interstitial lung disease, Raynaud's phenomenon, and destructive polyarthritis (Jo-1 syndrome).

Four other specific ANAs have potential clinical importance, although they are nonspecific:

1. *Anti-Ro/Sjögren's syndrome A (anti-Ro/SS-A)*—In women of childbearing age who have a known connective-tissue disease (e.g., SLE, MCTD, or early undifferentiated connective-tissue disease), a positive anti-Ro/SS-A is associated with an infrequent but definite risk of bearing a child with neonatal SLE and congenital heart block. Presence of this antibody also correlates with late-onset SLE and secondary Sjögren's syndrome. In patients who are ANA negative but have clinical signs of SLE, a positive anti-Ro/SSA increases the probability of diagnosing SLE. Anti-Ro/SSA occurs in 62% of ANA-negative SLE patients.
2. *Anti-La/Sjögren's syndrome B (anti-La/SS-B)*—In some patients, this antibody is a useful marker for the diagnosis of Sjögren's syndrome.[3]
3. *Anti-uridine-rich ribonuclear protein (anti-U$_1$RNP)*—A positive test in a patient with suspected MCTD increases the probability that this diagnosis is correct, even though the test is nonspecific.[4] On the other hand, a negative anti-U$_1$RNP in a patient with possible MCTD virtually excludes this diagnosis.
4. *Antihistone (nucleosome) antibodies*—These antibodies target the protein portions of nucleosomes, which are DNA-protein complexes comprising part of chromatin. These antibodies are present in virtually all cases of drug-induced lupus. In fact, the diagnosis of drug-induced lupus should be questioned in their absence. Most cases of drug-induced lupus are readily diagnosed because a commonly implicated drug (e.g., hydralazine, isoniazid, and procainamide) is being taken or a strong temporal relationship exists between drug initiation and the onset of SLE signs and symptoms. However, in some cases of potential drug-induced lupus, histone autoantibody testing can be helpful. Antihistone antibodies appear less commonly in other diseases, including adult RA, juvenile RA, autoimmune hepatitis, scleroderma, and others. There is some evidence that antihistone antibodies correlate with disease activity in SLE.

A positive ANA can also be found in otherwise healthy individuals. ANAs are also associated with various genetic and environmental factors (e.g., intravenous drug abuse), hormonal factors, and increased age. They also are associated with nonrheumatic diseases, both immunologically mediated (e.g., Hashimoto's thyroiditis, idiopathic pulmonary fibrosis, primary pulmonary hypertension, idiopathic thrombocytopenic purpura, and hemolytic anemia) and nonimmunologically mediated (e.g., acute or chronic bacterial, viral, or parasitic infections; neoplasm).

Quantitative Antinuclear Antibody Assay Results

Normal: Negative at 1:20 dilution, but varies among laboratories

Most laboratories use the indirect immunofluorescence ANA test (FANA) in initial ANA testing because it is a highly sensitive screening test for the presence of ANAs.[3] Although the FANA is positive in >95% of patients with SLE, it is also positive in at least 75–90% of patients with drug-induced lupus, MCTD, systemic sclerosis, polymyositis, dermatomyositis, and Sjögren's syndrome.[3] Laboratories usually report the ANA titer, which is the highest serum dilution that remains positive for ANAs. A very high concentration (titer >1:640) should raise suspicion for an autoimmune disorder but is not in itself diagnostic of any disease. In the absence of clinical findings, these patients should be monitored closely for the overt development of an autoimmune disorder. The finding of a low antibody titer (<1:80) in the absence of signs or symptoms of disease is of less concern, and such patients require less frequent follow-up than those with very high titers. False-positive ANAs are common in the normal population and tend to be associated with low titers (<1:40). Unfortunately, there is no consistent correlation between disease activity and ANA titer. When titers are high or considered positive, immunofluorescent staining patterns of the nucleus are assessed.

Qualitative Antinuclear Antibody Assay Results

The pattern of nuclear fluorescence after staining provides information that is limited but sometimes clinically useful. Different patterns of fluorescence correspond with the component(s) of the nucleus against which the patient's ANAs are directed. The four common immunofluorescent patterns are as follows:

1. *Homogeneous*—This pattern is seen most frequently in patients with SLE but can also be observed in patients with drug-induced lupus, RA, vasculitis, and polymyositis.
2. *Speckled*—This pattern is also seen most frequently in SLE but can appear in patients with MCTD, Sjögren's syndrome, progressive systemic sclerosis, polymyositis, and RA.
3. *Nucleolar*—This pattern is infrequently observed in patients with SLE but is more frequently seen in patients with polymyositis, progressive systemic sclerosis, and vasculitis.
4. *Nuclear rim*—This is the only pattern that is highly specific for any rheumatic disease and is observed predominantly (98%) in SLE patients.[4]

Patterns of immunofluorescence are less specific than the identification (or titer) of ANA to specific nuclear antigens. However, there are potential clinical applications for some ANAs associated with high disease specificity and low to moderate sensitivity. Table 18-1 summarizes the most frequently identified ANAs, their corresponding immunofluorescent staining patterns and targeted cellular material, and disease sensitivities and specificities.[3–6]

Antineutrophil Cytoplasmic Antibodies

As the name implies, antineutrophil cytoplasmic antibodies (ANCAs) are antibodies directed against neutrophil cytoplasmic antigens. Testing for ANCAs is important for the diagnosis and classification of various forms of vasculitis. In these disorders, the target antigens are proteinase 3 (PR3) and myeloperoxidase (MPO). Both antigens are located in the azurophilic granules of neutrophils and the peroxidase-positive lysosomes of monocytes. Antibodies that target PR3 and MPO are known as *PR3-ANCA* and *MPO-ANCA*.[7] There is an association between ANCA and three major vasculitic syndromes: Wegener's granulomatosis, microscopic polyangiitis, and Churg-Strauss syndrome.[8]

Wegener's granulomatosis is a vasculitis of unknown origin that can damage organs by restricting blood flow and destroying normal tissue. Although any organ system may be involved, the disorder primarily affects the respiratory tract (sinuses, nose, trachea, and lungs) and the kidneys. Many patients with active Wegener's granulomatosis have ANCAs. Although a positive ANCA test is useful to support a suspected diagnosis, the test is usually not used alone to diagnose this disorder. The ANCA test may be negative in some patients who have active Wegener's granulomatosis.

In patients with vasculitis, immunofluorescence after ethanol fixation reveals two characteristic patterns: cytoplasmic (*cANCA*) and perinuclear (*pANCA*). With cANCA, there is diffuse staining throughout the cytoplasm, which is usually caused by antibodies against PR3. The pANCA pattern is characterized by staining around the nucleus and perinuclear fluorescence. In vasculitis patients, the antibody causing this pattern is generally directed against MPO.

Although detection and identification of ANCAs is most useful in diagnosing various vasculitides, ANCAs have been reported in connective tissue diseases (e.g., RA, SLE, and myositis), chronic infections (e.g., cystic fibrosis, endocarditis, and HIV), and gastrointestinal diseases (e.g., inflammatory bowel disease, sclerosing cholangitis, and autoimmune hepatitis). Drugs that have been associated with false-positive ANCA reactions include hydralazine, propylthiouracil, penicillamine, and minocycline.[8]

Quantitative Assay Results

When used in the diagnosis of Wegener's granulomatosis, the specificity of PR3-ANCA is approximately 90%. The sensitivity of the test is about 90% when the disease is active and 40% when the disease is in remission. Thus, the sensitivity of PR3-ANCA is related to the extent, severity, and activity of the disease at the time of testing.

The utility of obtaining serial PR3-ANCA tests in assessing disease activity is controversial. Some data suggest that a rise in titers predicts clinical exacerbations and justifies increasing immunosuppressive therapy. However, data from the National Institutes of Health showed that changes in serial cANCA titers correlated with a change in disease activity in only 64% of patients.[8] A rise in PR3-ANCA titer preceded clinical disease relapse in only 24% of patients who had been in remission. Thus, serial ANCA testing probably has a small role in predicting relapse or assessing disease activity.

Higher titers of anti-MPO antibodies have been observed during active disease than during remission. Although titers have been observed to increase prior to disease relapse, no prospective study has demonstrated the usefulness of monitoring serial titers for predicting disease activity or initiating prophylactic treatment.

Qualitative Assay Results

The sensitivity and specificity of cANCA, pANCA, and anti-MPO tests for various diseases are listed in Table 18-2.[9] The presence of cANCAs denotes a spectrum of diseases ranging from idiopathic pauci-immune, necrotizing glomerulonephritis to extended Wegener's granulomatosis.[10] In most cases of vasculitis, renal disorder, and granulomatous disease, patient sera are negative for cANCAs.

The pANCA test has limited diagnostic value. A positive pANCA test should be followed by antigen-specific assays such as anti-MPO. In ulcerative colitis, the specificity of the pANCA test has been reported to be as high as 94%. However, with only moderate sensitivity and inconsistent correlation between titers and disease activity, pANCA screening may be of little value. Although sensitivity can reach 85% in primary sclerosing cholangitis, the pANCA test lacks specificity in the differential diagnosis of autoimmune hepatic diseases. In RA, pANCA may be related to aggressive, erosive disease. The sensitivity of the test increases in RA complicated by vasculitis, but its specificity remains low.

Complement

The complement system consists of at least 17 different plasma proteins that provide a defense mechanism against microbial invaders and serve as an adjunct or "complement" to humoral immunity. The system works by depositing complement components on pathologic targets and by the interaction of plasma proteins in a cascading sequence to mediate inflammatory effects such as opsonization of particles for phagocytosis, leukocyte activation, and assembly of the *membrane attack complex* (MAC).[11] Six plasma control proteins and five

TABLE 18-2

ANCA	SENSITIVITY	SPECIFICITY
cANCA	Extended Wegener's granulomatosis >90%; Limited Wegener's granulomatosis 70–85%; Microscopic polyarteritis 50%; Polyangiitis overlap syndrome 40%; Idiopathic crescentic glomerulonephritis 30%; Churg-Strauss syndrome 10%; Classic polyarteritis nodosa 10%	Wegener's granulomatosis disease spectrum 98% (extended Wegener's granulomatosis; limited Wegener's granulomatosis-microscopic polyarteritis; polyangiitis overlap syndrome; and idiopathic crescentic glomerulonephritis)
pANCA	Ulcerative colitis 60–75%; Crohn's disease 10–20%; Autoimmune chronic active hepatitis 60–70%; Primary biliary cirrhosis 30–40%; Primary sclerosing cholangitis 60–85%; Rheumatoid arthritis with Felty's syndrome 90–100%; Rheumatoid arthritis with vasculitis 50–75%; Rheumatoid arthritis 20–40%	Ulcerative colitis >90%; all others low
Anti-MPO	Idiopathic crescentic glomerulonephritis 70%; Churg-Strauss syndrome 70%; Microscopic polyarteritis 50%; Wegener's granulomatosis 20%; Classic polyarteritis nodosa 20%; Polyangiitis overlap syndrome 20%	Systemic vasculitis and/or idiopathic crescentic glomerulonephritis 94–99%

[a]Adapted from Reference 9.

Table 18-2. Disease Associations of Antinuclear Cytoplasmic Antibodies (ANCAs)[a]

integral membrane control proteins regulate this cascade. These proteins circulate normally in a precursor (inactive) form (e.g., C3 and C4). When the initial protein of a given pathway is activated, it activates the next protein (e.g., C3a and C4a) in a cascading fashion similar to that seen with clotting factors.

Activation of this system can occur through any one of three proteolytic pathways:

1. *Classical pathway*—This pathway is activated when IgM or IgG antibodies bind to antigens such as viruses or bacteria.
2. *Alternative pathway*—This is an evolutionary surveillance system that does not require the presence of specific antibodies.
3. *Lectin pathway*—Only recently described, this pathway is activated similarly to the classical pathway, but instead of antibody binding, mannose-binding protein (MBP) binds to sugar residues on the surface of pathogens.

Activation by any of the three pathways generates enzymes that cleave the third and fifth complement components (C3 and C5). A final common (or terminal) sequence culminates in the assembly of the MAC. Five proteins (C5 through C9) interact to form the MAC, which creates transmembrane channels or pores that displace lipid molecules and other elements, resulting in disruption of cell membranes and cell lysis.

Because the complement system is an important part of immune system regulation, complement deficiency predisposes an individual to infections and autoimmune syndromes. In disorders associated with autoantibodies and the formation of immune complexes, the complement system can contribute to tissue damage.

Serum complement levels reflect a balance between synthesis and catabolism. Hypocomplementemia occurs when the C3 or C4 concentration falls below its reference range. Most cases of hypocomplementemia are associated with hypercatabolism (complement depletion) due to activation of the immune system rather than decreased production of complement components (hyposynthesis). Most diseases associated with the formation of IgG- or IgM-containing circulating immune complexes can cause hypocomplementemia. Rheumatic diseases included in this category are SLE, RA with extra-articular disease, and systemic vasculitis. Nonrheumatic diseases associated with hypocomplementemia include subacute bacterial endocarditis, hepatitis B surface antigenemia, pneumococcal infection, gram-negative sepsis, viral infections (e.g., measles), recurrent parasitic infections (e.g., malaria), and mixed cryoglobulinemia.[11]

Because errors in interpretation of complement study results can occur, three important aspects should be considered when interpreting these results:

1. Reference ranges are relatively wide. Therefore, new test results should be compared with previous test results rather than with a reference range. It is most useful to examine serial test results and correlate changes with a patient's clinical picture.

2. Normal results should be compared with previous results, if available. Inflammatory states may increase the rate of synthesis and elevate serum complement protein levels. For example, some SLE patients have concentrations of specific complement components that are 2–3 times the upper limit of normal when their disease is clinically inactive. When the disease activity increases to the point that increased catabolism of complement proteins occurs, levels may then fall into the reference range. It would be a misinterpretation to conclude that these "normal" concentrations represent an inactive complement system. Consequently, serial determinations of complement levels may be more informative than measurements at a single point.

3. Complement responses do not correlate consistently with disease activity. In some patients, the increase and decrease of the complement system should not be used to assess disease activity.

Assessment of the complement system should include measurement of the total hemolytic complement activity by the complement hemolytic 50% (CH_{50}) test and determination of the levels of C3 and C4.

Complement Hemolytic 50%

Reference range: 100–250 IU/mL

The complement hemolytic (CH_{50}) measures the ability of a patient's serum to lyse 50% of a standard suspension of sheep erythrocytes coated with rabbit antibody. All nine components of the classical pathway are required to produce a normal reaction. The CH_{50} screening test may be useful when a complement deficiency is suspected or a body fluid other than serum is involved. For patients with SLE and lupus nephritis, serial monitoring of CH_{50} may be useful for guiding drug therapy.

C3 and C4

Reference ranges: C3, 72–156 mg/dL or 0.72–1.56 g/L; C4, 20–50 mg/dL or 0.2–0.5 g/L

Because C3 is the most abundant complement protein, it was the first to be purified and measured by immunoassay. However, C4 concentrations appear to be more sensitive to smaller changes in complement activation and more specific for identifying complement activation by the classic pathway. Results of C3 and C4 testing are helpful in following patients who initially present with low levels and then undergo treatment, such as those with SLE.

Acute-Phase Reactants

The concentration of a heterogeneous group of plasma proteins, called *acute-phase proteins* or *acute-phase reactants*, increases in response to inflammatory stimuli such as tissue injury and infection. Concentrations of C-reactive protein, serum amyloid A protein, alpha$_1$-acid glycoprotein, alpha$_1$-antitrypsin, fibrinogen, haptoglobin, prealbumin, ferritin, and complement characteristically increase, whereas serum transferrin, albumin, and transthyretin concentrations decrease. Their collective change is referred to as the *acute-phase response.*

In general, if the inflammatory stimulus is acute and of short duration, these proteins return to normal within days to weeks. However, if tissue injury or infection is persistent, acute-phase changes may also persist. Additionally, white blood cell (WBC) and platelet counts may be elevated significantly.

Rheumatic diseases are chronic and associated with varying severities of inflammation. The erythrocyte sedimentation rate (ESR) and C-reactive protein (CRP) are two tests that are of some value in estimating the severity of inflammation. They may also be useful for monitoring disease activity over time. Unfortunately, both tests are nonspecific and cannot be used to confirm or exclude any particular diagnosis.

Erythrocyte Sedimentation Rate

Reference range (Westergren method): 0–10 mm/hr for males; 0–20 mm/hr for females

The erythrocyte sedimentation rate (ESR) has been used widely as a reflection of the acute-phase response and inflammation for many years. The test is performed by placing anticoagulated blood in a vertical tube and measuring the rate of fall of erythrocytes in mm/hr. In rheumatic diseases, the ESR is an indirect screen for elevated concentrations of acute-phase plasma proteins, especially fibrinogen.[12] An elevated ESR occurs when higher protein concentrations cause aggregation of erythrocytes, causing them to fall faster.

A number of factors unrelated to inflammation may result in an increased ESR, including obesity, increasing age, and some drugs. The ESR also responds slowly to an inflammatory stimulus. Despite these limitations, the test remains in wide use because it is inexpensive, easy to perform, and a tremendous amount of data is available about its clinical significance in numerous diseases. The Westergren method of performing an ESR test is preferred over the Wintrobe method because of the relative ease of performing the former method in clinical or laboratory settings.

Correlation of serial Westergren ESR results with patient data may influence therapeutic decisions. Two rheumatic diseases, polymyalgia rheumatica and temporal arteritis (giant cell arteritis), are almost always associated with an elevated Westergren ESR. The ESR is usually >60 mm/hr and frequently >100 mm/hr in these disorders. During initial therapy or treatment initiated after a disease flare, a significant decrease or a return to a normal ESR usually indicates that systemic inflammation has decreased substantially. In the absence of clinical symptoms, an increased ESR may indicate that more aggressive therapy is needed. Disease activity can then be monitored by ESR results. Of course, if symptoms are present, they should not be ignored.

C-Reactive Protein

Reference range: 0–0.5 mg/dL or 0–0.005 g/L

C-reactive protein (CRP) is a plasma protein of the acute-phase response. In response to a stimulus, CRP can increase up to 1000 times its baseline concentration. Although CRP concentrations increase in response to tissue injury and infection, no specific CRP function has been identified. One suggested role is binding with necrotic cell membranes at inflammation sites, allowing phagocytes to adhere and activate the complement system. Because it more accurately reflects immune system activity, CRP may be a better test than the Westergren ESR.

With the advancement of technology, CRP is no longer reported as simply "present" or "absent." Serum levels can now be quantitated accurately by immunoassay or laser nephelometry. Most healthy adults have concentrations of <1 mg/dL by these methods. Moderate increases range from 1–10 mg/dL, and marked increases are >10 mg/dL. Bacterial infections are often associated with values above 10 mg/dL. As with the Westergren ESR, serial measurements of CRP are the most valuable, especially in chronic inflammatory diseases.

Currently, the routine use of CRP for the assessment of rheumatic diseases is limited. As with the ESR test, CRP concentrations generally increase and decrease with worsening and improving signs and symptoms, respectively. Nevertheless, CRP concentrations are not disease specific, nor are they part of the diagnostic criteria for any rheumatic disease. Unlike the ESR, the CRP test is difficult to perform without expensive equipment. However, concentrations are not affected by age, gender, or some other factors that may influence the ESR.

Recent clinical trials have found that CRP is also released in response to inflammatory markers present within atherosclerotic plaques. Using a new assay method called *high-sensitivity CRP (hs-CRP)*, data from several studies have shown a correlation between elevated levels and cardiovascular events in patients with coronary heart disease, independent of serum lipid concentrations. Some data indicate that hs-CRP levels may be more predictive of subsequent cardiovascular disease than LDL cholesterol levels in certain situations.[13] The American Heart Association recommends obtaining hs-CRP levels in patients at intermediate risk of a cardiovascular event (i.e., those whose Framingham multiple risk factor scoring projects a 10-year CHD risk in the range of 10–20%).[14] In these patients, an elevated CRP (>3 mg/L) is considered to confer high risk. A level of 1–3 mg/L is average risk, and <1 mg/L is low risk. Levels >10 mg/L should be disregarded for coronary risk prediction purposes and the patient should be evaluated for clear sources of systemic inflammation or infection. It is important to note that the units of measurement for the hs-CRP (*mg/L*) are different from those of the conventional CRP test (*mg/dL*). Because CRP levels fluctuate over time, the hs-CRP should be measured twice at least 2 weeks apart and the two values averaged. At the time of this writing, no clinical trials had been conducted to determine whether treating patients on the basis of elevated hs-CRP levels alone is beneficial or cost-effective. Thus, the precise role of hs-CRP testing as a predictor of cardiovascular disease awaits the results of further clinical studies.

Synovial Fluid Analysis

Synovial fluid is essentially an ultrafiltrate of plasma to which synovial cells add hyaluronate. This fluid lubricates and nourishes the avascular articular cartilage. Normally, synovial fluid is present in small amounts and is clear and acellular (<200 cells/mm³) with a high viscosity because of the hyaluronic acid concentration. Normal fluid does not clot because fibrinogen and clotting factors do not enter the joint space from the vascular space. Protein concentration is approximately one-third that of plasma, and glucose concentration is similar to that of plasma.

When performing arthrocentesis (joint aspiration), a needle is introduced into the joint space of a diarthrodial joint. With a syringe, all easily removed synovial fluid is drained from the joint space. Arthrocentesis is indicated as a diagnostic procedure when septic arthritis, hemarthrosis (blood within a joint), or crystal-induced arthritis is suspected. Furthermore, arthrocentesis may be indicated in any clinical situation, rheumatic or nonrheumatic, if the cause of new or increased joint inflammation is unknown. Arthrocentesis is also performed to administer intra-articular corticosteroids.

When arthrocentesis is performed, the synovium may be inflamed, allowing fibrinogen, clotting factors, and other proteins to diffuse into the joint. Therefore, the collected synovial fluid should be placed in heparinized tubes to prevent clotting and to allow determination of cell type and cell number.

TABLE 18-3

CHARACTERISTIC	NORMAL	NON-INFLAMMATORY	INFLAMMATORY	SEPTIC
Viscosity	High	High	Low	Variable
Color	Colorless to straw	Straw to yellow	Yellow	Variable
Clarity	Transparent	Transparent	Translucent	Opaque
WBC (/mm3)	<200	50–1000	1000–75,000	Often >100,000
PMN[b]	<25%	<25%	Often >50%	>85%
Culture	Negative	Negative	Negative	Often positive
Glucose (a.m. fasting)	≅ Blood	≅ Blood	<50 mg/dL lower than blood	>50 mg/dL lower than blood
Protein (g/dL)	<2.0	>3.5	>3.5	>3.5

[a] Adapted from Reference 15.
[b] WBC = White blood cell; PMN = Polymorphonuclear leukocyte.

Table 18-3. Synovial Fluid Classification[a]

If diagnostic arthrocentesis is indicated, the aspirated joint fluid should be analyzed for volume, clarity, color, viscosity, cell count, culture, glucose, and protein. Synovial fluid is subsequently reported as normal, noninflammatory, inflammatory or septic.[15] Table 18-3 presents the characteristics of four pathological types of synovial fluid. The presence and type of crystals in the fluid should be determined. The presence of crystals identified by polarized light microscopy with red compensation can be diagnostic (Table 18-4). (See Minicase 1.)

TABLE 18-4

CRYSTALS	SIZE (μm)	MORPHOLOGY	BIREFRINGENCE[b]	DISEASES
Monosodium urate	2–10	Needles, rods	Negative	Gout
Calcium pyrophosphate dihydrate (CPPD)	2–10	Rhomboids, rods	Positive (weak)	CPPD crystal deposition disease (pseudogout), osteoarthritis
Calcium oxalate	2–10	Polymorphic, dipyramidal shapes	Positive	Renal failure
Cholesterol	10–80	Rectangles with notched corners; needles	Negative or positive	Chronic rheumatoid or osteoarthritic effusions
Depot cortico-steroids	4–15	Irregular rods, rhomboids	Negative or positive	Iatrogenic postinjection flare

[a] Adapted from Reference 15.
[b] The property of birefringence is the ability of crystals to pass light in a particular plane. When viewed under polarized light, the crystals are brightly visible in one plane (birefringent), but are dark in a plane turned 90 degrees. Birefringence observed under polarized light can be categorized as "positive" and "negative" based on the speed at which rays of light travel through the crystals in perpendicular planes (at right angles).

Table 18-4. Morphology of Synovial Fluid Crystals Associated with Joint Disease[a]

Nonrheumatic Tests

The three most commonly performed groups of non-rheumatic tests performed in rheumatology are the complete blood count (CBC), serum chemistry panel, and urinalysis. These tests are not specific for any rheumatologic disorder, and abnormal results may occur in association with many rheumatic and nonrheumatic diseases. These tests are discussed from a more general perspective in other chapters.

MINICASE 1

N. S., AN 85-YEAR-OLD MAN, presented to the emergency department unable to bear weight on his right leg. Physical examination revealed a swollen, inflamed, and painful right knee without systemic signs or symptoms of infection. The patient was otherwise in good health except for several gout attacks over the past 10 years.

The right knee was aspirated and drained. Several drops of slightly cloudy, light yellow aspirate were placed on a slide and sent to pathology. The remaining aspirate was sent in heparinized tubes to the laboratory for Gram's stain, bacterial culture, cell count, and chemistry panel.

Examination of the slide revealed a mixture of needle-shaped, rhomboid or rod, and variably shaped crystals. The slide was then viewed under a polarizing light microscope with a first-order red plate compensator. Most crystals were weakly positive for birefringence.

After receiving the pathology report, the emergency department physician reviewed the preliminary laboratory results of the knee aspirate (see Tables 18-5 and 18-6 for reference values):

- 25,000 WBCs/mm^3.
- 55% polymorphonuclear leukocytes.
- 5 g/dL protein.
- No bacteria or other organisms were seen on Gram stain.

Question: What is the likely diagnosis in this patient? What additional laboratory studies should be performed?

Discussion: When the patient presented initially, septic arthritis would be high on the list of differential diagnoses. The absence of systemic signs and symptoms of infection does not rule out this condition. The aspiration of cloudy, yellow fluid from a red, swollen, and painful knee is consistent with infection and/or inflammation. Therefore, appropriate diagnostic tests were performed on the synovial fluid.

The patient's history of gout may have suggested a recurrent acute gouty attack as the most likely diagnosis. However, microscopic examination revealed a mixture of crystal shapes, and polarizing light microscopy distinguished their most likely chemical composition. Based on the weakly-positive birefringence findings and variable crystal shapes, the crystals were probably composed of calcium pyrophosphate dihydrate. Thus, the most likely diagnosis is calcium pyrophosphate deposition disease (pseudogout). In gouty arthritis, the monosodium urate crystals are needle-shaped and negatively birefringent. In both gout and pseudogout, phagocytosed crystals within polymorphonuclear leukocytes are usually observed in inflamed joints. The total synovial fluid leukocyte concentration is usually 15,000–30,000 cells/mm^3, often with up to 90% neutrophils.

Additional laboratory studies that should be obtained include a serum uric acid level to rule out gout and serum creatinine and blood urea nitrogen concentrations to assess kidney function. If the serum uric acid is elevated, consideration could be given to obtaining a 24-hr urine collection to determine if the patient is an overproducer or underexcretor of uric acid. These results could assist in the selection of prophylactic antihyperuricemic therapy, should that be considered desirable.

The CBC includes hemoglobin, hematocrit, red blood cell indices (MCV, MCH, and MCHC), white blood cell (WBC) count, WBC differential, and platelet count. Chronic inflammatory diseases such as RA and SLE are commonly associated with anemia (low hemoglobin and hematocrit). The RBC indices often indicate that the anemia is normochromic and normocytic; this is often referred to as *anemia of chronic disease*. Anemia may also be associated with a low MCV (microcytic anemia). Microcytic anemia accompanies chronic blood loss, which may occur as a result of drug therapy for rheumatic diseases (e.g., gastroduodenal hemorrhage from nonsteroidal anti-inflammatory drugs). Additional tests may be necessary to rule out iron deficiency anemia (e.g., stool guaiac, serum iron, and total iron binding capacity). The platelet count may be elevated in some disorders (thrombocytosis) and decreased in others (thrombocytopenia). Leukopenia may be present, and the WBC differential may reflect either increases or decreases in various cell elements. Leukopenia may be associated with Felty's syndrome and may also be caused by therapy with gold salts or immunosuppressive agents used to treat rheumatic diseases.

The chemistry panel may include baseline measurements of electrolytes (e.g., sodium, potassium, chloride, and carbon dioxide) and tests of hepatic and renal function. SLE may be associated with hepatic dysfunction, which can be assessed by determination of hepatic transaminases (aspartate aminotransferase [AST], alanine aminotransferase [ALT]), total and direct bilirubin, alkaline phosphatase, and gamma glutaryl transferase (GGT). Some drugs used in the treatment of rheumatologic disease may also cause hepatic injury. Chronically poor nutrition may result in low serum albumin and total protein levels. Renal function tests (usually the serum creatinine and blood urea nitrogen [BUN]) may provide evidence of renal involvement in patients with lupus nephritis.

The urinalysis with microscopic evaluation is useful in detecting proteinuria, hematuria, and pyuria, which may be seen in SLE and with use of drugs to treat rheumatologic disorders.

INTERPREATAION OF LABORATORY TESTS IN SELECTED RHEUMATIC DISEASES

Rheumatoid Arthritis in Adults

In clinical practice, the laboratory tests that are performed for a given patient depend on the clinical presentation and differential diagnosis.

Rheumatoid Factor

In patients with RA, affected diarthrodial joints have an inflamed and proliferating synovium infiltrated with T lymphocytes and plasma cells. Plasma cells in the synovial fluid generate large amounts of IgG RF and abnormally low amounts of normal IgG. However, plasma cells in the bloodstream of patients with RA produce IgM RF predominantly.[2]

TABLE 18-5

CRITERION	DEFINITION
1. Morning Stiffness	Morning stiffness in and around joints that lasts ≥1 hr before maximal improvement; must be present for at least 6 weeks
2. Arthritis of three or more joints	At least three joints simultaneously having soft tissue swelling or fluid (not bony overgrowth alone) observed by a physician[b]; must be present for at least 6 weeks
3. Arthritis of hand joints	At least one joint area swollen (as defined in 2) in wrist, MCP, or PIP joint; must be present for at least 6 weeks
4. Symmetric arthritis	Simultaneous involvement of the same joint areas (as defined in 2) on both sides of the body (bilateral involvement of PIPs, MCPs, or MTPs acceptable without absolute symmetry); must be present for at least 6 weeks
5. Rheumatoid nodules	Subcutaneous nodules over bony prominences or extensor surfaces or in juxta-articular regions, observed by a physician
6. Serum rheumatoid factor	Demonstration of abnormal amounts of serum rheumatoid factor by any method that has been positive in <5% of normal control subjects
7. Radiographic changes	Changes typical of rheumatoid arthritis on posteroanterior hand and wrist radiographs; must include erosions or unequivocal bony decalcification localized in or most marked adjacent to involved joints (not osteoarthritis changes alone)

[a] Adapted from Reference 16. Patients with four or more of the seven criteria are considered to have rheumatoid arthritis. Patients with two clinical diagnoses are not excluded.
[b] The 14 possible areas are right or left proximal interphalangeal (PIP), metacarpophalangeal (MCP), wrist, elbow, knee, ankle, and metatarsophalangeal (MTP) joints.

Table 18-5. American Rheumatism Association 1987 Revised Criteria for Classification of Rheumatoid Arthritis[a]

Approximately 60–70% of adults with RA have a positive RF titer, and most of those who are positive have titers of at least 1:320. Patients with RA have higher RF titers than individuals with most other nonrheumatic conditions. In patients with a positive RF, the titer generally increases as RA disease activity (inflammation) increases. Consequently, as the serum RF titer increases, the specificity of the test for the diagnosis of RA also increases.[2] Higher titers or serum concentrations suggest the presence of more severe disease than patients with lower levels and are associated with a worse prognosis.

A positive RF fulfills one of the American College of Rheumatology's classification criteria for RA[16] (Table 18-5). However, results of the RF test are always interpreted in light of the patient's medical history, symptoms, physical examination findings, and results of other diagnostic tests (e.g., x-rays). As outlined in Table 18-5, patients meeting at least four of the seven criteria are classified as having RA. The first four criteria must be present for at least 6 weeks. If patients satisfy four of the five clinical criteria for RA (#1 through #5 in Table 18-5), the RF test should not be performed. In this situation, a negative RF may mislead clinicians, and a positive test contributes nothing additional. RF testing should also not be used to screen patients with minimal or no symptoms. RF testing is most useful when the pretest likelihood of RA is neither very low nor very high.[17]

Although RFs are usually identified and quantified from serum samples, RA is a systemic, extravascular, autoimmune disease affecting the synovium. As a result, some RFs may be present in sites other than peripheral blood. IgG RFs are found in the synovial fluids of many patients with severe RA. IgA RF may be detected in the saliva of patients with RA or Sjögren's syndrome. The presence of IgE RF is correlated with extra-articular findings of RA.[2]

The majority of patients with RA are seropositive for RF, but some patients have negative titers. However, some of these patients may have non-IgM RF, predominantly IgG RF. Also, some seronegative patients convert to seropositive on repeat testing. A small percentage of adult RA patients (<10%) are considered to be truly seronegative. When compared with RF-positive patients, seronegative patients usually have milder arthritis and are less likely to develop extra-articular manifestations (e.g., rheumatoid nodules, lung disease, and vasculitis).

Because current treatment guidelines call for aggressive early treatment of rheumatoid arthritis—before end-organ damage—clinicians must be aware of the relationship between disease onset and RF development. Unfortunately, the RF test is least likely to be positive at the onset of rheumatoid arthritis, when it might be of the most help. Only 33% and 60% of patients who develop RF are seropositive during the first 3 and 6 months of disease activity, respectively.[17]

After RA has been diagnosed, RF titers are not routinely used to assess a patient's current clinical status or modify a therapeutic regimen. A specific titer or a change in titers for an individual does not correlate reliably with disease activity.

In summary, RF is not sensitive or specific enough to use as the sole laboratory test to diagnose RA.[18] Although it is present in the majority of patients with RA, it is negative in some patients with the disease. The RF is useful as a prognostic indicator, as RA patients with high RF titers generally have a more severe disease course.

Antinuclear Antibodies

Antinuclear Antibodies (ANAs) are usually negative in patients with RA. The frequency of positive ANAs in patients with RA is highly variable. As determined by indirect immunofluorescence, this frequency varies from 10–70%, depending on the substrate used and the titer considered positive. Regardless of frequency, a positive ANA test is generally associated with a low titer and a homogeneous pattern caused by antihistone antibodies.

Complement

The serum complement level is usually normal or elevated in RA. Complement elevations often occur as part of the acute-phase response. These increases parallel changes in other acute-phase proteins (e.g., CRP). Elevations of total hemolytic activity (CH_{50}), C3, and C4 are usually observed during active stages of most rheumatic diseases, including RA. The presence of circulating immune complexes in RA may lead to hypercatabolism of complement and acquired hypocomplementemia.

Acute Phase Reactants

As in other inflammatory diseases, the nonspecific ESR test is usually elevated in active RA. The level measured by the Westergren method is often 30 mm/hr or more. It usually decreases or normalizes when systemic inflammation decreases during initial treatment or after treatment for a disease flare. However, there is a large variability in response to treatment among individuals. Subsequent increases in disease activity will be mirrored by corresponding increases in ESR.

CRP levels may be elevated (approximately 2–3mg/dL) in adult RA patients with moderate disease activity. However, there is substantial individual variability, and 5–10% of such patients have normal values. Some patients with severe disease activity have levels of 14 mg/dL or higher.

Because of their nonspecificity, the ESR and CRP are of little use in distinguishing between RA and other rheumatic diseases such as osteoarthritis or mild SLE. These tests are more appropriate for monitoring disease activity in RA. Although the ESR is more commonly used, some studies have indicated that CRP levels are a better reflection of disease activity than the ESR. The role of acute-phase reactants in the assessment of RA progression and prognosis is currently under intense investigation.

Synovial Fluid Analysis

Arthrocentesis in early RA typically reveals straw-colored, turbid fluid with fibrin fragments.[15] A clot will form if the fluid is left standing at room temperature. There are usually 5000–25,000 WBC/mm³, at least 85% of which are polymorphonuclear leukocytes (PMNs). Complement C4 and C2 levels are usually slightly decreased, but the C3 level is generally normal. The glucose level is decreased, sometimes to <25 mg/dL. No crystals should be present, and cultures should be negative.

Nonrheumatic Tests

The CBC may reveal an anemia that is either normochromic-normocytic (anemia of chronic disease) or hypochromic-microcytic (MCV <80 µm³). Anemia of chronic disease is not associated with erythropoietin deficiency. Microcytic anemia is due to iron deficiency that may result from gastrointestinal blood loss associated with drug use (e.g., NSAIDs) or other causes. Further testing must be performed to identify the source of bleeding (e.g., stool guaiac testing and endoscopy).

The WBC count may show a slight leukocytosis with a normal differential. Eosinophilia (>5% of the total WBC count) may be associated with RF-positive severe RA. Felty's syndrome may be associated with granulocytopenia.

Thrombocytosis may be present in clinically active RA as part of the acute-phase response. As the disease improve spontaneously or as a result of drug therapy, the platelet count returns toward normal.

Serum chemistries may reveal low serum album and total protein levels because of poor nutrition and loss of appetite. Renal function, hepatic injury tests, and urinalysis should be normal.

Juvenile Rheumatoid Arthritis

The older term, *juvenile rheumatoid arthritis* (JRA), is gradually being replaced by the term *juvenile idiopathic arthritis* (JIA). The new term encompasses all of what has been called JRA in the past but also includes all other forms of childhood idiopathic arthritis. However, the traditional term JRA will be used in the remainder of this chapter.

The diagnosis of JRA is divided into three subsets based on symptoms and the number of involved joints[19]:

1. *Polyarticular onset*—This subset occurs in 30–40% of patients and involves five or more joints after 6 months. Symmetrical joint involvement is common, and the knees, wrists, and ankles are most frequently affected.

   Polyarticular onset JRA has no pathognomonic laboratory findings, but an elevated ESR (>40 mm/hr), anemia (hemoglobin <11 g/dL), and hypergammaglobulinemia may be observed. An elevated ESR is helpful in children who appear to have pauciarticular disease initially because these patients are likely to develop polyarticular disease within 6 months.

2. *Pauciarticular onset*—This subset occurs in about 50% of children with JRA and involves four or fewer joints after 6 months of illness. The knees and ankles tend to be involved; in 33–50% of these patients, the onset begins in a single joint, usually the knee.

3. *Systemic onset*—This subject of JRA accounts for 10–15% of cases and is characterized by fever that spikes once or twice daily and a migratory, measles-like rash. Hepatosplenomegaly, lymphadenopathy, and pleural or pericardial effusions are common. Arthritis can involve any number of joints and may first present at symptom onset or weeks to months later.

Rheumatoid Factor

RFs may be associated with JRA, although much less frequently than with adult RA. IgM RF is detected by latex agglutination testing in only 7–10% of JRA patients. A positive RF is rarely seen before the age of 10 and is present in fewer than 4% of children at disease onset. A positive RF in this age group is more likely to be associated with other disorders (e.g., MCTD and bacterial endocarditis) or laboratory error. It is most commonly seen when onset is late in childhood, predominantly in girls with late-onset polyarticular disease. Based on these observations, the RF is of little diagnostic value. In addition, seropositivity is frequently observed in other childhood connective-tissue diseases.

As in adult RA patients, most children who are seronegative for IgM RF (via latex agglutination testing) are actually positive when tested by the enzyme-linked immunosorbent assay (ELISA) for IgM, IgA, or IgG RF. In a substantial percentage of seronegative JRA patients, "hidden" IgM RF has been detected. Detection of IgM RF via latex agglutination occurs when IgG attached to latex particles binds unbound serum IgM RF. However, circulating IgM RF is already bound to IgG in the serum in the majority of patients with seronegative JRA. Therefore, the bound IgM RF is undetected—"hidden"—when latex agglutination is used.

Hidden IgM RF can be detected by latex agglutination after dissociation from serum IgG by acid-gel filtration. Due to the technical difficulty of this laboratory procedure, hidden RFs are not routinely detected, and their clinical significance remains unknown.[20]

Antinuclear Antibodies

Although a positive ANA is not part of official JRA diagnostic criteria, ANA testing may be useful clinically. JRA accounts for approximately 75% of all pediatric connective-tissue diseases; approximately 50–70% of children diagnosed with poly- or oligoarticular onset JRA demonstrate a positive ANA, making it a more useful test than the RF test. The staining pattern is usually homogeneous or speckled and diffuse, and the titer is usually low to moderate (≤1:256). The highest prevalence of ANA seropositivity (65–100%) is seen in young girls with oligoarticular onset JRA and uveitis.

The specificity of the ANA test in JRA patients is moderate; children diagnosed with SLE or scleroderma can also have a positive ANA. Clinically, the acute onset of SLE in children can resemble systemic-onset JRA. The diagnosis of SLE is likely to be made if the ANA test is positive, because the test is seldom positive (≤10%) in children with systemic-onset JRA.

Polyarticular- and pauciarticular-onset JRA cannot be easily differentiated from SLE. In most cases, additional characteristic signs or symptoms of SLE must develop before a conclusive diagnosis is possible.

Systemic Lupus Erythematosus

Antinuclear Antibodies

With current test methods, at least 95% of active, untreated patients with systemic lupus erythematosus (SLE) have a positive ANA. For patients presenting with rheumatic signs and symptoms (e.g., joint pain, joint swelling, and morning stiffness) and signs suggestive of SLE (e.g., butterfly rash, photosensitivity, oral ulcers, and discoid rash), a positive ANA test is considered one of the 11 possible SLE classification criteria established by the American College of Rheumatology (Table 18-6).[21,22] As with the RF test, results of an ANA test are always interpreted in light of a patient's clinical signs and symptoms.

The diagnostic criteria for SLE were developed as a guide for selecting a more homogeneous patient population for research studies. The diagnosis of SLE may be made if any four of the 11 classification criteria are present, serially or simultaneously, during any observation period. However, even if four criteria are fulfilled a clinician may elect not to diagnose SLE because of contradictory history and physical examination findings. Likewise, patients with only three classification criteria may have their signs and symptoms diagnosed as SLE when strong clinical suspicion is present.[5]

Two other highly specific tests for SLE are *anti-double-stranded DNA (anti-dsDNA)* and *anti-Sm*. The anti-dsDNA test is commonly used when the SLE diagnosis is questionable and the ANA titer is low or moderate with an immunofluorescent rim pattern. A positive anti-dsDNA test is very specific for, and essentially diagnostic of SLE (see Minicase 2). In contrast, testing for antibodies to *single-stranded DNA (anti-ssDNA)* has poor diagnostic specificity for SLE even though it is more sensitive (90%). Although this antibody appears to be important in the immunopathogenesis of SLE, the test has little clinical application because of poor specificity.

There is considerable evidence that antibodies to both dsDNA and ssDNA are important in the pathogenesis of lupus nephritis because they appear to correlate with its presence and severity. Titers of these antibodies tend to fall with successful treatment, frequently becoming undetectable during sustained remission. However, concentrations of anti-ds DNA may not predict long-term progression of lupus nephritis.[23–25]

An *anti-Sm* test may be done instead of an anti-dsDNA test if the ANA test is positive with a speckled pattern. Anti-Sm is an immunoglobulin specific against Sm, a ribonucleoprotein found in the cell nucleus. A positive anti-Sm is very specific for the diagnosis of SLE. Anti-Sm antibodies are detected in 30–40% of Asian or African SLE patients whereas only 10–20% of Caucasian SLE patients are positive.

MINICASE 2

J. A., A 50-YEAR-OLD MAN, presents to his family physician complaining of fever, sore throat, and "feeling run down" for 5 days. Even though he had stayed home from work for the past 5 days, his skin appeared to be slightly sunburned in sun-exposed areas.

His past medical history is significant for hypertension and a myocardial infarction 6 months ago complicated by arrhythmias afterward. He has a 20 pack-per-year smoking history. His family physician had referred him to a rheumatologist 11 months ago because of intermittent joint pain that was not characteristic of osteoarthritis. No diagnosis was made at that visit. The results of laboratory tests at that time indicated a low-titer rheumatoid factor (1:80) and a positive ANA rim pattern at a titer of 1:160.

His current medications (stable for the past 6 months) include enalapril, ibuprofen, procainamide, and one aspirin a day. He is allergic to penicillin and intolerant to erythromycin (stomach upset).

After her examination, the physician performed a rapid strep test (results negative) and throat culture and prescribed tetracycline. The patient continued to take tetracycline after his physician's office notified him of a positive throat culture for *Streptococcus pyogenes*.

Five days after starting tetracycline, the patient returned to his physician's office because of continued fever and malaise. His sore throat had resolved. Physical examination revealed a continued fever; slightly labored breathing without productive cough, signs of pneumonia, bronchitis, or congestive heart failure; and sunburned arms and neck. The patient mentioned that he had done light yard work, having forgotten that his antibiotic could make his skin sensitive to the sun.

When asked about his breathing, he indicated that he could not breathe deeply when he exerted himself because of chest pain. However, the pain was not like what he had during his heart attack. He stated that he had started taking more ibuprofen because his fingers and knees hurt.

Reluctant to put this patient on steroids, the physician asked him to stop taking tetracycline. She gave him a prescription for enough trimethoprim-sulfamethoxazole to complete 7 days of antibiotic therapy. Furthermore, she had blood drawn for a complete blood count (CBC) with differential, chemistry panel, rheumatoid factor (RF), and antinuclear antibodies (ANA). In addition, a second appointment was made with the rheumatologist.

The patient had completed his antibiotic course by the date of the rheumatology visit. Fever was still present, and all other signs and symptoms were unchanged except that his breathing was slightly more painful and labored and his sunburn was improved. Laboratory results obtained by the rheumatologist included

- A white blood cell (WBC) count of 2000 cells/mm^3 (reference range 4800–10,800 cells/mm^3) with 71% neutrophils (45–74%), 3% bands (3–5%), 20% lymphocytes (20–40%), 5% monocytes (2–8%), 1% eosinophils (0–4%), and 0% basophils (0–1%), and 0% metamyelocytes (0%).
- An unchanged rheumatoid factor titer (1:80).
- A high-titer ANA (1:320) rim pattern.
- A urine dipstick that was significantly positive for protein.
- Absence of antihistone antibodies.

Blood was drawn to identify the specific ANAs present; the results subsequently reported the presence of anti-double-stranded DNA antibodies.

Question: What are two likely diagnoses, which one is most likely, and what data support that diagnosis?

Discussion: This case demonstrates that it is often difficult to diagnose systemic lupus erythematosus (SLE). This patient's initial presentation was typical of an ongoing viral or bacterial infection. As a result of documented drug allergies and intolerances, tetracycline was a reasonable choice for the patient's bacterial infection. Moreover, his reaction to sunlight was not unexpected because of the concurrent antibiotic use. However, both fever and photosensitivity are potential presenting symptoms for SLE and drug-induced SLE, which are often recognized weeks to months after nonacute presentations.

The patient's previous arthritic symptoms occurred before procainamide was started, making drug-induced SLE less likely. Furthermore, antihistone antibodies were absent in this patient. These antibodies are present in >95% of cases of drug-induced SLE, particularly those taking procainamide (or hydralazine, chlorpromazine, and quinidine). Other autoantibodies are not usually seen in this situation. Although antihistone antibodies are seen in as many as 80% of patients with idiopathic SLE, these patients also have other autoantibodies, such as those against DNA.

Even though the first RF and ANA tests were positive, the patient was febrile, and photosensitivity was present prior to tetracycline ingestion. SLE was not diagnosed at that time. However, after completion of antibacterial therapy, symptoms continued and evidence of pleuritis occurred. Therefore, the family physician referred him to a rheumatologist.

With additional evidence of a lupus-like syndrome (leukopenia and proteinuria), a specific ANA test was ordered and anti-double-stranded DNA antibodies were detected. Based on the patient's symptoms, their time of presentation, and highly specific anti-double-stranded DNA antibodies, the diagnosis of idiopathic SLE was made.

Although drug-induced SLE was unequivocally ruled out, discontinuing procainamide (and changing to an alternative antidysrhythmic) may help alleviate some of the patient's symptoms. Additional studies that are needed to fully evaluate this patient include a chest x-ray to assess the nature and severity of the pleuritis (or possible pericarditis) and perhaps complement levels and an ESR.

To be useful in patient management, specific ANAs must correlate consistently with disease activity. The only test that may consistently fluctuate with disease activity is anti-dsDNA in patients diagnosed with SLE. Even in this situation, clinical and other laboratory findings are usually more consistent and more helpful than the anti-dsDNA test for patient management decisions.[5]

Complement

Total hemolytic complement levels (CH_{50}) are decreased at some point in most patients with SLE, but they are usually normal in individuals with discoid lupus. Complement levels decrease in SLE because of deposition of immune complexes in active disease (hypercatabolism). Complement depletion has been associated with increased disease severity, particularly renal disease. Analysis of various complement components has revealed low levels of C1, C4, C2, and C3. Serial determinations have demonstrated that decreased levels may precede clinical exacerbations.[11] As acute episodes subside, levels return toward normal.

The results of regularly scheduled complement tests have been used to guide decisions regarding immunosuppressive therapy of lupus nephritis. From a 10-year prospective study, findings in three consecutive reports (at 2, 5, and 10 years) positively correlated normalization of CH_{50} with histologic stabilization and improvement of lupus nephritis.

Despite the data described above, the utility of monitoring complement levels in patients with SLE is controversial. Although some authorities find routine testing to be of no value, others contend that complement determinations are useful in diagnosing SLE as well as in monitoring the treatment of patients with known disease.

Acute Phase Reactants

Serum ESR and CRP concentrations are elevated in many patients with active SLE, but many individuals have normal CRP levels. Those with acute serositis or chronic synovitis are most likely to have markedly elevated CRP levels. Patients with other findings of SLE, such as lupus nephritis, may have modest or no elevations.

Several studies have examined the hypothesis that elevations in CRP during the course of SLE result from superimposed infection rather than activation of SLE. In hospitalized patients, substantially elevated serum CRP levels occur most frequently in the setting of bacterial infection. Consequently, CRP elevations >6 to 8 mg/dL in patients with SLE (as well as other diseases) should signal the need to exclude the possibility of infection. Such CRP increases should not be considered proof of infection, because CRP elevation can be related to active SLE in the absence of infection.

Nonrheumatic Tests

Antiphosopholipid antibodies (i.e., *anticardiolipin antibodies* and the so-called *lupus anticoagulant*) can occur as an idiopathic disorder and in patients with autoimmune and connective tissue diseases such as SLE.[26] Anticardiolipin antibody and the lupus anticoagulant are closely related but different antibodies. Consequently, an individual can have one antibody and not the other. These antibodies react with proteins in the blood that are bound to phospholipid, a type of fat molecule that is part of normal cell membranes. Antiphospholipid antibodies interfere with the normal function of blood vessels by causing narrowing and irregularity of the vessel (vasculopathy), thrombocytopenia, and thrombosis. These changes can lead to complications such as recurrent deep venous thrombosis, stroke, myocardial infarction, and fetal loss. The presence of these antibodies may increase the risk of future thrombotic events. This clinical situation is referred to as the *antiphospholipid antibody syndrome (APS)*. The diagnosis of APS is made when an individual has an antiphospholipid antibody documented either by a solid phase assay (anticardiolipin) or by a test for an inhibitor of phospholipid-dependent clotting (lupus anticoagulant) along with a clinical event.[26] When APS occurs in patients with no other diagnosis, it referred to as primary APS. Patients who also have SLE or another rheumatic disease are said to have secondary APS.

Anemia is present in many patients with SLE. The CBC may reveal a normochromic-normocytic anemia (anemia of chronic disease) that is not associated with erythropoietin deficiency. Hemolytic anemia with a compensatory reticulocytosis may also occur due to antierythrocyte antibodies. This is one of 11 diagnostic criteria for SLE (Table 18-6) and occurs in approximately 10% of patients. The majority of patients also have a positive Coombs' test.

Leukopenia, also one of the SLE diagnostic criteria, is common but usually mild. It results primarily from decreased numbers of lymphocytes, which may be caused by the disease or its treatment. If the patient is not being treated with corticosteroids or immunosuppressive agents, ongoing immunologic activity should be suspected. A lymphopenia (<1500/mm³ on two or more occasions) is a diagnostic criterion for SLE. Thrombocytopenia due to antiplatelet antibodies may also occur; platelet counts may be <100,000/mm³.

The serum chemistry panel may reveal increased hepatic aminotransferases (AST, ALT) and alkaline phosphatase at the onset of disease. These elevations usually decrease as the disease improves with treatment.

The urinalysis with microscopic analysis may show proteinuria (>500 mg/24 hr) in about 50% of patients. Hematuria and pyuria may also occur. However, renal disease may exist in the presence of a normal urinalysis.

OSTEOARTHRITIS

Osteoarthritis (OA) is not generally considered to be an autoimmune disease. The synovium is normal, and the synovial fluid usually lacks inflammatory cells. While affected joints are painful, they are frequently not swollen or inflamed. There are no clinical laboratory tests that are specific for the diagnosis of OA. The RF test is negative, and serum chemistries, hematology tests, and urinalysis are normal. The ESR is usually normal but may be slightly increased if inflammation is present in patients with generalized or erosive OA. Synovial fluid analysis reveals nonspecific characteristics of mild inflammation, such as increased volume, low viscosity and a mild leukocytosis (WBC <2000/mm³). The primary use of laboratory tests when OA is suspected is to rule out other disorders in the differential diagnosis.

TABLE 18-6

CRITERION	DEFINITION
1. Malar rash	Fixed erythema, flat or raised, over the malar eminences, tending to spare the nasolabial folds
2. Discoid rash	Erythematous raised patches with adherent keratotic scaling and follicular plugging; atrophic scarring may occur in older lesions
3. Photosensitivity	Skin rash as a result of unusual reaction to sunlight, by patient history or physician observation
4. Oral ulcers	Oral or nasopharyngeal ulceration, usually painless, observed by a physician
5. Arthritis	Nonerosive arthritis involving two or more peripheral joints, characterized by tenderness, swelling, or effusion
6. Serositis	a) Pleuritis—convincing history of pleuritic pain or rub heard by a physician or evidence of pleural effusion OR b) Pericarditis—documented by electrocardiogram or rub or with evidence of pericardial effusion
7. Renal disorder	a) Persistent proteinuria >0.5 g/day or >3+ if quantitation not performed OR b) Cellular casts—may be red cell, hemoglobin, granular, tubular, or mixed
8. Neurologic disorder	a) Seizures—in the absence of offending drugs or known metabolic derangements (e.g., uremia, ketoacidosis, or electrolyte imbalance) OR b) Psychosis—in the absence of offending drugs or known metabolic derangements (e.g., uremia, ketoacidosis, or electrolyte imbalance)
9. Hematologic disorder	a) Hemolytic anemia—with reticulocytosis OR b) Leukopenia—<4000/mm^3 total on two or more occasions OR c) Lymphopenia—<1500/mm^3 on two or more occasions OR d) Thrombocytopenia—<100,000/mm^3 in the absence of offending drugs

10. Immunologic disorder[b]	a) Anti-DNA: antibody to native DNA in abnormal titer OR
	b) Anti-Sm: presence of antibody to Sm nuclear antigen OR
	c) Positive finding of antiphospholipid antibodies based on
	  1) an abnormal serum level of IgG or IgM anticardiolipin antibodies,
	  2) a positive test result for lupus anticoagulant using a standard method, or
	  3) a false-positive serologic test for syphilis known to be positive for at least 6 months and confirmed by Treponema pallidum immobilization or fluorescent treponemal antibody absorption test

11. Antinuclear antibody (ANA)	An abnormal titer of antinuclear antibody by immunofluorescence or an equivalent assay at any point in time and in the absence of drugs known to be associated with drug-induced lupus syndrome

For the purpose of identifying patients in clinical studies, a person shall be said to have SLE if any four or more of the 11 criteria are present, serially or simultaneously, during any interval of observation.
[a]Adapted from References 21 and 22.
[b]Modifications to criterion 10 were made in 1997.[22]

Table 18-6. 1982 Revised Criteria for Classification of SLE[a]

Fibromyalgia

Fibromyalgia is a descriptive term that connotes pain within tissues without attempting to define the pathogenesis of the pain.[27] According to the criteria for fibromyalgia established by an American College of Rheumatology (ACR) committee in 1990, an individual must have both a history of chronic widespread pain and tenderness at 11 or more of 18 specific tender point sites on physical examination.[28] However, many people who carry the clinical diagnosis of fibromyalgia do not meet these precise criteria.

Laboratory testing should be used prudently when evaluating patients with clinical features suggestive of fibromyalgia. A satisfactory patient assessment is usually obtained by history and physical examination and performance of routine laboratory tests, such as CBC and serum chemistry. Because the clinical features of hypothyroidism and polymyalgia rheumatica may resemble those of fibromyalgia, thyroid-stimulating hormone (TSH) and ESR are recommended when the diagnosis of fibromyalgia is being considered. Serologic tests such as ANA titers are not usually necessary unless there is strong evidence of an autoimmune disorder.

If the results of laboratory testing suggest a diagnosis other than fibromyalgia, a more directed evaluation is required. Individuals who actually have fibromyalgia are sometimes misdiagnosed with autoimmune disorders. This may be due to the common complaints of arthralgias, myalgias, fatigue, morning joint stiffness, and a history of swelling of the hands and feet. Conversely, patients with existing autoimmune diseases may suffer from symptoms suggestive of fibromyalgia. In fact, approximately 25% of patients with systemic inflammatory disorders such as SLE and RA also meet ACR criteria for fibromyalgia.

TESTS TO MONITOR ANTIRHEUMATIC DRUG THERAPY

Antirheumatic therapies can cause significant adverse reactions that are reflected in laboratory test results.[29–34] Normal test results may necessitate dose reduction, temporary discontinuation, or permanent withdrawal of the offending drug. The laboratory tests most commonly affected are the WBC count, platelet count, hepatic aminotransferases, total bilirubin, serum creatinine, BUN, and urinalysis (Table 18-7).

A decrease in WBC count (leukopenia) is considered to be clinically significant when the total count is 3000–3500 cells/mm^3 (3.0–3.5 × 10^9/L) or lower, because immune defenses are compromised. Leukopenia is due primarily to a relative and absolute decrease of neutrophils (neutropenia). Pancytopenia indicates a suppression of all cell lines, including WBC, red blood cells (anemia), and platelets (thrombocytopenia). Aplastic anemia indicates a complete arrest of blood cell production in the bone marrow.

Increases in hepatic aminotransferases of 2–3 times baseline may be clinically important. The most common abnormalities identified by urinalysis are proteinuria, hematuria, pyuria, and casts.

TESTS TO GUIDE MANAGEMENT OF HYPERURICEMIA AND GOUT

The serum uric acid and urine uric acid concentrations are the two most commonly used tests to diagnose gout and assess the effectiveness of its treatment.

Serum Uric Acid

Reference range: 3.4–7 mg/dL or 202–416 mmol/L for males >17 years old

2.4–6 mg/dL or 143–357 mmol/L for females >17 years old

Uric acid is the metabolic end-product of the purine bases of DNA. In humans, uric acid is not metabolized further and is eliminated unchanged by renal excretion. It is completely filtered at the renal glomerulus and is almost completely reabsorbed. Most excreted uric acid (80–86%) is the result of active tubular secretion at the distal end of the proximal convoluted tubule.[35]

As urine becomes more alkaline, more uric acid is excreted because the percentage of ionized uric acid molecules increases. Conversely, reabsorption of uric acid within the proximal tubule is enhanced and uric acid excretion is suppressed as urine becomes more acidic.

TABLE 18-7

DRUG	DISEASE	LABORATORY TEST	ADVERSE DRUG REACTION	INCIDENCE (%)
Methotrexate	RA[b]	CBC[b] with differential and platelet count	Leukopenia	0–3
			Pancytopenia	0–2
		Hepatic aminotransferases, bilirubin, serum albumin	Hepatotoxicity	4–21
		Monitor for infection	Infection, sepsis	Rare
Leflunomide	RA	CBC with differential and platelet count	Pancytopenia	<1
			Elevated aminotransferases	5–10
		Hepatic aminotransferases, bilirubin	Hepatic necrosis	Rare
Hydroxy-chloroquine	RA	CBC with differential and platelet count	Thrombocytopenia	0–6
		Urinalysis	Proteinuria	0–6
Sulfasalazine	RA	CBC with differential and platelet count	Leukopenia	0–3
		Hepatic aminotransferases	Hepatotoxicity	1–6
Injectable gold (gold sodium thiomalate and sodium aurothioglucose	RA[a]	CBC with differential and platelet count	Anemia	Variable
			Thrombocytopenia	1–3
			Leukopenia	<1
			Pancytopenia	<0.5
		Hepatic aminotransferases	Hepatotoxicity	4
		Urinalysis	Proteinuria	1
Oral gold (auranofin)	RA	CBC with differential and platelet count	Thrombocytopenia	0–1
			Leukopenia	0.5–1
		Hepatic aminotransferases	Hepatotoxicity	0–4
		Urinalysis	Proteinuria	0–3
Etanercept	RA	CBC with differential and platelet count	Pancytopenia, aplastic anemia	Rare
		Monitor for infection	Infection, sepsis	Rare
Infliximab	RA	Baseline tuberculin skin test CBC with differential and platelet count	Activation of tuberculosis	Rare
			Anemia, thrombocytopenia	Rare
		Monitor for infection	Infection, sepsis	Rare
Anakinra	RA	CBC with differential and platelet count	Neutropenia	8
		Monitor for infection		Rare
Adalimumab	RA	Baseline tuberculin skin test CBC with differential and platelet count	Activation of tuberculosis	Rare
			Leukopenia, pancytopenia	Rare
		Monitor for infection	Infection, sepsis	Rare
Cyclosporine	RA	BUN[b], serum creatinine, cyclosporine trough blood concentrations	Nephrotoxicity	25–38
		Serum potassium, uric acid	Hyperkalemia, hyperuricemia	Variable
		Hepatic aminotransferases, bilirubin	Hepatotoxicity	4–7
Cyclophos-phamide	RA	CBC with differential and platelet count	Leukopenia	5–40 (dose dependent)
		Urinalysis	Proteinuria, hematuria	8, 15–26
		Monitor for infection	Infection, sepsis	Rare
Azathioprine	RA	CBC with differential and platelet count	Leukopenia	0–32
		Hepatic aminotransferases	Hepatotoxicity	0–5
		Urinalysis	Proteinuria	2
		Monitor for infection	Infection, sepsis	Rare

Continued on next page

TABLE 18-7

DRUG	DISEASE	LABORATORY TEST	ADVERSE DRUG REACTION	INCIDENCE (%)
NSAIDs,[b] including aspirin	RA, SLE[b]	CBC with differential and platelet count	Anemia (due to gastroduodenal ulceration and blood loss)	Variable
		Hepatic aminotransferases	Hepatotoxicity	Rare
		BUN, serum creatinine; sodium, potassium	Nephrotoxicity; electrolyte disturbances	Rare
		Urinalysis	Proteinuria, hematuria, pyuria	Rare
Corticosteroids	RA, SLE	CBC with differential and platelet count	Anemia due to peptic ulceration and blood loss	Rare
		Serum sodium, potassium, bicarbonate	Electrolyte disturbances	Variable
		Serum calcium	Osteoporosis	Variable
		Blood glucose	Hyperglycemia	Variable
		Fasting lipid panel	Dyslipidemia	Variable
		Urinalysis	Glycosuria	Variable

[a]Adapted from References 29–34.
[b]RA = rheumatoid arthritis; SLE = systemic lupus erythematosus; CBC = complete blood count; BUN = Blood urea nitrogen; NSAIDs = nonsteroidal anti-inflammatory drugs.

Table 18-7. Routine Laboratory Tests to Monitor Patients Receiving Selected Drugs for Treatment of Rheumatoid Arthritis or Systemic Lupus Erythematosus[a]

In plasma at normal body temperature, the physicochemical saturation concentration for urate is 7 mg/dL. However, plasma can become supersaturated, with the concentration exceeding 12 mg/dL. In nongouty subjects with normal renal function, urine uric acid excretion abruptly increases when the serum uric acid concentration approaches or exceeds 11 mg/dL. At this concentration, urine uric acid excretion usually exceeds 1000 mg/24 hr.

Hyperuricemia

When serum uric acid exceeds the upper limit of the reference range, the biochemical diagnosis of hyperuricemia can be made. Hyperuricemia can result from an overproduction of purines and/or reduced renal clearance of uric acid. When specific factors affecting the normal disposition of uric acid cannot be identified, the problem is diagnosed as *primary* hyperuricemia. When specific factors can be identified (e.g., another disease or drug therapy), the problem is referred to as *secondary* hyperuricemia.

As the serum urate concentration increases above the upper limit of the reference range, the risk of developing clinical signs and symptoms of gouty arthritis, renal stones, uric acid nephropathy, and subcutaneous tophaceous deposits increases. However, many hyperuricemic patients are asymptomatic. If a patient is hyperuricemic, it is important to determine if there are potential causes of false laboratory test elevation and contributing extrinsic factors. In general, clinical studies have not shown that impaired renal function is caused by chronic hyperuricemia (unless there are other renal risk factors and excluding acute uric acid nephropathy resulting from tumor lysis syndrome). However, long-term, very high serum uric acid levels (e.g., ≥13 mg/dL in men and 10 mg/dL in women) may predispose individuals to renal dysfunction. This level of hyperuricemia is uncommon, and a conclusive link to renal insufficiency has not been established. Also, renal disease accompanying hyperuricemia is often related to uncontrolled hypertension. Correction of hyperuricemia has no measurable effect on renal function.[36]

Exogenous causes. Medications are the most common exogenous causes of hyperuricemia. The two primary mechanisms whereby drugs increase serum uric acid concentrations are (1) decreased renal excretion resulting from drug-induced renal dysfunction or competition with uric acid for secretion within the kidney tubules, and (2) rapid destruction of large numbers of cells from antineoplastic therapy for leukemias and lymphomas.

The reduction in glomerular filtration rate accompanying renal impairment decreases the filtered load of uric acid and causes hyperuricemia. A number of drugs cause hyperuricemia by renal mechanisms that may include interference with renal clearance of uric acid. These agents include low-dose aspirin, pyrazinamide, nicotinic acid, ethambutol, ethanol, cyclosporine, acetazolamide, hydralazine, ethacrynic acid, furosemide, and thiazide diuretics. Diuretic-induced volume depletion results in enhanced tubular reabsorption of uric acid and a decreased filtered load of uric acid. Salicylates, including aspirin, taken in low doses (1–2 g/day) may decrease urate renal excretion. Moderate doses (2–3 g/day) usually do not alter urate excretion. Large doses (>3 g/day) generally increase urate renal excretion, thereby lowering serum urate concentrations.

Many cancer chemotherapeutic agents (e.g., methotrexate, nitrogen mustards, vincristine, 6-mercaptopurine, and azathioprine) increase the turnover rate of nucleic acids and the production of uric acid. Drug-induced hyperuricemia after cancer chemotherapy, especially high-dose regimens, can lead to acute renal failure. Allopurinol is routinely administered prophylactically to decrease uric acid formation. In other clinical situations, drug-induced hyperuricemia may not be clinically significant.

The decision to continue or discontinue a drug that may be causing hyperuricemia is dependent on three factors: (1) the risk of precipitating gouty symptoms, based on the patient's past history and current clinical status; (2) the feasibility of substituting another drug that is less likely to affect uric acid disposition; and (3) the plausibility of temporarily or permanently discontinuing the drug. If the regimen of the causative drug must remain unchanged, pharmacologic treatment of hyperuricemia may be instituted.

Diet is another exogenous cause of hyperuricemia. High-protein weight-reduction programs can greatly increase the amount of ingested purines and subsequent uric acid production. If the average daily diet contains a high proportion of meats, the excess nucleoprotein intake can lead to increased uric acid production. Fasting or starvation also can cause hyperuricemia because of increased muscle catabolism. Furthermore, lead poisoning from paint, batteries, or "moonshine," in addition to recent alcohol ingestion, obesity, diabetes mellitus, and hypertriglyceridemia, is associated with increases in serum uric acid concentration. (See Minicase 3).

MINICASE 3

M. B. IS A 45-YEAR-OLD OBESE MAN who began a daily exercise program in an attempt to lose 50 lb. In addition, he began a high-protein liquid diet because he knew that "fatty foods are not healthy."

Two weeks later, he went to his family physician for his first complete physical examination in approximately 7 years. He told his physician not to tell him that he had to lose weight because he was already walking briskly for 1 hr 3 times a week and was watching his diet carefully. The only abnormal finding on physical examination was a high blood pressure (BP) of 150/95 mm Hg. After drawing blood for a CBC with differential and a full chemistry panel and obtaining a urine sample for urinalysis, the physician prescribed hydrochlorothiazide 25 mg once daily for hypertension. Three days later, the patient was notified that his laboratory results, including serum uric acid, were normal.

Two weeks later, M. B. returned on crutches to see his physician. He explained that he had injured his right foot 3 days prior. When taking his daily walk before sunrise, he had accidentally stubbed his right foot on a rock. Two nights ago, he had awakened with a fever and felt as if his right great toe was "in a vise while an ice-cold knife was being pushed into the joint."

Examination of the patient's right foot revealed abrasions on all five toes. The skin of the great toe appeared shiny, and the toe was swollen and warm to the touch. M. B. was also in obvious pain. Whitish fluid was oozing from a small wound on the dorsal aspect of the great toe. After anesthetizing the joint, the physician aspirated several drops of whitish fluid. He then performed a Gram stain and examined the fluid on a slide, finding needle-shaped crystals but no bacteria. He also ordered a serum uric acid level.

Question: What is this patient's likely diagnosis? What would constitute appropriate therapy?

Discussion: This patient probably experienced his first acute gout attack. Although his previous serum uric acid concentration was described as normal, one endogenous and two exogenous factors may have precipitated this attack. Hypertension is frequently associated with hyperuricemia. Also, the sudden change to a high-protein diet greatly increased his ingestion of purines, which are metabolized to uric acid. Finally, the patient was also started on hydrochlorothiazide, which is an inhibitor of the renal clearance of uric acid. The abrupt change in physical exertion probably did not contribute to the attack because it was low in intensity.

Although the patient attributed the condition to his traumatic toe-stubbing event, his physician noted that none of his other abraded toes appeared to be "infected." Examination of the synovial fluid using a polarizing-light microscope revealed monosodium urate crystals without bacteria (Table 18-6).

Treatment with a short course of anti-inflammatory doses of an NSAID would be appropriate therapy in this case. Although indomethacin in doses of approximately 50 mg 3 times a day for 5 days is a common regimen, other NSAIDs are also effective and may be associated with fewer adverse effects. Colchicine and oral corticosteroids are useful alternatives in certain situations. It may be advisable for the patient to discontinue hydrochlorothiazide for 2 weeks until the acute episode resolves.

The patient was told that his foot symptoms should greatly improve within 24–48 hr. After explaining the health risks of a high-protein diet, the physician convinced M. B. to begin a more balanced diet. The physician also informed the patient that if the serum uric acid concentration he ordered was highly elevated, he probably would add a drug to reduce the level.

Four days later, M. B. received a call from his physician and was told that his serum uric acid concentration was high at 9.8 mg/dL. His physician stated that he would not prescribe any additional treatment at this time but asked the patient to return in 2 weeks for a repeat blood test and re-evaluation of his BP.

Question: Why did the physician decide to take this action? Why did he delay antihyperuricemic therapy?

Discussion: After discontinuing M. B.'s hydrochlorothiazide and recommending a balanced low-fat diet, the physician decided to wait and see if the elevated serum uric acid concentration would decline without antihyperuricemic therapy (e.g., allopurinol, probenecid). In 2 weeks, he would consider starting such treatment if the repeat serum uric acid concentration was not near normal. Alternative therapy would also be considered for the patient's hypertension.

Some clinicians recommend only observation after the first attack of acute gouty arthritis, especially if the episode was mild and responded quickly to treatment, the serum uric acid concentration was only minimally elevated, and a 24-hr urine collection for measurement of uric acid concentration was not excessive (e.g., <1000 mg/24 hr on a regular diet). Patients who meet these criteria may never have a second attack or only experience a subsequent attack months or even years later.

On the other hand, patients, with a severe first attack associated with a high serum uric acid level (>10 mg/dL) or a 24-hr urinary uric acid excretion >1000 mg should probably receive prophylactic treatment immediately after resolution of the acute attack. The results of a 24-hr urine collection would be useful in determining whether the patient is an overproducer or underexcretor of uric acid and help to guide therapy with either allopurinol or probenecid, respectively.

Endogenous causes. Endogenous causes of hyperuricemia include diseases, abnormal physiological conditions that may or may not be disease related, and genetic abnormalities. Diseases include (1) renal diseases (e.g., renal failure); (2) disorders associated with increased destruction of nucleoproteins (e.g., leukemia, lymphoma, polycythemia, hemolytic anemia, sickle cell anemia, toxemia of pregnancy, and psoriasis); and (3) endocrine abnormalities (e.g., hypothyroidism, hypoparathyroidism, pseudohypoparathyroidism, nephrogenic diabetes insipidus, and Addison's disease).

Predisposing abnormal physiological conditions include shock, hypoxia, lactic acidosis, diabetic ketoacidosis, alcoholic ketosis, and strenuous muscular exercise. In addition, males and females are at risk of developing asymptomatic hyperuricemia at puberty and menopause, respectively.

Genetic abnormalities include Lesch-Nyhan syndrome, gout with partial absence of the enzyme hypoxanthine guanine phosphoribosyltransferase, increased phosphoribosyl pyrophosphate P-ribose-PP synthetase, and glycogen storage disease type I.

Hypouricemia

Hypouricemia is not important pathophysiologically, but it may be associated with low-protein diets, renal tubular defects, xanthine oxidase deficiency, and drugs (e.g., high-dose aspirin, allopurinol, probenecid, and megadose vitamin C).

Assays and Interferences with Serum Uric Acid Measurements

In the laboratory, the concentration of uric acid is measured by either the phosphotungstate colorimetric method or the more specific uricase method. With the colorimetric method, ascorbic acid, caffeine, theophylline, levodopa, propylthiouracil, and methyldopa can all falsely elevate uric acid concentrations. With the uricase method, purines and total bilirubin >10 mg/dL can cause a false depression of uric acid concentrations. False elevations may occur if ascorbic acid concentrations exceed 5 mg/dL or if hemoglobin exceeds 300 mg/dL (in hemolysis).

Urine Uric Acid Concentration

Reference range: 250–750 mg/24 hr or 1.48–4.46 mol/24 hr

In hyperuricemic individuals who excrete an abnormal amount of uric acid in the urine (hyperuricaciduria), the risk of uric acid and calcium oxalate nephrolithiasis increases. However, the prevalence of stone formation is only twice that observed in the normouricemic population. When a stone does form, it rarely produces serious complications. Furthermore, treatment can reverse stone disease related to hyperuricemia and hyperuricaciduria.

Pathologically, uric acid nephropathy—a form of acute renal failure—is a direct result of uric acid precipitation in the lumen of collecting ducts and ureters. Uric acid nephropathy most commonly occurs in two clinical situations: (1) patients with marked overproduction of uric acid secondary to chemotherapy-induced tumor lysis (leukemia or lymphoma); and (2) patients with gout and profound hyperuricaciduria. Uric acid nephropathy also has developed after strenuous exercise or convulsions.[36]

In hyperuricemia unrelated to increased uric acid production, quantification of urine uric acid excreted in 24 hr can help to direct prophylaxis or treatment. Patients at higher risk of developing renal calculi or uric acid nephropathy (patients with gout or malignancies) excrete 1100 mg or more of uric acid per 24 hr. Prophylaxis may be recommended for these patients; allopurinol should be used instead of uricosuric agents (e.g., probenecid) to minimize the risk of nephrolithiasis. Prophylactic therapy may be started at the onset of gouty symptoms.[36]

SUMMARY

Most specific rheumatologic laboratory tests are used in the diagnosis or management of patients with rheumatoid arthritis or SLE. When used alone, none of these tests is diagnostic for any particular disease. Positive results of RF testing are most commonly seen in patient with RA. Although higher concentrations of RF are associated with more severe disease, RF titers or concentrations are not used to assess disease severity or clinical response to treatment.

ANA testing is most frequently performed in SLE diagnosis. A positive ANA occurs in the majority of patients diagnosed with drug-induced lupus or MCTD. Anti-double-stranded DNA and anti-Sm are disease-specific for SLE.

cANCA is highly specific for the disease spectrum of Wegener's granulomatosis, and anti-MPO antibodies are highly specific for systemic vasculitis and/or idiopathic crescentic glomerulonephritis.

The most complete screen of complement activation includes measurements of C3, C4, and CH_{50}.

The degree of general systemic inflammation can be estimated with the Westergren ESR and CRP tests. In RA, polymyalgia rheumatica, and temporal arteritis, elevated ESRs may indicate the need for more aggressive drug therapy. Unlike the ESR, CRP does not appear to increase with age and may be useful in assessing potential infection in SLE patients.

RA may be associated with anemia of chronic disease and thrombocytosis. SLE is normally associated with anemia of chronic disease and thrombocytopenia and occasionally with hemolytic anemia. Proteinuria, hematuria, and pyuria are often seen on urinalysis in SLE patients with active disease. When RA or SLE patients begin antirheumatic drug therapy, laboratory tests must be performed regularly to monitor for adverse drug effects.

Patients with hyperuricemia are usually asymptomatic. Prophylaxis or treatment of gout, if initiated, is begun after the first attack. The severity and frequency of the attacks guide the decision. Allopurinol prophylaxis is recommended for patients at risk of forming renal calculi.

REFERENCES

1. Diamond B, Grimaldi C. B Cells. In: Ruddy S, Harris ED Jr, Sledge CB, et al., eds. *Kelley's Textbook of Rheumatology.* 6th ed. Philadelphia, PA: W. B. Saunders; 2001: 131–49.
2. Tighe H, Carson DA. Rheumatoid factor. In: Ruddy S, Harris ED Jr, Sledge CB, et al., eds. *Kelley's Textbook of Rheumatology.* 6th ed. Philadelphia, PA: W. B. Saunders; 2001: 151–60.
3. Peng ST, Craft J. Antinuclear antibodies. In: Ruddy S, Harris ED Jr, Sledge CB, et al., eds. *Kelley's Textbook of Rheumatology.* 6th ed. Philadelphia, PA: W. B. Saunders; 2001: 161–74.
4. White RH, Robbins DL. Clinical significance and interpretation of antinuclear antibodies. *West J Med.* 1987; 147:210–3.
5. Mills JA. Systemic lupus erythematosus. *N Engl J Med.* 1994; 330:1871–9.
6. Reichlin M. Antibodies to defined antigens in the systemic rheumatic diseases. *Bull Rheum Dis.* 1993; 42(8):4–6.
7. Stone JH, Rose BD. Clinical spectrum of antineutrophil cytoplasmic antibodies. In: Rose BD, ed. *UpToDate.* Wellesley, MA; 2003.
8. Calabrese LH, Duna G. Vasculitis associated with antineutrophil cytoplasmic antibody. In: Ruddy S, Harris ED Jr, Sledge CB, et al., eds. *Kelley's Textbook of Rheumatology.* 6th ed. Philadelphia, PA: W. B. Saunders; 2001: 1165–84.
9. Kallenberg CGM, Mulder AHL, Cohen Tervaert JW. Antineutrophil cytoplasmic antibodies: a still growing class of autoantibodies in inflammatory disorders. *Am J Med.* 1992; 93:675–82.
10. Kerr GS, Fleischer TA, Hallahan CW, et al. Limited prognostic value of changes in antineutrophil cytoplasmic antibody titer in patients with Wegener's granulomatosis. *Arthritis Rheum.* 1993; 36:365–71.
11. Ruddy S. Complement. In: Ruddy S, Harris ED Jr, Sledge CB, et al., eds. *Kelley's Textbook of Rheumatology.* 6th ed. Philadelphia, PA: W. B. Saunders; 2001: 185–93.
12. Ballou SP, Kushner I. Laboratory evaluation of inflammation. In: Ruddy S, Harris ED Jr, Sledge CB, et al., eds. *Kelley's Textbook of Rheumatology.* 6th ed. Philadelphia, PA: W. B. Saunders; 2001: 697–703.
13. Ridker PM, Rifai N, Rose L, et al. Comparison of C-reactive protein and low-density lipoprotein cholesterol levels in the prediction of first cardiovascular events. *N Engl J Med.* 2002; 347:1557–65.
14. Pearson TA, Mensah GA, Alexander RW, et al. Markers of inflammation and cardiovascular disease: application to clinical and public health practice: a statement for healthcare professionals from the Centers for Disease Control and Prevention and the American Heart Association. *Circulation.* 2003; 107:499–511.
15. Schumacher HR Jr. Synovial fluid analysis and synovial biopsy. In: Ruddy S, Harris ED Jr, Sledge CB, et al., eds. *Kelley's Textbook of Rheumatology.* 6th ed. Philadelphia, PA: W. B. Saunders; 2001: 605–19.
16. Arnett FC. Revised criteria for the classification of rheumatoid arthritis. *Bull Rheum Dis.* 1989; 38(5):1–6.
17. Shmerling RH, Delbanco T. The rheumatoid factor: an analysis of clinical utility. *Am J Med.* 1991; 91:528–34.
18. Shmerling RH, Delbanco TL. How useful is the rheumatoid factor? An analysis of sensitivity, specificity, and predictive value. *Arch Intern Med.* 1993; 153:137–8.
19. Cassidy JT. Juvenile rheumatoid arthritis. In: Ruddy S, Harris ED Jr, Sledge CB, et al., eds. *Kelley's Textbook of Rheumatology.* 6th ed. Philadelphia, PA: W. B. Saunders; 2001: 1297–313 .

20. Lawrence JM III, Moore TL, Osborn TG, et al. Autoantibody studies in juvenile rheumatoid arthritis. *Semin Arthritis Rheum*. 1993; 22(4):265–74.

21. Tan EM, Cohen AS, Fries JF, et al. The 1982 revised criteria for the classification of systemic lupus erythematosus. *Arthritis Rheum*. 1982; 25:1271–7.

22. Hochberg MC. Updating the American College of Rheumatology revised criteria for the classification of systemic lupus erythematosus. *Arthritis Rheum*. 1997; 40:1725.

23. Appel AE, Sablay LB, Golden RA, et al. The effect of normalization of serum complement and anti-DNA antibody on the course of lupus nephritis. *Am J Med*. 1978; 64:274–83.

24. Jarrett MP, Sablay LB, Walter L, et al. The effect of continuous normalization of serum hemolytic complement on the course of lupus nephritis. *Am J Med*. 1981; 70:1067–72.

25. Laitman RS, Glicklich D, Sablay LB, et al. Effect of long-term normalization of serum complement levels on the course of lupus nephritis. *Am J Med*. 1989; 87:132–8.

26. Lockshin MD. Antiphospholipid antibody syndrome. In: Ruddy S, Harris ED Jr, Sledge CB, et al., eds. *Kelley's Textbook of Rheumatology*. 6th ed. Philadelphia, PA: W. B. Saunders; 2001: 1145–52.

27. Clauw DJ. Fibromyalgia. In: Ruddy S, Harris ED Jr, Sledge CB, et al., eds. *Kelley's Textbook of Rheumatology*. 6th ed. Philadelphia, PA: W. B. Saunders; 2001:417–26.

28. Wolfe F, Smythe HA, Yunus MB, et al: The American College of Rheumatology 1990 Criteria for the Classification of Fibromyalgia. Report of the Multicenter Criteria Committee. *Arthritis Rheum*. 1990; 33:160–72.

29. Harris ED Jr. Clinical features of rheumatoid arthritis. In: Ruddy S, Harris ED Jr, Sledge CB, et al., eds. *Kelley's Textbook of Rheumatology*. 6th ed. Philadelphia, PA: W. B. Saunders; 2001: 967–1000.

30. Edworthy SM. Clinical manifestations of systemic lupus erythematosus. In: Ruddy S, Harris ED Jr, Sledge CB, et al., eds. *Kelley's Textbook of Rheumatology*. 6th ed. Philadelphia, PA: W. B. Saunders; 2001: 1105–23.

31. Schuna AS. Rheumatoid arthritis. In: DiPiro JT, Talbert RL, Yee GC, et al., eds. *Pharmacotherapy: A Pathophysiologic Approach*. 5th ed. New York, NY: McGraw-Hill; 2002: 1623–37.

32. American College of Rheumatology Ad Hoc Committee on Clinical Guidelines. Guidelines for monitoring drug therapy in rheumatoid arthritis. *Arthritis Rheum*. 1996; 39:723–31.

33. Schuna A, Megeff C. New drugs for the treatment of rheumatoid arthritis. *Am J Health-Syst Pharm*. 2000; 57:225–34.

34. Louie SG, Park B, Yoon H. Biological response modifiers in the management of rheumatoid arthritis. *Am J Health-Syst Pharm*. 2003; 60:346–55.

35. Hawkins DW. Gout and hyperuricemia. In: Dipiro JT, Talbert RL, Yee GC, et al., eds. *Pharmacotherapy: A Pathophysiologic Approach*. 5th ed. New York, NY: McGraw-Hill; 2002: 1659–64.

36. Wortmann RL, Kelley WN. Gout and hyperuricemia. In: Ruddy S, Harris ED Jr, Sledge CB, et al., eds. *Kelley's Textbook of Rheumatology*. 6th ed. Philadelphia, PA: W. B. Saunders; 2001: 1339–76.

Chapter **19**

CANCERS AND TUMOR MARKERS

Rebecca S. Finley

In most types of cancer, treatment is likely to be most successful if the diagnosis is made while the tumor mass is relatively small. Unfortunately, many common types of cancer (e.g., carcinomas of the lung, breast, and colon) are frequently not diagnosed until the tumor burden is relatively large and the patient has developed symptoms related to the disease. As the search for more effective treatments for cancer has intensified over the past 30 years, much effort and many resources have also been dedicated to elucidating new methods of detecting cancers earlier while the tumor burden is low and the patient is still asymptomatic. These efforts have led to improved radiologic and other diagnostic imaging as well as the identification of biologic substances, which occur in relation to the tumor and can be detected even at very low concentrations in the blood or other body fluids.

The term *tumor marker* is used to describe a wide range of proteins that are associated with various malignancies. Typically, these markers are either proteins that are produced by or in response to a specific type of tumor, or they may be other physiologic proteins that are produced in great excess of the normal concentrations by malignant cells. In either case, the concentration of the marker usually correlates with the volume of tumor cells (i.e., as the tumor grows, or the number of malignant cells increases, the concentration of the marker also increases). In other cases, the presence of such a biologic marker may be used to predict response to treatment or to monitor the effects of treatment. More recently, some tumor markers have been shown to be essential to the viability of tumors cells and have become targets for specific therapies.

This chapter describes tumor markers that are used clinically to detect cancers and the laboratory methods that are used to assess them. In addition the sensitivity, specificity and factors that may interfere with evaluation of these tests are discussed. For tumor markers that are widely used to screen for cancers or to assess response to treatment, the clinical applications are described.

OBJECTIVES

After completing this chapter, the reader should be able to

1. Define tumor markers, describe the characteristics of an ideal tumor marker, and discuss the usefulness of tumor markers in the diagnosis, staging, and treatment of malignant diseases.
2. List nonmalignant conditions or circumstances that may cause an increase in prostate specific antigen (PSA) and discuss how PSA may be used in diagnosing prostate cancer, including controversies.
3. List malignant and nonmalignant conditions that may cause an increase in carcinoembryonic antigen (CEA) and define the role of CEA in the management of colon cancer.
4. Describe how CA-125 may be used to diagnose and monitor ovarian cancer.
5. Describe how βhCG and AFP are used to diagnose and monitor germ cell tumors.
6. Discuss the role of estrogen and progesterone receptors and HER-2 in determining treatment decisions for breast cancer.

TUMOR MARKERS

Tumor markers may be found in the blood or other body fluids or may be measured directly in tumor masses or lymph nodes. They can be grouped into three broad categories: (1) tumor-specific proteins are markers that are produced only by tumor cells—these proteins usually occur as a result of translocation of an oncogene and may contribute to the proliferation of the tumor; (2) nonspecific proteins related to the malignant cells include proteins that are expressed only during embryonic development and by cancer cells; and (3) proteins that are normally found in the body but are expressed or secreted at a much higher rate by malignant cells than normal cells. In addition to the laboratory tests that are described in this chapter, it should also be remembered that abnormalities in other commonly used laboratory tests may provide some evidence that a malignancy exists. However, they are not related to specific tumors. For example, suppression of blood counts may represent infiltration of the bone marrow by tumor cells. Increased uric acid and/or LDH are frequently associated with large tumor burdens. Alkaline phosphatase is frequently elevated in patients with tumors of the biliary tract or the bone. Occasionally, tumors may also produce hormones in excessive amounts, such as adrenocorticotropin.

Clinical Uses for Tumor Markers

Tumor markers are used for several purposes including detection of occult cancers in asymptomatic individuals (i.e., cancer screening and early detection), determining the relative extent or volume of disease (staging), estimating prognosis, predicting responsiveness to treatment, and monitoring for disease recurrence or progression. Table 19-1 lists many of the commonly used tumor markers found in blood and their clinical applications. The characteristics of an ideal tumor marker are somewhat dependent on the specific application.

TABLE 19-1

		CLINICAL USE				
TUMOR MARKER	**MALIGNANT DISEASE**	**SCREENING ASYMPTO-MATIC**	**DIAGNOSTIC**	**STAGING OR PROGNOSIS**	**MONITOR TREATMENT (Outcome or Disease Recurrence)**	**OTHER CONDITIONS THAT ELEVATE**
Prostate Specific Antigen (PSA)	Prostate	X		X	X	Benign prostatic hyperplasia; prostatitis; prostate biopsy; urethral endoscopy; DRE
Carcino-embryonic Antigen (CEA)	Colon Pancreas		X	X	X	Hepatic cirrhosis; hepatitis; pancreatitis; peptic ulcer disease; hypothyroidism; ulcerative colitis; Crohn's disease
CA-125	Ovarian		X	X	X	Endometriosis; ovarian cysts; liver disease; pregnancy
Human Chorionic Gonado-tropin (HCG)	Germ cell of ovaries and testes; hyda-tidiform mole		X	X	X	Pregnancy; occasionally other types of cancer
CA 19-9	Pancreatic		X		X	Pancreatitis; gastric and colon cancer
Alpha Fetoprotein (AFP)	Hepatocellular Testicular (nonsemino-matous)		X	X	X	Pregnancy; hepatitis; cirrhosis; occasionally in pancreatic, gastric, lung and colon cancers

Table 19-1. Serum Tumor Markers in Clinical Use

Sensitivity and Specificity

In order for a tumor marker to be clinically useful, it must have a high degree of sensitivity and specificity. That is, presence of the marker should correlate with the presence of the tumor, and a negative test should indicate, with some certainty, that the patient does not have the cancer. Like many other laboratory tests, the measured concentrations of tumor markers in the blood may have a wide range in both diseased (i.e., patients with cancer) and healthy individuals. For tumor markers, it is more likely that the higher the concentration the more likely the patient has the disease. However, there is no absolute value that clearly delineates with 100% accuracy the presence of disease. The sensitivity of a test refers to its ability to identify patients who truly have the disease without classifying others who also have the disease as healthy (i.e., distinguish true positives).

$$\text{Sensitivity} = \text{true positives}/\text{true positives} + \text{false negatives}$$

Specificity, on the other hand, refers to the ability to identify those without the disease (i.e., true negatives).

$$\text{Specificity} = \text{true negatives}/\text{true negatives} + \text{false positives}$$

If the threshold abnormal value for a tumor marker is set very low, then it is likely that most individuals with the disease will fall into the abnormal range (high sensitivity). However, it is also likely that a significant number of healthy individuals will also be labeled as positive (low specificity). The predictive values of laboratory tests integrate the sensitivity or specificity of the test with the prevalence of the disease in the population and further aids clinicians in establishing the likelihood of disease.[4]

$$\text{Positive Predictive Value} = (\text{prevalence} \times \text{sensitivity})/(\text{prevalence} \times \text{sensitivity}) + ([1\text{-prevalence}] \times [1\text{- specificity}])$$

$$\text{Negative Predictive Value} = (1\text{-prevalence}) \times \text{specificity}/(1\text{-prevalence}) \times \text{specificity} + \text{prevalence} \times (1\text{-sensitivity})$$

Knowledge of the sensitivity, specificity and predictive values of tumor marker tests are particularly important when they are used to screen asymptomatic patients. If the tumor marker test is positive only in a portion of the patients that actually have the cancer or if the test is negative in patients who do have the disease, then diagnoses would be missed. In the case of malignant diseases, delay of the diagnosis until symptoms or other clinical findings actually appear may mean the difference between curable and incurable disease. Outcomes studies evaluating the usefulness of tumor marker testing in asymptomatic individuals must result in decreased mortality rates due to the disease, not just establishment of a diagnosis. On the other hand, false-positive tests not only cause a high level of anxiety, they also typically result in the performance of very costly and sometimes invasive, additional diagnostic tests.

Sensitivity and specificity are also important when tumor marker tests are used to monitor for recurrent disease in patients who have previously been treated for the cancer. A negative tumor marker test that is known to have a high degree of specificity will give the patient, their family, and their clinicians a great deal of comfort and sense of security that the disease has been eliminated. If the test has a lower degree of sensitivity, then it is likely that other screening and diagnostic tests will need to be performed at regular intervals to monitor for disease recurrence. In some cases, the presence of a positive tumor marker may be indication enough to resume cancer treatment. A decision to initiate or resume treatment should be made when there is a high degree of certainty that there is actual disease present because most cancer treatments are associated with significant toxicity and a small, but appreciable, mortality risk.

When tumor markers are used to assess the extent of disease or the presence of specific tumor characteristics (e.g., HER-2*neu*), the quantitative sensitivity may also be important in determining prognosis, appropriate diagnostic tests, and treatment options.

Accessibility

If a tumor marker test is to be used to screen asymptomatic individuals for cancer, both the individuals and their clinicians are more likely to include them if they do not necessitate painful, risky, or lengthy procedures to obtain the necessary fluid or tissue. Most clinicians request and patients willingly provide samples of blood, urine, or sputum in the course of regular physical examinations. However, if a test requires biopsy of other tissues or involves procedures that are associated with a significant risk of morbidity, patients and clinicians are likely only to consent to or include them in physical examinations if there is a high likelihood—or other evidence that supports the presence—of the disease.

Cost-Effectiveness

Widespread screening of asymptomatic individuals with a tumor marker test can be quite expensive. It is not surprising that insurance companies, health plans, and health policy decision-makers are also more likely to support the inclusion of these tests during routine physical examinations or other screening programs if health economic evaluations demonstrate that they may result in lower overall treatment costs and a positive benefit to society, such as prolongation of the patient's productivity.

Prostate Specific Antigen

Standard reference range: 0–4.0 ng/mL

Prostate specific antigen (PSA) is a protein produced by both malignant and normal (benign) prostate tissue that is secreted into the blood. The level of PSA in the blood increases with age and also with the size of the prostate. Serum levels of PSA can also be significantly elevated during nonmalignant prostate conditions including prostatitis and benign prostatic hyperplasia (BPH) and following manipulations of the prostate such as biopsy and endoscopic evaluation of the urethra.[2] Some men may also have transient increases in serum PSA following ejaculation. Although manipulation of the prostate during digital rectal examination (DRE) will increase secretion of PSA, at least one clinical study has shown that the elevation is not significant enough to influence the interpretation of the PSA.[3] However, in the course of physical examinations, it is recommended that blood for the PSA test be drawn prior to the DRE. If other significant manipulations have been done to the prostate such as biopsy or urethral endoscopy, a PSA test should not be done for at least 4 weeks. Similarly, the test should not be done for at least 4 weeks following resolution of prostatitis. BPH is the most common reason for elevation of serum PSA, and, therefore, only a biopsy of prostate tissue will differentiate between the benign condition and prostate cancer.

Several drugs, including the luteinizing hormone-releasing hormone agonists that are commonly used to treat prostate cancer (e.g., leuprolide) and antagonists and 5α-reductase inhibitors (e.g., finasteride) used to treat BPH, are known to decrease serum PSA levels. One report demonstrated that finasteride lowered PSA levels by an average of 50%.[5] For this reason, a baseline PSA level should be obtained prior to initiating finasteride therapy. A repeat PSA level approximately 6 months after the start of finasteride therapy can be used to assess the effect of treatment on the baseline PSA level. If, after multiplying this repeat PSA level by two, it exceeds the normal range, more extensive examination of the prostate including digital rectal exam and, possibly, biopsy should be used to rule out prostate cancer. Any significant increase in subsequent routine PSA levels should be further evaluated as well. Finally, a failure of PSA to decrease by 50% within 6 months after starting finasteride may be a sign of noncompliance.

Even though several nonmalignant circumstances may cause an elevation in PSA, a considerable amount of evidence supports that the level of PSA elevation does correlate with the probability of prostate cancer, especially when physical findings from the DRE are also suspicious. For example, Cooner et al.[6] demonstrated that the probability that a PSA level greater than 4.0 ng/mL was related to cancer increased from 25% in patients with a normal DRE to 62% in those with a positive or suspicious DRE.[6] Similarly, other investigators have made these associations.[7,8] Overall, the positive predictive value (i.e., the percent of cancer cases among those with PSA levels in the target range) of a serum PSA level between 4 ng/mL and 10 ng/mL is estimated to be 10–30% and the predictive value of a PSA above 10 ng/mL is believed to be 42–71%.[9] Conversely, the PSA levels are normal in about 30% of men with localized prostate cancer. Therefore, the PSA has only limited sensitivity (73–84%) and specificity (59–93%) when used alone.[10] The degree of elevation of PSA has also correlated with worsening pathological grading and prognosis in some series.

Prostate cancer is the most common cancer in American adult males, and it is the second leading cause of cancer deaths. It is well-documented that if prostate cancer is diagnosed and treated at an early stage, while it is still confined to the prostate, the survival rate is much higher than if the disease has progressed through the prostate capsule.[11,12] Despite the less than optimal sensitivity of the PSA test, it is widely used as a screening test in combination with DRE in asymptomatic men. However, this is considered controversial.[13,14] While the US Preventive Services Task Force (USPSTF) and the American College of Physicians currently recommend against the routine use of PSA as a screening tool for prostate cancer, the American Cancer Society recommends that men over age 50 with a life expectancy of at least 10 years should discuss the value of a PSA test with their health care provider.[15-17] The primary reason why the former groups do not support routine PSA testing is that routine screening has not demonstrated a clear cut reduction in mortality due to prostate cancer.[18-20] Clinicians who support routine PSA screening, however, cite evidence that PSA screening does reduce the risk of mortality due to prostate cancer and suggest that analysis of data from 1987 (when widespread screening using the PSA began) forward also supports this trend.[9,21,22]

Another argument against routine screening pertains to the evidence that some cases of prostate cancer found in asymptomatic men represent a slowly progressive or indolent disease, which is unlikely to progress to symptomatic or life-threatening illness. This diagnosis, which would not have produced signs or symptoms of the disease, is referred to as *overdiagnosis*. The concern regarding overdiagnosis is at least partially based on the demographics of prostate cancer, which increases in incidence with age and the realization that many of the elderly men would likely die of causes other than prostate cancer. Evidence that prostate cancer may be overdiagnosed is substantiated by the majority of primary care physicians in the US who routinely perform PSA testing in men over 80 years of age, even though these individuals are unlikely to benefit from treatment.[23] Detection of these cases would not alter mortality rates and could lead to invasive and costly treatments that may not be warranted. Nonetheless, many experts recommend widespread PSA screening in combination with DRE for men between the ages of 50 and 80. At the very least, patients should be informed of the potential benefits and risks associated with overdiagnosis and should be included in the decision regarding PSA screening. In addition, most agree that men who have a higher risk for prostate cancer, including African-Americans and men with close family members who have had prostate cancer, should be encouraged to receive routine screening beginning at an earlier age.[22]

Currently, a great deal of effort is underway to enhance the sensitivity and specificity of the PSA test. These include efforts to correlate the PSA level with the volume of the prostate gland (PSA density), the patient's age, and the rate of PSA increase over time (PSA velocity). In addition, some have suggested that the normal range of PSA should be ≤2.6 ng/mL and not ≤4 ng/mL.[16] Each of these is being evaluated as a potential method to differentiate an elevated PSA level due to BPH from cancer. Several groups have also demonstrated that men with a higher portion of PSA existing in the free form (not protein bound) were less likely to have prostate cancer than in those with less unbound PSA.[24,25] If the percentage of bound and unbound PSA are used to evaluate the test, serum samples must be processed and stored appropriately, and clinicians should be aware that different assays may yield varying results.[9]

In addition to its use as a screening tool for asymptomatic individuals, the PSA test is used to assess the effect of therapies and to monitor for recurrent disease following definitive treatments that have apparently rendered patients disease-free. A declining PSA level following initiation of cancer treatment (e.g., LHRH agonists including leuprolide) generally correlates with treatment response. In patients who were rendered disease-free by surgery or radiation, a rising PSA level often precedes clinical evidence of disease recurrence or relapse by months or even years.[26,27]

Prostatic Acid Phosphatase

Acid phosphatase synthesized by the prostate gland can be distinguished from acid phosphatases produced by other tissues in the body. It is called the *prostatic acid phosphatase* (PAP). Like PSA, PAP is elevated in prostatic cancer as well as benign conditions of the prostate. Prior to the availability of the PSA test, PAP was commonly used as a nonspecific method of monitoring patients after prostate surgery or other treatment. Because the PSA test is more sensitive and specific, it has largely replaced the PAP in this disease.

Carcinoembryonic Antigen

Normal range: <2.5 ng/mL nonsmokers; ≤5.0 ng/mL smokers

Carcinoembryonic antigen (CEA) is a protein that is found in the intestines, pancreas, and liver of fetal tissue. In healthy adults, the level of this protein is usually below 2.5 ng/mL. Serum CEA levels are also frequently elevated in patients with colon, breast, gastric, thyroid, or pancreatic carcinomas and a variety of nonmalignant conditions including hepatic cirrhosis, hepatitis, pancreatitis, peptic ulcer disease, hypothyroidism, ulcerative colitis and Crohn's disease. Occasionally, CEA is also elevated in patients with lung cancer. CEA levels are usually modestly increased in individuals who smoke, and the normal serum level in these individuals is usually considered to be <5.0 ng/mL. Nonmalignant conditions are usually not associated with CEA levels >10 ng/mL. However, many patients with malignant conditions will have CEA levels that greatly exceed 10 ng/mL.

Blood samples for CEA testing should be put in either red or lavender top tubes. Following separation of the serum (or plasma), the specimen can be refrigerated if it is to be assayed within 24 hr or frozen at –20 °C if the specimen is to be assayed later. Immunoassays from different manufacturers may provide different values, and, therefore, the same laboratory and assay should be used whenever possible for an individual patient.

CEA is most commonly used in the assessment of colon cancer. Unfortunately, this test does not have adequate sensitivity or specificity to make it a useful screening test for asymptomatic individuals. CEA may be elevated in a wide variety of conditions as noted above and may be negative in patients with widely metastatic disease. It is most commonly used in monitoring patients with a known history of colon cancer. Following detection of early stage colon cancer by screening tests such as fecal occult blood and colonoscopy or sigmoidoscopy with biopsy confirmation of suspicious areas, a baseline serum CEA level is usually measured to assess if the tumor produces excessive amounts of CEA. If the patient's CEA level is grossly increased, then the CEA level may be used to monitor the success of treatment or for evidence of tumor recurrence following successful treatment. Following surgical removal of a colon cancer, the CEA level should return to normal (<2.5 ng/mL) within 4–6 weeks. If the CEA level remains elevated beyond this point, it may indicate that either residual primary tumor or metastases are still present.

The CEA level also may provide some evidence of prognosis. The elevation of CEA level is consistent with extent of disease (stage), which often correlates with overall survival.[28,29] For patients with operable colon cancer (Stages: Dukes A, B, and C or AJCC I, II, or III), the CEA level should decline to below the 5 ng/mL level within 1 month following surgery if all tumor was successfully removed.[30] If the CEA remains elevated, there is a high likelihood that the tumor will recur, and many surgeons would even consider a second-look surgery at that time for identification and removal of residual disease.[31,32] Repeat assessment of the CEA level is strongly recommended at regular intervals following surgery to detect evidence of tumor recurrence. In many cases, the CEA level will start to increase long before there is clinical evidence of disease recurrence in the bowel or other metastatic site. A rising CEA should prompt aggressive diagnostic workup to detect sites of recurrent disease and initiation of appropriate therapy while the tumor burden is low. Most guidelines recommend that the CEA level be evaluated every 3 months during the first 2 years after surgery and then every 6 months thereafter.[33] When CEA levels are monitored in conjunction with other follow-up tests including periodic serum liver function tests and CT scans of the liver and colonoscopy, several studies have reported improved overall survival or other benefits including cost-effectiveness that they attribute to earlier detection of recurrent disease.[31,34]

Similarly, serial CEA levels are also used to monitor the effectiveness of chemotherapy for treatment of advanced colon cancer. Many clinicians that treat this disease have associated a 20% decrease of CEA with evidence of response. However, appropriate CT scans are necessary to confirm the extent of response.[35–37]

CA 125 Antigen

Normal range: <35 units/mL

The CA 125 antigen (cancer antigen 125) is a protein, which is usually found on cells that line the pelvic organs and peritoneum. It may also be detected in the blood of women with ovarian cancer and those with adenocarcinoma of the cervix or fallopian tubes. It may be elevated in nonmalignant conditions including endometriosis, ovarian cysts, liver disease, and pregnancy, as well as occasionally in many other types of cancer.[38] It is not, however, elevated by mucinous epithelial carcinomas of the ovaries. Levels of CA 125 also increase during menstruation and are lower at the luteal phase of the cycle.[39] Levels are lower in women who use systemic contraceptives and also decline following menopause.[40]

CA 125 is assessed using a blood sample placed in a red top tube. The sample should be refrigerated within 2 hr of collection. The level of CA 125 in the serum has been reported to correlate with the likelihood of malignancy, with levels >65 U/mL strongly associated with the presence of a malignancy. However, they should not be considered diagnostic.[41,42] Several studies evaluating serial levels of CA 125 in healthy women have shown that serum levels may start to rise 1–5 years before the detection of ovarian cancer.[41,43] It does not, however, have sufficient sensitivity to be recommended as a routine screening test for ovarian cancer in asymptomatic women. The sensitivity in early stage ovarian cancer (before symptoms are usually evident) is believed to be only approximately 60%, and, thus, many cases would not be detected.[38,41] However, some advocate that a rising serial CA 125 level could be used as a trigger to do more extensive (and often costly) screening tests in high-risk women.

Most often the CA 125 test is done to monitor for evidence of disease recurrence or residual disease in women who have undergone successful surgery for ovarian cancer.[44] This use, of course, would only be valuable in women whose tumors expressed CA 125 prior to surgery. For women who have undergone a tumor debulking surgery prior to chemotherapy, a level measured approximately 3 weeks after surgery correlates with the amount of residual tumor mass and is predictive of overall survival.[45] Serial levels during and following chemotherapy are used to monitor response to treatment, disease progression, and prognosis. Many women, however, with CA 125 levels that have returned to the normal reference range during treatment still have residual disease if a second-look laparotomy is done to pathologically evaluate the disease.[46] A more rapid decline of serum CA 125 during treatment has been associated with a more favorable prognosis.[44] Failure of the CA 125 level to decline may also be used to identify tumors that are not responding to chemotherapy and an increase usually indicates progression.[47,48]

CA 15-3

Normal range: <30 kU/L

CA 15-3 (cancer antigen 15-3) detects an antigen from human breast cancer. In addition to elevation in the serum of many women with breast cancer, it may also be elevated in lung cancer and other nonmalignant conditions including liver and breast disorders. The CA 15-3 test is not sensitive enough to use as a screening test for early stage breast cancer. This test may be useful in monitoring response to treatments in women with metastatic disease where no other reasonable measure of disease is feasible.[49]

Human Chorionic Gonadotropin

Normal range: < 3IU/L

Human chorionic gonadotropin (HCG) is a glycoprotein that is normally produced by the placenta during pregnancy, and the beta subunit is most commonly used as the determinant in both serum and urine tests for pregnancy. HCG is also commonly produced by tumors of germ cell origin including mixed germ cell or pure choriocarcinoma tumors of the ovaries and testis, extragonadal tumors of germ cell origin, and gestational trophoblastic disease (e.g., hydatidiform mole). Occasionally islet cell tumors and gastric, colon, pancreas, liver, and breast carcinomas also produce HCG. Patients with trophoblastic disease often produce irregular forms of HCG that may or may not be recognized by the various automated assays and false-positive HCG immunoreactivity has also been reported. Newer highly specific and highly sensitive immunoassays have improved the reliability of this test. Radioimmunoassays and the DPC Immulite HCG test have been reported to have the greatest accuracy.

In patients with testicular cancer, elevated levels of HCG may be present with either seminomatous (15–25%) or nonseminomatous disease (10–70%), depending on stage of disease), so the test is not sensitive enough to be used as a screening tool for asymptomatic patients.[44,50]

Most frequently, HCG is used to monitor response to therapy, including evidence of residual disease following surgery, and to monitor for evidence of disease progression or recurrence during or after treatment.[51] HCG has a half-life of only 18–36 hr, so serum levels decline rapidly following therapeutic interventions.[50]

CA 19-9

Normal range: <37 kU/mL

CA 19-9 is an oncofetal antigen expressed by several cancers including pancreatic (71–93% of cases), gastric (21–42% of cases), and colon (20–40% of cases) carcinomas. Serum for this test is collected in a red top tube, and the sample is frozen for shipping for analysis. The sensitivity of the test is not sufficient enough to be useful as screening test for early stage diseases.[49] It is primarily used to help discriminate benign pancreatic disease from cancer, to monitor for disease recurrence, and to determine the impact of treatment interventions.[52-54] An elevated CA 19-9 has also been associated with a poor prognosis of colon cancer.[52,55-57]

Alpha Fetoprotein

Normal range: <10ng/mL

Alpha fetoprotein (AFP) is a glycoprotein made in the liver, gastrointestinal tract, and fetal yolk sac. It is found in high concentrations in the serum during fetal development (~3 mg/mL) and following birth declines rapidly to <20 ng/mL. Serum for AFP evaluation should be collected in a red top tube and refrigerated until assayed using radioimmunoassay. It is elevated in about 70% of patients with hepatocellular carcinoma and 50–70% of patients with testicular nonseminomatous germ cell tumors and occasionally in other tumors such as pancreatic, gastric, lung, and colon cancers. Nonmalignant conditions that may be associated with increased levels of AFP include pregnancy, hepatitis, and cirrhosis. In patients with nonseminomatous germ cell tumors, the incidence of increased serum concentrations seems to correlate with the stage of the disease.[51] In some parts of the world, AFP is used as a screening procedure for hepatocellular carcinoma in patients who are positive for HBsAg, and, therefore, are at increased risk for hepatocellular carcinoma. In the US, however, AFP is used primarily to assist in the diagnosis of hepatocellular carcinoma (AFP >1000 ng/mL is seen in most patients with hepatocellular carcinoma).

AFP levels are also used to monitor patients with both hepatocellular carcinoma and germ cell tumors for disease progression or recurrence and to assess the impact of treatment interventions. The serum half-life of AFP is 5–7 days, and usually elevation of the serum level for more than 7 days following surgery is an indication that residual disease was left behind. Following successful treatment for nonseminomatous germ cell tumors of the testis, HCG and AFP are repeated every 1 or 2 months during the first year, every 2 or 3 months during the second year, and less frequently thereafter along with physical exams and chest x-rays. Increases in these serum tests are considered an indication for further treatment such as chemotherapy. Rising levels in patients receiving chemotherapy indicate that therapy should be changed, whereas declining levels predict a more favorable outcome.[58]

Estrogen and Progesterone Receptor Assays

The level of estrogen and progesterone receptors in biopsy tissue from breast cancers predicts both the natural history of the disease and the likelihood that the tumor will respond to hormonal manipulations. For over 25 years, it has been the standard of practice to evaluate breast cancer tissue for these protein receptors and to use that information in directing therapeutic interventions. The relative concentration of hormone receptors can be determined using very small amounts of tumor tissue. Each protein is measured using immunohistochemical methods, and values of less than 10 fmol/mg of protein in the biopsy are considered to be negative.[59] Positive estrogen receptor (ER) levels correlate with response to hormonal therapies including removal of the ovaries in premenopausal women or administration of an antiestrogen, such as tamoxifen, or an aromatase inhibitor such as anastrozole. In addition, estrogen receptor content in tumor biopsies also correlates with benefit from adjuvant tamoxifen therapy following surgical removal of the tumor. In women receiving tamoxifen for 5 years after surgery, the annual odds of disease recurrence may be reduced by 40–60%, and the annual odds of death may be reduced by 20–40%.[60]

HER-2

HER-2 (c-neu, HER2/neu) is a transmembrane glycoprotein member of the epidermal growth factor receptor family with intracellular tyrosine kinase activity. This group of receptors functions in the growth and control of many normal cells as well as malignant cells. The gene that encodes for HER-2 is c-erb B-2. About 20–40% of samples from human breast cancers exhibit amplification of c-erb B-2 or overexpression of HER-2.[61-63] Numerous studies have described the role of HER-2 in the prognosis and predictive value in breast cancer. However, the considerable variability in study design and the well-recognized heterogeneity of the disease itself have made interpretation difficult. A systematic review of this information led one group of investigators to conclude that overexpression of HER-2 is only a weak to moderate prognostic factor and should not be used to determine whether or not a woman should receive adjuvant therapy or whether endocrine therapy should be used. They did conclude that if adjuvant therapy is indicated, an anthracycline therapy is preferred, if not contraindicated, for HER-2 positive tumors.[63] It is well-established that HER-2 overexpression is predictive of a response to treatment with trastuzumab (Herceptin®), a monoclonal antibody against HER-2. Therefore, it is necessary to evaluate the tumor in order to select patients appropriate for trastuzumab therapy.[65,66]

A portion of the HER-2 receptor can dissociate from the cell and be detected in the serum. However, biopsies of the tumor are used to evaluate either gene amplification, overexpression of RNA, or overexpression of the protein. Several commercial assays have been recommended to aid in the selection of patients for trastuzumab therapy. The HerceptTest™ is an immunohistochemical assay that assesses overexpression of the HER-2 protein. The PathVysion™ is a fluorescence in situ hybridization assay that measures the number of HER-2 gene copies as a surrogate measurement for protein expression. Both of these assay methods score tumor specimens as 0, 1+, 2+, or 3+ with 3+ being the most strongly positive tumors for the HER-2 receptor. Scores of 2+ and 3+ have been required for enrollment in clinical trials and have correlated with beneficial response to trastuzumab.[65-68]

SUMMARY

In order to be clinically useful as a screening tool in asymptomatic individuals, tumor markers should be both sensitive and specific. Unfortunately, most of the tumor markers identified to date lack the sensitivity to be used in this capacity. In addition, many nonmalignant conditions cause elevations of these markers. Currently, only PSA is in widespread use as a screening tool when interpreted along with the results of a digital rectal exam. Today, tumor markers are most valuable when used to monitor for disease recurrence in patients who have undergone definitive surgery for cancers or to assess a patient's response to chemotherapy or other treatment interventions. In these situations, serial measurements of tests such as PSA for prostate cancer, CEA for colon cancer, HCG and AFP for testicular cancer, and CA 125 for ovarian cancer are considered standard in the follow-up care of patients with these malignancies.

REFERENCES

1. Lindblom A, Liljegren A. Tumour markers in malignancies. *Br Med J.* 2000; 320:424–7.
2. Nadler RB, Humphrey PA, Smith DS, et al. Effect of inflammation and benign prostatic hyperplasia on elevated serum prostate specific antigen levels. *J Urol.* 1995; 154:407–13.
3. Chybowski FM, Bergstralh EJ, Oesterling JE. The effect of digital rectal examination on the serum prostate specific antigen concentration: results of a randomized study. *J Urol.* 1992; 148:83–6.
4. Sacher RA, McPherson RA, eds. Principles of interpretation of laboratory tests. In: *Widmann's Clinical Interpretation of Laboratory Tests.* 11th ed. Philadelphia, PA: F. A. Davis, Co.; 2000: 4–9.
5. Guess HA, Heyse JF, Gormley GJ. The effect of finasteride on prostate-specific antigen in men with benign prostatic hyperplasia. *Prostate.* 1993; 22:31–7.

6. Cooner WH, Mosley BR, Rutherford CL, et al. Prostate cancer detection in a clinical urological practice by ultrasonography, digital rectal examination and prostate specific antigen. *J Urol.* 1990; 143:1146–52.

7. Ellis WJ, Chetner MP, Preston SD, et al. Diagnosis of prostatic carcinoma: the yield of serum prostate specific antigen, digital rectal examination and transrectal ultrasonography. *J Urol.* 1994; 152:1520–5.

8. Hammerer P, Huland H. Systematic sextant biopsies in 651 patients referred for prostate evaluation. *J Urol.* 1994; 151:99–102.

9. Carroll PR, Lee KL, Fuks ZY, et al. Cancer of the prostate. In: Devita VT, Hellman S, Rosenberg SA, eds. *Cancer Principles and Practice of Oncology.* 6th ed. Philadelphia, PA: Lippincott Williams & Wilkins; 2001: 1418–79.

10. Jacobs DS, DeMott WR, Oxley DK, eds. *Laboratory Test Handbook.* 2nd ed. Hudson, OH: Lexi-Comp, Inc.; 2002: 959.

11. Johansson JK, Holmberg L, Johansson S, et al. Fifteen-year survival in prostate cancer: a prospective population-based study in Sweden. *JAMA.* 1997; 277:467–71.

12. Aus G, Hugosson J, Norlen L. Long-term survival and mortality in prostate cancer treated with noncurative intent. *J Urol.* 1995; 154:460–5.

13. Etzioni R, Berry KM, Legler JM, et al. Prostate-specific antigen testing in black and white men: an analysis of medicare claims from 1991–1998. *Urology.* 2002; 59:251–5.

14. Legler JM, Feuer JM, Potosky AL, et al. The role of prostate-specific antigen (PSA) testing patterns in the recent prostate cancer incidence decline in the United States. *Cancer Causes Control.* 1998; 9:519–27.

15. U.S. Preventive Task Force. Guide to clinical preventive services. Alexandria, VA: International Medical Publishing; 1996.

16. U.S. Preventive Services Task Force. Screening for prostate cancer: recommendation and rationale. Clinical guidelines. *Ann Intern Med.* 2002; 37:915–16.

17. American Cancer Society. *Cancer Facts and Figures: 2002.* Atlanta, GA: American Cancer Society; 2002.

18. Hankey BF, Feuer EJ, Clegg LX, et al. Cancer surveillance series: interpreting trends in incidence, mortality, and survival rates. *J Natl Cancer Instit.* 1999; 91:1017–24.

19. Feuer EJ, Merrill RM, Hankey BR. Cancer surveillance series: interpreting trends in prostate cancer—Part II. Cause of death misclassification and the recent rise and fall in prostate caner mortality. *J Natl Cancer Instit.* 1999; 91:1025–32.

20. Etzioni R, Legler JM, Feuer EJ, et al. Cancer surveillance series: interpreting trends in prostate cancer—Part III. Quantifying the link between population prostate-specific antigen testing and recent declines in prostate cancer mortality. *J Natl Cancer Instit.* 1999; 91:1033–9.

21. Labrie F, Candas B, DuPont A, et al. Screening decreases prostate cancer death: first analysis of the 1988 Quebec prospective randomized controlled trial. *Prostate.* 1999; 38:83–91.

22. Rimer BK, Schildkraut J, Hiatt RA. Cancer Screening. In: Devita VT, Hellman S, Rosenberg SA, eds. *Cancer Principles and Practice of Oncology.* 6th ed. Philadelphia, PA: Lippincott Williams & Wilkins; 2001: 627–40.

23. Fowler FJ, Bin L, Collins MM, et al. Prostate cancer screening and beliefs about treatment efficacy: a national survey of primary care physicians and urologists. *Am J Med.* 1998; 104:526–32.

24. Stenman UH, Leinonen J, Alfthan H, et al. A complex between prostate-specific antigen and alpha 1-antichymotrypsin is the major form of prostate-specific antigen in serum of patients with prostate cancer: assay of the complex improves clinical sensitivity for cancer. *Cancer Res.* 1991; 51:222–6.

25. Partin AW, Catalona WJ, Southwick PC, et al. Analysis of percent free prostate-specific antigen (PSA) for prostate cancer detection: influence of total PSA, prostate volume, and age. *Urology.* 1996; 48:55–61.

26. Pollack A, Zagars GK, Kavadi VS. Prostate-specific antigen doubling time and disease relapse after radiotherapy for prostate cancer. *Cancer.* 1994; 74:670–8.

27. Zagars GK. Prostate-specific antigen as an outcome variable for T1 and T2 prostate cancer treated by radiation therapy. *J Urol.* 1994; 152:1786–91.

28. Harrison LE, Guillem JG, Paty P, et al. Preoperative carcinoembryonic antigen predicts outcomes in node-negative colon cancer patients: a multivariate analysis of 572 patients. *J Am Coll Surg.* 1997; 185:55–9.

29. Wiratkapun S, Kreamer M, Seow-Choen F, et al. High preoperative serum carcinoembryonic antigen predicts metastatic recurrence in potentially curative colonic cancer: results of a five-year study. *Dis Colon Rectum.* 2001; 44:231–5.

30. Minton JP, Martin EW. The use of serial CEA determinations to predict recurrence of colon cancer and when to do a second-look operation. *Cancer.* 1978; 42:1422–7

31. Graham RA, Wang S, Catalano PJ, et al. Postsurgical surveillance of colon cancer: preliminary cost analysis of physician examination, carcinoembryonic antigen testing, chest x-ray and colonoscopy. *Ann Surg.* 1998; 228:59–63.

32. Chu DZJ, Erickson CA, Russell P, et al. Prognostic significance of carcinoembryonic antigen in colorectal carcinoma. *Arch Surg.* 1991; 126:314–6.

33. Desch CE, Benson AB, Smith TJ, et al. Recommended colorectal cancer surveillance guidelines by the American Society of Clinical Oncology. *J Clin Oncol.* 1999; 17:1312.

34. Barillari P, Ramacciato GMC, Bovino A, et al. Surveillance of colorectal cancer: effectiveness of early detection of intraluminal recurrences on prognosis and survival of patients treated for cure. *Dis Colon Rectum.* 1996; 39:388–93.

35. Hine KR, Dykes PW. Prospective randomized trial of early cytotoxic therapy for recurrent colorectal carcinoma detected by CEA. *Gut.* 1984; 25:682–8.

36. Allen-Mersh TG, Kemeny N, Niedzwiedki D, et al. Significance of a fall in serum CEA concentration in patients treated with cytotoxic chemotherapy for disseminated colorectal disease. *Gut.* 1987; 28:1625–6.

37. Kouri M, Pyrhonen S, Kuusela P. Elevated CA 19-9 as the most significant prognostic factor in advanced colorectal cancer. *J Surg Oncol.* 1992; 49:78–85.

38. Jacobs I, Bast RC. The CA 125 tumour-associated antigen: a review of the literature. *Human Reprod.* 1989; 4:1–12.

39. Warner EA, Parsons AK. Screening and early diagnosis of gynecologic cancers. *Med Clin N Am.* 1996; 80:45–61.

40. Einhorn N, Sjovall K, Knapp RC, et al. Prospective evaluation of CA-125 levels for early detection of ovarian cancer. *Obstet Gynecol.* 1992; 80:14–8

41. Bast RC, Siegal FP, Runowicz C, et al. Elevation of serum CA125 prior to diagnosis of epithelial ovarian carcinoma. *Gynecol Oncol.* 1985; 22:115–20.

42. Eltabbakh GH, Belinson JL, Kennedy AW, et al. Serum CA-125 measurements >65 U/mL. Clinical value. *J Reprod Med.* 1997; 42:617–24.

43. Zurawski VR, Orjaseter H, Andersen A, et al. Elevated serum CA125 levels prior to diagnosis of ovarian neoplasia: relevance for early detection of ovarian cancer. *Int J Cancer.* 1988; 42:677–80.

44. Bidart JM, Thuillier F, Augereau C, et al. Kinetics of serum tumor marker concentrations and usefulness in clinical monitoring. *Clin Chem.* 1999; 45:1695–707.

45. Gadducci A, Zola P, Landoni F, et al. Serum half life of CA 125 during early chemotherapy as an independent prognostic variable for patients with advanced epithelial ovarian cancer: results of a multicentric Italian study. *Gynecol Oncol.* 1995; 58:42–7.

46. van der Burg MEL, Lammes FB, Verweij J. CA 125 in ovarian cancer. *Neth J Med.* 1992; 40:36–51.

47. Makar AP, Kristensen GB, Bormer OP, et al. Serum CA 125 level allows early identification of nonresponders during induction chemotherapy. *Gynecol Oncol.* 1993; 49:73–9.

48. Rustin GJ, Marples M, Nelstrop AE, et al. Use of CA-125 to define progression of ovarian cancer in patients with persistently elevated levels. *J Clin Oncol.* 2001; 15:4053–7.

49. Smith TJ, Davidson NE, Schapira DV, et al. American Society of Clinical Oncology 1998 update of recommended breast cancer surveillance guidelines. *J Clin Oncol.* 1999; 17:1080–2.

50. Cole LA, Shahabi S, Buter SA, et al. Utility of commonly used commercial human chorionic gonadotropin immunoassays in the diagnosis and management of trophoblastic diseases. *Clin Chem.* 2001; 47:308–15.

51. Bosl GJ, Geller NL, Chan EY. Stage migration and the increasing proportion of responders in patients with advanced germ cell tumors. *Cancer Res.* 1988; 48:3524–7.

52. Reiter W, Stieber P, Reuter C, et al. Multivariate analysis of the prognostic value of CEA and CA 19-9 serum levels in colorectal cancer. *Anticancer Res.* 2000; 20:5195–8.

53. Safi F, Schlosser W, Falkenreck S, et al. CA 19-9 serum course and prognosis of pancreatic cancer. *Int J Pancreatol.* 1996; 20:155–61.

54. Safi F, Schlosser W, Kolb G, Beger HG. Diagnostic value of CA 19-9 in patients with pancreatic cancer and nonspecific gastrointestinal symptoms. *J Gastrointest Surg.* 1997; 1:106–12.

55. Frebourg T, Bercoff E, Manchon N, et al. The evaluation of CA 19-9 antigen level in the early detection of pancreatic cancer. A prospective study of 866 patients. *Cancer.* 1988; 62:2287–90.

56. Halm U, Schumann T, Schiefke I, et al. Decrease of CA 19-9 during chemotherapy with gemcitabine predicts survival time in patients with advanced pancreatic cancer. *Br J Cancer.* 2000; 82:1013–6.

57. Kouri M, Pyrhonen S, Kuusela P. Elevated 19-9 as the most significant prognostic factor in advanced colorectal carcinoma. *J Surg Oncol.* 1992; 49:78–85.

58. Montgomery RC, Hoffman JP, Riley LB, et al. Prediction of recurrence and survival by post-resection CA 19-9 values in patients with adenocarcinoma of the pancreas. *Ann Surg Oncol.* 1997; 4:551–6.

59. Goss PE, Tye LM. Hormones and cancer. In: Tannock IF, Hill RP, eds. *The Basic Science of Oncology.* 3rd ed. New York, NY: McGraw-Hill; 1998: 263–94.

60. Early Breast Cancer Trialists' Collaborative Group. Tamoxifen for early breast cancer: an overview of the randomized trials. *Lancet.* 1998; 352:930.

61. Toner GC, Geller NL, Tan C, et al. Serum tumor marker half-life during chemotherapy allows early prediction of complete response and survival in nonseminomatous germ cell tumors. *Cancer Res.* 1990; 50:5904–10.

62. King C, Kraus M, Aaronson S. Amplification of a novel v-erbB-2 related gene in human mammary carcinoma. *Science.* 1985; 229:974–6.

63. Slamon DJ, Clark GM, Wong SG, et al. Human breast cancer: correlation of relapse and survival with amplification of the HER-2/neu oncogene. *Science.* 1987; 235:177–82.

64. Slamon D, Godolphin W, Jones L, et al. Studies of the HER-2/neu proto-oncogene in human breast and ovarian cancer. *Science.* 1989; 244:707–12.

65. Yamauchi H, Sterns V, Hayes DF. When is a tumor marker ready for prime time? A case study of c-erb B-2 as a predictive factor in breast cancer. *J Clin Oncol.* 2001; 19:2334–56.

66. Cobleigh MA, Vogel CL Tripathy D, et al. Multinational study of the efficacy and safety of humanized anti-HER2 monoclonal antibody in women who have HER2-overexpressing metastatic breast cancer that has progressed after chemotherapy for metastatic disease. *J Clin Oncol.* 1999; 17:2639–48.

67. Vogel C, Cobleigh M, Tripathy D, et al. First-line, non-hormonal treatment of women with HER2 overexpressing metastatic breast cancer with herceptin (trastuzumab, humanized anti-HER2 antibody). *Proc Am Soc Clin Oncol.* 2000; 19:17a, abstract.

68. Herceptin® package insert. San Francisco, CA: Genentech, Inc.; August 2002.

APPENDICES

CASE 1

CC: *"My heart feels like it's jumping out of my chest and I have trouble breathing."*

HPI:

T. J. is a 70-year-old male who presents to the ER with complaints of palpitations associated with occasional dizziness and dyspnea on exertion for the last 2 weeks. He was taking digoxin with apparent control of his atrial fibrillation and heart failure symptoms until about 10 days ago when he "ran out" and forgot to get a refill.

PMH:

Atrial fibrillation × 3 years
Mild CHF × 3 years
NIDDM × 5 years, controlled with diet
Chronic asthma × 8 years
HTN × 10 years

FH:

Father had HTN and died of a stroke at age 72; mother died of cancer at age 75; brother died of MI at age 62; and three children, alive and well.

SH:

T. J. is retired and lives alone. His wife died in a motor vehicle accident 2 months ago. T. J. claims to be having trouble managing his medications without the help of his wife. All of his children live out of state.

MEDS:

Digoxin 0.25 mg qam
Theo-Dur® 200 mg bid
Albuterol MDI 2 puffs qid prn
Atrovent® MDI 2 puffs bid
Inderal LA® 60 mg po qd
HCTZ 50 mg po qd

ALLERGIES:

NKDA

ROS:

No headache, blurred vision; complains of palpitations with feelings of lightheadedness and occasional chest pain on exertion; and occasional wheezing.

PE:

GEN: Pleasant man; in mild distress
VS: BP 135/83; HR155 (irregular); RR 20; T 98.5 °F; HT 5'8"; and WT 77 kg
HEENT: PERRLA, EIOMI, fundi benign, and TMs intact
NECK: Supple, no bruits, + JVD, and no lymphadenopathy or thyromegaly
CHEST: Diffuse wheezes bilaterally; rales at both bases
CV: Tachycardia with irregularly irregular rhythm without murmurs, gallops, or rubs
ABD: + BS, soft, and no organomegaly
LUNG: CTA bilaterally
EXT: 1+ pitting edema bilaterally
NEURO: A & O × 3; CN II-XII intact

LABS:

Sodium 137 mEq/L, potassium 4.0 mEq/L, Cl 102 mEq/L, CO_2 23 mEq/L, BUN 15 mg/dL, SCr 1.0 mg/dL, glucose 98 mg/dL, hemoglobin 14.0 g/dL, hematocrit 44%, WBC $5 \times 10^3/mm^3$, Plt $268 \times 10^3/mm^3$, MCV 77 μm^3, MCHC 29 g/dL, chol 160 mg/dL, and LDL 99 mg/dL. The serum digoxin concentration is nondetectable.

ECG:

Atrial fibrillation, ventricular rate 150

CXR:

Compatible with mild CHF

PROBLEM LIST

- Atrial fibrillation
- Mild CHF
- Asthma
- HTN-controlled
- NIDDM-controlled

Intravenous digoxin, 0.75 mg, is administered in divided doses over a 6-hr period and T. J. is admitted to the CCU for further care. The ventricular rate has slowed to 106, and a repeat cardiogram reveals an otherwise normal atrial fibrillation. A serum digoxin level is ordered by the resident 1 hr after the final dose of digoxin. The laboratory reports a digoxin level of 5 µg/L, using an enzyme immunoassay method.

QUESTIONS

1. What is your assessment of this digoxin serum concentration?

The digoxin level was drawn too early after administration of the last portion of the loading dose. Serum concentrations of digoxin do not reflect levels in cardiac tissue until at least 6–8 hr after a dose. The serum level of 5 µg/L is not surprising in this situation and should not be compared to the therapeutic range of digoxin, which is based on postdistribution serum concentrations of digoxin.

2. The resident is alarmed by the high digoxin level and is aware that patients have died with digoxin levels less than 4 µg/L. Even though the patient does not have any signs or symptoms of digoxin toxicity, the resident orders the administration of Digibind®. He orders a serum digoxin serum level 3 hr later in order to see if the digoxin level is decreasing. The level comes back as 85 µg/L. The resident wants to administer another course of Digibind®. How do you explain this digoxin concentration, and what do you advise?

First, the decision to administer Digibind® (digoxin immune Fab fragments) was based on a serum digoxin concentration that did not actually represent toxicity. This reinforces the need to always consider the patient's clinical condition in addition to the serum level. Second, the very much higher digoxin concentration of 85 µg/L reported by the lab is also not surprising. Shortly after administration of Fab fragments, the amount of circulating free digoxin decreases to near zero, but there is a rapid increase in concentrations of the Fab-digoxin complex. Most immunoassay methods measure both the free and Fab-bound digoxin. Thus, post-Digibind® digoxin levels measured by immunoassay may be as much as 20 times higher than the digoxin concentration prior to administration of the Digibind®.

The resident should be advised *not* to administer more Digibind®. (Surely the resident would have questioned this once he'd calculated that 65 vials of Digibind® would be needed based on the serum level of 85 µg/L. At more than $500/vial, this would have been a considerable expense.) The patient should be monitored for recurrence of the arrhythmia and continued signs and symptoms of the heart failure, since the pharmacologically active form of digoxin is now likely to be near zero.

3. What other explanations for an unusually high digoxin reading, without clinical signs of digoxin toxicity, might you have considered if you had not known about the administration of the Fab fragments?

Other than laboratory error, other interferences with digoxin measurements by immunoassay include digoxin metabolites, digitoxin, spironolactone and its metabolite, canrenone, administration of certain Chinese medicines, or ingestion of certain plants (oleander). None of these were consistent with T. J.'s medical history. Even if they were, the magnitude of interference could not possibly have explained a level as high as 85 µg/L. Another possible interference is endogenous digoxin-like immunoreactive substances (DLIS), but these substances are seen in neonates, pregnant women, and patients with liver or renal disease and might only be expected to increase digoxin readings by 3 µg/L, not to 85 µg/L.

Patients with hyperthyroidism are reported to be more resistant to digoxin and might tolerate somewhat higher digoxin serum concentrations. However, this patient does not have hyperthyroidism. Even if he did, hyperthyroidism would not protect him from digoxin toxicity if his level was 85 µg/L.

4. How and when should the patient be given digoxin again? What are your recommendations for monitoring serum levels?

The patient should not be re-digitalized until the Fab fragments have been eliminated from the body. This may require several days in this patient, who has good renal function. In the event that he has a recurrence of the CHF and/or atrial fibrillation with rapid ventricular response, intravenous inotropes such as dopamine or dobutamine, or vasodilators can be used temporarily. The loading dose may be administered again, followed by the oral regimen of 0.25 mg/day, since this dose rate was effective for this patient in the past. The clinical staff need to be reminded that serum levels of digoxin drawn prior to 6–8 hr after a dose do not reflect the true effect of digoxin. As long as the patient is responding to treatment, it would be best to wait until a new steady state is reached and draw a sample between 12 and 24 hr after the last dose. This level may be compared to the therapeutic range of 1–2 µg/L for this patient.

Janis J. MacKichan

CASE 2

CC: *"I've been feeling weak and unsteady on my feet and I can't seem to concentrate on my work over the last 2 weeks. I haven't had any more seizures, though."*

HPI:

J. P. is a 50-year-old female who was diagnosed 7 months ago with generalized tonic clonic seizures. After an initial trial with carbamazepine, she was switched to phenytoin. Her phenytoin regimen was gradually increased over time, with the final regimen of 320 mg/day initiated 2 months ago. At her clinic visit 1 month ago, she reported that she had 3 seizures that past month. The serum phenytoin level at that time was 17 mg/L; she did not report any side effects to the phenytoin. Valproic acid was added to her regimen at that visit. J. P. presents to the hospital outpatient clinic today for evaluation of her complaints.

PMH:

Generalized tonic-clonic seizures for 7 months; chronic essential hypertension for 10 years

FH:

Negative for epilepsy; three siblings—all alive and well

SH:

Patient states she stopped drinking her usual evening glass of wine when she was diagnosed with epilepsy. Patient has never smoked and denies use of illicit drugs.

MEDS:

ASA 325 mg po qd
Dilantin Kapseals® 160 mg 0800 and 2000
Depakote® tablet 500 mg 0800 and 2000
Atenolol 25 mg qam daily

ALLERGIES:

Carbamazepine—rash

ROS:

Patient complains of tiring easily, unsteadiness when walking, and inability to concentrate.

PE:

GEN: Pleasant Caucasian woman who appears very lethargic

VS: BP 139/75; HR 60; RR 13; T 98.4 °F; HT 5'7"; and WT 60 kg

HEENT: (-) gingival hyperplasia, PERRLA

CV: Normal S_1 and S_2, RRR, NSR, normal peripheral pulses

LUNG: CTA bilaterally

EXT: No clubbing, cyanosis, or edema; strength 4+

NEURO: Marked horizontal nystagmus on lateral gaze; broad-based gait with inability to stand in tandem position; CN II-XII intact

LABS:

Hemoglobin 14.5 g/dL, hematocrit 41.7%, RBC $4.75 \times 10^6/mm^3$, MCV 88.6 μm^3, MCHC 34.7 g/dL, WBC $5.4 \times 10^3/mm^3$, Plt $210 \times 10^3/mm^3$, sodium 138 mEq/L, potassium 4.1 mEq/L, Cl 99 mEq/L, CO_2 29 mEq/L, BUN 9 mg/dL, SCr 0.8 mg/dL, glucose 107 mg/dL, albumin 3.4 g/dL, ALT 25 U/L, AST 19 U/L [phenytoin]: 16 mg/L (last dose 3 hr ago), and [valproic acid]: 85 mg/L (last dose 3 hr ago).

PROBLEM LIST

- Suspected phenytoin toxicity
- Generalized tonic-clonic seizures
- Mild hypertension, controlled

QUESTIONS

1. *What are your expectations with regard to the valproic acid level: is it closer to a peak, a trough, or a* $C_{ss,avg}$*?*

   Depakote® tablets are not sustained-release products, rather they are delayed release. Thus, there is continued absorption into the next interval for between 1 and 6 hr. This level, drawn 3 hr after a dose, may reflect more of a trough than a peak level.

2. *What are your expectations with regard to the phenytoin level: is it close to a peak, a trough, or a* $C_{ss,avg}$*?*

   Phenytoin, given as the Dilantin Kapseal® product, is slowly released and slowly absorbed. Slow absorption, twice daily dosing, and a relatively long half-life suggest that concentrations of phenytoin will not fluctuate much during the interval. The difference between the dosing interval (12 hr) and peak time (5 hr, from product information) is only 30% of the drugs half-life, if the half-life of phenytoin is considered to be 24 hr at shortest. Using the table on page 130, this translates to a peak:trough ratio close to 1.2. Thus, peaks and troughs are very close to one another. This level could be considered to be a trough, a peak or a $C_{ss,avg}$.

3. *Were the samples for phenytoin and valproic acid drawn at a steady state?*

   The half-life of phenytoin for someone with population average Km and Vmax values is approximately 24 hr, and even higher for patients who have levels at the higher end of the therapeutic range, as this patient. However, the dose-rate of 320 mg sodium phenytoin was initiated 2 months earlier, and the steady state would be attained even if the patient's half-life was as long as 20 days.

   The half-life of valproic acid ranges as long as 18 hr in adults. Thus, steady state after initiation of therapy would have been reached in approximately 2 days. This patient has been taking valproic acid for 1 month. Therefore, she is certainly at a steady state.

4. *How might you explain the apparent symptoms of phenytoin toxicity at a total phenytoin concentration within the therapeutic range?*

   Valproic acid is known to displace phenytoin from albumin binding sites. This effect alone would result in lower total phenytoin concentrations with unchanged free phenytoin concentrations and no change in response. However, valproic acid has also been reported to inhibit phenytoin metabolism. Thus, concentrations of the pharmacologically active free phenytoin may be increased if this occurs. This combination of effect could result in similar or only slightly lower total phenytoin concentrations, yet increased unbound phenytoin concentrations. This effect of valproic acid on phenytoin makes the interpretation of total phenytoin concentrations very difficult.

5. *Determine the normalized phenytoin total level in this patient. What does this tell you?*

   An equation has been developed that allows normalization of phenytoin total concentration to what it would be if the binding of phenytoin were not unusual:

   Normalized PHT level = Measured PHT level + (0.01 × VPA level

   × Measured PHT level) = 16 mg/L + (0.01 × 85 mg/L × 16 mg/L) = 29.6 mg/L

   This means that in the absence of the displacement effect, a concentration of 29.6 mg/L would be measured. Comparing this to the usual therapeutic range of phenytoin (which can only be used for the situation of normal phenytoin binding or for normalized phenytoin concentrations), we see that this level is above the upper limit of 20 mg/L. Side effects to phenytoin are, therefore, not surprising.

6. *You recommend that a saliva sample be obtained using the method recommended by your hospital laboratory in order to confirm that this patient has an unusually high free phenytoin level. The hospital has previously ascertained that the ratio of saliva phenytoin concentration to unbound phenytoin concentration in serum is 1.1 using the EMIT® method. What precautions should you consider when obtaining this sample?*

   The specific method used by the hospital laboratory should be rigorously adhered to. Saliva may be stimulated by the chewing of Parafilm® or by placing citric acid crystals in the mouth, with careful attention to the amount that is used. Saliva from a particular salivary gland may be collected using special devices for this purpose. In any case, it is important that the possibility of retained drug in the mouth be considered. This sample is obtained more than 3 hr after the dose.

Therefore, you have the patient rinse their mouth thoroughly before starting collection, and you discard the first collection per your laboratory's guidelines.

7. *The saliva concentration is 3.2 mg/L. What do you predict the free phenytoin serum concentration to be, and how does this compare to the therapeutic range for unbound phenytoin concentrations in serum?*

Using the saliva:free phenytoin concentration ratio reported by your laboratory, we predict the free phenytoin concentration to be 3.2 ÷ 1.1 or 2.9 mg/L. The therapeutic range of unbound phenytoin concentrations (TRu) can be estimated by taking the therapeutic range of total concentrations (10 to 20 mg/L, which assumes normal binding) and multiplying by the normal unbound fraction of 0.1: 1 to 2 mg/L is the TRu. Thus, the free phenytoin concentration in this patient is clearly above the range of free concentrations considered to be *therapeutic* in most patients.

8. *The patient reports no additional seizures over the last month, suggesting that this combination of antiepileptic drugs is successful for this patient. The physician wishes to decrease the dose-rate of phenytoin to 60 mg tid in order to get her normalized phenytoin level back down to 17 mg/L. What would be the implications if the physician's recommendation is followed? What do you propose instead? Explain.*

The physician is using proportionality when determining the phenytoin dose-rate, which is inappropriate for this drug, which has nonlinear elimination behavior. By decreasing the dose-rate this much, the normalized phenytoin would likely drop to an ineffective range. You recommend a much more conservative decrease in the dose-rate, such as to 300 mg/day or possibly 290 mg/day. Methods are available to permit more accurate determinations of the dose-rate using a population average of the K_m.

9. *What measured total phenytoin levels might be considered therapeutic for this patient in the future?*

The following relationship between unbound concentration (Cu), total concentration (Ctot) and unbound fraction can be used for the following calculations using various rearrangements:

$$Ctot = Cu/fu$$

If it is assumed that the patient had normal phenytoin protein binding when the total phenytoin level of 17 mg/L was obtained 1 month ago, then we can assume the patient was not experiencing side effects at a free phenytoin concentration of 1.7 mg/L (Cu = 0.1 × 17 mg/L).

The unbound phenytoin fraction in this patient in the presence of valproic acid can be estimated using the estimated free phenytoin concentration of 2.9 mg/L and the measured total concentration of 16 mg/L: 2.9/16 = 0.18. As suspected, the patient's unbound fraction is unusually high due to displacement: 0.18 as compared to a normal of 0.1.

The total concentration of phenytoin in this patient associated with the target unbound level of 1.7 mg/L can now be calculated as follows, using the patient's current unbound fraction of 0.18: Ctot = 1.7/0.18 = 9.4 mg/L. Total concentrations in general associated with therapeutic unbound phenytoin concentrations of 1–2 mg/L would be calculated as Ctot = (1–2 mg/L)/0.18 = 5.6–11.1 mg/L for this patient.

10. *What would happen if a physician attempted to increase the dose-rate of phenytoin in order to get total levels within the usual therapeutic range of 10–20 mg/L? What precautions should be taken to assure this doesn't happen?*

Total concentrations of phenytoin in the range of 10–20 mg/L reflect supratherapeutic concentrations of the more pharmacologically important unbound phenytoin in this patient because of an unusually high unbound fraction. This patient will experience toxicity again if total levels are increased to within this range. A clear note should be written in the patient's chart to indicate the total concentration range that is more appropriate for this patient. The note should also indicate that the target therapeutic range of phenytoin should be 10–20 mg/L again if valproic acid is discontinued.

Janis J. MacKichan

CC: *R. M. is a 52 year-old male who presents to his primary care physician for routine follow-up. He has no current complaints.*

HPI:

R. M.'s last routine follow-up was 1 year ago with the same primary care physician. He has seen no specialists since that time.

PMH:

The patient reports a history of hypertension, for which he has been treated for 5 years with medication. He has no prior history of coronary artery disease and denies a history of myocardial infarction, angina, or cardiac surgery.

FH:

His older brother had angioplasty with stent placement at age 62. His father died of a myocardial infarction at age 70, with a history of diabetes (type 2) and dyslipidemia. His mother of age 77 is alive with hypertension and a history of breast cancer. His two children are alive and well.

SH:

R. M. smokes two packs per day and has a 60 pack-per-year history. He attempted to quit once, approximately 5 years ago, but failed. He admits to "social drinking" which he describes as one to two 12-ounce cans of beer on Fridays and Saturdays each week. He denies illicit drug use. He manages his own medications. He drinks 1–2 cups of coffee daily, with no other caffeine intake. His wife cooks meals at home for dinner, but he usually eats fast food for lunch. He frequently skips breakfast. He admits to ice cream or cheese consumption daily and uses whole milk at home. He has a high animal fat diet including hamburgers, fried chicken, sausage and steak. He states he "doesn't have a sweet tooth" and denies frequent intake of cookies, pies, or pastries. Exercise consists of regular yard work, but no formal exercise program.

MEDS:

Hydrocholorthiazide 25 mg po daily

ALLERGIES:

No known drug or food allergies

ROS:

No complaints; denies chest pain

PE:

GEN: WDWN WM in NAD; noted prominent central obesity

VS: BP 140/76; HR 88; RR 16; T 98.8 °F; HT 5'8"; and WT 90 kg. Abdominal circumference is 44 inches.

HEENT: Normal

CHEST: Lungs CTA

CV: RRR, (-) bruits, (-) murmurs, (+) S1, S2, (-) S3, S4

ABD: NTND, (+) BS

EXT: Pedal pulses equal bilaterally; no evidence of tendon xanthomas

LABS:

CBC and electrolytes within normal. BUN 16 mg/dL, creatinine 1.1 mg/dL, glucose 112 mg/dL, TSH 1.02 µU/mL, ALT 13 U/L, AST 14 U/L, and urinalysis negative. Total cholesterol 230 mg/dL, LDL 152 mg/dL, HDL 36 mg/dL, and TG 210 mg/dL.

PROBLEM LIST
• Hyperlipidemia
• Hypertension
• Metabolic Syndrome

QUESTIONS

1. *Low-density lipoprotein is the primary target of therapy due to strong evidence that patients with lower LDL lipoprotein levels have a decreased incidence of atherosclerosis. R. M.'s 10-year risk for coronary heart disease based on Framingham point scores is estimated at 25%. Based on his risk factors, what is your assessment of this patient's LDL cholesterol?*

R. M. has four risk factors for coronary heart disease (cigarette smoking, male age ≥45 years, hypertension, and HDL cholesterol <40 mg/dL). While he does have a family history of coronary heart disease, he does not have a family history of *premature* (male first-degree relative <55 years, female first-degree relative <65 years) coronary heart disease. Since R. M. has two or more risk factors, it is necessary to determine R. M.'s 10-year risk for coronary heart disease. Taking into consideration R. M.'s age, total cholesterol, HDL, systolic blood pressure, and smoking habit, his 10-year risk is estimated at greater than 20%. All patients with greater than 20% 10-year risk are considered as having a CHD risk equivalent, with a desired LDL goal of 100 mg/dL. Therefore, R. M.'s current LDL cholesterol of 152 mg/dL should be reduced to decrease his current cardiovascular risk.

2. *What information does non-HDL provide relative to this patient's hyperlipidemia? Is non-HDL useful in identifying cardiovascular risk?*

Once R. M.'s LDL is controlled, non-HDL will become a secondary target of therapy. Non-HDL takes into consideration both LDL and VLDL as atherogenic lipoproteins. Non-HDL should be considered in all patients with triglycerides between 200 and 499 mg/dL. R. M.'s current non-HDL cholesterol is 194 mg/dL (total cholesterol – HDL, or 230 mg/dL – 36 mg/dL). Since the desired non-HDL cholesterol is always 30 mg/dL over the LDL goal, R. M.'s desired non-HDL cholesterol is less than 130 mg/dL. Drug therapy should target LDL reduction first. Once the appropriate LDL reduction is obtained, then non-HDL should be assessed.

3. *In addition to lifestyle changes, the patient is given a prescription for simvastatin 20 mg daily. What laboratory tests should be obtained prior to initiating therapy?*

R. M. has had many of the necessary baseline laboratory tests already measured. Prior to initiating a statin, baseline lipid panel, transaminases (ALT and AST), and renal function tests are recommended. The lipid panel allows for monitoring of the drug effects on the lipid profile. Statin use is associated with hepatotoxicity, manifested as hepatic transaminase elevations. Since myopathy is more common in patients with renal insufficiency, renal function tests (BUN, creatinine) are helpful to determine if the patient is an appropriate candidate for the use of a statin. All of the above baseline values have already been obtained for R. M.

Additionally, a creatine phosphokinase level (CPK) is necessary at baseline. Myositis, or elevations in CPK with myopathy, may occur with statins. If a patient complains of muscle pain, CPK should be checked again. The drug should be discontinued if CPK is more than 10 times the upper limit of normal. Some patients have elevated CPK at baseline, and it is important to distinguish baseline elevations of CPK from CPK elevations due to the statin.

4. *When should liver function tests be obtained relative to the initiation of simvastatin?*

Transaminases, ALT and AST, are needed at baseline, at 6 weeks and at 12 weeks, then periodically during therapy. In some patients, the transaminase level may return to normal even with continuation of therapy. When the transaminase levels are more than three times the upper limit of normal, most clinicians discontinue the statin and wait for LFTs to return to normal. It is acceptable to rechallenge with a statin at that time.

5. *A follow-up lipid profile is ordered 6 weeks after the initiation of simvastatin. What is the expected effect of simvastatin on the lipid profile?*

Simvastatin is an HMG-CoA reductase inhibitor, or statin, which acts primarily to decrease LDL, but it may also lower triglycerides and raise HDL. Statins have been demonstrated to reduce major coronary events, CHD deaths, stroke, total mortality, and the need for coronary procedures. In clinical trials, simvastatin 20 mg usually decreases LDL cholesterol by 38%, total cholesterol by 28%, triglycerides by 19%, and increases HDL by 8%.[1]

6. *Hyperlipidemia can be due to a variety of causes, including other disease states. Based on the lab test results and history, does this patient have any disease-related secondary causes of hyperlipidemia?*

Secondary causes of hyperlipidemia include diabetes, hypothyroidism, obstructive liver disease, and chronic renal failure. Hypothyroidism is unlikely as this patient has a normal TSH of 1.02 μU/mL (normal 0.3–5.0 μU/mL). Liver function tests (e.g., ALT and AST) within normal limits, ruling out obstructive liver disease. Creatinine and urinalysis do not suggest nephropathy.

While R. M. does not have a history of diabetes, his fasting glucose (112 mg/dL) indicates impaired fasting glucose (>110 mg/dL). This value does not indicate that R. M. has diabetes, but rather suggests insulin resistance. In fact, R. M. has a number of lipid and non-lipid risk factors of metabolic origin, termed the *metabolic syndrome*. R. M. has abdominal obesity (waist circumference >40 inches), triglycerides ≥150 mg/dL, HDL cholesterol <40 mg/dL, and hypertension and a fasting glucose of >110 mg/dL. Metabolic syndrome enhances R. M.'s coronary heart disease risk, making it even more important to treat any identified abnormalities in the lipid profile.

7. *The patient has made changes in his diet and has increased exercise to walking twice weekly. He has attempted again to quit smoking but is still unsuccessful. He continues on simvastatin 20 mg daily. His lipid profile at 6 months is as follows: total cholesterol 175 mg/dL, LDL cholesterol 97 mg/dL, HDL cholesterol 38 mg/dL, and triglycerides 200 mg/dL. What is your assessment of the lipid profile? Should the drug therapy plan be changed? Justify your answer.*

The desired LDL reduction to a goal of less than 100 mg/dL has been achieved. However, R. M.'s non-HDL remains elevated. As in question 2, non-HDL becomes a secondary target of therapy once the appropriate LDL reduction has been achieved. R. M.'s non-HDL is 137 mg/dL (total cholesterol – HDL, or 175–38). The desired non-HDL cholesterol is less than 130 mg/dL. Reductions in non-HDL can be achieved through measures that either increase HDL or decrease trigylcerides. Statins increase HDL and lower triglycerides. Specific therapy targeting raising HDL or lowering triglycerides also includes the fibrates (gemfibrozil, fenofibrate or clofibrate) or nicotinic acid.

The choice of a particular agent would depend on the patient's tolerance of adverse effects and cost. Because R. M. has not been tried on any other lipid lowering agents, it would be appropriate to start any fibrate, nicotinic acid, or increase the dose of simvastain. Most clinicians would probably choose to add another agent to the regimen, as the desired LDL reduction has already been achieved with simvastatin. If nicotinic acid were chosen, a sustained-release formulation would likely be best tolerated.

Jill S. Burkiewicz

CASE 4

CC: *M. S. is a 46-year-old male who presents to the emergency department with severe substernal chest pain. He describes the chest pain as severe and crushing. The chest pain is not pleuritic in nature. He denies nausea and vomiting.*

HPI:

M. S. developed chest pain approximately a half-hour ago, peaking within a few minutes. He denies any history of chest pain.

PMH:

The patient reports a history of diabetes (type 2) for 10 years. He states he was controlled with diet for the first few years, but he has been on oral agents since. The patient reports a history of hypertension, for which he has been treated for 3 years with medications. He has no prior history of coronary artery disease and denies a history of myocardial infarction, angina, or cardiac surgery.

FH:

His mother died at age 68 of breast cancer. His father had a history of diabetes and diet of a myocardial infarction at age 75. He has two sisters with diabetes and two children who are alive and well.

SH:

He is married and works in an office. M. S. denies current or previous habit of cigarette smoking. He admits to up to one alcoholic drink daily, usually 3–4 times weekly. He denies illicit drug use and caffeine intake. He manages his own medications. He has no routine exercise. His diet primarily consists of fish, chicken, and vegetables, with occasional fried foods and dining out.

MEDS:

Metformin 500 mg po tid
Metoprolol 50 mg po bid

ALLERGIES:

He has no known drug or food allergies.

ROS:

Patient complains of severe substernal chest pain. He denies nausea and vomiting.

PE:

GEN: WDWN, obese BM, in apparent distress; diaphoretic and anxious

VS: BP 126/76; HR 98; RR 18; T 98.8 °F; HT 5' 8"; and WT 101 kg

HEENT: WNL, fundoscopic exam within normal limits

CHEST: Lungs CTA

CV: RRR, (-) carotid, abdominal or femoral bruits, (-) murmurs, (+) S1, S2, (-) S3, S4

ABD: NTND, (+) BS

EXT: Pedal pulses equal bilaterally, equal BP in arms/legs, (-) xanthomas

LABS:

CBC and electrolytes are within normal. BUN 20 mg/dL, creatinine 1.2 mg/dL, glucose (random) 240 mg/dL, hemoglobin A1C 8%, TSH 1.26 μU/mL, ALT 18 U/L, AST 20 U/L, and urinalysis negative. Lipid panel drawn the day of admission reveals total cholesterol 220 mg/dL, HDL 58 mg/dL, and TG 90 mg/dL.

ECG:

ECG reveals non-specific ECG changes. Cardiac enzymes (e.g., CK, CK-MB, and troponin) are elevated consistent with myocardial injury from non-ST segment elevation myocardial injury.

CXR:

CXR reveals normal heart size and clear lung fields.

PROBLEM LIST

- Acute myocardial infarction
- Hyperlipidemia
- Diabetes
- Hypertension
- Pain

QUESTIONS

1. *Which lipoprotein is the primary target to reduce this patient's cardiovascular risk? Based on an assessment of this patient's risk factors for coronary heart disease, what is the desired goal of this lipoprotein?*

   LDL is the primary target of therapy due to the atherogenic nature of LDL lipoproteins. In patients with coronary artery disease whose LDL cholesterol is lowered, there is evidence of angiographic regression in trials. All patients with either coronary heart disease or diabetes should have a goal LDL less than 100 mg/dL. While a direct measurement of LDL is not routinely performed due to tedious centrifugation technique required, LDL can be calculated when total cholesterol, HDL cholesterol, and triglyceride levels are available. If triglycerides are below 400 mg/dL, then LDL cholesterol = total cholesterol – HDL cholesterol – (triglycerides/5). Or, in M. S., LDL cholesterol = 220 – 58 – (90/5) = 144 mg/dL. This LDL value is above the desired goal of less than 100 mg/dL in a patient with coronary heart disease.

2. *What information does the HDL provide relative to the patient's hyperlipidemia? Is HDL useful in identifying the patient's cardiovascular risk?*

   HDL cholesterol is often termed the "good cholesterol" as it acts as an antiatherogenic particle. High levels of HDL (>60 mg/dL) are associated with cardioprotection, and low levels of HDL (<40 mg/dL) are associated with risk for coronary heart disease. Based on the NCEP ATP III recommendations, there is no specific goal for increasing HDL cholesterol in patients with low HDL. However, M. S. does not have elevated, or low HDL cholesterol. Though the entire lipid profile needs to be taken into consideration, the HDL value will not impact the degree to which LDL is lowered in M. S.

3. *The patient undergoes emergency angioplasty. The occlusion is stented with 0% residual stenosis. Follow-up exercise testing reveals normal LV size and mild inferior wall hypokinesis. Postmyocardial infarction, M. S. is started on a beta-blocker, ACE inhibitor, aspirin, and a hypolipemic agent. At discharge, he is counseled extensively on therapeutic lifestyle changes, including reduction in saturated fat and cholesterol intake along with initiation of moderate physical activity. M. S. may be counseled on replacing LDL-raising saturated fat from high-fat meats and whole-milk dairy products with LDL-lowering unsaturated fats such as olive oil. What lab tests would be useful for assessing the response to lifestyle changes? What is the expected impact of lifestyle changes on the lipid profile?*

   Monitoring of the fasting lipid profile (e.g., total cholesterol, triglycerides, LDL, and HDL) is necessary to determine the impact of therapeutic lifestyle changes. Therapeutic lifestyle changes are centered on both dietary change and weight reduction through physical activity. LDL reduction is the primary goal, but increases in HDL and decreases in triglycerides may also be noted with lifestyle changes. Reducing saturated fat in the diet to <7% of calories gives an approximate LDL cholesterol reduction of 8–10%, while an intake of <200 mg/day of dietary cholesterol would provide an additional 3–5% reduction in LDL. Since M. S. is overweight, a weight reduction by 10 pounds through moderate physical activity and dietary changes may provide an approximate LDL reduction of 5–8%. Due to the recent cardiovascular event, it is necessary to initiate drug therapy concomitantly with lifestyle changes. As such, it will be difficult to discern which changes in the lipid profile are due to lifestyle changes and which changes are due to the drug. If M. S. is able to adhere to the lifestyle changes, the above values give an estimate of the expected impact on LDL.

4. *When should the next fasting lipid profile be obtained relative to the start of lifestyle changes and initiation of drug therapy?*

   A fasting lipid profile should be obtained approximately 6 weeks after initiation of lifestyle changes and drug therapy. At that time, the effect of the drug in decreasing endogenous cholesterol synthesis and the effect of dietary changes to decrease cholesterol exogenous cholesterol sources will be evident.

5. *What effect does metoprolol have on the lipid profile? Should this drug be discontinued?*

    Beta-blocking agents, such as metoprolol, may cause increases in triglyceride concentrations and reduce HDL cholesterol concentrations. Agents with intrinsic sympathomimetic activity such as pindolol, do not have this effect. While it is important to realize the effect of antihypertensive agents on the lipid profile, agents that adversely affect the lipid profile should not be avoided in all patients with hyperlipidemia. Careful consideration of the patient-specific factors is warranted. For M. S., beta-blockers without intrinsic sympathomimetic activity are preferred treatment for hypertension due to documented decreases in mortality postmyocardial infarction.

6. *What effect does myocardial infarction have on the lipid profile? Can lipid values obtained during the acute phase of a myocardial infarction be used to guide treatment choices?*

    In persons admitted to the hospital for acute coronary syndromes or coronary procedures, lipid values may begin to decline in the first few hours after an event. The values may be significantly decreased by 24–48 hr and remain low for weeks following the event. Therefore, the lipid values obtained on the day of admission for M. S. may be lower than usual for him. However, these values are clearly elevated above our desired goals for M. S. Initiating treatment now, rather than waiting, may help prevent future cardiovascular events. These lipid values provide guidance for the initiation of therapy, but continued follow-up will be necessary.

7. *Postmyocardial infarction, M. S. is started on a beta-blocker, ACE inhibitor, aspirin, and a hypolipemic agent. Based on M. S.'s lipid profile, which hypolipemic medication would you recommend?*

    M. S.'s LDL cholesterol is elevated at 144 mg/dL, with a goal of less than 100 mg/dL. His HDL and triglycerides are at a desired level and do not need to be targeted with drug therapy. LDL reducing drug therapy includes a statin, bile acid sequestrant, and nicotinic acid. Due to their superior efficacy in reducing LDL cholesterol, evidence in reducing cardiovascular events, and safety profile, statins have become first-line therapy to treat elevations in LDL cholesterol. While bile acid sequestrants may provide 15–30% decrease in LDL, their use in achieving reductions of a magnitude of 30%, as needed for M. S., are limited by gastrointestinal tolerability. Nicotinic acid may provide LDL reductions of up to 25%. This may not provide enough LDL reduction for M. S., who needs a 30% decrease in LDL cholesterol to achieve is goal. Though nicotinic acid provides the additional benefit of decreasing triglycerides and increasing HDL, this is not needed for M. S. Therefore, a statin would provide the LDL reduction necessary. The choice of a particular agent would depend on the LDL reducing capabilities of individual agents, the patient's insurance drug formulary, and drug cost. It would be appropriate to use any agent that provides the appropriate LDL reduction.

REFERENCE

1. Zocor® (simvastatin) package insert. Whitehouse Station, NJ: Merck & Co., Inc.; 2002.

Jill S. Burkiewicz

CC: R. E., a 27-year-old male, was admitted to the surgical intensive care unit following emergency surgery for penetrating abdominal trauma.

CASE 5

HPI:

R. E. was in his usual good state of health until 2 days previously, when he was robbed and suffered three knife wounds to the abdomen. He was taken immediately to surgery for repair of the trauma including two areas of penetration of the ileum. His postoperative course has been uncomplicated. He was placed on broad spectrum antibiotics and has been receiving nothing by mouth and is on intermittent nasogastric suction for bowel rest.

PMH:

He has had asthma since he was a child, with no history of intubations required.

FH:

Noncontributory

SH:

He has smoked one pack of cigarettes per day for the past 10 years. He consumes occasional beer. He denies use of any illegal drugs.

MEDS:

Morphine 4 mg IV q 4 hr prn pain
Piperacillin-tazobactam 4/0.5 g IV q 8 hr
Heparin 7500 units subcutaneous q 12 hr
Salmeterol inhaler one puff q 12 hr
Albuterol inhaler two puffs q 4 hr prn
    shortness of breath
Furosemide 40 mg IV daily

ALLERGIES:

None known

ROS:

R. E. complains of incisional pain rated intermittently as 5 on a scale of 0 to 10. He complains of dry mouth.

PE:

GEN: Well-developed, well-nourished white male; currently in no distress

VS: BP 130/70; HR 90; RR 16; T 99 °F; HT 6'2"; and WT 85 kg

HEENT: No significant findings

CHEST: Lungs clear to auscultation

CV: Regular rate and rhythm; no abnormal heart sounds

ABD: Slightly distended with three areas of surgical repair; bowel sounds absent

GENIT: Normal

EXT: Normal

LABS:

Sodium 138 mEq/L (136–145 mEq/L), potassium 3.6 mEq/L (3.5–5.0 mEq/L), chloride 102 mEq/L (96–106 mEq/L), total carbon dioxide 34 mEq/L (24–30 mEq/L), serum creatinine (SCr) 1.0 mg/dL (0.7–1.5 mg/dL), and glucose 100 mg/dL (70–110 mg/dL). White blood cell (WBC) count 10,000 cells/mm^3 (4800–10,800 cells/mm^3), platelets 250,000/mm^3, hemoglobin 11 g/dL, and hematocrit 34%.

PROBLEM LIST

- S/P abdominal surgery
- Pain secondary to abdominal surgery
- Asthma, currently under control

QUESTIONS

1. *Based on the laboratory results provided, does an acid-base disorder appear to be present? What acid-base disorders are consistent with this result? What are potential causes? What additional laboratory tests are needed to more thoroughly assess the acid-base disorder?*

   The total carbon dioxide level (serum bicarbonate) is elevated. This is consistent with either metabolic alkalosis, renal compensation for respiratory acidosis, or a mixed acid base disorder. Without an arterial blood gas determination, it is not possible to conclusively differentiate between these possibilities. The patient history provides some possible causes of several acid-base disorders. Nasogastric suction causes loss of acid from the stomach and is a potential cause of metabolic alkalosis. Since the patient is not taking oral fluids and complains of a dry mouth, it is possible that he is dehydrated, which is also associated with metabolic alkalosis. However, he does not display hypotension, tachycardia, or other physical signs of intravascular volume depletion. He has a history of asthma and may be volume overloaded from IV fluids received during surgery, which could produce pulmonary edema. Both of these conditions could impair ventilation, leading to carbon dioxide retention and respiratory acidosis. However, the lung exam does not appear to support these as likely causes, as there is no evidence of wheeze or abnormal lung sounds suggesting asthma or pulmonary edema. In any case, an arterial blood gas determination is needed to definitively determine the patient's acid-base status.

2. *R. E. has an arterial blood gas determination which reveals a pH 7.47, PaO_2 98 mm Hg, $PaCO_2$ 45 mm Hg, and bicarbonate 32 mEq/L. What acid-base disorder is present?*

   Acid-base status should be determined by first evaluating the pH. R. E.'s pH is in the alkalemic range, suggesting that metabolic alkalosis, respiratory alkalosis, or a mixed acid-base disorder is present. Because the serum bicarbonate value is elevated, metabolic alkalosis is likely. The $PaCO_2$ is elevated, which eliminates the possibility of simple respiratory alkalosis (associated with a decreased $PaCO_2$). It is possible that a mixed acid-base disorder is present. This is assessed by comparing the degree of respiratory compensation in R. E. with that expected in simple metabolic alkalosis. In R. E., the serum bicarbonate is elevated by 8 mEq/L from the normal value of 24. The expected respiratory compensation in metabolic alkalosis is an increase in $PaCO_2$ of 4–5 mm Hg ($0.6 \times$ change in bicarbonate). R. E.'s $PaCO_2$ has risen by 5 mm Hg (from 40–45 mm Hg), the expected degree of compensation. Therefore, R. E. has a simple metabolic alkalosis.

3. *What is the most likely cause of metabolic alkalosis? How should this be managed?*

   The most likely cause of metabolic alkalosis in this patient is nasogastric suction, which removes hydrogen ions from the stomach. Over time, this can deplete the body of acid. If suction is still required as part of R. E.'s postoperative care, administration of medications that inhibit acid secretion in the stomach can prevent further loss of acid. Proton pump inhibitors (e.g., lansoprazole) or histamine-2 receptor antagonists (e.g., famotidine) are effective. The alkalosis will correct as the body produces acid from normal metabolism.

4. *What laboratory tests should be used to monitor resolution of R. E.'s metabolic alkalosis?*

   Unless the patient's status changes in a way that necessitates further diagnostic testing, additional arterial blood gases are not needed. The patient's serum bicarbonate (total carbon dioxide) level, obtained as part of typical electrolyte panels, can be monitored to assure that R. E.'s metabolic alkalosis resolves.

5. *R. E.'s nasogastric suction and heparin are discontinued. He is walking but still taking nothing by mouth. While walking, he becomes lightheaded and has to be helped back to bed. His blood pressure and heart rate are 120/60 mm Hg and 110 per minute supine and 100/50 mm Hg and 130 per minute sitting. His weight has dropped 10 kg over the past 24 hr and is now 5 kg below his admission weight. The morning's electrolyte panel reveals a serum bicarbonate of 33 mEq/L, potassium of 3.0 mEq/L, and chloride 92 mEq/L. Repeat arterial blood gases are done with pH 7.48, PaO_2 96 mm Hg, $PaCO_2$ 46 mm Hg, and bicarbonate 34 mEq/L. Why has the metabolic alkalosis not resolved? How should it be managed?*

R. E. still displays arterial blood gas results consistent with simple, compensated metabolic alkalosis. His physical exam and weight loss are consistent with intravascular volume depletion. This condition produces metabolic alkalosis by a variety of mechanisms. The most likely causes for volume depletion in R. E. are inadequate fluid intake and continued administration of furosemide. Presence of hypokalemia and hypochloremia produced by diuretics also contributes to metabolic alkalosis. R. E. should be treated with fluid repletion using intravenous normal saline supplemented with potassium chloride.

6. *R. E. responds to IV fluid and electrolyte replacement and the metabolic alkalosis resolves. Because of continued lack of oral intake he is started on total parenteral nutrition. His TPN formulation includes the following electrolytes in each liter: sodium 80 mEq, potassium 60 mEq, chloride 40 mEq, phosphate 20 mmol, and acetate to balance. After 5 days of TPN, R. E.'s metabolic acidosis recurs with pH 7.48 and serum bicarbonate 35. What is the cause?*

   It is most likely that R. E. has developed metabolic acidosis as a result of the TPN formulation. Acid-base balance is maintained in patients receiving TPN by providing the correct amounts of chloride and acetate as anions in the formulation. The liver converts acetate to bicarbonate. Providing an excessive amount of acetate and inadequate chloride can result in metabolic alkalosis.

7. *How should R. E.'s metabolic alkalosis be treated?*

   The relative amount of chloride in R. E.'s TPN should be increased. Based on the need to balance cations and anions in the formulation, R. E. is probably receiving approximately 80 mEq of acetate per liter with the current formulation, compared with only 40 mEq of chloride. Changing the formulation to include 80–100 mEq of chloride per liter should correct the alkalosis. The serum bicarbonate and chloride levels should be monitored closely and amounts of chloride and acetate adjusted to achieve normal levels.

   Thomas G. Hall

CASE 6

CC: A 65-year-old female, A. S., was admitted from the emergency department with a chief complaint of dysuria, fever, and back pain for the past 2 days.

HPI:

A. S. was in her usual state of health until 2 days ago when she noticed the onset of pain on urination and low back pain on arising. Later that day, she felt hot and her oral temperature was 100.5 °F. The symptoms continued to worsen at home, and she has spent the last 6 hr in bed. She now complains of dizziness and generalized weakness.

PMH:

She has a history of diabetes mellitus, obesity, and osteoarthritis.

FH:

She has history of breast cancer in her mother, maternal aunt, and sister.

SH:

A. S. is a previous smoker with a history of smoking 1 pack of cigarettes per day for 20 years, but she has abstained for the past 20 years. She consumes an occasional glass of wine. She denies use of any illegal drugs.

MEDS:

Glipizide 10 mg po q day
Alendronate 10 mg po q day
Black cohosh two capsules twice a day
Glucosamine-chondroitin two capsules twice a day
Ibuprofen 400 mg po every 6 hr as needed for joint pain

ALLERGIES:

None known

ROS:

She complains of sharp, burning pain on urination and sharp, constant pain in the lower back. She has recently begun to feel weak and unable to stay awake.

PE:

GEN: Well-developed, somnolent, moderately obese white female

VS: BP 80/40; HR 112; RR 16; T 102.2 °F; HT 5'4"; and WT 85 kg

HEENT: No significant findings

CHEST: Lungs clear to auscultation

CV: Tachycardic, regular rhythm, and no abnormal heart sounds

ABD: Slightly distended, minimal bowel sounds

GENIT: Moderate-severe costovertebral angle tenderness

EXT: Cool and pale

LABS:

Sodium 140 mEq/L (136–145 mEq/L), potassium 3.5 mEq/L (3.5–5.0 mEq/L), chloride 104 mEq/L (96–106 mEq/L), total carbon dioxide 14 mEq/L (24–30 mEq/L), SCr 1.5 mg/dL (0.7–1.5 mg/dL), glucose 300 mg/dL (70–110 mg/dL), and serum lactate 10 mEq/L (0.5–1.5 mEq/L). ABGs pH 7.17 (7.36–7.44), $PaCO_2$ 40 mm Hg (36–44 mm Hg), PaO_2 80 mm Hg (80–100 mm Hg), and serum bicarbonate 14 mEq/L (24–30 mEq/L). WBC count 15,000 cells/mm^3 (4800–10,800 cells/mm^3) with 50% segmented neutrophils, 20% band neutrophils, 20% lymphocytes, and 10% monocytes. Urinalysis revealed 4+ bacteria, more than 50 WBCs per high-power field, and WBC casts. Gram stain of urine revealed Gram-negative rods. Blood and urine bacterial cultures were sent.

PROBLEM LIST

- Urinary tract infection, probable pyelonephritis with urosepsis; piperacillin-tazobactam was started empirically
- Noninsulin dependent diabetes mellitus, currently out of control; sliding scale regular insulin was started
- Osteoarthritis, currently under control

QUESTIONS

1. *What is A. S.'s acid-base status at this time?*

   The pH of 7.17 is in the acidemic range. Because her bicarbonate concentration is low and the $PaCO_2$ is normal, A. S. must have metabolic acidosis. The fact that the $PaCO_2$ is not reduced to compensate for the low bicarbonate suggests that she has a mixed acid-base disorder, with combined respiratory acidosis and metabolic acidosis. Although the $PaCO_2$ is not elevated, as is expected in respiratory acidosis, pulmonary compensation for her metabolic acidosis is absent. This confirms the presence of respiratory acidosis. The mental status changes may be responsible for relative hypoventilation.

2. *How do other laboratory tests help to classify the acid-base disturbance and provide information regarding etiology?*

   In assessing the patient's metabolic acidosis, both the anion gap and serum lactate concentration are helpful. The anion gap is elevated (22 mEq/L) as is the lactic acid concentration. These elevations help to define the most likely causes of metabolic acidosis. In A. S., metabolic acidosis with an elevated anion gap and lactate concentration—in conjunction with a Gram-negative urinary tract infection and her clinical presentation—is most consistent with septic shock.

3. *A. S.'s mental status continued to deteriorate 12 hr after admission, and her respiratory rate dropped to 12/min. Chest film revealed diffuse pulmonary infiltrates. Repeat ABGs on room air were pH 7.07, $PaCO_2$ 50 mm Hg, PaO_2 55 mm Hg, and serum bicarbonate 14 mEq/L. She was taken to the intensive care unit and placed on mechanical ventilation with 100% oxygen. This patient's repeat blood gases 60 min later were pH 7.15, $PaCO_2$ 47 mm Hg, PaO_2 140 mm Hg, and serum bicarbonate 16 mEq/L. What acid-base disorder exists in this patient now?*

   A. S. now clearly has a mixed acid-base disorder. The low pH of 7.07 is evidence of an acidemia. Evaluation of the $PaCO_2$ and bicarbonate values reveals that the $PaCO_2$ is elevated, consistent with a respiratory acidosis, and the bicarbonate is low, consistent with a metabolic acidosis. A. S. displays a mixed respiratory and metabolic acidosis due to the septic shock producing lactic acidosis and deterioration of her mental status impairing ventilation, which superimposes respiratory acidosis.

4. *What do the two sets of blood gases in Question 3 imply about A. S.'s level of oxygenation?*

   The blood gases also provide important information about A. S.'s level of oxygenation. The PaO_2 of 55 mm Hg in Question 3 indicates that her blood is inadequately oxygenated. Her oxygen saturation at this level is less than 90%, in the steep portion of the Hgb–oxygen dissociation curve (see Figure 9-2, Chapter 9). Further decreases in PaO_2 will result in significant reductions in Hgb saturation and significant impairment in oxygen delivery to tissues.

   After initiation of mechanical ventilation with 100% oxygen, the PaO_2 rises dramatically. This increase is typical when the FiO_2 increases from 21% (room air) to 100%. At this point, her level of oxygen saturation is more than adequate. As long as measures are taken to ensure hemodynamic stability so that proper tissue blood flow is provided, tissue oxygen delivery should also be adequate.

5. *Do the results of the second set of ABGs in Question 3 indicate that A. S. needs increased or decreased mechanical ventilation?*

   The second set of blood gases in Question 3 also demonstrates inadequate correction of the respiratory acidosis. The pH is still low, but correction of the metabolic acidosis may take several hours even with appropriate therapy for sepsis. However, A. S.'s $PaCO_2$ is still elevated, indicating the presence of hypoventilation and respiratory acidosis. The mechanical ventilation should rapidly reverse this process. Since the $PaCO_2$ is still elevated despite ample time for correction, some alteration in mechanical ventilation is needed.

   Based on the ABGs, two changes are indicated in the ventilator settings. One change is a reduction in the inspired oxygen concentration, which should prevent the oxygen toxicity that occurs when FiO_2 exceeds 50% for prolonged periods. Oxygen toxicity is caused by production of oxygen free radicals with subsequent tissue damage in the lungs. Higher levels of FiO_2 and longer periods when FiO_2 exceeds 50% increase the risk for toxicity by depleting tissue antioxidants.

Oxygen toxicity in mechanically ventilated patients is manifested by reduced lung compliance and vital capacity, followed by increased difficulty in adequate oxygenation. In this patient, the percentage of inspired oxygen should be reduced to maintain adequate saturation of Hgb (90%) at the minimum of inspired oxygen concentration.

Another change in ventilator settings is that the minute ventilation rate should be increased to improve carbon dioxide excretion. This change can be accomplished by increasing the ventilation rate and/or the volume of air provided with each ventilation (the tidal volume).

6. *Over the next 24 hr, A. S.'s condition remained critical. She experienced a cardiac arrest and was successfully resuscitated with treatment including multiple doses of epinephrine and sodium bicarbonate. She was still receiving mechanical ventilation 24 hr later, but her hemodynamic status was stabilized. Her ABG's are pH 7.50, PaCO₂ 40 mm Hg, PaO₂ 100 mm Hg, and serum bicarbonate 30 mEq/L. What acid-base disorder does A. S. display now? What is the cause?*

A. S.'s pH of 7.50 is high, meaning that she is alkalemic. Her $PaCO_2$ of 40 mm Hg is normal, but her serum bicarbonate level is elevated at 30 mEq/L. This is consistent with a metabolic alkalosis. Metabolic alkalosis can occur following aggressive treatment of metabolic acidosis or cardiac arrest with sodium bicarbonate. In many cases, administration of bicarbonate to acutely raise pH can result in excessive bicarbonate stores. It can take a few days for the kidneys to remove the excess bicarbonate. In the case of patients who are mechanically ventilated, the level of $PaCO_2$ is regulated by the ventilator settings. This may prevent the process of normal respiratory compensation, as is seen in this case.

Thomas G. Hall

CC: *"I'm here for a blood pressure check."*

CASE 7

HPI:

A. H. is a 47-year-old Hispanic woman who comes to the pharmacist-managed diabetes clinic for a follow-up blood pressure check and evaluation of her diabetic therapy. She also complains of nervousness and diaphoresis. Her blood glucose logbook indicates that she has been monitoring her blood glucose levels twice a day (before breakfast and dinner) with a range of 140–200 mg/dL. She reports adherence to an 1800-calorie meal plan and 40 minutes of walking on a treadmill every morning.

PMH:

Type 2 diabetes mellitus (diagnosed 2 years ago)

FH:

Maternal grandmother had DM; father had emphysema; no family history of CAD

SH:

A. H. is married, a secretary at a college, and is active in church and a social club. She denies tobacco use (stopped 10 years ago) and consumes about two to three alcoholic drinks per week.

MEDS:

Glipizide 10 mg po bid
Rosiglitazone 8 mg po daily
Conjugated estrogen 0.625 mg po daily
ASA 81 mg po daily

ALLERGIES:

None

ROS:

A. H. denies nausea, constipation, diarrhea, signs or symptoms of hypoglycemia, paresthesias, and dyspnea. She reports occasional blurry vision.

PE:

GEN: WDWN mildly obese, woman in NAD

VS: BP 120/70; HR 80; RR 18; T 38.6 °C; HT 5'2.5"; and WT 82.2 kg

SKIN: Dry appearing skin and scalp; (-) rashes or lesions

HEENT: PERRLA, EOMI, and R&L fundus exam without retinopathy; AV nicking

NECK: (-) thyroid nodules or goiter; (-) lymphadenopathy

CV: RRR, no m/r/g, normal S_1, S_2; (-) S_3 or S_4

ABD: NT/ND

LUNG: Clear to A&P

GENIT/RECT: Deferred

EXT: Carotids, femorals, popliteals, and right dorsalis pedis pulses 2+ throughout, left dorsalis pedis 1+; feet show thick calluses on MTPs

NEURO: DTRs 2+ throughout; feet with normal sensation (5.07 monofilament)

LABS:

March 23

$$\begin{array}{c} 139 \quad | \quad 102 \quad | \quad 33 \\ \overline{} \diagdown 200 \\ 4.3 \quad | \quad 22 \quad | \quad 1.8 \end{array}$$

UA (+) protein, (110 mg/24 hr), (-) blood, (-) ketones, AST 9 IU/L, and ALT 12 IU/L.

Sept 23

Fasting plasma glucose 140 mg/dL, Ca 9.8 mg/dL, phosphate 3.3 mg/dL, AST 10 IU/L, ALT 13 IU/L, alkaline phosphate 43 IU/L, T. bili 1.0 mg/dL, TSH 1.2 µU/mL, RT_3U 24%, FT_4 16 pmol/L, free T_4 0.7 ng/dL, RBC $5.2 \times 10^6 mm^3$, WBC 6.0×10^3 mm^3, Tchol 210, trig 190, HDL 30, and LDL 142.

QUESTIONS

1. *What additional test (s) would assist in assessing this patient's glycemic control?*

   Glycosylated hemoglobin will assist the clinician in the assessment of glycemic control over the last 2–4 months. During the 120 day lifespan of a red blood cell, (RBC) nonenzymatic glycosylation occurs, a process in which glucose adheres to hemoglobin moieties of the cell.

   Therefore, the A1C reflects glycemic control over the last 3–4 months. However, this lab test must be interpreted with caution. Patients who have diseases with chronic or episodic hemolysis (e.g. sickle cell anemia) may have low A1C levels caused by the presence of young RBCs that carry less A1C. The A1C may be falsely elevated or low during pregnancy. Therefore, this test should not be used to assess glycemic control during pregnancy.

2. *Based on the laboratory data provided what changes if any, would you make in this patient's antidiabetic drug therapy?*

   Bedtime insulin should be considered to achieve glycemic control. Metformin is not an option in this patient since serum creatinine level >1.5 mg/dL.

3. *Based on the laboratory values obtained, what other therapeutic interventions should be made at this time to decrease this patient's risk of complications associated with diabetes mellitus?*

   The patient's urinalysis is positive for protein. Obtain another urinalysis for microalbumin. An ACEI or ARB should be initiated if microalbumin is >30 mg/dL.

4. *What information (e.g., signs, symptoms, and laboratory values) indicates the presence of hyperthyroidism?*

   Although the patient presents with signs of hyperthyroidism (e.g., nervousness and diaphoresis), the normal free thyroxine, TSH, and thyroxine index rule out hyperthyroidism. The depressed resin uptake is consistent with increased TBG levels observed in patients with acute hepatitis, pregnant women, or persons taking estrogen, oral contraceptives, or tamoxifen. TBG and bound T_4 levels are increased by estrogens. Therefore, total serum T_4 measurements will be falsely elevated. Thyroid tests will return to normal within 4 weeks after discontinuation of the estrogen.

   Eva M. Vivian

CC: *A. C. is a 74-year-old African American male with a 3-year history of type 2 diabetes mellitus, hypertension, and dyslipidemia. He lives alone. He does not monitor his glucose readings at home. He is concerned about his frequent urination throughout the day and night, which has increased over the last 6 days. He denies any nausea or vomiting, but states he hasn't had much of an appetite lately. "I'm just not feeling like myself lately." His daughter accompanied him to the doctor's office because she felt he has been acting weird lately.*

HPI:

Hypertension and high cholesterol for 3 years

PMH:

Hypertension, DM, hyperlipidemia

FH:

A. C.'s father died of heart attack at age 51; mother is still alive and well

SH:

A. C. smokes one pack of cigarettes per day and drinks two to three shots of whiskey on the weekend with friends.

MEDS:

Glipizide 5 mg po twice a day
Simvastatin 20 mg po daily at bedtime
Hydrochlorothiazide 50 mg po daily
ASA 325 mg po daily

ALLERGIES:

Penicillin (hives)

ROS:

Patient complains of frequent urination and fatigue over the last month.

PE:

GEN: WDWN mildly obese, elderly African American; disoriented and confused

VS: BP 120/60 (dropped to 95/50 when sitting); HR100; RR 20; T 39 °C; HT 5'9.5"; and WT 82.2 kg

SKIN: Turgor poor, mucous membranes dry

HEENT: PERRLA, EOMI, R&L fundus exam without retinopathy; AV nicking

NECK: (-) thyroid nodules or goiter; (-) lymphadenopathy

CV: RRR, no m/r/g, normal S_1, S_2; (-) S_3 or S_4

ABD: NT/ND

LUNG: Clear to A&P

GENIT/RECT: Deferred

EXT: Carotids, femorals, popliteals, right dorsalis pedis pulses 2+ throughout, and left dorsalis pedis 1+; feet show thick calluses on MTPs

NEURO: DTRs 2+ throughout; feet with normal sensation (5.07 monofilament)

HEENT: No significant finding

CHEST: Lungs clear to auscultation

CV: RRR, (-) bruits, (-) murmurs (-) S3 or S4, carotids bilaterally palpable

EXT: Unremarkable

LABS:

Sodium 139 mEq/L, (136–145 mEq/L), potassium 4.6 mEq/L (3.5–5.0 mEq/L), chloride 102 mEq/L, total CO_2 24 mEq/L, BUN 50 mg/dL (8–20 mg/dL), creatinine 3.0 mg/dL (0.7–1.5 mg/dL), glucose 715 mg/dL, pH 7.39 (7.36–7.44), bicarbonate, 26 (24–30 mEq/L), ketones (negative), alkaline phosphate 70, AST 18, and ALT 20.

QUESTIONS

1. *Based on the subjective and objective data provided, what is the most likely diagnosis for this patient? And what signs and symptoms support the diagnosis?*

   HHS is secondary to uncontrolled type 2 DM. This patient is over 60 years of age, and HHS occurs most frequently in the elderly population. He complains of symptoms >5 days. He has decreased skin turgor, dry mucous membranes, tachycardia (HR 100), and orthostatic hypotension (a fall of systolic blood pressure of 20 mm Hg after 1 min of standing), which is consistent with dehydration. He is lethargic, confused, and disorientated (HHS patients are generally more dehydrated). Therefore, mentation changes are more commonly seen than in DKA. The elderly often have an impaired thirst mechanism that increases the risk of HHS. This patient has lost fluids over a long period of time.

2. *What lab values suggest HHS?*

   The plasma glucose level is >600 mg/dL, bicarbonate concentration is normal, and pH normal. Negative ketone bodies <2+ in 1:1 dilution confirms the diagnosis of HHS. Ketones are present in the blood and urine of patients with DKA. Insulin deficiency is less profound in HHS. Therefore, lipolysis resulting in the production of ketone bodies does not occur.

3. *What is this patient's osmolarity?*

   The osmolality is a measure of the number of osmotically active ions or particles present per unit of solution. It represents the total number of particles, not the weight of the particles. The particles that are used to determine serum osmolality are sodium, glucose, and urea. Serum osmolality is usually 280–295 mOsm/kg. This patient's serum osmolarity: estimation formula $(2 \times 143) + (715/18) + 50/3 = 342$ mOsm/kg.

4. *What could have precipitated this disorder?*

   Massive fluid loss due to prolonged osmotic diuresis secondary to hyperglycemia, as well as the thiazide diuretic-hydrochlorothiazide 50 mg qd may have precipitated the onset of HHS.

5. *What measures should be taken in this patient?*

   The patient should be rehydrated with oral fluids since he has no complaints of gastrointestinal discomfort. Insulin should be administered. Although this patient's sodium and potassium are within normal limits, the presence of orthostatic hypotension is consistent with decreased intravascular volume, causing hemoconcentration of sodium and potassium. Potassium shifts out of cells when the pH of the blood is acidic due to an increased influx of hydrogen ions. The total potassium concentration appears normal because potassium has shifted from the intracellular compartment to the circulation. These levels may decline when the patient is rehydrated with fluids. Potassium replacement will probably be required. Phosphorus is also within normal limits but may decrease after rehydration and insulin.

   Decreased intravascular volume has led to hemoconcentration of hematocrit and BUN. BUN is also elevated due to decreased renal perfusion (prerenal azotemia), although intrinsic renal causes should be considered if serum creatinine is also elevated.

6. *What other interventions should be taken to prevent risk of complications associated with DM?*

   A fasting lipid panel should be obtained. This patient's goal LDL is <100 mg/dL, goal HDL is >45 mg/dL, and goal triglycerides is <150 mg/dL. The patient's simvastatin dose can be increased to achieve this goal. Blood pressure should be monitored (goal <130/80 mmHg) closely. A urinalysis for the presence of microalbumin should be performed to identify incipient nephropathy. Once glucose levels are below 200 mg/dL, the addition of another oral agent should be considered. Evaluation of renal function is required after HHS has resolved. If serum creatinine is >1.5 mg/dL, rosiglitazone or bedtime insulin should be considered to achieve glycemic control. Metformin is not an option in patients with serum creatinine levels >1.5 mg/dL.

   Eva M. Vivian

CC: *"I have neck and chest pain."*

CASE 9

HPI:

J. D. is a 60-year-old white man who presents to the emergency department (ED) with complaints of neck and chest pain that started 3 hr earlier today. The pain was pressure-like, was rated 7–8/10 in severity (sometimes radiated to the left scapula), and lasted 5–10 minutes and then returned again. He denies any shortness of breath, dizziness, palpitations, diaphoresis, nausea, or vomiting. While in the ED, J. D. experienced another episode of neck/chest pain associated with diaphoresis, which was partially relieved by nitroglycerin. The patient had a stress test performed one year ago with normal findings. A coronary angiogram performed 6 years ago revealed normal coronary arteries.

PMH:

Hypercholesterolemia; s/p tonsillectomy in 1995

FH:

His father has polycythemia.

SH:

J. D. is married with three children and lives with his family. He is a retired electrician with a+30 pack-per-year history of smoking, which he quit 3 years ago. He denies alcohol or illicit drug use.

MEDS:

Simvastatin 20 mg po qpm
Enteric coated aspirin 325 mg po qd

ALLERGIES:

NKDA

ROS:

Neck pain with some chest pressure

PE:

GEN: A& O × 3; in NAD
VS: BP 101/54; HR 78; RR 16; T 37.2 °C; HT 5'6"; and WT 79.8 kg
HEENT: Normocephalic, PERRLA
NECK: Supple, (-) JVD
CV: RRR, normal S_1,S_2, (-) murmurs
LUNGS: CTA
ABD: Soft, NT, (+) BS
EXT: (-) edema, +2 pulses
NEURO: No focal deficits

LABS:

```
135 | 101 | 15
            < 91
3.8 | 23  | 0.8
```

```
        16.3
10.34 <       < 274
         45
```

ECG:

NSR, LVH, (-) ST-T changes

LABS:

Ca^{+2}: 8.6 mg/Dl, cholesterol 284 mg/dL, LDL 198 mg/dL, HDL 38 mg/dL, TG 241 mg/dL, PT 10.8 sec, INR 1.0, and aPTT 35.9 sec.

Hospital Day	Time	CK (32–237 U/L)	CK-MB (0–5.0 ng/mL)	CK-MB Index (0.0–6.0%)	Troponin I* (ng/mL)
1	1950	79	1.9	2.4	0.22
2	0500	1719	119.4	6.9	42.8
	1600	1082	64.9	6.0	45.6

Median values for (1) apparently healthy person ≤0.07 ng/mL; (2) noncardiac related disorder <0.10 ng/mL; (3) diagnostic cutoff for AMI patients 1.5 ng/mL; and (4) confirmed MI 7.6 ng/mL.

QUESTIONS

1. *What initial findings in this patient's diagnostic and laboratory tests are consistent with acute coronary syndrome (ACS)?*

The triad of diagnostic criteria for AMI is symptoms of chest pain, ECG, and elevated biochemical markers. Symptoms include neck and chest pressure-like pain, rated 7–8/10 in severity with diaphoresis and radiation to the left scapula. The ECG is not diagnostic of AMI at this point— no T wave abnormalities, ST-segment elevation or depression, or Q waves are detected. Initially, none of the markers were elevated. However J. D.'s symptoms started 3 hr prior to presentation, and the release kinetics of both CK-MB and troponin I are such that the levels begin to rise between 3–12 hr after onset of AMI. Because the clinical presentation is highly suspicious of a cardiac etiology for the chest pain, a second set of markers was drawn and the levels were assessed 6–12 hr after onset of symptoms.

Another option would be to check myoglobin or CK-MB2 isoform levels since they are released earlier after AMI and their concentrations start to rise in the peripheral circulation between 1–4 hr post-MI. Relying on a single test of CK, CK-MB, or myoglobin is not prudent because of the lack of cardiac specificity of these lab tests. In this case, for example, myositis or rhabdomyolysis secondary to simvastatin intake may lead to elevation in the aforementioned biochemical markers. To the contrary, troponin I is a sensitive and highly cardiac specific biochemical marker and may be used as the only marker to diagnose AMI when drawn at appropriate times from time of onset of chest pain.

2. *Based on the symptoms, ECG findings, and biochemical markers, what type of ACS is this patient experiencing? Justify your answer.*

This patient is experiencing NSTEMI. The symptoms are consistent with anginal pain. Because the biochemical markers are elevated, myocardial infarction is most likely rather than unstable angina. ECG did not show any ST-segment elevation.

Wafa Y. Dahdal

CC: *"I have chest pain."*

HPI:

J. K. is a 68-year-old Caucasian man who present to the emergency department (ED) with complaints of chest pain that started earlier today. This is the first time he experiences such pain. The pain started suddenly, was nonradiating, and was rate 7/10 in intensity. The patient did not identify any aggravating factors, and the pain was not reproducible by pressure. He measured his blood pressure (192/120) and took one of his wife's medications. Pain was not associated with shortness of breath, dizziness, diaphoresis, nausea, or vomiting.

PMH:

N/C

FH:

N/C

SH:

JK is a retired engineer and lives with his wife. He denies tobacco, alcohol, or illicit drug use.

MEDS:

None

ALLERGIES:

NKDA

ROS:

Unremarkable except for chest pain

PE:

GEN: A& O × 3; in NAD
VS: BP 116/80; HR 62; RR 12; T 37.1 °C; HT 6'2"; and WT 243 lb
HEENT: PERRLA, EOMI
NECK: Supple, (-) JVD, (-) lymphadenopathy
CV: RRR, normal S_1S_2, (-) M/G/R
LUNGS: CTAB
ABD: Soft, NT, (+) BS, (-) organomegaly
EXT: (-) edema
NEURO: CN II-XIII intact; no focal deficits noted

LABS:

$$\begin{array}{c} \dfrac{134}{3.8} \bigg| \dfrac{100}{20} \bigg| \dfrac{16}{1.0} \bigg\langle 125 \end{array}$$

$$11.21 \bigg\rangle \dfrac{17.7}{49} \bigg\langle 222$$

Ca^{+2}: 9.1 mg/dL

INR 1.0; aPTT 32.6 sec

Lipid panel (hospital day 2 @ 0500): Cholesterol 248 mg/dL; LDL 198 mg/dL; HDL 38 mg/dL; and TG 241 mg/dL.

ECG:

(In the ED): ST-segment depression in leads V_1 to V_4 consistent with anterior wall MI

CXR:

(In the ED): Normal cardiac markers; no evidence of pulmonary congestion

LABS:

Hospital Day	Time	CK (32–237 U/L)	CK-MB (0–5.0 ng/mL)	CK-MB Index (0.0–6.0%)	Troponin I* (ng/mL)
1	1930	396	21.1	5.3	3.0
2	0500	681	55.3	8.1	21.73
	1049	644	44.5	6.9	14.14
3	0455	396	13.7	3.5	12.78
4	0455	248	5.2	2.1	4.86

*Median values for (1) apparently healthy person ≤0.07 ng/mL; (2) noncardiac related disorder <0.10 ng/mL; (3) diagnostic cutoff for AMI patients 1.5 ng/mL; and (4) confirmed MI 7.6 ng/mL.

QUESTIONS

1. *What laboratory abnormalities are consistent with acute coronary syndrome (ACS) in this patient?*

   At presentation, all biochemical markers (CK, CK-MB, and troponin I) are elevated beyond the upper limits of normal. The initial CK-MB index is 5.3%, which is less than the diagnostic cutoff for a cardiac etiology for CK elevation versus noncardiac etiologies. Used alone, this may lead to uncertain attribution of the chest pain to a cardiac etiology or to inaccurate differentiation between UA and AMI. Cardiac specific troponin I is highly sensitive and is more specific to myocardial damage. The initial troponin is elevated beyond the diagnostic cutoff for AMI (1.5 ng/mL), which leads to a more confident and accurate diagnosis of AMI. Based on the patient's chest pain symptoms, ECG changes, and the elevated biochemical markers, the diagnosis is NSTEMI.

2. *Based on the following plot of biochemical markers elevation vs. time for J. K., which would be an appropriate test to assess for myocardial ischemia if he presented 3 days post-onset of symptoms?*

   Troponin I is the ideal marker in this situation since the CK-MB and the CK levels are superimposed at 1 × the AMI cutoff limit (CK-MB index is 3.5%). Like troponin I, both CK and CK-MB begin to rise 3–12 hr after AMI and peak at 24 hr. However, CK and CK-MB return to normal concentrations in 2–3 days while troponin I remains elevated for 5–10 days afterwards.

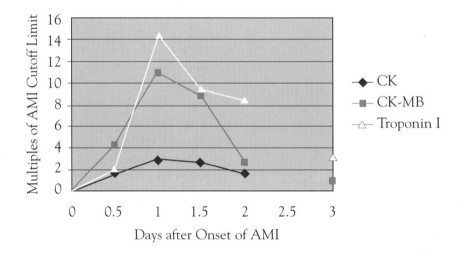

Wafa Y. Dahdal

CC: *R. S. is a 51-year-old man who presents to the emergency department complaining that his foot hurts so much that he can't get his shoe on.*

CASE 11

HPI:

He has severe pain in his right great toe that started after he returned from a business convention two days ago. The pain has been persistent and increasing since the initial morning and has awakened him from sleep two nights in a row. He states that it is difficult to even put weight on his right foot without experiencing excruciating pain. He has been taking acetaminophen 500 mg, 2 tablets qid since the onset of pain without significant relief.

PMH:

Hypertension for 5 years; seasonal allergic rhinitis, worse in the spring and fall; and dyslipidemia

FH:

Both parents are deceased. Father had hypertension and diabetes and died of renal failure. Mother died of ovarian cancer. Patient has no siblings.

SH:

R. S. is employed as a manager for a local department store; the job is primarily sedentary, and he does not attempt to exercise regularly. He smokes one pack of cigarettes/day and has one to two martinis with dinner and occasionally during lunch. He is divorced and lives alone.

MEDS:

Hydrochlorothiazide 25 mg po once daily
Fexofenadine 60 mg/pseudoephedrine 120 mg extended-release tablets, 1 tablet po twice daily as needed
Atorvastatin 10 mg once daily
Acetaminophen 500 mg, 2 tablets po qid since onset of foot pain

ALLERGIES:

No known drug or food allergies

ROS:

No headache, dizziness, rhinorrhea, sneezing, itching, or generalized swelling or tenderness in the joints; no chest pain or shortness of breath; and no nausea, vomiting, diarrhea

PE:

GEN: Well-developed, well-nourished man grimacing in pain and taking care not to put weight on his right foot

VS: BP 138/86; HR 89; RR 24; T 100.3 °F; HT 5'11"; and WT 98 kg

HEENT: Pupils equal, round, and reactive to light; no AV nicking, hemorrhages, or exudates

CHEST/THORAX: Lungs clear to auscultation and percussion

CV: RRR, normal S_1 and S_2, (-) S3 or S4; (-) murmurs; carotids palpable bilaterally

ABD: Obese; nontender, nondistended; (+) bowel sounds; no hepatosplenomegaly

GENIT/RECT: No rectal masses; normal prostate; stool guaiac (-)

EXT: The right first MTP joint is swollen, warm, erythematous, and very tender to the touch. The ankle and remaining digits on that foot are normal. The left foot is normal. There are no other joint abnormalities.

NEURO: Patient is alert and oriented to person, place, and time; cranial nerves II through XII are intact. No focal abnormalities.

LABS:

Hemoglobin 15.2 g/dL, hematocrit 46%, WBC 12.0×10^3/mm³ with 60% neutrophils, 3% bands, 36% lymphocytes, and 1% eosinophils. Sodium 142 mEq/L, potassium 4.1 mEq/L, chloride 100 mEq/L, total CO_2 22 mEq/L, BUN 12 mg/dL, creatinine 1.0 mg/dL, and glucose 101 mg/dL. Uric acid 11.5 mg/dL, erythrocyte sedimentation rate (Westergren) 22 mm/hr. Urinalysis: Negative.

OTHER TESTS:

X-ray right great toe: Some soft tissue swelling; normal joint spaces; and no evidence of fracture or trauma.

Right great toe synovial fluid aspirate: Abundant PMNs and intracellular monosodium urate crystals.

PROBLEM LIST

- Hyperuricemia with probable gout
- Hypertension, controlled with thiazide diuretic
- Hyperlipidemia treated with statin; repeat fasting lipid panel at next routine visit
- History of seasonal allergic rhinitis

QUESTIONS

1. *Which of the available serum laboratory tests can be used to make the presumptive diagnosis of acute gouty arthritis in this patient?*

   The presumptive diagnosis of gout is often made on the basis of the clinical presentation and the presence of hyperuricemia (serum uric acid level >7 mg/dL). However, serum uric acid levels can be normal at the time of an acute attack, and the presence of hyperuricemia alone is not always associated with gouty arthritis.

2. *What is the value of obtaining a synovial fluid aspirate of the affected joint in this patient who has classic clinical findings of gout as well as hyperuricemia?*

   Even though the clinical presentation and serum uric acid level suggest gout as the underlying disorder, needle aspiration of the acutely inflamed joint(s) is necessary to confirm the diagnosis. A number of other disorders may closely mimic the symptoms of gout (e.g., acute septic arthritis, other crystalline-associated arthropathies, and psoriatic arthritis). When examined using polarized light microscopy, the presence of needle-shaped, strongly negative birefringent monosodium urate crystals within neutrophils is pathognomonic of gout.

   The synovial fluid in gout is also characterized by the presence of inflammatory cells, with a white blood cell count ranging from 5000 to $50,000 \times 10^3/mm^3$, predominantly neutrophils.

3. *This patient was treated with a 5-day course of a nonsteroidal anti-inflammatory medication for acute gouty arthritis and referred to his physician for a 24-hr urine collection for uric acid. Why is this test useful if the diagnosis of gout has already been made?*

   Oral nonsteroidal anti-inflammatory drugs, colchicine, or corticosteroids are usually effective in relieving the acute gouty episode within several days, but they have no effect on reducing elevated serum uric acid levels. Patients with chronic hyperuricemia who have one attack of gout are predisposed to subsequent attacks as well as to the development of uric acid nephropathy, nephrolithiasis, and tophaceous gout. A 24-hr urine collection for measurement of uric acid is valuable for assessing the risk of nephrolithiasis, determining whether the patient is an overproducer or underexcretor of uric acid, and in deciding which hypouricemic regimen to use chronically to prevent future attacks and complications of gout.

   If hyperuricemic patients who are maintained on a regular diet excrete more than 800 mg of uric acid per day, this suggests that the patient is overproducing uric acid. In this situation, an agent that decreases synthesis of uric acid is preferred. Hyperuricemic patients who excrete less than 600 mg of uric acid per day on a regular diet are considered to be underexcretors of uric acid.

4. *This patient's 24-hr urine collection revealed the presence of 1050 mg of uric acid per 24 hr. If prophylactic therapy is considered to be indicated, what drug and dosage regimen would provide optimal therapy?*

   Allopurinol (a xanthine oxidase inhibitor) is the drug of choice in individuals who have been shown to be overproducers of uric acid. It is also the drug of choice in patients with uric acid kidney stones, to prevent tumor lysis syndrome in patients receiving cancer chemotherapy associated with high nucleic acid turnover, and in individuals with severe renal impairment. The initial allopurinol dose is 100 mg once daily, with subsequent weekly dosage increases to 300 mg po once daily. The dosage must be reduced in the presence of renal impairment.

   If this patient had been found to be an underexcretor of uric acid, a uricosuric agent such as probenecid could be used if renal function was adequate. Adequate urine volume must be maintained (at least 1500 mL/day) to prevent urate crystal deposition in the kidneys. Probenecid is ineffective in patients with severe renal impairment and should not be used to prevent tumor lysis syndrome in patients undergoing cancer chemotherapy.

5. *How should the allopurinol therapy be monitored for efficacy and adverse effects?*

A measurable decrease in serum uric acid levels may be observed within 2–3 days after the start of therapy. Normal serum urate levels are usually achieved within 1–3 weeks. Although urine uric acid levels will also decline, it is generally not necessary to repeat the 24-hr urine collection. The magnitude of the decrease in serum uric acid is dose-dependent to a certain degree. The allopurinol dose can be increased to a maximum of 800 mg/day in patients not achieving a satisfactory response with the standard dose. The serum uric acid will increase slowly to pretreatment levels if therapy is discontinued.

The adverse effects of allopurinol include skin rash, occasional gastrointestinal symptoms (nausea, vomiting, abdominal pain), increased frequency of acute gouty attacks at the start of therapy (due to mobilization of tissue urate stores), hepatic injury, leukopenia, and rarely agranulocytosis and aplastic anemia. Periodic liver and renal function tests should be performed. Some clinicians monitor a complete blood cell count periodically, especially during the first few months of therapy. A complete blood cell should be obtained if clinical signs or symptoms of myelosuppression develop.

6. *At the time of initial presentation, was this patient taking any medications that could affect his serum uric acid level?*

Thiazide diuretics (e.g., hydrochlorothiazide) are associated with elevated serum uric acid levels and can precipitate attacks of acute gouty arthritis. Because these diuretics are weak acids and are secreted by the proximal renal tubules (as is uric acid), there may be competition for renal excretion. The magnitude of this effect is dose dependent, and chronic administration increases the serum uric acid level in many patients. Loop diuretics may also cause hyperuricemia by inhibiting renal excretion of uric acid and perhaps due to volume contraction and the resultant increased uric acid reabsorption in the proximal tubules.

7. *Does the patient have any concurrent disease states that are associated with increased risk for the development of acute gouty arthritis?*

Comorbidities present in this patient that have been shown to be associated with hyperuricemia and gout include hypertension, obesity (primarily truncal), and dyslipidemia (hypertriglyceridemia and low HDL cholesterol). Other comorbidities with a similar association that are not present in this patient include type 2 diabetes mellitus and coronary atherosclerotic heart disease.

Terry L. Schwinghammer

CC: *L. N., a 52-year-old woman, presents to the ambulatory care clinic for follow-up of her complaints of fatigue, weakness, decreased appetite, muscle aches, and pain and stiffness in her hands.*

CASE 12

HPI:

The patient states that the stiffness and pain in her hands have increased during the 3 months since her last visit despite adherence to twice daily naproxen. She reports that there is now some redness and swelling around the joints of her hands. The joint stiffness is worse in the morning after she arises, but she slowly "loosens up" throughout the morning. She is beginning to have difficulty performing ordinary tasks without pain, such as opening jars and using hand tools at home and at work.

PMH:

Patient has hypertension (5 years), currently well-controlled on diet and medications. She has a history of depression, treated with sertraline. She had a cholecystectomy 10 years ago

FH:

Mother had RA and diabetes; died of breast cancer in her 70s. Father had HTN, diabetes, and renal failure. The patient has one sister who lives out of state.

SH:

Patient is an elementary school teacher. She is married and has two grown children. She does not smoke cigarettes but has one or two glasses of wine per week during dinner. She adheres to a no-added-salt diet to help control her blood pressure. She goes on a long walk "on most days" in an attempt to keep fit and control BP.

MEDS:

Hydrochlorothiazide 25 mg po once daily
Lisinopril 20 mg po once daily
Sertraline 50 mg once daily
Naproxen 500 mg twice daily as needed
Multiple vitamin 1 tablet daily

ALLERGIES:

Sulfa → skin rash

ROS:

Pain and stiffness in both hands; no pain reported in shoulders, elbows, wrists, hips, knees, ankles, or feet. Also complains of fatigue, especially during the late afternoon. Some loss of appetite despite a good overall mood. No nausea, vomiting, diarrhea, stomach/abdominal pain, or blood in stool. Reports some small weight loss (<5 lb.). Denies headache or chest pain.

PE:

GEN: Well-developed, well-nourished woman in mild discomfort

VS: BP 126/84; HR 72; RR 16; T 99.4 °F; HT 5'6"; and WT 55 kg

HEENT: Head normocephalic, atraumatic; pupils are equal, round, and reactive to light; extraocular movements intact; funduscopic exam not performed

NECK: Supple; no JVD or thyromegaly; no lymphadenopathy

CHEST/THORAX: Clear to auscultation and percussion

CV: RRR, normal S1 and S2; no S3 or S4; no murmurs, rubs, or gallops

ABD: Nontender, nondistended; bowel sounds present

GENIT/RECT: No masses; guaiac (–) stool

EXT: Redness, warmth, tenderness, and swelling of 2nd, 3rd, and 4th proximal interphalangeal (PIP) joints bilaterally; the distal interphalangeal (DIP) and metacarpophalangeal (MCP) joints appear normal; there is decreased grip strength bilaterally; and there is some minor tenderness and decreased range of motion of both wrists; no Boutonniere deformity, ulnar deviation, or subcutaneous nodules noted; and the remainder of the exam was normal

NEURO: Alert and oriented to person, place, and time; cranial nerves II through XII are intact; and there are no focal abnormalities

LABS:

Hemoglobin 11.5 g/dL, hematocrit 36%, WBC 5.3×10^3/mm³, platelets 380×10^3/mm³; MCV 90 fL, MCH 32 pg/cell, MCHC 33%, reticulocytes 0.8%; sodium 139 mEq/L, potassium 4.2 mEq/L, chloride 102 mEq/L, total CO_2 24 mEq/L, BUN 12 mg/dL, creatinine 0.8 mg/dL, glucose 120 mg/dL (random); AST 24 IU/L, ALT 28 IU/L, alkaline phosphatase 90 IU/L, total bilirubin 1.0 mg/dL, and albumin 4.4 g/dL; erythrocyte sedimentation rate (Westergren method) 48 mm/hr, rheumatoid factor (+) 1:1280, antinuclear antibody (-); C-reactive protein 11 mg/dL.

OTHER TESTS:

Hand x-ray: There is soft-tissue swelling of the PIP joints bilaterally; no erosions, decalcification, or joint space narrowing.

PROBLEM LIST

- New-onset rheumatoid arthritis
- Hypertension, well controlled with diet and medications
- History of depression, treated with sertraline

QUESTIONS

1. *Which one of the available laboratory tests can be most helpful in establishing the diagnosis of rheumatoid arthritis in this patient?*

   An abnormally high serum rheumatoid factor titer is one of the seven criteria established by the American Rheumatism Association for the classification of rheumatoid arthritis. Rheumatoid factors are immunoglobulins that are directed abnormally against the Fc portion of IgG. Because these immunoglobulins do not recognize IgG as "self", the presence of RFs in the blood indicates an autoimmune process. A titer of ≥1:160 is generally is considered to be positive. Patients with rheumatoid arthritis usually have RF titers of at least 1:320. As the titer increases, the specificity of the test for RA also increases. When tested by a method that has been shown to be positive in <5% of normal control subjects, approximately 70–90% of patients with rheumatoid arthritis have a positive RF titer. Although some patients with rheumatoid arthritis do not have a positive titer (so-called seronegative rheumatoid arthritis), some of these patients convert to seropositive upon repeat testing. A small percentage of adult patients with rheumatoid arthritis (<10%) are truly seronegative. It is important to note that a positive rheumatoid factor is not specific for rheumatoid arthritis; other disorders that may be associated with a positive titer include Sjögren's syndrome, systemic lupus erythematosus, progressive systemic sclerosis, polymyositis/dermatomyositis, some infectious diseases (e.g., endocarditis, and tuberculosis), and some other nonrheumatologic disorders (e.g., pulmonary fibrosis, hepatic cirrhosis, and sarcoidosis).

2. *What information does the erythrocyte sedimentation rate provide? How does its usefulness for diagnosing rheumatoid arthritis differ from the rheumatoid factor test?*

   The erythrocyte sedimentation rate (ESR) is a commonly-used but nonspecific test that indicates the presence of an ongoing generalized inflammatory process. The Westergren method is used more commonly than the Wintrobe ESR because of relative ease in performing the procedure. Because it is nonspecific, the ESR is not diagnostic of any given disease.

3. *The hematology tests for this patient indicate a mild anemia. Because myelosuppression is a potential toxicity of some disease-modifying antirheumatic drugs, should the patient be tested and treated for anemia caused by iron, B$_{12}$, or folic acid deficiency?*

   It is not uncommon to observe a mild to moderate anemia associated with rheumatoid arthritis. In addition, this patient is taking naproxen that, like other nonsteroidal anti-inflammatory drugs, has been associated with gastritis and gastrointestinal bleeding and ulceration. However, evaluation of the red blood cell (Wintrobe) indices in this patient indicate that the patient's anemia is normochromic and normocytic (i.e., the MCV, MCH, and MCHC are normal). This "anemia of chronic disease" is characteristic of the anemia that is seen with rheumatoid arthritis. In other anemias, the RBC indices would be expected to show microcytosis (iron deficiency, chronic GI bleeding) or macrocytosis (B$_{12}$ or folate deficiency). Furthermore, this patient's stool is guaiac-negative, making ongoing GI hemorrhage less likely. A more complete evaluation of the cause of anemia should be conducted if there are other laboratory or clinical indications that it may be due to something other than rheumatoid arthritis.

4. *If this patient is started on an effective disease-modifying antirheumatic agent, what will be the effect of therapy upon the ESR and RF tests?*

   In general, laboratory monitoring is of little value of assessing an individual patient's response to antirheumatic drug therapy. The effectiveness of therapy is more precisely evaluated by careful questioning of the patient about improvement or worsening of symptoms. The caregiver must also perform a thorough physical examination and perhaps other tests (e.g., x-rays) to assess improvement or worsening of joint manifestations, constitutional symptoms, and development of extra-articular complications such as rheumatoid nodules, vasculitis, pulmonary fibrosis, and pericarditis. Evaluation of serial ESR results may be useful, because the ESR generally declines as the inflammatory process is brought under control. Similarly, subsequent rises in ESR may indicate a disease exacerbation.

5. *Is this patient taking any medications that may cause a false-positive antinuclear antibody (ANA) test? What are the most common medications that cause this effect?*

   No, this patient is not taking any medications that are likely to cause a false-positive ANA test. Over 35 drugs have been known to cause this effect; they may also be associated with a condition that includes SLE symptoms, called drug-induced lupus. The symptoms usually disappear when the medications are discontinued. The medications most closely associated with this effect include hydralazine, isoniazid, and procainamide. Based on this patient's history, it is conceivable (though it seems unlikely) that hydralazine could eventually be used to treat her hypertension. If that were to occur, the possibility that a false-positive ANA might occur would have to be kept in mind.

6. *This patient has an elevated C-reactive protein (CRP) value (reference range 1–3 mg/dL). Does an elevated CRP carry any potential significance other than as a marker for a generalized inflammatory process?*

   CRP is an inflammatory marker that is often elevated in rheumatoid arthritis and other inflammatory disorders, infection, and trauma. Because it is nonspecific, it is usually no more helpful than the ESR in diagnosing rheumatic conditions. Recent studies have found that CRP is also released in response to inflammatory markers present within atherosclerotic plaques. When using a new high-sensitivity CRP (hs-CRP) test, data from several clinical studies have shown a correlation between elevated hs-CRP levels and cardiovascular events in patients with coronary heart disease, independent of serum lipid concentrations. In fact, some studies indicate that hs-CRP levels may be more predictive of subsequent cardiovascular disease than LDL cholesterol levels. The American Heart Association now recommends obtaining hs-CRP levels in selected patients. At the time of this writing, no clinical trials had been conducted to determine whether treating patients on the basis of elevated hs-CRP levels alone is beneficial or cost-effective. Thus, the exact role of hs-CRP testing as a predictor of cardiovascular disease awaits the results of further clinical studies.

7. *Because this patient has had an inadequate response to NSAID therapy after a trial of regular use for 3 months, the decision is made to continue naproxen and start the disease-modifying antirheumatic drug methotrexate in order to prevent joint erosions and potentially arrest the disease process. What initial dose should be recommended, and how should the therapy be monitored to detect or prevent adverse effects?*

   The usual starting dose of methotrexate is 7.5 mg given as a single dose once weekly. An alternative regimen is to give the totally weekly dose as a divided dose of 2.5 mg every 12 hr for 3 doses. The maximum recommended dose is 20 mg once weekly. The dose should be reduced to the lowest effective dose once a response has been achieved.

   In addition to gastrointestinal adverse effects (e.g., nausea, stomatitis, GI discomfort, diarrhea, vomiting, and anorexia), abnormal laboratory findings may include elevation of hepatic enzymes and myelosuppression (leukopenia, thrombocytopenia, anemia). Renal insufficiency may delay excretion of the drug, increasing the risk of myelosuppression.

   Baseline laboratory tests that should be obtained before starting therapy should therefore assess hepatic, bone marrow, and renal function. These tests include AST, ALT, alkaline phosphatase, serum albumin, total bilirubin, hepatitis B and C serologies, complete blood cell count with platelets and differential, and serum creatinine. Once therapy is begun, it is prudent to repeat the complete blood cell count with platelets, ALT, albumin, and serum creatinine periodically (e.g., every 1–3 months).

   Terry L. Schwinghammer

CC: *D. J. is an 8-year-old male, who was admitted to the emergency room from a local pediatric long-term care facility with c/o pain, tenderness, and decreased movement to his right leg.*

HPI:

D. J. sustained a fall at the long-term care facility when he was being moved from his bed to his wheel chair.

PMH:

Born at 40 weeks gestational age, D. J. suffered a traumatic birth with severe perinatal asphyxia. He subsequently developed seizures during his stay in the neonatal nursery. Seizures were controlled by the combined anticonvulsant therapy of phenobarbital and phenytoin. As a result of his asphyxia at birth, D. J. developed spastic cerebral palsy and severe neurodevelopmental delay. He was transferred to the long-term care facility at 6 months of age and has been a resident there ever since. At 2 years of age an attempt was made to discontinue phenytoin, but D. J. had an episode of status epilepticus. Therefore, he has remained on phenobarbital and phenytoin since that time. At 6 years of age D. J. was diagnosed with gastroesophageal reflux disease (GERD), which has been controlled with antacids.

FH:

Noncontributory

SH:

Noncontributory

MEDS:

Phenobarbital elixir 40 mg (10 mL) po bid
Phenytoin suspension 50 mg (2 mL) po tid
Alternagel® 5 mL po qid

ALLERGIES:

No known drug allergy; allergic to strawberries

PE:

GEN: Underdeveloped, small-for-age male, sleeping, and in no apparent distress

VS: BP 105/69; HR 90; RR 22; T 98.6 °F; HT 124 cm (25th percentile for age); and WT 20 kg (<5th percentile for age)

HEENT: No significant findings

CHEST: Pigeon breast deformity; slightly palpable enlargement of costochondral junctions

CV: RRR, (-) murmurs

ABD: No significant findings

EXT: Redness in right leg, 10 cm below knee; pain on movement; left leg: unremarkable

LABS:

Sodium 140 mEq/L, potassium 3.8 mEq/L, chloride 102 mEq/L, total CO_2 28 mEq/L, BUN 12 mg/dL, Cr 0.4 mg/dL, glucose 97 mg/dL; calcium 8.0 mg/dL (normal for children: 8.8–10.8 mg/dL); and albumin 2.8 g/dL (normal for children 7–19 years: 3.7–5.6 g/dL).

OTHER TESTS:

Preliminary x-ray findings: Fracture of right tibia; osteomalacia and bone changes consistent with rickets.

PROBLEM LIST

- Fracture of right tibia
- Hypocalcemia
- Probable rickets
- Hypoalbuminemia
- Seizure disorder, currently controlled with phenobarbital and phenytoin
- GERD, currently controlled with antacids
- Spastic cerebral palsy
- Neurodevelopmental delay

QUESTIONS

1. *The preliminary x-ray findings and the physical findings of the pigeon breast deformity (i.e., the sternum and adjacent cartilage appear to be projected forward) and the palpable enlargement of costochondral junctions (rachitic rosary sign) are compatible with the diagnosis of rickets. However, rickets is diagnosed by both radiologic and chemical findings. Hypocalcemia may occur in patients with rickets. What other laboratory tests are required in order to diagnose rickets in this patient?*

   Serum calcium may be low or normal in patients with rickets, depending on the etiology. The primary causes of rickets in the United States are: vitamin D deficiency (with secondary hyperparathyroidism), primary phosphate deficiency, and end-organ resistance to 1,25-dihydroxy-vitamin D. In patients with vitamin D deficiency, serum calcium concentrations can be normal or low, phosphorus concentrations are usually low, and alkaline phosphatase activity is elevated. In patients with primary phosphate deficiency, serum calcium is normal, serum phosphorus is low, and alkaline phosphatase is elevated. In patients with end-organ resistance to 1,25-dihydroxy-vitamin D, serum calcium is low, serum phosphorus may be low or normal, and serum alkaline phosphatase is elevated.

   To properly diagnose rickets in this patient, a serum phosphorus and alkaline phosphatase are needed. A serum magnesium should also be obtained since hypomagnesemia may cause hypocalcemia.

2. *What other laboratory test should be drawn to better assess this patient's calcium status?*

   This patient also has hypoalbuminemia. A total serum calcium measures all three forms of extracellular calcium: complex bound, protein bound, and ionized. In patients with low albumin, the concentration of ionized calcium will be increased for a given total serum calcium concentration. Equations can be used to "correct" total serum calcium measurements for low concentrations of serum albumin, but these equations have limitations and may not be precise. Thus, in patients with low albumin, an ionized serum calcium should be obtained.

3. *Due to your recommendations from # 1 and # 2 above, the following lab tests results are obtained:*
   - Ionized calcium: 4.1 mg/dL (normal for infants–adults: 4.8–4.92 mg/dL)
   - Phosphorus: 2.1 mg/dL (normal for 4–11 years old: 3.7–5.6 mg/dL)
   - Mg: 1.8 mg/dL (normal for 2–14 years of age: 1.5– 2.3 mg/dL)
   - ALT: 55 U/L (normal for children and adults: 1–30 U/L
   - AST: 63 U/L (normal for children and adults: 0–35 U/L
   - Alkaline Phosphatase: 674 U/L (normal for children 2–19 years of age: 100–320 U/L)

   What is your assessment of these laboratory values?

   Ionized calcium and serum phosphorus are both low and serum alkaline phosphatase is high, all of which are consistent with a diagnosis of rickets. Serum magnesium is normal for age. ALT and AST are slightly elevated.

4. *The patient is admitted to the hospital and his leg fracture is cast. His medications prior to admission are continued and he is started on oral supplements of calcium (as calcium glubionate), phosphorus (as potassium phosphate) and Vitamin D (as ergocalciferol). How frequently should this patient's serum calcium, phosphorus and alkaline phosphatase be monitored?*

   Since significantly low concentrations of either calcium or phosphorus may cause seizures, it would be important to closely monitor this patient's serum calcium and phosphorus. Although it will take a while for both to be corrected to normal values, measurement several times weekly is needed at first to make certain they are not decreasing further. Once calcium and phosphorus begin to rise, they can be monitored less frequently. However, the rate of rise should also be assessed, because hypercalcemia and hyperphosphatemia can occur. This would be due to the increased oral intake of calcium and phosphorus and the effects of vitamin D. It should be noted that nutritional rickets and osteomalacia are usually treated with vitamin D therapy for 6–12 weeks.

Evidence of radiographic healing of rickets may begin to be seen within 2–4 weeks. However, alkaline phosphatase levels will take longer to decrease to normal levels. Alkaline phosphatase may be measured weekly until a significant decline is observed and less frequently thereafter.

5. *How did this patient's medications prior to admission affect his serum phosphorus, calcium, and liver enzymes?*

    This patient is receiving an aluminum-containing antacid, which will bind phosphorus in the gastrointestinal tract. This resulted in decreased absorption of phosphorus and contributed to this patient's low serum phosphorus.

    Enzyme inducing anticonvulsants, such as phenobarbital and phenytoin, will increase the metabolism of vitamin D and may result in a deficiency of vitamin D with a resultant anticonvulsant-induced osteomalacia and rickets.

    Both the aluminum-containing antacid and the anticonvulsants contributed to this patient developing rickets and thus to the elevated serum alkaline phosphatase.

6. *What other factors contributed to this patient's development of rickets?*

    Due to this patient's other medical conditions, he is nonambulatory and resides at a long-term care facility. Thus, he may have a lack of exposure to sunlight and, therefore, a lack of vitamin D.

    This lack of vitamin D would also contribute to the development of rickets.

7. *How would you modify this patient's drug therapy?*

    The aluminum-containing antacid (Alternagel®) should be discontinued and replaced with a calcium containing antacid (e.g., calcium carbonate). The amount of calcium in this new antacid should then be subtracted from the calcium supplement that was started in the hospital, so that the total daily dose of calcium stays the same. Alternatively, the total dose of calcium supplement can be given as calcium carbonate. Discontinuing the aluminum-containing antacid will result in a greater amount of phosphorus absorbed enterally. This will then require a decrease in the oral supplement of phosphate (depending on serum phosphorus concentrations).

Donna M. Kraus

CASE 14

CC: G. N. is a 2-day-old female who is currently in the neonatal ICU being treated with antibiotics for suspected sepsis. This morning G. N. began having rhythmic clonic twitching of her lower extremities, fluttering of her eyelids, and repetitive chewing movements.

PMH:

G. N. was born at 39 weeks gestation to a mother with prolonged rupture of membranes (>72 hr). On the day of her birth, G. N. was admitted to the neonatal ICU with an elevated temperature, tachycardia (HR 153) and low WBC count (3.5×10^3 cells/mm^3). Blood and urine cultures were obtained and antibiotics were started to treat her possible sepsis. Culture results are still pending.

FH:

Noncontributory

SH:

Noncontributory

MEDS:

Ampicillin 85 mg IV in 25 mL D5W as IV rider q 8 hr (75 mg/kg/day)

Gentamicin 8.5 mg IV in 25 mL D5W as IV rider q 12 hr (5 mg/kg/day)

ALLERGIES:

No known allergies

PE:

GEN: Normal size for age, well-nourished with intermittent movements consistent with seizure activity

VS: BP 76/46; HR 125; RR 35; T 98.8 °F; HT 49 cm (50th percentile for age); and WT 3.4 kg (50th percentile for age)

HEENT: Occasional episodes of fluttering of eyelids

CHEST: No significant findings

CV: RRR, no murmurs

ABD: No significant findings

EXT: Upper extremities: no significant findings; lower extremities: episodes of rhythmic clonic twitching

LABS:

Sodium 120 mEq/L, potassium 3.9 mEq/L, chloride 98 mEq/L, total CO_2 20 mEq/L, BUN 8 mg/dL, Cr 0.8 mg/dL, and glucose 87 mg/d/L.

PROBLEM LIST

- Seizures
- Hyponatremia
- Possible sepsis (r/o sepsis)

QUESTIONS

1. *What is the most likely cause of this patient's seizure activity and electrolyte imbalance?*

   Electrolyte imbalance is a common cause of neonatal seizures. As in adults, hyponatremia may cause seizure activity in neonates and occurs when the ratio of water to sodium is increased. The total body content of sodium in patients with hyponatremia may be low, normal or high, and the volume status may be hypovolemic, euvolemic or hypervolemic.

   There are many causes of hyponatremia, but the most likely cause in this patient is the extra D5W that the patient received with her antibiotics. Dilutional hyponatremia may occur in neonates and young infants when medications are administered in excess fluids, such as IV riders of 5% dextrose in water. These patients are more prone to water overload due to their lower glomerular filtration rate and their limited ability to excrete water. Medications for these patients should be diluted in smaller amounts of IV fluid, so that excess fluid is not administered.

   To better define this patient's sodium and volume status, G. N.'s total fluid intake and output, type of IV fluids administered, changes in body weight, and other laboratory data need to be assessed. In addition, other causes of hyponatremia, such as meningitis and SIADH, should be ruled out.

2. *What other laboratory tests should be obtained to further assess this patient's seizure disorder?*

   Although the most likely cause of this patient's seizure activity is her low serum sodium, serum calcium, phosphorous, and magnesium should also be assessed, as other electrolyte abnormalities can also cause seizure activity.

3. *The clinicians appropriately treat G. N.'s symptomatic hyponatremia with hypertonic saline and closely monitor her serum sodium. G. N.'s antibiotics are no longer being given as IV riders and are being administered in an appropriate amount of IV fluid. Her seizure activity is now controlled. G. N.'s serum calcium, phosphorous and magnesium are found to be within the normal range for her age. Later that day, G. N. experienced a prolonged episode of apnea with hypoxia and respiratory arrest. G. N. is intubated and placed on mechanical ventilation. Her blood culture results come back positive for a gram-negative bacteria (identification pending). The next morning (day 3 of life), the following laboratory results are obtained:*

   LABS: Sodium 133 mEq/L, potassium 5.7 mEq/L, chloride 100 mEq/L, total CO_2 19 mEq/L, BUN 14 mg/dL, Cr 1.2 mg/dL, glucose 83 mg/d/L, serum albumin, 2.9 g/dL, and total bilirubin, 16 mg/dL.

   PROBLEM LIST: Sepsis, renal dysfunction, and hyperbilirubinemia.

   Which of the above laboratory results should be used to assess the safety of G. N.'s gentamicin therapy?

   Aminoglycoside antibiotics may cause nephrotoxicity, with elevations in serum creatinine and BUN. G. N.'s serum creatinine has increased from 0.8 mg/dL to 1.2 mg/dL, and her BUN has increased from 8 mg/dL to 14 mg/dL in 24 hr. However, G. N. has only been receiving gentamicin for a short time, and aminoglycoside nephrotoxicity in newborns receiving appropriate doses of gentamicin rarely occurs. A more likely reason for G. N.'s increase in BUN and serum creatinine is renal dysfunction due to the prolonged episode of hypoxia and respiratory arrest. Hypoxia decreases the delivery of oxygen to the tissues and can result in damage to internal organs, including the brain, kidney, and liver. This patient's hypoxia may have caused renal injury resulting in the increase in serum creatinine and BUN.

4. *How frequently should G. N.'s serum creatinine be monitored?*

It may take several days after G. N.'s hypoxic insult for serum creatinine to reach its maximum value. During this time, renal function is very unstable. G. N.'s serum creatinine should be frequently monitored (e.g., 1–2 times per day) to better assess her worsening renal function. Once it stabilizes, serum creatinine could be monitored daily.

It should be noted that although serum potassium is still within the normal range for newborns (3.7–5.9 mEq/L), a significant rise from 3.9–5.7 mEq/L has occurred. One would expect serum potassium to increase further in this patient due to her renal dysfunction. Serum potassium, therefore, should be monitored closely and appropriate treatment of hyperkalemia should be readily available.

5. *Will G. N.'s antibiotics interfere with the determination of serum creatinine?*

Ampicillin and gentamicin are not noted to produce false elevations in serum creatinine. However, many of the cephalosporin antibiotics (e.g., cefoxitin, cephalothin, and cefazolin) may cause a false increase in serum or urine creatinine, depending on the specific assay used.

6. *Does G. N. have any medical problems which might interfere with the determination of serum creatinine?*

G. N. has hyperbilirubinemia, which may interfere with the determination of serum creatinine. With certain analytical techniques, bilirubin may produce falsely low creatinine measurements. In this case, the hospital lab should be contacted to determine which assay for serum creatinine is being used and whether bilirubin will interfere.

Other common neonatal conditions (which G. N. does not have) such as lipemia and hemolysis may also interfere with serum creatinine determinations.

7. *Given G. N.'s current medical conditions, what drug therapy recommendations do you now make?*

It is imperative to optimally treat G. N.'s sepsis. Her culture results are positive for a gram-negative organism, and she has had an episode of apnea with respiratory arrest. Due to the seriousness of this infection, meningitic doses of appropriate antibiotics should be used until meningitis can be ruled out. The hospital lab should be contacted to see if the gram-negative organism has been identified and if sensitivities are known. The antibiotics should be changed based on the organism's sensitivities and safety profile of the antibiotics to which the organism is sensitive.

Since gentamicin can be nephrotoxic and this patient already has renal dysfunction, an antibiotic with a lower risk of nephrotoxicity should be selected if possible. Gentamicin is eliminated via the kidney and if it must be used, gentamicin serum concentrations should be obtained and the dose adjusted accordingly. The dose of other antibiotics commonly used in neonates (such as ampicillin) must also be adjusted in patients with renal dysfunction.

In addition to renal dysfunction, the patient's hyperbilirubinemia should also be taken into consideration when selecting antibiotics. For example, ceftriaxone, a third generation cephalosporin, can displace bilirubin from albumin binding sites. It also may cause sludging in the gall bladder and cholelithiasis. Therefore, it should not be used in neonates with hyperbilirubinemia.

Donna M. Kraus

A 51-year-old woman was admitted to the hospital with the diagnosis of rectal bleeding, necessitating surgical consultation and endoscopic examination. She had a long standing history of alcohol abuse. Physical examination findings revealed a cachectic appearing female with spider hemangiomas, petechial hemorrhages, and asterixis. The patient was taking cimetidine and phenytoin. She denied taking any over the counter medications. The patient was noted to be positive for antiphospholipid antibody syndrome (APLABS) for which she had been on oral anticoagulant therapy with warfarin for prevention of thromboembolism—having suffered prior thromboembolic episodes due to her APLABS (cerebrovascular accident as well as deep venous thrombosis). Additionally, her past medical history was noted for having systemic lupus for which she was taking chronic steroid therapy and rheumatoid arthritis.

On admission, warfarin was discontinued. Surgical consultation recommended "bowel rest," bed rest, and "avoidance of over anticoagulation"—recognizing her continued need for anticoagulant therapy. She underwent lower endoscopic examination revealing no acute site of bleeding. Continued workup confirmed a diagnosis of pseudomembranous colitis—an inflammatory gastrointestinal disease. The patient's inpatient hospitalization was complicated by a nosocomial infection resulting in a diagnosis of pneumonia.

Her history was significant for several risk factors predisposing her to the potential of venous thromboembolism (VTE): her age was >40; she had previous episodes of VTE; and she had an embolic stroke. The diagnosis of APLABS placed her at heightened risk for thromboembolic complications. She was placed at bed rest for greater than 3 days.

It was elected by the Internal Medicine Teaching Service physicians to place her on continuous infusion of unfractionated heparin to be monitored by activated partial thromboplastin time (aPTT) determinations—though her baseline value was noted to be elevated—before implementation of unfractionated heparin.

After joining the rounding team the morning after her admission, it was noted by the pharmacists and pharmacy students that several things had to be considered, which gave rise to change in her drug therapy armamentarium prompting change from continuous infusion unfractionated heparin to low-molecular-weight heparin:

1. The patient was at heightened risk of thromboembolic complications for several reasons:

    a. The patient was greater than 40 years of age.

    b. The patient was nonambulating.

    c. The patient has significant history of previous thromboembolic risk putting her at additional risk for subsequent disease.

    d. The patient was diagnosed with pseudomembranous colitis and inflammatory bowel disease.

    e. The patient had a past medical history of rheumatoid arthritis.

    f. The patient developed nosocomial pneumonia.

    g. The patient had APLABS. Efforts to use the aPTT test to appropriately follow unfractionated heparin treated patients are inappropriate and fraught with error, as our team had already discovered. The aPTT responsiveness was extremely variable but did not accurately reflect her true anticoagulant status relative to unfractionated heparin.

The pharmacists discussed with the rounding team of physicians options available to address her ongoing risk of embolic events as well as VTE for now being hospitalized, bedridden, and at considerable risk given her concomitant risk factors and disease states. Given our concerns for the patient needing adequate anticoagulant protection, which required no aPTT monitoring, and her past medical history as well as her present medical condition (e.g. pneumonia), a recommendation for low-molecular-weight heparin subcutaneously administered once-daily was made. This recommendation was based on a study by Sammama et al. appearing in *The New England Journal of Medicine* in which a similar patient population (heart failure, acute respiratory failure, acute infectious disease, inflammatory bowel disease, and rheumatologic disorders) showed statistically significant decrease in venous thromboembolism when compared to placebo-randomized patients. Meta-analyses of the medical literature reveal a statistically significant lessened incidence of hemorrhagic complication as well as a 33% reduction in the potential of thrombocytopenia for low-molecular-weight heparin when compared to unfractionated heparin drug therapy. Finally, Anti-Xa heparin level serum drug concentrations may be monitored in patients with renal impairment, morbid obesity, or in any patient for which there is concern regarding potential accumulation based on either body habitus or other concomitant disease states.

The physicians heeded the advice of the pharmacists accompanying them on rounds and wrote orders for nonpharmacologic as well as appropriate pharmacologic prophylaxis against embolic events and VTE, requiring no routine laboratory monitoring via the aPTT.

The following laboratory parameters were determined for this 51-year-old female:

Laboratory Study	Normal Results	Patient Results
PT	10–13 sec	14.8 sec
INR	–	1.49
aPTT	21–45 sec	54 sec
CBC		
Hgb	14–18 g/dL	11 g/dL
Hct	42–52%	33%
Platelet count	140,000–440,000/μL	87,000/μL
MPV	7–11 fL	19 fL
AST	8–42 IU/L	85 IU/L
ALT	3–30 IU/L	25 IU/L
Albumin	3.5–5 g/dL	1.4 g/dL
Anti-Xa heparin level	Not detected at baseline	0.3–0.7 U/mL at 6 hr

QUESTIONS

1. *What specific test(s) may be performed to assess the pertinent patient findings from the physical examination? How might these tests relate to normal hemostasis?*

    Specific studies for bleeding disorders include the PT/INR and aPTT; they should be used as a preliminary screening for this 51-year-old female. Her elevations above baseline are consistent with coagulopathies common in patients who have APLABS.

    Platelet count determination and general hematologic values (Hgb and Hct) are consistent with physical examination findings (petechial hemorrhages), revealing the patient to be thrombocytopenic and anemic. As expected, the lowered platelet count and higher platelet volume demonstrate the inverse relationship that typically exists when thrombocytopenia occurs (MPV section). Liver function tests (LFTs) would further substantiate the suspected etiology of the patient's petechial hemorrhages. The typical AST/ALT "split" (i.e., a doubling of the AST relative to ALT) is consistent with the patient's history of alcohol abuse.

    These findings suggest liver impairment and, when paired with the patient's albumin, indicate the possibility of clotting abnormalities (demonstrated objectively by his prolonged PT and aPTT). Additionally, the APLABS can similarly account for prolonged aPTT results obtained at baseline before introduction of heparin.

    With this patient, history is important. Cimetidine and phenytoin have been associated with thrombocytopenia, which could also account for petechial hemorrhages. She denies using aspirin, but many patients unknowingly ingest it in over-the-counter products such as brand-name aspirin and cold preparations.

    For prophylaxis or treatment against venous thromboembolism in patients who do not have renal impairment, morbid obesity, or in any patient for which there is no concern regarding potential accumulation based on either body habitus or other concomitant disease states, the anti-Xa heparin level does not need to be drawn. An appropriate anti-Xa heparin level for patients receiving LMWH for venous thromboembolism prophylaxis or treatment would be 0.3–0.7 U/mL drawn at peak.

James B. Groce III, Julie B. Leumas

CC: *P. T. is a 19-year old college student who presents to the hospital emergency department with a high fever (up to 103.5 °F at home), a stiff neck, vomiting, a rash, decreased tolerance to light, and "the worst headache of my life."*

HPI:

Six hr prior to admission, P. T. started to have body and joint aches and started to develop a severe headache. Within hours, she developed a high fever, a purple rash, and began to have shaking chills and a stiff neck. She then became very lethargic and was brought in to the ED by her roommate when she began to vomit and complain of photophobia.

PMH:

No significant history

FH:

Father has a history of high blood pressure. Mother has no significant history.

SH:

P. T. does not smoke and has a history of occasional alcohol use (last drink 7 days ago).

MEDS:

Loestrin® qd as directed

ALLERGIES:

Sulfa rash

ROS:

Patient complains of headache, stiff neck, rash, photophobia, vomiting, lethargy, arthralgias, and myalgias.

PE:

GEN: Lethargic, well-developed female in apparent distress and discomfort
VS: BP 90/60; HR 104; RR 22; T 39.8 °C; HT 5'3"; and WT 62 kg
HEENT: PERRLA, decreased ROM neck (stiff)
CHEST/THORAX: Lungs clear to auscultation
CV: RRR; (–) bruits, (–) murmurs
ABD: Distended abdomen, + bowel sounds
GENIT: No significant findings
EXT: Petechial skin rash covering all extremities

LABS:

Sodium 138 mEq/L, potassium 3.9 mEq/L, chloride 108 mEq/L, CO_2 content 20 mEq/L, BUN 10 mg/dL, SCr 0.9 mg/dL, glucose 98 mg/dL, CBC with differential, hemoglobin 13.5 g/dL, hematocrit 34%, platelets 315,000/mm^3, and WBC 23,500/mm^3 with 70% PMNs, 23% bands, 6% lymphocytes, and 1% monocytes. Cerebrospinal fluid analysis: protein 200 mg/dL, glucose 35 mg/dL. WBCs 1200 cells/mm^3 with 99% polys and 1% lymphs. Gram stain and culture: Pending.

OTHER TESTS:

CT scan head: No significant findings.

PROBLEM LIST

- Acute bacterial meningitis

QUESTIONS

1. *What signs, symptoms, laboratory parameters, and test results are consistent with a diagnosis of meningitis in this patient?*

    This patient has all of the classic symptoms of acute bacterial meningitis. She has a sudden onset of high fever, stiff neck, arthralgia and myalgia, photophobia, vomiting, lethargy, and a petechial skin rash (characteristic finding in a particular type of meningitis). In terms of laboratory findings, she has an elevated peripheral WBC with a prominent left shift, as well as abnormal CSF findings consistent with bacterial meningitis (high protein, low glucose, and high WBC with neutrophilic predominance).

2. *Based on the patient age, history of illness, and infection type, what is the most likely causative organism of this patient's infection?*

    This patient is a college student with acute bacterial meningitis. The most common causative organisms of bacterial meningitis in this setting include *Streptococcus pneumoniae* and *Neisseria meningitidis*. Based on the history of a petechial skin rash in this patient, the most likely infecting organism is *Neisseria meningitidis*.

3. *What are the factors that should be considered when choosing empiric antibiotic therapy for the treatment of meningitis?*

    The factors that should be considered when choosing an antibiotic in a patient with acute bacterial meningitis include probable or known infecting organism, probable or known antibiotic susceptibilities, age of the patient, end organ function of the patient, concomitant disease states, concomitant medications, and patient allergies. The most important antibiotic factor for effective treatment of meningitis is the ability of the antibiotic to penetrate the blood brain barrier sufficiently to provide high enough drug concentrations in the CSF in order to successfully eradicate the infecting bacteria. It is crucial to have an understanding of which antibiotics are able to penetrate through the blood brain barrier and into the cerebrospinal fluid (CSF) in the presence or absence of inflamed meninges in order to assure appropriate antibiotic treatment.

4. *What antibiotic regimen would be most appropriate to empirically treat this patient's acute bacterial meningitis?*

    Even though the patient's presenting signs are more indicative of bacterial meningitis due to *Neisseria meningitidis*, empiric therapy should be chosen based on all of the most likely organisms (including *Streptococcus pneumoniae*) until the culture results are available since meningitis is a life-threatening infection. An empiric antibiotic regimen should have excellent activity against both organisms and be able to penetrate the CSF. In addition, in the treatment of meningitis, maximal antibiotic doses are utilized to maximize penetration into the CSF. Based on known national and regional susceptibility data, empiric therapy should probably begin with intravenous vancomycin therapy, since it has activity against *Streptococcus pneumoniae* isolates (including penicillin-resistant *S. pneumoniae*) and ceftriaxone for coverage of *Neisseria meningitidis*. A reasonable starting dose of vancomycin in this patient would be 1000 mg IV every 12 hr, and ceftriaxone should be given at a dose of 2 grams every 12 hr. Therapy can be changed to a more directed antibiotic regimen once the results of the culture and susceptibility are available.

Questions 5–7: Within the ensuing 24 hr, the results of the CSF Gram stain culture become available. The Gram stain contains many WBCs and many Gram-negative cocci, and the culture is growing *Neisseria meningitidis* susceptible to penicillin and ceftriaxone.

5. *Based on the culture and susceptibility results, what is the most appropriate antibiotic therapy for the treatment of this patient's Neisseria meningitidis meningitis?*

    Now that the culture and susceptibility results are available, the patient's antibiotic regimen can be changed to a more directed therapeutic agent. Based on the activity against the organism as well as established efficacy in the treatment of serious meningococcal infections, the patient's therapy should be changed to penicillin G 3 million units IVPB every 4 hr. It is not necessary to maintain the patient on vancomycin and ceftriaxone since only *Neisseria meningitidis* grew from the culture and it is susceptible to penicillin (with penicillin being the drug of choice).

6. *What is the appropriate length of therapy for the treatment of acute bacterial meningitis due to Neisseria meningitidis?*

The appropriate length of antibiotic therapy for the treatment of acute bacterial meningitis due to *Neisseria meningitidis* is usually 7–10 days. The whole course of antibiotics is administered parenterally. She may require a longer course of therapy because of the presence of disseminated meningococcemia (petechial rash).

7. *How do you monitor the response to treatment in a patient with meningitis?*

In a patient who is responding to antibiotic therapy for the treatment of acute bacterial meningitis, the signs and symptoms of infection should resolve (fever, headache, photophobia, arthralgias, myalgias, and vomiting). Her stiff neck should begin to resolve and her rash should dissipate over time. The white blood cell count should also decrease to normal values. Follow-up cultures are usually not performed in patients receiving treatment for acute bacterial meningitis, unless the symptoms or clinical condition of the patient worsens.

Sharon M. Erdman, Keith A. Rodvold

CASE 17

CC: G.G. *is a 48-year-old white male who presents to the hospital complaining of pain, worsening redness, and cloudy drainage from a wound on his right upper extremity.*

HPI:

Ten days prior to admission, G. G. was involved in a work-related accident with a forklift, which led to a deep laceration on his right upper arm. The patent sought medical attention at the local emergency department where the wound was irrigated and closed. The patient was sent home with a prescription for Augmentin® 875 mg bid for 5 days. Three days after the antibiotic was discontinued, the patient began noticing increased pain, erythema, and purulent discharge from the wound site. The patient presented to the ED this morning when he developed a fever, and he was subsequently admitted to the hospital to await an Infectious Diseases and Orthopedic Consult.

PMH:

High blood pressure for 5 years

FH:

Father has a history of peripheral vascular disease. Mother's history is unremarkable.

SH:

Patient smokes one and a half packs of cigarettes per day for the last 10 years (30 pack-per-year history).

MEDS:

Lisinopril 20 mg po daily

ALLERGIES:

No known drug or food allergies

ROS:

Patient complains of pain, erythema, and purulent discharge from wound site.

PE:

GEN: Alert, well-developed, slightly obese male complaining of right arm pain and malaise

VS: BP 150/90; HR 84; RR 16; T 38.8 °C; HT 6'1"; and WT 102 kg

HEENT: No significant findings

CHEST/THORAX: Lungs clear to auscultation

CV: RRR; (-) bruits, (-) murmurs

ABD: Distended abdomen, + bowel sounds

GENIT: No significant findings

EXT: Right axillary lymphadenopathy; 3 cm margin of erythema surrounding the 5 cm closed wound; area is warm and painful to the touch; and the distal 1 cm of the wound site is now open with purulent discharge

LABS:

Sodium 142 mEq/L, potassium 4.5 mEq/L, chloride 110 mEq/L, CO_2 content 24 mEq/L, BUN 12 mg/dL, SCr 1.1 mg/dL, glucose 98 mg/dL, ESR 90 mm/hr, CBC with differential, hemoglobin 15.8 g/dL, hematocrit 44%, platelets 295,000/mm³, WBC 18,500/mm³ with 84% PMNs, 3% bands, 10% lymphocytes, and 3% monocytes. Gram stain results of wound drainage: Many white blood cells and many gram-positive cocci in clusters. Culture of wound drainage: Pending.

OTHER TESTS:

Right upper extremity radiograph: Periosteal elevation and bony destruction of the right humerus consistent with osteomyelitis.

PROBLEM LIST

- Acute osteomyelitis of right humerus
- High blood pressure

QUESTIONS

1. *What signs, symptoms, laboratory parameters, and test results are consistent with a diagnosis of osteomyelitis in this patient?*

   This patient experienced trauma to his right upper extremity over 10 days ago. He originally sought medical treatment in which the ED MD irrigated his traumatic wound, closed it with sutures, and prescribed a 5 days course of antibiotics. Once the antibiotics were stopped, the patient began experiencing increased pain, warmth, redness, and discharge from the wound site. The labs reveal an increase in WBC and ESR, which are consistent with an infectious process. The x-ray of his arm reveals periosteal elevation, which is consistent with osteomyelitis. And lastly, the gram stain from the wound discharge is showing many WBCs and gram-positive bacteria.

2. *Based on the patient history, infection type, and Gram stain results, what is the most likely causative organism of this patient's infection?*

   This patient sustained a traumatic injury through the skin of his arm, which has led to the development of osteomyelitis. The most common causative organisms in this setting include *Staphylococcus aureus* and *Streptococcus pyogenes*. Based on the Gram stain results of the wound drainage culture, the likely infecting organism is *Staphylococcus aureus*.

3. *What are the factors that should be considered when choosing empiric or directed antibiotic therapy for the treatment of osteomyelitis?*

   The factors that should be considered when choosing an antibiotic for an individual patient include infection type, site of infection, probable or known infecting organism, probable or known antibiotic susceptibilities, age of the patient, end organ function of the patient, concomitant disease states, concomitant medications, and patient allergies. One of the most important antibiotic parameters for effective treatment of osteomyelitis is that the antibiotic must penetrate the bone sufficiently in order to successfully eradicate the infecting bacteria. There are only a few antibiotics that achieve adequate bone concentrations.

4. *What antibiotic regimen would be most appropriate to empirically treat this patient's presumed Staphylococcus aureus osteomyelitis?*

   Empiric therapy should be chosen based on the regional or hospital-wide susceptibilities of the potential infecting organism. Since it is suspected that the patient has *Staphylococcus aureus* as the causative pathogen, an empiric antibiotic agent should be chosen that has excellent activity against *S. aureus*. Based on recent national and regional susceptibility studies, it is known that approximately 45% of *S. aureus* are resistant to ß-lactam antibiotics (e.g., are Methicillin-resistant *Staphylococcus aureus* or MRSA). Therefore, empiric therapy should probably begin with intravenous vancomycin therapy, since it has activity against virtually all *Staphylococcus aureus* isolates. Therapy can be changed to a more directed approach once the results of the culture and susceptibility are available. A reasonable starting dose of vancomycin in this patient would be 1000 to 1250 mg IV every 12 hr.

Questions 5–7: Over the next few days, the appearance of the patient's arm worsened, requiring him to go to the operating room for surgical debridement of his humerus bone. Cultures from the wound discharge and bone both grew *Staphylococcus aureus* susceptible to oxacillin, cefazolin, trimethoprim-sulfamethoxazole, clindamycin, linezolid, and vancomycin.

5. *Based on the culture and susceptibility results, what is the most appropriate antibiotic therapy for the treatment of this patient's Staphylococcus aureus osteomyelitis?*

   Now that the culture and susceptibility results are available, the patient's antibiotic regimen can be changed to a more directed therapeutic agent. Based on the activity against the organism as well as efficacy in the treatment of serious infections due to *Staphylococcus aureus*, either Nafcillin 2 grams IV every 4 hr or Cefazolin 2 grams IV every 8 hr can be chosen. It is not necessary to maintain the patient on vancomycin since the organism is not MRSA.

6. *What is the appropriate length of therapy for the treatment of acute osteomyelitis?*

   The appropriate length of antibiotic therapy for the treatment of acute osteomyelitis is usually 4–6 weeks (28 to 42 days) based on the response to therapy. The course of antibiotics is usually started with intravenous therapy. Patients may occasionally be switched to oral therapy if the infection is responding and an appropriate oral formulation of the drug (or alternative) is available.

7. *How do you monitor the response to treatment in a patient with osteomyelitis?*

   In a patient who is responding to antibiotic therapy for the treatment of osteomyelitis, the signs and symptoms of infection should resolve (pain, fever, tenderness, and discharge), the wound should close and heal without drainage, the white blood cell count and ESR should decrease to normal values, and abnormalities present on the initial radiograph should disappear. Follow-up cultures are usually not performed in patients receiving treatment for osteomyelitis.

Sharon M. Erdman, Keith A. Rodvold

CC: *H. T. is a 26-year-old female who just finished graduate school. She had no medical complaints when she presented for a pre-employment physical exam. As she related, the examination itself was normal, but several days later she was told that she had "abnormal liver tests," and was referred to a specialist.*

CASE 18

HPI:

She stressed that she felt "great," and wondered, "What all the fuss is about?" She denied having ever been told she had any problems with her liver. She was on no medications, vitamins, or herbal preparations. She stated she only drank alcohol on weekends and then only one or two drinks an evening. She denied having received blood products or the use of illicit drugs. She had not traveled outside of the Northeast. Presently, she was living alone and noted that none of her friends or colleagues had any liver problems.

PMH:

She had her appendix removed at age 15. There were no other medical problems reported.

FH:

There was no family history of liver disease.

SH:

She does not smoke. Alcohol was (as above) limited to weekends.

MEDS:

None

ALLERGIES:

No known drug or food allergies

ROS:

The patient felt fine. Her last menstrual period was 2 weeks ago.

PE:

GEN: Well-developed, well-nourished white female in no apparent distress
VS: BP 120/76; HR 74; RR 16; T 98.6 °F; HT 5'8"; and WT 70 kg
HEENT: No significant findings; no evidence of scleral icterus
CHEST/THORAX: Heart and lungs normal
ABD: No evidence of organomegaly or ascites; no masses, tenderness, guarding, or rigidity; normal bowel sounds
GENIT: Normal examination
EXT: Unremarkable

LABS:

Hemoglobin 13.5 g/dL, hematocrit 38%, WBC $8.4 \times 10^3/mm^3$, MCV 90 fL, ALT 135 IU/L, AST 168 IU/L, bilirubin 0.8 mg/dL, alkaline phosphatase 68 IU/L, amylase 95 IU/L, lipase 1.4 U/mL, AND glucose 80mg/dL. Prothrombin time, albumin, and total proteins were normal.

PROBLEM LIST

- Elevated aminotransferases

QUESTIONS

1. *Into which category, cholestatic or hepatocellular, would these numbers fit?*

   The presence of normal bilirubin and alkaline phosphatase would tend to exclude cholestatic causes of abnormal liver function tests. The elevated aminotransferases, ALT and AST, would suggest hepatocellular disease.

2. *What, if anything, can we tell about the status of her liver? Does she have cirrhosis?*

   The level of aminotransferases does not correlate with the pathologic picture. With these aminotransferase levels, this patient could have anything from the mildest inflammation in her liver to advanced cirrhosis. However, the absence of physical findings suggesting cirrhosis (edema, ascites, jaundice, muscular wasting, spider telangiectasias, palmar erythema, and asterixis) would suggest that advanced cirrhosis is unlikely. Similarly, the presence of normal tests for liver synthetic function (protime, albumin) are also encouraging.

3. *What could cause these tests to be abnormal, and what would the next step in her workup entail?*

   Establishing a diagnosis in an asymptomatic patient with abnormal liver function tests can be challenging as the differential diagnosis is extensive. Quite often in a case such as this, the diagnosis is that of a fatty liver or fatty liver with inflammation, referred to as NASH (nonalcoholic steato-hepatitis). Viral infections; exposures to medications/drugs; inherited forms of liver disease (Wilson's disease or hemochromatosis); occupational exposure to toxins; alcohol use; drug abuse; HIV; and autoimmune diseases are all in the differential diagnosis. The best initial approach is to check for viral hepatitis with appropriate markers, rule out other forms of liver diseases with appropriate serologies, and to review the patient's history in more detail.

   In this patient additional laboratory data showed negative HbsAg, negative HbcAb, negative total hepatitis A antibodies, normal iron studies, normal ceruloplasmin level (to exclude Wilson's disease, an inherited disease of copper metabolism), negative ANA and antismooth muscle antibody (to rule out certain types of autoimmune hepatitis), and a positive hepatitis C antibody level. HIV serology was negative.

4. *What would the next step be in evaluating this patient for Hepatitis C?*

   The ELISA test used to screen for HCV (often referred to as a hepatitis C antibody test) is relatively inexpensive and has a high sensitivity but relatively poor specificity; this makes it a good screening test but requires that a positive result be confirmed by a more accurate test. Thus, positive HCV ELISA results are followed up by a confirmatory test, either a RIBA or detection of HCV RNA by PCR testing. In this case the RNA PCR test showed a high viral count, thus confirming Hepatitis C. Of note is that most patients with hepatitis C will not have any symptoms, and most cases are "picked up" on routine physical examinations or when people attempt to donate blood.

5. *How did she get the Hepatitis C?*

   Some studies have suggested that up to 40% of patients with hepatitis C will have no clear history explaining how they may have caught this illness. Hepatitis C is generally transmitted via blood, and common means of transmission include sharing needles, transfusions with blood or blood products (prior to the time when blood was screened for Hepatitis C [1990]), cocaine use (apparently associated with increased nasal ulceration and bleeding and subseqent bloody contamination of the "straws" used), and nonsterile piercing. Hepatitis C can be spread sexually, although the incidence of spread in monogamous heterosexual relationships seems low, and spread in such relationships may be related to sharing razor blades, and nail clippers.

   When questioned in more detail, she related that during the summer of her sophomore year in college she and her boyfriend had snorted cocaine at several parties with shared straws. She has not been in touch with her boyfriend and had no idea whether or not he had or developed any liver problems.

6. *What should be done next?*

Initiating therapy in patients with newly diagnosed hepatitis C is always a challenge. A long discussion on how to avoid spreading this disease and implications for her future life are crucial. Alcohol seems to potentiate this virus and is best avoided. It is known that a large percentage of patients with asymptomatic hepatitis C can develop cirrhosis, liver failure, or hepatocellular carcinoma. Therapy (generally with interferon and ribavirin) should be considered, unless there are specific contraindications.

Prior to administering such therapy, it is important (if not done) to check a quantitative PCR to determine viral load, and to determine the genotype of the hepatitis C virus as this will influence the duration of therapy (for example, type 1 patients will receive 12 months of therapy, and types 2 and 3 will be offered 6 months of therapy), and the likelihood of cure (much higher for genotypes 2 and 3). Given that this patient does not have antibodies to hepatitis B or A, she should be vaccinated for both of these as these infections can be especially severe in patients with chronic liver disease. The role of liver biopsy is becoming increasingly controversial in the setting of newly diagnosed hepatitis C. Advantages include the exclusion of cirrhosis (and, thus, excluding the need to screen for hepatocellular carcinoma) and providing some information as to the severity of the disease, as well as ruling out the possibility of other concurrent liver ailments.

7. *What was the outcome in this patient?*

She received vaccines for hepatitis B and A. Her genotype was 2a, and after much discussion in terms of side effects and relative benefit, she underwent a 6-month course of therapy with pegylated interferon and ribavirin. Although she reported increased fatigue, anorexia, and a flu-like illness with these medications, she tolerated them well. Subsequent serum RNA levels have been undetectable by PCR, and her ALT and AST returned to normal and have stayed there.

Joshua D. Farkas, Paul Farkas, Douglas K. Hyde

CASE 19

CC: R. J. is a 48-year-old woman who presented to her doctor after her boyfriend had told her she was looking "yellow." On questioning she noted some increasing fatigue recently, as well as some mild generalized itching.

HPI:

She was not aware of any liver problems in her past. She denied having received blood or blood products. Currently she drinks one glass of wine a night, and she denied the use of any medications, vitamin supplements, or herbal preparations. There had been no recent travel, and working as a receptionist she had no known toxin exposure. She denied any abdominal discomfort, change in her bowel movements, or darkening of her urine. Five years ago she had her navel pierced, "by a friend," and had developed a localized infection, which had healed with antibiotics. She had three tattoos, but felt fairly confident that all had been done under sterile conditions. While in college she had experimented briefly with cocaine, but she denied using parenteral narcotics. She had had multiple sexual partners in the past, but she was not aware that any of them had had liver disease.

PMH:

She related no history of other illness or surgeries.

FH:

Noncontributory

SH:

None

MEDS:

None

ALLERGIES:

No known drug or food allergies

ROS:

Other than increased fatigue and some mild itching, she felt well and denied any other problems.

PE:

GEN: Well-developed, well-nourished white female who appeared slightly jaundiced

VS: BP 140/84; HR 88; RR 18; HT 5'5"; and WT 65 kg

SKIN: Slightly jaundiced; no spider telangiectasias

CHEST/THORAX: Normal heart and lung examinations

ABD: No organomegaly, ascites, tenderness, guarding, rebound, or rigidity; midline pierced umbilicus without evidence of infection; three tattoos on lower abdomen and upper thighs

GENIT: Normal examination

EXT: Unremarkable; no edema

LABS:

Hemoglobin 14 g/dL, hematocrit 42%, WBC $8.0 \times 10^{23}/mm^3$, indices normal. BUN, creatinine, and glucose normal. AST 44 IU/L, ALT 56 IU/L, alkaline phosphatase 728 IU/L, GGTP elevated to 4 times normal, total bilirubin 4.1 mg/dL, albumin 3.0 g/dL, and prothrombin time normal.

PROBLEM LIST

- Elevated liver function tests (aminotransferases, ALP, GGTP)
- Fatigue
- Pruritus

QUESTIONS

1. *Into which category, cholestatic or hepatocellular, would these numbers fit?*

   With relatively normal (or mildly elevated ALT and AST) but pronounced elevations in the alkaline phosphatase and GGTP values, cholestatic diseases are suggested.

2. *In general terms, what would be the differential diagnosis?*

   Generally, cholestasis can be divided into two broad categories: intra- and extrahepatic. Extrahepatic cholestasis is due to anatomic biliary obstruction outside of the liver, and possible causes include stones blocking the bile ducts, cancer of the bile ducts, head of pancreas, ampulla, sclerosing cholangitis, or other forms of stricturing cholangitis (as seen in HIV), which can involve both intra- and extrahepatic bile ducts. Intrahepatic cholestasis is related to problems in the liver cells or the smaller bile ducts within the liver. Possible causes include drugs, viral hepatitis (especially type A), alcoholic hepatitis, HIV associated liver diseases, autoimmune liver disease, sclerosing cholangitis, and primary biliary cirrhosis (although some of these—notably viral hepatitis, alcoholic liver disease, and autoimmune liver disease—are generally accompanied by a hepatocellular component, which seems to be lacking in this patient.) Alcoholic liver disease is often suggested by an elevated AST/ALT ratio, elevated MCV, and disproportionately elevated GGTP. It can also be seen in cholestasis of pregnancy or benign recurrent cholestasis.

3. *How may we distinguish intra- from extrahepatic cholestasis?*

   Dividing causes of cholestasis along the lines of intrahepatic vs. extrahepatic is a convenient approach because extrahepatic causes may often be diagnosed by radiologic imaging due to their macroscopic nature, whereas intrahepatic causes may require lab testing or liver biopsy. The hallmark of extrahepatic cholestasis, especially in the face of jaundice, is dilated bile ducts due to "damming" up behind the obstruction. Imaging methods to detect this would include ultrasound (echo) of the abdomen, CT scanning, or MRI/MRCP (magnetic resonance imaging or magnetic resonance cholangio-pancreatography). Endoscopic retrograde cholangiopancreatography (ERCP) or the injection of contrast into the bile ducts via a special endoscope is also of use, but it is associated with some risk and is generally not used to help sort out between intra- and extrahepatic cholestasis. However, it may be invaluable once a diagnosis of extrahepatic cholestasis is established in order to determine the etiology and permit resolution (removing stones impacted in the duct) or palliation (putting stents above strictures or dilating strictures). In this patient, an abdominal ultrasound was done and showed normal liver, biliary system, and pancreas.

4. *What is the approach to intrahepatic cholestasis in this patient?*

   In this patient some of the most likely causes, drugs and toxins, have been excluded. With her history of multiple risk factors for HIV, hepatitis C, and hepatitis B (multiple sexual partners, cocaine use, and piercings), these diseases need to be excluded. Generally, hepatitis B and C will present as hepatocellular diseases rather than cholestatic, but there can be exceptions. HIV is associated with multiple forms of liver disease, both cholestatic and hepatocellular. Aside from the patient's current illness, it is also important (in the face of her risk factors) to screen for these diseases because of other implications a positive result could have on the patient's general health and medical management. In this patient serologies for HIV, hepatitis B, and hepatitis C were all negative. This patient had her last period within the past two weeks, and a serum pregnancy test was normal, excluding cholestasis of pregnancy. Markers of autoimmune hepatitis, ANA and antismooth muscle antibodies, were negative. One would wonder about the extent of her previous alcohol use (generally understated by patients). Ultimately a test for primary biliary cirrhosis, the AMA (antimitochondrial antibody) was positive at a high titer.

5. *What is the significance of a positive AMA titer in the face of cholestasis?*

   This combination would strongly suggest the diagnosis of primary biliary cirrhosis. AMA positivity, especially at low titers, is not entirely specific and can be seen in chronic viral hepatitis. In this patient a liver biopsy served to confirm the diagnosis, and while confirming the diagnosis of PBC, it showed no indication of alcoholic liver disease.

6. *What is the management of primary biliary cirrhosis?*

   There is no specific therapy for PBC. Some have used colchicine, methotrexate, and ursodeoxycholic acid in treating this disease. Additionally, attention needs to be directed to the fat soluble vitamins—A, D, E, and K—as there can be deficiencies in these patients, especially with respect to vitamin D and an increased risk of bone problems. Itching may occur in cholestatic patients and seems to respond to resolution of the cholestasis (not possible in this case) or treatment with cholestyramine or ursodeoxycholic acid. In more severe cases, rifampin, naltrexone, phenobarbital, or plasmaphoresis may be of value.

7. *What about this patient's fatigue?*

   Fatigue is a nonspecific syndrome often associated with advanced liver disease. Interestingly, PBC is associated with many other autoimmune diseases including celiac sprue, rheumatoid arthritis, Sjögren's, and hypothyroidism. In this patient, work-up for hypothyroidism was normal with a normal TSH and thyroid profile.

   Joshua D. Farkas, Paul Farkas, Douglas K. Hyde

Therapeutic Ranges of Drugs in Traditional and SI Units[a]

Drug	Traditional Range	Conversion Factor[b]	SI Range
Acetaminophen	>5 mg/dL toxic	66.16	>330 µmol/L toxic
N-Acetylprocainamide	4–10 mg/L	3.606	14–36 µmol/L
Amitriptyline	75–175 ng/mL	3.605	180–720 nmol/L
Carbamazepine	4–12 mg/L	4.230	17–51 µmol/L
Chlordiazepoxide	0.5–5.0 mg/L	3.336	2–17 µmol/L
Chlorpromazine	50–300 ng/mL	3.136	150–950 nmol/L
Chlorpropamide	75–250 µg/mL	3.613	270–900 µmol/L
Clozapine	>250–350 ng/mL	0.003	0.75–1.05 µmol/L
Cyclosporine	100–200 ng/mL[c]	0.832	80–160 nmol/L
Desipramine	100–160 ng/mL	3.754	170–700 nmol/L
Diazepam	100–250 ng/mL	3.512	350–900 nmol/L
Digoxin	0.9–2.2 ng/mL	1.281	1.2–2.8 nmol/L
Disopyramide	2–6 mg/L	2.946	6–18 µmol/L
Doxepin	50–200 ng/mL	3.579	180–720 nmol/L
Ethosuximide	40–100 mg/L	7.084	280–710 µmol/L
Fluphenazine	0.5–2.5 ng/mL	2.110	5.3–21 nmol/L
Glutethimide	>20 mg/L toxic	4.603	>92 µmol/L toxic
Gold	300–800 mg/L	0.051	15–40 µmol/L
Haloperidol	5–15 ng/mL	2.660	13–40 nmol/L
Imipramine	200–250 ng/mL	3.566	180–710 nmol/L
Isoniazid	>3 mg/L toxic	7.291	>22 µmol/L toxic
Lidocaine	1–5 mg/L	4.267	5–22 µmol/L
Lithium	0.5–1.5 mEq/L	1.000	0.5–1.5 µmol/L
Maprotiline	50–200 ng/mL	3.605	180–720 µmol/L
Meprobamate	>40 mg/L toxic	4.582	>180 µmol/L toxic
Methotrexate	>2.3 mg/L toxic	2.200	>5 µmol/L toxic
Nortriptyline	50–150 ng/mL	3.797	190–570 nmol/L
Pentobarbital	20–40 mg/L	4.419	90–170 µmol/L
Perphenazine	0.8–2.4 ng/mL	2.475	2–6 nmol/L
Phenobarbital	15–40 mg/L	4.306	65–172 µmol/L
Phenytoin	10–20 mg/L	3.964	40–80 µmol/L
Primidone	4–12 mg/L	4.582	18–55 µmol/L
Procainamide	4–8 mg/L	4.249	17–34 µmol/L
Propoxyphene	>2 mg/L toxic	2.946	>6 µmol/L toxic
Propranolol	50–200 ng/mL	3.856	190–770 nmol/L
Protriptyline	100–300 ng/mL	3.797	380–1140 nmol/L
Quinidine	2–6 mg/L	3.082	5–18 µmol/L
Salicylate (acid)	15–25 mg/dL	0.072	1.1–1.8 mmol/L
Theophylline	10–20 mg/L	5.550	55–110 µmol/L
Thiocyanate	>10 mg/dL toxic	0.172	>1.7 mmol/L toxic
Valproic acid	50–100 mg/L	6.934	350–700 µmol/L

[a]Also see Table 16-5 in Chapter 6.
[b]Traditional units are multiplied by conversion factor to get SI units.
[c]Whole blood assay.

Nondrug Reference Ranges for Common Laboratory Tests in Traditional and SI Units[a]

Laboratory Test	Reference Range Traditional Units	Conversion Factor	Reference Range SI Units	Comment
Alanine aminotransferase (ALT)	0–30 IU/L	0.01667	0–0.50 µkat/L	SGPT
Albumin	3.5–5 g/dL	0.00	35–50 g/L	
Ammonia	30–70 µg/dL	0.587	17–41 µmol/L	
Aspartate aminotransferase (AST)	8–42 IU/L	0.01667	0.133–0.700 µkat/L	SGOT
Bilirubin (direct)	0.1–0.3 mg/dL	17.10	1.7–5 µmol/L	
Bilirubin (total)	0.3–1.0 mg/dL	117.10	5–17 µmol/L	
Calcium	8.5–10.8 mg/dL	0.25	2.1–2.7 mmol/L	
Carbon dioxide (CO_2)	24–30 mEq/L	1.000	24–30 mmol/L	Serum bicarbonate
Chloride	96–106 mEq/L	1.000	96–106 mmol/L	desirable
Cholesterol (HDL)	>10 mg/dL	0.026	>1.55 mmol/L	desirable
Cholesterol (LDL)	100 <130 mg/dL	0.026	<3.36 mmol/L	males
Creatine kinase (CK)	25–90 IU/L (males) 10–70 IU/L (females)	0.01667	0.42–1.50 µkat/L 0.17–1.17 µkat/L	females adults
Serum creatinine (SCr)	0.7–1.5 mg/dL	88.40	62–133 µmol/L	
Creatinine clearance (CrCl)	90–140 mL/min/1.73 m²	0.017	1.53–2.38 mL/sec/ 1.73 m²	
Folic acid	150–540 ng/mL	2.266	340–1020 nmol/L	GGTP
g-Glutamyl transpeptidase	0–30 U/L (but varies)	0.01667	0–0.50 µkat/L (but varies)	
Globulin	2–3 g/dL	10.00	20–30 g/L	fasting
Glucose (fasting)	<110 mg/dL	0.056	6.1 mmol/L	males
Hemoglobin (Hgb)	14–18 g/dL 12–16 g/dL	0.622	8.7–11.2 mmol/L 7.4–9.9 mmol/L	females
Iron	50–150 µg/dL	0.179	9–26.9 µmol/L	TIBC
Iron-binding capacity	250–410 µg/dL	0.179	45–73 µmol/L	LDH
Lactate dehydrogenase	100–210 IU/L	0.01667	1667–350 nmol/L, 1.7–3.2 µkat/L	Lactic acid
Serum lactate (venous)	0.5–1.5 mEq/L	1.000	0.5–1.5 mmol/L	
Serum lactate (arterial)	0.5–2.0 mEq/L	1.000	0.5–2.0 mmol/L	
Magnesium	1.5–2.2 mEq/L	0.500	0.75–1.1 mmol/L	
5′ Nucleotidase	1–11 U/L (but varies)	0.01667	0.02–0.18 µkat/L (but varies)	
Phosphate	2.6–4.5 mg/dL		0.85–1.48 mmol/L	
Potassium	3.5–5.0 mEq/L	1.000	3.5–5.0 mmol/L	
Sodium	136–145 mEq/L	1.000	136–145 mmol/L	
Total serum thyroxine (T_4)	4–12 µg/dL	12.86	51–154 nmol/L	Total T_4
Triglycerides	<150 mg/dL	0.0113	<1.26 mmol/L	Adults >20 yo
Total serum triiodothyronine (T_3)	78–195 ng/dL	0.0154	1.2–3.0 nmol/L	Total T_3
Urea nitrogen, blood	8–20 mg/dL	0.357	2.9–7.1 mmol/L	BUN
Uric acid (serum)	3.4–7 mg/dL	59.48	202–416 µmol/L	

[a]Some laboratories are maintaining traditional units for enzyme tests.

Glossary of Medical Terms: Contextual Definitions

Abscess—Localized, walled-off collection of pus (white blood cells and cellular debris).

Absorption, drug—Extent of drug transfer from one body compartment (e.g., intestines) to another (bloodstream).

Accuracy—Degree of correlation of results between assay being investigated and alternative (usually standard) assay in analyzing patient samples.

Acetylcholine—Chemical released from nerve endings responsible for stimulating other nerves, muscles, and glands; neurotransmitter.

Acidemia—Abnormally acidic blood (pH <7.35).

Acidosis—Process causing acidemia; pH is often less than 7.35 but may be higher if compensation mechanisms are effective.

Actin—Protein in muscle tissue that acts with myosin to allow muscle contraction and relaxation.

Action potential—Changes in electrical potential across muscle or nerve cell when triggered by an appropriate stimulus leading to cellular contraction.

Addison's disease—Adrenal gland dysfunction resulting in low or no output of hormones such as cortisone and aldosterone.

Agglutination—Endpoint of process used in certain assays. Clumping of cells (e.g., blood cells and bacteria) due to presence of antibodies. Use of known antigen (usually attached to latex particles) allows detection and identification of antibody in serum or other fluid (e.g., cerebrospinal fluid).

Aggregation—Clumping of cells due to electrostatic charges, commonly used to describe one of the steps in platelet plug formation.

Alkalemia—Abnormally alkaline blood (pH >7.45).

Alkalosis—Process causing alkalemia; pH is often greater than 7.45 but may be lower if compensation mechanisms are effective.

Amyloidosis—Generic term for group of clinically and biochemically diverse disease states characterized by deposition of insoluble fibrillar protein (including prealbumin or transthyretin) in extracellular space.

Analyte—Component intended to be measured in collected body fluid or tissue.

Anemia—Decrease in hemoglobin concentration or red blood cell count.

Angiotensin—Vasoconstrictor and stimulator of aldosterone secretion; formed from interaction of angiotensinogen (present in blood) and renin (released from kidneys); active form is angiotensin II.

Antibody—Protein produced by body in response to exposure to foreign proteins. As part of body's defense against invasion, antibodies help to increase efficiency of phagocytes and to activate complement.

Anticoagulant—Additive that prevents a blood specimen from clotting.

Antigen—Foreign substance (e.g., bacteria, toxins, or proteins) that causes formation of antibodies.

Antipyretic—Having the ability to decrease elevated body temperatures. Examples are aspirin, ibuprofen, acetaminophen, and prednisone.

Apparent distribution mass—Mass or weight of body into which a drug apparently distributes; derivative of volume of distribution.

Artifact—False or spurious reading of laboratory test results caused by substance not usually present in specimen or assay equipment.

Assay—Test measuring concentration or activity of analyte.

Asterixis—Flapping tremor of fingers when arms and hands are outstretched; usually seen with hepatic encephalopathy and hypercapnia.

Ataxia—Incoordination of muscle action, usually without loss of muscle power; seen with excessive alcohol and phenytoin.

Atherosclerosis—Hardening of arteries with deposition of fat along inner arterial walls.

Atrophy—Reduction in size; can be normal physiological process (e.g., due to aging) or caused by disease.

Autoimmune—Specific humoral or cell-mediated immune response directed against constituents of body's own tissue.

azo-—Word root relating to nitrogen.

Azotemia—Excessive concentration of nitrogenous substances (e.g., blood urea nitrogen) in blood.

Azoturia—Excessive concentration of nitrogenous substances (e.g., blood urea nitrogen) in urine.

Bacilli—Rod-shaped bacteria (singular form: bacillus).

Bacteremia—Presence of bacteria in blood.

Bacteria—Single-celled procaryotic organisms that lack chlorophyll but have cell wall (unlike human cells).

Basal—Rate of process when body is at rest. For example, basal energy expenditure (also called basal metabolic rate) refers to amount of energy the body requires when at rest.

Benign prostatic hypertrophy—Noncancerous enlargement of prostate, usually seen in older men.

Bioavailability—Extent of drug absorption from gastrointestinal tract into bloodstream.

B lymphocyte—Thymus-independent, mononuclear white blood cell that is product of lymphoid tissue and participates in humoral immunity; also known as B cell.

Canaliculi—Very small ducts or channels; often refers to tiny bile ducts in liver between hepatocytes.

Carpopedal—Relating to both hands and feet.

Catabolism—Breakdown of tissue or protein in body; opposite of anabolism.

Catalyst—Substance that increases velocity of chemical reaction.

Catecholamine—Neurotransmitter that contains catechol ring and is produced by adrenal medulla or nerve cells. Examples are epinephrine, norepinephrine, and dopamine.

Celiac disease—Intestinal malabsorption, characterized by diarrhea, malnutrition, and predisposition to bleeding. Treatment is gluten-free diet.

Cerebrospinal fluid—Fluid that occupies a space between the arachnoid membrane and pia matter; formed by choroid plexuses of cerebral ventricles and serves as fluid buffer for central nervous system, as reservoir for regulating contents of cranium, and as mechanism for exchange of nutrients and gases of nervous system. It may be a specimen in tests to assess integrity of central nervous system.

Cheyne-Stokes respiration—Rhythmical (periodic) rapid and shallow breathing occurring in grave conditions of central nervous system, heart, and lungs and during severe intoxication.

Chief cell—Cell in stomach lining; secretes pepsin and extrinsic factor aiding in digestion.

Choreiform—Usually relating to involuntary "spastic," purposeless movements that can be symptoms of chorea or side effects of central nervous system drugs.

Chromatin—Deoxyribonucleic acid attached to protein structure base.

Chromatography—A method by which drugs or biochemicals are separated or purified in order to quantify them without interference from other bodily chemicals.

Chromogen—Chemical substance that imparts color to specimen. This color may be made by substance intended for measurement in an assay or by unintended substance (interferent) such as noncreatinine chromogens (e.g., ketones and cefoxitin). A large number of interferents decreases an assay's specificity.

Chromophore—Chemical group that gives color to compound.

Chronotropic—Affecting rate; usually used in context of heart rate. See Inotropic.

Chvostek's sign—Spasm of facial muscles elicited by tapping the facial nerve in the region of the parotid gland; associated with hypocalcemia.

Circadian—Relating to cycle of physiological events encompassed by a 24-hr day.

Cirrhosis—Disease characterized histologically by fibrosis and nodular formations in liver.

Clinical—Pertaining to patient. Throughout this book, clinical connotes information (symptoms and signs) that is readily obtainable from, or apparent in, patients (history and physical examination) in contrast to information obtained from tests or procedures.

Cocci—Sphere-shaped bacteria (singular form: coccus).

Coefficient of variation—In statistics, standard deviation of series expressed as percentage of arithmetic mean of series; used in measuring assay performance. The smaller the coefficient of variation, the more likely it is that the test result is accurate.

Complement—Group of nine proteins. When activated by antibody, they sequentially bind to cell membranes, causing cell lysis.

Conjugation (metabolism)—Combining one compound with another to form a third (often a more water-soluble compound), which is more readily eliminated by body.

Contagium—Any microorganism, virus, or infectious matter producing or transmitting disease.

CREST—Indolent subgroup of systemic sclerosis historically referred to as acrosclerosis. CREST is acronym for calcinosis, Raynaud's phenomenon, esophageal hypomotility, sclerodactyly, and telangiectasia.

Culture—Quantity of microorganisms (e.g., bacteria and fungi) growing in artificial nutritive medium.

Cushing's disease—Disease characterized by adrenal gland hypersecretion of hormones such as cortisol (cortisone); manifests as truncal obesity, moonface, edema, hypertension, striae, and electrolyte imbalances.

Cuvette—Glass container having well-defined optical properties; used to hold solution being analyzed for color changes or light-scattering properties.

Cyanosis—Bluish coloration of skin and mucous membranes that results from excessive unoxygenated hemoglobin in blood; usually sign of respiratory disease.

Cytosol—Colloidal solution that comprises cellular fluid outside nucleus.

Defervescence—Lowering of elevated body temperature (fever); often seen when antibiotic therapy is effective in treating infection.

Demographic—Relating to statistical study of population's specific characteristics (e.g., age, weight, height, sex, and health).

Depolarization—An electrical phenomenon that represents the decrease in the differential ionic charges across muscle or nerve cell from the resting state. The intracellular space becomes more positively charged than the extracellular space leading to cellular activation and contraction.

Diabetes mellitus—Metabolic disorder characterized by hyperglycemia caused by absolute or relative lack of insulin.

Diarthrodal—Relating to joints that are normally freely movable.

Disseminated—Spread throughout entire body or particular organ.

Disseminated intravascular coagulation—Excessive activation of coagulation system, resulting in clotting at multiple sites. Rapid consumption of clotting factors may then result in bleeding; also called consumptive coagulopathy.

Dose—With regard to pharmacokinetics, the amount of drug given at the beginning of a dosing interval.

Dosing interval—With regard to pharmacokinetics, the period of time between administration of drug doses.

Dose rate—Rate at which drug is administered during chronic administration. For example, 1000 mg per day.

Duodenum—First portion of small bowel beginning at pylorus and extending for about 12 in.

Dyscrasia, blood—Abnormal generation or production of one or more blood cell types; usually refers to inadequate formation of red blood cells, white blood cells, or platelets.

Dysrhythmia—Abnormal cardiac rhythm.

Dysuria—Discomfort or pain upon urination.

Ecchymosis—Appearance of bruises caused by blood leakage into skin.

Eclampsia—Toxic condition of late pregnancy characterized by increasing blood pressure, seizures, and, ultimately, coma.

Ectopic—In area other than its normal location. A heart beat originating from somewhere other than SA node is an example.

Electrocardiography—Recording of the electrical activity of the heart on an electrocardiogram

Electrophoresis—Separation of differently charged particles (often protein) by passing an electric current through mixture on support medium. Molecules move toward electrodes at different rates, depending on their charge and molecular configuration and on physical properties of support medium.

Elution—Separation of substance from adsorbent material (e.g., chromatography column) by extraction or washing with solvent.

Embolism—Blood clot that travels from one vascular location to distant site.

-emia—Suffix relating to blood.

Endemic—Any disease that is constantly prevalent in a particular area, sometimes in varying degrees.

Endocarditis—Condition characterized by inflammation of endocardium, particularly valves; usually due to bacterial infection.

Endogenous—Of or relating to substances normally found within body (e.g., urea, ammonia, or potassium).

Enzyme-linked immunosorbent assay (ELISA)—Procedures where enzyme activation indicates that immune reaction has occurred. Usually the enzyme is attached to an antibody. When it reacts with its antigen, the antibody undergoes changes that activate the enzyme. Indicator system employs enzyme substrate. Also available as enzyme-multiplied immunoassay technique (EMIT) and enzyme immunoassay (EIA).

Enzyme-multiplied immunoassay (EMIT)—See Enzyme-linked immunosorbent assay.

Erythropoiesis—Production of erythrocytes.

Euthyroid—Relating to normally functioning thyroid gland.

Euthyroid sick state—Decreased total serum thyroxine (T_4) level in seriously ill patient.

Exogenous—Of or relating to substances not normally found within body (e.g., drugs).

Exophthalmos—Abnormal protrusion of eyeball; seen in hyperthyroidism.

Extracellular—Outside of cells; includes interstitial and intravascular spaces.

False negative—Test result that is negative when it should be positive (i.e., disease tested for is actually present).

False positive—Test result that is positive when it should be negative (i.e., disease tested for is not present).

Fibronectin—Subendothelial structure that accompanies collagen. When these structures are exposed to circulation following injury, they cause a potent platelet adhesion reaction.

First-order (or linear)—Refers to the elimination pattern of a drug when elimination processes are not becoming saturated.

Fluorophore—Compound emitting wavelength of light longer than light it absorbs. This phenomenon results in fluorescence.

Fulminant—Coming on suddenly with great severity.

Gestational diabetes—Onset of glucose intolerance during pregnancy.

Giant cell arteritis—Vascular disease that typically manifests as headache and involves inflammation of carotid arteries; also known as temporal arteritis.

Glanzmann's thrombasthenia—Genetic (autosomal-recessive) disorder associated with normal clotting factors, normal platelet count, abnormal platelet function, and severe congenital bleeding.

Glomerulus—Filtering unit of nephrons of kidneys.

Gluconeogenesis—Formation of glucose from noncarbohydrates, such as protein or fat.

Glucose intolerance—Inability of body to process glucose properly; usually leads to hyperglycemia.

glyc-—Word root relating to carbohydrates.

Glycogenolysis—Hydrolysis of glycogen to glucose

Glycolysis—Process of carbohydrate breakdown into smaller molecules.

Glycosuria—Presence of glucose in urine.

Goiter—Enlargement of thyroid gland.

Gram negative—Microorganisms that are decolorized by alcohol during Gram staining process. They appear pink under microscope. Examples are—*Escherichia coli, Pseudomonas, Haemophilus, Klebsiella, Salmonella, Neisseria,* and *Bacteroides* species.

Gram positive—Microorganisms that retain stain during Gram staining process. They appear purple under microscope. Examples are *Streptococcus, Staphylococcus, Listeria, Clostridia,* and *Peptococcus* species.

Granulocytopenia—Decrease in number of granulocytes below normal range.

Granulocytosis—Increase in number of granulocytes above normal (reference) range.

Half-life—Time needed for original amount or concentration to be reduced to 50%. With drugs, half-life usually refers to time needed for serum concentration to fall from 20 to 10 μg/ml, for example.

Hapten—Part of antigen containing structure that determines its immunologic specificity.

Haptoglobin—Plasma protein that binds hemoglobin set free from erythrocytes to plasma.

Hemagglutination—Clumping of red blood cells.

Hemarthrosis—Hemorrhage into joint.

Hematoma—Collection of extravasated blood often caused by trauma or coagulopathy.

Hematopoietic—Pertaining to production of erythrocytes.

Hemochromatosis—Genetic disorder characterized by excessive deposition of hemosiderin and hemofuscin in some organs.

Hemodynamics—Study of blood movement and forces (pressures) concerned therein.

Hemolysis—Breakdown of red blood cells.

Hemolytic—Destructive of erythrocytes.

Hemolytic uremic syndrome—Disease characterized by acute microangiopathic hemolytic anemia, thrombocytopenia, and renal failure. It is most common in early childhood and in pregnant and postpartum women. See Uremic syndrome.

Hemolyzed—Serum or plasma that is pink-tinged due to the release of hemoglobin from hemolyzed red blood cells.

Hemostasis—Arrest of blood escaping from vessels.

Hepatic—Of or relating to liver.

Homeostasis—System of control mechanisms used by body to maintain normal balance of given substance or state.

Human chorionic gonadotropin—Gonad-stimulating hormone stimulated by anterior pituitary. Its secretion increases dramatically after pregnancy; elevated concentrations can be detected as early as 4 days after missed menses. It is, therefore, the basis for most pregnancy tests.

Humoral—Pertaining to body fluids or substances contained in them.

Hydrostatic pressure—Pressure exerted by pumping of blood by heart. Hydrostatic pressure is roughly equivalent to arterial blood pressure but increases in standing person as one measures from the heart level to feet. It tends to push fluid out of vessels toward interstitial tissue.

Hyper-—Prefix meaning above normal or excessive.

Hyperaldosteronism—State of excessive aldosterone secretion by adrenal cortex.

Hyperglycemia—Abnormally high glucose concentration in blood.

Hyperplasia—Abnormal increase in number of cells in given tissue. For example, gingival hyperplasia involves gums.

Hyperpyrexia—Abnormally high fever (for given disease).

Hypersegmented—When referring to nucleus of granulocytes, nucleus has more lobes (segments) than usual; seen in some deficiency states.

Hyperthyroid—Condition that develops from excess of thyroid hormone activity.

Hypo-—Prefix meaning below normal or deficient.

Hypochromic—Referring to erythrocytes that appear more lightly colored than usual because of decreased amounts of hemoglobin.

Hypoglycemia—Abnormally low glucose concentration in blood.

Hypophosphatasia—Rare genetic disease of bone mineralization where serum alkaline phosphatase is about 25% (0–40%) of normal, serum phosphorus is normal, and serum and urine phosphoethanolamines are elevated.

Hypothyroidism—Condition that develops from deficiency of thyroid hormone activity.

Hypovolemia—Inadequate volume of blood in body.

Iatrogenic—Any disorder caused by clinician, practitioner, or drug.

Ileum—Terminal portion of small intestine.

Immunofluorescence assay—Any technique where a fluorescent marker is attached to one of the immune reactants. In *direct* testing, fluorescein or similar label is attached to a specific antibody that identifies the location of its specific antigen in tissue or in a specimen. In *indirect* testing, the label is attached to an antiglobulin serum, which reacts with human antibody molecules. The fluorescent antiglobulin marker shows that an antigen-antibody reaction has occurred in the test system. The indirect method is used to reveal whether or not a fluid contains antibody.

Immunoglobulin—See Antibody.

Infarction—An inadequate blood flow to a part of the body secondary to constriction or blockage of the supplying artery.

Inotropic—Related to the contraction of heart muscle (e.g., positive inotropic agents increase the force of contractions of the heart muscle).

Insensible loss—Small, gradual loss of body fluid that is not readily appreciated with naked eye. Examples include sweat and respiratory water vapor.

Interferent—Component of collected sample of body fluid or tissue, other than analyte, that falsely alters final results.

Interstitial—Fluid between cells or tissue; extracellular fluid excluding fluid in blood vessels.

Intracellular—Fluid within cells; opposite of extracellular.

Intrinsic factor—Protein produced in stomach that is necessary for intestinal absorption of vitamin B_{12}.

Ischemia—An inadequate blood flow to a part of the body secondary to constriction or blockage of the supplying artery.

Jodbasedow effect—Development of hypothyroidism in previously euthyroid patient as result of exposure to increased quantities of iodine.

-kal-—Word root relating to potassium.

Leukocytosis—Increased concentration of circulating white blood cells; often associated with infection or inflammation.

Lipemia retinalis—Whitish cast in vascular bed of retina due to light scattering by triglyceride particles in blood.

Lipemic—Serum or plasma that appears milky due to the presence of excessive lipids.

Lumen—Internal space of tube or tubule through which fluid flows; used commonly in reference to airways, kidney tubules, and blood or lymph vessels.

Maceration—Softening of tissue by action of liquid (e.g., effect on anal skin by persistent diarrhea).

Macrocyte—Erythrocyte that is larger than normal.

Macrophage—Phagocytic cell in organs such as spleen, liver, and lungs.

Macroscopic—Visible by naked eye without microscope.

Mast cell—Cell that has membrane binding sites for IgE and contains granules of histamine and other substances important in causing symptoms of immediate hypersensitivity reactions.

Megakaryocyte—Giant white blood cell in bone marrow that gives rise to platelets.

Megaloblast—Nucleated erythrocyte distinct from normal nucleated erythrocyte precursors; found in bone marrow and peripheral blood in vitamin B_{12} and folic acid deficiencies.

Mesenteric—Relating to fold of peritoneum connecting small intestine with posterior abdominal wall.

Metabolite—Result of hepatic transformation of a drug or chemical. Metabolites of drugs may be inactive or active.

Microcytic—Referring to erythrocytes that are smaller than normal.

Microscopic—Not visible by naked eye without microscope.

Mineralocorticoids—Corticosteroids (e.g., aldosterone) secreted by adrenal cortex. They cause sodium retention and potassium loss.

Minimal bactericidal concentration—See Chapter 17.

Minimal inhibitory concentration—See Chapter 17.

Mixed connective-tissue disease—Rheumatological diagnosis associated with symptoms commonly seen separately in systemic sclerosis, rheumatoid arthritis, polymyositis, and systemic lupus erythematosus. Symptoms are bonded together by presence of antiribonucleoprotein antibodies.

Mononucleosis—Disorder produced by infection by Epstein-Barr virus; characterized by fever, sore throat, malaise, swollen lymph glands, enlargement of liver and spleen, and typical rash.

Morbidity—Unhealthy state; untoward effects of disorder or drug.

Morphologic—Referring to form or appearance.

Myeloproliferative—Increase of cellular elements of bone marrow.

Myocardium—The muscular tissue of the heart.

Myoglobin—Pigment in muscle that is similar to hemoglobin in action. It acts as oxygen reservoir within muscle fibers.

Myosin—Protein in muscle tissue that acts with actin to allow muscle contraction and relaxation.

-natr-—Word root pertaining to sodium.

Nephelometry—Determination of solute concentration by measurement of light-scattering properties of molecules in suspension. Degree of light scattering is proportional to molecule's concentration.

Nephron—Functional unit of kidneys.

Nephrotic syndrome—Disorder where glomerular lesions cause enhanced permeability to proteins; characterized by heavy loss of serum proteins to urine and low serum albumin.

Neuroglycopenia—Abnormally low glucose concentration in central nervous system; usually associated with hypoglycemia and manifests as confusion, seizures, and/or coma.

Neurohypophysis—Posterior lobe of pituitary gland; secretes antidiuretic hormone and oxytocin.

Nonlinear (or Michaelis Menton)—Refers to elimination pattern of a drug when enzymatic metabolism starts to become saturated.

Nucleic acid—Either deoxyribonucleic acid (DNA) or ribonucleic acid (RNA).

Nystagmus—Involuntary rhythmic movement of eyeballs.

Occult—Hidden; referring to blood in specimen that can be discovered only by chemical tests or microscopy.

Oliguria—Diminution in urine production or excretion.

Oncotic pressure—Osmotic pressure developed at vascular capillary membrane by plasma proteins (e.g., albumin) that tends to hold fluid in bloodstream; also called colloid osmotic pressure.

Osmolality—Measure of pressure caused by solute concentration difference between opposite sides of semipermeable membrane.

Osmolar gap—Difference in osmolality between two compartments (e.g., intracellular and extracellular fluids).

Osteoblast—Bone cell responsible for bone production.

Osteoclast—Bone cell responsible for bone resorption and removal.

Osteolytic—Relating to promotion of bone dissolution.

Osteomalacia—Disease characterized by softening of bone, usually from vitamin D deficiency; seen in uremic syndrome.

Ototoxicity—Damage to function of ears.

P wave—The electrocardiogram recording of the electrical activity of the heart leading to atrial depolarization and contraction.

Parasite—Organism that lives on surface of or within another organism and, by so doing, causes harm to that organism.

Parietal cell—Cell in stomach that produces gastric acid and intrinsic factor.

Parotid gland—Salivary gland, below and in front of the external ear. It produces amylase (ptyalin), which aids in initial breakdown of starches.

Pathogenic—Producing disease.

Pathognomonic—Information that definitively distinguishes one pathophysiological process, etiology, or diagnosis from another. For example, a theophylline concentration of 25 µg/mL without clinical signs of toxicity is not pathognomonic for theophylline toxicity.

Peak (drug concentration)—Maximum concentration during a drug dosing interval.

Pelvic inflammatory disease—Disease of female reproductive organs, commonly caused by infection due to gonococci or chlamydia.

Performance, assay—Tests used to determine overall usefulness of assay; may include testing for precision, accuracy, specificity, sensitivity, and substrate stability.

Petechiae—Small, pinpoint, purplish-red spots on skin caused by intradermal leakage of blood.

Phagocyte—Cell that ingests and digests microorganisms or other cells and foreign particles.

Pharmacokinetics—Study of the time course of drug concentrations in the body after drug administration.

Pheochromocytoma—Tumor (usually benign) of adrenal medulla that secretes excessive catecholamines into blood; manifests primarily as hypertension.

Pickwickian syndrome—Disorder characterized by chronic alveolar hypoventilation, somnolence, polycythemia, hypoxemia, and hypercapnia; occurs in morbidly obese patients when excessive fat apparently limits movement of lungs.

Plasma—Aqueous component of blood consisting of 92% water and 8% solids (e.g., albumin, globulin, fibrinogen, clotting factors, minerals, nutrients, waste products, and enzymes).

Plasma cell—Terminally differentiated B lymphocytes that are devoted entirely to antibody production.

Pluripotential—Purported ability of certain stem cells to differentiate into numerous types of blood cell precursors.

Polydipsia—Excessive thirst; often associated with diabetes.

Polymorphonuclear cell—Cell containing nucleus with many lobes. Granulocytes are polymorphonuclear cells.

Polymyalgia rheumatica—Self-limited syndrome characterized by proximal joint and muscle pain, high erythrocyte sedimentation rate, malaise, low-grade fever, weight loss, and fatigue.

Polymyositis—Rheumatic disease characterized by interstitial inflammatory infiltrates of skeletal muscle, increased creatine phosphokinase, and symmetrical, proximal limb weakness.

Polyphagia—Excessive hunger; associated with diabetes.

Polyuria—Excessive excretion of urine resulting in profuse micturition.

Porphyria—Condition producing increased concentrations of any heme precursor.

Postantibiotic effect—Effect of some antibiotics (e.g., ciprofloxacin) against certain bacteria, characterized by inhibition of growth hours after antibiotic concentrations fall below minimal inhibitory concentration.

Postprandial—After a meal.

Precision—Degree of variation of assay results when known specimens are tested repeatedly in one run or over several days.

Preeclampsia—Syndrome of nausea, vomiting, headache, dyspnea, and albuminuria; precedes onset of true eclampsia (hypertensive toxemia associated with seizures and coma).

PR interval—Part of electrocardiogram between onset of atrial activity (P wave) and ventricular activity (QRS complex); indicator of conduction between two chambers.

Prodrome—Advanced clinical finding indicating approach of disease.

Prostacyclin—Prostaglandin metabolite in vascular tissue that is potent vasodilator and inhibitor of platelet aggregation.

Pseudopod—Temporary protrusion of outer membrane of ameba, platelet, etc.

Purpura—Confluent petechiae and/or ecchymoses.

Pyelonephritis—Inflammation of kidneys (usually caused by bacterial infection) that may be accompanied by flank pain and tenderness, bacteriuria (often bacteremia), pyuria, and fever.

Pyuria—White blood cells in urine.

QRS complex—Electrocardiogram recording of the electrical activity of the heart leading to the ventricular depolarization and contraction.

Radionuclide—Atom or type of atom with unstable nucleus that spontaneously decays to a more stable form while emitting radiation; also called radioisotope. Radionuclides used in scintigraphy are technetium-99m pyrophosphate and thallium-201.

Raynaud's phenomenon—Intermittent vasospasm in fingers or toes leading to blanching; brought on by cold and sometimes by emotion.

Renal—Pertaining to kidneys.

Repolarization—An electrical phenomenon that represents the recovery of the resting state electrical potential across muscle or nerve cell. The intracellular space becomes more negatively charged than the extracellular space, leading to cellular relaxation.

Retention time—Time between when compound is injected and its characteristic band emerges from chromatographic column.

Rhabdomyolysis—Disintegration or dissolution of muscle associated with elevated serum creatine phosphokinase and excretion of myoglobin in urine.

Rheological—Relating to study of (blood) flow.

Scintigraphy—Process of acquiring a scintigram—image of radioactivity distribution obtained with scintillation camera after internal administration of radionuclide; used in diagnosis of myocardial infarction.

Scleroderma—Multisystem disorder characterized by "hidebound" fibrotic skin, vascular lesions, and residual atrophy with fibrosis of multiple organs; now called progressive systemic sclerosis.

Sensitivity—Lowest quantity of substance that an assay can measure accurately. Also see Chapter 1 for meaning with qualitative tests.

Serological—Relating to (tests) detecting, identifying, and or quantifying antibodies (immunoglobulins) or antigens from serum; most useful in evaluating viral infections and (auto) immune diseases.

Serum—Aqueous portion of blood containing all plasma substances except fibrinogen and clotting factors. See plasma.

S3 heart sound—Low-pitched extra heart sound that occurs during rapid ventricular filling; also referred to as S_3 gallop. It may occur normally in children and young adults. In older patients, however, it is usually produced by ventricular failure.

S4 heart sound—Low-pitched extra heart sound that occurs when atria contracts against noncompliant ventricle; also referred to as S_4 gallop. Noncompliance is usually the result of reduced ventricular wall distensibility or increased ventricular volumes. This physical sound is associated with hypertension.

Sjögren's syndrome—Diagnostic triad of dry eyes, dry mouth, and presence of rheumatic disease (usually rheumatoid arthritis). It is a chronic autoimmune disorder characterized by lymphocytic infiltration of lachrymal and salivary glands. Diagnosis of its primary form is confirmed by minor salivary gland biopsy and presence of circulating autoantibodies.

Solute—Substance dissolved in solvent.

Specificity—Degree of assay cross-reactivity with unintended substances as opposed to substance being tested. Also see Chapter 1 for meaning with qualitative tests.

Specimen—Sample of tissue or fluid (e.g., sputum, stool, or urine) to be tested.

Spherocyte—Red blood cell that is more spherical and fragile than normal. Spherocytosis is a hereditary disease in which there is excessive hemolysis.

Spirochete—Spiral-shaped microorganism (e.g., Treponema).

Steady state (drug concentration)—See Chapter 6.

Subluxation—Sprain or incomplete dislocation.

Supernatant—Floating on surface of liquid.

Susceptibility, bacterial—Propensity of bacteria to be killed by antimicrobial agent.

Synovium—Tissue lining nonarticulating surfaces inside joint capsule of movable joint that maintains integrity of synovial fluid by supplying nutrients and clearing wastes.

Systemic—Referring to entire body (in contrast to—"local").

T wave—Electrocardiogram recording of the electrical activity of the heart leading to ventricular repolarization and relaxation.

Tachypnea—Abnormal breathing rate (respiratory rate) seen in patients with obstructive lung disorders, acidosis, etc.

Tetany—Syndrome manifested by muscle twitching, cramps, and convulsions; often due to hypocalcemia.

Therapeutic drug monitoring—Use of drug concentrations to optimize drug therapy for individual patients.

Therapeutic range—See Chapter 6.

Third spacing—Abnormal accumulation of fluid outside intravascular and intracellular spaces. An example is ascites.

Thrombocythemia—Increase in number of circulating blood platelets.

Thrombocytopenia—Decrease in number of platelets below normal (reference) range.

Thrombocytosis—Unusually large number of platelets in blood.

Thromboplastin, tissue—Complex mixture of substances in vascular intima that are released with vascular injury; initiating factor in extrinsic system for clotting.

Thrombosis—Development of blood clot.

Tinnitus—Ringing in ears.

T lymphocyte—Thymus-influenced leukocyte that helps B lymphocytes make antibodies, destroy cells infected with virus, activate phagocytes to destroy engulfed pathogens, and control the level and quality of the immune system.

Trigeminal neuralgia—Disease of trigeminal nerve typically characterized by sharp, shooting pains in jaw and face.

Trough—Minimum concentration during a drug dosing interval.

Trousseau's sign—Hand spasms and contortions after inflation of blood pressure cuff on arm; may indicate hypocalcemia.

Turbidity—Cloudiness; often refers to serum or urine.

Ultrafiltrate—A sample that is filtered through a membrane. A plasma ultrafiltrate does not contain plasma proteins.

Urea—Chief nitrogenous component of urine and principal end-product of protein metabolism; NH_2-CO-NH_2.

Uremic syndrome—Symptom complex associated with end-stage renal failure; characterized by headache, vertigo, vomiting, blindness, and, later, convulsions and coma; once believed to be due to excess urea in blood. Patients develop metabolic acidosis, electrolyte imbalances, hypertension, congestive heart disease, anemia, and osteomalacia.

-uria—Suffix relating to urine.

Uricosuric—Relating to ability to increase uric acid excretion in urine.

Urticaria—Allergic skin reaction also known as hives.

Uveitis—Inflammation of iris, ciliary body, and choroid of eye.

Vagus nerve—Tenth cranial nerve; cholinergically innervates heart, lungs, esophagus, stomach, small intestine, liver, gallbladder, pancreas, and upper portions of colon and ureters.

Volume of distribution, drug—Volume of body tissue into which drug apparently distributes; not a real body space.

Von Willebrand factor and disease—Part of factor VIII molecule responsible for platelet adhesion and function; also called factor VIII/vWF. The disease is a genetic (autosomal-dominant) deficiency of this factor, manifesting as bleeding.

Whole blood—A sample specimen that contains red blood cells and plasma

Wilson's disease—Rare, hereditary liver disease where copper accumulates in liver and ultimately causes cirrhosis.

Wolf-Chaikoff effect—Iodide-induced hypothyroidism.

Xanthoma—Yellow skin plaque due to lipid deposition.

Blood Collection Tubes: Color Codes, Additives, and Appropriate Sample Volumes[a,b]

CAP COLOR	ADDITIVE(S)	NUMBER OF TUBE INVERSIONS AT COLLECTION	LABORATORY USE AND COMMENTS[d]
Red	None	0	For serum determinations in chemistry, serology, and blood banking
Lavender	Liquid potassium EDTA Freeze-dried sodium EDTA	8 8	For whole-blood hematology determinations; inversions prevent clotting
Light blue	0.105 *M* sodium citrate 0.129 *M* sodium citrate	8 8	For coagulation determinations on plasma; inversions prevent clotting; some tests may require chilling
Royal blue	Heparin sodium Sodium EDTA None	8 8 0	For trace element, toxicology, and nutrient determinations; not for chromium, manganese, aluminum and selenium
Green	Heparin sodium Lithium heparin Ammonium heparin	8 8 8	For plasma determinations in chemistry; inversions prevent clotting; used for arterial blood gases, ammonia (on ice), and electrolytes
Orange	Thrombin	8	For stat serum determinations in chemistry; inversions ensure clotting within 5 min.
Gray	Potassium oxalate/ sodium fluoride Sodium fluoride Lithium iodoacetate Lithium iodoacetate/ heparin Heparin sodium	8 8 8 8 8	For glucose, lactate, alcohol, and bicarbonate determinations; glycolytic inhibitors stabilize glucose for ≤24 hr at room temperature (iodoacetate) and for ≤3 days with fluoride; oxalate and heparin give plasma samples—without them, samples are serum; for lactate (on ice)
Brown	Sodium heparin	8	For lead determinations; inversions prevent clotting
Gold	Clot activator and gel for serum separation	5	Serum separator tube for serum determinations in chemistry; inversions ensure mixing of clot activator with blood and clotting within 30 min.
Light green	Lithium heparin and gel for plasma separation	8	Plasma separation tube for plasma determinations in chemistry; inversions prevent clotting
Yellow	Sodium polyanetho-esulfonate (SPS)	8	For blood culture specimen collections in microbiology; inversions prevent clotting

[a]Compiled from (1) 1990 company literature (Becton Dickinson, Rutherford, NJ 07070) on Vacutainer collection systems; (2) Jacobs DS, Kasten BL Jr, Demott WR, et al., eds. Laboratory Test Handbook. St. Louis, MO: Lexi-Comp/Mosby; 1988; (3) National Committee for Clinical Laboratory Standards. Procedures for handling and processing of blood specimens, H18-A. Villanova, PA: 1989; and (4) editor's experience. NA = not applicable; EDTA = ethylenediaminetetraacetic acid.

[b]Colors and additives are specific only for Vacutainer tubes with Hemogard closure or stoppers from Becton Dickinson. Other types and brands may vary.

[c]If known, that volume of blood required to avoid spurious results due to inappropriate ratio of anticoagulant to specimen. In general, tubes with liquid additives should be filled.

[d]In general, specimens should not be chilled before delivery to the laboratory unless specified otherwise. Exceptions include lactic acid, blood gases, pyruvate, gastrin, ammonia, parathyroid hormone, catecholamines, and possibly activated partial thromboplastin time. Stoppers should not be removed outside the laboratory, because specimens may be oxidized, volatile, or contaminated by bacteria. Serum or plasma should be separated from contact with cells within 2 hr of collection unless specified otherwise.

INDEX

Note: The following symbols indicate whether the information is part of a table (t), figure (f), minicase (mc), or glossary (g). Material within QuickViews is not indexed.

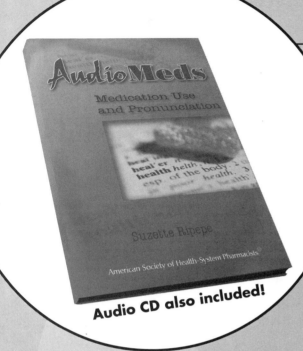
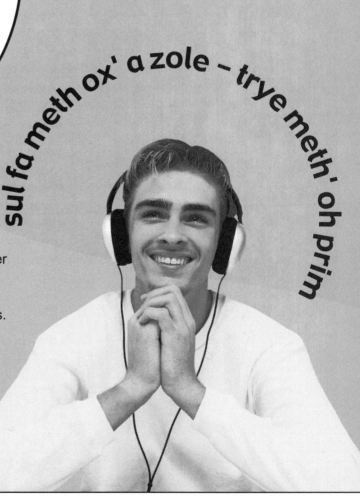
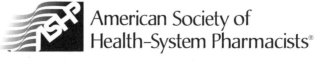